The World's Greatest Treasury of

HEALTH SECRETS

From the Editors of
Bottom Line Publications

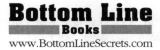

www.BottomLineSecrets.com

10 9 8 7 6 5 4 3

Bottom Line® Books publishes the advice of expert authorities in
many fields. The use of this material is not a substitute for
health, legal, accounting or other professional services. Consult a
competent professional for answers to your specific questions.

Telephone numbers, prices, offers and Web sites listed in this book are accurate
at the time of publication, but they are subject to frequent change.

Library of Congress Cataloging-in-Publication Data
The World's Greatest Treasury of Health Secrets
p.cm.
Includes index.
ISBN 0-88723-268-X

Bottom Line® Books is an imprint of
Boardroom® Inc.
281 Tresser Blvd., Stamford, CT 06901

Printed in the United States of America

Contents

6 • HEALTH SECRETS FOR WOMEN

7 • THE HEALTHY FAMILY

8 • REDUCE STRESS, LENGTHEN LIVES

9 • HOSPITAL AND SURGERY AWARENESS

10 • HEALTH SECRETS FOR MEN

11 • FOOD AND NUTRITION TIPS FOR A HEALTHIER YOU

12 • VITAMINS AND MINERALS SAVVY

13 • FOR A HEALTHY SEX LIFE

14 • GROWING OLDER—HEALTHIER

22 • NATURAL WAYS AND HERBAL SOLUTIONS

23 • HEALTH CARE SMARTS

24 • EMOTIONAL HEALTH MEANS A HAPPIER YOU

25 • NEW WAYS FOR THE 21ST CENTURY

INDEX 485

1

Best of Bests

The Time/Health Connection

Stephan Rechtschaffen, MD
Omega Institute for Holistic Studies

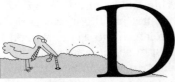

Do you have enough time in your life? When I pose this question to people attending my wellness seminars, only one or two people say *yes*—out of 50 or more.

The others—like most of us—suffer from "time poverty." These individuals are so busy trying to go faster, do more and buy more that they never get a chance to just experience being alive.

Inevitably, time poverty leads to psychological stress…and to stress-related ailments like heart disease, diabetes, fatigue, insomnia and high blood pressure.

THE HISTORY OF TIME

Most of us are so used to living by the clock that we think we *must* live by the clock. But the modern clock wasn't invented until the 16th century. Even the hourglass didn't see wide use until the 13th century.

Without clocks to control them, our ancestors experienced time as a series of moments defined by *nature's* pace—not as an endless parade of deadlines.

We *can* return to this wonderful sense of timelessness. I've developed a technique called *timeshifting*. This technique helps demonstrate that your experience of time is under your control. It lets you transform time from your master into your servant.

People come to my seminars expecting tips on time management. What they don't realize is that "managing" time only turns up the speed on the treadmill of life.

What I teach is *time awareness*. It's not about being more efficient. It's about slowing down and focusing on one thing at a time. It's

Stephan Rechtschaffen, MD, founder and president of the Omega Institute for Holistic Studies, 150 Lake Dr., Rhinebeck, NY 12572. He is author of *Timeshifting: Creating More Time to Enjoy Your Life*. Doubleday.

a process governed by a single rule—*live life in the now.*

FIND YOUR OWN RHYTHM

The rhythms that rule our lives are not fixed, though they may seem to be. It's just that our *internal* rhythms have fallen into sync with the rhythms of the world around us.

This process by which internal rhythms synchronize with external rhythms is called *entrainment.*

Timeshifting involves becoming aware of these external rhythms. Then you can *choose* to entrain with a slow, peaceful rhythm...or stay in sync with the rhythms of your environment, but in a more relaxed way.

FEEL YOUR EMOTIONS

Right now, put aside this article and spend a few minutes doing nothing—no TV, no books or magazines, no chitchat.

How did you feel? When I ask my seminar participants, the usual answers are "anxious," "guilty" or "sad." Sound familiar?

Good news: If you allow yourself to "stay with" your sorrow, rage, anxiety, etc., these negative emotions quickly lose their "charge." You'll feel free—and no longer compelled to replay old issues in your mind.

EXPAND THE MOMENT

I like to tell the story of the Zen monk and the tigers. To elude a hungry tiger, a monk climbed halfway down a cliff, until he was hanging by a branch above a ledge that held... a second tiger.

Beside the branch grew a strawberry bush. With his free hand, the monk picked a berry, popped it into his mouth and thought, "How delicious!"

Try to be like the monk. Consciously expand each moment of your life, free of regret about the past (tiger #1) or fear of the future (tiger #2). Remember—in the present there is no stress.

TIMESHIFTING EXERCISES

●**Develop rituals that help you stay "in the moment."** Let the ringing of a telephone signal you to pause and take a deep breath before answering...or gaze at a favorite photo when you feel anxious. One acquaintance of mine keeps a prism on her desk to look at when she feels worried. *Other rituals to cultivate.*

●**Do one thing at a time**, giving it your full attention. Pause for a few minutes after finishing one task before beginning another.

●**Take several three- to five-minute "mini breaks"** during the day to focus on your breathing. Slowly fill your lungs, then slowly release the air. Imagine watching your breath as it goes in and out.

Close your eyes and relax. Notice how your body feels. What does the room smell like? What sounds do you hear?

●**Get to meetings early** so you can compose yourself before others arrive.

●**Learn to timeshift in the midst of "busyness."** While waiting for a phone call or standing in line, shift into the present.

●**Create time boundaries.** Each day, set aside some time to devote entirely to yourself. During this period—ideally 15 minutes or so before work or after dinner—permit no meetings, no phone calls, no worries.

●**Honor the mundane.** We tend to focus on the day's highlights—a business luncheon, going to the movies, meeting someone for a date, etc. But to get the most out of life, we must learn to treasure mundane events, too.

If you're sweeping the floor, for example, bring full attention to the act. Notice the play of your muscles, the floor's appearance, the sound the broom bristles make, etc.

●**Create spontaneous time.** One of the happiest days of my life came during a forced layover in New Delhi, after my flight was postponed for 24 hours. I felt as if the day had been given to me, free of responsibilities or goals.

Nothing in particular happened that day, but the *spontaneity* of it all made it seem magical.

Paradoxically, I now *schedule* spontaneous time. You can, too. Open your date book to a day three weeks hence, and pencil in your own name. Set aside a few hours for an unplanned drive...or for just lying in bed.

●**Create time retreats.** Once a year, spend a week or more doing something extraordinary. I'm not talking about a jam-packed vacation, but a retreat into nature—anything that lets you shift to a slower rhythm.

Whatever your retreat involves, it should help you entrain to a slower, more peaceful pace.

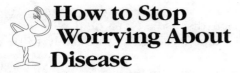

How to Stop Worrying About Disease

Carla Cantor, coauthor, with Brian Fallon, MD, of *Phantom Illness: Shattering the Myths of Hypochondria.* Houghton Mifflin. Cantor lives with her husband and two children in Maplewood, NJ.

Everyone worries about getting a serious illness *sometime*. But when occasional concern turns into a morbid obsession that interferes with daily life—it represents a more serious psychological problem.

Hypochondria is surprisingly common. One in 10 people who visit doctors' offices have the disorder to some degree...and three out of four patients have emotional problems that exacerbate their physical symptoms.

Unfortunately, few primary-care doctors take hypochondria seriously. Psychotherapists, too, have a poor track record. As a result, the majority of hypochondriacs suffer needlessly.

Good news: The outlook for hypochondriacs who get proper treatment is now excellent—thanks to psychoactive drugs, along with refinements in cognitive-behavioral and psychodynamic therapy.

WHAT CAUSES HYPOCHONDRIA

Hypochondriacs are *not* feigning illness. Their symptoms are *real*—but it's their interpretation of these symptoms that is unbalanced.

Everyday aches and pains are—to the hypochondriac—evidence of serious illness.

Hypochondria usually begins in the 20s or 30s—I was a college freshman when my hypochondria struck—although it can develop at any age. The condition is often portrayed as a woman's disorder, but it's just as common among men.

Single people seem to be especially susceptible. Psychologists theorize that's because they spend more time alone—and solitude encourages obsession about one's own health.

Some researchers believe that hypochondria has a biological basis—a pattern of neural "misfiring" in the brain that makes the individual unusually sensitive to physiological sensations.

Upbringing may also be a factor. Studies show that children of hypochondriac parents go to the emergency room more often—and show more disability and suicidal behavior—than children from normal families.

Presumably, the children are simply mimicking their parents' behavior.

It has also been theorized that parents who are overprotective unwittingly cause their children to grow up to be excessively vigilant about their health.

Others believe that hypochondria is simply a strategy for coping with emotional trauma—the death of a loved one, divorce, etc. The emotional pain caused by such trauma is so overwhelming that the person "buries" it under an obsession with disease.

EFFECTIVE MEDICATIONS

Though Prozac and related drugs have FDA approval for treating depression and obsessive-compulsive disorder (OCD), they are also effective against hypochondria.

In a study, 70% of hypochondriacs who took Prozac daily improved after 12 weeks.

Typical dosage: 60 to 80 mg a day. That's a bit higher than the 20 to 40 mg used to treat depression.

PSYCHOTHERAPY

Two forms of therapy are especially helpful...

●**Cognitive-behavioral therapy.** Patients learn to recognize the irrational statements they make to themselves...and learn new ways to interpret and respond to their symptoms.

With the therapist's help, patients confront the discomfort that arises in the absence of repeated trips to the doctor, endless discussions of symptoms and other rituals...and learn to replace them with alternative methods of relaxation—breathing techniques, relaxation exercises and cognitive strategies.

For referral to a cognitive-behavioral therapist in your area, contact the American Psychiatric Association (APA), 1400 K St. NW, Washington, DC 20005 (888-357-7924). *www.psych.org.*

●**Psychodynamic therapy.** In this form of therapy—the traditional "talk cure"—patients explore how their fear of disease might serve an emotional function, such as avoiding other painful feelings and conflicts. They receive support in confronting these conflicts and finding constructive ways to deal with them.

For more information on psychodynamic therapy, contact the APA (see previous page).

WHO SHOULD SEEK HELP

Seek help if you answer "yes" to any of these four questions…

●**When you hear about an illness,** do you fear you have it?

●**Do you often ask family and friends** to reassure you that you're not ill?

●**Are you obsessed with one particular disease?**

●**Do you "doctor shop"**—go from doctor to doctor, rejecting one diagnosis after another?

If you suspect you may have hypochondria, consult a therapist with training and experience in treating the disease.

MORE HELPFUL RESOURCES

●**Obsessive-Compulsive Foundation**, 337 Notch Hill Rd., North Branford, CT 06471 (203-315-2190).

●**New York State Psychiatric Institute**, 1051 Riverside Dr., New York 10032 (212-543-5000).

Creating Your Medical Family Tree To Save Your Life

Victor Herbert, MD, JD, professor of medicine and chief of the hematology and nutrition research laboratory at the VA Medical Center in the Bronx, NY. He is coauthor of *The Healing Diet: How to Reduce Your Risks and Live a Longer and Healthier Life if You Have a Family History of Cancer, Heart Disease, Hypertension, Diabetes, Alcoholism, Obesity, Food Allergies.* Macmillan.

If you have only a vague idea of your family's medical history, you may be setting yourself up for needless health problems.

All chronic diseases—including asthma, rheumatoid arthritis, multiple sclerosis, heart disease and cancer—have a hereditary component. Knowing that you carry the gene for a particular disease gives you a chance to prevent that disease…or to deal with it at its earliest stage, when it's more likely to be curable.

The key to gaining this invaluable knowledge is making a brief history of ailments that run in your biological family. A medical family tree is simple to create. More important, it pays off.

Example I: One of my patients, a 20-year-old man, discovered a family history of *hemochromatosis*, an often deadly disease in which the body absorbs too much iron. When a blood test showed that he suffered from a mild iron overload, he corrected the problem by donating blood on a monthly basis and giving up his daily iron supplement.

Example II: After her mother died of ovarian cancer, a 31-year-old woman put together a medical family tree. Using it, an oncologist determined that this woman and her sisters each had a 50% chance of developing ovarian cancer, too. So far, aggressive screenings and dietary strategies have kept the sisters cancer-free.

Example III: Another tree revealed a genetic link between five female relatives stricken with autoimmune disorders, including lupus, rheumatoid arthritis and a condition called Boeck's sarcoid. A dietician's question revealed that each woman had been taking alfalfa pills and vitamin E—both of which bring out latent genetic autoimmune disorders. When they stopped taking the supplements, symptoms gradually disappeared in four of the five women.

These are *not* isolated cases. In a 1988 study, 25,000 medical trees were responsible for identifying 43,000 individuals at high risk for hereditary ailments—and who were great candidates for preventive treatment.

It's easy to collect data on your immediate relatives, but don't stop there. Go back as many generations as possible—even if you must do some digging.

Don't worry if the information you unearth is inexact or incomplete. Anything that adds to the big health picture of your family could be helpful.

GATHERING INFORMATION

Make a list of all your living biological relatives…and any friends, neighbors, coworkers, etc., who can provide information on those who have died. If your family is small, interview relatives by phone.

Or, consider holding a family reunion—and add your tree-making project to the agenda.

Helpful resources: Medical records and death certificates can be obtained from doctors and hospitals, as well as from bureaus of vital statistics and state and county archives.

In addition, you can send a self-addressed, stamped, business-sized envelope to the National Genealogical Society (4527 17 St. N., Arlington, VA 22207) for more information.

CREATING YOUR TREE

Get a piece of sturdy paper, measuring at least 36 inches wide and 30 inches long. Fold it into fourths, horizontally. Each section will represent a single generation.

If you plan to cover more than four generations, get bigger paper and fold it into more sections—or attach additional sheets.

Spread the paper flat on a table. In the bottom section, tape the health questionnaires on your children and/or those of your siblings.

In the section just above, tape your questionnaire and those of your spouse and spouse's siblings.

Above your own information, place your parents' and their siblings' information, and so on.

Position all the remaining questionnaires so that they branch outward and upward in the traditional family tree pattern.

Too much work? You can purchase a ready-made chart from the National Genealogical Society…or create your own using a computer program such as the PC-compatible *Family Tree Maker* (Genealogy.com, 800-548-1806). *www. familytreemaker.com.*

HOW TO USE YOUR TREE

Once your chart is complete, take it to your doctor. Ask him/her to study it for patterns of disease through the generations—and to identify family members who may be at risk.

Good news: Discovering that you are likely to carry the gene for a particular disease does not necessarily mean you will develop it. In many cases, a simple blood test will pinpoint your degree of risk.

Example: If breast cancer runs in your family…*and* your percentage of body fat is 20% or more above mean desirable body fat for your sex and age…*and* your blood test shows elevated lev-els of estrogen, your doctor may order more rigorous tests and frequent checkups.

Almost certainly, the doctor will also recommend lifestyle modification. Whether a genetic predisposition leads to disease—or is suppressed—is at least partly determined by diet, exercise, smoking and other controllable factors.

Many genetic disorders, such as diabetes and some cancers, are triggered in part by obesity. Other conditions may be prevented by following a particular diet.

Example: If colon polyps run in your family, you should be examined regularly by a gastroenterologist…and eat a calcium-rich diet. Such a diet has been shown to help suppress polyps and colon cancer.

Once your family medical tree has alerted you and your doctor to a possible predisposition, controlling your lifestyle and getting regular checkups will give you the best chance of beating the genetic odds.

Secrets to Staying Healthy—and Happy—While Traveling

Karl Neumann, MD, editor and publisher of *Traveling Healthy*, 108-48 70 Rd., Forest Hills, NY 11375. He is also coeditor of *The Business Traveler's Guide to Good Health While Traveling.* Chronimed Publishing.

No matter what your destination or why you're traveling, fatigue, stress, an upset stomach or worse can spell disaster for your trip.

Fortunately, the wear and tear of travel can be kept to a minimum with simple advance planning.

Here are some easy ways to make your travel more comfortable—and healthful…

SELF-CARE CHECKLIST

Your chief consideration when packing for a trip is where you're going, how long you'll be away and what the climate is like at your destination. But no matter what sort of trip you're planning, bring along a well-stocked self-care kit. It should be easily accessible in your carry-on luggage and should contain some or all of the following…

•**Antacid.** Familiar store-bought remedies such as Maalox, Mylanta, Gelusil, Tums or Rolaids combat the stomach upset, heartburn and abdominal cramping sometimes caused by unfamiliar food or drink—or overindulgence in either.

•**Diarrhea remedy.** Over-the-counter preparations like Imodium AD, Kaopectate or Pepto-Bismol are all effective at stopping diarrhea. Tablets are easier to take along on a trip, although the liquid forms of these medications usually offer faster relief.

•**Laxative.** On the road, constipation is often more of a problem than diarrhea.

Reason: Your diet while traveling is apt to lack high-fiber foods. Also, it may be difficult while you are traveling to maintain a regular exercise routine. Take along some Metamucil, Fibercon or Senokot just in case.

•**Antihistamine.** The over-the-counter medication Benadryl is effective against a host of potential allergens and irritants and is well-tolerated by most people. If you have to stay alert, ask your doctor to prescribe Claritin. It causes little or no drowsiness.

•**Antibiotic.** For tooth abscesses, severe bronchitis, festering skin wounds or other stubborn bacterial infections, ask your doctor to prescribe an antibiotic in advance.

Caution: Antibiotics should be used *only under a doctor's supervision.* Call your doctor at home for instructions if you need to use one.

•**Motion sickness remedy.** Dramamine or Bonine tablets are effective medicines.

Caution: Dramamine and Bonine can cause drowsiness. Avoid them if you have to stay alert.

•**Athlete's foot remedy.** Be sure to include antifungal foot powder or solutions like Lotrimin, Micatin or Tinactin in your travel kit, since showers in hotel rooms and fitness centers are not always fungus-free.

Also helpful: Rubber thongs to wear in the shower.

•**Sunscreen, sunglasses and a wide-brimmed hat.** These are a must for travel to sunny places or if you intend to be outdoors for extended periods of time.

Important: Your sunscreen should have an SPF of at least 15 and should guard against both UVB and UVA rays.

•**Insect repellent.** Look for one that contains 20% to 30% DEET.

•**Aspirin, acetaminophen or ibuprofen.**

•**A decongestant, as well as a supply of facial tissues.**

You might also want to bring along a basic first-aid kit containing an antibacterial cream or ointment, bandages, gauze, thermometer, scissors and tweezers.

If you wear corrective lenses, pack a spare pair of contacts or eyeglasses—plus your prescription.

If you intend to swim in unchlorinated water, take along a remedy for swimmer's ear, an infection marked by redness, itching and pain of the outer ear canal. I recommend an over-the-counter preparation called Vosol.

FIGHTING JET LAG

Anytime you fly across several time zones, you disrupt the body's circadian rhythms. The resulting jet lag should be thought of not as a special problem, but as another form of manageable stress. *Ways to control it:*

•**Avoid drinking alcohol during your flight.** Alcohol is a depressant, and can aggravate lethargy and fatigue, two classic symptoms of jet lag. It can also cause restlessness, which can disturb your sleep or keep you from sleeping altogether. And because it acts as a diuretic, alcohol can leave you feeling dehydrated.

•**Limit your consumption of caffeine.** Like alcohol, caffeine is a diuretic that can leave you feeling dehydrated and out of sorts. Too much caffeine can also cause nervousness, anxiety, tremors and insomnia.

•**Drink plenty of water.** Studies have shown that even slight dehydration can cause listlessness and fatigue and can even make you prone to mental errors—symptoms similar to those of jet lag.

Bear in mind that you may be dehydrated even *before* departure.

Reason: Your eating and drinking patterns may be erratic in the hours before your flight. Breathing dry cabin air only increases this dehydration and its enervating effects. To stay hydrated, drink plenty of water or other nonalcoholic beverages before and during your flight—one eight-ounce glass every two to three hours. Don't wait until you feel thirsty—by then you may already be dehydrated.

SAFE FOOD AND DRINK

Regions of the world fall into three "tiers":

- **Europe, North America and Australia.**

- **Israel and the Caribbean.**

- **The rest of the Middle East, most of Africa, the Far East** and other developing regions.

Anytime you travel to the second or third tier, you must be especially vigilant about what you eat and drink. *Self-defense:*

- **Eat cooked food while it is still hot.** Make sure meats are well-done. Throughout developing countries, undercooked beef and pork are major sources of tapeworms and other parasites. Likewise, all poultry, seafood and vegetables should be fresh and thoroughly cooked.

- **Avoid peeled fruits** and those with broken skin. Watch out for raw vegetable salads, too. They can be contaminated with bacteria from the food preparer's hands or from the water used to rinse the vegetables.

- **Avoid custards, pastries and other baked desserts.** These foods are often contaminated with microbes that trigger gastric distress, especially if improperly refrigerated.

Exception: Served hot from the oven, these foods are generally safe. If you want dessert, stick to wrapped candy or fresh fruit that you peel yourself.

- **Stick to bottled or canned beverages.** Don't use ice cubes, which might be contaminated. Avoid milk, milk products and foods that are prepared with them unless you are positive that they have been properly pasteurized.

- **Avoid bread that has been left in open baskets**—it may have been exposed to flies and other disease-bearing insects. If you're not certain whether bread has been properly stored, remove the crust and eat only the *interior* of the loaf.

WATCHING OUT FOR INFECTIOUS DISEASES

If you are planning a trip to the tropics, get immunizations *at least one month before your departure*. Frantic, last-minute efforts to obtain shots only compound the ordinary stress occasioned by an overseas journey. And multiple immunizations require several shots over a period of days or weeks.

A 24-hour hotline run by the Centers for Disease Control and Prevention (CDC) (404-639-3534) provides recorded messages outlining immunization requirements and recommendations for international travel.

To avoid malaria, ask your doctor about taking prophylactic drugs. Some must be taken one week before you travel to ensure that adequate blood levels of the drug are reached before you arrive—and that any adverse reactions occur before you leave for your trip.

How to Read Your Body's Messages

Martin Rush, MD, a psychiatrist in private practice for more than 30 years who lives in Middletown, OH. He is author of *Decoding the Secret Language of Your Body.* Fireside.

Many physical problems, from mere discomfort to chronic pain to serious illness, have psychological as well as physical roots.

Of course, viruses, bacteria, muscle strain and other physical factors play a large role in making us feel awful. However, these troublemakers are more likely to do damage if we are also troubled by distressing emotions—such as fear, anger, guilt or sadness.

The problem isn't the negative *emotions* themselves—everyone feels them at one time or another. It's *repressing* these emotions that gets our bodies into the act. When we stuff our feelings inside instead of expressing them, the body's response is to send a physical signal—which can't be ignored so easily.

In my 30-plus years as a family physician and then as a psychiatrist, I've noticed that when people identify the stressful situation that preceded a physical symptom—and then talk about the feelings associated with that situation—the physical problem often goes away and their emotional burden lightens as well.

I do not mean to trivialize illness, nor do I claim that talking about your feelings is a substitute for good medical treatment. Physical problems are very real and may well require physical intervention. But if the emotional roots of a problem are neglected, the issue will keep showing up in the body—in one way or another—until it's resolved.

DECODING YOUR BODY'S LANGUAGE

How do you uncover the hidden emotions that are behind a physical problem? Try thinking back on the stresses that were present in your life just before the illness occurred...or simply review recent events that might have upset you.

Since you might not recognize certain situations as upsetting, it's a good idea to have a friend (or therapist) help you with this step. Others may spot connections you missed.

Once identified, get those painful feelings off your mind (and body) by talking about them.

If you have trouble identifying the source, pick up clues from the physical location of the problem. Although each person's situation is unique, I have observed a number of common themes in my patients (and myself).

COLD HANDS AND FEET

When hands and feet get cold or numb, it's usually because the nervous system has signaled the arteries to contract, reducing blood supply to the extremities. What causes this to occur? I've noticed that the phenomenon often seems to strike people who are reluctant to "reach out" for their desires—they're afraid of getting the very thing they want.

Example I: The old cliché about brides or grooms getting "cold feet" isn't just an expression—it's a genuine physical phenomenon that expresses the conflict between the longing for connection and the fear of responsibility.

Example II: When I took up skiing in my 50s, my feet and hands got so icy cold—no matter how many layers of socks and mittens I wore—that I couldn't enjoy myself. As I thought about the issue, I remembered that although I had always longed to learn to ski, this pastime had been beyond my family's means. I realized that I was terrified of enjoying the kind of carefree pleasure that was denied my parents.

As I faced this conflict, I became more relaxed...and now I'm quite comfortable on the slopes!

SORE THROAT

For many people, the throat is where they store tension when they have been slighted, insulted or otherwise rejected. These wounds to the spirit create an urgent need for reassurance, comfort and love.

On a primitive level, we associate those yearnings with food—and especially the security we felt as nursing infants.

Years later, when we feel rejected, the throat contracts instinctively, as though to re-create that old feeling of comfort. But when comfort isn't forthcoming, the protective mucus that lines the back of the throat dries up, leaving the area vulnerable to incoming germs.

When your feelings are hurt, say so—to yourself, to the person who hurt you (if appropriate)...and to other people, if the insult was serious. Be sure the people you tell about the incident can be depended upon to respond with the kindness and reassurance you crave.

BOWEL TROUBLE

Constipation, spastic colon and other problems related to elimination tend to be associated with holding in "nasty" feelings—anger, spitefulness, jealousy, disappointment—because we're afraid people won't like the "real" us.

Hemorrhoids—small ruptures that can occur when the anal sphincter muscles become so tight they disrupt circulation—are another expression of this conflict.

Example: A woman in one of my psycho-therapy groups was plagued with constipation. No one in the group had ever heard her raise her voice. Encouraged to talk about her childhood, she described growing up as the middle sibling and learning to keep her feelings to herself in order to avoid confrontation. As an adult, she continued to squelch her own needs in favor of tending to the demands of her husband and children. As she became more comfortable discussing her feelings freely with the group, she gradually learned to stand up for herself, and constipation ceased to be a problem.

LOWER BACK PAIN

Carrying too much weight can cause the muscles supporting the back to go into spasm, leading to acute or chronic pain. The excess weight can be physical or emotional—when we feel overburdened and want someone to take care of us for a change.

Example: A middle-aged man developed back trouble after his aging mother came to live with him and his wife. He loved his mother and wanted to help her, but having her join the household and arranging for her care put him under a great deal of stress. He didn't want to hurt her feelings by airing his complaints—and he also felt selfish and guilty about resenting her.

When he was finally able to talk to his wife about his feelings, he no longer felt as though he were carrying the burden alone. Once his back didn't need to speak for him, the pain lessened dramatically.

HOW TO DEAL WITH HIDDEN FEELINGS

Though many people do find therapy valuable, you don't necessarily have to talk to a therapist to discharge these emotions. A friend, relative, colleague or member of the clergy can be just as helpful—if that person can be counted on to be supportive.

You may not even need a long, drawn-out ranting session. Often it's enough simply to acknowledge the previously buried feeling ("That made me really mad") and have someone affirm your reaction ("I can see why you felt that way").

If you're concerned about wearing out your friends or being viewed as a complainer, spread the burden around. Mention the issue briefly to a few different people. You'll feel better each time you talk about it.

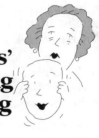

Dr. Joyce Brothers' Secrets of Winning The Ever-Changing Game of Life

Joyce Brothers, PhD, the nationally renowned psychologist. She is author of numerous books, including *How to Get Whatever You Want Out of Life*. Ballantine Books.

I don't believe in luck. I believe that good fortune comes through hard work and preparation, so that you are able to take advantage of life's big opportunities when they present themselves to you.

However, there are steps you can take to ensure that your efforts are well placed and you can recognize opportunities when they appear.

CLARIFY YOUR ASPIRATIONS

The first and most important step is to discover what you really want out of life. Before dreams can come true, you have to identify them.

This, of course, is one of the most difficult discussions you'll ever have with yourself. Most of us find identifying our goals and aspirations too broad to ponder and too difficult to answer.

In fact, most people know what they want out of life—*on a subconscious level*. The goal is to bring the knowledge up to our conscious levels, where it can be articulated and achieved.

Helpful: Quick—ask yourself right now what you want most in the world and, without stopping to think, write down the first three things that come into your head. Read your list, and put it away.

Repeat the process weekly for six weeks. At the end of six weeks, take out all the lists and study your answers. You will find a pattern—the responses that repeat themselves are your dreams.

If that doesn't show you what you want most in the world, you will at least have a much clearer idea.

MASTER THE ART OF POWER READING

Almost every goal we set involves improving ourselves through studying material with which we are unfamiliar. The ability to read and retain what you need to know in a hurry is the basic tool for getting what you want.

The problem is that few people have efficient techniques for absorbing written materials, so progress is slow. Here is my five-step strategy—it works no matter what you want to study.

• **Get an overview.** Whether it's one document or a stack of books, rapidly skim the material. If you don't need to absorb the material overnight, decide how many days you can devote to it. Then divide the text into even amounts.

• **Divide each day's material into three equal parts.** Plan to spend the most time on the second part. Since our brains learn most easily at the beginning and end of a study session, the middle section will give you the most trouble.

• **Internal command.** As you read the first part, tell yourself that when you're done, you're going to close the book and recite what you've read. This internal command sets your mind so you can concentrate better.

• **Turn over the material when you've finished the first part.** The goal is to recite aloud the essence of what you've read. I suggest turning over the material because we tend to be unconscious cheaters.

• **Recite aloud the major points of what you just learned.** Even better, write them down while you're reciting. There's a direct relationship between senses and memory. The more ways your brain senses something, the better you remember it. When you finish, check your work against the material to be sure you are right—or to see what needs more work.

Important: When reciting material, pause for a few seconds between sections. Otherwise, new information won't be retained.

Repeat steps three, four and five with the remaining sections.

CREATE A POSITIVE "HALO EFFECT"

What psychologists call the *halo effect* has nothing to do with goodness or godliness. It has to do with your aura and how it affects other people's first impressions of you.

The impression you leave with others who could be helpful to you will create a halo effect that radiates out to color their opinion of everything you do in the future.

Five rules for creating a great impression with others…

• **Appear knowledgeable and smart.** Before meeting new people, determine what subjects are likely to come up in conversation and learn as much as you can about those subjects. The goal isn't to appear as a know-it-all but as someone who is informed and well read.

• **Avoid smoking**, excessive drinking and other bad habits. All create a negative impression and shift the focus away from you and to your habit.

• **Be on time.** Not only is lateness discourteous, it makes people think you don't value their time. Lateness is a sure way to create a negative halo effect.

• **Get the person's name right**, and use it a few times while speaking.

• **Don't talk too much**—or interrupt the person speaking. There is a great deal of power in silence, especially if you are attentive to the person speaking.

LEARN THE SUBTLE ART OF FLATTERY

No matter how successful people become, nearly everyone has an inferiority complex. So when you tell people they are talented, marvelous or brilliant, they will appreciate the compliment and be much more likely to do things for you.

The most effective flattery always comes from the heart. The best compliments come from people who truly believe what they are saying and recognize areas of real interest to the person being flattered.

Learn to appreciate aspects of other people's personalities or work. Be confident enough in yourself to recognize *their* strengths.

Secondhand flattery is also tremendously effective.

Example: "Greg told me that everyone over in your office is excited about the new project you started. Congratulations."

STRIVE TO BECOME ENGROSSED IN YOUR WORK

In every endeavor, there are moments of magic experienced by people who are acting with total involvement. This peak experience —similar to the high long-distance runners experience—is what psychologists call *flow*.

To achieve this state, avoid doing what is easy. Instead, focus on challenging yourself, and work at it as intensely as you can.

But don't pick an overwhelming challenge that exceeds your limits. Choose the kind that stretches you and pushes your limits.

You must also set aside a significant span of uninterrupted time. It is virtually impossible to switch into a flow state in less than half an hour. It is *absolutely* impossible to do so if you are bedeviled by interruptions.

Use It...or Lose It Physically...Mentally

Martin Groder, MD, a Chapel Hill, NC, psychiatrist and business consultant. He is author of *Business Games: How to Recognize the Players and Deal with Them.* Boardroom Classics.

The longer you neglect your talents and special skills that were developed over the years, the harder it is to restore them and the less likely you'll be able to bring them back to their old levels of excellence. Once you've reached the point of no return, you probably won't even make the effort.

The deterioration of our abilities occurs due to disuse, and this law applies equally to both your mental and physical abilities—to chess as well as to tennis.

WHY WE LOSE IT

Much of the decline in strength and stamina that we blame on age is actually due to the disuse cycle. Slow down, and it gets harder to pick up the pace again—so the natural tendency is to slow down even more.

Activities as diverse as shooting pool, playing the piano, speaking a foreign language or responding sexually are coordinated by complex interactions of nerve cells in the brain.

When you practice, these neurons actually grow microscopic filaments to connect to one another. It's a process known as *arborization*. When you stop practicing, these connections wither away.

Every time you learn new skills or master fresh areas of knowledge, neurons secrete growth hormones that foster arborization, thus stimulating their own growth and the growth of their neighbors.

BRAIN DRAIN

Part of the brain is devoted to learning, striving to meet challenges and dealing with frustration, while another part takes care of establishing habits and routines. Let one part atrophy, and its functions are taken over by the areas that are used more.

When you stop challenging yourself and expanding your skills, that part of your brain goes quiet and brain activity shifts to its humdrum mode. The more you let yourself become stodgy and fail to challenge yourself, the harder it is to reactivate that part of your brain.

Motivation is often a major victim of this process. Once you let your skills decay, it's harder to feel excited.

Example: Playing piano poorly...or not seeing results from exercising...isn't very rewarding, so you're sorely tempted to let the activity slide altogether rather than make the effort to correct the situation or merely stay at a level that matches your abilities.

A LITTLE PRACTICE

Finding the time to maintain skills in the midst of our busy lives may seem an elusive goal. But it's important to remember that in midlife or beyond, you get the most benefit from the first small effort. By practicing your skills, even just a little each week, you will be able to exercise the capacities that are important to you.

Practicing many of your skills just a little bit is more important than concentrating on just one or two.

How much practice is enough? There's no universal rule, but when it comes to physical exercise, a workout every other day for 20 to

40 minutes appears to be enough to keep you in shape…and healthy.

In music, too, it appears that a half-hour to one hour of practice every other day will maintain a significant level of skill.

So—using what you don't want to lose at least two to three times a week for a half-hour to an hour is a good minimum for which to strive.

MAKE PRACTICE COUNT

To ensure the time you devote to maintaining your skills is well spent, take yourself, your talents and your strengths seriously enough to optimize the conditions for fruitful practice. *Here's how to do it…*

●**Use the right equipment.** If you're walking to maintain fitness, get good walking shoes. Want to hone your piano-playing skills? Get the piano tuned. It will make the experience more rewarding and increase the odds you'll keep doing it.

●**Make practice enjoyable.** Some people like to walk, run or bike alone…while others need to feel the support of fellow strivers in a gym or health club. Ask yourself what works best for you.

Example: Will sharing your essays with others motivate you to keep writing? Join a workshop or organize a writers' group on your own.

●**Find your level of practice and stick with it.** Some people want to keep their skills sharp in a relaxed way, without strain, as an enjoyable leisure pursuit. Others prize the exhilaration of feeling themselves tested and stretched.

Let your personal preference guide you in choosing whether you practice your skills for fun or find opponents who will force you to stretch.

●**Know your limits.** A big mistake many people make when practicing is falling into the "pro" trap. They don't bother practicing their skills because they know they won't ever become the champions they so admire.

Admire those who have achieved excellence, but don't model yourself after them. Realize your limitations, and remind yourself that the goal is to keep your abilities alive, not to conquer the world.

BE KIND TO YOURSELF

Attitude plays a big role in how well you perform and whether you stick to your practice regimen. A positive outlook fuels your determination to keep your capacities sharp, while negativity kills motivation. *Helpful…*

●**Be generous and accepting toward yourself**, particularly if you're trying to retain or regain competence in an area where you were once highly skilled.

●**Accept the role of a student**, even if your endeavor is something at which you once excelled.

●**Don't match your performance against memories** of a younger self at the peak of your powers…at a time when lots of practice had honed your skills.

●**Be a kindly, patient teacher or coach to yourself**, the kind who throws the ball to a kid a thousand times before the child learns to catch it properly. Summon up thoughts of past mentors. Enlist patient, supportive companions who will encourage you.

Important: Keep bad coaches and negative role models out of the picture. Listen for that nasty self-critical inner voice—we all have one—and silence it. Avoid "friends" who will sap your confidence.

PRACTICE PEOPLE SKILLS

The abilities you need to get along with others—communicating, working as part of a team, compromising, making helpful judgments instead of destructive criticisms—also need practice to stay sharp.

If you work at home, as increasing numbers of people do today, you may lack the day-to-day interaction that maintains these parts of your personality.

Solitude is important as well. People who are constantly surrounded by others—mothers who have young children…anyone who works in a busy office and comes home to a lively house—can lose the capacity for quiet and reflection.

12 Quick and Easy Things You Can Do to Improve Your Health

Harold H. Bloomfield, MD, a psychiatrist in private practice in Del Mar, CA. He is coauthor of *The Power of 5*. Rodale Press.

No more excuses. Here are ways to boost your health and happiness—*in five minutes or less*.

1. Inhale an energizing scent. Research suggests that lemon and peppermint scents are energizing. To exploit this finding, have an occasional cup of lemon or peppermint tea…or chew peppermint gum. Keep a bottle of peppermint and/or lemon extract to sniff…add a couple of drops to a small scent dispenser…or experiment with potpourri containing other energizing scents such as pine, jasmine, lavender or orange.

2. Sip ice water. It keeps your cells hydrated *and* helps you burn calories. *Reason:* Whenever you drink something cold, your body raises your metabolism to keep your body temperature from falling. That process burns calories—eight 16-ounce glasses of ice water will burn an extra 200 calories per day.

Strategy: Start the day with eight to 16 ounces of ice water. Sip a 16-ounce glass every hour or two, keeping one next to you at work and at home. All told, you should drink eight glasses a day. Finish up by 7 p.m.—to avoid having to use the bathroom after you go to bed.

3. Practice "one-breath" meditation. You don't have to spend years mastering meditation. This one-breath method is a powerful, straightforward relaxation technique that can be practiced anytime, anywhere. Try it whenever you feel fatigued or out of sorts.

What to do: Sit in a comfortable chair. Straighten your back, relax your shoulders and take a deep breath. Let the air "open" your chest. Imagine it filling every cell in your body. Hold the breath for a moment, then exhale, releasing every bit of tension.

Also helpful: One-touch relaxation. Place your fingertips just in front of your ears. Inhale and clench your teeth. Hold for five seconds. Exhale, and let your jaw muscles go loose.

Repeat this exercise three more times, using half the original tension, then one-fourth, then one-eighth. Then take a deep breath, press your fingertips against your jaw, let it go slack and say, *Ah-h-h-h*. Imagine you are breathing out tightness.

4. Minimize noise at home and at work. Loud or irritating sound creates severe emotional and physical tension. Fortunately, many aggravating noises can be silenced.

Strategy I: Place foam pads under blenders and other kitchen appliances…and under printers, typewriters and other office machines.

Strategy II: Before buying an air conditioner or another potentially noisy appliance, compare noise levels of different brands. Use noise-absorbing insulation around dishwashers.

5. Bask in bright light. Most people get a powerful surge of energy from sunlight or bright indoor light. Try moving your desk chair closer to a window…or, better yet, take a five-minute outdoor walk every few hours.

Also helpful: Each day, get five minutes of nonpeak sun (before 10 a.m. or after 3 p.m.) without sunscreen or sunglasses to enjoy the full mood-lifting effects of sunlight.

Indoors, replace incandescent or fluorescent bulbs with full-spectrum "daylight" bulbs from a lighting or health-food store. *Cost:* $7 to $9 for bulbs, $12 to $20 for tubes.

6. Do abdominal exercise. Use this technique while sitting at your desk or while stuck in traffic. Sit up straight. Place hands on hips with thumbs pointing toward your back. Exhale slowly and completely, pushing the last air out forcefully with your lower abdominals.

Repeat up to 10 times a day. You might try one or two stomach-flattening sessions just before meals, at stoplights on your commute or each time you sit down at your desk. These exercises are great muscle toners for the lower abdomen.

7. Perform mental "cross-training." Cross-training is the process by which you "stretch" your mind in as many different directions as possible by engaging in a variety of mental and physical activities. Word puzzles and other games are an easy way to perform

13

this cross-training. Pick a random sentence from the newspaper, then rearrange the words to make a new sentence…play Scrabble or do crossword puzzles…challenge a friend to chess or checkers.

8. Cook with "nutriceuticals." These are vegetables, herbs and spices that have specific healing properties…

•**Garlic and onions** boost the immune system, helping prevent colds.

•**Basil, cumin and turmeric** help prevent cancer of the bladder and prostate.

•**Black pepper, jalapeños, hot red peppers and mustard** all boost your metabolism for several hours. That helps burn fat.

•**Cinnamon** helps metabolize sugar, keeping your blood sugar levels steady.

9. Check your reading posture. Poor posture—leaning over a desk, for instance—can cause tension headaches, vision problems and pain in the jaw and/or neck.

Self-defense: Bring reading material up to your field of vision or use a book stand to hold a book at the proper angle. If you spend a lot of time on the telephone, get a headset. Don't cradle the phone between ear and shoulder.

10. Do trigger-point therapy. Wherever you feel tense, feel for a tight band of muscle tissue—a trigger point. Press or squeeze it with light to moderate pressure. Continue pressing for five to 10 seconds, then release.

11. Curb indoor pollution. Whenever possible, keep your windows open. All gas appliances should be checked annually and properly vented to the outside to limit their output of carbon monoxide. Use exhaust fans in the bathroom, kitchen and garage whenever you use these rooms. Make your home and office smoke-free.

12. Do absolutely nothing. "Lyming" is the Caribbean art of doing nothing—without feeling guilty about it. Try lyming frequently to give your brain time to process all the information it receives over the course of a day.

Helpful: Take a five-minute "mental vacation" every few hours. Picture your favorite beach or other getaway place. The idea is to escape the rat race briefly—but completely.

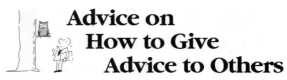

Advice on How to Give Advice to Others

Jeswald C. Salacuse, dean of the Fletcher School of Law and Diplomacy at Tufts University in Medford, MA. He is author of *The Art of Advice: How to Give It and How to Take It*. Times Books.

There is an art to giving advice. When you have mastered the art, people will listen to what you say…and come back for more. Both you and those who consult you will benefit from the relationship.

BENEFITS OF ADVISING OTHERS

Professionals are paid very well for their expert advice. But there are other reasons for giving advice.

•**Parents advise their children** out of love and concern for their welfare.

•**Senior managers counsel junior executives** because of idealism, friendship and good sound business. Just knowing that other people want your advice boosts your own self-esteem.

ADVISING IS AN ART

To be a good adviser it is not enough to provide information, no matter how accurate. You must be able to form relationships with others that can help them find the best solutions to their specific problems.

Example: A good parent knows what his/her children should do—and must be able to talk to them in a way that shows he understands their concerns.

HOW TO GIVE ADVICE

Good advice is the product of a three-step process…

•**Understand the other person's particular problem and objectives.** Your goal is not to demonstrate your own superior wisdom, but to help someone else solve his problem. To do that, always listen closely to what the other person says. Try to discover how he got into the current situation…exactly what problem he wants you to help him solve…how he hopes to benefit from your advice.

To help another person open up to you: Break the ice by starting off with something relevant about yourself…encourage him to discuss the problem in his own way…don't interrupt… don't anticipate…never suggest a solution before you understand the problem.

Example: An unhappy wife tells you about her husband's inattention and prolonged absences from home and asks your advice. Don't immediately tell her to change all the house locks, empty out the joint checking account and call a divorce lawyer. If you draw her out some more, you may find that she really wants to rebuild her relationship with her husband, whose troubled business is threatened with bankruptcy.

Important: Understand your precise role. Before you start dispensing advice, make sure the other person really wants it. He may just be looking for a sympathetic listener.

If the other person wants your advice, determine whether you are qualified to give it.

Ask yourself: Do I have the knowledge, skills and time I need to help this person?

Example: Martha often helps other people fill in standard tax returns. While helping a recently widowed friend, she discovers a tax problem outside her experience. Martha should not just go ahead and guess what her friend should do. She should tell her to get professional assistance. If the friend has never dealt with financial matters, Martha could help her find the right adviser.

● **Identify and evaluate the options and explain them as clearly as possible.** Don't try to be a solo performer—and don't always apply your favorite solution to a particular problem. You may know more about the technical details of the problems other people face…but they know better than you how well any proposed solution will fit them.

Example: If a couple about to retire asks your advice, don't automatically tell them to sell their big house, invest the profits and move to a small condo. They may prefer, for instance, to keep the house so they can put up many relatives and friends who come to visit.

● **Let the other person make the decision.** After you give your best advice to the person who consulted you, remember that he—not you—will have to live with the consequences.

That does not mean you wash your hands of any responsibility. In most cases, you should leave the decision entirely up to the

person who asked your advice. But it is appropriate for you to intervene in the decision if he asks explicitly what you would do…or wants to do something immoral or very risky …or does not understand the likely outcome of a particular choice.

ETHICAL RULES OF ADVISING

Do no harm. The person who has chosen you as an adviser thinks you will be able to help him.

Make sure before you give any advice that following it will not cause him harm. Give pure advice. Your job is to help someone else make the right decision, not to benefit yourself.

A good adviser is loyal to his client and committed to giving the best advice. He shows respect to the person who consulted him, is careful to use his full attention and skill to find the best solution and is reliable in keeping his promises.

Important: As an adviser, you need your own adviser—someone trustworthy to give you counsel on difficult problems.

KNOW WHEN TO STOP

When you have given the advice the other person needs to solve his problem, step aside. *Reasons to quit:*

● **The individual who approached you has reached the goal he originally sought.** Make sure you understand the goal clearly from the very beginning of the task.

Example: If your children ask your opinion about a house they are thinking about buying, do not assume that if they purchase it they will want your unsolicited advice on how to furnish it.

● **You are in over your head.** If this happens to you, explain the problem frankly—like Martha in the earlier example, who agreed to help her friend with her taxes but then found that the job exceeded her knowledge and her capabilities.

● **Your situation changes.** You may want to retire from the role of advice-giver or just don't have the time or energy needed to keep advising someone.

If he is continuously relying on your advice, give him adequate notice that you are no longer available and—if he really needs good advice

—try to steer him to someone who can take your place.

BOTTOM LINE

People who ask for your advice are really paying you a compliment. They are showing very high regard for your expertise and judgment. Make sure you repay it by giving the best advice possible.

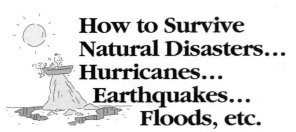

How to Survive Natural Disasters... Hurricanes... Earthquakes... Floods, etc.

Betsy Shand and Janice McCann whose company, House Calls, Etc., helps people prepare for disasters. They are authors of *Surviving Natural Disasters.* House Calls Books.

If you think that you'll never be hit by a natural disaster, you're not alone. That's what people thought in Los Angeles before the last earthquake...and in the Northwest before the catastrophic floods.

Reality: There's hardly a home in the country that is truly safe from some type of disaster, ranging from major catastrophes, such as a major flood, to relatively minor emergencies, such as electrical blackouts and freak snow storms.

Good news: Elaborate survival procedures aren't necessary. Commonsense precautions go a very long way in avoiding loss of property and life.

Though the list of precautions might seem long, they can be taken over a period of weeks or months. And once the measures are in place, there's little left to do except cope with the next disaster with greater peace of mind.

EMERGENCY PROVISIONS

Think of weathering a disaster as a little like camping out in your own home, where electricity and water have been cut off. *Store in a closet or other convenient location...*

●**Food that can be eaten with little or no preparation**, such as peanut butter, whole-grain crackers, baby food, powdered milk and cold cereal.

●**Several gallons of water**, which you can buy in bottles at the supermarket.

●**Food and water** for a pet if you have one.

●**A first-aid kit** that contains not just the standard items such as bandages and iodine—but also scissors, needles and thread and several days' supply of whatever medication you're currently taking. Kits can be bought from the Red Cross, camping-supply shops and most drugstores.

●**Flashlights with batteries stored separately** so they'll stay fresh.

●**Cash.** If electricity goes out, banks and Automatic Teller Machines will not be working.

●**An extra pair of eyeglasses** or contact lenses.

●**A ladder and basic tools**, including a crowbar, screwdriver, saw and hammer.

Keep a full or nearly full tank of gas in your car. The last experience you want is seeing an empty gas gauge while you're racing to escape rising flood waters. (Don't store gasoline outside your car's tank.)

DOCUMENT DEFENSE

Since disasters often destroy homes and their contents, store copies of important documents and vital information with a trusted friend. *Examples...*

●**A copy of your insurance policy** and the phone number of your agent.

●**Your attorney's name and number.**

●**A list of health problems**, medication and your doctor's number.

●**The location of your safe-deposit box** and an extra key.

●**Banking information**, such as Certificates of Deposit and checking account numbers.

As a rule, choose an out-of-town friend to hold these items since a neighbor's house may be just as vulnerable as yours. Keep change for a pay phone on hand. Moreover, local phone service often goes down in a disaster while long-distance is still operating. An out-of-town contact person can then take and relay messages if family members are separated.

DISASTER TRAINING

First-aid training does more than let you help the injured. It also builds up a sense of confidence that can be vital in getting you through a disaster. The Red Cross, YMCAs, YWCAs, community centers and many hospitals offer courses in first aid. Courses in preventing and surviving fires are offered by most fire departments. But even if you don't take a course, make your own plan to evacuate in case of fire. *Key elements of the plan…*

• **Install smoke alarms and/or sprinklers.** (Insurance companies often lower their rates on homes with sprinklers.)

• **Store towels, water and a rope ladder** under your bed. In case of fire, you can often buy lots of escape time by soaking towels in water and stuffing them under doors to block incoming smoke.

• **Keep fire extinguishers in appropriate places.**

• **Sleep with the doors closed.**

• **Plan an evacuation procedure**, and practice it periodically, just as you'd go through a fire drill.

Beware of items that can become hazardous in a disaster…

• **Difficult-to-see power lines** that have fallen or are dangling.

• **Water pipes, electricity lines and gas mains** in your home. Ask utility companies to show you how to shut them off. That's what to do if water is leaking, if you smell gas or if you suspect an electrical problem after a disaster.

NEIGHBORHOOD TEAMS

Organize a neighborhood disaster committee whose members can come to each other's aid in the event of an emergency. Working as a team, neighbors can often save a home if, for example, the owners are away and a gas main has ruptured.

Many residents have skills or equipment that can be invaluable in a disaster.

Examples: Doctors, carpenters, plumbers or neighbors with generators or cellular phones.

Key: A system that lets homeowners signal their postdisaster status to the rest of the neighborhood. Pin large white, yellow or red ribbons to your door or other conspicuous location.

White means all is okay. Yellow indicates residents are fine but need some assistance. Red signals an emergency and the immediate need for help.

THE RIGHT INSURANCE

Few events are more disheartening than surviving a disaster only to discover that insurance won't cover your property loss. *To avoid the problem:*

• **Buy a homeowner's policy** that covers the *replacement* of your home and contents. Many policies cover only the current value. That means if a Regency chair is destroyed in a fire, insurance pays only the *current* value of a chair, not the replacement value of the antique.

• **Choose an insurance policy that pays your living expenses** for an adequate period of time for putting your house back in living condition.

• **To document the value of your home and its contents**, keep all receipts for items you buy. Then photograph or videotape your possessions, or consider hiring a professional appraiser to put a price on items for which you don't have receipts. *Cost:* About $200 for most households. If you don't have a video camera, rent one from a local video store.

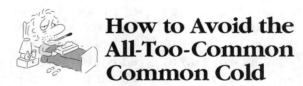

How to Avoid the All-Too-Common Common Cold

David A.J. Tyrrell, MD, who has been studying the common cold for more than 35 years. Now a health care consultant, Dr. Tyrrell is the former director of the Common Cold Unit of the Medical Research Council in Salisbury, England.

We hear reports of all kinds of remedies for the common cold, from sucking on zinc lozenges to rubbing garlic on your clothes. To find out what medical science has to say about such remedies, we talked to Dr. David A. J. Tyrrell, one of the world's foremost experts on the common cold.

•What causes colds? Colds are caused by any of several hundred different viruses specially adapted to grow in the nose (*rhinoviruses* and *coronaviruses*). That's why it has proven impossible—so far—to make a reliable vaccine. We simply haven't been able to come up with one that's effective against all the viruses.

Smokers are particularly vulnerable to colds. Tobacco smoke dries out the mucus membranes lining the mouth and nose, impairing their ability to fend off viruses. Moderate drinkers (those who have the equivalent of one glass of wine a day) seem to be less susceptible.

One thing that does not affect your risk of catching a cold is being cold. Over the years, there have been various studies in which volunteers got soaked in cold baths or stood out in the rain. These people did not catch colds at a higher rate than people who stayed warm and dry.

This doesn't mean it's a good idea to go out in wintry weather without warm clothing. Being cold can precipitate bacterial pneumonia and other serious ailments.

•How do colds spread? Scientists disagree on this. Many think the virus spreads when a person inhales tiny virus-laden droplets of mucus and saliva liberated by the sneeze of an infected person. Some evidence suggests that it's possible to catch a cold simply by being close (within a yard or so) to an infected person.

Other scientists think the virus spreads via hand-to-hand contact…or by touching an object recently touched by an infected person, then touching the germ-laden hand to the face.

•What can I do to avoid colds? Since we can't count on others to stay at home when they're ill, it pays to avoid sitting or standing near anyone you suspect has a cold…and to watch where you put your hands.

•Does vitamin C prevent colds? Despite its popularity, vitamin C has never been proven either to prevent or cure colds. Study after study has found no real difference in the incidence, duration or severity of colds between people who took vitamin C (up to

3,000 milligrams a day) and those who did not take C.

•What about flu shots? They prevent certain types of influenza but won't keep you from catching a cold.

•Does psychological stress increase my vulnerability to colds? Absolutely. Several years ago, I did a series of studies in collaboration with Sheldon Cohen, PhD, a Carnegie Mellon University psychologist. We found that people who had recently been through a stressful experience—job loss, the death of a close relative or even desirable forms of stress like getting married—were more prone to colds than other individuals.

We found an almost twofold difference in infection rates among the most- and least-stressed individuals.

•What's the best way to treat a cold? While there's no way to cure the common cold, there are ways to make the symptoms more bearable…

•Drink liquids to keep mucus membranes moist.

•Soothe a sore throat with warm, sweet drinks, such as tea with honey. Or gargle with salt water.

•Inhale water vapor from a steam kettle or a hot bath or shower to help clear nasal passages. A hot bath is relaxing as well.

•Keep air moist with a humidifier or a kettle.

•What about over-the-counter medications? Take aspirin, acetaminophen or ibuprofen to reduce pain and fever. Aspirin should not be given to children under 12 because of the risk of Reye's syndrome. Aspirin can cause stomach upset, and acetaminophen occasionally causes liver damage. Ibuprofen has a good safety record, although it, too, can cause stomach upset.

A decongestant containing *ephedrine* constricts dilated blood vessels, reducing swelling and secretion of mucus. It's best to take this drug in nose drops or nasal spray, because the effect will be localized. Taking any drug orally exposes the entire body to its effects. Never use a nasal decongestant spray or drops for more than a week. If you do, you risk a "rebound" reaction, in which congestion worsens and the body becomes dependent on the drug.

●Should I see a doctor if I have a cold? In most cases, that's unnecessary. But if symptoms persist for more than a week, or you have high fever or a pus-like nasal secretion, you may have developed a bacterial infection on top of your cold. In such cases, see a doctor immediately. Ask if you need antibiotics—which, by the way, are *ineffective* against colds.

Children under age three, elderly people and those with lung or heart trouble are at greater risk of potentially deadly complications. They should notify a doctor at the first sign of anything more than a very mild cold.

The doctor should also determine whether you have a cold or the flu. A mild case of flu is often indistinguishable from a cold...and a severe cold may resemble the flu. Although both are characterized by sore throat, runny nose and cough, influenza usually involves muscle aches, headache and high fever.

The antiviral drugs *rimantidine* (Flumadine) and *amantidine* (Symadine) and the newer drugs *oseltamivir* (Tamiflu) and *zanamivir* (Relenza), an inhaled medication, can hasten recovery from influenza. However, they're effective only if taken soon after the onset of symptoms.

●Is it okay to exercise with a cold? There's no evidence that exercise prolongs or exacerbates a cold. Indeed, some people say they feel better afterward. But don't push yourself if you feel terrible.

●Are any popular home remedies helpful? Many old-fashioned remedies do seem to reduce discomfort, even if they don't actually get rid of the cold. For example, warm liquids like chicken soup soothe the throat, while the rising steam loosens up mucus. And tea made with ginger or another fragrant herb helps settle an upset stomach.

Menthol—mixed with hot water to make steam or rubbed in gel form on the upper lip —seems to clear clogged nasal passages.

Zinc lozenges, the herb *echinacea* and homeopathic products are said to be helpful in

treating colds. But at this point, their effectiveness has not been proven.

●What about those mechanical devices that blow hot air up the nose? There's no evidence that these hair-dryer-like devices do much good. They may relieve some symptoms, but they won't make your cold go away.

You can derive the same benefit by inhaling the steam from a bowl of soup or hot water.

How to Stop Sinusitis

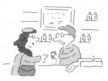

Juan C. Guarderas, MD, senior associate consultant in the division of allergic diseases at the Mayo Clinic in Jacksonville, FL.

If you have a stuffy nose for more than a week or two, you may not be suffering from a cold—but from sinusitis. That's an inflammation or infection of the sinuses, the hollow spaces in the bones near the nose.

Among other functions, the four groups of sinuses warm and humidify air on its way from the nostrils to the lungs. A lining of mucus keeps the sinuses moist.

When everything's working right, tiny hairs called *cilia* sweep mucus from the sinuses down into the nose. But when the passages connecting the nose and the sinuses are congested—such as during a cold or allergy attack—the sinuses may fail to drain. Bacteria and/or fungi multiply in the trapped mucus, causing infection.

Sinusitis can lead to persistent cough or bronchitis—and can exacerbate existing cases of asthma. In rare cases, it can result in a life-threatening infection of the eyes or brain.

SYMPTOMS AND CAUSES

Sinusitis is usually marked by severe congestion...headache...mild fever...pain in the face or teeth...and a thick yellowish-green nasal discharge that continues all day and night. Some sinusitis sufferers are sensitive to shifts in barometric pressure—for example, on plane flights or during changes in the weather.

The common cold, in contrast, is characterized by watery white or yellow mucus that clears up as the day goes on. Allergies are often accompanied by itching and watering eyes.

Most cases of sinusitis occur during or shortly after a cold. Other cases are caused by allergies...tobacco smoke or other respiratory irritants...mouth infections...or anatomical problems, such as nasal polyps or a deviated septum, that obstruct sinus drainage.

Forty percent of cold-related sinus attacks get better without treatment as sinuses begin to drain again. But sinusitis often becomes chronic, creating long-term changes in the delicate lining of the sinus (the *mucosa*).

Chronic sinusitis may damage the cilia or acidify the mucus, leading to further irritation and inflammation. Over time, repeated bouts of sinusitis can permanently narrow the opening of the sinuses into the nose.

TREATING ACUTE SINUSITIS

The standard treatment for acute sinusitis is a course of antibiotics lasting 10 to 14 days... plus oral decongestants and nasal spray.* Antihistamines are not recommended. They're too drying.

Caution: Using over-the-counter decongestant nasal sprays for more than five days can produce a "rebound" effect, in which the sprays themselves cause the nose to clog up.

With antibiotics, it's important to take the full course—even *after* you start feeling better. Otherwise, you create prime breeding conditions for drug-resistant bacteria.

Another good treatment for acute sinusitis is *saline irrigation*. When done under a doctor's supervision, it can be highly effective at reducing nasal and sinus congestion.

What to do: Each morning, fill a clean, narrow-tipped plastic squeeze bottle with a mixture of one teaspoon salt to one pint lukewarm water. As you lean over a sink, squirt the solution into your nose until it's all gone. The solution will drain out. Be sure to clean the container and tip after each use.

*Most doctors recommend over-the-counter decongestant sprays like Afrin or NeoSynephrine...saline sprays like Ocean...or prescription steroid sprays like *beclomethasone* (Beconase).

TREATING CHRONIC SINUSITIS

Chronic sinusitis is harder to treat. In addition to decongestant sprays and pills, a three-week course of antibiotics is often helpful. If there's still no improvement at that point, see an allergist or otolaryngologist.

To pinpoint the source of your sinus trouble, this doctor may recommend an X ray or CT scan...or perform endoscopy.

Via this simple procedure—done in the doctor's office—the doctor can determine whether you have nasal polyps or another anatomical obstruction. If so, surgery to remove polyps or to widen the sinus opening slightly may be helpful.

If your sinusitis is diagnosed as allergy-related, it may be necessary to avoid dust, animal dander and other allergens.

Nasal medications such as steroid inhalers may also provide some relief.

If you've had sinus trouble in the past and want to avoid recurrence, take precautions whenever you have a cold—to keep it from turning into a sinus attack.

Use decongestants and nasal irrigation...and avoid flying, scuba diving and other activities that involve rapid changes in air pressure.

Indigestion...How to Be Rid of It Forever!

Henry D. Janowitz, MD, a gastroenterologist affiliated with Mount Sinai Medical Center in New York City. He is author of *Indigestion*. Oxford University Press.

Indigestion affects millions of Americans each year. This catch-all term encompasses a wide array of complaints—from "acid stomach," belching, nausea, bloating and distention...to much more serious problems, such as peptic esophagitis, gallstones and stomach cancer.

The leading source of gastrointestinal distress is heartburn, technically known as acid reflux. At one time or another, nearly all of us have experienced this burning sensation behind the breastbone. Often it's accompanied by a rush of highly acidic fluid into the back of the throat, leaving an unpleasant burning sensation there as well. Reflux occurs when the movement of food and digestive juices in the digestive tract causes stomach acid to back up into the esophagus.

Reflux may also arise from defects in the esophageal sphincter—the muscular "gateway" between the esophagus and the stomach.

This problem may be caused by a hiatal hernia—a weakness in the diaphragm, the muscular wall that separates the abdominal cavity from the lungs. *Other possible reflux triggers:*

•**Caffeine and cigarettes.** Both cause excessive secretion of stomach acid.

•**Fatty foods.** Fats are hard to digest, so fatty foods stay in the stomach longer than carbohydrates or proteins.

•**Alcohol.** While it doesn't induce reflux directly, it can cause erosion, swelling and inflammation of the stomach lining.

•**Ulcers.** Scar tissue from previous duodenal or peptic ulcers sometimes blocks the passage of food through the stomach.

•**Diabetes and viral infections.** They interfere with stomach motility by several mechanisms, including direct injury to nerves leading to the stomach or encouragement of overgrowth of intestinal bacteria.

Untreated reflux can cause chronic inflammation of the esophagus (esophagitis), a serious disorder marked by hoarseness, bleeding, pain, scarring, difficult swallowing, nausea and frequent awakening at night.

ANOTHER COMMON COMPLAINT

Nonulcer dyspepsia (NUD) is another common stomach complaint.

Symptoms: Gnawing stomach pain, nausea and vague acidity. These symptoms often mimic those of a peptic ulcer, although the stomach is otherwise normal.

Sometimes NUD is marked more by a feeling that the stomach is not emptying quickly enough. Food seems to linger too long, leading to fullness, swelling and gassiness. These symptoms can begin well before a meal is over…or up to two hours later.

No one knows exactly what causes NUD, but studies point to disturbances in the muscular action of the stomach, duodenum or esophagus.

RX FOR TROUBLED STOMACHS

While Maalox, Mylanta, Tums, Rolaids and other over-the-counter antacids are often helpful, it's better to *prevent* indigestion in the first place. *Prevention strategies:*

•**Eat three square meals a day.** Or, if you prefer, eat several small, light meals. Never skip breakfast or lunch with the intention of "making up for it" at the end of the day. Stuffing yourself at one sitting only increases pressure inside the stomach—and with it, the possibility of reflux.

•**Don't lie down too soon after eating.** Reflux is more likely to occur when you're lying down. So avoid late-night snacks and "siestas" during the day.

If you must sleep immediately after eating, be sure to keep your chest elevated. Put several pillows under your head, insert a foam wedge under your mattress or put the head of the bed on blocks.

If you crave a late-night snack, try drinking a cup of herbal or decaffeinated tea—fluids leave the stomach faster than solids.

•**Take steps to avoid constipation.** It raises abdominal pressure, making reflux more likely. Eat fiber-rich foods…drink plenty of fluids… exercise regularly…avoid tight belts or girdles …and keep excess weight off.

•**Avoid greasy or highly seasoned foods.** *Examples:* Curries, Szechuan dishes and dishes made with chili powder. If you've experienced indigestion after eating such foods in the past, be especially careful to avoid them in the future.

BEYOND SELF-HELP

If your discomfort persists, seek professional help. To help the doctor make an accurate diagnosis, prepare a detailed account of symptoms—how long you have had them and under what circumstances.

Example: A gnawing or burning pain above the navel within one to three hours after eating can signal an ulcer. A thorough checkup should consist of a general physical exam, a blood and stool test and an upper GI series with barium in the stomach and esophagus.

In order to clearly see the esophageal lining, the doctor may perform an upper GI *endoscopy,* in which he will use a viewing probe called an *endoscope.*

Some prescription remedies are designed to reduce the irritating effects of reflux by suppressing stomach acidity or neutralizing the acid already secreted. Others clear the esophagus, strengthen its sphincter muscle and help empty the stomach—in the proper direction.

A class of drugs called *histamine 2 blockers,* along with newer antacid medications such as Prilosec, stop production of hydrochloric acid in the stomach—especially overnight when it is most likely to accumulate and back up. The histamine 2 blockers Pepcid, Tagamet and Zantac are available over-the-counter, and help the pain of heartburn.

If tests confirm full-blown esophagitis, caffeine, tobacco and alcohol must be strictly forbidden, along with aspirin and other nonsteroidal anti-inflammatory drugs (NSAIDs). The suggestions on diet and sleep must also be followed rigorously, and prescription medications must be continued for months even after all symptoms have disappeared.

The most striking new information about stomach ulcers is the discovery that the bacterium *H. pylori,* if present, must be eliminated by antibiotics to ensure lasting healing of the problem.

THE BRAIN-GUT CONNECTION

The brain is intimately linked to the stomach, esophagus and small bowel through a direct "rapid transit" system of nerve pathways —as well as through the slower, more indirect route of chemical "messengers," or hormones.

Such connections help explain why stress and emotional upset affect our digestive health so dramatically. Emotional disturbances change the brain's chemical activity, which in turn sends distress signals back to the gastrointestinal tract.

Your ability to tolerate stomach problems depends in large measure upon your disposition. For reasons unknown, some people have an unusually low tolerance for disturbances of the GI tract, whether these disturbances are caused by reactions to food, psychological stress or illness.

In such cases, stress management, relaxation, guided imagery and other behavioral modification techniques are often helpful. Thus, a consultation with a psychologist or other mental health professional is often a vital part of any "cure" for a troubled stomach.

Cosmetic Surgery... The Best Solutions

Kimberly Henry, MD, a plastic and reconstructive surgeon in private practice in Greenbrae, CA. She is coauthor of *The Plastic Surgery Sourcebook.* Lowell House.

Cosmetic surgery means more than nose jobs and breast implants. There are now hundreds of different procedures designed to take care of everything from wrinkles and scars to sagging skin and loose jowls.

FURROWED BROW

Deep vertical lines between the eyebrows can usually be eliminated with *BoTox,* a toxin derived from the same microbe that causes the deadly ailment botulism.

Injected between the brows, BoTox paralyzes the facial muscle causing the wrinkles. The procedure takes about 10 minutes. Results last for three to six months. *Cost:* $500 per injection.

TIRED-LOOKING FACE

Although collagen injections work well for isolated facial wrinkles, they are not very effective for a face that is "tired-looking" all over. The best remedy for such a face is usually laser therapy.

Laser light causes collagen in the skin to shrink, eliminating wrinkles for about nine years. That's how long it takes facial wrinkles to form.

Several different kinds of lasers are now in use. For mild wrinkling, the best bet is the newly approved *erbium* laser. It combines good results with a brief recovery period.

The skin is red for three or four days. You can go back to work within a week. *Cost:* $1,000 to $3,000.

Avoid: Dermabrasion and chemical peels. These once-popular treatments for removing facial wrinkles yield unpredictable results. They can also cause scarring or lightening of the skin.

DEEP WRINKLES OR SCARRING

For acne scars or *deep* wrinkles caused by years of smoking and/or sun exposure, the best approach is once again laser therapy. But instead of the erbium laser, it's better to use the more powerful *carbon dioxide* laser.

Carbon dioxide laser therapy takes only 90 minutes, but the recovery period often lasts up to 10 days.

During the first week of this postoperative period, it's a bit like having a bad sunburn. The skin peels and crusts over. Pain medication is often needed. After seven to 10 days, the crust falls off, leaving behind new, pink skin. *Cost:* $3,000 to $6,000.

SAGGING JOWLS OR NECK WATTLES

For loose skin on the face or neck, the best treatment is a face-lift or neck-lift. In this four-hour operation, the surgeon makes an incision in front of and behind the ears.

Then he/she lifts the skin off the underlying muscles and fat of the face and tugs it back till it's snug.

Face-lifts are done on an outpatient basis. The recovery period lasts seven to 10 days. At that point, the stitches are removed, and you can return to normal activity. *Cost:* $5,000 to $25,000.

Good news: A new variant of the traditional face-lift procedure reduces the slight risk of nerve damage associated with the older procedure. *Supra-platysmal* face-lift involves repositioning only the superficial layers of skin.

The surgeon repositions the cheek fat and removes some fat around the jaw. *Cost:* $3,300.

Since neither type of face-lift can completely eliminate wrinkles, many patients opt to have laser therapy six weeks or so after the face-lift.

FLABBY HIPS, THIGHS AND ARMS

With America's obesity problem continuing unabated, liposuction has become the most popular cosmetic surgery procedure.

In conventional liposuction, the surgeon sucks out fat using a thin tube (*cannula*) inserted through the skin. Most surgeons now use *tumescent liposuction*, in which fluids containing essential salts and sugars along with a local anesthetic and *epinephrine* to control bleeding are injected into the area being suctioned.

Unlike conventional liposuction, tumescent liposuction allows safe removal of *lots* of fat—up to 22 pounds at a time. *Cost:* $1,500 per site.

Some surgeons are starting to use *ultrasonic* liposuction instead. It involves use of a special probe that "melts" fat before it's sucked out of the body.

ENLARGED BREASTS IN MEN

The standard approach to this problem is to make an incision around the outside of the nipple and then cut away the excess fat with a scalpel.

This method generally yields good results, especially when used in combination with liposuction. *Cost:* $2,000 to $3,000.

FINDING A GOOD COSMETIC SURGEON

Picking a surgeon certified by the American Board of Plastic Surgery is not enough. You must also look for a surgeon who has…

• **Treated someone you know,** with good results and

• **Performed the same procedure several times.**

Best strategy: Consult two or three cosmetic surgeons. Listen to their recommendations, and see how your personalities mesh.

For a list of board-certified plastic surgeons in your area, contact the national referral service of the American Society of Plastic Surgeons at 888-4-PLASTIC. *www.plasticsurgery.org.*

All About Dizziness

Brian Blakley, MD, PhD, associate professor of otolaryngology and director of the dizziness clinic at Wayne State University School of Medicine in Detroit. He is coauthor of *Feeling Dizzy: Understanding and Treating Dizziness, Vertigo and Other Balance Disorders.* Macmillan Books.

In the absence of other symptoms, occasional mild dizziness is nothing to worry about. But see a doctor right away if dizzy spells recur…if they're severe enough to force you to lie down…or if they're accompanied by…

- **Double vision.**

- **Incontinence.**

- **Arm and/or leg weakness.**

- **Difficulty with speaking or swallowing.**

- **Severe headache.**

These symptoms are suggestive of stroke, brain tumor, aneurysm or another potentially life-threatening problem.

COMMON TYPES OF DIZZINESS

- **A mild turning sensation.** Caused by almost any systemic ailment, including transient ischemic attacks, multiple sclerosis...even AIDS.

Some women have mild turning during menstruation—or as a side effect of hormone replacement therapy or menopause.

- **Imbalance.** This swaying or wobbling feeling can be caused by flu, infection, arthritis, compression of the spinal cord, diabetes or another metabolic disorder.

Imbalance can also be caused by alcohol abuse, depression or anxiety (rapid breathing reduces the flow of oxygen to the brain)...or by certain medications, including cough medicines and blood pressure drugs.

- **Vertigo.** This sensation of spinning often accompanies migraine headaches and many diseases.

- **Feeling of faintness.** This is often a result of *postural hypotension,* the brief period of reduced blood pressure that occurs when someone abruptly stands or sits up.

Several medications can contribute to postural hypotension, including antihypertensives, antihistamines, sedatives and antipsychotics.

With proper treatment, most cases of dizziness disappear. However, some cases resist treatment—including those that are caused by multiple sclerosis, AIDS and menstruation. In these cases, the patient simply has to learn to live with the problem.

EAR AND BRAIN DISORDERS

Persistent dizziness not linked to an underlying illness usually involves brain or inner ear trouble.

- **Benign paroxysmal positional vertigo** (BPPV) occurs when a person moves his head in a certain position—typically when he lies on his back, then rolls quickly to one side.

BPPV itself isn't life-threatening, but it can be deadly if it occurs while driving an automobile or standing up.

BPPV in people under 50 is often caused by head trauma. Even a light bump can be enough. In people over 50, BPPV can occur after illness, or be caused by degeneration of the nerves in the middle ear. In some cases, BPPV appears for no apparent reason.

- **Vestibular neuronitis** is sudden vertigo that occurs a few days or weeks after recovery from a viral infection. Often it's accompanied by nausea and/or vomiting. *Likely cause:* Inflammation of the vestibular nerve, which connects the brain and inner ear.

- **Ataxia** is a loss of coordination. It's usually caused by the death of brain cells, although it can also be caused by vitamin deficiencies or heavy drinking. Most common among elderly people, it often comes on gradually, and is generally irreversible.

- **Ménière's disease** is a set of related symptoms, including vertigo attacks...roaring, ringing or hearing loss in one ear...a feeling of fullness in the ear. Most cases are caused by fluid buildup in the inner ear.

Ménière's usually strikes between the ages of 30 and 50. Symptoms tend to recur, lasting an hour or more at a time. They range from mild to debilitating.

- **Ear infection** that causes fluid to accumulate in the middle ear can cause everything from mild imbalance to severe vertigo.

GETTING GOOD TREATMENT

There's no easy way to test the balance mechanisms in the ear and the brain, so your doctor may have trouble pinpointing the cause of your dizziness. If he/she fails to take a complete medical history...or does not take your dizziness seriously...or has little experience with dizziness, find another doctor.

Best: An otolaryngologist or neurologist working in a dizziness clinic. For the name of one near you, call the American Academy of Otolaryngology–Head and Neck Surgery. 703-836-4444.

Doctors use several tests to check for inner ear damage. The tests I use most often are the hearing test (audiogram) and two more specialized tests, *electronystagmography* (ENG) and the *rotary chair exam.*

ENG looks at eye movements caused by electrical stimulation of the vestibular system. The rotary chair exam measures eye movements as the patient sits in a computer-controlled rotating chair.

The best antidote for inner ear ailments is *time.* Inner ear damage usually heals within a few weeks or months. Fluid buildup from ear infection also tends to disappear in a few weeks.

Even persistent nerve damage usually stops causing dizziness after several months. The brain simply learns to re-sort incoming information (much as it adjusts to the rocking of a ship).

Vestibular neuronitis often persists until the underlying inflammation clears up. That can take years—though medicine, bed rest and rehabilitation exercises are helpful.

Dizziness may be *permanent* in those suffering from ataxia, multiple sclerosis or other central nervous system disorders.

Treatment for Ménière's disease may involve surgery to relieve accumulation of fluid, but diuretics and/or steroids can provide significant relief.

If you do have surgery, make sure the surgeon is certified in otolaryngology. *To check credentials:* Contact the American Board of Medical Specialties, 866-ASK-ABMS, *www.abms.org.* Dizziness usually subsides within eight weeks of surgery.

In some cases of dizziness, the mild sedative *meclizine* (Antivert) brings short-term relief. *Scopolamine* is even more effective...but also causes more side effects, including drowsiness and dry mouth. *Caution:* These drugs should be used for no more than a week or two, during severe episodes.

REHABILITATION EXERCISES

Many people with dizziness benefit from rehabilitation exercises. These speed the brain's adaptation process by enhancing neural connections in the inner ear. In fact, rehabilitation exercises are helpful for most balance problems, with or without a doctor's supervision. *Two helpful exercises:*

Horizontal head rotations: Sit down. Face forward. Turn your head to the right, then the left, going back and forth. Start slowly and increase the speed of rotation of your head as much as you can in 20 seconds. Repeat for the other side.

Vertical head rotations: Sit down. Face forward. *Position I:* Turn your head 45 degrees to the right. *Position II:* Move the top of your head from its vertical position so that your left ear moves toward your left knee and your head is horizontal. Alternate between positions 1 and 2 as fast as you can for 20 seconds. Repeat for the other side.

These exercises should be repeated two to three times in each session. Three sessions per day should be performed.

How to Win the Chronic-Pain War

Norman Marcus, MD, diplomat of the American Board of Pain Medicine...president of the International Foundation for Pain Relief...and medical director of the New York Pain Treatment Program at Lenox Hill Hospital. Dr. Marcus is author of *Freedom from Pain.* Simon & Schuster.

If you suffer from headaches, back pain, neck pain or joint pain that persists for more than six to eight weeks, you may be experiencing chronic pain.

The good news is that now you can do more than just put up with it.

ORIGINS OF CHRONIC PAIN

The body requires about six weeks to heal following major injuries—broken bones, surgical incisions, etc. The pain associated with those injuries, however, can be felt long after the body has healed.

The acute or short-term pain that immediately follows an injury is directly related to how much damage the body has sustained. But pain that persists longer than might be expected following such conditions is chronic pain—and it is *not* related to the amount of damage that was sustained.

For years, chronic pain has been thought of as a disease itself and, therefore, the favored approach was managing the pain rather than looking for a cause of the pain.

CAUSES OF CHRONIC PAIN

Muscles are the major cause of chronic pain. They produce pain in four ways.

Emotional stress is the chief culprit that makes us tense our muscles without even being aware of it. Not surprisingly, all the day-to-day stress we experience affects the body. You tense your muscles, and you feel pain. And that pain may travel to different parts of the body.

Most chronic pain should not be seen as evidence of disease. It may, however, serve as your barometer of tension. The other causes for muscle pain are weaknesses and stiffness, spasm and trigger points.

HOW TO REDUCE CHRONIC PAIN

●**Tune in to what your body is telling you.** If you are experiencing persistent pain, you have a problem and should get help. Unfortunately, many doctors may not be able to help with your back or neck pains.

Reason: Although about 80% of the human body is made of muscle, most doctors are not taught a "hands-on" approach to examining muscles or evaluating the possible effects of muscle tension, weakness or spasm. As a result, muscle-related pain may not be recognized by your doctor or managed appropriately.

If previous pain-management strategies have not worked for you, look for a doctor who has expertise in muscle-related pain. Screen potential doctors to see if they incorporate evaluation and treatment of muscles in their pain-management regimens.

●**Stop thinking of the pain as a disease.** It will be more difficult to get rid of your pain if you make it the focus of a lot of worry and concern.

Try to carry on with as many normal daily activities as you can. Don't be afraid of movement, even if it's a little uncomfortable. Movement is necessary for chronic pain sufferers because muscle inactivity worsens the pain.

●**Begin a moderate exercise program.** This does not mean taking strenuous aerobics classes…or jogging five miles a day. In fact, both types of exercise should be avoided.

Better: Start a walking or swimming program, beginning with a modest distance and gradually increasing your goal as you feel more comfortable. Work with your doctor to develop the appropriate regimen for you. Work up to 30 to 40 minutes of exercise, three or four times a week.

Always remember that a proper exercise program starts with relaxation techniques such as meditation…then limbering and stretching prior to the initial exercise…followed by a cool-down period, which ends with relaxation again.

In addition to helping you stretch and strengthen, the process will help your mind release tension and stress, the major causes of chronic muscle-related pain.

If your pain is associated with danger signs—fever, chills, night sweats, headaches and malaise—it could indicate an underlying disease or potentially serious problem. You should consult your doctor.

IDEAL EXERCISE

●**Walk outdoors.** When you walk, you go a little faster, a little slower, take a bigger step, then a smaller step. That's natural for the body and a great way to exercise to eliminate chronic pain. Don't worry about the speed at first. Increase your distance by about 20% every few days. Aim to walk two to three miles each day.

●**Use a stationary bike** with the seat adjusted so you can extend your legs a little less than full extension. A stationary bike offers a good aerobic workout—if it is done with minimal tension at first and slowly built up in difficulty. If your back hurts on an upright bike, try a recumbent one.

●**Cross-country ski machines** offer a great workout if you are fit enough.

●**Swimming is terrific.** But if you have back pain, doing multiple laps with a crawl may result in overarching your back, causing more pain. If you have back pain, the back stroke and the side stroke are safer.

EXERCISES TO AVOID

●**Do not use any type of exercise machine that forces your body** into awkward positions to which you are not accustomed.

•Do not overdo any muscle-strengthening exercise. Three to four repetitions of any movement is sufficient. Then you should move on to the next exercise. You may return to any of the completed exercises for another set but only if you are completely free of pain.

•Avoid stair-step exercises. They can produce pain and soreness from the repetition of one movement. These leg exercises involve only ascending—not descending—motion for an aerobic workout. It's better and cheaper to simply walk up and down a staircase.

•Avoid exercising on treadmills, since they also force you to repeat the same motion at the exact same pace over and over again. The body is not made to handle that type of repetitive motion.

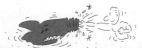

Beating Arthritis Pain

Jason Theodosakis, MD, assistant clinical professor of medicine and director of the preventive medicine residency program at the University of Arizona College of Medicine in Tucson. He is coauthor of *The Arthritis Cure: The Medical Miracle that Can Halt, Reverse and May Even Cure Osteoarthritis.* St. Martin's.

The 16 million Americans who suffer from osteoarthritis* tend to rely on aspirin, ibuprofen and other nonsteroidal anti-inflammatory drugs (NSAIDs) to control their pain.

But NSAIDs do nothing to treat the underlying condition. Consequently, arthritis pain tends to worsen with time. In addition, NSAIDs can trigger a host of troublesome side effects, including digestive problems and high blood pressure.

Worst of all, new evidence suggests that NSAIDs can *aggravate* arthritis by blocking synthesis of *proteoglycans*, key molecules that help draw much-needed water into dry, damaged joints.

Breakthrough: Daily use of two nutritional supplements—*glucosamine* and *chon-*

*Osteoarthritis is one of 100 different kinds of arthritis. It is caused by the degeneration of the cartilage lining the joints.

droitin—controls pain, boosts joint mobility and helps undo the cartilage damage that is the hallmark of osteoarthritis.

Glucosamine and chondroitin work together to block the action of cartilage-destroying enzymes...promote the flow of water and nutrients into cartilage...and boost the activity of cartilage-producing cells called *chondrocytes*. The supplements have been proven effective in studies around the world...

•In a double-blind study conducted in Portugal, 40 arthritis patients were given either 1.5 grams (g) of glucosamine or 1.2 g of ibuprofen a day. Ibuprofen's pain-reducing effect faded after two weeks. Glucosamine relieved pain for the study's full eight-week duration.

•A double-blind study of 80 arthritis patients in Milan, Italy, found that 1.5 g a day of glucosamine reduced symptoms by 73% after 30 days. Patients who were given a placebo experienced only a 41% reduction in symptoms.

•In a 1992 French study, 120 people with knee or hip arthritis were given chondroitin or a placebo. After three months, the chondroitin group reported significantly less pain than the placebo group.

I can personally vouch for the effectiveness of glucosamine and chondroitin. Five years ago, my osteoarthritis—the result of chronic sports injuries—became so bad that I was forced to use crutches and a wheelchair.

After a search of the medical literature on arthritis uncovered several references to glucosamine and chondroitin, I began taking both supplements. My symptoms diminished within two weeks...and disappeared within four weeks. Several months later, a medical exam revealed that the cartilage in my joints had actually repaired itself.

USING THE SUPPLEMENTS

Glucosamine and chondroitin are available at drugstores and health-food stores. They're available without a prescription, but it's best to use them under the supervision of a sports medicine specialist, a rheumatologist or an orthopedic surgeon.

How much of each supplement should you take every day? That depends upon your body weight. *I use these guidelines...*

Less than 120 pounds: 1,000 milligrams (mg) glucosamine...800 mg chondroitin.

Between 120 to 200 pounds: 1,500 mg glucosamine...1,200 mg chondroitin.

More than 200 pounds: 2,000 mg glucosamine...1,600 mg chondroitin.

I tell my patients to divide each dose into halves, taking the first half in the morning, the second half in the evening—preferably with food.

As their arthritis pain subsides, I have them reduce the dosage. Symptoms generally begin to diminish within six weeks.

Important: Potent as these supplements are, they are only part of an effective arthritis treatment regimen. Here are the other key components.

ANTIOXIDANTS

Since the cartilage damage associated with arthritis is caused in part by cell-damaging *free radicals*, I urge my patients to take daily antioxidants. The "ACES" antioxidants are particularly effective at controlling free radicals...

●**Vitamin A**...5,000 international units (IU) a day.

●**Vitamin C**...4,000 mg a day.

●**Vitamin E**...400 IU a day.

●**Selenium**...200 micrograms (mcg) a day.

It's also a good idea to eat foods rich in *bioflavonoids*. These compounds make *collagen* —the tough protein that is a primary constituent of cartilage—stronger and less prone to inflammation.

Bioflavonoid sources: Green tea, berries, onions, citrus fruits and pitted fruits, such as cherries and plums.

REGULAR EXERCISE

Walking, swimming and other forms of exercise are key elements of any arthritis regimen.

Exercise boosts production of synovial fluid, the nutrient-rich "broth" that lubricates the joints. It also strengthens the muscles, tendons and ligaments that support the joints...extends your range of motion...and boosts your flexibility.

Challenge: Finding an exercise that won't trigger additional pain. I often refer my arthritis patients to a physical therapist. He/she can tailor a fitness regimen to suit your specific needs—and limitations.

To find a physical therapist in your area, contact the American Physical Therapy Association at 800-999-2782 or online at *www.apta.org*.

Caution: People who bill themselves only as "personal trainers" often lack the training required to work safely and effectively with arthritis patients.

BODY MECHANICS

Some cases of arthritis are caused by misaligned joints or other "body mechanics" problems. Such problems place undue stress on the joints, causing cartilage to break down.

To identify body mechanics problems, I often ask my arthritis patients to have a biomechanical analysis. That involves taking a close look at how they walk, work and move about.

A typical analysis involves videotaping your movements and/or using electronic "force plates" to measure forces on the soles of your feet as you walk.

Once problem areas are pinpointed, you'll be shown how modifying your movements can reduce the mechanical stresses on your joints.

Example: A woman with severe arthritis pain in her ankle was told by three different doctors that she had to give up tennis. She was also informed that she needed surgery to stabilize the joint.

Her gait *appeared* normal, but a biomechanical analysis showed that it was putting unusual stress on her right knee, ankle and foot. She spent a few hours learning how to walk correctly and bought a different pair of shoes. Within two weeks, her pain was gone.

Biomechanical analysis is available from sports medicine doctors and practitioners who have completed a fellowship in sports medicine. It costs $100 to $1,000, depending on the equipment used.

WEIGHT LOSS

Each step you take subjects your knee and hip joints to forces that are 2.5 to 10 times your body weight. That's why it's essential to stay slim if you want to control arthritis pain.

Example: The knees of a 200-pound man must bear up to one ton of weight whenever he squats or walks downstairs.

If you're overweight, take steps to lose the excess weight. If your weight is normal, make sure it stays that way.

Beating Joint Pain

David S. Pisetsky, MD, PhD, professor of medicine and immunology at Duke University Medical Center in Durham, NC, and medical adviser to the Arthritis Foundation, 1314 Spring St., Atlanta 30309. He is author of *The Duke University Medical Center Book of Arthritis.* Fawcett Columbine.

A sudden twinge in an elbow, shoulder, knee or another joint is probably *not* arthritis. Most forms of arthritis develop slowly, striking first in the hands.

Instead, you've probably irritated the soft tissue around the joint. This ailment—really a family of ailments including bursitis, tendinitis and carpal tunnel syndrome—calls for a slightly different approach to treatment than arthritis.

Soft-tissue inflammation is not a natural consequence of aging. Most cases can be traced to excessive exercise...or to a job-related activity involving repetitive motion. The pain is usually apparent within 24 hours of overuse. It can range from a dull ache to shooting pain.

COMMON SOFT-TISSUE INJURIES

•**Rotator cuff tendinitis** affects the tendons that hold the shoulder joint in place. Common among swimmers and other athletes, this ailment can make it hard to get dressed or lie down.

•**Shoulder bursitis**—very common among gardeners and house painters—is caused by repeated pressure on shoulder *bursae*, fluid-filled "cushions" that protect the joints. It becomes painful to move the arm away from the body.

•**Tennis elbow** strikes carpenters, gardeners, mechanics, dentists...and tennis players who use poor form or a tightly strung racket. The pain makes it hard to shake hands or lift a briefcase.

•**Carpal tunnel syndrome** is an inflammation of tissue surrounding the median nerve of the hand. Symptoms include weakness, pain, burning or aching in the wrist and/or hand. Usually caused by repeated hand motions, like those used by checkout clerks, seamstresses and computer operators.

•**Prepatellar bursitis** involves inflammation of the bursa in front of the kneecap (patella). It is common in people who must stand or kneel for extended periods. The pain is rarely severe.

•**Shin splints** involve pain in the front of the lower leg. Most cases are caused by repetitive exercise—especially running on hard surfaces. This can injure muscle and tendon tissue.

•**Achilles tendinitis**—inflammation of the Achilles tendon—is common among basketball and squash players and runners (especially those who run on concrete or in flimsy shoes). Symptoms include pain, swelling and tenderness in the heel.

•**Plantar fasciitis** involves a tear in the ligament connecting the arch to the heel. It causes a burning pain on the sole of the foot and the heel, making it painful to walk or stand on your toes. Common among runners.

•**Trochanteric bursitis** is inflammation of the bursa near the hip. Symptoms include pain in the hip and thigh, especially when you walk, rise from a chair or lie on the affected side.

FINDING OUT WHAT AILS YOU

If you experience sudden pain, tenderness or swelling in a joint, consult a doctor at once. His/her initial examination of you should include...

•**Complete medical history.** Tell the doctor what preceded the injury, including whether the problem is chronic or an isolated case.

•**Physical exam of the joint.** The doctor should manipulate your limb to see if and how your range of motion is limited.

•**Review of systems.** Asking about symptoms in different systems of the body, such as fever or weight loss, is the only way to be sure there is no underlying illness, such as gout or joint infection.

The doctor may x-ray the joint—to check for swelling and anatomical abnormalities, such as worn cartilage. If a more detailed picture is needed, he/she may order an MRI scan.

Most cases of soft-tissue inflammation can be treated by a primary-care physician.

Caution: With doctors under increasing pressure from insurers, soft-tissue injuries often get superficial treatment—a recommendation of rest and a prescription for anti-inflammatory drugs. This works in some cases, but it's also how short-term problems can turn into chronic joint ailments.

If your pain doesn't respond to treatment within a few weeks, consult an orthopedist or rheumatologist.

FIRST-LINE TREATMENT

First, it's essential to stop whatever activity caused the injury in the first place, at least until the inflammation has healed.

Your doctor may choose to put the joint in a sling for a few days. Immobilization should be done only when absolutely necessary, however…and then only for a few days. *Reason:* It can cause muscle weakness.

An ice pack often helps during the first 24 to 48 hours after the onset of pain. Once the pain subsides, you can use a hot water bottle, heating pad or hot bath to improve joint mobility.

For pain and swelling, doctors often recommend aspirin or another nonsteroidal anti-inflammatory drug (NSAID)—typically *ibuprofen* (Motrin), *naproxen* (Aleve) or *indomethacin* (Indocin). Indomethacin is especially popular because of its effectiveness and rapid action.

Acetaminophen (Tylenol) is not a NSAID. It works on pain—but not inflammation. It may not be effective for overuse injury.

For maximum effectiveness, NSAIDs must be taken in high doses. Since these doses can cause stomach upset, bleeding and other side effects, NSAID therapy requires close supervision by a doctor.

STEROIDS AND PHYSICAL THERAPY

If NSAIDs fail to reduce the inflammation, your doctor may inject the affected bursa with cortisone or another steroid. Though effective, steroids can cause increased vulnerability to infection and other side effects.

Some doctors give steroids right away. I prefer to wait at least 10 days to see what effects rest and NSAIDs have.

Physical therapy is also very helpful. I start my patients on gentle "range-of-motion" exercises as soon as possible. Your doctor can show you one or more that are appropriate for your injury.

Some soft-tissue injuries stem from improper joint movements, which are often caused by muscle weakness. In such cases, I recommend strength training.

If you're new to strength training, consider hiring a physical therapist for a few sessions—to be sure you're using proper form. Do *not* begin strength training without a doctor's supervision.

To find an accredited therapist in your area, contact the American Physical Therapy Association at 800-999-2782.

SURGERY

For chronic or severe joint pain—especially in older people—orthopedic surgery may be the only option. Several procedures are used, from minimally invasive arthroscopic surgery to full-blown joint reconstruction. *Cost:* Several thousand dollars.

PREVENTING RECURRENCES

If exercise caused your injury, you may be able to return to your former level of intensity —but only gradually, over several months… and only after carefully analyzing the mechanical problems that caused the injury in the first place.

If the inflammation stemmed from an anatomical problem, consider replacing the offending activity with one your body can better handle. Switch from running to cycling, for example, or replace tennis with swimming.

For job-related tendinitis or bursitis, ask your doctor to refer you to an occupational therapist. He will carefully analyze your work movements and find ways to reduce stress on your joints.

A switch in equipment often helps. *Examples:* Wearing shoes with good cushioning and firm heel support…playing with a light, shock-absorbent tennis racket…using a cushioned pad when kneeling…and using a raised, padded bar to support your wrists when typing.

Beating Migraines

Fred Sheftell, MD, president of the American Council for Headache Education, and director of the New England Headache Center, Stamford, CT. He is author of *Headache Relief for Women.* Little Brown.

Migraine isn't just any headache. It's a severe, throbbing pain that can keep you home from work, disrupt your family life…and leave you with significant disability.

Migraines are *very* common. In fact, they affect 18% of women and 6% of men in the US. Without treatment, they can recur year after year.

A typical migraine…

…occurs on one side of the head.

…is of moderate to severe intensity.

…interferes with daily activity.

…is exacerbated by physical activity like coughing, walking or climbing stairs.

…is accompanied by nausea, vomiting or sensitivity to light and sound.

Most migraine sufferers (migraineurs) can recognize what's called a *prodrome* in the 24 hours leading up to a migraine—sudden depression or exhilaration, increased or decreased appetite, disruptions in sleep, etc.

About 15% of migraine sufferers "see" flashing lights or strange shapes just before the headache hits. Such hallucinations are known collectively as an *aura.*

There's no easy way to tame migraines. But when migraineurs get good medical care and take an active role in their treatment, nine out of 10 can reduce a once debilitating problem to a minor inconvenience.

WHAT TRIGGERS MIGRAINES

A migraine starts with abnormal electrical activity in the cerebral cortex, the thinking part of the brain. It spreads quickly to the hypothalamus and the midbrain.

Levels of the brain chemical *serotonin* rise and then drop sharply, making blood vessels swollen and inflamed.

Though the migraine predisposition is inherited, most *individual* attacks are triggered by either dietary or environmental factors…

• **Alcohol** (especially beer and red wine).

• **Erratic meal and/or sleep schedules.**

• **The artificial sweetener *aspartame*** (NutraSweet).

• **The flavor enhancer *monosodium glutamate*** (MSG).

• **Processed meats** and other foods containing the preservatives nitrates or nitrites.

• **Aged cheeses**, freshly baked bread, chopped liver and other foods that contain the amino acid *tyramine*…and chocolate, which contains *phenylethylamine.*

• **Perfume or cigarette smoke.**

• **Caffeine withdrawal.** To avoid trouble, it's best to have no more than one five-ounce cup of coffee a day.

• **Psychological stress.** Most migraines occur when the period of stress is *over.* That's why migraines are common *after* exams or holidays.

HOW TO PREVENT ATTACKS

The first step in controlling migraines is to keep a "headache diary." Record the frequency and severity of your attacks…as well as the foods you consumed during the 24 hours prior to each attack. *Other key strategies:*

• **Maintain a regular schedule.** Eat at the same times each day. Keep consistent sleep hours seven days a week. Don't "sleep in" on weekends.

• **Take vitamin supplements**—vitamin E, 400 international units (IU), twice a day…vitamin B-2, 400 milligrams (mg) a day…vitamin B-6, 50 mg a day. Vitamin supplements help stabilize levels of estrogen and serotonin.

• **Schedule "nurturing" time** during which you listen to music, read, play with your dog or cat, etc.—anything you find enjoyable and relaxing.

• **Practice a relaxation technique** like yoga, meditation, deep breathing or biofeedback once or twice a day for 15 minutes.

Deep breathing: Loosen your clothing and sit in a quiet place. Breathe in as you count to five, then out to the count of five. Silently repeat to yourself, "Breath in relaxation, breath out tension."

Biofeedback: With this high-tech relaxation aid, you're hooked up to a unit that measures skin temperature or muscular tension. With practice, you learn to raise the temperature or loosen the muscle. Either way, your body relaxes.

When traveling: Give yourself plenty of time to pack. Don't carry heavy bags using a neck or shoulder strap. Avoid alcohol during airplane flights.

● **Exercise regularly.** Physical activity relieves stress and boosts levels of *endorphins*, the body's pain-relieving chemicals. At least three times a week, have a moderate, *noncompetitive* workout. Competitive exercise boosts your stress level.

MOST EFFECTIVE MEDICATION

If migraines persist despite these lifestyle changes, *daily* medication may prove helpful.

Over-the-counter (OTC) painkillers like acetaminophen, aspirin, ibuprofen and naproxen are often effective in *treating* an attack. If you do not respond to one of these, "combination" analgesics like Excedrin or Anacin may help. These products combine aspirin or acetaminophen with caffeine, which constricts swollen blood vessels and enhances pain relief.

If OTC remedies don't work, ask your doctor about Tylenol with codeine…Fiorinal (aspirin plus a mild sedative)…and Midrin (acetaminophen plus a muscle relaxant and a drug to shrink swollen blood vessels).

For *preventing* attacks, daily use of the beta-blockers *propranolol* (Inderal) and *nadolol* (Corgard) is often effective. The calcium-channel blocker *verapamil* (Calan, Verelan) and antidepressants such as *amitriptyline* (Elavil), *nortriptyline* (Pamelor) and *fluoxetine* (Prozac) are also effective.

Although *methysergide* (Sansert) is often effective, it can scar the lungs, kidneys and heart. If it must be used for more than five months, periodic chest X rays, MRI scans of the kidneys and other tests should be performed to make sure no harm is taking place.

What about alternative remedies? Some migraineurs get relief from a daily dose of the anti-inflammatory herb *feverfew*, which is available at health-food stores. Others get relief from fish oil supplements.

Caution: Fish oil can increase cholesterol to dangerous levels. It should be taken only with a doctor's supervision.

TO THE RESCUE

● **Acupressure** offers relief to some migraineurs. At the first sign of a headache, press the web between your thumb and index finger, on the same side as your headache, for five minutes.

● **Sumatriptan** (Imitrex) is the biggest advance in migraine care in more than a century. One self-injection relieves most migraines within 60 minutes. The pill form is also effective, but it takes longer.

Beware: Don't use sumatriptan if you have heart disease—it narrows blood vessels. If you're at risk for heart disease (men over 40, family history of heart attack, smoking, blood pressure over 140/90, cholesterol over 220), the doctor may want to administer the first dose in the office, and check your electrocardiogram.

A sensation of pressure in the chest after a dose of sumatriptan is common. But if the drug causes chest *pain*, discontinue it.

● **Dihydroergotamine** (Migranal) is as effective as sumatriptan but takes longer to work. Inhaled and injectable versions of dihydroergotamine (DHE) and sumatriptan are very helpful when vomiting makes it impossible to keep pills down.

Living Cancer-Free

Sidney J. Winawer, MD, chief of the gastroenterology and nutrition service at Memorial Sloan-Kettering Cancer Center and professor of medicine at Cornell University Medical College, New York. He is coauthor of *Cancer Free: The Comprehensive Cancer Prevention Program.* Simon & Schuster.

The medical staffs of cancer centers continually witness the agony of patients and their families when a diagnosis of advanced cancer is delivered. I believe the great tragedy in all this is that nine out of 10 cancer cases could have been prevented.

HOW TO DO IT

Cancer may soon surpass heart disease as America's number-one killer. However, that doesn't have to happen if Americans…

•**Reduce fat consumption to 20%** of total daily calories.

•**Increase fiber intake to 25 to 30 grams a day** to reduce the risk of colon cancer.

•**Avoid tobacco in all forms.** This would prevent most of the 165,000 cancer deaths attributed to tobacco use each year. Smoking causes high rates of carcinoma of the lungs, mouth, throat, larynx, esophagus, bladder, kidneys, pancreas and cervix.

•**Drink much less alcohol.** Seventeen thousand cancer deaths each year are caused by alcohol abuse.

•**Practice safe sunning habits.** This would reduce melanoma and other skin cancers by 90%, saving more than 8,000 lives a year.

CONTRACT AGAINST CANCER

People think that because they feel well, they *are* well. But cancer typically lurks in the body for 10 to 30 years before it surfaces. *Exceptions:* Rapidly progressing forms, such as acute leukemia and certain brain tumors.

Conflicting reports confuse the public. It's not easy to weigh the results of an individual research study against prior medical evidence. While you wouldn't know it from the media, no single effort—such as eating garlic or having an annual Pap smear—is enough to prevent cancer.

Many people sign service contracts for their computers and regularly have their cars tuned up. Yet they don't do the same for their bodies.

ASSESSING YOUR CANCER RISK

Chances are you already practice some preventive measures. Expand on those measures by formulating and following a comprehensive game plan.

Bonus: Most of the recommendations that follow will also help to protect you against heart disease, diabetes, emphysema and other serious diseases while promoting vital, active, healthy living.

Before you make a plan, first determine your likelihood of developing cancer. *It hinges on four factors:*

•**Family health history.** Your risk of disease is increased if a close blood relative has ever had prostate, lung, breast, ovarian or colorectal (colon and rectum) cancer. The risk increases according to the person's generation as compared with yours, the number of relatives with the same kind of cancer or a related type of cancer and whether the disease developed at an age earlier than average for that type of cancer.

To find out about your family history, ask your family and their close friends about your relatives' health histories and, for those who have died, the cause of death. Death certificates, which list the official cause of death (but are not always reliable), are available for about $10 to $15 from the vital records division of the state department of health, generally located in the capital city of the state where the person died.

If necessary, your doctor can help you obtain medical records and hospital discharge summaries for deceased relatives.

List all the information in a notebook—to review with your doctor. You'll be helping the future generations as well.

Some people who learn that they have a family history of cancer adopt a fatalistic attitude. Since cancer will get them anyway, they shrug, why fight it?

On the contrary: It is precisely the person with a high genetic risk who may gain most from living a healthful life. Preventive measures, such as changes in lifestyle, can override a genetic predisposition. Your doctor might suggest that you undergo different screening tests, for example, or be tested for specific types of cancer at an earlier age than most people.

Genetic counseling: The Hereditary Cancer Institute, Department of Preventive Medicine, Creighton University School of Medicine, 2500 California Plaza, Omaha 68178, 800-648-8133. There's also a clinical genetics counseling service at Memorial Sloan-Kettering Cancer Center, 1275 York Ave., New York 10021, 212-434-5149.

●**Personal health history.** Having a complete rundown of your own health history will help your doctor weigh your cancer risks.

Examples: Diabetes increases the risk of developing malignancies in the uterus and ovaries. Breast cancer risk is higher among women who have never been pregnant or who had their first pregnancy after age 30.

●**Environment.** The list of known or suspected carcinogenic materials is growing. If you are retired, describe your previous workplace to your doctor. If you have a hobby that involves fine wood dust or paint, pesticides (used more by homeowners than by farmers) or other chemicals, you should always wear a closely fitting mask and work with plenty of ventilation.

Test your home for radon, a radioactive gas that causes the second-highest number of cases of lung cancer a year (smoking is first).

Surprising: Excess radon seeps out of the ground into nearly one in 15 US homes. Start with a test kit from the hardware store. If results are positive, hire a professional.

●**Lifestyle.** This very significant category includes activities within your control…

   ●**Exposure to the sun.**
   ●**Tobacco and alcohol use.**
   ●**Diet.**
   ●**Physical fitness.**

ENLIST YOUR DOCTOR'S HELP

Armed with all this information, your doctor can evaluate your cancer risk and help you plan a path to prevention. A crucial step is determining which tests to undergo, as well as when and how often to schedule them. If you're deterred by expense, inconvenience or fear, think how relieved you would be if you stopped a symptomless slow-growing cancer in its tracks.

Example: A colonoscopy—in which a flexible tube is inserted into the colon via the rectum for the doctor to look through—is less uncomfortable than many people think. In a 15- to 20-minute exam, the doctor may find polyps that can be easily removed, eliminating this common source of colon cancer.

AVOID STRESS

The role of stress in cancer prevention is only beginning to be understood. We know that stress—especially in combination with other risk factors—weakens the immune system and affects the secretion of hormones. Reducing stress may be as important as exercise, nutrition and regular checkups.

Items high on a well-known list of life stressors…retirement, moving and having a grown child leave home. Highest of all is the loss of a spouse. To reduce the negative effects of stress, find zest in life.

Take ballroom dancing lessons…join a bird-watching group or a walking club…volunteer at a library or museum…meditate. Studies indicate that people who are busy, relaxed and happy are less likely to develop cancer than those who are bored, stressed and depressed.

Booklets, such as *Cancer Tests You Should Know About: A Guide for People 65 and Over*, as well as other publications on specific types of cancer, are available free of charge from the Cancer Information Service at the National Cancer Institute. 800-422-6237.

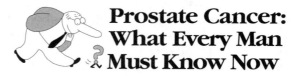

Prostate Cancer: What Every Man Must Know Now

E. Roy Berger, MD, a medical oncologist and prostate cancer specialist affiliated with North Shore Hematology-Oncology Associates, East Setauket, NY. He is coauthor of New Guidelines for Diagnosing and Treating Prostate Cancer. *Health Education Literary Publisher.*

For such a small gland, the prostate causes big trouble. This year alone, 200,000 men will be diagnosed with prostate cancer.

The disease kills almost as many men as breast cancer kills women.

SCREENING IS ESSENTIAL

Little is known about what *causes* prostate cancer, although men who eat a high-fat diet seem to be at greatest risk. That's why *screening* is essential.

Caught in its early stages, prostate cancer can usually be cured with surgery or radiation, and possibly helped by drug therapy. Key, of course, is catching the tumor *before* it spreads.

Self-defense: Once a year, starting at age 50,* all men should undergo...

•**Digital rectal examination** (DRE). The doctor inserts a finger into the rectum to feel the prostate gland for nodules or firmness suggestive of cancer.

•**Prostate-specific antigen test.** This blood test measures levels of prostate-specific antigen (PSA), a protein secreted by the prostate. Elevated PSA levels suggest the need for further evaluation.

It's important to realize that PSA levels increase with age. A level that's normal for a man of 80, for instance, may suggest prostate cancer in a man of 45.

For men 51 or older, a level above 3.5 suggests the need for further tests. Above age 70, the cutoff is 6.5.

GETTING A PROPER BIOPSY

If your PSA is high, or if the digital exam reveals a suspicious lump, it's prudent to have the prostate biopsied.

Problem: Some doctors take just one or two tissue samples. To be sure to find any tumor (and to estimate its size), however, the doctor must take at least six tissue samples.

OTHER IMPORTANT TESTS

Some prostate tumors grow fast, others slowly. A slow-growing tumor might cause no trouble for years—without any treatment. A virulent tumor calls for immediate, aggressive intervention.

Science has yet to find a foolproof method for telling one type of tumor from the other. However, a tumor's *Gleason score* can help you pick appropriate treatment. The Gleason score is an indication of how "aggressive" the cancer cells are.

Two other tests are often helpful when making the treatment decision...

•**Ploidy analysis**—how much DNA the tumor contains. A tumor that has either more or less DNA than normal is likely to spread.

•**Polymerase chain reaction (PCR) test.** This test can show whether the tumor has spread long before other tests.

*Start screenings at age 40 if your father or brother had prostate cancer or if you are African-American. Risk is significantly higher among these men.

WATCHFUL WAITING

If tests indicate that the tumor is small and slow-growing, treatment may be unnecessary.

As long as PSA levels stay low and the tumor grows slowly, "watchful waiting" may be appropriate. All you have to do is have a checkup every two months, including a DRE and PSA test.

Watchful waiting is generally more reasonable for a man of 70—who is likely to die of other causes before a sluggish tumor causes any trouble—than a 50-year-old.

THE CASE FOR SURGERY

If the cancer is confined to the prostate, surgical removal of the gland—a procedure called *radical prostatectomy*—is sometimes curative. Following surgery, up to 70% of men become impotent. Up to 5% become incontinent.

Innovation: *Nerve-sparing prostatectomy.* In this procedure, the surgeon is careful not to sever the delicate nerve bundles next to the prostate that control erection. Nerve-sparing prostatectomy is a trade-off. You're less likely to become impotent, but there's more risk that some cancerous tissue will remain.

WHAT RADIATION HAS TO OFFER

In traditional radiation therapy, a machine zaps the prostate with high-intensity X rays.

For cancer limited to the prostate, this *external beam radiation* (EBR) may be as effective as surgery. Unlike prostatectomy, it doesn't involve weeks of recovery.

Up to 50% of men who undergo radiation therapy become impotent. Incontinence is generally not a problem.

Brachytherapy is a form of radiation that is sometimes performed on an outpatient basis. In this procedure, tiny "seeds" of radioactive iodine or palladium are implanted within the prostate.

Since brachytherapy causes less damage to surrounding tissues, the impotence rate is only about 15%, the incontinence rate close to 0%. Brachytherapy delivers more radiation to the tumor.

Seed radiation seems to be just as effective as prostatectomy at curing the disease.

HORMONE THERAPY

For prostate cancer that has spread to other tissues, prostate surgery and radiation are unlikely to extend life.

In such cases, the best strategy is to block action of *testosterone* and *dihydrotestosterone*. Secreted primarily by the testicles and adrenal glands, these male hormones spur growth of prostate cancer cells—wherever they appear in the body.

Doctors can "shut down" the testicles by administering drugs called *LHRH agonists*...or by surgically removing them in a procedure called *orchiectomy*.

Doctors also prescribe the drugs *flutamide* (Eulexin) or *bicalutamide* (Casodex), which block hormonal action at the cellular level. This combined hormone therapy is the treatment of choice for metastatic prostate cancer.

In a study of men with metastatic cancer, those who got combined therapy lived 1½ years longer than those who got single hormone therapy. Combined therapy is also used —with surgery or radiation—to treat cancer limited to the prostate.

EXPERIMENTAL APPROACHES

In *cryotherapy*, the prostate is destroyed by freezing. Even with a highly skilled surgeon, this experimental therapy often causes impotence. Since it's never been widely used, there are no long-term survival statistics.

Research suggests that *modified citrus pectin*, a powder derived from citrus fruit, helps stop prostate cancer from spreading. But this potential lifesaver won't be ready for several years.

SUPPORT GROUPS

Any man with prostate cancer should find out about support groups in his community. To find a support group or cancer specialist in your area, contact Patient Advocates for Advanced Cancer Treatments (PAACT) at 616-453-1477, *www.paactusa.org*.

With all the treatment options, any man with prostate cancer should consult *three* doctors—a urologic surgeon, a medical oncologist and a radiation specialist familiar with brachytherapy.

Colon Cancer Self-Defense Essentials

Peter McNally, DO, chief of gastroenterology at Eisenhower Army Medical Center in Augusta, GA, and a spokesperson for the American College of Gastroenterology, 4900 B South 31 St., Arlington, VA 22206. He is author of the medical textbook *GI/Liver Secrets*. Hanley & Belfus.

Colon cancer kills more people than any other malignancy except lung cancer. One American in 20 will develop colon cancer in his/her lifetime—usually after age 50.

Tragically, 90% of colorectal cancers could be avoided through early detection.

DETECTION MEANS PREVENTION

Colon cancer doesn't just come out of nowhere. Most cases develop from a polyp, a premalignant growth on the lining of the colon.

Periodic screening offers a way to spot tumors early...and to find and remove polyps while they're still benign. It takes five to 10 years for a polyp to turn cancerous. *Here's what to do...*

●**Age 40 to age 50.** Have an annual *digital rectal exam* (DRE). The doctor inserts a gloved finger into the rectum and feels for suspicious growths.

●**After age 50.** Each year, have a DRE and a *fecal occult blood test*. In this test, you'll be asked to put a smear of stool on a specially treated card on three successive days, while following a special diet.

If the test shows blood—or if you're at high risk for colon cancer—the doctor will examine the full length of your colon with a long, flexible viewing scope (colonoscope). Any polyp that is found is removed during the procedure.

Because *colonoscopy* can cause discomfort, you will probably be given an intravenous sedative like Demerol or Valium.

Undergo *flexible sigmoidoscopy* every three years unless you've had a recent colonoscopy. Using a short, flexible tube inserted into the rectum, the doctor inspects the lower one-fourth of the colon. That's where most tumors develop.

The procedure causes only mild discomfort, so it's usually done without sedation.

WHO IS AT HIGH RISK

Colon cancer runs in families. Your risk is above average if one or more first-degree relatives (parents or siblings) has had the disease.

In such cases, it's prudent to have a flexible sigmoidoscopy every three to five years, starting at age 35.

A rare hereditary condition known as *familial adenomatous polyposis* dramatically raises your risk of colon cancer. If genetic tests reveal that you have this condition—in which hundreds of polyps form in the colon—screening should begin in adolescence.

If you've had one polyp removed, you're likely to develop more. Have a colonoscopy every three years.

Ulcerative colitis and Crohn's disease are also associated with an elevated risk. Anyone who has either condition for 10 years or more should have an annual colonoscopy.

REDUCING RISK WITH DIET

Colon cancer is rare in regions where vegetables and grains make up the bulk of the diet. It's common in the US and other Western nations where the diet is largely based on meat.

Implication: A diet rich in fruits, vegetables, beans and whole grains prevents colon cancer. The American Cancer Society recommends at least five servings of these foods each day.

While it's hard to determine exactly which components of this healthy diet are protective, research has zeroed in on several candidates…

●**Low fat.** There is a clear link between dietary fat and colon cancer. Fats boost the body's production of bile acids, which promote rapid cell growth.

●**High fiber.** The indigestible part of plant-based foods, fiber moves food through the bowel quickly—reducing its contact with carcinogens and bile acids.

Wheat bran is more protective than fruit and vegetable fiber. Oat bran has little impact on colon cancer risk, though it does reduce cholesterol levels.

Get at least 25 grams (g) of dietary fiber per day—from whole grain cereals and breads and vegetables, fruits and beans.

●**Calcium.** Some studies suggest that calcium protects the colon by neutralizing bile acids and fatty acids.

Consume at least 1,000 milligrams (mg) of calcium each day—ideally through diet, not supplements.

●**Antioxidants.** Low blood levels of vitamins C and E and beta-carotene seem to confer an increased risk of colon cancer.

Eat lots of citrus fruits and dark-green and yellow vegetables—these are the best sources of antioxidants.

WHAT ELSE MAY HELP

●**Exercise.** A sedentary lifestyle increases the risk of colon cancer. Like fiber, physical activity reduces the risk by hastening the passage of waste through the body. It also stimulates blood flow to the colon.

Walk briskly or do some other exercise at least 30 minutes, three days a week.

●**Nonsteroidal anti-inflammatory drugs** (NSAIDs). As several studies have shown, individuals who take aspirin or ibuprofen regularly for years face a reduced risk of colon cancer.

Unfortunately, there is not enough evidence to justify taking aspirin or NSAIDs strictly for cancer prevention.

●**Estrogen.** Preliminary studies suggest that postmenopausal women who take estrogen are less likely to develop colon cancer than similar women who don't take estrogen.

WATCH OUT FOR SYMPTOMS

See a doctor at once if you experience changes in bowel habits…blood in the stool…rectal pain…and/or recurrent abdominal cramps.

The earlier cancer is detected, the better the chance for cure.

Often-Overlooked Causes of Chronic Fatigue

Ronald L. Hoffman, MD, director of the Hoffman Center for Holistic Medicine in New York City. He is author of *Tired All the Time: How to Regain Your Lost Energy.* Pocket Books.

If you feel tired all the time, you have lots of company. Each year, Americans make 500 million visits to the doctor seeking treatment for fatigue.

Many people who frequently feel tired fear they have the debilitating condition *chronic fatigue and immune dysfunction syndrome* (CFIDS).

If your fatigue has persisted for more than six months or is accompanied by sleep disturbances, joint pain, headaches, inability to concentrate or short-term memory loss, you may indeed have CFIDS.

In such cases, it's best to seek treatment from a CFIDS specialist. For a list of specialists in your area, contact the CFIDS Association of America, Box 220398, Charlotte, NC 28222. 800-442-3437, *www.cfids.org.*

Good news: Only about 10% of my patients with fatigue actually have CFIDS. The rest are suffering from "garden variety" fatigue, caused by too little sleep or exercise, poor dietary habits or other easily correctable problems.

THYROID PROBLEMS

Many cases of chronic fatigue are caused by over- or underproduction of thyroxine. That's the thyroid hormone responsible for regulating how energy is consumed by the body's cells.

Overactive thyroid: Symptoms of hyperthyroidism include fatigue, anxiety, insomnia, heart palpitations and bulging eyes. This condition is treated with thyroxine-blocking drugs... or with surgery or radioactive iodine to destroy the thyroid gland.

Underactive thyroid: Suspect hypothyroidism if you feel depressed or lethargic, chill easily, are gaining weight or suffer from premenstrual syndrome (PMS), muscle aches, dry skin, eczema, hair loss, low libido, a hoarse throat or frequent colds or flu.

If you're experiencing any of these symptoms, it's a good idea to check your basal body temperature. Insert a thermometer under your armpit as soon as you awaken, before getting out of bed. Record results for three consecutive mornings.

A basal temperature of 97.4 degrees or lower suggests hypothyroidism. Your doctor can give you a blood test to confirm your suspicions.

Most doctors treat hypothyroidism with synthetic thyroxine (*Synthroid*). However, some patients show more improvement when they take *natural* thyroid hormone (derived from beef or pork).

If Synthroid doesn't relieve your symptoms, ask your doctor to consider that alternative.

ADRENAL INSUFFICIENCY

Anyone whose fatigue is accompanied by malaise, frequent illness, allergies or low blood pressure or sugar may be making too little of the adrenal hormone *dehydroepiandrosterone* (DHEA).

Adrenal insufficiency is usually caused by autoimmune disease...or by adrenal gland damage stemming from long-term use of cortisone.

If a blood test reveals low levels of DHEA, you might need to take it in pill form.

In Europe, DHEA has long been used to boost immune function and combat fatigue—though few American doctors have much experience with the drug.

To find an endocrinologist familiar with DHEA, call the American College for Advancement in Medicine, 949-583-7666.

DIABETES

Adult-onset diabetes is an often-overlooked source of persistent fatigue. To rule out this condition, ask your doctor for a *fasting blood glucose test*.

The normal range of insulin is 80 to 100 mg per deciliter of blood. If you fall above that range, eating a special diet and getting regular exercise can help lower blood sugar levels. That should boost your energy.

HORMONAL PROBLEMS

In men, some cases of chronic fatigue are caused by abnormally low levels of testosterone. Men suffering from this problem (which can be spotted with a simple blood test) can boost their energy levels by taking testosterone supplements.

Hormone problems can cause fatigue in women, too. But tests for hormone imbalances in women are often inaccurate.

Instead of relying on a blood test, women should suspect hormone problems if…

•**Their fatigue is cyclical,** getting worse prior to menstruation and improving afterward.

•**They experience weight gain** of more than five pounds prior to each period.

•**They perpetually crave sugar,** spicy foods or chocolate.

•**They experience migraines** or breast tenderness when taking birth-control pills.

To treat hormone-related fatigue, women should reduce their consumption of alcohol, meat and dairy products…eat more dietary fiber and less sugar and refined foods…take supplements of *gamma linolenic acid* (GLA).

GLA is found in primrose oil, borage oil and black currant seed oil, available at health-food stores.

Women with extreme PMS-related fatigue should ask their doctor about having a *Meyer's cocktail* once a month. That's an intravenous drip of calcium, magnesium, and vitamins B and C.

FOOD ALLERGIES

Chronic, mild food allergies can cause fatigue. Suspect allergies if you have dark circles under your eyes…are frequently irritable…feel foggy or depressed…or have frequent infections or dry skin.

Cravings for particular foods or cycles of energy and fatigue also suggest food allergies —especially to wheat and dairy products. These foods can cause the body to produce an energy-sapping morphine-like substance.

Consider a medically supervised fast of one to four days, to see if your energy increases. Add foods back to your diet only with the doctor's permission.

ENVIRONMENTAL TOXINS

If you can't find another source of fatigue, you may be suffering from exposure to indoor pollutants. *Usual culprits:*

•**Benzene.** In linoleum and degreasers.

•**Formaldehyde.** In carpets and drapes.

•**Lead.** In tap water and house paint.

•**Mercury.** In dental fillings and in some house paints.

•**Nitrogen dioxide.** Released by kerosene heaters, gas stoves and furnaces.

•**Trichloroethylene.** Used in dry cleaning.

Have your home tested for environmental toxins. For companies that test air and water, look under "Laboratories–Testing"—in the *Yellow Pages.* One reputable firm is RCI Environmental, 17754 Preston Rd., Suite 101, Dallas 75252. 972-250-6608.

If toxins *are* a problem, install carbon-based water and air filters. Make sure your home is well-ventilated so that fumes can escape. Fill your home with house plants to help filter the air.

Your doctor should test your blood for chemical markers of contaminants…and your hair for lead, mercury and other toxic metals. If traces of toxins are found, ask him/her about adding selenium, vitamin E, beta-carotene, garlic and sodium alginate to your diet. They help rid the body of toxic metals.

For more information on environmental toxins, contact the Human Ecology Action League, Box 29629, Atlanta 30359. 404-248-1898.

THE ROLE OF SUGAR

In many cases, fatigue is the result of eating too much sugar. Sugar and refined carbohydrates make your blood sugar rise. This signals the pancreas to produce insulin. Too much insulin leads to *hypoglycemia* (low blood sugar), which causes extreme fatigue.

If you suspect hypoglycemia, ask your doctor for an oral *glucose-tolerance test.* If, during the test, you experience heart palpitations, mental confusion or extreme fatigue, or feel dizzy or shaky, suspect a sugar problem—even if your doctor says your blood sugar levels are normal.

Treatment is simple—stop eating sugar. *Also helpful:* Eating six small meals instead of the usual three big meals. Small, frequent meals help stabilize blood sugar levels.

Finally, ask your doctor about taking ergogenic (energy-generating) dietary supplements, including vitamin B-15…L-carnitine…octacosanol, a wheat germ extract…ginseng.

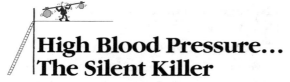

High Blood Pressure… The Silent Killer

Vincent Friedewald, MD, clinical assistant professor of medicine at Baylor College of Medicine in Houston. He is author of *Ask the Doctor: Hypertension.* Andrews and McMeel.

High blood pressure is the most overlooked health problem in the US. Only 14 million of the estimated 70 million Americans who have it are getting adequate treatment.

The rest may *feel* fine, but they're at increased risk for stroke, heart attack, kidney failure and other ailments.

To find out more about detecting and treating this "silent killer," we spoke with prominent cardiologist Dr. Vincent Friedewald…

●**When is blood pressure considered high?** Any pressure above 120/80 is high. We used to think that only the second (diastolic) number mattered. Now we know that the first (systolic) reading is important, too.

Hypertension is ranked in stages…

Stage	Systolic	Diastolic
1	140 to 159	90 to 99
2	160 to 179	100 to 109
3	180 to 209	110 to 119
4	210 or higher	120 or higher

●**My blood pressure is only slightly elevated. Is that cause for concern?** Even Stage 1 hypertension can cause serious health problems. I believe that everyone should try to maintain a pressure of 120/80 or lower.

●**What causes high blood pressure?** We don't know the full story. However, blood pressure is a reflection of how hard your heart is pumping…and of the size of your *arterioles,* special blood vessels that act as gatekeepers between the arteries and the capillaries, the tiniest blood vessels.

Arterioles dilate or narrow according to nerve signals from the brain, which bases its "decisions" on feedback from nerve endings near the heart. These nerve endings constantly monitor your blood pressure.

This feedback loop boosts your pressure when you exercise or undergo psychological stress and lowers it when you're asleep or relaxed.

In hypertension, blood pressure is *consistently* higher than it should be—whether you are stressed or relaxed.

Ninety percent of people with high blood pressure have *primary* (essential) hypertension. This condition seems to be largely hereditary, although excess weight, lack of exercise, high salt intake, alcohol consumption and age can also play a role.

●**What about the other 10% of cases?** They're the result of other ailments—typically kidney disease, thyroid or adrenal gland problems or sleep apnea. Once the underlying disease is diagnosed, blood pressure can usually be controlled.

●**How do I know if I have high blood pressure?** Have a doctor measure it…or buy and use your own blood-pressure monitor. *Cost:* $25 to $30. Ask your doctor to make sure it's properly calibrated.

A *single high* reading—especially a diastolic reading *above* 90 or a systolic reading *above* 140—may be cause for concern. However, it does *not* necessarily mean you have hypertension.

A single measurement may not be representative of your blood pressure throughout the day. And about one in five people who visit the doctor exhibit high blood pressure *simply because they're nervous.*

Your doctor must be careful to distinguish real hypertension from this "white-coat" variety. Aggressive treatment of white-coat hypertension can be dangerous.

To tell if your blood pressure is *consistently* high, you must take several readings—preferably over a period of days or weeks.

If you are diagnosed with hypertension, your doctor should follow up with a thorough physical exam. This exam should include an electrocardiogram, a urinalysis and blood tests for…

- Blood lipids
- Glucose
- Calcium
- Potassium
- Complete blood count
- Uric acid
- Creatinine

●**What can I do to lower my blood pressure?** If it's just a bit high, you can probably nudge it down into the safe range by making a few lifestyle changes…

●**Cut back on alcohol.** Alcohol in any form raises blood pressure. Have no more than one ounce a day—the amount in two beers, a glass of wine or a jigger of whiskey.

●**Exercise more.** Get 30 to 60 minutes every day of moderate activity—walking, jogging, bicycling, etc. Becoming fit can lower your blood pressure by six to seven points.

●**Lose weight.** Overweight people who reduce their body weight by 5% to 10% often experience a significant drop in blood pressure.

●**Quit smoking.**

●**Reduce sodium intake.** Some people are salt-sensitive, others aren't. My advice is to stop using a salt shaker…and to avoid processed foods, which account for two-thirds of daily salt intake.

●**Is there any special diet that can help?** In addition to restricting your salt intake, try to eat calcium- and potassium-rich foods (especially fruits, grains and vegetables). These minerals promote excretion of sodium.

Being a vegetarian also seems to lower blood pressure. Vegetarians not only eat more fruits and veggies than their meat-eating peers, but are also thinner. Some people swear by magnesium supplements, fish oil, garlic and other purported pressure-lowering remedies. But there's no hard evidence that these products have any beneficial effect.

●**When is it appropriate to treat hypertension with drugs?** If you're more than a few points above normal, your doctor will probably prescribe antihypertensive medication *in addition to* lifestyle changes.

There is now a wide variety of effective antihypertensives…

●**Diuretics** remove sodium and water from the bloodstream, shrinking blood volume and dilating arteries. Diuretics are especially effective in African-American and elderly individuals… and in individuals whose blood pressure is salt-sensitive. Diuretics can deplete potassium levels, so any patient taking them should have his/her potassium levels carefully monitored.

●**Beta-blockers** reduce the force of each heartbeat and block the release of hormones that boost blood pressure. Beta-blockers can cause fatigue, insomnia and sexual problems. They should be avoided by those with asthma or heart failure.

●**ACE inhibitors** slow key chemical interactions in the bloodstream that lead to hypertension. Relatively free of side effects, they can cause coughing and—rarely—swelling of the face and limbs.

●**Calcium-channel blockers** have been in the news recently because one *short-acting* form of *nifedipine* (Procardia, Adalat) has been linked to heart attack. Some doctors are questioning using calcium-channel blockers as a first-line treatment for hypertension because they do not appear to provide the protective benefits of diuretics, beta-blockers and ACE inhibitors.

●**Can hypertension be cured?** Once you have essential hypertension, it never goes away. You'll have to monitor your blood pressure on a regular basis for the rest of your life. However, with a combination of lifestyle changes and well-tailored medication, most people can bring their pressure down to safe levels.

Lifesaving Breakthroughs In Stroke Treatment

Thomas Brott, MD, professor of neurology and director of the Stroke Research Center at the University of Cincinnati Medical Center. He helped develop one of the most successful citywide emergency stroke treatment programs in the US.

Not long ago, stroke was considered untreatable. There was little doctors could do for the half-million Americans each year who suffer this devastating neurological problem.

Now: Armed with a new "clot-busting" medication, doctors can prevent much of the brain damage caused by the most common form of stroke.

We spoke recently with Thomas Brott, MD, about the new developments in stroke care...

●**What are the new drug treatments we've been hearing about?** The first approach is to use a genetically engineered anticoagulant called *tissue-plasminogen activator* (TPA) to dissolve stroke-related blood clots. This brings oxygen to brain cells whose oxygen supply has been cut off by clots.

In the second approach, doctors treat brain cells with *neuroprotectors*. These experimental drugs prevent the "cascade" of chemical reactions that kill brain cells subjected to brief periods of oxygen starvation.

●**How effective are these treatments?** The jury is still out on neuroprotectors, but studies suggest that TPA increases the chance for total or near-total recovery from a stroke by 35% to 55%.

The hitch is that TPA works well only if it's given within three hours of the onset of the stroke. Since there was little they could do anyway, doctors used to take a "wait-and-see" approach to stroke. Now that effective treatments are available, doctors and patients alike should treat stroke as a medical emergency— just like heart attack.

●**How can I be sure to get prompt, effective treatment, should I suffer a stroke?** Know the telltale symptoms of stroke— and make sure anyone you live with knows them, too.

Typical symptoms include a loss of balance or coordination...a sudden inability to walk... numbness or weakness, particularly on one side of the body...and blurred or decreased vision, particularly in one eye or on one side of the visual field of each eye.

If the language area of the brain is affected, there may be an inability to speak, slurred speech or difficulty understanding what's being said.

If even *one* of these symptoms is present, call 911 immediately.

●**Is there any special procedure that should be followed?** To determine what type of stroke the patient has suffered, doctors should order a *computed tomography* (CT) scan of the head within one hour.

Five out of every six stroke patients have what is known as an *ischemic* stroke. It's caused by a blood clot that blocks the flow of blood to the brain.

The other likely possibility is *hemorrhagic* stroke. It's caused by the rupture of a blood vessel in the brain.

If the CT scan and other tests indicate that the patient has had an ischemic stroke, doctors should administer TPA right away.

●**Is TPA widely available?** Virtually every hospital pharmacy in the US now has TPA. But not every emergency room is staffed with doctors skilled at administering the drug.

TPA is *very* tricky to use. About 6% of people who get it experience bleeding in the brain. And—TPA is off-limits to many patients with high blood pressure...those taking *warfarin* (Coumadin) or another blood thinner...and those who have problems with their platelet count or blood sugar levels.

●**When will neuroprotective drugs be available?** Several neuroprotective drugs are now in Phase III clinical trials (the last hurdle before FDA approval).

Other promising neuroprotective agents— including *aptiganel, nalmefene, citicoline* and *anti-ICAMA-1 antibodies*—may still be years off.

●**Are any other promising treatments on the way?** Other stroke drugs currently in Phase III trials include the clot-dissolving drug *prourokinase* and *ancrod*, a blood thinner derived from pit viper venom.

Another promising treatment involves temporarily reversing the direction of blood flow in the large veins of the body. Researchers hope that this "retrograde" blood flow therapy will be even more effective than TPA at dislodging clots from blood vessels within the brain.

●**Who is at greatest risk for stroke?** Risk for stroke goes up with age—doubling each decade after age 55. You can't do anything about your age, of course, but if you have any of the risk factors for stroke, ask your doctor about treating the underlying disorder.

You should also ask your doctor about taking aspirin or another blood thinner.

Evidence suggests that aspirin therapy reduces the risk for stroke—especially in those who have the heartbeat abnormality known as *atrial fibrillation.*

●**What are the risk factors for stroke?** High blood pressure (140/90 or higher)...elevated cholesterol...atrial fibrillation...diabetes...previous heart attack...and cholesterol deposits in the carotid arteries in the neck. A doctor can check for such blockages using ultrasound.

For Serious Medical Emergencies

Stephan Lynn, MD, director of the department of emergency medicine at St. Luke's/Roosevelt Hospital Center in New York City. Dr. Lynn is also author of *Medical Emergency!* Hearst Books.

When a serious health emergency strikes, our first instinct is to panic. That's because most of us don't know what to do in such a situation. *Here are the most serious medical conditions—and what to do until help arrives...*

HEART ATTACK

Chest pain is the most common symptom of a heart attack, which occurs when an artery is blocked by a blood clot. This stops blood flow to the heart and damages the cardiac muscle.

Symptoms: Crushing pain in the middle of the chest, which may radiate to the jaw, neck, shoulders, back or arms...shortness of breath ...sweating...nausea and/or vomiting.

How to help yourself or someone else: If the symptoms last longer than three to five minutes and are particularly severe or aren't relieved by antacids...

●**Call an ambulance.** Never drive yourself to the hospital since there is a strong possibility that you may pass out. Paramedics can provide early medical care—most ambulances carry defibrillators, the machines that can restore a normal heart rhythm and prevent death.

●**Take an aspirin.** It's been shown to limit damage from a heart attack.

●**Lie down, breathe slowly and keep calm.** Anxiety and activity can increase heart damage.

STROKE

As the name implies, a stroke hits suddenly —when a blood clot or hemorrhage affects the brain, preventing blood and oxygen from circulating.

Symptoms: Unexpected numbness and weakness that usually affects one side of the body...vision disturbances...an inability to speak.

How to help yourself or someone else: Have the person sit down immediately so he/she doesn't fall...call an ambulance...make sure the airway is open by tilting the head back and the chin up.

SHORTNESS OF BREATH

Many conditions can cause severe shortness of breath—pneumonia...asthma...inhalation of toxic fumes or smoke...bronchitis...an airway obstruction...a blood clot in the lungs...or a heart attack.

Symptoms: Nostrils that open wide...an Adam's apple that moves up when you inhale... the need to use neck muscles to breathe...discomfort when you inhale...gasping...dizziness and/or fainting.

How to help yourself or someone else: Call an ambulance, which will supply you with oxygen while taking you to the hospital...sit with your head elevated...breathe slowly and deeply...remain calm.

ALLERGIC REACTION

A serious allergic reaction can occur after eating certain foods, receiving an injection, taking a drug or getting an insect bite or sting. Many times the cause is unknown.

Symptoms: Severe or sudden hives, itching or a rash...flushed skin...swollen tissues around the mouth and in the airway...breathing difficulties such as wheezing...physical weakness... nausea...dizziness and/or collapse.

How to help yourself or someone else: Call an ambulance. If you have a known allergy and carry an *epinephrine* injection, immediately give yourself a shot or have someone else do it.

If you don't have *epinephrine*, take an antihistamine. *Diphenhydramine* (Benadryl) can be bought without a prescription. Apply ice to the affected area to reduce the swelling and itching. Lie down.

FRACTURE

It can be difficult to distinguish a mere sprain from a more serious fracture without an X ray.

Symptoms: Fractures are signaled by intense pain or swelling, an inability to use a body part—hip, wrist, arm, shoulder, ankle, leg—or an obviously misshapen or broken extremity or body part.

How to help yourself: When in doubt go to a hospital emergency room. While you're in transit, follow the *RICE* procedure if you can...

Rest...

Ice the injury to reduce swelling...

Compression. Wear an elastic bandage around the extremity to provide support...

Elevate the body part so blood and other fluids won't pool there.

Important: If you're not in severe pain or don't obviously have a break, you can do the RICE procedure for 24 to 48 hours and see if the injury improves. If you do not notice any improvement, see a doctor.

How to help someone else: Don't move or bear weight on the injured part. You may make a splint out of a rolled-up magazine. If there is severe pain, multiple injuries or bleeding, call an ambulance.

AT THE EMERGENCY ROOM

Gaining appropriate attention and priority in the emergency department depends upon "planning for your emergency" and carefully communicating with personnel once you are there.

●**Create a list that you can always carry with you.** Include your medical problems, your medications and your allergies, as well as your name, address and phone number and your insurance information.

●**Know how to call an ambulance in your community** and which emergency rooms are best for your special needs.

●**Communicate effectively by speaking slowly**...telling the doctor or nurse exactly what happened to you. Don't expect that medical personnel will already know what's wrong or why.

●**Understand that a triage nurse** will determine the order in which you will be seen based upon his/her assessment of your medical needs compared with those of others who are waiting.

Easy Ways to Save Big Money on Prescription Drugs

Donald L. Sullivan, RPh, PhD, a Columbus, OH, pharmacist and author of *The Consumer's Guide to Generic Drugs: The Complete Reference Book for Anyone Using Prescription Drugs*. Berkley Books.

No doubt you already know that you can often save on costly medications by asking your doctor for a prescription for generic equivalents. *Here are five more cost-cutting tricks...*

●**Ask for free samples.** Doctors are deluged with drug samples from manufacturers—but they don't always distribute these samples to their patients.

Ask, and you may get a week or more of a pricey drug for free.

Caution: Check expiration dates. Forgo samples that have been sitting around the doctor's office for too long.

●**Use mail order**—but only when appropriate. Buying prescriptions by mail can be an economical, convenient way to purchase drugs. But you should know that many mail-order pharmacies use nonpharmacists to fill prescriptions.

While a pharmacist does do a final check, the volume of drugs being processed is very high—and mistakes are possible.

Going the mail-order route also means you lose the benefit of a face-to-face meeting with your pharmacist—who can warn you about drug interactions or answer your questions on the spot.

Bottom line: If you want to use mail order, do so only with drugs you're familiar with—ideally, drugs you must take on a long-term basis. That way, you reduce your risk of taking the wrong drug or falling victim to unforeseen drug interactions.

●**Don't let your insurance company impose limits** on prescription length. If your doctor writes a prescription for a 90-day supply of pills, your insurer may approve only a 30-day supply.

Limiting your prescription in this manner helps the insurer cut costs...but costs you money and extra trips to the drugstore.

Loophole: If you need 90 days of pills but your insurer covers only 30 days, ask your doctor to substitute "take as directed" instead of "take once a day" on the prescription form.

That makes it hard for the insurance company to calculate how many pills comprise a 30-day supply. You'll be able to get the full 90-day supply filled.

Caution: Find out how often the drug should be taken, and write it yourself on the bottle.

●**Avoid time-release formulations.** Many prescription drugs are available in both time-release and non-time-release forms. Time-release pills are more convenient because they don't have to be taken as often as their "plain" counterparts. But they're also more costly.

●**Look into patient-assistance programs.** Under such programs—offered by most pharmaceutical makers but rarely publicized—individuals short on cash because of job loss or another financial setback may qualify for free prescription medication.

In most cases, all that's required is your doctor's certification that you're unable to afford a costly but necessary medication.

Call the manufacturer directly to find out if a particular drug is available through such a program—and what the terms are.

The Importance of Support Groups for Chronic Illness

David Spiegel, MD, professor of psychiatry and behavioral sciences and director of the Psychosocial Treatment Laboratory at Stanford University School of Medicine in Stanford, CA. He is author of *Living Beyond Limits: New Hope and Help for Facing Life-Threatening Illness.* Fawcett Columbine.

If you're suffering from arthritis, diabetes, cancer or another serious or chronic illness, participating in a support group can boost your emotional and even your physical well-being.

Unfortunately, few people who could benefit from participating in a group do so.

Some of us shy away from support groups because we fear we'll be too embarrassed to discuss our problems with strangers. Of course, members of a support group don't remain strangers for long.

Others view support groups as a source of emotional "hand-holding" for people who are weak or insecure.

In fact, group participants spend little time feeling sorry for each other. They help one another face their problems head-on—*and it really pays off.*

WHAT THE RESEARCH SHOWS

●**Breast cancer.** In a study at Stanford University, 86 women with advanced (metastatic) breast cancer were randomly assigned to one of two groups.

One group received standard medical care. The other group got identical care *plus* weekly sessions with a support group. At the end of the first year, women who had participated in the support group felt less anxious and depressed than the women who had not participated in the group. They also reported half as much physical pain as the other women.

Long-term follow-up showed something even more remarkable—that the support group participants lived an average of 18 months longer.

●**Malignant melanoma.** University of California at Los Angeles researchers conducted a randomized trial of 80 melanoma patients.

The 40 patients assigned to the control group received standard medical care. The other 40 patients in the experimental group got standard medical care—and they participated in weekly support group sessions.

When tested six weeks later, the experimental group reported less anxiety and depression than the control group. Six years later, 10 members of the control group had died. Only three of the experimental group had died.

●**Diabetes.** A 1992 University of Chicago study found that male diabetics who participated in support groups were less depressed than similar men who did not participate in support groups.

HEIGHTENED IMMUNITY

What accounts for these dramatic findings? One theory is that the social support created by a group boosts the immune system by reducing the psychological stress associated with serious illness, and is known to interfere with immunity.

This theory is supported by the UCLA study, which found unusually high levels of immune system cells called *natural-killer cells* in patients who participated in support groups.

MUTUAL ENCOURAGEMENT

Support group members also encourage each other to take better care of themselves physically. Some act as advocates for one another, making sure they get access to information and proper treatment.

Groups fight isolation by giving members a chance to talk to people who understand what they're going through—this at a time when family and friends may not know what to say.

Finally, support groups help people find meaning in their suffering. Because the group gives them an opportunity to use their own experiences to help others, many patients feel that some good has come from a bad situation.

FINDING THE RIGHT GROUP

If your doctor or a hospital social worker is unable to steer you to a group, call the American Self-Help Clearinghouse at 973-326-6789. *Web site: www.selfhelpgroups.org.*

The group's facilitator should be knowledgeable about group dynamics as well as about your specific illness and its treatment.

Look for a group headed by a doctor, psychologist, nurse or social worker. Fees should be reasonable—no more than $40 per person per session.

If you can't find a group near you, start your own. Post a notice at a hospital, clinic or church, seeking members who are dealing with the same illness. At the same time, start your search for a facilitator.

Many successful groups are run by their members (and have no leader). However, a professional facilitator is best equipped to handle members who get upset, try to dominate the discussion or keep avoiding important issues.

FOR MAXIMUM BENEFIT

You'll get the most out of your group by making a point to attend every session. It's much easier to establish a trusting environment if all of the participants commit themselves to showing up for the sessions.

Do not feel obliged to speak up. Realize, however, that you will get more from a group the more you talk about what you are going through...and the better you are at listening to other members.

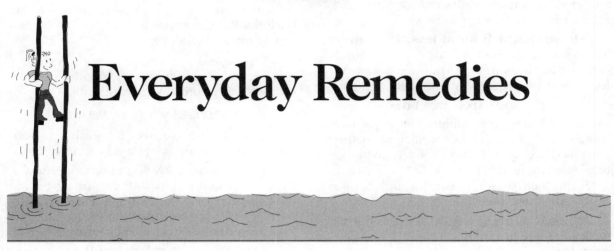

2

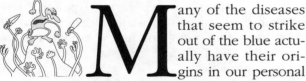

Everyday Remedies

The Ultimate Guide to Infectious Disease

Winkler G. Weinberg, MD
Southeast Permanente Medical Group

Many of the diseases that seem to strike out of the blue actually have their origins in our personal habits. *Here's how to protect yourself and your family from infectious illnesses…*

WASH YOUR HANDS

Colds and flu are contracted not by being *near* a coughing, sneezing person, but by *touch*.

Self-defense: Wash your hands as soon as possible after touching someone who's ill… after touching something an ill person has touched…and just periodically when you're living or working with an infected individual.

Until you wash up, don't touch your eyes or nose. Those are the main entry points for cold

viruses. For times when no sink is handy, carry a supply of alcohol-based wipes.

PREPARE FOOD CAREFULLY

Much of the meat and eggs in the supermarket are tainted with *salmonella*.

Escherichia coli (E. coli) is present in up to 4% of ground beef, pork, poultry and lamb. It's also found in unpasteurized milk and juice and other beverages.

To prevent food poisoning…

● **Refrigerate food immediately after preparing or serving it.** If it's been sitting out for more than an hour, throw it away.

● **Avoid steak tartare and raw or undercooked eggs.** Steer clear of Caesar salad and homemade eggnog and mayonnaise. If *any*

Winkler G. Weinberg, MD, chief of infectious diseases for Atlanta-based Southeast Permanente Medical Group, and director of a consortium for research on infectious diseases. He is author of *No Germs Allowed! How to Avoid Infectious Diseases at Home and on the Road.* Rutgers University Press.

yolk from a contaminated egg remains liquid, salmonella can survive.

●**Wash utensils or surfaces that have been in contact with raw meat or eggs** before using them again.

●**Drink only *pasteurized* milk and juice.**

●**Avoid bottom-feeding fish.** Grouper, red snapper, amberjack and barracuda can harbor *ciguatera*, a disease-causing toxin.

●**Steam shellfish for at least 15 minutes.** Thorough steaming takes care of E. coli and other infectious agents that are commonly found in clams, oysters and mussels.

GUARD AGAINST TICK BITES

Most tick bites are benign. But since Lyme disease and other tick-borne illnesses can be hard to detect and treat, it's best to avoid getting bitten in the first place.

During tick season (April through the first frost), take these precautions…

●**When walking in wooded or grassy areas,** wear long-sleeved shirts and long, loose-fitting pants tucked into socks.

●**Use insect repellent containing DEET.** A 30% concentration is best. Put it on your clothing *and* any exposed skin.

●**If you have outdoor pets, use tick-killing powder or spray.** Your veterinarian can recommend a good brand.

●**Check yourself for ticks daily.** Have a family member check your scalp and other hard-to-see areas. Look closely—some ticks are the size of a pinhead.

If you find a tick, do *not* remove it with alcohol, petroleum jelly or a lighted match. These methods can cause the tick to regurgitate under your skin, raising your chance of illness.

Better: Using tweezers, gently grasp the tick and pull steadily *outward* at the same angle the tick is facing.

Keep the tick in a jar of alcohol, so it can be identified later if you develop a bull's-eye rash or other suspicious symptoms.

PREVENT URINARY INFECTIONS

Women who are prone to urinary tract infections (UTIs) should consider using a birth con-

trol method other than the diaphragm. Spermicidal jellies and foams used with a diaphragm create an environment hospitable to bacteria.

Women should also urinate after intercourse to flush out infection-causing bacteria. UTIs are rare among men.

AVOID PARASITES IN WATER

In most areas, tap water is chlorinated to kill bacteria. But chlorination does not kill *Cryptosporidium* and other parasites.

Self-defense: If you have poor immunity, boil water for one minute or install a reverse-osmosis water purifier under your sink.

BE CAREFUL WHILE TRAVELING

Check with a doctor well in advance of your trip and get any recommended vaccinations.

In the US, Canada, Western Europe, Australia, New Zealand and Japan, food and water are usually safe. In other regions, eat only fully cooked or freshly peeled foods. Bring your own water…or drink carbonated beverages or wine.

Watch out for ice cubes and the mixers in mixed drinks.

To purify water: Boil it for at least one minute. Or—add 2% tincture of iodine (five drops per quart of water), and let it sit for at least an hour. This method is good for suspect tap water and water from a stream or lake.

If you visit an area where malaria and/or other insect-borne diseases are endemic, wear light, loose-fitting clothing and mosquito netting…use DEET spray…and stay indoors as much as possible.

LEGIONNAIRE'S DISEASE

Smokers, elderly people and individuals taking immunosuppressant drugs are at risk for Legionnaire's disease.

The bacteria that cause Legionnaire's are often found in shower heads, air conditioning systems and cooling towers—in the US and abroad.

Self-defense: Stay as far away as possible from cooling towers. And—before using an unfamiliar shower, sterilize the shower head by running the water at its hottest setting for five minutes.

Everything You Need to Know About Bacteria!

Linda Gooding, PhD, professor of microbiology and immunology at Emory University School of Medicine, Atlanta.

Though bacteria are often viewed as agents of disease, many of the billions of microorganisms dwelling inside our bodies are essential for good health.

"Friendly" bacteria—such as the lactobacillus and bifida cultures in yogurt—inhibit growth of yeast and other disease-causing organisms. There's even evidence that friendly bacteria help lower cholesterol levels.

Problem: Each time you take an antibiotic, you kill bacteria in your body—friendly and unfriendly alike. That raises your risk of diarrhea, yeast infection and food sensitivity.

Bacteria are also killed by cortisone, prednisone, birth-control pills, antacids—even stress.

To the rescue: A family of supplements known as *probiotics*. These blends of bacteria and rice or milk powder repopulate the bowel with friendly bacteria.

In a study at Long Island Jewish Medical Center, women who ate a daily cup of yogurt had fewer vaginal infections than women who didn't eat yogurt. The effect would have been even *more* significant had the women taken probiotics.

To keep your intestinal flora healthy, I recommend eating yogurt regularly. Most brands contain active cultures. Check labels if you're unsure.

Take probiotics in *addition* to yogurt if you have high cholesterol or chronic yeast infections…while traveling…or while taking antibiotics, steroids, birth-control pills or antacids.

Probiotics, available at health-food stores, cost $12 to $15 for 30 capsules. Pick a brand that contains at least one billion live organisms per gram. Be sure to check the package's expiration date.

How to Stay Healthy on Your Next Airplane Flight

Adriane Fugh-Berman, MD, a Washington, DC-based medical researcher who specializes in women's health and alternative medicine. She is author of *Alternative Medicine: What Works.* Williams & Wilkens.

Any long trip is tiring. But air travel can also cause health problems—colds and other respiratory infections, aches and pains, jet lag and even a potentially fatal condition known as *pulmonary embolism*. Fortunately, there are easy ways to prevent each of these problems.

COLDS

It's easy to catch cold while traveling by air. That's because the air inside most jets is recirculated. And so are the airborne germs.

Sitting far away from someone with a cough doesn't help. Since you're in a confined space, you're almost equally likely to be exposed to germs whether the source of the germs is 20 rows away or right next to you.

Making matters worse, the humidity inside a modern jetliner is usually 10% or lower. That's less humid than desert air. By drying the mucous membranes lining your nose, mouth and respiratory tract, low humidity makes it easy for viruses and bacteria to get a foothold.

To fend off "airliner germs," some people have resorted to wearing surgical masks during flights. I don't recommend that. But I do recommend boosting your immune system. The day before, the day of and the day after your departure, swallow one-half dropperful of *echinacea* tincture…along with 2,000 milligrams (mg) of vitamin C (divided into two 1,000 mg doses).

Drink 16 ounces of water or juice just before boarding the plane…and 12 ounces *each hour* while you're in the air. You might want to bring your own water bottle, in case the flight attendants are too busy to serve you.

BACKACHE AND NECK PAIN

Support your lumbar spine by placing a rolled blanket behind your back. If you plan to doze, a U-shaped neck pillow makes a big difference. I

49

prefer *inflatable* pillows, since they take up less space in your carry-on bag. They cost about $10 and are available at luggage stores.

Two exercises are also helpful...

●**Shoulder circles.** Shrug your shoulders up and down, then roll them forward and back.

●**Head circles.** Tilt your head to the side, ear toward shoulder. Hold briefly, then raise your head back to center. Tilt to the other side, then return to center. Drop your chin to your chest, hold briefly, then return your head to its normal position. Tilt your head back, hold, then return to center.

JET LAG

The best way I've found to fight jet lag is to reset your biological clock with melatonin after your arrival. Two hours before your new bedtime, take 1 to 3 mg. Take it the next two days, too, if you have trouble adjusting to your new schedule. Exposure to natural daylight after your arrival will also help you adjust.

PULMONARY EMBOLISM

Hours of sitting almost motionless slows your circulation, raising your risk for pulmonary embolism. In this potentially deadly condition, a blood clot forms in the leg, then breaks away and travels to the lung—where it can interfere with the body's oxygen supply.

To keep blood from pooling in your lower extremities, take periodic walks during the flight. As you walk about the cabin, occasionally stand on your toes, then rock back on your heels.

If the seat belt sign is on, do the following exercises in your seat...

●**Heel rocks.** Sit with your back straight and feet flat on the floor. Lift your heels, then rock back on them. Then alternately flex and point your toes.

●**Leg lifts.** Press down on your left thigh with your left hand, and lift your thigh against this resistance. Repeat 20 times. Switch sides and repeat.

Water Therapy for Common Ailments

Dian Dincin Buchman, PhD, a New York City-based lecturer on water therapy and other alternative therapies. She is author of several books, including *The Complete Book of Water Therapy*. Keats Publishing.

Ice packs, hot and cold compresses, medicated baths and other forms of water therapy were mainstays of folk medicine for centuries.

Today, high-tech medicine has eclipsed water-based treatments. Yet these treatments—safe, inexpensive and easy to use—remain valuable tools for easing discomfort caused by common ailments.

MEDICATED BATHS

We all know how relaxing a warm bath can be. But not everyone realizes that even *greater* benefits can be reaped by adding natural ingredients to the water.

●**Apple cider vinegar.** Add a cup to bathwater, and splash a handful over your shoulders, back and chest. That will invigorate you when you're fatigued.

This technique also helps restore the skin's germ-killing natural acidity, which is continually washed away by bathing.

To soothe poison ivy or sunburn, add *two* cups of vinegar.

●**Bran.** A bran bath eases itching, soothes dermatitis or other skin irritations and eliminates scaly patches.

Sew several handfuls of wheat or oat bran into a cheesecloth pouch. Soak the pouch in hot water for several minutes, then place in a tub filled with tepid water. Squeeze the pouch until the water turns milky.

●**Pine extract.** One capful in a warm bath helps open clogged pores, speeds healing of rashes and relieves muscle fatigue.

Pine extract is available at drugstores and health-food stores. Do not confuse it with pine *cleanser*, which will irritate the skin.

SALT MASSAGE

This energizing technique tones tissues, relieves stress and fatigue...and can help you ward off a cold.

Sit on the edge of a tub filled with warm water. Pour salt into a cupped hand. Slowly add water to the salt until you make a thick paste.

Using firm, circular motions, rub the paste over your body. Then rinse off the paste with a brief soak in the tub...or sponge it off with cold water. Be careful not to rub salt onto sores, cuts, etc.

HAND BATH

To ease writer's cramp, soak hands in hot water. To warm cold hands, soak them alternately in hot water (three minutes) and cold water (30 seconds). Repeat several times, ending with cold water.

Caution: Don't leave hands in cold water for more than a few minutes at a time.

COLD-WATER TREADING

Fill the tub ankle-deep with cold water. Holding onto a firmly anchored rail, march in place for a few seconds or minutes (as long as you can comfortably tolerate). Then rub your feet briskly with a towel.

Done twice daily, this technique creates a remarkable sense of well-being...and is great for relieving exercise-related leg cramps. Some believe that it builds resistance to disease as well.

Done at night, cold-water treading promotes sound sleep—yet it has an eye-opening effect when done in the morning.

COMPRESSED

To prevent or relieve headache pain, fold a washcloth in half, dip it in ice water and wring it out. Place it on your head or neck. Rewet it every few minutes to keep it cold.

To relieve a sore throat or laryngitis, fold a cotton cloth in thirds, wet it with cold water and wring it out. Wind it once around the neck and fasten with a safety pin. Over the cloth, wrap a wool scarf.

Leave this wrap in place as long as you like. With the cold trapped against the skin by the wool, the body continues to divert more warming blood to the area—helping break up congestion.

How to Feel and Look Younger

David Ryback, PhD, an antiaging/stress reduction consultant in Atlanta. He is author of *Look 10 Years Younger, Live 10 Years Longer*, which is available in editions for men and for women. Prentice Hall.

Practice stretching each morning. Regular stretching helps you feel more flexible and, as a result, you will feel and look younger. By stretching, you relax your muscles, and movements become more graceful and youthful.

●**Stand up straight.** By maintaining good posture, you'll look 10 pounds thinner. Practice in front of the mirror, and you'll notice that your stomach looks flatter, your torso appears longer and thinner—and you don't have that old, tired, hunched look.

●**Exercise at least 15 minutes a day.** Physical activity alleviates depression and improves your mood. It also sends more blood to the skin, giving your complexion a healthy, rosy, youthful glow.

●**Eat more fruits and vegetables.** A vegetarian or even a semivegetarian diet that includes lots of fruits, vegetables and grains will help you maintain a stable energy level. By eating sensibly, you can quickly increase your energy level and feel younger.

●**Reduce stress.** If left unchecked, stress puts unnecessary wear and tear on your body's internal organs and causes you to look tired and years older.

How to Break Bad Habits

William Knaus, EdD, author of *Change Your Life Now: Powerful Techniques for Positive Change*. John Wiley & Sons.

To break a problem habit, you need to create a *will to change*—not an attempt to restrain yourself. Self-restraint against bad habits rarely works.

Example: Dieters usually gain back the weight they have lost. But a *will to change* is a command effort that allows experimenting with change, accepting its difficulty and moving ahead again even after inevitable backsliding.

Helpful: Deflect your attention from the habit to something else.

Example: Keep a pitcher of water in the refrigerator. Whenever you have a habit urge—of any kind—pour and slowly sip two glasses of ice water. This will often allow time for the urge to pass.

Simple Solutions For Incontinence

Kristene E. Whitmore, MD, clinical associate professor of urology at the University of Pennsylvania in Philadelphia. She is coauthor of *Overcoming Bladder Disorders.* HarperPerennial.

More than 13 million Americans have trouble controlling their bladders.

Urinary incontinence is *not* a disease. It's a symptom of an underlying problem—diabetes, stroke, multiple sclerosis (MS), Parkinson's disease or even chronic bladder infection.

Obese people face heightened risk for incontinence. So do smokers and women—especially those who have recently had a baby. Passage of the baby through the birth canal often damages the abdominal muscles responsible for holding and releasing urine.

In men, incontinence is usually a result of nerve damage caused by surgery to treat prostate enlargement or cancer.

Good news: Incontinence can often be prevented—or controlled. If you're incontinent—or worried that you might become incontinent—avoid caffeine, alcohol, spicy foods, chocolate, artificial sweeteners and other bladder irritants...urinate before and after intercourse to expel infection-causing bacteria...and drink lots of water.

Do *not* drink large quantities of water at one time, however. Doing so causes the bladder to fill too rapidly. Have one sip every five to 10 minutes throughout the day.

Women: To keep pelvic floor muscles strong, do Kegel exercises.

Women with recurrent bladder infections should take a cranberry pill with each meal. The pills contain compounds that keep infection-causing bacteria from sticking to bladder walls.

Cranberries and cranberry juice also contain these compounds—but at lower levels.

Men: Ask your doctor about taking a zinc supplement and saw palmetto extract. Both have been shown to prevent or relieve prostate enlargement.

TYPES OF INCONTINENCE

Four out of five cases of incontinence can now either be cured or made better. The first step is to identify which of the four types is involved...

●**Stress incontinence** is associated with a weakness of the urinary sphincter, the circular valve-like muscle around the bladder neck and urethra that controls the flow of urine.

Coughing, laughing, etc., exert more pressure on the bladder than the sphincter can contain, and urine spills out.

Usual causes: Abdominal or pelvic surgery, childbirth, estrogen deficiency. Certain drugs, including alpha blockers and diuretics, make matters worse.

●**Urge incontinence** occurs when "overexcited" nerves cause involuntary contraction of bladder muscles. You have a sudden urge to urinate—but can't reach a toilet in time.

Usual causes: Parkinson's disease, multiple sclerosis, bladder infection, the bladder disorder *interstitial cystitis*, spinal cord problems, chemotherapy.

●**Overflow incontinence** occurs when weak bladder muscles or a urinary obstruction makes it hard to empty the bladder. Urine eventually overflows, like water over a dam.

Usual causes: Diabetes, enlarged prostate in men, prolapsed (dropped) bladder or uterus in women. The problem can also be caused by over-the-counter cold and allergy medications... or by the decongestant *pseudoephedrine*.

●**Functional incontinence** is a transient problem associated with stool impaction, restricted mobility, vaginal irritation and other conditions.

BLADDER TRAINING

The aim of bladder training is to empty the bladder *on schedule*—so that urine won't build up to the point where an accident occurs.

At first, urinate every 90 minutes. Gradually lengthen the interval between trips to the bathroom—up to three hours—until you find a schedule that's safe and convenient.

Helpful: A "voiding diary." For two to three days in a row, record how often you urinate—and when leakage occurs. Review the diary with your doctor.

KEGEL EXERCISES

Most people with stress or urge incontinence get partial relief if they strengthen the urinary sphincter. *To do Kegel exercises:*

• **Identify the muscle you want to train.** It's the same muscle used to control a bowel movement. If you have trouble identifying it, place a finger in your vagina (if you're a woman) or anus (if you're a man). Practice squeezing only the muscle around your finger.

• **For the first three to six days,** squeeze the muscle for three seconds at a time.

• **Over the next few weeks,** gradually build up till you can tighten the sphincter for 10 seconds at a time. Relax the muscle for 10 seconds after each contraction. Do 50 every day.

BIOFEEDBACK AND WEIGHTS

Biofeedback uses a special tampon, inserted in the vagina or rectum, to help you identify the muscles that need to be strengthened. The tampons are available by prescription.

Women whose incontinence is caused by weak abdominal muscles often benefit from vaginal "weight training." Cone-shaped weights are held in the vagina for 15 minutes, twice a day, as you go about your daily activities.*

HELPFUL MEDICATIONS

Drug therapy brings faster relief than do the nondrug approaches outlined above—but it often causes side effects.

Best approach: Start taking the medication when you begin bladder training, diet and Kegel exercises. Gradually wean yourself off the drugs as the non-drug methods start to work.

*To locate a store in your area that sells Fem-Tone weights, call 800-422-8811.

• **Oxybutinin** (Ditropan), *propantheline* (Norpanth), tricyclic antidepressants like *imipramine* (Tofranil) are good for stress and urge incontinence. Side effects include dry mouth, constipation and dry skin.

• **Diet pills** containing *pseudoephedrine* are good for stress incontinence. Side effects include anxiety, insomnia, sweating. Do not use if you have high blood pressure.

• **Estrogen** is useful for women who develop mixed incontinence after menopause. However, since it can promote breast and uterine cancer, it should be taken only after a thorough discussion of these risks with a doctor.

THE SURGICAL OPTION

When other treatments fail to provide relief from incontinence, surgery may be the answer.

Several different forms of surgery are available, depending upon the exact nature of the problem and its severity.

Hemorrhoid Self-Defense

Mayo Clinic Health Letter, 200 First St. SW, Rochester, MN 55905.

Eat high-fiber foods—fresh fruits, vegetables and whole grains…drink plenty of water—at least six cups a day…stay active, which reduces pressure in anal and rectal veins that results from being in one position too long. Regular exercise also helps prevent constipation.

Prevention and Treatment of Common Foot Problems

Suzanne M. Levine, DPM, a clinical podiatrist at New York Hospital–Cornell Medical Center in New York City. She is author of *My Feet Are Killing Me!* (Fawcett), *Walk It Off* (Plume) and *50 Ways to Treat Foot Pain* (Signet).

Eighty-seven percent of Americans have foot trouble—bunions, corns, calluses, foot odor, etc. Despite their prevalence, however, such problems are *not* inevitable. Most can be prevented via a simple five-step foot-pampering regimen…

- **Soak your feet at the end of each day.** Use lukewarm water along with Dr. Scholl's Soap 'n Soak Instant Foot Bath or another product containing *sodium bicarbonate*. This compound lowers the skin's acidity, rendering it less susceptible to fungus and calluses.

After soaking, dry your feet thoroughly—especially between your toes.

- **Massage moisturizer into your heels after each soak.** Moisturizer will help prevent skin fissures and calluses. These problems are common in summer—especially if you wear open-heeled shoes.

- **Use foot powder twice a day.** After soaking at night and then again in the morning, dust your feet with Quinsana Deodorant Foot Powder or another product containing the perspiration-fighting agent *benzethonium chloride*.

Foot powder is especially beneficial during summer months, when foot perspiration is a big problem.

- **Inspect your toenails once a week.** If they need trimming, cut them straight across using a long-handled nail clipper. Each time you trim your nails, scrub your toes and the soles of your feet to remove calluses.

For dry skin, use Kerasal or another foot mask containing *salicylic acid* or another "keratolytic agent." This rids the feet of excess keratin, a moisture-repelling protein found in skin.

- **Do nightly foot exercises.** Before going to bed, spend a few minutes picking up a pencil with your toes…pressing on an imaginary accelerator pedal with each foot…and using your toes to trace the outlines of letters of the alphabet on the floor.

Nightly foot exercises help minimize the foot swelling that inevitably occurs during the day.

BUNIONS

These bony protuberances on the sides of the feet are caused by ill-fitting shoes and/or hereditary factors. They can lead to painful calluses, osteoarthritis and/or hammertoes.

Self-defense: Wear loose-fitting shoes. New shoes should be purchased at midday, when the feet are slightly swollen. Make sure there's a thumb's-width space between the front of the shoe and your longest toe.

To reduce redness and swelling: Use ice around the bunion.

Finger test: If a whitish area appears when you press down on a bump, you may not be suffering from a bunion but from bursitis, a condition that requires medical attention.

CORNS

These areas of yellowish, thickened skin atop or between the toes can be quite painful. They're usually caused by friction and pressure on the foot.

Self-defense: Soak your feet in water containing Epsom salts. Afterward, apply moisturizer and cover the area with plastic wrap. After 15 minutes, remove the plastic and use a pumice stone to smooth out the corn.

Also helpful: Orthotics or foam insoles. Orthotics, which are custom-made, cost $350 or more—but are usually covered by insurance. Insoles are available at drugstores for less than $15.

HAMMERTOES

This problem—twisted or misshapen toes that may overlap each other—is common among people who have high arches.

Self-defense: Relieve pressure on the toes by wearing shoes with wide toes…and by covering corns with corn pads, lamb's wool or bandages. In severe cases, outpatient surgery may be necessary.

HEEL SPURS

These bony growths protruding downward from the heel bones are typically caused by rapid weight gain…or from playing tennis or another sport that places pressure on the heels.

Heel spurs are often confused with *plantar fasciitis*. This condition is usually caused by excessive stress or pressure on the plantar fascia, the protective tissue under the soles of the feet.

Self-defense: Put foam or felt pads in the heels of your shoes…or purchase insoles to help raise the arches of the feet.

Each time pain strikes, elevate your foot and apply an ice pack to the heel for 20 minutes.

Over-the-counter painkillers are effective against both heel spurs and plantar fasciitis.

Also helpful: Exercises that stretch the Achilles tendons. Once a day, try picking up marbles with your toes…or lifting your toes while the soles of your feet are planted firmly on the ground.

COLD FEET

This condition usually stems from foods, drugs and/or behaviors that cause impaired circulation—caffeinated foods and beverages …appetite suppressants…and smoking.

Self-defense: Stop smoking. Cut down on caffeinated foods and beverages. Switch shoes at least once a day, wearing shoes of different heel heights. Shift your weight back and forth while standing. Each night, take a bath in lukewarm water.

Once a day, do these three circulation-boosting exercises…

Exercise #1: Cross your legs at your ankles, then try to pull them apart as you simultaneously resist. Hold for one minute. Switch sides, and hold again.

Exercise #2: Place the balls of your feet on a telephone book, with your heels resting on the floor. Push up and down. This exercise may be done sitting or standing for one minute.

Exercise #3: Lie on the floor with your feet pressed flat against the wall. For about one minute, "climb the walls" using your feet.

TOENAIL FUNGUS

This condition (*onychomycosis*) can lead to warped and discolored toenails.

Self-defense: Make a paste with lukewarm water and baking soda. Rub it on the affected area daily. Rinse and dry.

Also helpful: Wear cotton socks…change shoes twice a day…and use antibacterial drying powder and foot deodorant. Avoid garlic and other spicy foods if they cause your feet to perspire.

Do *not* use opaque nail polish. It darkens the nail bed, making it vulnerable to fungal growth.

If symptoms persist, ask your doctor for the oral medication *itraconazole* (Sporonox).

ATHLETE'S FOOT

Most cases are caused by *Candida*, the same yeast that causes vaginal infections, and/or by *T. rubrum*, another type of fungus.

Self-defense: Keep feet dry. Change socks at least once a day. Avoid colored socks—some are made with dyes that promote growth of fungus. Use Tinactin, Halotex or another antifungal ointment or spray containing a broad-spectrum antifungal agent of the *azole* family.

FOOT ODOR

This condition is caused by bacteria that thrive on moist, sweaty skin. It can also be caused by eating spices, which can cause sweat glands to become overactive.

Self-defense: Cut back on spicy foods, and keep feet dry. Change shoes at least once a day. Air them out after each wearing.

Also helpful: Dr. Scholl's Deodorant Foot Powder and Johnson & Johnson's Odor-Eaters.

Heel Pain Relief

Carol Frey, MD, associate professor of orthopedic surgery at the medical school of the University of Southern California in Los Angeles.

Store-bought pads relieve heel pain more effectively than custom-made inserts. Researchers gave foot stretching exercises to 200 people suffering from a heel condition called *isolated proximal plantar fasciitis.*

In addition, they provided different cushioning devices ranging from off-the-shelf rubber and silicon cushions and insoles costing between $9 and $40 to custom-made orthotic arch inserts costing between $300 and $500.

Stretching plus the store-bought devices helped 81% to 95% of the sufferers. But when combined with orthotics, stretching relieved less than 70%.

Medicine Cabinet Must-Haves

Timothy McCall, MD, a Boston internist, author of *Examining Your Doctor: A Patient's Guide to Avoiding Harmful Medical Care.* Citadel Press. He is a regular commentator on the public radio program Marketplace, and can be found on the Web at *www.drmccall.com.*

Every medicine cabinet should have the following basics…

- **Acetaminophen** or aspirin for pain and fever.

- **An antihistamine** for hives or other allergic reactions.

- **Triple-antibiotic ointment,** adhesive bandages, gauze, tape for minor wounds.

- **Ipecac syrup** to induce vomiting in certain types of poisoning.

- **Ace bandages** for strains and sprains.

- **Thermometer.**

- **Pointed tweezers** for splinters.

Extend the Life of Athletic Shoes

Carol Frey, MD, associate professor of orthopedic surgery, University of Southern California, Los Angeles.

Air shoes out for 24 hours after each use… pull out the insoles and stuff them with newspapers or paper towels and place in a well-ventilated area…never leave shoes in the sun or a hot car…never toss them into a washing machine.

Also: Don't try to resuscitate worn-out shoes by adding new insoles. Most shoe breakdowns occur in the midsole—the wedge of cushioning between the outsole and the upper. Insoles are designed to provide support, not replace the midsole.

Emergency Ice Packs

Peter Bruno, MD, internist for the New York Knicks basketball team.

If ice cubes aren't available, use a bag of frozen peas. It will hug body contours, easing pain and helping to heal.

Important: Wrap the bag in a cloth to prevent ice burn…apply for 10 minutes at a time.

CPR to the Rescue

Richard O. Cummins, MD, professor of medicine, University of Washington, Seattle.

Rescuers should start CPR before calling 911 when trying to resuscitate a child or a young adult. Clear the airway, do one minute of breath/chest compressions, *then* call 911. With individuals over age 30, call 911 first.

Reason: An older person whose heart stops is probably experiencing ventricular fibrillation. This heart condition requires prompt treatment by emergency personnel. But a young person whose heart stops usually has only an obstructed airway—which can be cleared by anyone with minimal training. If you lack CPR training, call 911 first, then return to the victim and try to help.

Music Fights Insomnia

Gail C. Mornhinweg, PhD, ARNP, associate professor of nursing, University of Louisville, KY. Her six-month study of 25 adults with insomnia was published in *Journal of Holistic Nursing,* 2455 Teller Rd., Thousand Oaks, CA 91320.

Patients who had trouble sleeping were given two cassette tapes—one of Baroque music, the other of New Age music. After listening to the tapes at bedtime, all but one of the patients said they fell asleep faster and slept longer than usual.

Also: Sleeplessness returned on nights when the patients did not listen to music.

How to Reduce Your Risk of Cancer

David Alberts, MD, director of Cancer Prevention and Control at the Arizona Cancer Center in Tucson.

Reduce your risk of colorectal cancer by eating a diet high in fiber and calcium. Ninety people at risk for colorectal cancer were given varying doses of calcium and wheat bran fiber supplements.

Result: The high-fiber group (13.5 g per day) produced 52% less bile acid than did the low-fiber group. Those who consumed the most calcium (15,000 mg) had a 35% reduction in bile acid production.

Theory: Fiber and calcium soak up these cancer-promoting acids. One ounce of Kellogg's All-Bran contains 10 g of fiber…and one cup of milk contains 300 mg of calcium.

Can't Sleep?

Mark R. Pressman, PhD, associate director, Sleep Disorders Center, The Lankenau Hospital and Medical Research Center, Wynnewood, PA. His study of 80 patients was published in *Archives of Internal Medicine*, 515 N. State St., Chicago 60610.

Sleep disorders often go undiagnosed. If you awaken repeatedly at night to use the bathroom, see a doctor to rule out the possibility that you're waking because of a sleep disorder. In a study, 79% of patients who *thought* they were getting up to urinate were actually being awakened by sleep apnea, snoring or leg movements.

Good news: Most sleep disorders can be successfully treated.

Help for People Who Can't Fall Asleep

Rituals of Healing: Using Imagery for Health and Wellness by Jeanne Achterberg, PhD, psychologist and body-mind researcher, Big Sur, CA. Bantam Books.

Simply telling your body to sleep probably will not work. Instead, try *active imaging*, where you use images to bring you to sleep.

Examples: Imagine a calming, repetitive scene, like waves at the seashore. Or let your mind drift into the memory of what it feels like to go to sleep.

Remember your usual sleeping position, and allow yourself to feel your body floating or moving downward into a comfortable, restful state.

Elevation and Breathing

Norman H. Edelman, MD, consultant for scientific affairs, American Lung Association, 1740 Broadway, New York 10019.

People with breathing disorders feel better if they move to a lower elevation. The lower the elevation, the more oxygen is in the air and the easier oxygen is transferred to blood. Some people who live at high elevations will benefit from moving to sea level.

Control Pet Allergies

Martha V. White, MD, director of research, Institute for Asthma & Allergy, Washington Hospital Center, 106 Irving St. NW, Washington, DC 20010.

Keep the pet outside, off the furniture and out of your bedroom. In most cases, it is the saliva and dander—the dead skin that flakes off and travels through the air—not the pet hair that causes the allergy problem. Also consider washing your dog or cat daily with water. Avoid frequent shampooing—it can release dander more quickly.

Feeling Forgetful?

Barry Gordon, MD, PhD, behavioral neurologist, cognitive neuroscientist and experimental psychologist at Johns Hopkins University, Baltimore, and author of *Memory: Remembering and Forgetting in Everyday Life.* MasterMedia.

Boost your memory by deciding what you need to remember most and focusing on it ...paying close attention to anything you want to memorize...learning to remember in little bits over time, not trying to remember a large amount of information at once.

Also helpful: Designate a *memory spot* in your home where you leave things, so you don't have to bother remembering where you put the car keys...or use a pocket notebook or file cards to help jog your memory.

Does Drinking Coffee Help Control Hay Fever?

Vincent Tubiolo, MD, fellow of allergy and immunology, Harbor-UCLA Medical Center, Torrance, CA.

In a study, hay fever sufferers given 400 mg of caffeine (equal to 18 ounces of coffee) reported a 51% reduction in symptoms, compared with a 19% reduction in those given a placebo. Caffeine blocks nasal inflammation caused by hay fever.

Trap: Caffeine can raise blood pressure and heart rate. This study is *not* an excuse for hay fever sufferers to drink more coffee.

All About Home Testing

Rosemary Soave, MD, infectious disease specialist, and associate professor at New York Hospital–Cornell Medical Center, New York City.

Home diagnostic tests are reasonably accurate. Be sure to follow directions carefully.

To protect yourself: If you do not understand something, call the toll-free number on the package, or ask your pharmacist or doctor before using the test...always read the directions carefully before starting a test...check the packaging to make sure the test has not passed its expiration date...store temperature-sensitive test kits in a dark area away from heat and sunlight. *Also:* When doing a timed test, use a watch that clearly shows seconds.

Bee Sting First Aid

Recommendations from the American Academy of Allergy, Asthma and Immunology, 611 E. Wells, Milwaukee 53202.

Remove the stinger if it is visible by scraping gently with a butter knife or credit card. Do not squeeze the area and pull with tweezers or fingers—that can release more venom.

After removing the stinger, wash the area with soap and water and apply a cold pack to reduce pain and swelling.

Though rare, serious allergic reactions to bee stings occur within minutes. If the person who has been stung collapses, develops hives or swollen lips or eyes or has trouble breathing, call 911 immediately.

For Heartburn Relief...

M. Michael Wolfe, MD, associate professor of medicine, Harvard Medical School, and coauthor of *The Fire Inside: Extinguishing Heartburn and Related Symptoms.* W.W. Norton.

Use lozenges, sucking candy or gum. These stimulate saliva, which contains a natural antacid that helps relieve heartburn. Do not lie down for three hours after eating a meal. More acid is pumped into the stomach when lying down. Elevate the head of your bed with three- to six-inch blocks so you sleep on a slight incline. Propping your head on pillows will not help.

Drink Up!

Food and You by the editors of *Prevention* magazine Health Books. Rodale.

To drink your recommended 64 ounces of water each day…

• **Drink a glass as soon as you wake up**— to replenish fluids lost during sleep.

• **Have a glass of water before any meal or snack** to help control your appetite.

• **Buy a 64-ounce container and fill it every day**—then keep it near you, on your desk at work or the kitchen table at home, so you can see how much you are drinking.

• **To have chilled water all day**—freeze a partially filled plastic bottle overnight, then top it off with more water in the morning.

Three Quick Massages

Donna DeFalco, massage therapist, writing in *American Health*, 28 W. 23 St., New York 10010.

Anchor your thumbs behind your ears and make circles on your scalp with your fingers.

Knead the palms of your hands with the opposite thumbs, starting where the hand joins the wrist and working toward the spaces between the bones of the fingers.

Close your eyes and place your ring fingers just below your eyebrows, near the bridge of the nose. Press gently, slowly increasing the pressure for five seconds, release, and repeat twice more.

Headache Prevention

Robert Ford, MD, director, Ford Headache Clinic, Birmingham, AL.

Taking five minutes to relax at the very first sign of trouble can help stop a headache.

Examples: If you're stopped at a red light, progressively relax your left leg, from toes to buttock, while your right foot stays on the brake pedal. *At the office:* Close your eyes for one minute every hour and take long, deep breaths.

At the first sign of a headache: Rub your hands together to create heat, then gently press the heels of your hands onto your eyelids. Close your eyes and give your face, scalp and neck a brief massage. Look away at a distant point—or stare at your hands for a minute.

Avoiding Headache Triggers

Bob Niklewicz, PT, MA, a physical therapist in private practice in Rohnert Park, CA.

A headache can be triggered by holding the neck in one position for a prolonged period—such as when working on a computer, driving or even bird-watching.

Self-defense: If you're prone to headaches, ask your doctor to help you pinpoint neck strain or other headache triggers.

Also helpful: Learn deep breathing and other relaxation techniques. Use good posture when standing or sitting.

Headache Relief

John G. Arena, PhD, director of the pain evaluation and intervention program at the Department of Veterans Affairs Medical Center, Augusta, GA.

Relaxation of the neck and shoulder muscles is the best way to relieve tension headaches. A study found that people who learned to relax their trapezius muscles reduced the intensity and duration of headaches by at least half. Relaxing these muscles proved far more effective than relaxing the forehead or using relaxation methods to relax all the other muscles of the body.

59

The headache sufferers taught themselves how to relax the neck and shoulder muscles by mental means until they discovered what worked best for them.

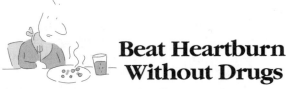

Beat Heartburn Without Drugs

Marvin Lipman, MD, chief medical adviser, Consumers Union, writing in *Consumer Reports on Health*, 101 Truman Ave., Yonkers, NY 10703.

Avoid foods that can trigger it—alcohol, chocolate, peppermint, spearmint and fat. Avoid caffeine in foods and over-the-counter pain medications. Avoid carbonated drinks. *Also:* If you are overweight, lose weight…if you smoke, quit.

For nighttime heartburn: Raise the head of your bed on four- to six-inch blocks, or use a wedge-shaped support to elevate the upper half of your body. Do not lie down with a full stomach.

For Better Driving With Arthritis…

Tammi Shlotzhauer, MD, a clinical instructor of medicine, University of Rochester Medical Center, a rheumatologist in group practice and author of *Living with Rheumatoid Arthritis*. Johns Hopkins University Press.

Stop frequently to get out and stretch in order to prevent stiffness and soreness.

Consider having lever aids installed on door and ignition keys, to make them easier to turn …and adding grab handles on the ridge of the roof inside the car to make entry and exit easier.

Keep medicines in the glove compartment, not the trunk, to avoid exposure to extreme temperatures…and carry snacks and a beverage so you can take the medicines on schedule. In cold weather, have someone warm up the car before you get into it.

Arthritis in the Kitchen

Arthritis: Stop Suffering, Start Moving by Darlene Cohen, certified movement therapist, San Francisco. Walker & Co.

If your fingers and wrists are stiff, it is tempting to do kitchen tasks with your upper arms, shoulders and upper back. But this can cause neck and shoulder aches.

Better: Look at kitchen chores as a way to exercise those joints and improve their mobility. But find ways to do the chores that do not strain painful areas too much.

Example: Use an extra-heavy, high-quality, sharp knife for chopping and cutting. Its weight can make it easier to cut without using a painful amount of wrist pressure.

Homemade Heating Pad

Allison Scheetz, MD, instructor of medicine, and David Mathis, MD, assistant professor of medicine, Mercer University School of Medicine, Macon, GA.

Fill a tube sock with uncooked rice, knot the top, then microwave on high for three minutes.

This creates a pad that will mold easily around any painful joint and hold its heat for about one hour—without risk of burns.

To Stop a Nosebleed…

Earl Schwartz, MD, spokesperson, American College of Emergency Physicians, Winston–Salem, NC.

Pinch nostrils and hold them together for five minutes. Tilt the head back only a little…not enough for blood to run down the throat. If the bleeding does not stop in five minutes, continue pinching nostrils for another seven minutes. If bleeding still continues, call your doctor.

Better Dandruff Shampoo Use

Richard Berger, MD, clinical professor of medicine, University of Medicine and Dentistry of New Jersey, Robert Wood Johnson Medical School, New Brunswick, NJ.

Apply shampoo twice. Leave the first application on your hair for one to two minutes, then rinse and relather. Leave the second application on your hair for three to five minutes. That is how long the medication needs to work.

For serious dandruff problems: Ask your doctor about Nizoral, a potent antidandruff shampoo available over-the-counter.

Tongue Scraping

Ray Wunderlich, MD, a physician in private practice in St. Petersburg, FL. A specialist in preventive and nutritional medicine, he is author of *Natural Alternatives to Antibiotics.* Keats Publishing.

Cleaning the top of your tongue twice a day with a scraping device is a simple, inexpensive way to control even the most stubborn cases of bad breath...and to prevent infections in and around your mouth.

Every day, infectious bacteria, viruses, fungi and yeast—along with food particles and cellular debris—collect on the rough surface on the back of the tongue.

From this "staging area," these microorganisms launch infections that cause tooth decay, gum disease, sore throats and colds, as well as bad breath.

Why not simply clean the tongue with a toothbrush? That's far less effective at removing microorganisms, and it can cause gagging.

For best results, use a plastic tongue scraper, such as the one manufactured by Oolitt. Bend it in a U-shape, with the open end of the U pointing away from you and the serrated edge against your tongue.

Starting at the back of your tongue on the right side, sweep the serrated edge forward until it reaches the tip. Rinse any debris off the scraper, and sweep repeatedly until no more "gunk" is being collected. Then switch to the left side and repeat.

Do this twice a day, after breakfast and at bedtime, just before brushing your teeth. Rinse the tongue scraper after each use with 3% hydrogen peroxide.

If your dentist or local drugstore doesn't sell one, you can purchase a variety of easy-to-use Oolitts for all ages from Oolitt Advantage, Inc., P.O. Box 273653, Tampa, FL 33688. 813-496-9917, *www.oolitt.com. Cost:* $11.70 for a one-year supply (six scrapers), includes shipping and handling.

Better Toothbrushing

Michael W. Davis, DDS, a dentist in private practice in Brunswick, ME.

Slip the plastic spool from a roll of adding machine paper over the toothbrush handle. This enlarges the gripping surface, making brushing easier.

Avoid Bad Breath

Jon Richter, DMD, founder, Center for Breath Disorders, Philadelphia.

Clean your tongue with a tongue scraper or plastic teaspoon with the bowl pointing down...eat fibrous foods like apples...use breath mints or chewing gum to promote saliva flow.

Common causes of bad breath: Postnasal drip from a cold or allergy...mouth dryness—a side effect of many antihistamines and other medications...dieting, since less frequent eating slows saliva flow...sulfur-containing foods, such as garlic, onions, broccoli and cabbage...heredity—some people simply have more mouth odor than others...and hormonal changes, especially just before a menstrual period.

Jaw Pain Relief

Irwin Mandel, DDS, chief dental adviser, Consumers Union, Yonkers, NY, and professor emeritus, Columbia University–School of Dental & Oral Surgery, New York.

Relieve jaw pain caused by *temporomandibular disorder* (TMJ) by giving your jaw a rest during painful episodes. Eat soft foods, and avoid extreme jaw movements like those involved in gum chewing, wide yawning, eating thick sandwiches and singing loudly. Apply moist heat or ice packs—whichever feels better—to the chewing muscles along the sides of the face. Keep a detailed pain diary to help you identify triggers and avoid them. It can help, when your mouth is closed, to keep your lips together and teeth apart.

Bike Helmet Fact

Diane Thompson, epidemiologist, Harborview Injury Prevention and Research Center, Seattle, who led a study of more than 3,000 cyclists treated for injuries at seven hospitals.

Bike helmets prevent injuries even in big collisions.

Study: Wearing a helmet reduces the risk of head injury by 69%...the risk of severe brain injury by 74%...and the risk of eye, ear, nose and forehead injuries by 65%. Helmets are important for all age groups.

 # Quick Cures

Tim Clark, executive editor of *The Old Farmer's Almanac* for more than 20 years. The *Almanac* is published each September in four regional editions.

For hiccups: Briefly apply ice to the side of the neck—to interrupt the reflex that causes hiccups.

When craving sweets: Rinse your mouth with one teaspoon of baking soda dissolved in a glass of warm water. Do not swallow. Craving should disappear immediately.

Painless Adhesive Bandage Removal

Kathryn Marion, editor, *The Reality Check Gazette*, 8667 Sudley Rd., Manassas, VA 22110.

Soak a cotton ball in baby oil and wipe it around the sides of the bandage. In about 10 minutes, the adhesive will be softened—making bandage removal easy and painless.

Neck Pain Relief

Robert A. Lavin, MD, assistant professor of physical medicine and rehabilitation, Johns Hopkins Medical Institutions, Baltimore, whose study was published in *Archives of Physical Medicine and Rehabilitation.*

To ease neck pain, sleep on a water pillow. Volunteers who slept on pillows with adjustable water-filled pouches for two weeks reported better sleep and less pain when they awoke than those who slept on down-filled, foam or roll pillows. Water pillows are available from selected home/health care stores. *Cost:* About $50.

Natural Air Filters

Bonnie Wodin, owner of Golden Yarrow Landscape Design, a garden consulting firm, Box 61, Heath, MA 01346.

Houseplants can serve as natural air filters. They can remove indoor air pollutants such as carbon monoxide and formaldehyde.

Best: Aloe vera, Chinese evergreen, elephant-ear philodendron, English ivy, ficus, golden pothos, corn plant, peace lily and spider plant.

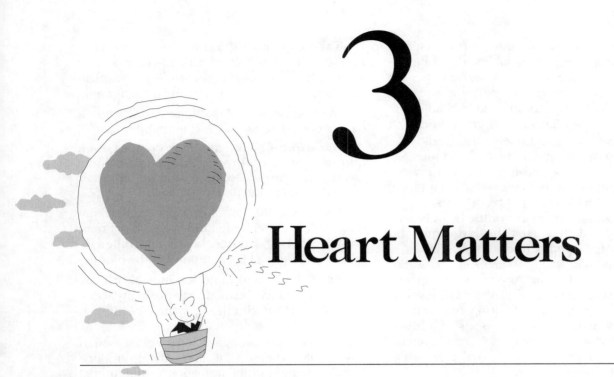

3

Heart Matters

It's Never Too Late to Start Taking Care of Your Heart

Harvey B. Simon, MD
Harvard Medical School
Massachusetts General Hospital

Some people mistakenly believe that if they've had bad health habits all their lives, it won't help to change now. But you can prevent—and in some cases even reverse—damage to your heart...no matter how old you are. And since heart disease is the number-one killer in America, it makes sense to do what you can to prevent it.

FOUR MAJOR LIFESTYLE CHANGES

The changes that can make an enormous difference in preventing heart disease...

●**Stop smoking.** Smoking is the greatest risk factor for coronary artery disease. It increases the chance of heart attack by 250%.

Even if you've smoked for years, stopping will improve your health. Heart rate and blood pressure will return to normal, and the risk of heart attack will fall until it matches that of people who never smoked.

●**Reduce blood cholesterol.** The most effective way to do this is by watching your diet. It isn't just cholesterol in food that raises levels in blood, it's the saturated fat—which stimulates the body to produce its *own* harmful cholesterol. The average American gets 37% of daily calories from fat. A much healthier level would be 30% or 15%.

Helpful: New food labeling regulations make it easier to estimate the fat content of the foods you eat.

Cholesterol reduction diet: Cut back on desserts and animal products—eggs, meat,

Harvey B. Simon, MD, department of internal medicine and preventive cardiology at Massachusetts General Hospital in Boston. He is on the faculties of Harvard Medical School and the Massachusetts Institute of Technology and is a founding member of the Harvard Cardiovascular Health Center...and author of *Conquering Heart Disease*. Little, Brown.

cheese and other whole dairy products. Increase your intake of vegetables, dried beans and whole grains. Switch from using butter or margarine in cooking to small amounts of olive oil, which appears to reduce "bad" LDL cholesterol but not "good" HDL cholesterol.

●**Exercise.** Exercise benefits the cardiovascular system by strengthening the heart muscle, improving circulation, raising HDL and lowering LDL cholesterol, reducing stress on arteries and fighting the formation of blood clots.

The best kind of exercise for the heart is aerobic—the kind that uses the large muscle groups for prolonged periods of time.

Examples: Biking, swimming, fast walking, running, stair climbing, rowing, racquet sports.

You're exerting yourself at the right level if you work up a sweat but don't feel out of breath. Any amount of exercise is helpful— even an hour a week. But you'll reap greater benefits if you work up to a total of at least three to four hours a week.

●**Lower your blood pressure.** One-fourth of American adults—and half of those over age 60—have high blood pressure, also known as hypertension. High blood pressure strains the heart muscle and damages the arterial wall, making people with hypertension more than twice as likely as others to have heart attacks.

The best way to lower blood pressure is to get the correct amount of minerals in your diet…

●**Reduce sodium.** Aim for less than 1,500 milligrams of sodium per day. Check food labels for sodium content. Sodium comes in many guises—the familiar table salt, as well as baking powder, baking soda, monosodium glutamate and soy sauce. Snack foods and processed foods tend to be especially high in sodium.

●**Increase potassium and calcium.** Many fresh fruits and vegetables are rich in potassium, including bananas, dates, oranges, cantaloupe, apples, raisins, potatoes, winter squash, lima beans, beets and broccoli. Healthful calcium-rich foods include skim milk, broccoli, spinach, fish and soybean products—particularly tofu.

OTHER WAYS TO HELP YOUR HEART

In addition to these four basic lifestyle changes for heart health, research suggests several other behaviors that may help to prevent heart disease…

●**Take aspirin.** Aspirin reduces blood clotting and has been shown to lower risk of a second heart attack. It's possible that aspirin may help to prevent a first heart attack as well.

Recommended dose: One baby aspirin a day, or one adult aspirin tablet every other day.

Caution: Check with your doctor before taking aspirin regularly. People who have ulcers, excessive bleeding or who are on other medications may need to avoid aspirin.

●**Eat fiber.** Numerous studies suggest that water-soluble fiber—the kind found in oat bran and also barley, prunes, beans and other legumes—reduces LDL cholesterol in the blood.

●**Eat fish.** Two to three servings of fish per week can reduce heart disease risk by about 40%. *Exception:* Shellfish, which is high in cholesterol.

Fish contains omega-3 fatty acids, which lower LDL and raise HDL, and may also reduce blood clotting and inflammation in the arterial walls.

●**Avoid secondhand cigarette smoke.** "Passive" smoking is thought to cause up to 35,000 deaths from heart attack in the US each year. At highest risk are people who live with someone who smokes or who work in smoke-filled environments. Try to reduce exposure as much as possible—ask smokers to consider your safety…or even leave the room when someone is smoking, if you must.

●**Take antioxidant vitamins.** There's some evidence that vitamins C, E and beta-carotene —which seem to fight the dangerous effects of unstable molecules in the body called free radicals—lower the risk of heart disease.

If you take supplements, stick to moderate doses—1,000 milligrams of vitamin C, 400 international units of vitamin E and 10,000 international units of beta-carotene.

Caution: One study found that smokers who took beta-carotene supplements had a higher rate of death from lung cancer—so until further research is done, smokers should probably avoid these supplements.

●**Learn to cope with stress.** The link between emotional strain and heart disease is difficult to prove. But if you're prone to anxiety or depression, learn more about stress-fighters—yoga, meditation, deep breathing or psychotherapy. You will be helping your heart —and you'll certainly enjoy life more.

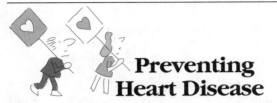

Preventing Heart Disease

Harvey B. Simon, MD, associate professor of medicine at Harvard Medical School, Boston. He is author of *Conquering Heart Disease: New Ways to Live Well Without Drugs or Surgery.* Little, Brown.

How can you minimize your risk of heart disease? Most Americans are already familiar with the basics…

●**Don't smoke.** Tobacco-induced heart damage causes 150,000 fatal heart attacks a year.

●**Eat less fat** (especially saturated fat). Less fat means lower cholesterol levels and reduced risk of obesity.

●**Watch your blood pressure.** A reading toward the high end of the normal range (135 over 85, for example) is not too bad, but one in the low-normal range (120 over 70 or lower) is better.

●**Get regular exercise.**

If you're already making these efforts, terrific. But there's much *more* you can do to protect yourself.

WHAT CAUSES HEART DISEASE

Heart disease occurs via a three-step process:

Step 1: **Levels of LDL (bad) cholesterol get too high**…and/or levels of HDL (good) cholesterol fall too low.

Ideally, your total cholesterol should be under 200. Your level of HDL should be at least 35. Your ratio of total cholesterol to HDL cholesterol should be 4.5 to 1 or lower.

Step 2: **The arterial lining is injured**—usually via smoking or by having high blood pressure or blood sugar levels. This injury facilitates the entry of cholesterol from the blood into the artery wall.

Step 3: **A blood clot forms.** The growing cholesterol deposit disrupts the flow of blood. That causes blood clots to form. Eventually, a clot blocks the artery, causing a heart attack.

Lesson: A comprehensive heart disease prevention program must take aim at each step.

EAT LESS SALT

If you have hypertension, the less salt you eat, the lower your blood pressure is likely to be. And the lower your blood pressure, the smaller your risk of heart disease.

Tossing the salt shaker is a good start. But 75% of the sodium in a typical diet comes from salt that is hidden in processed foods.

Self-defense: Read labels. A bowl of canned soup can have up to 1,200 milligrams (mg) of sodium. That's half the 2,400-mg-per-day level recommended by health experts.

MORE POTASSIUM AND CALCIUM

Potassium has just the opposite effect of sodium—more means reduced blood pressure. But there's no evidence to suggest that blood pressure can be lowered by taking potassium supplements.

Better: Increase your intake of potassium-rich foods, such as bananas, oranges, dates, lima beans and potatoes.

Calcium also seems to play a key role in lowering blood pressure. For instance, blood pressure levels tend to be unusually low among people who live in areas with hard (calcium-rich) water and among those who eat lots of dairy products.

Lesson: If you are concerned about your blood pressure, eat more nonfat dairy products, dark green vegetables and tofu (bean curd). *Also:* Ask your doctor about taking Tums or another calcium supplement.

GET MORE DIETARY FIBER

Dietary fiber helps prevent heart disease by lowering cholesterol, blood pressure and blood sugar.

Sadly, most Americans get only one-third of the recommended 30 daily grams (g) of fiber.

Sources of dietary fiber: Beans, beets, prunes, citrus fruits and grains. It's a good idea to start your day with a breakfast cereal containing at least 10 g of fiber per serving.

EAT FISH TWICE A WEEK

Heart disease is quite uncommon among people who eat lots of fish. Certain unsaturated fatty acids unique to fish are thought to be responsible for this protective effect.

I urge my patients to eat at least four ounces of fish a week. *Best:* Rich, oily species like bluefish, mackerel, tuna and salmon.

What about fish-oil supplements? There's little evidence that they're beneficial.

ALCOHOL AND ASPIRIN

Study after study has proven that an *occasional* drink raises levels of HDL cholesterol. Men whose HDL is below 30 should consider having one or two drinks daily (one if you're a woman). One drink equals a glass of wine, a shot of distilled spirits or 12 ounces of beer.

Low-dose aspirin therapy—one-half tablet a day—is proven to prevent heart attacks in those who have heart disease.

Aspirin may also be beneficial for individuals *at risk* for heart disease. That includes men over 50 and postmenopausal women. There's no evidence that aspirin therapy is beneficial to people with healthy hearts.

Caution: If you're allergic to aspirin, have ulcers or are prone to digestive bleeding, aspirin therapy is *not* for you.

CONSIDER TAKING ANTIOXIDANTS

Cholesterol damages arteries when it has been oxidized, via a chemical reaction analogous to rusting.

Fortunately, the body has enzymes that prevent oxidation by "mopping up" the unstable molecules (free radicals) that cause oxidation. Three antioxidant nutrients—vitamins C and E and beta-carotene—give this natural defense system a big boost, especially when taken in *combination.*

Sufficient levels of beta-carotene can easily be obtained by eating green and yellow vegetables, and vitamin C is abundant in citrus fruits. But it's hard to get much vitamin E from dietary sources, so I recommend taking a daily supplement.

WHAT ABOUT OTHER SUPPLEMENTS?

There's been much less research on chromium than on the "big three" antioxidants. But in one study, volunteers took 200 micrograms of the mineral three times a day.

Result: Levels of protective HDL cholesterol rose by 16%. That translates into a 20% reduction in the risk of heart disease.

If your HDL level is below 30, and it cannot be raised via weight loss, exercise or moderate alcohol consumption, ask your doctor about taking chromium supplements.

Important: *Glucose tolerance factor* (GTF) seems to be safer than the more popular supplement, *chromium picolinate.*

In another study involving more than 15,000 physicians, researchers found that those whose blood contained high levels of the amino acid *homocysteine* were more likely to have a heart attack. Homocysteine seems to damage artery walls and promote clotting.

To keep homocysteine levels down: Take a daily supplement containing vitamins B-6 and B-12 and folic acid.

MEDICAL TESTS

Your blood pressure, cholesterol and blood sugar should be checked each time you have a physical exam. That's once every year for people 50 or older and once every two to three years for people 35 to 49 years of age.

I'd also suggest an electrocardiogram with each checkup. Stress tests aren't necessary unless you're having chest pains or other heart disease symptoms.

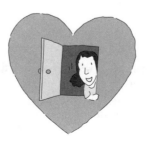

Eating Right for a Healthy Heart and Long Life

Joe D. Goldstrich, MD, former medical director of the Pritikin Longevity Center in Santa Monica, CA, and a physician in private practice in Pacific Palisades, CA. He is author of *Healthy Heart, Longer Life*. Ultimate Health Publishing.

Researchers have identified three mechanisms by which to lower the risk of developing heart disease…

•**Lower the amount of LDL (bad) cholesterol in the blood.** An LDL level in excess of 100 confers an increased risk for heart disease.

•**Block *oxidation* of LDL cholesterol.** LDL cholesterol is benign until it has been oxidized. Only then can it be incorporated into obstructions along the walls of the coronary arteries. These obstructions are called *plaques*.

•**Control blood clotting.** Heart attacks occur when a plaque fissures or cracks, triggering formation of clots that block the flow of blood to the heart.

How do you set these mechanisms into motion? Regular exercise, avoiding smoking and keeping your blood pressure and weight under control are essential. But that's only the beginning…

HEART-PROTECTIVE FOODS

A diet low in saturated fat reduces levels of LDL cholesterol. In addition, certain foods have *extra* power to protect the heart…

•**Olive oil.** While it's a good idea to reduce consumption of *all* kinds of dietary fat (including oils), substituting olive oil for other oils helps keep your heart healthy.

The monounsaturated fats in olive oil reduce levels of LDL cholesterol while raising levels of HDL (good) cholesterol.

What makes monounsaturated fats superior to the polyunsaturated fats found in most other vegetable oils? They don't facilitate the conversion of cholesterol into its oxidized form.

•**Nuts.** Almonds and pistachios contain the same kind of monounsaturated fats found in olive oil. While nuts are too fatty to eat all the time, an occasional snack of almonds or pistachios could be beneficial to your heart.

•**Garlic.** In addition to reducing LDL and raising HDL, garlic helps prevent blood clotting.

If you don't like the taste of garlic—or worry about bad breath—take garlic capsules.

•**Fish.** Numerous studies have shown that the omega-3 oils in certain kinds of fatty fish (salmon, cod, sea bass, tuna, etc.) inhibit blood clotting and lower the risk for sudden cardiac death.

Try to eat fish at least once a week. Fish oil capsules can be rancid, and rancid oil *boosts* the oxidation of cholesterol.

•**Soy foods.** Tofu, miso soup, textured vegetable protein (TVP) and other soy products lower levels of LDL cholesterol. Researchers suspect that a compound in soy called *beta-sitosterol* is responsible for soy's cholesterol-lowering effect.

•**Red wine.** Any form of alcohol raises HDL cholesterol and reduces clotting. Red wine has additional benefits—if consumed in moderation (no more than two glasses a day). It contains clot-inhibiting *bioflavonoids* and *resveratrol*, a powerful antioxidant that guards cholesterol from oxidation.

VITAMIN SUPPLEMENTS

•**Vitamin E.** A potent antioxidant, vitamin E keeps LDL cholesterol from turning into its toxic form. Ask your doctor about taking 400 to 800 international units (IU) on a daily basis.

Of the many forms of vitamin E now available, capsules containing *d-alpha tocopherol succinate* are best. These capsules don't go rancid. Oil-filled vitamin E capsules sometimes do.

•**Vitamin C.** This antioxidant vitamin protects the smooth tissue that lines the coronary arteries against microscopic injuries caused by high blood pressure, smoking and high cholesterol. It's these injuries that are thought to provide a beachhead for plaques.

Studies suggest that a daily dose of at least 500 milligrams (mg) of vitamin C is best.

Since the usual form of vitamin C (ascorbic acid) can cause stomach irritation, it's better to get your C in the form of *calcium ascorbate* or *magnesium ascorbate*.

•**B Vitamins.** B-6, B-12 and folic acid all reduce blood levels of *homocysteine*. High levels of this clot-promoting amino acid are linked to heart disease.

It's best simply to take daily doses of the B vitamins. I usually recommend 100 mg of B-6 …500 micrograms (mcg) of B-12…and 800 mcg of folic acid.

●**Carotenoids.** Beta-carotene is the best-known member of this family of antioxidants.

Studies suggest that another carotenoid called *lycopene* also offers protection against heart disease. Tomatoes are an excellent source of lycopene.

It's best to get your carotenoids in their natural form—red, yellow or leafy green vegetables. If you'd like to take carotenoids in supplement form, pick a supplement containing "natural mixed carotenoids."

MINERAL SUPPLEMENTS

●**Selenium.** This mineral is the raw material used by the body to make the antioxidant enzyme *glutathione*. People who take selenium supplements face a reduced risk for both heart disease and cancer. The usual dose is 200 mcg a day.

●**Chromium.** It helps keep levels of blood sugar in balance. Elevated blood sugar spurs the body to secrete insulin, and chronically high insulin levels can lead to obesity, high blood pressure and high triglycerides. All boost heart disease risk.

I advise my patients to take 200 mcg of *chromium picolinate* or *chromium polynicotinate*. These natural forms of chromium are safe and readily absorbed.

●**Magnesium and potassium.** Magnesium helps lower blood pressure by relaxing the tiny muscles that line blood vessel walls. Potassium lowers blood pressure by replacing sodium, a known provoker of high blood pressure.

The best way to get these minerals is from fruits and vegetables. Bananas and citrus fruits are especially good sources.

Heart Disease and Weight

Leslie Katzel, MD, PhD, associate professor of medicine at the University of Maryland School of Medicine, Baltimore.

If you are overweight, a key to reducing heart disease is losing weight. A study of men found that when they lost an average of 18 pounds over nine months, their risk of heart disease fell by 40%. Researchers found that this benefit did not automatically follow from simply changing the composition of the diet. It was necessary to lose weight by eating less, changing to fat-free and low-fat foods and/or exercising.

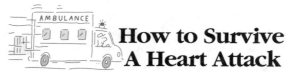 # How to Survive A Heart Attack

William Cole, MD, director of the Coronary Care Unit at New York Downtown Hospital, and associate professor of medicine at New York University Medical Center, both in New York City.

Heart attack kills 600,000 Americans each year, making it the number one cause of death. But for every fatal heart attack, many more heart attacks do not prove fatal.

Why do some people succumb while others survive? To find out, we spoke with Dr. William Cole, a cardiologist who directs one of the busiest coronary care units in the US.

We can learn important lessons from heart attack survivors, according to Dr. Cole…

DON'T IGNORE SYMPTOMS

When lay people envision a heart attack (*myocardial infarction*), they tend to picture someone clutching at the chest, falling to the floor and losing consciousness. This scenario actually describes *cardiac arrest*, when the heart stops beating. The typical heart attack is far less dramatic.

Problem: Heart attack sufferers are often stoic. When they have chest pain or other symptoms suggestive of heart trouble, they think, *It must be something I ate.*

Plenty of securities traders have sought treatment at my hospital only after being carried off the floor of the stock exchange. Many had endured chest pain for hours.

Why the delay in seeking treatment? In most cases, the individual was too frightened even to consider the *possibility* of a heart attack...or reluctant to risk embarrassment by calling an ambulance only to find out the problem was heartburn.

These individuals wait until they're in agony before seeking help. By the time they reach the emergency room, irreversible damage has often been done.

The most common symptom of heart attack is pain in the chest. But in some cases there is no pain—just a sensation that has been described as "someone sitting on the chest." The pain may radiate up the neck and down the arms.

Other symptoms: Sudden sweating, shortness of breath, tightness in the jaw or nausea.

In some cases, these signs occur several days before an attack. Because the sensations wax and wane, patients are tempted to ignore them. That's a *big* mistake.

Those at obvious risk for heart disease—smokers, overweight people and individuals with high blood pressure or elevated cholesterol—should be especially alert to these signals.

But heart attacks also strike—and kill—people with *no* known risk factors. If you or someone you know notices even mild symptoms, call a *doctor at once.*

GET TO THE HOSPITAL QUICKLY

If treatment is initiated during the first "golden" hour following a heart attack, mortality is only 1% to 5%. After four to five hours of delay, the mortality rate climbs to 12%.

Just 10 to 15 years ago, the death rate associated with heart attack victims who reached the hospital alive was 15% to 20%. Doctors could do little more than administer oxygen and morphine—to make the patient more comfortable.

Now: The death rate for these patients is 5% to 7%. Doctors have "clot-busting" drugs that actually restore blood flow to the heart. But the patient must still reach the hospital right away.

Helpful: Call 911 first. Then have someone call your doctor so he can alert the hospital that you're on your way. If the cardiac care team is expecting you, you'll be treated without delay.

GET AGGRESSIVE TREATMENT

Since the early 1980s, heart attack patients have received *thrombolytic therapy*—intravenous drugs that dissolve blood clots. The most effective clot-busters are *tissue plasminogen activator* (TPA) and *streptokinase.*

In addition, nearly all heart attack patients receive aspirin (to thin the blood) and *heparin* (to prevent arteries from re-closing).

While thrombolytic treatment has brought about a significant decline in heart attack mortality, we can do *much* better. Studies suggest that a surgical procedure known as *acute angioplasty* is even more effective than clot-busting drugs.

In this procedure, an X ray called an *angiogram* is used to pinpoint the blocked coronary artery. Then a small balloon is inserted into the artery through a catheter. The balloon is inflated, pushing aside the blockage and restoring blood flow to the heart.

Problem: Not all hospitals are equipped to perform angioplasty. If you must choose between two hospitals a similar distance away, ask to be taken to the one that is better equipped to do acute angioplasty. If this choice would prolong your trip by 15 minutes or more, it's probably better to go to the closer hospital.

PREPARE FOR EMERGENCIES

If a patient is at high risk of cardiac arrest, it's a good idea for his family members and co-workers to know cardiopulmonary resuscitation (CPR). In fact, *everyone* should learn CPR.

High-risk patients include people who have had prior episodes of cardiac arrest...have a weak heart muscle as a result of a prior heart attack or bypass surgery...or have a history of life-threatening irregularities in the heartbeat (arrhythmias).

These patients might also want to consider asking their doctor about purchasing their own defibrillator. That's the twin-paddled device doctors use to shock the heart into a normal rhythm.

Paramedics usually carry defibrillators, and many sports arenas have begun keeping their own units on the premises.

New, "smart" models are simple enough to be used by almost anyone—even without training. When placed on the victim's chest, these devices automatically monitor arrhythmias and—if necessary—administer a shock.

Unfortunately, the expense—thousands of dollars—puts personal defibrillators out of the reach of many patients.

Some high-risk patients have been fitted with *implantable* defibrillators. *Cost:* About $20,000.

A Benefit of Having Friends

Blair Justice, PhD, professor of psychology, University of Texas–Houston School of Public Health and author of *Who Gets Sick.* J.P. Tarcher.

People who live isolated lives—without hugs, handshakes or other physical contact—are as likely to develop heart disease as those who smoke, eat high-fat diets and don't exercise.

Theory: Close connections with other people relieve stress and boost immunity. And—sharing one's troubles is a healthier coping mechanism than overeating, drinking or smoking.

Helpful: Regularly discuss what's going on in your life openly with your spouse…a friend …or a family member.

Heart Trouble Predictor

James A. Blumenthal, PhD, professor of medical psychology at Duke University Medical School, Durham, NC.

Mental stress tests help predict who is likely to have heart trouble, over and above physical stress tests. Researchers measured the blood flow in the hearts of 126 people undergoing mental stress tests such as solving difficult math problems rapidly. They found that 27% of those who showed an abnormal response to

mental stress suffered a cardiac event within the next five years—more than twice the rate of those who showed a normal response.

Longer Life

Data from the *American Journal of Epidemiology.*

The approximate number of years you can add to your life by adopting good habits that reduce the risk factors that lead to coronary heart disease…

- **Avoid diabetes** ....8 years
- **Exercise regularly** ....5.5 years
- **Avoid hypertension** ....5 years
- **Don't smoke** ....3 years
- **Maintain healthy weight** .....2 years

Warning Signs of Angina Pectoris

Richard Helfant, MD, clinical professor of medicine, division of cardiology, University of California at Irvine, 101 The City Dr., Bldg. 53, Rm. 100, Orange, CA. He is author of *Women, Take Heart.* Putnam.

Tightness, pressure, heaviness or constriction in the center of the chest are warning signs of angina pectoris. Discomfort may start in the shoulders—more often on the left—or spread to shoulders from the center of the chest…then move down the arms or into the neck or jaw. Chest discomfort is diagnosed as angina pectoris when symptoms are caused by physical activity, and usually disappear within minutes after activity stops.

Warning: Angina pectoris is the most common initial symptom of heart disease in women. If you have symptoms, see your doctor immediately.

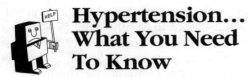

Hypertension... What You Need To Know

Marvin Moser, MD, clinical professor of medicine at Yale University School of Medicine in New Haven, CT. He is author of *Week by Week to a Strong Heart* (Avon Books) and *Heart Healthy Cooking for All Seasons* (Pocket Books).

Some doctors have begun to rethink long-held views about the link between diet and blood pressure, thanks to two studies...

●**A study conducted by Michael H. Alderman, MD,** at Albert Einstein College of Medicine in the Bronx, New York, suggested that sodium restriction may not be beneficial—and could even be harmful—to people with high blood pressure.

●**A study sponsored by the National Institutes of Health** (NIH) showed that a low-fat diet rich in fruits and vegetables could lower even moderately high blood pressure without the need for medication.

To sort through these and other findings in the field, we sat down with one of the country's leading hypertension specialists, Dr. Marvin Moser...

●**Are the new studies valid?** Dr. Alderman's study did find that heart attacks were more common among hypertensives who ate very little sodium than among those who ate lots of sodium.

But the vast majority of the study's 2,900 participants consumed moderate levels of sodium...and showed no increased incidence of heart attack at all.

There are other potential problems with the study, including a lack of data on the specific treatments used. Given this fact—plus the fact that other studies have consistently shown that a low-sodium diet reduces the risk of hypertension by about 25% and may lower blood pressure if it is high—I don't think Dr. Alderman's study should be considered in treatment decisions.

●**If the study was flawed, why did it get so much publicity?** Because the Salt Institute—the leading lobby for the salt industry—is try-ing to use the study in an attempt to persuade the National Heart, Lung and Blood Institute (NHLBI) to change its long-standing recommendations regarding sodium consumption.

NHLBI guidelines call for consuming no more than 2.4 grams (g) of sodium per day. That's the amount contained in about 6 g of table salt (about 1¼ teaspoons).

The average American eats 10 g to 15 g of salt each day—the equivalent of two to three teaspoons.

●**Then what is the bottom line regarding salt and high blood pressure?** For someone with normal blood pressure, a low-sodium diet may not lower blood pressure by more than one to two points. This is a small number for an individual, but it could have a big impact on public health.

If everyone followed the NHLBI guidelines, the incidence of stroke would drop by approximately 7%.

●**Isn't it hard to stick to a low-sodium diet?** Not at all. I tell my patients that they can help keep their pressure in check by going easy on salt used in cooking and at the table... and by minimizing their consumption of chips, canned soups, corned beef, hot dogs and other salty foods.

●**What about salt substitutes?** These products—which substitute potassium for sodium—are a great way to limit sodium consumption. But potassium tastes bitter.

Fortunately, a salt substitute called Cardia Salt Alternative tastes like ordinary salt. Ounce for ounce, it contains half the sodium, along with extra potassium and magnesium, which are believed to have a small but possibly beneficial effect on blood pressure.

●**What about the NIH study?** I believe the study is valid. It found that people who stick to a low-fat diet and consume lots of fruits and vegetables generally experience a seven- to 10-point drop in blood pressure.

●**What explains the effectiveness of such a diet?** Fruits and vegetables contain lots of potassium. Many doctors now believe that it's not sodium alone, but the ratio of potassium to sodium in the diet that affects blood pressure.

Ideally, we should all be consuming potassium and sodium in a one-to-one ratio. The best way to do this is to avoid salty foods, as I mentioned, and to eat as many high-potassium vegetables and fruits as possible.

The best sources of potassium are baked potatoes and fruit—especially oranges and orange juice, cantaloupe and bananas.

You could take potassium supplements, but this would be rather expensive, since you would need several pills a day.

●**Does the NIH study suggest that lifestyle modification alone is enough to control high blood pressure?** For most cases, the answer is no.

If you follow a healthy diet, get regular exercise, reduce your alcohol intake and avoid smoking, you'll cut your risk for heart disease and reduce the likelihood that you'll *develop* high blood pressure.

But when it comes to reducing *existing* high blood pressure, these strategies alone generally aren't enough. Three out of four people with hypertension (defined as having a blood pressure of 140/90 or higher) must take antihypertensive medication.

For patients with mildly elevated blood pressure, I usually give lifestyle changes a couple of months to work before turning to medication. In severe cases, I generally prescribe medication right away.

●**Which blood pressure medication is most effective?** Two classes of drugs have been tested and proven to reduce long-term complications and mortality in people with high blood pressure—diuretics and beta blockers.

Diuretics, in particular, are underprescribed. Most antihypertensive drugs work better when used in combination with diuretics.

The long-term data on a third class of antihypertensive medication, ACE inhibitors, aren't in yet. My guess is that they'll demonstrate reduced mortality as well.

This may or may not be true for the fourth group of blood pressure drugs—calcium channel blockers. In fact, short-acting channel blockers such as *nifedipine* (Procardia) seem to make matters worse.

Surprisingly, doctors prescribe calcium channel blockers more than any other blood pressure-lowering drug. Perhaps that's because calcium channel blockers are heavily promoted by the drug companies that make them.

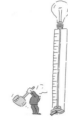

High Blood Pressure Mistakes Can Easily Be Avoided

Thomas Pickering, MD, professor of medicine at New York Hospital–Cornell Medical Center and director of the hospital's Blood Pressure Center, in New York City. He is author of *Good News About High Blood Pressure*. Simon & Schuster.

Elevated blood pressure is a major risk factor for heart attack and stroke, along with smoking and high cholesterol.

With proper treatment, high blood pressure (hypertension) can be controlled.

Sadly, doctors and patients alike often err in their efforts to do so…

***Mistake:* Ignoring systolic pressure.** Blood pressure is expressed as two numbers. The first represents *systolic* pressure—arterial pressure when the heart contracts. The second represents *diastolic* pressure—arterial pressure between beats. Normal blood pressure is defined as any pressure below 140/90.

Because the first studies linking heart disease with hypertension focused on diastolic pressure, doctors long assumed that just the second number was important.

Now we know that systolic pressure is an even bigger factor in heart disease than diastolic pressure.

***Mistake:* Treating strictly by the numbers.** At what level does hypertension become so dangerous that treatment is required? Some doctors insist on treating any pressure of 140/90 or higher. Others wait until pressure rises above 160/95.

But no magic number applies to everyone. When deciding whether treatment is needed, your *overall* risk of heart disease and stroke is what's important.

A 65-year-old diabetic with high cholesterol might need antihypertensive medication for a pressure of 140/90. A healthy 35-year-old with a pressure of 150/95 can probably forgo treatment.

***Mistake:* Relying on pressure readings taken in the doctor's office.** Blood pressure fluctuates throughout the day. One in five patients labeled hypertensive actually has "white-coat" hypertension. Because of anxiety, their pressure reads high at the doctor's office —but is normal under other conditions.

White-coat hypertension usually requires no treatment, although it should be followed up.

To avoid needless treatment, I recommend *home monitoring.* This involves taking your own pressure two to three times a day to get a more complete picture of your blood pressure.

Home blood pressure readings are usually about five points lower than clinic readings.

When home monitoring gives equivocal results, I suggest *24-hour monitoring.* A Walkman-like device worn on the waist and attached to a blood pressure cuff on the arm automatically records blood pressure at 30-minute intervals.

***Mistake:* Using an unreliable blood pressure monitor.** Many monitors designed for home use are unreliable. However, we have found that Omron monitors *are* reliable.*

Before using your monitor, have your doctor calibrate it. Have your doctor check your technique, too.

***Mistake:* Failing to rule out secondary hypertension.** Most high blood pressure is *primary* hypertension—there's no single underlying cause. In roughly 5% of all cases, however, high blood pressure is *secondary* to kidney disease, an adrenal gland tumor or another ailment. In such cases, it's essential to treat this underlying cause.

Your doctor should examine you carefully and do key diagnostic tests. *Two tests are especially important...*

●**Echocardiogram**, a noninvasive ultrasound exam, shows if hypertension has caused the heart to become enlarged. If it has, medication is usually required.

*If you have access to the World Wide Web, read more about home blood pressure monitors at *www.bloodpressure.com.*

●**The ankle-arm index test** is simple— but often neglected. Blood pressure should be roughly the same whether measured at the arm or the ankle. A lower reading at the ankle suggests a blocked artery in the leg. Such a blockage calls for aggressive treatment to lower pressure.

The ankle-arm test is especially important for people over 65.

***Mistake:* Being too quick to begin drug therapy.** When pressure is only modestly elevated—150/100, for example—and there is no sign of kidney damage or heart enlargement, I generally recommend six months of lifestyle modification—weight loss, proper diet, exercise. Only if these *nondrug* strategies fail to lower the pressure do I prescribe antihypertensive medication.

Weight loss is the most important lifestyle change. If you are overweight, your pressure should drop five points for every 10 pounds you lose.

***Mistake:* Drinking alcoholic beverages.** The finding that moderate drinking cuts the risk of heart disease has led many to act as if there were no downside to drinking. *There is.*

Alcohol can raise blood pressure significantly. Five or more drinks a day boosts systolic pressure by about five points...diastolic by about three. I urge my patients to have no more than two drinks a day—preferably of wine.

***Mistake:* Not exercising properly.** After vigorous exercise, blood pressure stays low for hours. And getting into shape will *permanently* reduce your blood pressure and your risk of heart disease.

I recommend at least 20 minutes of running, biking, walking, etc., at least four days a week.

For strength training, weight machines are safer than free weights—because muscular contractions, which raise blood pressure, are not sustained as long with the machines. Push-ups and other calisthenics are OK.

***Mistake:* Thinking that cutting back on salt will do the trick.** Only about half of all hypertensives are salt-sensitive. Their pressure drops if they cut back on salt and other sources of sodium. For the other 50%, avoiding salt makes no difference.

To find out if your blood pressure is affected by salt, avoid salt altogether for four weeks. See if there's any change.

Mistake: **Ignoring potassium.** There's now solid evidence that dietary potassium lowers blood pressure. Potassium-rich foods include bananas, oranges, beans, squash and sunflower seeds.

Watch out for potassium *supplements.* They can raise blood levels of potassium so high that dangerous disturbances in heart rhythm can result.

Mistake: **Ignoring the effects of other drugs.** Blood pressure can be raised by many prescription and over-the-counter drugs.

Examples: Pseudoephedrine, a decongestant found in many cold and allergy pills...and nonsteroidal anti-inflammatory drugs (NSAIDs) like *ibuprofen* (Advil).

If you take high doses of NSAIDs, ask your doctor about taking aspirin or acetaminophen instead. To set up an effective antihypertensive regimen, your doctor must know *all* the drugs you're taking.

Mistake: **Staying on medication indefinitely.** Most individuals who need pressure-lowering drugs must take them for life. *But not everyone.* Once a patient's blood pressure is under control, I try withdrawing medication. In many cases, the pressure stays down.

Alter your blood pressure medication regimen only under medical supervision—and with careful home monitoring. If pressure rises again, resume treatment.

Borderline Blood Pressure Risk

Christopher J. O'Donnell, MD, MPH, cardiologist and epidemiologist, Framingham Heart Study, Framingham, MA. His analysis of health data on 18,682 men 40 to 84 years of age was published in *Circulation*, 6720 Bertner St., Houston 77030.

Even borderline high blood pressure raises the risk for stroke and heart attack. Patients with *borderline isolated systolic hypertension—* systolic pressure (the "upper" number) between 140 and 159 and diastolic pressure (the "lower" number) 90 or below—had a 42% higher risk of stroke, 56% higher risk of dying from heart disease and a 26% greater chance of having a heart attack.

Systolic pressure represents blood pressure during contractions of the heart. Diastolic pressure is that between beats.

Best Place to Take Your Blood Pressure

Clarence E. Grim, MD, professor of cardiovascular medicine and director of the high blood pressure treatment center, Medical College of Wisconsin, Milwaukee. To learn how to take your blood pressure, consider ordering the video *A Skill for Life.* Shared Care.

Blood pressure readings taken at home are more accurate than readings taken in a doctor's office. The stress of being in a doctor's office (white-coat syndrome) can send blood pressure soaring—by as much as 23%.

Helpful: A home blood pressure monitor is available in most drugstores. Take readings three times a day (morning, afternoon, evening) for one week. Average your readings before your next doctor appointment.

Angioplasty Trap

James G. Jollis, MD, assistant professor of medicine, Duke University Medical Center, Durham, NC. His review of 97,000 Medicare patient records was presented at a meeting of the American Heart Association.

Many cardiologists perform too few angioplasties to meet national standards.

Trap: Up to 6.8% of patients treated by inexperienced doctors suffer complications—including fatal ones. Only 4.6% of patients whose angioplasties are done by experienced surgeons develop such complications. To meet standards set up by the American College of Cardiology, a cardiologist must perform at least 75 angioplasties a year. Half of all cardiologists perform 40 or fewer a year.

Lesson: If you're scheduled for angioplasty, ask your cardiologist about his/her level of experience.

How Effective Are Implantable Defibrillators?

Eleanor Schron, RN, project director, National Heart, Lung and Blood Institute, Bethesda, MD. Her study of 1,016 patients suffering from severe heartbeat abnormalities was presented at a meeting of the North American Society for Pacing and Electrophysiology.

Implantable defibrillators are very effective. In a study, patients with an irregular heartbeat who were implanted with one of the cassette-tape-sized devices were 38% less likely to die than similar patients who relied solely on drug therapy. The defibrillator—which shocks the heart back to life after cardiac arrest—proved so superior to drugs that the study was stopped early. Up to 1,500 lives could be saved a year if patients who chose drug treatment instead received a defibrillator.

Beating Heart Disease: When Surgery Is Necessary...and When It's Not

Steven F. Horowitz, MD, chief of cardiology at Beth Israel Medical Center, and professor of medicine and nuclear medicine, Albert Einstein College of Medicine, both in New York City.

When fatty deposits narrow the arteries in your heart, the consequences can be deadly.

Reduced blood flow starves the heart of oxygen, causing an often severe form of chest pain called *angina.* You tire easily and may be unable to exercise. And your risk of heart attack is dramatically increased.

A technique known as *coronary artery bypass graft* (CABG) surgery has proven very effective at creating a detour around these potentially deadly blockages. But any form of surgery—especially open-heart procedures like CABG—is risky. In fact, 1% to 2% of individuals who undergo bypass surgery die in the hospital.

The risk is especially great for diabetics and hypertensives...and those who have already sustained a heart attack or have had previous bypass surgery.

Good news: Blocked coronary arteries can often be opened up via drug therapy...or less invasive surgical procedures—even lifestyle changes.

EVALUATING THE BLOCKAGE

If you develop chest pain or excessive shortness of breath upon exertion, or if you have other symptoms of coronary artery disease, your doctor will probably schedule some non-invasive diagnostic tests...

•**Stress electrocardiogram** (cardiac stress test) monitors the heart's electrical activity during strenuous exercise.

•**Thallium scans and positron emission tomography** (PET) check to see if certain areas of the heart are deprived of oxygen-rich blood.

If tests suggest significant blockage, your doctor will probably recommend angiography.

In this low-risk procedure, a narrow tube (catheter) is inserted through an incision in the groin and threaded up to the coronary arteries. Special dye injected through the catheter renders coronary arteries visible on X-ray equipment.

DRUG THERAPY

If the blockage is severe, your doctor may recommend immediate surgery. In most cases, however, the first treatment is medication...

•**Nitroglycerin** (Monoket, IMDUR). Tiny pills containing this time-tested drug can be placed under the tongue at the first sign of angina...or supplied all day long via a skin patch or pills. It relaxes veins, diminishing the amount of blood returned to the heart. This allows the heart to work less. It also relaxes coronary arteries.

●**Beta-blockers** (Lopressor, Tenormin, Inderal). These oral drugs limit the heart's response to adrenaline in the bloodstream. Since the heart pumps more slowly, it needs less oxygen.

●**Calcium-channel blockers** (Calan, Procardia, Cardizem). This family of oral medications relaxes arteries and lowers blood pressure. Some of these medications should not be used by those with heart failure. Short-acting *nifedipine* (Procardia) probably shouldn't be used at all with coronary disease.

Three other groups of medications may also be helpful…

●**Aspirin** may reduce the risk of heart attack by preventing platelets from sticking together and forming clots.

●**A.C.E. inhibitors** (Capoten, Vasotec, Prinivil) are especially valuable in treating or preventing heart failure after a heart attack.

●**Cholesterol-lowering drugs** (niacin, Mevacor, Zocor, Pravachol, Questran) work primarily by lowering "bad" LDL cholesterol and, in some cases, raising "good" HDL cholesterol.

If your angina worsens despite drug therapy, your doctor will probably recommend bypass surgery or angioplasty.

ANGIOPLASTY

In this procedure, a catheter is used to introduce a tiny balloon into the coronary arteries. The balloon expands to squash the fatty deposits blocking the arteries.

If blockages aren't too numerous or severe enough to necessitate bypass, and drugs really aren't doing the trick, then angioplasty may be appropriate.

Angioplasty involves less pain and risk than bypass surgery. You may be out of the hospital in a few hours—at most a couple of days…and back to full activity shortly thereafter.

Drawback: In up to 50% of cases, the artery closes again—often within six months— and the procedure must be repeated.

In recent years, a variation on angioplasty has become popular. After the blocked artery is opened, a mesh reinforcing tube called a stent is inserted. With a stent, the chance of the artery closing again is cut by 50%.

CORONARY BYPASS

In bypass surgery, the chest is opened, the ribs are spread and the heart is cooled to a standstill while a heart-lung machine takes over. Blood vessels "harvested" from the leg or chest are grafted onto the coronary arteries in such a way that they carry blood around the blockage.

Bypass surgery is the only reasonable option if tests reveal obstruction of the left main coronary artery. Bypass is also the best bet if three or more coronary arteries are blocked and function of the left ventricle is diminished.

Bypass surgery requires at least four days of hospitalization, and several weeks of recuperation at home. It may take two to four months before you can resume a full, active life. The grafts generally stay open for five to 15 years but may close earlier.

LIFESTYLE MODIFICATION

We all know that a low-fat diet, exercise and stress reduction can help prevent heart disease. These strategies can also relieve angina —even reverse coronary artery disease.

You may have heard of the program developed by Dr. Dean Ornish, of the Preventive Medicine Research Institute in Sausalito, CA. His program is *not* a substitute for bypass or angioplasty if you have life-threatening artery blockage…or if you have unstable angina that does not respond to medication.

But for patients in the "gray zone" where neither Coronary Artery Bypass Graft (CABG) nor angioplasty offers any clear advantages, lifestyle intervention may be the best option.

The program involves…

●**A very low-fat vegetarian diet.** To reduce total fat to 10% of calories, participants learn to cook without oil or other forms of fat. The American Heart Association recommends that 30% of calories come from fat—but that's too high.

●**Aerobic exercise.** Brisk walking, jogging, stair-climbing or biking, at least three hours a week.

●**Yoga, stretching and meditation**—for an hour a day. Facilitates deep relaxation.

●**Group therapy.** To teach people ways to express their emotions and improve their relationships.

For the first three months, program participants come in three times a week for exercise, diet counseling, stress reduction and group therapy. For the next nine months, they come once a week.

By then, they have incorporated the diet, exercise and stress-reduction into their lives.

What to Do When The Doctor Says Bypass Surgery

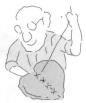

Fredric J. Pashkow, MD, medical director of cardiac rehabilitation at The Cleveland Clinic Foundation. He is author of *Fifty Essential Things to Do When the Doctor Says It's Heart Disease* and *The Woman's Heart Book.* Plume.

Since its introduction in 1967, coronary artery bypass graft (CABG) surgery has enabled thousands of people to survive severe coronary artery disease.

Coronary artery disease (atherosclerosis) occurs when fatty deposits form in the coronary arteries, restricting flow of oxygen-rich blood to the heart. Over time, atherosclerosis may lead to a form of chest pain called *angina* …or to heart attack.

In bypass surgery, doctors reroute blood flow around arterial blockages, using blood vessels grafted from another part of the body, usually a leg.

The procedure has become so common that people tend to forget just how serious it is.

One surgeon slices open the chest, cracking the breastbone (sternum) to reach the heart, while another "harvests" the arteries or veins to be grafted. The heart is stopped for several hours as doctors attach the grafts.

Bypass surgery generally requires a hospital stay of four or more days, plus a one-month convalescence.

Bypass surgery is often the best therapy for heart disease, but it is not the *only* approach. *Other options to consider:*

LIFESTYLE MODIFICATION

As Dr. Dean Ornish and other researchers have shown, a low-fat diet (10% of calories from fat) can slow the progress of atherosclerosis—and in some cases reverse it. This approach is very effective when combined with cholesterol-lowering drugs called *statins.*

Drawback: The low-fat diet doesn't always work. And such a diet is hard to follow. Only about 15% of patients are motivated enough to stick with it.

ANGIOPLASTY

This procedure costs less and is less invasive than open-heart surgery. Often, the patient can go home the same day.

The surgeon inserts a catheter into a tiny incision in the leg and threads it into the coronary artery. A balloon on the tip is then inflated to flatten the plaque against the artery wall, widening the artery and easing the flow of blood.

Drawback: About 25% of the time, angioplasty has to be repeated to eliminate plaques that recur—sometimes within six months of the original operation.

To prevent recurrence, some cardiologists now use *stents*—tiny metallic tubes inserted into the artery to keep it open.

KEYHOLE SURGERY

This experimental procedure is a less invasive variant of conventional bypass surgery. Instead of cracking the chest, the surgeon makes a small incision between the ribs. Using an endoscope, he/she removes the *internal thoracic artery* from the chest and grafts it onto the coronary artery.

For *accessible* blockages, keyhole surgery should prove just as effective as CABG. But it's still too early to know its exact success rate.

WHICH APPROACH IS BEST?

Can you get by using one of these less invasive approaches? *The answer depends on several factors…*

•**Condition of the heart.** If the heart can pump enough blood despite the blockages, bypass surgery can probably be avoided.

Bypass surgery is preferable if the heart has been weakened by heart attack.

77

●**Location and number of blockages.** The more severe and numerous the blockages, the greater the need for bypass surgery.

Bypass is preferable to angioplasty if blockages are "upstream" (close to the point where the arteries branch off of the aorta)...if the patient has one or more blockages of the *left main coronary artery*...and/or if two or all three coronary vessels are blocked.

●**Level of chest pain.** If angina isn't relieved by medication, bypass is probably the best option.

Angioplasty may be more appropriate if the patient has had just one tiny heart attack, with minimal damage to the heart...has just started to experience angina...or is highly motivated to follow a low-fat diet and regular exercise regimen.

If your doctor recommends bypass, consult a bypass surgeon *and* a cardiologist who specializes in angioplasty.

WHAT TO DO *BEFORE* SURGERY

Anyone who decides to have bypass surgery can increase the chance of a successful operation by doing the following...

●**Find a good surgeon.** He should be board-certified in cardiothoracic surgery. In addition, he should perform at least 150 bypass operations each year. Fewer than that, and he may lack the necessary expertise.

Some patients are uncomfortable asking a surgeon about these details. But good surgeons are happy to share this information—and you want only the best. If the surgeon seems defensive, find another one.

●**Check out the hospital.** It should perform at least 200 bypass operations a year, with a death rate of less than 1.5%.

The hospital should be accredited by the Joint Commission on Accreditation of Healthcare Organizations (JCAHO). To inquire about a hospital's status, call JCAHO at 630-792-5800.

●**Stop smoking.** Smoking in the 10 days before surgery increases the risk of pneumonia and other surgical complications.

●**Avoid aspirin.** If you take aspirin on a regular basis (to prevent heart attack, for instance), ask your cardiologist about stopping temporarily. Doing so will reduce the risk of excessive bleeding during and after surgery.

●**Rethink diet and exercise habits.** Doctors once thought that bypass surgery would allow patients to carry on their high-fat, low-exercise lives as before. That's simply untrue. To keep your newly grafted vessels healthy, you must keep fat intake low and get regular exercise.

If you have diabetes: Ask your doctor about "tight control" of your blood sugar before surgery. The better you manage your diabetes, the lower your risk of postoperative infection.

It's essential to continue to monitor your cholesterol level after surgery—and take steps to control it with diet, exercise, stress management and—if necessary—cholesterol-lowering medication.

Better Bypass Surgery

Frederick St. Goar, MD, clinical assistant professor of cardiology, Stanford University, Stanford, CA. For more information on port access surgery, contact the Stanford University Department of Cardiothoracic Surgery, 300 Pasteur Dr. CVRB 5247, Stanford, CA 94305.

Recovery is faster with a procedure called "port access" coronary artery bypass graft surgery than with ordinary bypass surgery. In conventional surgery, the surgeon must make a 12-inch incision in the chest. Port access surgery requires only one three-inch and two one-inch incisions.

New Surgical Procedure For Heart Failure Sufferers

Anthony P. Furnary, MD, associate director, Albert Starr academic center, St. Vincent Hospital, Portland, OR. His 12-month study of cardiomyoplasty in 68 heart failure patients was published in the *Journal of the American College of Cardiology*, 415 Judah St., San Francisco 94122.

Cardiomyoplasty involves transplanting muscle tissue from the patient's own back to the ventricles of the failing heart. A pacemaker-like device implanted at the same time stimulates the transplanted tissue to contract, assisting the heart as it pumps. Cardiomyoplasty is especially promising for older patients who fail to respond to less drastic treatments, yet who have other medical problems that disqualify them for a heart transplant.

Open-Heart Surgery Breakthrough

Karl Krieger, MD, professor of cardiac surgery, New York Hospital–Cornell Medical Center, New York City.

Open-heart surgery can now be performed without multiple transfusions. The drug *erythropoetin* boosts red cell count prior to surgery, while *aprotinin* helps stop postoperative bleeding.

More: The surgeon uses a machine to collect blood lost during surgery, then transfuses it back into the patient. Ordinarily, open-heart surgery requires up to four units of blood—and each carries a chance of being tainted with a disease-causing virus. If you're scheduled for surgery, ask your doctor about these strategies.

Saving Your Heart Without Bypass Surgery ...Without Angioplasty

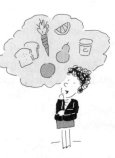

John A. McDougall, MD, director of the McDougall Program for controlling heart disease at St. Helena Hospital in Santa Rosa, CA. He hosts the nationally syndicated television program "McDougall" and is author of *The McDougall Program for a Healthy Heart*. Dutton.

For anyone with heart disease—even for anyone at *risk* for heart disease—it may seem as if time is running out.

But having treated thousands of heart patients in my clinic over the past 10 years, I know that there is time to recover cardiovascular health in nine out of 10 cases. This can usually be accomplished *without* angioplasty or bypass surgery.

Anyone eager to prevent or cure heart disease must learn to avoid fatty foods and other dietary "poisons."

I'm often asked, "How often can I eat steak and eggs without hurting my heart?" I reply, "How often can you smoke without any ill effects on your body?" The only honest answer to both questions is *never*.

DRAMATIC CHANGES ARE POSSIBLE

Most of the people who participate in my two-week program are seriously ill. Many have already had a heart attack. Others take medication for chest pain (angina) or high blood pressure.

By the time they leave our clinic, most have significantly lowered their cholesterol and blood pressure...and stopped taking medicine. The vast majority go on to live full lives.

This remarkable transformation involves three simple steps...

●**Eliminate *all* excess fat from your diet.** That means substituting fruits, vegetables and grains for red meat, chicken, dairy products, eggs, oils, cakes and candies and refined and processed foods.

●**Get daily aerobic exercise.** Patients in my program are required to walk for at least 30 minutes a day.

●**Learn to manage psychological stress** — without resorting to overeating or other self-destructive behavior. Massage, meditation and group discussion are all effective ways to do this.

THE SKINNY ON FAT

The typical American gets a whopping 40% of his daily calories in the form of fat. It's this fat that clogs the coronary arteries with the fatty streaks (plaques) that cause heart attack.

Dietary fat endangers your heart by...

●**Causing red blood cells to clump.** That slows circulation, reduces oxygen in the blood and raises blood pressure.

●**Creating new plaques** and making them prone to rupture.

●**Causing existing plaques to grow.**

●**Causing abnormally rapid clotting of the blood.** That can lead to arterial occlusion if a new plaque bursts.

79

●**Causing release of hormone-like compounds.** Called *prostaglandins,* these compounds boost the clumping effect.

To keep plaques from forming, the American Heart Association (AHA) suggests limiting daily fat intake to 30% of calories. Yet studies show that even at this level of fat intake, new plaques *continue* to form. Amazingly, the AHA stands by its misguided recommendation.

HOW HEART ATTACKS OCCUR

Many people think that a heart attack occurs when an *old* plaque grows so big that it occludes a coronary artery.

Actually, most heart attacks occur following the rupture of a *newly formed* plaque—which contains liquid fat and cholesterol.

This rupture leaves a wound on the artery wall—which is quickly capped with a blood clot. This clot can grow quickly, becoming so large that it occludes the artery and stops blood flow to the heart.

The implication? Heart attacks can occur even when the coronary arteries are relatively plaque-free. As I tell my patients, you play Russian roulette *each time you eat a fatty meal.*

THE MCDOUGALL PROGRAM

My diet separates foods into three categories…

●**Eat all you want.**

●**Brown rice**, wheat, corn, oatmeal and other whole grains.

●**Whole-grain products**, including noodles, breads, pancakes and waffles. Make sure they contain no fats or oils.

●**Potatoes and yams.**

●**Squash.**

●**Peas**, lentils, lima beans and string beans.

●**Green and yellow vegetables.**

●**Cucumbers**, onions, peppers and tomatoes.

●**Beets**, carrots, turnips and other root vegetables.

●**Mild spices and herbs.**

●**Eat in moderation.**

●**Fruit**, fruit juice and dried fruit (up to three servings a day).

●**Sugar** and artificial sweeteners.

●**Salt.**

●**Alcohol.**

●**Fatty plant foods**, including nuts, peanut butter and tofu.

●**Avoid.**

●**Red meat**, poultry, fish, seafood, eggs, milk and milk products like butter, cheese, yogurt and sour cream. Even *nonfat* dairy products should be avoided. They contain proteins that can trigger an artery-damaging immune response.

I allow fatty foods *only* on special occasions—eggs on Easter…turkey on Thanksgiving …cake on your birthday.

●**Cooking oil.** Instead, use a nonstick pan or wok. Sauté with water, soy sauce, wine, tomato juice, lemon or lime juice or Worcestershire sauce.

When baking, replace the oil in the recipe with half the amount of applesauce, mashed bananas or soy yogurt.

●**Sulfites.** These preservatives, used in wines and in salad bars, can cause an allergic reaction.

When buying packaged food, read labels carefully. Avoid products containing fats and oils, including monoglycerides, diglycerides and/or hydrogenated or partially hydrogenated fats or oils. Before making long-term dietary changes, discuss your nutritional needs with a doctor or dietician.

ONE MAN'S STORY

Charles Schaefer of Santa Rosa, CA, suffered his heart attack at age 46.

After undergoing balloon angioplasty, he was told he would probably need bypass surgery. At the time, his cholesterol was 220—average for Americans. His weight and blood pressure were normal, too.

After leaving the hospital, he went on my diet. His cholesterol immediately fell to 180. He then visited my office, and I put him on a cholesterol-lowering drug that brought his level down to 150. He also began walking or bicycling several times a week.

Four years later, treadmill stress tests show that his coronary arteries are wide open. His heart is healthy, and he feels in better shape than ever.

"If I had stayed on the rich American diet," says Mr. Schaefer, "I would not be alive today."

Bypass Surgery Dangers Are Real

Dennis Mangano, PhD, MD, a physician at the San Francisco Veterans Affairs Medical Center and director of the McSPI International Research Group.

Heart bypass surgery leads to stroke and other brain damage more often than people realize—one out of 15 patients who undergo surgery and one out of six patients over age 75 will suffer serious damage.

Greatest risk: Older patients…women…prior stroke sufferers…people with diabetes or hypertension.

Prior to surgery: Make sure your surgeon uses techniques designed to reduce stroke risk—echocardiography (to locate the safest place for instrumenting the main artery) and drugs to prevent blood pressure drops—and pays attention to the temperature of fluids used to re-warm the heart and brain. Your surgeon should check for evidence of stroke within 90 minutes of the operation…and consider aggressive treatment for complications.

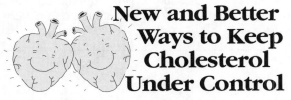

New and Better Ways to Keep Cholesterol Under Control

Daniel Rader, MD, director of preventive cardiology at the University of Pennsylvania Health System in Philadelphia.

For decades now, cardiologists have been warning us that a high level of *low-density lipoprotein* (LDL, or "bad") cholesterol means an increased risk of heart attack.

In the US, the average total cholesterol level is 210…the average LDL cholesterol level about 140.

But a growing consensus of doctors now believe that these average levels may be *too high* to ensure a healthy heart.

Each year, more than 800,000 Americans suffer their first heart attack. And—many of these people have average cholesterol readings.

Doctors now think that your level of LDL cholesterol should ideally be no higher than 130. At that level, the fatty arterial deposits (plaques) that cause heart attacks are less likely to form.

LOWERING ELEVATED LEVELS

If your LDL cholesterol is 130 or higher…

•**Switch to a diet low in fat.** The average American gets 37% of his/her calories from fat. To lower the amount of fat in your diet, eat less meat and more fruits and vegetables…substitute nonfat milk for whole milk…and eat more oat bran and other forms of soluble fiber. *Also:* Ask your doctor about taking *psyllium* (Metamucil).

Saturated fat should account for no more than 10% of your daily caloric intake.

The body uses dietary fat to make cholesterol. Few people realize it, but eating too much fat is worse for your heart than eating too much cholesterol. It's okay to eat eggs once or twice a week.

•**Get more exercise.** Aerobic exercise—at least 20 minutes, three or four times a week—brings moderate reductions in LDL cholesterol.

Exercise also increases levels of *high-density lipoprotein* (HDL) cholesterol. That's the "good" form associated with reduced heart attack risk.

DO YOU NEED DRUG THERAPY?

What if your LDL cholesterol level is 160 or above despite a good diet and exercise regimen? Cholesterol-lowering medication may be appropriate—if you smoke, have high blood pressure or diabetes and/or have a family history of heart attack. Even in the absence of these risk factors, drug therapy may be appropriate.

Three tests can give you information about your risk…

•**Lipoprotein (a) test.** High levels of this blood component—often represented as Lp(a)—have been linked to heart attack. Normal Lp(a) levels are 20 or lower.

•**Homocysteine test.** Individuals with high levels of this amino acid in their blood are prone to heart attack. Your homocysteine level should be 10 or lower. Folic acid supplements help reduce levels of homocysteine.

•**Ultrafast computed tomography (CT) scan.** This 20-minute noninvasive test can check your coronary arteries for calcium. Calcified plaques are a sure sign of heart disease—and may predict future risk of heart attack.

If these tests suggest an elevated risk, your doctor may recommend cholesterol-lowering medication.

WHICH DRUG IS BEST?

The most widely used cholesterol-lowering drugs are the "statins." Your doctor may recommend a statin, such as *pravastatin* (Pravachol) or *simvastatin* (Zocor). These two have been shown in large-scale studies to reduce heart attack rates.

Your doctor may also recommend high doses of the vitamin *nicotinic acid* (niacin). Although it is quite effective at lowering cholesterol, niacin can cause facial flushing and elevated blood sugar or uric acid. People taking it must be closely monitored by a doctor.

HDL AND TRIGLYCERIDES

Low levels of HDL cholesterol are associated with increased risk for heart attack. If your HDL level is less than 35, ask your doctor what you can do to raise it.

Studies suggest that HDL can be raised by niacin therapy...moderate alcohol consumption (one or two drinks a day)...and vigorous exercise.

A triglyceride level of 250 or higher is associated with increased heart attack risk, although high triglycerides pose less of a threat than high cholesterol.

Triglyceride levels can usually be lowered via weight loss, exercise and a diet low in fat and—especially important—sugar.

If you have high triglycerides, ask your doctor about substituting fresh fruit for fruit juices, which are extremely high in sugar.

ALTERNATIVE APPROACHES

People who eat lots of fish have a lower risk of heart disease. But there's no evidence that fish oil capsules have the same effect. In some people, they actually *raise* LDL.

Fish oil capsules can help reduce extremely high triglycerides (over 1,000). If you have high triglycerides, ask your doctor if fish oil capsules are appropriate. Heavy consumption of garlic has been shown to bring modest reductions in cholesterol. But garlic *pills* have not been shown to work. There's no harm in taking them, but don't substitute them for proven cholesterol-lowering medication.

ALREADY HAD A HEART ATTACK?

If you have had a heart attack or have heart disease, your LDL cholesterol should be less than 100. There is a good chance you may need medication to reach this goal.

Doctors are beginning to think that medication may be appropriate for virtually all heart attack survivors. A study published in *The New England Journal of Medicine* suggests that they are right. In this study, more than 4,000 heart attack survivors with average LDL cholesterol levels were given *pravastatin* or a placebo. Over the next five years, those who received pravastatin suffered 24% fewer heart attacks than those who got the placebo.

Lesson: If you've had one heart attack, reducing your cholesterol can reduce your risk of another—even if your cholesterol level is not elevated. Your new target for LDL cholesterol should be 100 or lower. Currently, only one in four heart patients achieves this level.

Bottom line: Reducing cholesterol levels prevents heart attacks. If diet and exercise don't do the job, medications are effective and very safe.

For a Better Echocardiogram

Nelson B. Schiller, MD, director, echocardiography laboratory, Moffitt-Long Hospitals, San Francisco.

For a better ultrasound exam of the heart (echocardiogram), ask the doctor about squeezing a tennis ball during the procedure. Doing so boosts blood pressure and heart rate, making it easier for the doctor to spot heart and circulatory system problems. Doctors commonly use echocardiograms to gauge damage to the heart following a heart attack.

Aspirin and Anger

Murray A. Mittleman, MD, DPH, an instructor at Harvard Medical School and a physician at Deaconess Hospital, Boston.

Aspirin may reduce the risk of heart attacks for angry people. A study of 1,623 people found that angry people were more than twice as likely to suffer a heart attack within two hours after feeling angry than they were at other times.

The connection between anger and heart attacks was not found, however, in members of the group who took aspirin regularly.

It has long been recommended that people take one aspirin tablet (or half a tablet daily) to reduce heart attack risk. Aspirin makes heart attacks less likely by minimizing the chance of formation of potentially dangerous blood clots.

Researchers think that the same works to counteract the effects of adrenaline and other anger-generated stress hormones that make clots more likely to form.

Better than Aspirin

Michael Gent, DSc, director, clinical trials methodology group, Hamilton Civic Hospitals Research Centre, Hamilton, Ontario, Canada. His study of 19,185 volunteers who had suffered heart attack, stroke or clogged arteries in their legs was published in *The Lancet*, 42 Bedford Square, London, WC1B 3SL.

The blood thinner *clopidogrel* is better than aspirin at warding off heart attack and stroke. Clopidogrel cuts the risk of new heart attacks and strokes by one-third, compared with one-fourth for aspirin.

More: Volunteers who took this drug were less likely to suffer gastrointestinal bleeding than those who took aspirin. The drug may be appropriate for patients with heart disease and/or peripheral arterial disease.

Heart Health Trap

Bruce Yaffe, MD, an internist in private practice, 121 E. 84 St., New York 10028.

If your doctor has prescribed Procardia or Adalac for you, make sure it is the long-acting form.

The FDA now requires that older, short-acting forms of these calcium channel blockers for high blood pressure or angina carry a warning label because some studies have linked them to an increased risk of heart attack.

These studies have little relevance for people taking the newer, long-acting forms. The newer calcium channel blockers control hypertension by keeping a steady level of the drug in the body, rather than allowing the amount to fluctuate rapidly, which may be dangerous.

Work Hours May Be Hazardous

Ichiro Kawachi, MD, PhD, assistant professor of medicine, Harvard Medical School, Boston.

In a study, risk of heart attack was 70% higher among nurses who worked rotating shifts than among co-workers who worked regular hours.

Likely culprit: Stress resulting from disruption of the body's daily biological clock. This causes release of stress hormones such as epinephrine, norepinephrine and cortisol. In turn, these hormones raise blood pressure, reduce glucose tolerance and increase wear and tear on the cardiovascular system.

Cholesterol Drug Benefits

James Shepherd, MD, professor of pathological biochemistry at The Royal Infirmary, Glasgow, Scotland.

The cholesterol-reducing drug *pravastatin* may prevent heart attacks in men who have elevated cholesterol levels but no history of heart disease.

Researchers in Scotland studied more than 6,000 apparently healthy men between age 45 and age 64 with high cholesterol levels. Those who took the drug suffered 28% fewer deaths from heart disease, and 31% fewer nonfatal heart attacks, than a similar group that took a placebo.

Helping Blood Vessels Work Properly

David G. Harrison, MD, a professor of medicine at Emory University, Atlanta.

A study of people with high cholesterol found that their artery walls didn't expand when they were supposed to (e.g., after exercise). After researchers gave these patients cholesterol-lowering drugs for nine months, they found that the artery walls began to dilate properly and blood pressure had dropped. Arteries that don't open properly prevent blood from moving through the body quickly enough in times of stress, and are associated with heart attacks and other cardiovascular problems.

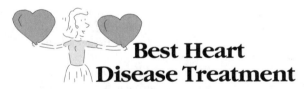

Best Heart Disease Treatment

Nanette Kass Wenger, MD, professor of medicine at Emory University School of Medicine, 69 Butler St. SE, Atlanta 30303.

Individually prescribed programs of exercise and diet and other risk-reduction programs reduce mortality rates among heart disease victims by 25%—but fewer than one-third of patients who could benefit from such programs are enrolled in them.

Why: Many doctors fail to refer appropriate patients because they do not know of local programs, and many patients have inadequate insurance coverage. Exercise programs pose no health risk even for older patients.

Useful: A free booklet, *Recovering from Heart Problems Through Cardiac Rehabilitation*, #96-0674 is available by contacting the Agency for Healthcare Research and Quality at 800-358-9295, *www.ahrq.gov.*

Easy Disease Risk Reducer

Ralph S. Paffenbarger, Jr., MD, professor emeritus of epidemiology at Stanford University School of Medicine, Stanford, CA.

A follow-up of the famous 1978 study of 20,000 Harvard alumni confirmed its findings that middle-aged and older men who exercised moderately had half as many heart attacks as their contemporaries who did not exercise.

A Smoke-Free World

Alan Blum, MD, associate professor of family medicine at Baylor College of Medicine, Houston. Dr. Blum is the founder of Doctors Ought to Care (DOC), an antismoking group long recognized for its service to public health.

More than 46 million people have successfully stopped smoking. Most people who succeed in giving up smoking do so only after making three to five attempts, so failing once or twice is no reason to give up. After stopping, health improves no matter how long you've smoked or how old you are. The extra risk of heart disease that results from smoking decreases by 50% within one year, then continues to drop to zero after 15 years. And after five years, the risk of stroke faced by former smokers drops to the level faced by persons who have never smoked.

Timing Is Critical

Charles Hennekens, MD, chief of preventive medicine at Brigham and Women's Hospital, Boston.

Taking an aspirin during—or very soon after—a heart attack reduces the risk of death significantly. A study of more than 17,000 patients worldwide found that those who took aspirin within 24 hours of the first symptoms were 23% less likely to die from a heart attack than those who did not.

When aspirin was taken along with the clot-dissolving drug *streptokinase*, the death rate dropped by 42%. It is believed that aspirin prevents production of prostaglandins, substances that encourage blood to clot and block blood vessels that carry vital oxygen to the damaged heart.

Height and Heart Disease

Donna Parker, ScD, an epidemiologist in the division of health education at Memorial Hospital of Rhode Island, Pawtucket, who recently completed a study of more than 6,500 people.

Men over five-feet, 10-inches have an 80% lower risk of heart disease than men under five-feet, five-inches.

Possible reasons: Poor childhood nutrition—or prenatal nutrition—may stunt growth and affect adult health. Also, arteries in the hearts of shorter people are narrower, possibly increasing blockage risk.

Self-defense: Short men should focus on controllable risks—smoking, blood pressure, exercise, diet, weight. Results were inconclusive for shorter women—but they should be similarly cautious.

Average height: Around five-feet, nine-inches for men...five-feet, four-inches for women.

Even a Little Is Too Much

James Shepherd, MD, professor and head, department of pathologic biochemistry, University of Glasgow (Scotland) School of Medicine. His five-year study of 6,595 men 45 to 64 years of age with cholesterol levels of 250 to 300 was published in *The New England Journal of Medicine*, 10 Shattuck St., Boston 02115.

Until recently, most doctors agreed that cholesterol-lowering drugs should be reserved only for patients at highest risk for heart disease.

Finding: Otherwise healthy patients with mildly elevated cholesterol who took *pravastatin* (Pravachol) had 31% fewer heart attacks than those who got a placebo.

Test Results Can Vary

Glen Griffin, MD, former primary care physician who now writes and lectures on following a low-fat diet and coauthor of *Good Fat, Bad Fat: How to Lower Your Cholesterol and Beat the Odds of a Heart Attack.* Fisher Books.

Cholesterol test results can vary. Factors affecting results include illness and pregnancy.

Helpful: Have your doctor perform two or more tests before you make any major lifestyle changes.

Important: Cholesterol testing should include a determination of your HDL ratio—the ratio of total cholesterol to HDL ("good") cholesterol. A healthy ratio is *under four*. This measure is a much better predictor of heart disease risk than overall cholesterol readings.

Exercise and Heart Attack

Wayne Chandler, MD, associate professor of laboratory medicine, University of Washington, Seattle, who led a study of 44 men and women around age 66.

Men and women who biked, walked or jogged three times a week over a period of six months were less likely to suffer blood clots—and potentially fatal heart attacks—than those who did only flexibility exercises.

Their blood was also less likely to clot in the morning, the time of day when heart attacks are most likely to occur. This study may be the first to finally explain exactly how exercise helps prevent heart attacks.

Also: Those whose fitness levels improved the most during the study were least likely to suffer blood clots, but benefits vanished once they stopped their regular exercise routine.

More Harm than Good?

William E. Boden, MD, chief, medical service, Veterans Affairs Healthcare Network of Upstate New York, Syracuse. His study of 920 heart attack survivors was presented at a meeting of the American College of Cardiology.

A common heart test does more harm than good for survivors of one type of heart attack. *Angiography*—an X-ray procedure in which a catheter is threaded into the heart—may be too invasive for survivors of non-Q-wave heart attacks.

Study: The death rate among non-Q-wave heart attack survivors who underwent angiography was 34% higher than the rate among those who received a noninvasive heart test instead. Physicians can distinguish a Q-wave heart attack from a non-Q-wave heart attack via a simple electrocardiogram (EKG).

Hooray! Heart Help!

Tomas A. Salerno, MD, chief of cardiothoracic surgery at Buffalo General Hospital, Buffalo, NY.

One type of operation may allow many patients with failing hearts to avoid transplants and enjoy near-normal lives.

The operation, developed by Randas J.V. Batista, MD, a Brazilian surgeon working in a primitive rural hospital, involves removing a slice of muscle from the left ventricle of patients with severely enlarged hearts. This surgery enables the remaining part of the heart to pump more effectively. US physicians who have observed the procedure in Brazil are exploring how it can be improved via high-tech medical techniques.

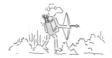

Hunting Danger

Susan Haapaniemi, MS, exercise physiologist, William Beaumont Hospital, Royal Oak, MI.

The excitement of spotting the prey can trigger a heart attack in hunters with clogged arteries. In a study of 25 hunters, spotting a deer caused the hunters' heart rates to soar. One hunter's heart rate shot up from 78 to 168 beats per minute—and he was seated.

Self-defense: Get in shape before hunting season begins…rest frequently while hunting…avoid tobacco, caffeine and alcohol…and hunt with a buddy. *Also:* Hunters and nonhunters alike should wear bright orange when venturing into the woods during deer season.

Personality Danger

Mark Goodman, PhD, behavioral medicine specialist, and George Moran, MD, chief of cardiology, Union Memorial Hospital, Baltimore. Their 18-month study of 41 angioplasty patients was published in *Mayo Clinic Proceedings*, Room 660, Siebens Bldg., 200 First St. SW, Rochester, MN 55905.

Heart patients with Type A (hostile) personalities are more likely to need repeat angioplasties.

Background: More than one-third of heart patients who undergo angioplasty to open a blocked coronary artery eventually need to have the procedure repeated—because the artery closes back up. This process is called *restenosis*.

Study: Type A patients were 2.5 times more likely to experience restenosis than their calmer counterparts. *Theory:* Type A people have high levels of adrenaline in their blood. Adrenaline causes arteries to constrict.

Needed: Further study to determine if Type A patients can use relaxation techniques to reduce their risk of restenosis.

Mother's Diet and Heart Disease Link

David J. P. Barker, MD, PhD, director, Medical Research Council Environmental Epidemiology Unit, University of Southampton, Southampton, England.

Your risk of heart disease and other illnesses is linked to your mother's diet during pregnancy. An undernourished mother is more likely to give birth to a small baby. Small birth size is linked to insulin resistance (a condition that can lead to diabetes)…high blood pressure…and two major risk factors for heart disease—elevated triglycerides and low levels of HDL (good) cholesterol.

Fish Oil and Heart Attacks

Christine M. Albert, MD, research fellow, Brigham and Women's Hospital, Boston.

Fish seems to fight heart attack. In a study, men who ate fish at least once a week were 50% less likely to die of coronary artery disease than men who ate fish less than once a month. The more fish they ate, the lower their risk.

Theory: Compounds in fish—probably omega-3 fatty acids—are beneficial to the heart. *However:* Fish oil capsules may not benefit the heart, since they don't contain all the compounds found in fish.

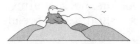

Cutting Heart Attack Death Risks

Arthur Moss, MD, professor of medicine, University of Rochester Medical Center in Rochester, NY, leader of the study of almost 200 heart attack survivors, published in *The New England Journal of Medicine,* 10 Shattuck St., Boston 02115.

Implanted heart defibrillators could cut the risk of death by 50% for people who survive a first heart attack and have erratic heartbeats. The battery-powered implants work like the external defibrillators routinely used by emergency personnel—they shock the heart back into normal rhythm during a cardiac arrest.

Beta-Blockers and Heart Attacks

Stephen Soumerai, ScD, associate professor of ambulatory care and prevention at Harvard Medical School and Harvard Pilgrim Health Care, Boston. His study was published in the *The Journal of the American Medical Association.*

Older heart attack patients who were given *beta-blockers* lived longer. A five-year study of 5,300 Medicare patients found that those who used beta-blockers after heart attacks were 43% less likely to die within two years than those who did not. Researchers believe that if physicians prescribed beta-blockers for all eligible patients, it would save about 7,000 lives per year. The heart-slowing beta-blockers cost only about $3 per month, compared with $30 to $50 per month for the more frequently prescribed —but less effective—calcium channel blockers.

Garlic and Cholesterol Link

Manfred Steiner, MD, PhD, professor of medicine, East Carolina University School of Medicine, whose study was published in the *American Journal of Clinical Nutrition.*

When otherwise healthy men who had high cholesterol took garlic supplements for six months, their cholesterol levels dropped 5% or more. The supplements contained seven grams of aged garlic—equivalent to 10 to 15 grams of cooked garlic or two cloves of fresh garlic.

Possible explanation: Garlic reduces LDL ("bad") cholesterol, although it had no effect on HDL ("good") cholesterol.

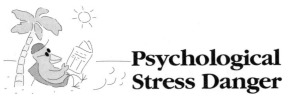

Psychological Stress Danger

Debra K. Moser, DNSc, RN, assistant professor of nursing, Ohio State University, Columbus. Her nine-month study of 86 heart attack survivors was published in *Psychosomatic Medicine*, 428 E. Preston St., Baltimore 21202.

Severe stress in the aftermath of a heart attack increases the chance of complications. All heart attack survivors experience some anxiety, but some are more anxious than others.

Study: Patients who felt more anxious following a heart attack were 4.9 times more likely to suffer angina, heart spasms, another heart attack or dangerous heart rhythms than their less anxious counterparts. Almost 20% in this high-anxiety category suffered complications, compared with 6% of low-anxiety patients.

Theory: Severe anxiety causes the body to produce *catecholamines* and other stress-related chemicals that thicken the blood.

Helpful: Unrestricted visiting with friends and family...and relaxation therapy.

Triglyceride Levels

Michael Miller, MD, assistant professor of medicine, University of Maryland Hospital, Baltimore. His study of triglyceride levels in 492 men and women was presented at a meeting of the American Heart Association.

Safe triglyceride levels may not be so safe after all. Current guidelines call for triglycerides to be no higher than 200. But a study found that people with levels between 100 and 200 had twice the risk of dying from a heart attack as those with levels below 100. They were also twice as likely to require bypass surgery or another procedure to clear blocked coronary arteries.

To keep triglyceride levels down: Get regular exercise...minimize consumption of sugar and saturated fat...and boost intake of omega-3 fatty acids. Sources of omega-3 fatty acids include sardines, mackerel, tuna, fish oil capsules and flaxseed oil.

Stroke Risk Reduction

Gregory W. Albers, MD, director, Stanford Stroke Center, Stanford University Medical Center, Palo Alto, CA. His study of atrial fibrillation in 309 elderly patients was published in *Archives of Internal Medicine*, 515 N. State St., Chicago 60610.

To cut their risk of stroke, individuals experiencing irregular heartbeat (atrial fibrillation) should usually be treated with blood thinners like aspirin or *warfarin* (Coumadin). In a study, 82% of these patients were found to be at high risk for stroke, yet only 64% were being treated with either drug. Many doctors are hesitant to prescribe the drugs because they are not prepared to do the necessary monitoring of patients and/or they fear bleeding complications.

Early Treatment Is Best

Eric Topol, MD, chairman, department of cardiology, The Cleveland Clinic, Cleveland, OH.

Starting treatment earlier could reduce heart attack deaths by 15%. On average, treatment now starts almost three hours after the onset of symptoms.

Self-defense: If you have symptoms of a heart attack, seek treatment immediately.

Danger symptoms: Pain or pressure in the chest that lasts more than a few minutes...pain radiating to shoulders, neck or arms...lightheadedness...nausea...shortness of breath.

4

Your Doctor and You

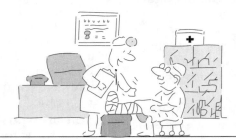

The Smart Way to Pick a Physician

Timothy McCall, MD

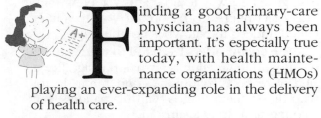Finding a good primary-care physician has always been important. It's especially true today, with health maintenance organizations (HMOs) playing an ever-expanding role in the delivery of health care.

In most HMOs and other managed-care plans, your primary-care doctor acts as the "gatekeeper." He/she decides when you can see a specialist, get physical therapy, be hospitalized, etc.

Since HMO doctors receive financial incentives to keep costs down, it's important to find someone who'll balance the insurance company's desire to maximize profits with your own health needs.

How do you find a good doctor? Whether you belong to an HMO or have traditional insurance

coverage, much of the conventional wisdom is misguided.

Some experts say to choose a doctor on the strength of her credentials. It is sensible to find out where your doctor went to medical school and whether she's board-certified. But a doctor who went to a prestigious medical school like Johns Hopkins, may have graduated last in her class. You might be better off with someone who excelled at the Medical College of Who-Knows-Where. Credentials can be misleading.

Other experts say it's best to ask friends and family members to recommend a doctor. That's not always a good idea.

Most people are pretty good at judging bedside manner, and that's important. But some doctors with a pleasant manner don't practice good medicine. Few people are equipped to judge a doctor's medical judgment and skills.

Timothy McCall, MD, a Boston internist, author of *Examining Your Doctor: A Patient's Guide to Avoiding Harmful Medical Care*. Citadel Press. He is a regular commentator on the public radio program Marketplace, and can be found on the Web at *www.drmccall.com*.

A more reliable way to find a good doctor is to get a recommendation from a medical insider. If you know someone who works in a hospital or clinic, that person probably knows the scuttlebutt about local doctors—which ones are good and, more important, which ones you should avoid.

Once you've found a few good prospects, how do you narrow the field?

Conventional wisdom says to interview each doctor until you find one you feel comfortable with. Many physicians will agree to a brief "get acquainted" session. It's not a bad idea. You may learn a bit about a doctor's bedside manner and maybe even her medical philosophy.

Ultimately, though, it's not the doctor's credentials or reputation or what she says that matters. What matters is how well she practices. Contrary to popular belief, just about anyone can judge that.

Start by reading up on any condition you're diagnosed with and any drug you're prescribed. The more you know, the better your ability to assess a doctor's knowledge and skills.

Probably the easiest thing to determine is whether the doctor is spending enough time with you.

A careful interview and a thorough physical exam are the foundation of good medical practice—and they take time. So do explaining things and answering questions.

Since clinics and HMOs are pressuring doctors to spend less time with their patients, I believe the amount of time a doctor spends with you is the best single indication of how concerned she is with your welfare. A doctor who's willing to buck the system to give you the time you need may also be more likely to go to bat for you if your insurer tries to deny you a needed service.

The process of evaluating a doctor should be ongoing. There's only so much you can find out about a doctor before your first appointment. Over time you'll learn much more.

It's like choosing a job or a college. You make your best guess, but you often don't know what you've got till you've had it for a while.

How to Get the Most from Your Doctor–Patient Relationship

Bernard Lown, MD, professor emeritus of cardiology at Harvard University School of Public Health and a senior physician at Brigham and Women's Hospital, both in Boston. He is author of *The Lost Art of Healing.* Houghton Mifflin.

Does your doctor really care about you …or just treat you? As a doctor with more than 40 years of experience, I can attest to the fact that a good doctor–patient relationship greatly reduces the anxiety associated with being sick. It also improves the likelihood that you'll get good medical care.

Lesson: It pays to examine a doctor's demeanor at least as carefully as you examine the diplomas hanging in his/her office.

Here are seven signs that you've come to the right office…

• **You talk with the doctor *before* disrobing.** If upon arriving for your first appointment, you are led to an exam room and asked to take off your clothes, you're at a patient "mill"—not a doctor's office.

Your first meeting with the doctor should be in his private office—while you are fully clothed. His initial goal should be to put you at ease. The best way to do that is via a few minutes of conversation. Forcing you to shiver naked under a thin gown is not the way.

• **The doctor offers his hand to you.** Extending a hand in greeting is a small but significant sign of respect. I wouldn't condemn a doctor who didn't shake hands with his patients, but it counts as a strike against him.

Similarly, does the doctor assume that it's fine to call you by your first name? Doing so is a sign of disrespect. A good doctor asks his patients what they wish to be called—then respects their wishes.

• **The doctor is on time.** A doctor may want you to *think* he's late because he has given priority to patients sicker than you. That's rarely the case.

Consistent lateness is inevitably the result of poor management, overbooking and/or arrogance—an indifference to the time of others. A good doctor shows respect for his patients by seeing them on time.

•The doctor is not interrupted by phone calls. Your doctor's concentration is broken every time he answers his secretary's buzz. I've forbidden my assistant to interrupt me except for a dire emergency. A good doctor responds to phone calls between patients.

•The doctor is optimistic. A doctor's mood influences not only a patient's emotional status, but also his/her medical outcome. Words can either heal or harm, and a good doctor knows this.

Your doctor should be upbeat no matter what your condition. There's always *something* that can be done to help—even if it's just to lessen your anxiety. I tell my patients that they no longer have to worry about their illness because I'll be the one taking over that duty from now on.

•The doctor takes a careful history. Seventy-five percent of the information needed to make an accurate diagnosis comes from taking a careful and detailed patient history.

This makes sense. While a doctor may know a great deal about a particular illness, he knows little about how that illness manifests itself in you. Only you can reveal that, and only if he pays attention to what you tell him.

Your doctor should question you closely not only about your medical condition, but also about your work, social relationships and any other aspects of your life that might be affecting your health. Taking a good medical history is the single most important sign of good doctoring.

•You *feel* cared for. Each time you leave your doctor's office, you should feel better emotionally, if not physically. You should feel that the doctor took your concerns seriously and answered all your questions.

The doctor should talk in terms you can understand, but you should never get the feeling you're being talked down to.

Mostly, you should have confidence in the doctor not just because of his expertise, but because he's another human being who has made a commitment to care for you.

HOW'S YOUR DOCTOR?

If you've broken your foot and the best orthopedist in town is gruff and rushed, so be it. Since you'll be under his care only for a limited period of time, his expertise is more important than his personality.

But I wouldn't be so quick to excuse a difficult demeanor in my primary care physician.

If your doctor doesn't meet all the criteria listed above, let him know. You might even give him a copy of this article—just to get the conversation going.

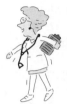

How to Get The Best Care From Your Doctor

Richard L. Sribnick, MD, an internist in private practice in Columbia, SC. He is coauthor of *Smart Patient, Good Medicine: Working with Your Doctor to Get the Best Medical Care*. Walker & Co.

Although conscientious doctors try to provide good care for all patients, they tend to do their best work for patients with whom they have good rapport.

The doctor-patient relationship, like any other, requires effort to make it work. *Here's how...*

•Speak clearly and concisely when describing your symptoms. Though a physical exam and lab tests may follow, the first—and often critical—ingredient for an accurate diagnosis is how well you describe your symptoms.

A good description reduces the risk of misdiagnosis...and helps you avoid needless diagnostic tests and surgical procedures.

Helpful: Prepare your spiel ahead of time —in writing. If you wait until you're half-clothed in the doctor's office, you may have a hard time expressing your thoughts clearly. *Four key issues:*

•When did the problem first appear?

•Where is it located? Be specific. "Pain in the temples" is better than "a headache."

•How does it feel? Is it a stabbing pain? Throbbing? How often does it occur? How long does it last?

91

•**What** brings it on or makes it worse? What relieves it? What other symptoms occur at the same time?

If you have several problems, list all of them as soon as the doctor walks into the examination room. Let *him/her* decide which to pursue first.

Say you've been experiencing chest pain. How do you describe your symptoms to the doctor?

Wrong: "My chest feels funny sometimes at work. It's probably just stress."

A busy doctor may dismiss this problem as trivial, and not investigate further.

Right: "I feel like there's a fist tightening in the center of my chest. This chest pressure began several weeks ago and lasts for a couple of minutes each time. I first noticed it after walking up two flights of stairs at work. I felt better after I stopped to rest."

Such a description will alert the doctor to the possibility of heart disease, and the need for diagnostic tests like angiography.

•**Be calm—but not stoic.** If you don't look like you're in pain, the doctor may fail to appreciate just how much it hurts. If you make light of a symptom, he is likely to do so as well.

Important: Share your concerns. If you fear that your headaches are being caused by a brain tumor, for instance, say so. But do so *after* you've described your symptoms. That way, the doctor's thinking won't be biased.

Whatever you do, *don't* panic. If you do, the doctor may be tempted to order needless tests and procedures to comfort you.

•**Adopt a positive attitude.** Some patients exhibit a negative, almost accusatory attitude when talking to the doctor. It's an attitude exemplified by statements such as, "I want my money's worth here, and I don't want you to cut any corners."

Such an attitude puts the doctor on the defensive. That can lead to hostility, and it's hard for a doctor to provide good care when he's mad at you.

If you tend to leave your doctor's office feeling shortchanged of time or attention, you may need another doctor.

If you have this feeling with several different doctors, odds are you need a new *attitude*. Discuss the situation with a friend whose judgment you respect.

•**Don't put up with rudeness.** If you feel you've been treated poorly by the doctor or his staff, let him know. Just be sure to do so diplomatically. Make it clear that your purpose is problem-solving, so you can work better together.

Wrong: "Why do I always have to wait? Isn't my time important too?"

Right: "How can I minimize the time I have to wait?"

Always wait until the *end* of your visit to voice any complaints. That way, the doctor can turn his full attention to your medical problem—without being distracted by his own defensiveness.

•**Take steps to avoid frustration.** Minimize waiting for appointments by scheduling routine visits for the first slot after the doctor's lunch hour.

If that slot is unavailable, ask for the first appointment in the morning.

If the doctor agrees to "work you in" between appointments, ask in advance how long you'll have to wait. That will give you a sense of control—and reduce your frustration.

Phone strategy: Unless it is a true emergency, don't expect to speak with the doctor right away.

Tell the receptionist you would like the doctor to call you as soon as it's convenient.

In an emergency, of course, don't hesitate to ask the nurse to interrupt the doctor.

Prescription refills: Call during office hours, not on evenings or weekends. Call from home or work—not the pharmacy. Ask the doctor or nurse approximately when the prescription will be phoned in.

•**Show your appreciation.** Like everyone else, doctors want to feel good about their work…and they have affection for patients who express their appreciation for their efforts.

Don't be afraid to say "thank you" to your doctor. A simple note can really make a doctor's day—and improve the quality of your care.

How to Get the Most From Your HMO

Timothy McCall, MD, a Boston internist, author of *Examining Your Doctor: A Patient's Guide to Avoiding Harmful Medical Care*. Citadel Press. He is a regular commentator on the public radio program Marketplace, and can be found on the Web at *www.drmccall.com*.

If you're not already enrolled in a health maintenance organization (HMO) or other managed-care plan, you may be soon. Three-quarters of American workers are enrolled in some form of managed care (HMO, PPO, POS) plan.

The number in traditional fee-for-service insurance is decreasing every year, and even these plans increasingly incorporate managed care features.

The rules are very different in this new system. To get good care, you must understand how managed care works and adjust your approach accordingly.

The first thing to understand is how the financial incentives for doctors have changed. Under the fee-for-service system, insurance companies paid doctors for every service rendered. Each time doctors stuck in a needle, ran a cardiogram or took out someone's tonsils, they were paid.

Unfortunately, doctors responded to this arrangement by doing millions of needless tonsillectomies and other procedures. As a result, medical costs skyrocketed, with health care consuming a larger and larger chunk of the GNP.

HMOs came along and changed the way doctors are paid. Although they use dozens of different systems, the bottom line in most plans is this—*the less the doctor does, the more money he or she makes*.

It's increasingly common for doctors to receive a flat monthly fee for every patient under their care. Under this arrangement, known as *capitation*, the cost of lab tests, procedures and other care comes out of the doctor's pocket. If the doctor orders an $80 X ray, $80 is deducted from his paycheck.

Frequently, HMOs give bonuses and assess monetary penalties according to how much the doctor spends. For example, many HMOs reward doctors who limit the number of patients they hospitalize or who minimize referrals to expensive specialists. Using a technique known as "economic credentialing," managed-care plans terminate doctors who spend too much on patients.

To further limit costs, HMOs set up barriers to care. Under most managed-care plans, you can't see a specialist without being referred by your primary care doctor. Visits to the emergency room require pre-authorization. And it can take weeks—even months—to get an appointment.

Given these new realities, here's how to protect your interests. If you're thinking of joining an HMO or are already enrolled, learn as much as you can about the plan. Read the membership materials carefully. If possible, talk to current and former members about their experiences with the HMO in question.

Since your primary care doctor functions as the "gatekeeper"—blocking or granting access to specialists—choosing a good gatekeeper can be vital. You want someone who, if necessary, will appeal on your behalf if you need a special test or an extra day in the hospital. It's often hard to tell much about a doctor from the brochures, so again, talk to other members, even people you bump into in the waiting room.

If you feel you're being unjustly denied services you need, don't be afraid to fight for them. If politely making your case to your doctor doesn't work, try appealing to an administrator. All HMOs have formal grievance procedures.

Finally, the more you can learn about any medical conditions you have, the better position you'll be in to assert yourself. HMO doctors have a difficult time saying no to reasonable, well-informed patients.

Don't forget, though, much of the medical care we've come to expect really isn't necessary. Sometimes you really don't need that $80 X ray.

How to Get the Very Best Possible Medical Care

Peter H. Berczeller, MD, former professor of clinical medicine, New York University School of Medicine, New York City. A practicing internist from 1960 until his retirement in 1992, he is author of *Doctors and Patients: What We Feel About You.* Macmillan.

Visiting the doctor can be a stressful experience—whether the visit is for a routine checkup or to diagnose a troubling symptom. And with so much negative press about health care these days, anxiety among patients seems to be at an all-time high. Soaring costs, needless tests, faulty diagnoses and uncaring doctors are but a few of the chief complaints patients have today.

As a result, there's growing tension—even hostility—between doctors and patients.

In some cases, this tension is beneficial to patients—as when it motivates them to take a more active role in their treatment, for example. In other cases, doctor–patient tension leads patients to act in ways that are self-defeating and detrimental to their care.

Here's how to be a better patient—and how to bring out the very best in your physician…

●**Choose a doctor who is emotionally accessible.** Ideally, you want someone who conveys a sense of genuine concern, interest and involvement…and in whom you feel you can confide.

Do *not* select a doctor solely for his/her technical expertise. If I had a choice between a genius doctor and one who was merely competent but warm and humane, I'd pick the latter.

Reason: Easy, open communication between doctor and patient is essential both to the diagnosis and the healing process.

●**Tell your doctor all your concerns.** If it's your first visit, come prepared to give a complete medical history. If your records are on file with another doctor, make sure they've been transferred to the new doctor. On subsequent visits, report in detail any symptoms or changes you've experienced since your last visit. If you tend to be forgetful, bring a written list of all your concerns to your appointment.

●**Dress and behave appropriately.** Although the doctor is working for you, it's important to treat him with respect. Proper attire and courteous behavior not only are polite, but they can enhance your care. When I was seeing patients, I have to admit that I tended to listen just a little bit better when the patient was nicely dressed and well-spoken.

Proper attire and courteous behavior on the part of both the doctor and the patient help to dignify their interaction—entirely appropriate, given the serious nature of what patients and doctors talk about.

●**Tell the doctor if you're dissatisfied with your medical care.** Being honest and direct helps clear the air and puts your relationship on a better footing.

Some patients keep their negative thoughts to themselves, fearing that complaining will simply antagonize the doctor…and that he will retaliate by providing inferior care. Such thinking is misguided. In fact, because good communication is critical to receiving good health care, there's nothing most doctors like more than an open, honest patient.

Bonus: By revealing your inner feelings, you'll make it easier for your doctor to help you cope with the anxiety or helplessness that often accompanies illness. In other words, telling your doctor how you feel is a little like undergoing psychotherapy.

●**Don't expect your doctor to be perfect.** Doctors are human, and they make mistakes. While a big mistake is reason to find a new doctor, inconsequential ones are no cause for alarm.

Solution: You and your family must be assertive, vigilant and actively involved in your care. Politely question all medications given to you. Any allergies you have should be detailed in your medical record—but be sure to mention them to the doctor just in case.

If you're to be hospitalized, ask friends and relatives to watch out for you. Tell them to alert the doctor or nurse if they notice you don't look right.

●**Don't be put off if your doctor sometimes appears uncertain.** Far from being a liability, a doctor's uncertainty can be very helpful—it can even lead to better care. The best doctors don't try to project a sense of omniscience. Rather, they realize that there's always something else they can learn...and that there's always room for improvement in their performance.

●**Know when to get a second opinion.** An unusual physical finding, a lab test that doesn't make sense, an unexpected worsening of your condition—all suggest the need for a second opinion.

Problem: Some patients are too timid to seek one, fearing that doing so will offend their doctor. While some doctors are defensive about the prospect of an outside consultation, most are perfectly happy if the patient wants to seek another opinion.

Other patients are too *quick* to seek a second opinion—sometimes seeking one even before the first one has been rendered. I think it's best to wait until your doctor has had a chance to make a diagnosis and plan a treatment strategy.

Give your doctor a chance to set the scene properly—to find order in the random set of symptoms and findings and to give your condition a name.

To do this, a doctor must order appropriate diagnostic tests and observe you over a period of time. Hard as it is to believe, there's a logic and rhythm to each illness. Some take weeks or even months to identify—even if your doctor is first-rate.

There's simply no substitute for the imagination, enthusiasm and—most important—the concern that comes from a conscientious doctor who has been involved in your care from the outset. That's why the timing of other opinions is so critical.

●**Don't let family members become obstacles to your treatment.** Loved ones are invaluable as sources of emotional support. But too often they get in the way of your treatment—by interfering with the doctor's decisions...or by being hostile toward the doctor in a misguided attempt to show love for you.

A doctor who asks family members to leave a patient's room is not trying to demonstrate his power. Chances are, he simply wants an opportunity to form his own impression of the patient—without outside interference.

It's surprising just how much information can be obtained from a patient if there's nobody there to speak for him.

●**Develop a solid, caring relationship with one doctor.** While it's sometimes necessary to "fire" a doctor or to get a second opinion, some patients run from doctor to doctor haphazardly. *Skipping from doctor to doctor...*

●**Makes you easy prey for quacks** and other practitioners eager to exploit your obvious anxiety and subject you to needless tests and expensive treatments.

●**Delays your diagnosis.** The workup required for a diagnosis usually begins anew each time a new doctor is consulted.

●**Leads you to get the diagnosis you want to hear**—rather than the diagnosis that's most accurate.

For true healing to occur, a one-on-one, caring relationship with your doctor is essential. You should maintain this relationship with a primary doctor even if your condition necessitates consulting a specialist...or getting a second opinion.

Doctors are not magicians. Leaving one—especially someone who has a good track record with you—and seeking out another is not usually the answer. The new "magician" will probably not cure you any more quickly, and switching mid-illness will probably cause even more delay in making you better.

Questions to Ask When Your Doctor Recommends a Specialist

Charles Inlander, president of The People's Medical Society, a patient advocate organization, 462 Walnut St., Allentown, PA 18102. He is author of several books, including *The People's Medical Society Health Desk Reference.* Hyperion.

Finding the best medical specialist takes more than just getting a name and phone number from your doctor. *Steps to take...*

●**First ask your doctor why you are being referred to this particular specialist.**

Trap: Referrals are often professional courtesies. This may mean that a fellow colleague isn't likely to contradict your doctor's recommendations or that you may not be getting the name of the best person to confirm a diagnosis or treat your condition.

Important: Find out if your doctor knows the specialist's success rate in treating your problem. This is basic information that your doctor should know about the doctor to whom he is referring you.

●**Ask your doctor for a list of all the likely medical causes of your condition before you seek another opinion.** Similar symptoms can exist for different problems. Find out from your doctor the most likely causes of your problem...and the most remote causes. This information will help you when you seek another opinion.

Example: Hearing loss can indicate that you have damage to the eardrum—or a brain tumor. But the specialists who can diagnose and treat these conditions are in different fields. One is an ear, nose and throat specialist...and the other one is a neurologist or a neurosurgeon.

You can save yourself a lot of time and money by learning—and prioritizing—all your options before you shop around.

●**Once you have a diagnosis, find out how many times the specialist has treated your kind of problem within the last year.** Volume is critical, although the ideal volume depends on the problem being treated. For common problems, such as heart surgery, a specialist should treat hundreds of people a year. For rarer conditions, 10 to 20 cases is acceptable.

If the specialist's office is reluctant to share this information, consider seeking treatment elsewhere.

●**Get the name of a specialist who can give you a second opinion.** Up to 80% of second opinions on *treatments* don't agree with the first. Twenty percent of second opinions disagree with *diagnosis.* That's why it's important to seek several opinions.

If you have trouble finding someone, call the national headquarters of that specialty's association for a few names.

If you live in a rural or suburban area that doesn't have a concentration of specialists with the breadth of experience you need, it's worth it to get in the car or on the plane and go somewhere that does.

●**Find out if there are other treatment options.** Get a treatment plan from each doctor whom you see for an opinion. Then phone a prominent medical school in your state and ask to speak to the person who chairs the department under which your problem falls—for example, the orthopedic surgery department if surgery has been recommended for a knee injury. He/she may be willing to tell you about recent medical advances in the field. You can also do your own research through a local medical school library or an online medical database.

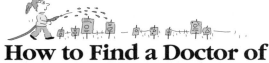

How to Find a Doctor of Alternative Medicine

For a free referral to an alternative doctor in your area, contact the American College for Advancement in Medicine, Box 3427, Laguna Hills, CA 92654. Include a self-addressed, stamped, business-sized envelope.

Is Your Doctor Listening?

Robert A. Murden, MD, associate professor of clinical medicine, Ohio State University, Columbus. His six-month study of 818 subjects was published in *Medical Care,* 227 E. Washington Sq., Philadelphia 19106.

Doctors aren't good at listening to patients their own age. If your doctor seems to be a poor listener and he/she is roughly your age, consider looking for a new physician who is significantly younger or older.

Better Doctor–Patient Communications

Timothy McCall, MD, a Boston internist, author of *Examining Your Doctor: A Patient's Guide to Avoiding Harmful Medical Care.* Citadel Press. He is a regular commentator on the public radio program Marketplace, and can be found on the Web at *www.drmccall.com.*

Don't be intimidated by your doctor's manner. Decide what you want to talk about before your appointment—and make a list if necessary. Maintain eye contact with your doctor, both to show that you're participating in the process and to encourage the doctor to deal more directly with you. Don't let your doctor avoid answering your questions or make insensitive comments that go unchallenged. If your efforts to improve communications fail, consider finding another doctor.

The Right Way to Talk to Your Doctor

Timothy McCall, MD, a Boston internist, author of *Examining Your Doctor: A Patient's Guide to Avoiding Harmful Medical Care.* Citadel Press. He is a regular commentator on the public radio program Marketplace, and can be found on the Web at *www.drmccall.com.*

While most people know that it's important to talk to the doctor, what they really focus on are diagnostic tests like X rays, blood analyses and electrocardiograms.

If a doctor fails to order tests, many people believe that he or she hasn't taken their complaints seriously.

But studies have shown that in three out of four cases good doctors arrive at an accurate diagnosis just by talking with their patients. The physical exam yields another 12% of diagnoses. Lab tests and X rays account for only about 11%.

Even when tests do lead to a diagnosis, often it's information gleaned from the interview that enabled the doctor to decide which tests were necessary.

The beauty of the medical interview is that it's inexpensive and—unlike medical tests—it has no undesirable side effects. Time spent talking also builds rapport—and that in itself can be very therapeutic.

To get the most from the patient interview, the doctor must devote enough time to it. Unfortunately, physicians are under increasing pressure from insurance administrators and health maintenance organizations to cut down the length of office visits. As a result, many doctors have begun to skimp on the interview. But good doctors resist the pressure and spend the time to do the job right.

Doctors and patients alike have a role to play in making the most of their time together.

Doctors must use good interview techniques. The first rule is to allow the patient to talk without needless interruption. Sounds simple enough. But one study found that, on average, doctors listened to their patients for only 18 seconds before interrupting. Once interrupted, patients rarely return to what they had intended to say. As a result, important clues are lost.

It's also poor technique if the doctor attempts to control the conversation by barraging you with yes or no questions. This tactic results in less accurate information and missed diagnoses. Doctors should favor open-ended questions like, *What's bothering you?* or *Is there something you're worried this might be?*

Smart patients help their doctors get the most from the interview by preparing for their appointments. Before you go in to see your doctor, plan what you'd like to cover. Write down all your questions, but be realistic. It's impossible to cover a whole laundry list in a few minutes. Stick with those items of greatest importance to you. If you can't cover everything you need to, schedule a return visit.

If you're going in to have a specific symptom evaluated, ask yourself: When did it start? When does it happen? How long does it last? Is there anything that makes it better or worse? Have I ever had anything similar?

If the problem is pain, try to pinpoint its location in your body. Is the pain sharp? Crampy? Does it feel like pins and needles?

Honesty and openness are vital to a good medical interview. Unfortunately, doctors and patients tend to avoid embarrassing topics like sexuality and incontinence. Steering away from such areas can compromise your medical care.

Sexual difficulties, for example, can provide important clues to such problems as diabetes, thyroid disorders and medication side effects. And in this age of AIDS, knowledge of a patient's sexual habits can help the doctor recognize early symptoms and—more important —teach the patient how to avoid becoming infected in the first place.

Considering the importance of the medical interview, maybe it's time you had a little talk with your doctor.

Is There Something Your Doctor Isn't Telling You?

Timothy McCall, MD, a Boston internist, author of *Examining Your Doctor: A Patient's Guide to Avoiding Harmful Medical Care.* Citadel Press. He is a regular commentator on the public radio program Marketplace, and can be found on the Web at *www.drmccall.com.*

Doctors depend upon their patients to be open and honest in discussing their health concerns. But there are a few things that some doctors prefer their *patients* didn't know.

Here's what your doctor may not be revealing to you:

●**"I've been sued for malpractice."** Many doctors who have been sued—even repeatedly —continue to practice without their patients having any idea. Most malpractice settlements are shrouded in secrecy by agreements that prevent the information from ever becoming public. Since doctors may not want to reveal past disciplinary actions against them either, you may want to check out information collected by the Public Citizen health research group.

This consumer advocacy group publishes information on disciplinary actions against doctors. To obtain a report on actions taken against doctors in your state, contact the group at 202-588-1000 or online at *www.citizen.org.* The report costs $20.

●**"I'm years out of date."** Medical information is mushrooming so fast that no doctor can keep up completely. But some doctors do a better job than others.

To tell if your doctor is up-to-date, learn as much as possible about any condition you're diagnosed with. Start with consumer health guides and articles in magazines and newsletters. For more information, spend time at your local library or do research on the Internet. You'll be able to spot doctors who are dangerously behind the times.

The federal government and hundreds of consumer organizations provide free or low-cost health information. And, for a fee, private health research firms will provide you with a detailed report on your ailment.

●**"The HMO pays me a bonus for not referring you to a specialist."** Most health maintenance organizations and other managed-care plans give doctors financial incentives for keeping costs down. Doctors get bonuses for such things as reducing the number of referrals to specialists, keeping patients out of the hospital and cutting down on MRI scans and other expensive services.

Since it's hard to learn this information from the plans themselves, I recommend discussing the matter with your employer's benefits manager.

If that doesn't work, ask your doctor directly. You might say, "It's not that I don't trust you, Dr. Smith, but I've been reading a lot about HMOs lately and would appreciate knowing if the doctors have any financial incentives to limit certain services." Some plans forbid doctors from revealing how they're paid. If your doctor says he or she cannot tell you, that's a bad sign.

●**"I'm not what I claim to be."** A study in *The New England Journal of Medicine* revealed that many doctors who call themselves specialists have never had the required training or passed the rigorous exam required for board certification. In teaching hospitals medical students sometimes fool patients by introducing themselves as "Dr. So and So."

To find out if a particular doctor is certified, call the American Board of Medical Specialties (866-ASK-ABMS). Better HMOs and hospitals generally check the credentials of their doctors—but it certainly doesn't hurt for you to check, too.

If you're hospitalized, insist that anyone rendering care tell you his name and training. This will help you spot poorly trained aides who—in an attempt to cut costs—hospitals are now substituting for registered nurses.

What you don't know—and what your doctor may not be telling you—could indeed hurt you. Unless you do your homework.

Protect Yourself From Your Doctor's Financial Interests

Marc A. Rodwin, PhD, JD, associate professor of law and public policy at Indiana University in Bloomington. He is author of *Medicine, Money and Morals: Physicians' Conflicts of Interest*. Oxford University Press.

We trust our doctors to make our health the highest priority—to "do the right thing" when ordering tests, prescribing drugs, etc. In taking the Hippocratic Oath, they swore to do just that.

Like the rest of us, however, doctors must earn a living. And sometimes the treatment a doctor prescribes—or withholds—has a direct bearing on his/her own financial well-being.

DOCTORS, HOSPITALS AND LABS

Some doctors have a financial stake in a diagnostic lab, hospital or another local health-care facility. Others don't have a direct stake—but have a close relative who does.

With such an arrangement, each referral the doctor makes is, effectively, a self-referral. Each time he orders a $1,000 MRI exam or puts you in the hospital, he turns a profit—or turns a profit for someone to whom he's closely tied.

Such an arrangement tempts doctors to order needless tests, recommend needless operations and hospitalizations, etc.

Or doctors may be tempted to send you to a hospital that handles their bills or provides them with other perks—even when another hospital is better equipped to treat your specific ailment. Doctors who have a financial stake in a health-care facility make referrals to it more often than doctors who lack such an interest, studies have shown.

Self-defense: Ask your doctor, "What financial ties or other arrangements do you have with the lab (or hospital) you're sending me to?" The fewer ties, the better.

In areas with few doctors, it may be impractical to reject a doctor simply because he owns a share of a local diagnostic lab. You may not have a choice. Or—your illness may require immediate attention, leaving you little time to consider other options.

But if you have a choice, a doctor's financial ties are a factor to consider—along with his training, reputation, etc.

NEEDLESS PROCEDURES

Doctors who work under the traditional "fee-for-service" system get paid for each service they render to patients. With such a setup, it's always in a doctor's financial interest to do more procedures—not fewer.

Most doctors manage to resist the obvious temptation to perform needless surgery, order superfluous diagnostic tests, etc. But the profit motive can—and sometimes does—cloud clinical judgment.

Self-defense: If your doctor recommends endoscopy, hysterectomy, catheterization or another invasive diagnostic test or elective (non-emergency) surgery, get a second opinion. Find a physician with no ties to your doctor—ideally someone who practices at another hospital.

DRUG COMPANY GIFTS

For almost any illness, a range of treatment options is available. But drugmakers spend millions of dollars on marketing campaigns designed to convince doctors that drug therapy is the best route.

And—each drugmaker spends millions on advertisements designed to convince doctors to use its drug. These efforts don't end at advertising.

Kickbacks are illegal. But drugmakers find other ways to ensure that doctors think of their products when they reach for a prescription pad.

Usual approach: Showering doctors with inexpensive gifts such as pens embossed with the name of the drug being promoted...or coffee and danish in the doctors' lounge.

But drug companies have also been known to offer doctors...

- **All-expenses-paid weekends** at resorts hosting "educational seminars" on new drugs.
- **Super Bowl tickets.**
- **Cash payments** for participating in "market research."

Bottom line: The drug your doctor prescribes may be the one he's been persuaded to prescribe. That might not be the cheapest drug or the most effective one for your condition.

Self-defense: If you have a chronic condition such as arthritis or asthma, find out which drug (or nondrug therapy) is best for you. Explore all of the alternatives.

Conduct research at your local library or on the World Wide Web...consult a drug reference book such as Dr. Sidney M. Wolfe's *Worst Pills Best Pills II* (Pantheon)...and/or contact the National Self-Help Clearinghouse (212-817-1822) to locate a support group in your local area.

Once your research is done, ask the doctor, "What makes the drug (or treatment) you've chosen a better choice than other drugs (or treatments) that are available?" Be sure to inquire about any possible side effects.

PERILS OF MANAGED CARE

Most health maintenance organizations (HMOs) pay doctors a monthly fee for each patient, rather than for each service. The doctor is paid the same sum whether he sees you once a year or 20 times. Performing procedures or scheduling follow-up visits means that he does more work without getting paid more.

This arrangement—called *capitation*—keeps costs down by encouraging doctors to provide *less care.* The risk, of course, is that a doctor might withhold care a patient needs.

HMOs also limit spending via *risk sharing.* Here, the doctor and the HMO share the financial risk for the cost of services. Risk sharing discourages doctors from making referrals, ordering tests, hospitalizing patients or recommending costly treatments.

Lawsuit: A woman claimed risk sharing discouraged her doctor from ordering a biopsy despite her symptoms of breast cancer. By the time her cancer was diagnosed, it had spread.

Self-defense: Ask your doctor, "What percentage of your income depends on risk sharing incentives and bonuses?" The larger the percentage, the more likely his judgment will be compromised.

To Take Charge of Your Medical Care...

Richard N. Podell, MD, clinical professor of family medicine, Robert Wood Johnson Medical School, New Providence, NJ. He is author of *When Your Doctor Doesn't Know Best.* Simon & Schuster.

Choose a doctor whose office hours fit your schedule—and who is available by phone. Research your symptoms before an appointment and prepare a list of questions. Take notes on the answers. Keep a journal with dates of shots, illnesses, aches and pains to help pinpoint problems more quickly. Ask to see your records and have them explained to you.

To Control Your Medical Costs...

Charles Inlander, president of The People's Medical Society, a patient advocate organization, 462 Walnut St., Allentown, PA 18102. He is author of several books, including *The People's Medical Society Health Desk Reference.* Hyperion.

Negotiate with your doctor to keep charges in line. Find out what other doctors in your area charge for the same procedure. Make mention of your research to your doctor and ask him/her to accept the rate charged by his peers.

Also: Work out fees for regular treatments —for instance, a charge only for a shot when you need one regularly, instead of an extra charge for an office visit each time. And—try to get flat rates for some procedures, such as being charged one price for having several moles removed instead of a rate per mole.

GPs Often Err When Prescribing Psychiatric Drugs

Cecilia P. Kane, MD, department of psychiatry, Emory University School of Medicine, Atlanta.

General practitioners (GPs) may not keep up with the trends in prescribing psychiatric medications...or they may prescribe dosages that are too high or too low.

Shocking: Of 145 *diazepam* (Valium) prescriptions dispensed by general practitioners at one hospital, 43% were for patients over 65—even though the drug is not recommended for older patients.

To Prevent High Blood Pressure in The Doctor's Office

Claude Le Pailleur, MD, clinical cardiologist, Hôpital Necker, Paris. His study of 42 adults with high blood pressure was published in *Behavioral Medicine*, 1319 18 St. NW, Washington, DC 20036.

Limit conversation with your doctor before he/she takes your blood pressure.

Background: Many people whose blood pressure is normal at other times experience a sudden rise in pressure at the doctor's office. *Cause:* Anxiety associated with interacting with the doctor. This "white coat" effect—named for the doctor's garb—makes it hard to get an accurate reading.

Study: Hypertensive patients who talked with the doctor before having their blood pressure checked had a sudden rise in blood pressure. This effect was more drastic during discussions of stress and disease than during chitchat. During periods of silence, blood pressure rapidly fell.

Dirty Hands and Doctors

William R. Jarvis, MD, chief, investigation and prevention branch, Hospital Infections Program, Centers for Disease Control and Prevention, Atlanta.

Doctors wash their hands between patients only 50% of the time. Dirty hands spread everything from colds, flu and diarrhea to pneumonia and toxic shock syndrome.

Self-defense: Always make sure your doctor washes his/her hands before touching you.

Medical Hygiene

Jeffrey Jones, MD, associate professor of medicine, Michigan State University College of Medicine, East Lansing. His study and survey were published in the *Annals of Emergency Medicine*, 11830 Westline Industrial Dr., St. Louis 63146.

Dirty stethoscopes may be spreading illness. In a test of 150 stethoscopes, 133 were found to harbor staphylococcus bacteria. Asked how often they cleaned their stethoscopes, 48% of doctors said daily or weekly...37% said monthly...and 14% said once a year or *never*. While there have been no reported cases of infection spreading via dirty stethoscopes, outbreaks of drug-resistant bacteria have been linked to germ-laden blood pressure cuffs...thermometers...latex gloves...even doctors' white coats.

At greatest risk: Patients with burns or open wounds. Always ask if the doctor has cleaned his/her stethoscope.

Is Your Doctor Up-to-Date?

Charles Inlander, president of The People's Medical Society, a patient advocate organization, 462 Walnut St., Allentown, PA 18102. He is author of several books, including *The People's Medical Society Health Desk Reference*. Hyperion.

Find out if he/she has been certified or recertified by calling the American Board of Medical Specialties, 866-ASK-ABMS.

Ask the doctor how he completes the *continuing* medical education requirements imposed by all states. Find out if your doctor teaches or does research at a local medical school—which would make him more likely to have current knowledge.

MDs and Continuing Education

99 Questions You Should Ask Your Doctor and Why by Paul Keckley, PhD, president of a health care market research firm in Nashville. Rutledge Hill Press.

Continuing medical education is crucial to a doctor's ability to maintain his/her skill and training in the latest medical research and procedures. Ask your doctor how many hours of continuing medical education credits he averages in a year. And do your own research in areas of particular concern to you—then bring the material to your doctor's attention in case he has not seen it.

Plan Ahead for Medical Emergencies

Managing Your Health Care: Making the Most of Your Medical Resources by Martin Gipson, PhD, professor of psychology at University of the Pacific, Stockton, CA, who has been treated for kidney cancer since 1989. Pathfinder Publishing.

Ask your doctor where to call and where to go to in case of emergency. Anticipate medical-care needs before the weekend—do not ignore symptoms during the week that might become emergencies on the weekend. If communicating with doctors by phone, describe symptoms yourself—not through someone else—if possible.

Prescription Danger

Daniel Albrant, PharmD, president, Pharmacy Dynamics, a health care consulting company in Arlington, VA.

When writing prescriptions, few doctors take into account the patient's weight.

Trap: Most of the standard dosages are calibrated for a 155-pound person.

Example: A 130-pound person needs 10% to 15% less medication. Taking too much can cause nausea, drowsiness—or worse.

Self-defense: If you weigh less—or more—than 155 pounds, talk to your doctor to make sure he/she is prescribing the proper dosage.

When to Look for A New Doctor

John Connolly, EdD, former president, New York Medical College, and author of *How to Find the Best Doctors, Hospitals, HMOs for You and Your Family*. Castle Connolly Medical Ltd.

If your doctor has a poor bedside manner...is vague or evasive with explanations...is never on schedule...can't make a diagnosis...orders too many tests...discourages you from seeking a second opinion...doesn't protect patients' privacy...has an unpleasant office staff.

Women and Their Doctors

Lila Wallis, MD, a clinical professor of medicine at Cornell University Medical College and a former president of the American Medical Women's Association, Alexandria, VA.

Women must be more aggressive about their own health care. Studies show that some male doctors are not as attentive to the needs of their female patients as they are to the needs of their male patients. This does not mean that women should only see female doctors.

Vital for women: Come to your appointments prepared with questions...fill out the health questionnaire thoroughly…make notes of the doctor's answers to your questions as well as any advice…and be sure the doctor explores all the options for treating a particular problem.

Helpful: If a doctor has taken a course on *women's* health.

Easier Dental Visits

Thomas McGuire, DDS, dentist specializing in preventive care, president of Tooth Fitness, Grass Valley, CA, and author of *Tooth Fitness: Your Guide to Healthy Teeth.* St. Michael's Press.

For less stressful dental visits, plan to go before noon, when you can expect to have more energy. Take an aspirin an hour before the appointment to head off minor pain. Bring a book to pass time in the waiting room, and keep your mind occupied. Work out a stop signal with the dentist and assistant so you can let them know if you're feeling pain. Divert your attention by raising your foot or arm a few inches from the chair and holding it there. Concentrating on that makes it hard to focus on the dental procedure.

How to Tell a Good Dentist from a Bad One

Marvin J. Schissel, DDS, vice president of the New York chapter of the National Council Against Health Fraud, 8639 Woodhaven Blvd., Woodhaven, NY 11421. He is coauthor of *The Whole Tooth: What You Must Know to Find a Good Dentist, Keep Healthy Teeth, and Avoid the Incompetents, Quacks, and Frauds.* St. Martin's Press.

How do you tell a good dentist from a bad one? Here's what to look for…and look *out* for.

THE TIME FACTOR

At each checkup, your dentist should spend about 30 minutes examining your teeth and removing the plaque and mineral deposits known as tartar.

Filling a cavity could take 15 to 60 minutes, depending on the extent and location of the decay.

Also: A good dentist does not shuttle back and forth between his/her patients.

This might enable him to squeeze in a few more patients, but can a dentist who flits about the office really focus on his work? Not very likely.

TREATING GUM DISEASE

Gum disease is caused by bacteria that breed in "pockets" between the gum and the root of each tooth. Your dentist should measure the depth of these pockets using a *periodontal probe.* If your dentist fails to do so, remind him.

The best way to prevent gum disease—and to treat mild cases—is via meticulous scaling (scraping) of tartar and plaque, which harbor the disease-causing organisms.

But some dentists save time by having their patients *self-treat* gum disease by gargling at home with hydrogen peroxide and baking soda.

Problem: There's no evidence that peroxide/baking soda is more effective than ordinary brushing. It will not remove tartar.

THE EQUIPMENT FACTOR

Just because a dentist has the latest equipment does *not* mean that he provides cutting-edge care. In fact, some impressive gadgets have little impact on the level of care.

Example I: Some dentists show their patients video close-ups of areas of decay using an *intraoral camera.* This system provides dramatic pictures. But too often unscrupulous dentists use the camera to persuade patients to have unnecessary work.

Example II: Some dentists use a *Cavitron* to dislodge tartar from under the gum line. This device, which blasts tartar with high-frequency vibrations, can save time when the buildup is heavy. But even if he uses a Cavitron, a good dentist always finishes tartar removal by hand.

THE TRUTH ABOUT FILLINGS

For years "holistic" dentists have urged patients to have their old silver fillings (which contain mercury amalgam) replaced with fillings made of plastic composite.

These practitioners maintain that mercury leaches out of silver fillings, poisoning the body and causing multiple sclerosis and other diseases.

Yet there is no solid evidence linking silver fillings to health problems. A very few people are allergic to mercury, but they rarely develop anything more than a rash.

If a filling cracks or falls out, of course, it must be replaced. But steer clear of any dentist who urges you to replace intact fillings for health reasons.

Composite fillings blend in with the tooth color, so they're good for teeth in the front of the mouth. But amalgam costs less and lasts longer than composite, so it's still the best choice for out-of-sight fillings.

NEEDLESS EXTRACTIONS

Even badly decayed teeth can usually be saved with fillings or crowns (perhaps in conjunction with a root canal procedure).

But these time-intensive procedures are often poorly reimbursed by dental insurance companies. Consequently, some unscrupulous dentists save time by simply pulling such teeth.

If your dentist recommends pulling a tooth, ask him why the tooth cannot be saved. If you're not convinced by the explanation, get a second opinion.

5

The Truth About Medicines

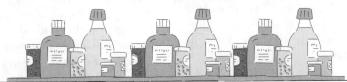

Where to Get Information On the Drugs You Take

Timothy McCall, MD

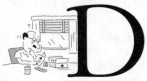rug side effects represent more than just an annoyance. They're one of the most frequent causes of hospitalization in the US. Some of these side effects occur as a result of a mistake by a doctor or pharmacist. Others occur when patients take their medicines incorrectly. Either way, your best protection is to learn as much as possible about every drug you're prescribed.

Ideally, your doctor would give you all the drug information you need. But that doesn't always happen. Many patients leave the doctor's office without knowing even the most basic information—such as how many times a day to take the drug or whether it should be taken with food.

Under managed care, the drug information problem is only getting worse. The length of the average doctor's appointment continues to decrease, with many appointments now lasting less than 10 minutes. That means the doctor has less time to explain things.

Good doctors still make the effort. When you walk out of the office, you should know the generic *and* brand names of any drug you've been prescribed. You should also know the dosage, how to take it and what to do if you miss a dose.

The doctor should also explain common side effects, as well as the symptoms that suggest a serious problem—and what to do if they appear.

Many doctors and clinics now offer patient handouts that explain medications. They're a great idea as long as they're written in plain English—and if they aren't used as a substitute for the brief question-and-answer session that should be a part of every doctor's appointment.

Timothy McCall, MD, a Boston internist, author of *Examining Your Doctor: A Patient's Guide to Avoiding Harmful Medical Care.* Citadel Press. He is a regular commentator on the public radio program Marketplace, and can be found on the Web at *www.drmccall.com.*

Another good source of drug information is your pharmacist. He should be able to answer virtually all drug-related questions. Be sure to ask him for the "package insert" that comes with the drug. Although the typical insert is written in nearly impenetrable "medicalese," look through it anyway. Keep it around, too, in case you develop a problem later on.

Be sure to list for your doctor and pharmacist *every* medicine you're taking. That goes for over-the-counter and herbal preparations, too, since these can interact—sometimes in deadly fashion—with prescribed drugs. What *they* don't know could hurt you.

Have all your prescriptions filled at one pharmacy—ideally one with a computerized prescription system. That way, your entire medication history—including any drug allergies you might have—will be contained within a single file. This makes it easy for your pharmacist to spot any potential drug interaction or allergic reaction.

Managed care is affecting pharmacists as well as doctors. Independent drugstores, which often provide the most personalized attention, are being squeezed out by the big chains and mail-order houses, which offer HMOs deep discounts. Chain stores and mail-order drugs may save you money. However, you probably won't get much drug information. That means you must do more homework. Fortunately, several good consumer guides to drugs are available.

Recommended: Dr. Sidney M. Wolfe's *Worst Pills, Best Pills* (Pantheon), Dr. James Long's and Dr. James Rybacki's *The Essential Guide to Prescription Drugs* (HarperCollins) and Joe and Teresa Graedon's *The People's Pharmacy* (St. Martin's Press).

You can also get reliable drug information via the Internet. If you have access to the World Wide Web, here are two sites to try: RxList at *www.rxlist.com* and the US Pharmacopeia on the InteliHealth site at *www.inteli health.com*.

Important Drugs for Glaucoma, Cancer, Diabetes

Jack M. Rosenberg, PharmD, PhD, professor of clinical pharmacy and pharmacology at Long Island University (LIU), and director of the International Drug Information Center, both in Brooklyn, NY. Also participating in the interview were Lorraine Cicero, a research fellow at the Center, and Satyapal Pareddy, adjunct assistant professor of drug information at LIU.

Several years ago, the Food and Drug Administration approved a number of drugs for the treatment of diabetes and glaucoma...plus a drug that boosts the effectiveness of cancer chemotherapy.

CANCER

Many anticancer drugs are highly toxic to the heart. This risk of heart damage keeps doctors from giving the high doses that are sometimes needed to destroy a malignancy.

Good news: A drug called *dexrazoxane* (Zinecard) helps counteract this cardiotoxicity. So people with breast cancer, liver cancer or another serious malignancy will be able to take high-dose chemo—*without* a heightened risk of heart disease.

DIABETES

People with adult-onset diabetes who cannot control the disease with a special diet usually resort to Micronase, Diabeta or another drug that boosts the body's insulin output. When these oral medications don't work, diabetics have always had to opt for daily insulin injections.

Two oral drugs make shots unnecessary even for people with hard-to-control diabetes. *Acarbose* (Precose) slows carbohydrate digestion, keeping blood sugar levels steady. *Metformin* (Glucophage) slows the conversion of stored starch into sugar. It also helps the body use its own insulin more effectively. These medications can be combined with standard antidiabetic medications for a double-barreled effect.

Many people experience stomach upset when they begin taking Precose, but this usually disappears in time.

Glucophage, too, can cause digestive distress, though lowering the dose often helps. It can also interfere with the absorption of vitamin B-12 and folic acid. People taking the drug should ask their doctor about taking vitamin supplements.

GLAUCOMA

A drug called *dorzolamide* (Trusopt) is great news for the millions of people with glaucoma. That's the potentially blinding disease marked by increased pressure in the eye.

The usual glaucoma treatment—eyedrops containing beta-blocker drugs like *timolol* (Timoptic)—is quite effective at lowering eyeball pressure. But beta-blockers don't always work. People with asthma shouldn't use them at all.

Trusopt limits the secretion of the fluid that accumulates in the eyeball. It's just as effective as beta-blockers—and much less likely to cause troublesome side effects. Used together, the two drugs may bring pressure down to normal when neither works alone.

Side effects: Burning or stinging in the eye, blurred vision, dryness, sensitivity to light.

Marijuana Can Be Effective Medicine

John P. Morgan, MD, professor of pharmacology at the City University of New York Medical School in New York City. He is coauthor of *Marijuana Myths, Marijuana Facts.* Lindesmith Center.

Marijuana is an effective treatment for several serious medical conditions. Nine states—Alaska, Arizona, California, Colorado, Hawaii, Maine, Nevada, Oregon and Washington—and the District of Columbia have taken steps to legalize medical marijuana within their borders.

But federal laws still make it a crime to possess or use marijuana—whether it's for recreational or medical purposes.

Medical marijuana expert John P. Morgan, MD, explains the health benefits of marijuana...

●**For which ailments is marijuana effective?** Marijuana has been clinically proven to be excellent therapy for...

●**Nausea and vomiting.** People undergoing cancer treatment can get fast relief from these common side effects of chemotherapy.

●**Muscle spasms.** Marijuana can relieve spasms in multiple sclerosis patients and individuals with spinal cord injuries.

●**Glaucoma.** Marijuana reduces pressure within the eyes. It can help prevent eye damage as well as discomfort.

●**AIDS-related "wasting."** Marijuana is an excellent appetite stimulant. It can reverse malnutrition and the extreme weight loss (cachexia) associated with AIDS.

Anecdotal evidence suggests that marijuana helps with migraines, insomnia and chronic pain.

●**Given these benefits, why isn't medical marijuana widely used?** Along with heroin and LSD, marijuana is classified as a Schedule I substance. That means that it is considered dangerous and without medical value. Reclassifying it as a Schedule II drug would allow doctors to prescribe it under controlled conditions.

But until federal laws change, the average patient considers marijuana too risky...and the average doctor is unwilling to recommend it.

●**Do people get "high" when using marijuana as medicine?** Regular smokers of marijuana tend to develop a tolerance to the high.

●**Is marijuana addictive?** Few people who use medical marijuana develop a physical or psychological dependence on it.

In a recent study, researchers found marijuana no more addictive than caffeine.

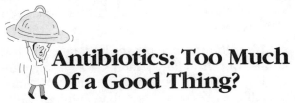

Antibiotics: Too Much Of a Good Thing?

Timothy McCall, MD, a Boston internist, author of *Examining Your Doctor: A Patient's Guide to Avoiding Harmful Medical Care.* Citadel Press. He is a regular commentator on the public radio program Marketplace, and can be found on the Web at *www.drmccall.com.*

The development of antibiotics in the 1940s was one of the biggest breakthroughs in medical history. Many infections that had been deadly—pneumonia, meningitis, dirty wounds, tuberculosis—suddenly could be treated.

Unfortunately, antibiotics proved so effective in treating these *bacterial* infections that many doctors started to prescribe them for colds and other *viral* infections—for which antibiotics are completely ineffective.

Doctors should know better—but they are often only too willing to oblige their patients, who often request antibiotics.

One study found that doctors prescribed antibiotics for two out of three patients with colds. Some gave antibiotics to virtually every cold sufferer who walked in the door.

Needless antibiotics waste billions of dollars. And when you take an antibiotic you don't need, you risk side effects ranging from yeast infections to life-threatening allergic reactions. And as you may have heard, the rampant overuse of antibiotics is fueling the development of drug-resistant bacteria.

Many antibiotics that were once highly effective have now been rendered useless—and the problem is getting worse all the time. We risk returning to an age in which there is no effective treatment for certain infections.

The key, of course, is to use antibiotics only when you really need them. That way, they'll be more likely to work. *Here's what I recommend:*

●**Don't ask your doctor for antibiotics.** Given how often antibiotics are overprescribed, if your doctor says you don't need one, chances are you don't. If your condition worsens, you can always return.

●**If antibiotics are prescribed, take the full course of pills.** Many patients stop taking antibiotics when they feel better. That's a big mistake. If the infection is not quite eradicated, the bugs are likely to develop resistance.

●**If you find any leftover antibiotics in your medicine chest, throw them out.** Some people who fail to finish a course of antibiotics save their leftover pills, thinking they can use them later for another illness.

But taking antibiotics before you see the doctor thwarts his efforts to diagnose you. You probably won't have enough pills to treat an infection properly anyway.

●**Take antibiotics for a sore throat *only* if you get a clear diagnosis of strep.** If you have a sore throat, your doctor should order a throat culture—and prescribe antibiotics only if the culture indicates Group A streptococcus bacteria. In adults, fewer than 10% of sore throats are caused by strep.

●**If you're over age 65 or have a chronic illness, get a pneumococcal pneumonia vaccine.** The *Pneumovax* vaccine prevents the leading cause of bacterial pneumonia—which is one of the leading causes of death.

●**When you get sick, listen to your body.** Many of the requests I get for needless antibiotics come from people who refuse to slow down when they get sick. When you're ill, you need rest. If you go to work when you're not up to it, you risk infecting your coworkers and staying sick longer. You probably won't get much work done either.

●**Don't let a doctor prescribe antibiotics without examining you in person.** In these days of cost-cutting, HMOs and some doctors now try to cut costs by having you *not* come in for a visit. Instead, they'll offer you a prescription for an antibiotic—often one that isn't needed—over the phone. This strategy is convenient for doctors and patients—and good for business. In general, though, it's lousy medical care.

Medication Errors Can Be Avoided...Easily

Joe Graedon, coauthor of *The People's Guide to Deadly Drug Interactions* and *The People's Pharmacy: Completely New and Revised.* St. Martin's Press.

Each year, mistakes involving prescription and over-the-counter drugs cost the US economy $20 billion in hospitalization expenses...and kill 140,000 people in this country alone.

Here's how to avoid "medication misadventures"—taking the wrong drug...overdosing... suffering a drug-induced allergic reaction, etc.

INTERACTING WITH YOUR DOCTOR

Before every doctor's appointment, jot down in order of importance all your medical concerns and/or symptoms. If you suspect that a rash or any other new symptom is drug-related, make that a priority. Such a problem could be life-threatening.

Most doctors have a limited amount of time to spend with their patients, so it is essential to start with the most urgent problem. If you ramble on about several other problems, the doctor may interrupt you—or you may get sidetracked—before you reach the important one.

Occasionally, psychological stress caused by seeing a doctor makes it hard to "take in" everything the doctor says. In such cases, take along a tape recorder. That way, you can record the doctor's comments and review them when you're more relaxed.

Important: Be as diplomatic as possible when making your recording. Let the doctor know that you simply want to avoid any confusion following his/her instructions.

Alternative: Ask a friend or family member to accompany you to your appointments. Have him/her take written notes regarding the doctor's instructions.

NEW PRESCRIPTIONS

Before accepting any new prescription, provide your doctor with the following information…

• **A complete list** of all prescription, over-the-counter (OTC) and recreational drugs you take, including vitamins, cold remedies, alcohol and tobacco.

• **Any allergy or sensitivity** you may have to any food or drug.

• **Any special diet** that you may be following.

• **Any condition** for which you are already receiving a doctor's care.

Women: Let the doctor know if you are pregnant or attempting to become pregnant.

Ask the doctor for written information about the drug, its side effects and how to take it. If possible, read this literature before you leave the office—but ask for a copy to take home with you.

Questions to ask: Are there any precautions or warnings of which you should be aware? Should you avoid certain foods, drugs or vitamin supplements while taking the medication?

Failure to get answers to these questions can cause serious problems—even death.

Example: A family of antidepressants called MAO inhibitors (Marplan, Nardil and Parnate) is extremely dangerous when taken in combination with certain other antidepressants…with cheese or soy sauce…or with OTC cold preparations or diet aids (Acutrim and Dexatrim).

Never take any medication without knowing its purpose. Is the drug intended to alleviate symptoms? If so, which symptoms? Is it intended to cure an ailment? Which ailment?

Get explicit instructions about how the medication is to be taken. A simple "three times a day" is inadequate. Find out the correct dosage and at what times of day the drug should be taken.

Ask if the medication should be taken with food or on an empty stomach.

What if you miss a dose? Should you take the dose as soon as you think of it? Or should you simply skip that dose and "double up" on the next one?

Your doctor should double-check for potential interactions between your new prescription and any medications you're already taking. He should not rely on his memory. Instead, he should consult a reference text or a computer program.

If the relevant information isn't on hand, ask your doctor to telephone the drug manufacturer. It is also a good idea to buy a reference book to double-check drug information.

If you experience any unexpected side effects once you begin taking a new medication, let your doctor know right away. Have your doctor tell you which side effects or symptoms require immediate attention.

Caution: Do not stop taking the medication without consulting your doctor. Abruptly stopping certain medications can trigger irregular heart rhythms, convulsions or even heart attack.

AVOIDING PHARMACY MISTAKES

Some patients routinely ask their doctor to "phone in" their prescriptions to a pharmacy.

Doing so can be a big mistake—especially when a new prescription is involved.

Reason: Drug names often sound alike—especially when heard over the telephone in a noisy drugstore. The ulcer medication *Zantac*, for instance, can easily be confused with the antianxiety medication *Xanax*.

Your doctor should provide you with a written prescription form. This form should be printed clearly, in English, including the drug's brand and generic names, along with detailed instructions. Abbreviations should not be used.

Do not accept sloppy handwriting. In a survey, more than half of pharmacists acknowledged that a doctor's sloppy handwriting had caused them to make prescription errors.

Example: One patient who was supposed to get the anti-inflammatory drug *Tolectin* was instead given *Tolinase*, a diabetes drug. She developed pseudosulinoma, a serious condition that mimics excess insulin production.

Bottom line: If you can't read the prescription, odds are the pharmacist won't be able to either.

To further minimize errors, make sure your prescription is filled by the pharmacist. Because they have less training than pharmacists, pharmacy technicians are more prone to errors. If you're not sure who is filling your prescription, ask.

Finally, visit your pharmacy between the hours of noon and 3 p.m. In most drugstores, that's the slowest time of day. Avoid having a prescription filled immediately before or after work. That's the busiest time of day.

DRUG INTERACTION SELF-DEFENSE

Use one pharmacy for all your family's prescriptions. That way, you can be certain that the pharmacist is familiar with all your medications…and alert to potential interactions.

If possible, find a pharmacy that uses a computerized patient profile system to track the various medications family members are taking. Ask the pharmacist to check the computer for potential interactions. Be prepared to wait —or come back at another time—if the pharmacist needs to check your prescription with your doctor.

Your pharmacist should also check your new prescription for possible interactions with alcohol…or with OTC medications. Such interactions can cause big problems…

Example I: The antibiotic *tetracycline* can be rendered inactive by a single Tums tablet.

Example II: Even small quantities of alcohol can cause a serious reaction in someone taking an antihistamine, tranquilizer, sedative or pain reliever.

Like your doctor, your pharmacist should provide instructions on how to take the drug, potential side effects and any foods or drugs to avoid.

How to Measure Dosages

Michael Leff, editor, *Consumer Reports on Health*, 101 Truman Ave., Yonkers, NY.

Use a real measuring spoon to portion out medicine—not a tableware spoon. Tableware spoons may hold from *half*…to twice as much as a measured spoon.

The Eight Most Common Medication Mistakes… And How to Avoid Them

Harold Silverman, PharmD, a pharmacist and healthcare consultant in Washington, DC. He is author of *The Pill Book: The Illustrated Guide to the Most Prescribed Drugs in the United States*. Bantam.

Many people unwittingly reduce the effectiveness of the drugs they take—or worse, cause themselves great harm —by mishandling their pills. *The most common drug traps and how to avoid them…*

Trap #1: Failing to double-check your prescription. Drug-dispensing mistakes are rare, but they do occur.

In his/her haste, a doctor may prescribe the wrong drug or dosage. The pharmacist may misread the doctor's handwriting…or reach for the wrong bottle of pills when filling your prescription.

Self-defense: Before handing the prescription form to the pharmacist, jot the drug name and dosage on a piece of paper.

When you pick up the bottle of pills, compare the label with your note. If you suspect a mistake, call your doctor.

Also, consider keeping a copy of *The Pill Book* (Bantam) or *Physicians' Desk Reference* (Medical Economics) on hand. These books contain photos of pills.

Trap #2: **Being unaware of a drug's side effects.** Doctors are supposed to tell patients about a drug's possible side effects. But they don't always do so—because they don't want to "scare" their patients.

Prescription drugs can cause a variety of troublesome side effects, including sexual problems like diminished sex drive, impotence and retrograde ejaculation (in which semen is ejaculated "backward" into the bladder). If you are unaware that your medication is causing such a problem, you may worry yourself sick.

Self-defense: Before taking *any* newly prescribed drug, ask your doctor and pharmacist about side effects.

If you experience a problem, ask about taking a lower dose or switching to a substitute.

Trap #3: **Taking one drug that interacts with another.** Nine out of 10 pharmacies now have sophisticated drug-dispensing software that screens for drug interactions.

Each time you come in with a new prescription, the pharmacist runs a computer check. If the drug interacts with any other drug you're taking, the pharmacist alerts you.

But such systems work only if you have all your prescriptions filled at one pharmacy.

If you patronize different drugstores, you risk subjecting yourself to side effects and/or not receiving the drug's full benefits. You may even fail to discover that you have two prescriptions for the same drug from different doctors—and are double-dosing yourself.

Self-defense: Stick to one pharmacy. If you're taking several drugs and are uncertain about interactions, ask your pharmacist or doctor

for a "brown bag" session. Put all the drugs you take in a bag, and bring it in. Review the name and dosage of each drug, and what each is for.

Be sure to schedule your brown bag session in advance. Otherwise, the pharmacist or doctor may be too busy to spend enough time with you.

Trap #4: **Combining certain prescription and nonprescription drugs.** In recent years, several drugs that used to be available only by prescription have gone on sale over-the-counter (OTC).

This cuts costs for consumers, but it makes it harder for doctors to monitor their patients for potentially dangerous drug combinations.

Example I: In rare cases, nonsteroidal anti-inflammatory drugs (NSAIDs) like *ibuprofen* (Motrin), *naproxen* (Aleve) and *ketoprofen* (Orudis) can cause kidney damage. If you have kidney disease, avoid large doses. Don't take them on a long-term basis.

Example II: The acid blocker *cimetidine* (Tagamet) interacts with the antidiabetes medication *sulfonylurea…benzodiazepine* tranquilizers like Valium…and calcium channel blockers like Adalat and Procardia.

Self-defense: If you're taking a medication on a long-term basis, ask your doctor if any OTC drugs interact with it.

Or—buy your OTC drugs where you have your prescriptions filled, and check with your pharmacist before taking the two together.

Trap #5: **Storing drugs incorrectly.** No doubt you have already heard that heat and humidity degrade drugs. Yet most of us continue to store our medications in the bathroom—the hottest, most humid room in the house.

Even if you cannot discern any degradation, your pills probably are becoming less potent.

Self-defense: Store all prescription and OTC drugs in a cool, dry spot—your bedroom closet, for example (or in the refrigerator, if the drug is supposed to be refrigerated).

If you have children in your house, make sure to keep the drugs out of their reach.

Trap #6: **Failing to have the dosage adjusted after a major change in body weight.** If you lose a lot of weight, a once-correct dose may become a harmful overdose. Conversely, a significant weight gain may lead to under-dosing.

Self-defense: If you lose or gain more than 10% of your body weight, alert your doctor so that he can adjust your dosage accordingly.

Trap #7: Using prescription drugs without medical supervision. Many people hang on to unused pills, thinking they will save a few bucks—and a trip to the pharmacy—if they get sick again.

Yet even if you get the same symptoms again, prescribing to yourself in this fashion is dangerous. Your new symptoms could stem from a different ailment—which calls for different treatment.

Self-defense: If you have pills left over after taking a course of medication, discard them. If you insist on hanging on to unused pills, at least call the doctor and get his approval before using them.

Trap #8: Disobeying the doctor's orders. When it comes to prescription medications, an amazing number of people simply don't follow their doctor's directions.

Some patients take more medication than was prescribed—on the erroneous "more-is-better" theory. Others take less than the doctor ordered—in a misguided effort to avoid side effects. Doctors call such behavior "patient noncompliance."

Self-defense: Take all medications according to instruction. If you have trouble remembering to do so, devise a plan to jog your memory at the appropriate times.

Jot down your dosing schedule in your date book…carry your pill box in your pants pocket as a constant reminder…or pick up a combination pill box/alarm at your local pharmacy.

If you miss a dose, check with your doctor or pharmacist about what to do. In some cases, it's best to continue with your regimen as if you hadn't missed a dose. In others, it's better to "double up" on a subsequent dose.

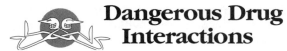

Dangerous Drug Interactions

Joseph Graedon, one of the country's foremost experts on drug interactions. He has served as a consultant to the Federal Trade Commission on nonprescription drug advertising and as a member of the advisory board of the University of California (San Francisco) Drug Studies Unit. He is author, with Teresa Graedon, PhD, of many books on health topics, including *The People's Guide to Deadly Drug Interactions* and *The People's Pharmacy: Completely New and Revised.* St. Martin's Press.

Every year, thousands of people combine drugs they are taking with other medications or foods that produce negative reactions. In most cases, they weren't aware there would be a problem, since the medications and foods seemed harmless.

Here are just some of the most common hazardous drug interactions—and what you can do to protect yourself and your family from harm.

DRUG/FOOD INTERACTIONS

No doubt your pharmacist has cautioned you to avoid taking certain antibiotics with dairy products. This combination can reduce the effectiveness of the medications.

But many pharmacists and doctors are unaware of some unusual drug/food interactions. *Foods that could cause problems with some medications:*

●**Grapefruit and grapefruit juice** contain compounds that can interact powerfully with medications—and cause devastating side effects.

Example: Blood pressure medications, such as Procardia and Adalat *(nifedipine)* and Plendil *(felodipine)*, are dangerous when combined with grapefruit, resulting in higher blood levels of blood pressure medications. Symptoms may include facial flushing, nausea, dizziness, confusion, palpitations or irregular heartbeat.

●**Green, leafy vegetables,** such as broccoli, brussels sprouts and cabbage reduce the effectiveness of the blood thinner Coumadin *(warfarin)*, a commonly prescribed blood thinner that prevents blood clots. These foods are rich in vitamin K, which helps the blood to clot. Coumadin, meanwhile, works by counteracting vitamin K's clotting action.

Consuming a small amount of vitamin K–rich foods daily probably won't pose a problem. But if you usually skip these vegetables and then overindulge, at a Chinese restaurant, for example, you reduce the drug's effectiveness and put yourself at risk for a blood clot or stroke.

●**Oatmeal and other high-fiber foods** may interfere with the absorption of Lanoxin (*digoxin*), a drug prescribed to control an irregular heart rhythm, which can lead to blood clots and stroke. Take Lanoxin two or three hours before or after eating high-fiber foods.

●**Salt substitutes** are used by people with high blood pressure. But they contain high amounts of potassium. If consumed with potassium-sparing diuretics such as Aldactone (*spironolactone*)—which are prescribed for high blood pressure or congestive heart failure—they can cause potassium levels to soar, increasing the risk of cardiac arrest.

●**Licorice and Lanoxin**—or a diuretic like Lasix (*furosemide*)—can lead to low levels of potassium, causing irregular heart rhythms and cardiac arrest. One piece of licorice probably won't hurt—but regular handfuls of licorice could be deadly.

PRESCRIPTION DRUG INTERACTIONS

●**Antibiotics vs. blood thinners.** Antibiotics like Flagyl and Protostat (*metronidazole*) can cause problems when taken with the blood thinner Coumadin. The antibiotics prevent the body from purging Coumadin, and if Coumadin levels get too high, life-threatening bleeding could occur.

If you are taking both metronidazole and Coumadin, you must be monitored carefully by your physician and have frequent blood tests.

●**Antibiotics vs. antihistamines.** Macrolide antibiotics such as *clarithromycin*, *erythromycin* and *azithromycin* can boost blood levels of the antihistamine Hismanal (*astemizole*) to dangerous—and potentially lethal—levels.

Rx/OTC DRUG INTERACTIONS

Don't assume over-the-counter (OTC) medications are risk-free. Teamed with certain prescription drugs, some can cause complications. *Examples...*

●**Pain relievers.** Aspirin...Advil and Nuprin (*ibuprofen*)...Aleve (*naproxen*)...and Orudis KT (*ketoprofen*) can reduce the effectiveness of beta blockers, such as Inderal (*propranolol*) and Lopressor (*metoprolol*), which are prescribed to treat high blood pressure.

If this happens, blood pressure can rise, increasing the risk of heart attack and stroke. If you are taking a beta blocker, check with your doctor before adding a pain reliever. If your doctor prescribes a beta blocker and aspirin, he/she should monitor your blood pressure.

●**Antacids** can inhibit the absorption of the heart and blood pressure medications Capoten (*captopril*) and Tenormin (*atenolol*), as well as Lanoxin.

And the activated charcoal added to counteract gas may reduce the effectiveness of a number of drugs, including tricyclic antidepressants such as Elavil (*amitriptyline*) and the diabetes medications Diabinese (*chlorpropamide*) and Tolinase (*tolazamide*).

●**Allergy and cough/cold remedies** that contain *pseudoephedrine*, *ephedrine* or *phenylephrine* should not be combined with a monoamine oxidase inhibitor antidepressant like Nardil (*phenelzine*) or Parnate (*tranylcypromine*). Your blood pressure could soar, leading to a hypertensive crisis and stroke.

GUARDING AGAINST INTERACTIONS

●**Make your doctors aware of the prescription and OTC drugs you are taking** and have your doctors check for interaction potential. Ask them to consult drug reference books and/or computer reference programs before you leave the office.

●**Have all prescriptions filled at a single pharmacy,** preferably one that keeps computerized data on all your medications and can zero in on possible interactions. Tell your pharmacist about OTC drugs you are taking.

●**Make a list of key questions to ask.** When a new drug is prescribed, don't assume doctors and pharmacists are aware of every drug interaction—or if they are, that they will remember to alert you. List the following questions and give copies to your doctor and pharmacist to fill out independently. If one contradicts the other, speak with both to get the correct answer.

- What is the medication's name?
- What is the dose?
- What time(s) should I take it?
- Should I take it with food? After eating? Before eating? How long?
- Should I avoid any foods?
- Are there vitamins or supplements I should avoid? Increase?
- Are there any precautions or warnings I should know about?
- Are there any contraindications that would make this drug inappropriate?
- What other prescription medicines should I avoid?
- Are there any OTC remedies I should avoid?
- What side effects are common with my medicine?
- Are there any side effects that are so serious you would want to know about them immediately?

If your doctor or pharmacist tells you that a drug won't interact adversely with another medication or food, don't assume that no interactions exist. Though rare, life-threatening interactions can go undetected by drug companies, the medical establishment and the Food and Drug Administration for months or even years after a drug hits the market.

So...if you experience any strange symptoms that cannot be easily explained, ask your doctor to contact the drug's manufacturer and file a report with the FDA.

Over-the-Counter vs. Prescription Drugs

Patricia Wilson, Wilson & Associates, a benefits consulting firm in Rosemont, PA.

While over-the-counter (OTC) drugs are generally less expensive than prescription drugs, insurance plans that cover all or part of the cost of prescription medications often make these drugs cheaper for plan participants than comparable uncovered OTC products.

Example: Two hundred milligrams a day of the heartburn medication *cimetidine* can cost as little as $60 per year for HMO members, while a year's worth of the over-the-counter drug Tagamet HB can cost $110 or more.

More than 50 prescription drugs have made the switch to drugstore shelves since 1972, and dozens more are being considered for approval by the Federal Drug Administration this year.

Finish All Prescriptions

Ted Ferry, EdD, professor emeritus, Institute for Safety and Systems Management, University of Southern California, and author of *Home Safety Desk Reference*. Career Press.

Do not stop taking a medicine once you feel better—unless your doctor says it's okay. Prescription drugs often help you feel better before the underlying illness is cured. The end of symptoms does not necessarily mark the end of the disease.

Expiration Date Alert

Timothy McCall, MD, a Boston internist and author of *Examining Your Doctor: A Patient's Guide to Avoiding Harmful Medical Care.* Citadel Press. He is a regular commentator on the public radio program Marketplace, and can be found on the Web at *www.drmccall.com.*

Some medicines, like codeine, become more potent with age, while others lose effectiveness. Taking out-of-date medicine is an ineffective way to try to save money.

To make medicines last as long as possible: Do not store them in the bathroom. Bathroom moisture and germs can cause medicines to deteriorate prematurely.

Kids' Medication Overuse

James A. Taylor, MD, director of the pediatric center, University of Washington, Dept. of Pediatrics, Seattle 98195.

More than half the three-year-olds in a major survey had taken at least one over-the-counter drug in the past 30 days.

Bottom line: Many children suffer side effects from the colorings, flavorings and alcohol in some kids' medicines. And—parents waste money on inappropriate drugs.

Prescription Drug Self-Defense I

Rosemary Soave, MD, infectious disease specialist and associate professor at New York Hospital–Cornell Medical Center, New York.

To be sure your prescriptions are filled correctly, have your doctor note the purpose of the drug on the prescription, in addition to its name.

Reason: Many drugs have similar names, and some doctors' handwriting can be difficult to decipher.

Prescription Drug Self-Defense II

Charles Inlander, president of The People's Medical Society, a patient advocate organization, 462 Walnut St., Allentown, PA 18102. He is author of several books, including *The People's Medical Society Health Desk Reference.* Hyperion.

Mistakes on prescriptions are made *17 million* times a year. *To ensure that you don't take the wrong medication...*

When your doctor prescribes a drug, have him/her write down—on a separate piece of paper from the prescription—the exact name of the drug...dosage...number of times a day you should take it...and any side effects you should call to his attention. When you fill the prescription, compare the label with the doctor's note—and talk with your doctor about any discrepancies.

Caution: Mail-order or managed-care companies sometimes substitute drugs. Get your doctor's approval before you take a substitute.

Tell your doctor about all medications you use regularly—including over-the-counter drugs.

How to Save on Your Medicines

Rick Doble, editor, *$avvy Discount$ Newsletter*, Box 96, Smyrna, NC 28579.

Buy double-strength pills (if your doctor will prescribe this way) and cut them in half with a pill cutter. Pill cutters cost about $5.

● **Compare prices**—and include a discount mail-order pharmacy in comparison.

● **Always ask for generic medications.** When refilling a prescription, ask if a generic is now available. New ones come on the market regularly.

Aspirin? Tylenol? Advil? None of the Above?

Timothy McCall, MD, a Boston internist and author of *Examining Your Doctor: A Patient's Guide to Avoiding Harmful Medical Care.* Citadel Press. He is a regular commentator on the public radio program Marketplace, and can be found on the Web at *www.drmccall.com.*

Deciding on a pain reliever can be tough. Advertisements that tout one drug's advantages while slamming the competition are about as objective as political commercials.

For treating fever, headaches or routine aches and pains, different over-the-counter (OTC) painkillers are of similar effectiveness. But there are important differences.

● **Aspirin** is the least expensive OTC painkiller. But it's also the most likely to cause stomach upset. This can range from trivial indigestion to life-threatening hemorrhages.

No doubt you've heard that low doses of aspirin, taken regularly, help prevent heart attack and colon cancer. While aspirin does offer some protection against these ailments—other pain relievers don't—it also appears to raise the risk of bleeding into the brain (hemorrhagic stroke).

Aspirin therapy to prevent heart attacks is appropriate for people over age 50 with cardiac risk factors (high blood pressure, high

115

cholesterol, etc.). I usually recommend a daily dose of 81 mg (one "baby" aspirin tablet). Of course, you should check with your doctor.

●**Ibuprofen** (Advil, Motrin) and other newer nonsteroidal anti-inflammatory drugs (NSAIDs) are less likely than aspirin to upset the stomach. Ibuprofen is especially good for menstrual pain. But these drugs—including *naproxen* (Aleve) and *ketoprofen* (Orudis KT) —are by no means perfectly safe.

Each year, an estimated 10,000 Americans are hospitalized for intestinal bleeding caused by newer NSAIDs. One thousand die of such bleeding. These drugs can also cause kidney problems and reduce the effectiveness of some blood pressure medicines.

●**Acetaminophen** (Tylenol) is probably the safest OTC pain pill. But it's not entirely harmless. As Advil commercials correctly point out, drinking more than three alcoholic beverages a day while taking acetaminophen can cause liver damage. But if you drink that much alcohol and take ibuprofen or aspirin, your risk of a fatal intestinal hemorrhage also climbs.

For certain individuals, some drugs are better choices…

●**Anyone with a history of ulcers** should avoid aspirin and other anti-inflammatory drugs. Acetaminophen is usually a better choice.

●**Anyone with chronic hepatitis or another liver problem** should avoid acetaminophen. Aspirin or ibuprofen is better.

●**Heavy drinkers** should avoid regular use of all pain relievers. If one is needed, it should be taken at the lowest effective dose—and taken as infrequently as possible. Of course, the best bet is to cut back on drinking.

●**Elderly people** should generally stick to acetaminophen for treating minor aches and pains. Taking aspirin to prevent heart attack is a separate matter—one that should be discussed with a doctor.

●**For children,** acetaminophen and ibuprofen are safer than aspirin. When kids with influenza are given aspirin, they can develop a devastating illness called Reye's syndrome.

Whichever pain pill you choose, remember to use it sparingly. All drugs cause side effects.

If you do need a pain pill, forget all the marketing hype. Generic aspirin, acetaminophen and ibuprofen are every bit as effective as Bayer, Tylenol and Advil.

Painkiller Danger

William L. Henrich, MD, professor of medicine, Medical College of Ohio, Toledo, and chairman of the Consensus Conference on Analgesics, National Kidney Foundation.

Aspirin and acetaminophen, taken together over a long period of time, can cause kidney failure.

Self-defense: Avoid combination painkillers, such as Excedrin and Vanquish…and do not "mix and match" analgesic tablets. The National Kidney Foundation has called for a ban on over-the-counter cough, cold and headache remedies that contain both painkillers.

Insomnia and Painkillers

S. Lori Brown, PhD, MPH, research scientist officer, Food and Drug Administration, Rockville, MD. Her study was published in the *Journal of the American Geriatrics Society*.

Insomnia can be caused by over-the-counter painkillers that contain caffeine. *Examples:* Aspirin-free Excedrin and Anacin. In a study of 2,885 patients, those who took caffeinated formulations of aspirin and acetaminophen were nearly twice as likely to report sleep problems as those taking similar noncaffeinated analgesics.

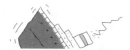

Tablets vs. Liquids

Malcolm Robinson, MD, clinical professor of medicine, University of Oklahoma, Oklahoma City. His study of 65 heartburn sufferers was published in *Gastroenterology*, American Gastroenterology Association, 7910 Woodmont Ave., 7th Floor, Bethesda, MD 20814.

Researchers compared Tums E-X and Mylanta Double Strength tablets with the liquid antacids Mylanta II and Extra Strength Maalox. *Result:* The tablets were more effective at controlling heartburn and acid reflux.

Theory: When chewed, tablets mix with saliva to create a protective film that adheres to the esophagus longer than swallowed liquids do. *Also:* Chewing promotes production of saliva, which contains natural acid-fighting substances.

Economical Cholesterol Control

J. David Spence, MD, director, Stroke Prevention and Atherosclerosis Research Centre, Robarts Research Institute, London, Ontario, Canada.

The cholesterol-lowering drug *colestipol* (Colestid) can be used more economically *and* more effectively when mixed with the natural fiber supplement *psyllium*. Patients who took half (2.5 g) their usual dosage of colestipol, plus 2.5 g of psyllium, had greater declines in the all-important cholesterol-to-HDL ratio than when they took colestipol alone. Fewer side effects were reported with the mixture, too. Consult your doctor first.

Cholesterol Controversy

Bruce Yaffe, MD, an internist and gastroenterologist in private practice, 121 E. 84 St., New York 10028.

The benefits of cholesterol-lowering drugs far exceed any cancer risk. Some research suggested that long-term use of two main classes of drugs, *fibrates* and *statins,* might lead to an increased risk of cancer. For people with greatly elevated cholesterol, that fear may be dwarfed compared to the immediate risk of a heart attack. Many years of experience show that the drugs cut heart attacks by 40%.

Aspirin Reduces Colon Cancer Risk

Edward Giovannucci, MD, assistant professor of medicine, Harvard Medical School, Boston. His review of health questionnaires completed by 121,701 women in 1976 was published in *The New England Journal of Medicine*, 10 Shattuck St., Boston 02115.

But the beneficial effects become apparent only after a decade or more of taking the drug. After 10 years, women who consistently took two or more aspirin tablets a week had a slightly lower risk of colon cancer than other women. After 20 years, the risk was nearly halved.

Important: Consult your physician before taking aspirin to reduce your risk of colorectal cancer.

Drug Scare Reality

Ralph E. Small, MD, professor of pharmacy and medicine, Medical College of Virginia Hospital, Box 980533 MCV, Richmond, VA 23298.

Prescription drug scare resulted from news reports that 25% of older Americans are taking drugs that could hurt rather than help them.

Reality: The risk is exaggerated—most problems with prescription drugs result from failing to follow doctor's instructions. In a small number of cases, drugs also may have adverse effects when taken in combination with over-the-counter remedies or other drugs that your doctor does not know you are taking.

Important: Always consult your doctor or pharmacist before combining any medicines.

Testosterone Patch Is Available

Adrian Dobs, MD, associate professor of medicine and director of clinical studies, The Johns Hopkins Medical Institutions, Baltimore.

A testosterone patch can be used to treat men with *hypogonadism*—a condition in which the body produces too little testosterone, often leading to impotence and osteoporosis. Approved by the Food and Drug Administration, the patch is placed on the upper arm, abdomen, back or thigh—and releases the testosterone continuously. The patch is sold under the brand name *Androderm*—by prescription only. *More information:* See your doctor.

Daily Headache Syndrome

Robert Sheeler, MD, staff physician at the Mayo Clinic, Rochester, MN.

Daily use of aspirin, acetaminophen, ibuprofen or other analgesics can create a rebound effect called daily headache syndrome.

Alternatives: Ice packs, heat, massage, relaxation therapy or other nondrug means. Use medications sparingly for more troublesome headaches.

All About Rebound Headaches

Joel Saper, MD, FACP, director, Michigan Head–Pain and Neurological Institute in Ann Arbor.

Rebound headaches are becoming more common as people rely on over-the-counter (OTC) medications without consulting their doctors. OTC headache drugs can create headache rhythms that can only be controlled with ever-increasing doses.

Result: A form of addiction that requires detoxification. No other treatment will work until these medicines are eliminated.

Self-defense: Follow label directions carefully. Most specify not to use OTC medications for more than 10 days to relieve pain or more than three days to control fever—unless directed by a doctor…check ingredients carefully. Long-term use of these drugs for more than two days a week on a regular basis makes you vulnerable to the rebound potential.

Don't Self-Medicate

Stuart Levy, MD, director, Tufts University's Center for Adaptation Genetics and Drug Resistance, Boston, and author of *The Antibiotic Paradox: How Miracle Drugs Are Destroying the Miracle.* Plenum Press.

Don't take antibiotics prescribed for someone else—or even your own leftover pills.

Danger: Overuse of antibiotics has caused drug-resistant strains of bacteria—making antibiotics powerless against many infectious diseases.

Important: If you have an infection, ask your doctor to confirm that it is bacterial and that you need antibiotics.

Antidepressant Danger

Joe Graedon, coauthor of *The People's Guide to Deadly Drug Interactions* and *The People's Pharmacy: Completely New and Revised.* St. Martin's Press.

Common foods can cause headaches, fever, visual disturbances, confusion and a dangerous rise in blood pressure when eaten by individuals taking a prescribed antidepressant.

Self-defense: Avoid tyramine-containing foods while taking a monoamine oxidase (MAO) inhibitor—even for several weeks after you stop taking the drug. Tyramine-containing foods include avocados, bananas, bologna, broad beans, aged cheese, caviar, chicken liver (stored), miso soup, meat concentrate (in gravy), pepperoni, pickled herring, salami, summer sausage, soy sauce, wines (Chianti and vermouth) and yeast extract (marmite).

Attention Arthritis Sufferers

Guidelines from the American College of Rheumatology and the Arthritis Foundation, Atlanta.

The osteoarthritis drug of choice is *acetaminophen*, found in Tylenol. It has surpassed aspirin in popularity as an arthritis treatment because doctors say it is less likely to cause serious side effects.

Osteoarthritis treatment guidelines recommend first treating the disease with acetaminophen—then talking with your doctor about stronger drugs if the acetaminophen does not provide adequate pain relief.

Also helpful: Exercise to strengthen muscles...proper diet to maintain weight at a level that does not place extra stress on joints.

Break the Strep-Throat Cycle

Gary Ruoff, MD, family physician and researcher, Westside Family Medical Center, Kalamazoo, MI.

Take the *full course* of antibiotics prescribed by your doctor.

Most people use just enough antibiotics to relieve symptoms, then stop. This may result in symptomless infections that cause hidden damage (rheumatic fever)...a recurrence of the strep throat...or the transmission of strep throat to someone else.

Ulcerative Colitis and Nicotine Therapy

William J. Sandborn, MD, director of inflammatory disease research, Mayo Clinic, Rochester, MN. His four-week study of 64 nonsmoking colitis patients was published in *Annals of Internal Medicine*, Independence Mall West, Sixth St. at Race, Philadelphia 19106.

Ulcerative colitis patients often benefit from nicotine therapy. Doctors have long observed that smokers rarely develop this chronic inflammation of the colon and rectum...and that nonsmokers with colitis often go into remission when they *start* smoking.

Study: Among patients who wore a nicotine patch, 39% showed improvement after four weeks, compared with 9% on a placebo patch. Many of the patients did not respond to *sulfasalazine* (Azulfidine), steroids and other conventional colitis drugs.

Lesson: If you have colitis, ask your doctor about using a nicotine patch.

Former Smokers and Nicotine Gum...

Harlan Krumholz, MD, assistant professor of cardiology at Yale University School of Medicine, New Haven, CT, and author of *No If's, And's or Butts: The Smoker's Guide to Quitting*. Avery Publishing Group.

Nicorette gum should be used to help smokers quit. It should not be used to provide a long-term smoke-free source of nicotine—one of the most addictive drugs around. And don't expect that chewing this gum is enough to quit.

Most important: Making a commitment to quit...combined with as many other strategies as possible, including group therapy, visualization exercises and support of family, friends and doctors. *Note:* While there are some risks associated with nicotine gum, the risks from smoking are far greater.

Seizure Relief

Michael Privitera, MD, associate professor of neurology, University of Cincinnati Medical Center.

The drug *topiramate* (Topamax) helps prevent seizures in the 30% of epilepsy patients who fail to respond to *phenytoin* (Dilantin) and other traditional antiseizure drugs. Topiramate reduces seizures by as much as 75% in some epilepsy patients. Side effects—including dizziness and coordination problems—largely disappear over time. About 30% of epilepsy patients—a total of 650,000 in the US—continue to suffer seizures despite the use of traditional antiseizure drugs.

Aspirin Therapy and Stomach Problems

Judith P. Kelly, MS, epidemiologist, Slone Epidemiology Unit, Boston University School of Medicine, Brookline, MA.

Enteric-coated and buffered aspirin tablets are no easier on the stomach than plain aspirin. It's now popular to take an aspirin a day to help prevent heart attack. In a study, users of "aspirin therapy" were three times as likely to be hospitalized for stomach bleeding as those who didn't take aspirin regularly. They were equally likely to suffer bleeding no matter what kind of aspirin they took.

To avoid stomach trouble: Talk to your doctor about taking one-quarter tablet (or one baby aspirin)…and taking it with food.

Grapefruit Juice Danger

Paul B. Watkins, MD, director, Clinical Research Center, University of Michigan, Ann Arbor.

Grapefruit juice boosts the body's absorption of certain pills. The effect is especially pronounced with some sedatives and blood pressure drugs.

Self-defense: If you are already taking your medication with grapefruit juice—and are having no problems—you can continue to do so. But do not start drinking grapefruit juice with a sedative or a blood pressure medication without first talking with your doctor.

Channel Blockers and Cancer Link

Marco Pahor, MD, associate professor of preventive medicine, University of Tennessee, Memphis. His study of calcium channel blocker use in 5,000 people over 71 years of age was published in *The Lancet*, 42 Bedford Square, London WC1B 3SL, England.

Short-acting versions of this popular class of blood pressure drugs have been linked to cancer, as well as to stomach bleeding and heart attack. In one study, short-acting *nifedipine* (Procardia) raised cancer risk 72% in patients who took it.

Self-defense: If you're taking Procardia, ask your doctor about switching to a beta blocker or a diuretic. Even if you're taking a longer-acting calcium channel blocker like long-acting *nifedipine* (Procardia XL) or *amlodipine* (Norvasc), it's a good idea to talk to your doctor.

Asthmatics and Inhalers

James Donahue, PhD, epidemiologist, Brigham and Women's Hospital, Boston, whose study of 16,941 health maintenance organization enrollees was published in *The Journal of the American Medical Association*, 515 N. State St., Chicago 60610.

Asthmatics who use inhaled steroids are *half* as likely to be hospitalized as those who use other—or no—medications. Inhaled steroids are most beneficial when used to treat persons with severe asthma.

Asthma Trap

Barbara P. Lukert, MD, director, Osteoporosis Clinic, University of Kansas Hospital, Kansas City.

Inhaled corticosteroids—often used to treat asthma—interfere with bone metabolism and may cause bone loss.

Self-defense: If you must take corticosteroids, ask your doctor about countering these side effects.

Possibilities: A daily diet containing at least 1,500 mg calcium…regular exercise…a low-salt diet. Evaluate estrogen levels for women and testosterone levels for men. *Also:* Ask your doctor about the antileukotriene asthma medications such as *zafirlukast* (Accolate). One glass of milk contains 300 mg calcium.

Shingles Treatment

Richard J. Whitley, MD, professor of pediatrics, microbiology and medicine, University of Alabama, Birmingham. His 21-day study of 208 volunteers 50 years of age or older was published in the *Annals of Internal Medicine*, Independence Mall West, Sixth St. at Race, Philadelphia 19106.

Shingles respond well to the prescription drugs *acyclovir* (Zovirax) and *prednisone* (Deltasone). Blisters caused by this ailment (herpes zoster) healed faster in patients given the two-drug combination, compared with those given placebos.

Who Should Get the Hepatitis A Vaccine?

William S. Kammerer, MD, consultant, division of executive and international internal medicine, Mayo Clinic, Jacksonville, FL.

Travelers under 50 should get the vaccine (Havrix, VAQTA) if they expect to take two or more extended trips to Russia, Eastern Europe and/or tropical, developing countries within the next 10 years. If you'll be going only once, and plan to stay 10 days or fewer, *gamma globulin* injections represent a cheaper, though slightly less effective, alternative. Travelers 50 or older should speak with their physician. The vaccine is given in two injections, six to 12 months apart. *Cost:* About $50 to $75 per dose.

Cut Your Risk of Getting an Ulcer

Robin I. Russell, MD, PhD, chief of gastroenterology, Glasgow Royal Infirmary, Glasgow, Scotland. His study of 285 arthritis patients was published in the *New England Journal of Medicine*, 10 Shattuck St., Boston 02115.

To avoid stomach trouble, arthritis patients who use aspirin for pain should ask their doctor about also taking prescription-strength *famotidine* (Pepcid).

Study: Ulcer risk fell by more than 50% when aspirin users also took Pepcid.

Caution: Over-the-counter famotidine (Pepcid AC) won't prevent ulcers…and might mask ulcer symptoms until they become severe.

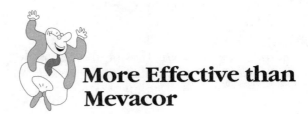

More Effective than Mevacor

Donald B. Hunninghake, MD, director, Heart Disease Prevention Clinic, University of Minnesota, Minneapolis.

The cholesterol-lowering drug *Atorvastatin* (Lipitor) is more effective than *lovastatin* (Mevacor) and other common "statin" drugs in cases where both LDL (bad) cholesterol and triglycerides are elevated. Patients with high LDL and high triglycerides face a greater risk of heart disease than those with high LDL and normal triglycerides.

Study: Atorvastatin reduced LDL levels by as much as 60% and triglycerides by 30% to 40%, and raised HDL (good) cholesterol levels by 6% to 10%.

121

Better Bowel Movements

Ervin Y. Eaker, Jr., MD, associate professor of medicine, University of Florida College of Medicine, Gainesville.

Severe constipation can sometimes be eased with the common gout drug *colchicine*. In a preliminary study, patients took oral colchicine for six weeks.

Result: The average number of bowel movements rose from two to six a week. Bloating, pain and nausea also dropped dramatically. If ongoing research corroborates these findings, colchicine could become the drug of choice for severe constipation.

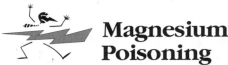

Magnesium Poisoning

Bruce Yaffe, MD, internist and gastroenterologist in private practice, 121 E. 84 St., New York 10028.

Magnesium poisoning from antacids can occur in people who take large doses for a long time. Magnesium is also found in many laxatives and some pain relievers.

People most at risk: Those with improperly functioning kidneys...older people, since kidney function generally declines with age...people who have had intestinal surgery...those taking medicines that slow intestinal transit...anyone with longtime diabetes.

Self-defense: Use only the recommended amount of medicines that contain magnesium. If those doses do not help, do not increase them—see your doctor.

Medical History Danger

Thomas J. Romano, MD, PhD, rheumatologist in private practice in Wheeling, WV.

Don't forget about over-the-counter (OTC) medications if your doctor asks what drugs you take.

Common mistake: Thinking that OTC medications aren't "real" drugs. In fact, OTC drugs can affect the action of prescription drugs.

Example: One arthritis sufferer stopped responding to a prescription painkiller after she began taking a daily vitamin A pill. Two months after laying off the vitamin A, she once again got relief from the painkiller.

6

Health Secrets for Women

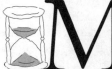

The Secrets of a Happy, Healthy Menopause

Wulf H. Utian, MD, PhD
Case Western Reserve University

Most women alive today will spend more than a third of their lives in their postmenopausal years. Menopause is often associated with uncomfortable symptoms like hot flashes, vaginal dryness and mood swings…and possibly a heightened risk of heart disease and osteoporosis.

Good news: There are now many ways to minimize the ill effects of menopause.

LIFESTYLE CHANGES

Without a doubt, the three most important ingredients for health before, during and after menopause are…

●**Proper diet.** Diet can do a great deal to prevent age-related ailments like heart disease, cancer and osteoporosis. By *proper*, I mean mostly fruits, vegetables and grains, and minimal fat, salt and sugar. If your eating habits aren't perfect, take a daily multivitamin.

To reduce your risk of osteoporosis, starting at menopause increase your consumption of calcium to 1,500 mg a day. And be sure to get at least 400 international units (IU) of vitamin D —from dairy products, vitamin supplements and/or sun exposure. (The skin makes vitamin D when exposed to the sun.)

Vitamin D boosts the body's absorption of calcium. One cup of milk contains about 300 mg of calcium and 100 IU of vitamin D.

●**Exercise.** Besides staving off heart disease and osteoporosis, regular workouts improve mood and overall well-being.

Best: "Weight-bearing" aerobic activities like walking, dancing, running, cross-country skiing and cycling…along with weight lifting.

Wulf H. Utian, MD, PhD, professor and chairman of reproductive biology at Case Western Reserve University School of Medicine in Cleveland. He is coauthor of *Managing Your Menopause*. Fireside Books.

123

Try to fit in at least three 20-minute sessions a week.

●**Good habits.** Hot flashes can often be controlled by stopping smoking and limiting intake of alcohol, caffeine and spicy foods.

ALTERNATIVES TO HRT

If you choose not to go on hormone-replacement therapy (HRT), there are other options for relieving problems associated with menopause…

●**Alendronate** (Fosamax). When approved by the FDA, this drug was the first nonhormone remedy for osteoporosis.

In two large studies, alendronate was given in conjunction with daily calcium supplements. *Result:* Bone density increased by 8% at the hip and spine. The rate of fractures fell by 63%.

●**Calcitonin-salmon** (Miacalcin). This nasal spray is another option for osteoporosis. It's good for women who are more than five years past menopause and who have low bone mass. Two two-year studies have proven that the drug quickly increases bone mineral density in the spine, more slowly in the forearm or hip.

For maximum effectiveness, it must be taken with at least 1,000 mg of calcium and 400 IU of vitamin D a day.

●**Progestin.** If your only problem is hot flashes, oral progestin (without estrogen) may help. But it won't help other menopause symptoms…and it may boost your risk of heart disease.

●**Relaxation.** Biofeedback, deep breathing, yoga and meditation can all be used to reduce the intensity of hot flashes.

●**Vaginal lubricants.** If you experience vaginal discomfort during intercourse, Replens or K-Y Jelly can help. *Also helpful:* Having sex on a regular basis.

A PROMISING TREATMENT

The combination of a twice-daily slow-release fluoride tablet and 400 mg of calcium has been shown to reduce spinal fractures by 70% among women suffering from osteoporosis…and build bone mass in the hip and spine at the rate of 2% to 6% a year.

FDA approval of slow-release fluoride is expected soon.

UNPROVEN REMEDIES

Some doctors believe that megadoses of vitamins E and C reduce menopause symptoms and cut the risk of heart disease and cancer. Vitamin E may also relieve hot flashes and vaginal dryness. However, their role in treating menopause symptoms remains unproven, especially when taken in supplement form. I don't recommend them.

Likewise, there's a lot of hype about herbal remedies like *dong quai, sarsaparilla, red clover* or *damiana*—but there's no evidence that any of these work.

 # The Great Hormone Debate

Christiane Northrup, MD, a physician in private practice in Yarmouth, ME, and former clinical assistant professor of obstetrics and gynecology at University of Vermont College of Medicine in Burlington. She is the author of *The Wisdom of Menopause.* Bantam Doubleday Dell.

Joyce Kakkis, MD, assistant professor of obstetrics and gynecology at the University of California-Irvine. She is in private practice in Long Beach, CA, specializing in HRT, and is the author of *Confessions of an Estrogen Evangelist.* KMG, Inc.

Recent media reports have stressed the dangers of hormone replacement therapy. But two eminent gynecologists, who have researched hormone therapy for themselves, say it's a bit more complicated.

Doctors have long recommended hormone replacement therapy (HRT) to not only prevent hot flashes and other menopausal symptoms, but also to curb the risk for heart disease and osteoporosis.

But when researchers recently halted a major study on the benefits of HRT, millions of women were forced to re-evaluate their options for controlling menopausal symptoms.

After five years of study, researchers at the Women's Health Initiative (WHI) found that women who took a daily tablet of synthetic estrogen and synthetic progesterone had a 26% higher rate of breast cancer, a 29% higher rate of heart attack and a 41% higher rate of stroke than those taking a placebo. As a result of these findings, the 16,608 women being studied were instructed to stop taking the medications—immediately.

Is this the last word on HRT? For answers, we interviewed two leading experts in women's health—physicians who have addressed these questions for themselves and for their patients.

Christiane Northrup, MD, age 53, is menopausal (complete cessation of periods) and favors the use of natural treatments for menopausal symptoms.

Joyce Kakkis, MD, age 46, is perimenopausal (the years preceding menopause, when periods become irregular) and favors the use of HRT.

Here's what each doctor says about the current issues surrounding HRT…

DR. NORTHRUP

●**What is your opinion of the WHI study?** I felt that the study had major flaws from the outset. Women took a pill consisting of estrogen made from the urine of a pregnant mare, in combination with a chemically synthesized form of the hormone progesterone.

In all the years of human evolution, except for about the last 50, these chemicals have never been introduced into human bodies. And this so-called medicine—prescribed at the same dosage for millions of women, whether they weighed 110 or 210 pounds —was supposed to reduce the risk for heart disease, osteoporosis and other chronic degenerative diseases in the majority of women who took it. Given that the hormone dosages weren't individualized and didn't match those found in human females, I'm not surprised that there were adverse consequences.

●**Do you ever recommend HRT?** Yes. Some perimenopausal and menopausal women need hormones to control symptoms or feel their best. Working with her doctor, a woman should have her hormone levels checked and then decide what she needs. Some women's bodies, like mine, make adequate levels of hormones. Others don't. Some women feel best on HRT, while others don't. Women who have had their ovaries removed often need HRT for a few years.

If hormones are recommended, they should be *bio-identical*. This means they are chemically identical to the hormones manufactured in a woman's body, not patented animal versions or synthetic substitutes, which are so widely used today. And the doctor should check hormone levels every year, since a woman's body changes.

For myself, I wouldn't hesitate to use hormones if I needed them, but since my hormone levels are adequate and I don't have any health problems, I do not take them. Instead, I use natural alternatives to control my menopausal symptoms.

●**What do you use in place of HRT?** Soy does nearly everything HRT does without any of the side effects. I use soy to help control symptoms, such as hot flashes. Soy can also help control insomnia, dry skin and hair, depression and vaginal dryness, as well as strengthen the bones and heart.

The active ingredient in soy is *isoflavones,* a plant-derived "phytoestrogen" that acts like the estrogen found in the body. Do not take isolated soy isoflavones in pill form. Recent studies have shown that large amounts may increase breast cancer risk. Eat soy foods, including edamame (soybeans), soy milk, soy burgers and tofu.

●**How do you protect yourself against heart disease, bone loss and other age-related conditions?** In addition to eating soy, I follow some simple strategies. To build bones, I lift weights two to three times per week. Each day, I take 1,200 milligrams (mg) of calcium, 800 mg of magnesium and 400 mg to 800 mg of vitamin D—and get 15 minutes of sunlight without sunscreen in either the early morning or late afternoon. (I wear sunscreen the rest of the day.) To protect my heart, I take a brisk, 30-minute walk five times a week and eat a heart-healthy diet, including at least five daily servings of colorful fruits and vegetables.

DR. KAKKIS

●**What is your opinion of the WHI study?** I think the negative results of the WHI were overstated. By analyzing 10,000 of the study subjects on HRT, researchers found that eight additional women developed breast cancer or had a stroke and seven additional women developed heart disease each year, compared with those not taking HRT.

In light of these findings, should *everyone* stop HRT? I don't think so. Also, most experts think that women who get breast cancer within 10 years of starting HRT have a pre-existing condition that was simply accelerated by HRT. In other words, HRT is not the cause of their cancer.

The study also showed some benefits of HRT. Among the women analyzed, six fewer developed colorectal cancer and five fewer suffered hip fracture each year. Should women with a family history of colon cancer and osteoporosis stop HRT? I don't think so.

Finally, quality-of-life issues—hot flashes, insomnia, irritability and depression—were not addressed by this study. I do not intend to stop taking hormones on the basis of the WHI results, nor am I advising my patients to stop.

●**What's the best way to take HRT?** By using the lowest effective dose, which minimizes the risks. Typically, I start my patients at 25% to 50% of the standard dose of HRT. Then I monitor symptoms every six weeks and gradually increase the dosage only if the lower level is not working. The therapy is individually designed for each woman.

To get this type of treatment, a woman needs to work with a doctor who is familiar with the various options available for HRT. These include gels, creams, patches, pills and suppositories, as well as lower doses and "compounded" formulations, custom-blended by a compounding pharmacist.

If you don't find such a doctor, you're likely to be stuck with a standardized formulation that may not be right for you. The North American Menopause Society (NAMS) lists physicians who know about the latest in HRT. *To find a physician in your area:* Consult the NAMS Web site at *www.menopause.org.*

Once you've found the right doctor, you need to have blood tests to determine your hormone levels. Afterward, you should be re-evaluated by your doctor to see whether the therapy is working and to have it adjusted if it is not.

●**What do you take?** I take birth-control pills to control my perimenopausal symptoms. I'm still fertile, so the Pill acts as a contraceptive while providing the needed mix of hormones to prevent hormonal fluctuations for a perimenopausal woman my age. I intend to go from the Pill to low-dose HRT, and to take it for the rest of my life.

●**Do you use any natural remedies?** I eat edamame. It makes a delicious dish after 10 minutes of steaming. I have three, one-cup servings a week to control my perimenopausal symptoms.

I also take 800 international units (IU) of vitamin E to help control hot flashes and 1,500 mg a day of calcium (500 mg per meal) to reduce muscle cramps, stabilize my mood and strengthen my bones.

Estrogen Trap

Graham Barr, MD, fellow, Channing Laboratory, Brigham and Women's Hospital, Boston.

Estrogen replacement therapy (ERT) may contribute to asthma. *Recent finding:* Menopausal women on ERT have an 80% higher risk of developing asthma than women not taking hormones. *Theory:* Estrogen affects cells involved in the body's allergic or inflammatory response. *Important:* Women considering estrogen therapy should discuss these findings with their physicians. Asthma risk must be weighed against the potential benefits of ERT.

Wrinkle Remover

Stephen E. Chiarello, MD, a dermatologist in private practice in Port Charlotte, FL.

A "hand-sanding" technique lets doctors remove wrinkles without the high cost of the usual technique (laser resurfacing).

Called *manual dermasanding,* the technique involves injecting the wrinkled area with topical anesthetics. Wrinkles are then buffed away using a sandpaper-like material.

Strategies for Avoiding Troublesome Breast Cysts

Christiane Northrup, MD, assistant clinical professor of obstetrics and gynecology, University of Vermont College of Medicine, at Maine Medical Center, Portland. She is author of *Women's Bodies, Women's Wisdom.* Bantam Books.

Breast cancer gets lots of media attention—and rightly so. But far more common is *fibrocystic breast disease.* At some point during their lives, 70% of women develop the fluid-filled, tender or painful breast lumps that characterize this condition.

We asked University of Vermont gynecologist Christiane Northrup, MD, to answer the most common questions about breast cysts…

●**What causes breast cysts?** During ovulation and just prior to menstruation, fluctuating hormone levels can cause breast cells to retain fluid—resulting in cysts.

An estrogen/progesterone imbalance also appears to promote cyst development, but doctors don't know exactly how—or why.

In some cases, cysts are linked to abnormally high levels of estrogen. This is usually caused by eating too much fat.

Other women develop breast cysts despite having normal estrogen levels. *Good news:* The lumps usually disappear following menopause.

●**How can I tell a tumor from a cyst?** Cysts typically feel like a bunch of peas or grapes just under the skin. A painful lump is nearly always a cyst. Cancerous lumps are generally not tender.

●**Is breast cancer more common among women who get breast cysts?** In the 1970s, a few studies indicated that this might be the case. But subsequent research at the National Cancer Institute found that the vast majority of fibrocystic breast disease diagnoses did *not* involve an increased risk of cancer.

Exception: About 1% of women with fibrocystic breasts have *ductal atypia.* These abnormal breast cells sometimes turn cancerous.

●**If I discover a lump in my breast, what should I do?** Have your doctor examine it at once. He/she may want to obtain additional tests, such as a mammogram, sonogram or needle aspiration/biopsy.

If the lump contains fluid, odds are it's a cyst. It should disappear once the fluid is removed.

●**Are certain women more likely to get breast cysts?** Fibrocystic breasts are more common among women who are sensitive to caffeine…and those who have heavy periods, severe menstrual cramps and/or premenstrual syndrome.

●**The lumps in my breasts are very painful. What can I do for relief?** First, avoid all sources of caffeine. That goes for chocolate and caffeinated soft drinks, as well as coffee and tea. And don't overlook over-the-counter painkillers and diet aids. Many contain caffeine.

To keep your estrogen levels in check, adopt a low-fat, high-fiber diet. This diet should contain no dairy products…and should be high in whole grains, fruits, vegetables and beans. If dairy products are your primary source of calcium, be sure to take calcium supplements. After three months, add dairy foods back into your diet to see if they make a difference.

●**Are nutritional supplements helpful?** Many women get at least partial relief by taking a daily multivitamin or a daily pill containing 400 to 600 international units (IU) of vitamin E.

Also helpful: Selenium (24 to 32 micrograms a day)…vitamin A (1,000 to 5,000 IU a day)…capsules of evening primrose oil, flaxseed oil or black currant seed oil (500 mg four times a day).

●**A friend of mine suggests that I try massage. Is that helpful?** Yes. Massage relieves discomfort by dispersing excess fluid to the lymph glands, where it's channeled out of the body.

What to do: Rub your hands together until they are warm, then massage each breast in concentric circles about 30 times. Use both hands, with your fingertips meeting in the middle. Move clockwise on the right breast, counterclockwise on the left breast.

For persistently painful breast cysts, I often recommend self-treatment with topical iodine. Iodine seems to affect estrogen's ability to bind to breast cells.

Apply iodine tincture in a three-inch-square patch to your upper thigh or lower abdomen. If the iodine stain fades within a few hours, apply it to another area of the upper thigh or lower abdomen.

Repeat these applications as long as they continue to fade within a few hours. When you can see a slight stain that persists for 24 hours, stop the treatment.

Easy Relief for Hot Flashes

Gregory L. Burke, MD, professor and vice chair, department of public health services, Bowman Gray School of Medicine, Winston–Salem, NC.

Try eating more soy. In a study, menopausal women who added 20 grams (g) of soy powder a day (about four tablespoons) to their diets reported reduced severity of hot flashes and night sweats.

Bonus: Their cholesterol levels also fell.

Theory: Soy contains *isoflavones*, compounds that mimic the beneficial effects of estrogen without its risks. Estrogen-replacement therapy raises the risk of breast and ovarian cancer. Soy powder, available at health food stores, can be added to juice, cereals and other foods.

Breast Cancer and Abortions

JoAnn Manson, MD, codirector of women's health, Brigham & Women's Hospital, Harvard Medical School, Boston.

The risk of breast cancer does *not* appear to be increased by abortion. This conclusion is based on a comprehensive study in which researchers studied the histories of 1.5 million Danish women born between 1935 and 1978. Because Danish law requires registration of all births, abortions and cancer cases, this study avoided reporting bias found in earlier studies in which some women who had undergone abortions may not have disclosed that fact to researchers. This bias may explain results in some earlier studies that suggested a link between abortion and breast cancer.

Evaluating Breast Lumps

Ellen Mendelson, MD, director, Breast Diagnostic Imaging Center of the Western Pennsylvania Hospital, Pittsburgh.

A technique for evaluating breast lumps—*high-resolution ultrasound imaging*—can reduce the need for biopsies by 40%. This equipment is used in many breast imaging centers. Ultrasound can be used to distinguish lumps that are fluid-filled and not cancerous from those that are solid and require further evaluation. Solid masses with thin, sharp, smooth margins are often benign...those with jagged edges or irregular shapes may be malignant.

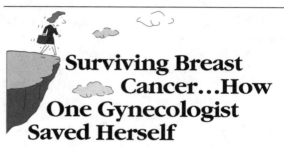

Surviving Breast Cancer...How One Gynecologist Saved Herself

Barbara Joseph, MD, an obstetrician and gynecologist in private practice in Stamford, CT. She is author of *My Healing from Breast Cancer: A Physician's Personal Story of Recovery and Transformation.* Keats Publishing.

In April 1991, 36-year-old Barbara Joseph, MD, was nursing her eight-week-old son when she felt a lump in her left breast. Days later, the 36-year-old obstetrician-gynecologist was diagnosed with advanced (Stage III) breast cancer.

At first Dr. Joseph was gripped by panic. But she knew that this was only the beginning of her journey...so she took a deep breath and started to investigate her treatment options.

Ultimately, Dr. Joseph underwent selected conventional treatment, including surgery and chemotherapy. But she gives equal credit for her recovery to her use of holistic medical strategies.

Dr. Joseph spoke with us about how women should respond to a diagnosis of breast cancer...

•**Don't rush into treatment.** By the time a tumor is big enough to be seen on a mammogram, odds are it's been forming for six to eight years. Breast cancer in general is not an emergency situation.

When I was diagnosed, part of me wanted to start treatment the next day. But you need not act the next day—or even the next week. Better to spend a few days or weeks considering all your options.

●**Find the right doctor.** Your diagnosis may have been made by your gynecologist or internist. But when it comes to breast surgery, you'll want a surgeon—perhaps one who specializes in treatment of the breast.

You may also need to consult a *medical oncologist* (a cancer specialist who administers chemotherapy)…and/or a *radiation oncologist* (who administers radiation therapy).

The doctor's credentials are important, but they aren't the only thing to consider.

You must feel comfortable with the treatment plan recommended by the doctor…and with the doctor's ability to communicate and listen.

Is he/she compassionate? Do you have rapport with him/her? Will he/she support you in your treatment decisions—even if they're not all conventional ones?

Do not just jump into the first treatment suggested. *Always* get a second opinion.

●**Learn as much as you can about breast cancer.** Talk to your doctors and read everything you can get your hands on.

In addition to my own book, I recommend Dr. Susan Love's *Breast Book* and *Breast Cancer: What You Should Know (But May Not Be Told) About Prevention, Diagnosis and Treatment* by Steve Austin, MD, and Cathy Hitchcock.

Another source of up-to-date information is the Y-ME National Breast Cancer Organization (800-221-2141).

●**Consider breast-sparing surgery.** We now know that *lumpectomy* (removal of just the lump) plus radiation is just as effective as *mastectomy* (removal of the entire breast).

Yet lumpectomy isn't always possible.

If the tumor lies in the center of the breast, for example, mastectomy may be better.

These are also matters you should research —and discuss with your surgeon.

●**Do not leave the treatment decision up to your doctor.** You may be overwhelmed by all your options, but ultimately it's you who must decide.

Taking charge of the decision process empowers you emotionally—and physically. A study by Dr. Steven Greer showed that breast cancer patients who exhibited a fighting spirit were twice as likely to be alive 15 years later than those who felt hopeless.

●**Rethink your lifestyle.** Although it's hard to prove, I am convinced that cancer is the body's response to a host of insults that it's been subjected to over the years.

That includes dietary fat and pesticide residues in food…air and water pollution… psychological stress…and repressed anger.

Unless you take steps to eliminate these things, your cancer is likely to recur.

Up to 60% of all cancers in women are related to diet. A woman who eats traditional American fare tends to ingest huge amounts of carcinogens—pesticides, preservatives and other additives as well as cancer-causing partially hydrogenated oils.

Women's breasts are particularly sensitive to these toxins. That's because many toxins are soluble in body fat—and breast tissue is composed of a large percentage of fat.

Since my diagnosis, I've chosen to eat only organic foods (grown without pesticides). My diet also incorporates some of the principles I learned through my study of *macrobiotics*. It consists largely of grains, plant-based proteins and sea vegetables (kelp, nori, etc.) and is free of dairy products.

I also eat lots of soy—miso, tofu and tempeh. These foods contain phytochemicals that are breast-protective.

●**Join a support group.** I believe that repressed anger and other negative emotions disrupt the healing process.

Individual and/or group therapy can help you develop the emotional strength you need to stop investing your energy in old resentments—so that you can move on and live in the present.

The evidence for this is compelling. In one study, conducted by David Spiegel, MD, of

Stanford University, women with Stage IV breast cancer who attended weekly group therapy sessions survived twice as long as those who didn't attend—even though both groups received the same medical treatment.

To find a support group in your area, contact the Cancer Care Counseling Line (800-813-4673) or the Y-ME National Breast Cancer Organization. Or simply network with other breast cancer patients. Women heal by nurturing one another, and support groups foster this process.

●**Take nutritional supplements.** Foods are the best source of cancer-fighting nutrients. But certain supplements can make a crucial difference—especially if chemotherapy has left you too weak to eat properly.

Ask your doctor (or a nutritionist) about taking…

●**Daily multivitamins/multiminerals.**

●**Antioxidants.** Each day, I take beta-carotene and vitamins C and E.

●**Flaxseed oil.** Each day, I add one to two tablespoons of a product called Udo's Choice. It provides essential fatty acids.

Milk and Breast Cancer Connection

Neal Barnard, MD, president of Physicians Committee for Responsible Medicine, 5100 Wisconsin Ave., Washington, DC 20016. He is author of *Eat Right, Live Longer*. Harmony Books.

Milk has been connected to breast cancer through a growth hormone given to cows. The more milk you drink, the greater the risk.

Problems in children: Diabetes, anemia and colic.

Problems in adults: Arthritis, cataracts, anemia, infertility in women and ovarian cancer.

Best alternative sources of calcium: Dark green, leafy vegetables like broccoli, kale and collards (not spinach)…beans…calcium-fortified foods.

Avoid calcium wasters: Animal protein—including beef, poultry and fish…caffeine…salt…tobacco…a sedentary lifestyle.

Surprising High Heels Benefit

Suzanne Levine, DO, clinical adjunct podiatrist, New York Hospital–Cornell Medical Center, New York.

High heels can relieve heel and arch pain, often experienced by women after pregnancy or weight gain. They take pressure off those painful areas and move it to the ball of the foot.

Helpful: Wear heels of different heights at different times of the day to stretch muscles and tendons. The highest heel should be two-and-a-half inches tall. Also, avoid very thin heels.

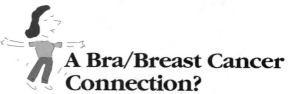

A Bra/Breast Cancer Connection?

Adriane Fugh-Berman, MD, a Washington, DC-based medical researcher who specializes in women's health and alternative medicine. She is author of *Alternative Medicine: What Works*. Odonian Press.

Do brassieres cause breast cancer? Will switching to undershirts decrease your risk? Probably not. Although Singer and Grismaijer, the husband and wife coauthors of *Dressed to Kill* (Avery), maintain that the bra/breast cancer link is supported by scientific evidence, their "study" of this evidence is full of holes.

The bra/breast cancer theory was born several years ago in Fiji, when Grismaijer found a lump in her breast. Around the same time, her husband noticed the red marks on her body from her bra…and became convinced that the bra was to blame for her lump.

Grismaijer did not have the lump biopsied. Instead, she embarked on a regimen of exercise, organic vegetarian food, purified water, herbs and vitamin supplements—and complete bralessness.

Guess what? The lump disappeared. But attributing its disappearance to not wearing a bra—as Grismaijer does—is ridiculous.

There's a good chance that the lump was benign. Grismaijer was pregnant when the lump was found, and hormonal changes during pregnancy are known to cause lumps.

After interviewing more than 4,000 women with and without breast cancer, the authors concluded that wearing a bra for more than 12 hours a day significantly increases the risk for breast cancer.

Unfortunately, this "finding" was unwarranted. Their study was conducted in a haphazard manner—without adherence to fundamental principles of scientific research. For example, no effort was made to ensure that the women in the two groups were similar in age, family history, medical history and other known risk factors for breast cancer.

The study was of such poor quality that it would have been disqualified from being published in a reputable medical journal. I'm afraid that's why it was packaged as a paperback book and directed at consumers instead of doctors.

The bottom line? There is simply no evidence that bras cause breast cancer. Fortunately, there are other things women can do to reduce their risk...

●**Eat more soy foods.** Tofu, tempeh, miso and soy milk all contain plant estrogens (phytoestrogens). These weak hormones inhibit the body's own production of estrogen, which may provide the "fuel" for breast cancer growth.

Neither soy oil nor soy sauce contain significant amounts of phytoestrogens.

●**Eat cruciferous vegetables.** Broccoli, cauliflower, brussels sprouts and kale affect estrogen metabolism in a beneficial way.

●**Think twice about estrogen-replacement therapy.** It's reasonable to use estrogen temporarily to treat hot flashes and vaginal dryness. But in general, long-term estrogen therapy is not a good idea. Estrogen can increase the risk of breast cancer.

●**Avoid pesticides.** Some pesticides contain estrogen-like compounds. Eat organic food whenever possible...and peel or wash all fruits and vegetables.

●**Eat a low-fat diet.** There is reason to believe that an extremely low-fat intake (less than 20% of calories from fat) is protective.

●**Exercise.** Women who exercise aerobically for more than three hours a week have a lower risk of developing breast cancer.

What about mammograms? They do not prevent breast cancer, but they reduce the risk of death from breast cancer by helping to find tumors in their early, treatable stages.

Smart Sports Bra Buying

James Dolan, MD, gynecological oncologist, Lutheran General Cancer Care Center, Park Ridge, IL.

Look for a bra made from soft fabric, especially in the nipple area...straps should be wide enough to support without digging into shoulders...avoid seams across the nipple area and bras with hook fasteners, which can chafe ...make sure that it won't ride up in the back or restrict arm movement. Be certain the chest band will stay in place and not roll up.

Most Breast Lumps Are Normal

Christiane Northrup, MD, assistant clinical professor of obstetrics and gynecology, University of Vermont College of Medicine, at Maine Medical Center, Portland. She is author of *Women's Bodies, Women's Wisdom*. Bantam Books.

Human breast tissue is naturally very lumpy. But 20% of women who are between the ages of 25 and 50 have fibrocystic changes that produce unwanted, often painful lumps. These lumps are usually benign...but they can mask early detection of breast cancer.

Self-defense: Wear a supportive bra to minimize your discomfort...cut your salt intake to reduce swelling from water retention...perform breast self-examinations monthly...and see a doctor to make sure a lump is normal and not potentially troublesome.

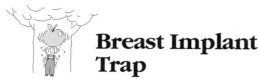

Breast Implant Trap

Sherine E. Gabriel, MD, associate professor of medicine and epidemiology, Mayo Clinic, Rochester, MN. Her review of medical records of 749 breast implant recipients was published in *The New England Journal of Medicine*, 10 Shattuck St., Boston 02115.

One in four women who has breast implant surgery needs repeat surgery within eight years.

Usual reasons: Formation of hard tissue around the implant...ruptured implant...infection...chronic pain...nipple necrosis (tissue death).

Such complications are more common with implants put in following breast cancer (34% at five years) than with those put in for cosmetic reasons (12% at five years).

When to Schedule A Mammogram

Pamela A. Propeck, MD, radiologist, associate professor, department of radiology, University of Wisconsin, Madison.

Schedule mammogram appointments well in advance. It can take as long as eight weeks to get a routine mammogram screening. *Reasons:* Low reimbursement rates by insurers have caused many imaging centers to cut back services or close...and more women have mammograms annually instead of every two years.

Large Women and Mammograms

Matthew J. Reeves, PhD, State Chronic Disease Epidemiologist, Michigan Dept. of Community Health, Lansing, MI.

Annual mammograms are particularly important for larger women.

A study of almost 3,000 women with breast cancer found that among women who detected their own cancer, the tumors were larger and more advanced among overweight women.

The findings suggest that larger women are less likely to find small lumps by self-examination techniques than smaller women, making it more important for them to get regular mammograms.

The best chance of detecting breast cancer at an early stage for women of all weights is to obtain regular mammograms along with regular exams by your doctor.

Antiperspirants and Mammograms

Daniel Kopans, MD, director, Breast Imaging Division, Massachusetts General Hospital, and associate professor of radiology, Harvard Medical School, both in Boston.

Antiperspirants can interfere with mammography. They contain aluminum and/or other metals that can be mistaken for suspicious calcium deposits. Deodorants don't interfere—because they contain no metal.

Other substances that interfere with mammography: Lotions, oils, powders and zinc oxide, often used by women with large breasts to treat chronic irritation.

Incontinence and Exercise Connection

Ingrid Nygaard, MD, assistant professor of obstetrics and gynecology, University of Iowa, Iowa City. Her study of 18 women 33 to 73 years of age was published in the *Journal of Reproductive Medicine*, 8342 Olive Blvd., St. Louis 63132.

One in three women experience incontinence while working out.

Helpful: A tampon worn in the lower vagina—to support the urethra. Fifty-eight percent of women who tried this remedy reported no urine leakage during aerobic exercise. Wet the tampon to ease insertion—and to prevent vaginal dryness.

Urinary Incontinence Advance

Jane Miller, MD, assistant professor of urology, University of Washington Medical Center, Seattle.

A disposable urethral insert significantly reduced incontinence in 98% of women who participated in a study. When inflated, the balloon-tipped device rests at the neck of the bladder, blocking the flow of urine. To urinate, the woman pulls the attached string to deflate the balloon, then removes the device. The insert must initially be fitted by a doctor.

Sold under the name *Reliance*, the device is now available in most drugstores.

Osteoporosis Advance

Robert R. Recker, MD, professor of medicine and director, Osteoporosis Research Center, Creighton University School of Medicine, Omaha.

A prescription drug called *alendronate* (Fosamax) cut the incidence of vertebral fractures by nearly 50% among women with osteoporosis. During a three-year study, only 18% of women on alendronate suffered more than one fracture, compared with 68% of women given a placebo.

A Mile a Day...

Study of 238 postmenopausal women by Elizabeth Krall, USDA Agricultural Research Service, Washington, DC.

Walking as little as a mile a day can delay osteoporosis up to seven years.

Background: Most women lose 3% to 6% of their bone mass annually during the five years surrounding menopause. A study found that walking will delay osteoporosis significantly. Women who walked regularly took four to seven years longer to lose as much bone as women who did not walk at all.

Cancer and Chemotherapy

Bernard Fisher, MD, distinguished service professor of surgery, University of Pittsburgh.

All breast cancer patients can benefit from chemotherapy. For years, chemotherapy has been the standard treatment for all *node-positive* tumors and *node-negative* tumors that are *estrogen-receptor negative*. But *node-negative, estrogen-receptor-positive* tumors traditionally have been treated with the drug *tamoxifen* (Nolvadex) alone.

Finding: After five years, 90% of patients with such tumors who underwent chemotherapy were cancer-free. Only 84% of patients on tamoxifen alone remained cancer-free after five years.

Weight Loss May Not Be Good for Some

Jean Langlois, ScD, an investigator in epidemiology at the National Institute on Aging, Bethesda, MD.

Women over 50 who lose a lot of weight increase their risk of hip fractures. A study of women age 67 and older found that those who lost 10% or more of their weight after age 50 doubled their chances of breaking a hip. Physicians suggest that overweight 50-year-old women should strive to reach an appropriate weight and then stay at that level, because heart disease, associated with being overweight, is more dangerous than hip fractures. But they should take calcium and vitamin D supplements to help strengthen bones and prevent osteoporosis.

Hot Summer Days And Premature Labor

Shoghag Lajinian, MD, assistant professor of obstetrics–gynecology, State University of New York Health Science Center, Brooklyn. Her analysis of New York City's heat index and admissions for preterm labor was presented at a meeting of the American College of Obstetricians and Gynecologists, 409 12th St. SW, Washington, DC 20024.

Hot summer days can trigger premature labor. Women were twice as likely to begin contractions on the hottest days of the year as on the coldest.

Theory: Heat and dehydration boost the body's production of the hormones *oxytocin* and *antidiuretic hormone*. These compounds play a role in inducing contractions.

Self-defense: Women at risk—those between 24 and 36 weeks of pregnancy—should stay out of the heat and drink plenty of liquids to prevent dehydration.

Depression–Osteoporosis Link

David Michelson, MD, medical officer, National Institute of Mental Health, Bethesda, MD. His study of bone density in 48 women, average age 41, was published in *The New England Journal of Medicine*, 10 Shattuck St., Boston 02115.

Depression raises a woman's risk of osteoporosis. Bone density in young women who had suffered depression was 6% to 14% lower than in women who had never been depressed.

Theory: Depression boosts synthesis of the stress hormone *cortisol*, which has been linked to bone loss.

Breast-Feeding Benefit

Burris Duncan, MD, professor of pediatrics, pediatrics department, University Medical Center–Arizona Health Sciences, Tucson. His study of 1,013 infants was published in *Pediatrics*, 141 Northwest Point Blvd., Elk Grove Village, IL 60009.

Breast-fed infants experience fewer ear infections than those who are bottle-fed. Infants who nurse exclusively during their first four months have half as many ear infections as bottle-fed babies…and 40% fewer infections than those who were breast-fed but had supplemental feedings prior to four months. At least some of the beneficial effects last a full year, even if breast-feeding is stopped.

Pregnancy and Smoking

Carolyn D. Drews, PhD, associate professor of epidemiology, Emory University, Rolling School of Public Health, Atlanta. Her study of the mothers of 221 children with mental retardation and 400 other mothers in a control group was published in *Pediatrics,* 141 Northwest Point Blvd., Elk Grove Village, IL 60009.

Pregnant women who smoke as few as five cigarettes per week are 50% more likely to give birth to children with mental retardation. The more a woman smokes during pregnancy, the greater the likelihood that her child will have mental retardation. Smoking during pregnancy has been linked to low birth weight, higher infant mortality and lower intelligence in children. This is the first study to link smoking and mental retardation. If these numbers are accurate, mental retardation could have been prevented in one-third of the children whose mothers smoked during pregnancy.

Folic Acid's Role in Pregnancy

William F. Rayburn, MD, chief of maternal–fetal medicine and professor of obstetrics and gynecology, University of Oklahoma College of Medicine, Oklahoma City.

Folic acid supplements are worth considering for all women of reproductive age. This B vitamin helps prevent brain and spinal column defects in newborns. To prevent such defects, women should begin taking 400 micrograms a day at least one month prior to conception…and continue for at least three months afterward.

Problem: If women start taking folic acid supplements *after* learning they are pregnant, it may be too late for the nutrient's beneficial effects in preventing birth defects.

Morning Sickness Self-Defense

Miriam Erick, MS, RD, nutritionist at Brigham and Women's Hospital, Boston, and author of *Take Two Crackers and Call Me in the Morning: A Real-Life Guide for Surviving Morning Sickness.* Grinnen-Barrett Publishing Co.

Avoid smells that commonly trigger nausea—coffee, perfume/cologne, rotting garbage, pet foods, hot foods, body odors.

● **Don't watch food commercials on TV.**

● **Be wary of public transportation and driving in stop-and-go traffic.** Jerky motion can add to nausea.

● **Avoid visual motion**—such as a fast-paced music video—which can increase nausea.

● **Drink at least 10 cups of water or liquids daily** or eat foods with high water content, since adequate hydration reduces nausea.

Pregnancy and Thinking

T. Murphy Goodwin, MD, associate professor of obstetrics and gynecology, University of Southern California Medical Center, Los Angeles.

Pregnancy dulls women's thinking. In a study, women scored as much as 20% lower on intelligence tests during their last month of pregnancy than they did after giving birth.

Weakest areas: Remembering new information and tracking more than one piece of information at a time.

The Truth About "Post-Baby Blues"

John Studd, MD, DSc, consultant gynecologist, Chelsea and Westminster Hospital, London. His study of 61 women with postpartum depression was published in *The Lancet*, 42 Bedford Square, London WC1B 3SL, England.

Because of a drop in estrogen levels following childbirth, one in 10 new mothers experiences depression. Sadness can last for months, and severe cases can lead to suicide.

Good news: Estrogen skin patches eliminated depression within three months in 80% of new mothers. Most of those who wore *placebo* patches stayed depressed for at least four months.

Bladder Pain Relief

Vicki Ratner, MD, an orthopedic surgeon in private practice in San Jose, CA. An interstitial cystitis sufferer, she is cofounder of the Interstitial Cystitis Association, Box 1553, Madison Square Station, New York 10159.

Bladder pain caused by the mysterious disorder *interstitial cystitis* (IC) can be controlled with an oral medication called *pentosan polysulfate* (Elmiron). Sufferers say the pain is like having broken glass inside the bladder. The only drug previously approved to treat IC, *dimethyl sulfoxide* (DMSO), had to be administered into the bladder via a catheter. It was inconvenient and unpleasant.

Study: Pentosan helped about 38% of sufferers who took it three times a day. Ninety percent of the 500,000 people who have IC are women.

How Reliable Are Pregnancy Ultrasound Exams?

Sheryl Burt Ruzek, PhD, MPH, professor of health education, Temple University, Philadelphia.

Although they can provide valuable information about a developing fetus, ultrasound scans are prone to misinterpretation. For example, doctors often identify anatomical defects where none actually exist...or fail to spot actual defects.

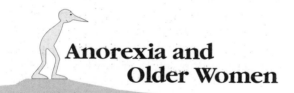

Anorexia and Older Women

Paul L. Hewitt, PhD, associate professor of psychology, University of British Columbia, Vancouver, Canada. His study of 10 million death records over a five-year period (1986 to 1990) was presented at the International Congress of Psychology in Montreal.

Only 25% of those who die of this eating disorder fit the stereotype of the young, overachieving woman.

Reality: Four out of five of those who die of anorexia nervosa are 45 years of age or older.

Female Athletes and Knee Injuries

Laura Huston, MS, researcher, department of orthopedic surgery, University of Michigan, Ann Arbor, who led a study of 140 men and women of varying fitness levels.

Female athletes suffer eight times more knee injuries than male athletes.

Reason: In female athletes, the quadriceps (the muscles at the front of the thigh) are generally stronger than their hamstrings (the muscles at the back of the thigh). This imbalance stresses the knee, causing injury.

Simple self-defense: Strengthen hamstrings by jumping rope for a few minutes three times a week.

Bone Density Study

Ethel Siris, MD, professor of clinical medicine, College of Physicians and Surgeons, Columbia University, New York City.

Bone thinning is grossly undiagnosed in women over age 50. In a recent study of more than 200,000 seemingly healthy women age 50 or older, 40% were found to have low bone density. Seven percent suffered from full-fledged osteoporosis. In the following year, the women with low bone density suffered broken bones at twice the rate of those with normal bone density. Those with osteoporosis did so at four times the rate.

Women and Calcium

Ethel S. Siris, MD, director, osteoporosis program, Columbia–Presbyterian Medical Center, New York City.

Few women get enough calcium. The recommended intake is 1,000 mg for women 25 to 50 years of age and for women over 50 who take estrogen. For women 50 or older who are not taking estrogen and for all women over 65, 1,500 mg is recommended. Eight ounces of milk (or yogurt) contains about 300 mg of calcium.

Getting Enough Minerals

Barbara S. Levine, RD, PhD, director, Calcium Information Center, New York Hospital–Cornell Medical Center, New York City.

Women taking calcium to ward off osteoporosis should be sure to get enough magnesium, too. The body aims to keep the two minerals in balance. Without enough magnesium, calcium is simply excreted.

Surprising: Up to 70% of women are magnesium-deficient.

Helpful: If you're already taking calcium supplements, ask your doctor about adding a magnesium supplement (200 mg a day)…or about eating more magnesium-rich foods like green, leafy vegetables, whole-grain breads, fortified cereals, soybeans, tofu, milk or yogurt.

Incontinence and Smoking

Richard C. Bump, MD, associate professor of obstetrics and gynecology, Duke University Medical Center, Durham, NC. His study of 606 women was published in the *American Journal of Obstetrics and Gynecology*, 11830 Westline Industrial Dr., St. Louis 63146.

Women smokers—even those who had kicked the habit—were two to three times more likely to suffer from incontinence than women who never smoked.

Theory: Harsh, persistent coughing permanently damages pelvic muscles that control urine flow. Animal studies have found that nicotine constricts the bladder, causing unintentional urine leakage.

How Women Can Outwit The Sneaky Malignancy That Killed Gilda Radner

M. Steven Piver, MD, chief of gynecologic oncology, and director of The Gilda Radner Familial Ovarian Cancer Registry, both at Roswell Park Cancer Institute, Elm and Carlton Streets, Buffalo 14263. He and Gilda Radner's former husband, actor Gene Wilder, are the authors of *Gilda's Disease*. Prometheus.

In the autumn of 1985, comedienne Gilda Radner began experiencing fatigue, abdominal cramps, intestinal gas and distension and shooting pains down her thighs.

Gilda consulted gynecologists, gastroenterologists, holistic doctors—even an acupuncturist. All reassured her that her symptoms were harmless.

The doctors were wrong. Gilda's symptoms got worse. Finally, on October 23, 1986, after extensive testing, she was diagnosed with ovarian cancer.

Over the next three years, Gilda underwent four operations, plus agonizing bouts of chemotherapy and radiation. Nothing worked. She died on May 20, 1989.

Gilda's story is tragic. Even more tragic is the fact that her case of missed and delayed diagnosis is typical of ovarian cancer.

Many of the 26,000 American women diagnosed with the disease each year go months or even years without a diagnosis. The longer it takes to get a correct diagnosis, the smaller the chance of survival.

RISK FACTORS

Ovarian cancer is a sneaky and often deadly disease—one doctors frequently fail to consider when rendering a diagnosis. It is easily confused with many other conditions, including uterine fibroids and colitis.

None of Gilda's doctors suspected ovarian cancer until it was too late, even though she had all the classic risk factors. *Gilda…*

●**Ate a high-fat diet.** Dietary fat has been implicated in many cancers, including cancer of the breast, ovaries and colon.

●**Was childless.** Some cases of ovarian cancer are associated with ovary damage caused by

137

years of repeated ovulation. The more times a woman ovulates, the greater her risk.

●**Used fertility-boosting drugs.**

●**Used personal hygiene products containing talcum powder.** Many soaps, deodorants, condoms and contraceptive diaphragms contain talc. Asbestos-like talc particles travel through the cervix and then line the uterus and fallopian tubes, slowly poisoning the ovaries.

●**Had several relatives with ovarian or breast cancer.** The gene for ovarian cancer can be inherited from the mother's or father's side.

THE FAMILY CONNECTION

Women can inherit a predisposition to ovarian cancer *even if none of their relatives had the disease*. That is, women with a family history of certain other types of cancer (breast, colon or prostate) are at increased risk for ovarian cancer.

GENETIC TESTING

It's now possible to be tested for BRCA1 and BRCA2, two of the genes that predispose women to breast and ovarian cancer. In most cases, however, testing is pointless unless you have at least two close relatives with ovarian cancer.

Even then, genetic testing is of limited value. Knowing that you're at increased risk for ovarian and breast cancer causes anxiety…and it doesn't really help you prevent either disease, unless you have your ovaries and breasts surgically removed.

TELLTALE SYMPTOMS

Ovarian cancer is often thought of as a disease that produces no symptoms until it's too far advanced to be cured. That's untrue—although the symptoms tend to be "nonspecific" and thus easy to misinterpret.

In addition to the abdominal and gastrointestinal symptoms Gilda experienced, these symptoms include fever and back pain.

Any woman who experiences one or more of these symptoms for three or more weeks should consult her primary-care doctor or gynecologist. Do *not* wait for the doctor to think of ovarian cancer as a possible diagnosis. Ask to be checked for it right away.

In addition to a pelvic exam, this checkup should include…

●**Blood test for CA125.** This protein is elevated in about 50% of cases of early ovarian cancer and about 95% of cases of advanced ovarian cancer.

●**Vaginal ultrasound exam.** By placing the probe *inside* the vagina, rather than on the abdomen as is traditionally done, the doctor can obtain a better picture of the ovaries.

If the doctor uncovers anything suspicious, he/she should perform a transvaginal sonogram using color-flow Doppler technology (an advanced form of ultrasound).

He should also perform a CT scan of the abdomen and/or a laparoscopy. That's a surgical procedure in which the doctor inserts a viewing scope through a small incision in the abdomen.

GETTING EFFECTIVE TREATMENT

The key to surviving ovarian cancer is getting a prompt diagnosis…and aggressive treatment by a doctor specializing in the disease. For referral to a *gynecologic oncologist* in your area, contact the Gynecologic Cancer Foundation at 800-444-4441.

Most cases of ovarian cancer are treated via removal of the ovaries, plus chemotherapy.

Recently, it was found that women who take a combination of the drugs *paclitaxel* (Taxol) and *cisplatin* (Platinol) live almost three times longer (38 months) than women who undergo standard chemotherapy (25 months).

When the disease is diagnosed early, the five-year survival rate approaches 95%. When it is diagnosed in later stages, survival is reduced to 5% to 30%.

HOW TO PROTECT YOURSELF

In addition to eating a low-fat diet and avoiding talc, women should take these precautions…

●**Get regular checkups.** Women without a family history should have an annual pelvic exam, starting at age 18. Women with a family history of ovarian cancer should have a pelvic exam, CA125 test and a transvaginal ultrasound twice yearly, starting at age 25.

●**If you use birth control, consider taking the Pill.** Oral contraceptives prevent damage to the ovaries that occurs during the childbearing years.

Women who take the Pill for four years have a 40% reduction in their risk for ovarian cancer. Ten years of use cuts the risk by 80%—and the protection lasts for 15 years after you stop taking it.

In women with a strong family history of ovarian cancer, use of the Pill can reduce their risk to that of women who do not have a family history of the disease.

● **Get pregnant...and breast-feed your children.** Pregnancy and breast-feeding interrupt ovulation, cutting your risk by 40%.

● **Consider surgical sterilization.** Having your "tubes tied" stops ovulation, reducing risk by 71%.

● **If you have a strong family history of ovarian cancer,** consider having your ovaries removed. If you're over 40 and scheduled for a hysterectomy, it's prudent to have your ovaries removed along with your uterus—even if you don't have a family history of the disease.

Any woman with two or more close relatives who had ovarian or breast cancer should consider enrolling in The Gilda Radner Familial Ovarian Cancer Registry. Call 800-682-7426 ...or point your Web browser to *http://rpci. med.buffalo.edu/clinic/gynonc/grwp.html.*

Weight-Loss Health Trap

Jean Langlois, ScD, epidemiologist, who published a study of more than 3,600 women, age 67 and older, National Institute on Aging, Bethesda, MD.

Women who become too thin can endanger their well-being.

Reason: Women who go to extremes to eliminate fat from their bodies often go too far. Researchers have found that in healthy women, body fat should be between 16% and 26% of total weight—with the ideal being about 20%.

Quick way to see if weight is in healthy range: Use the hip-to-waist ratio. Pass a tape measure around your body, and cross the navel. Jot down the result. Then pass the tape around your buttocks to measure your hips. Divide the waist measurement by the hip measurement. If the result is below 0.85, you are in

good shape. If it is higher than 1.0, you are heavy and need to lose weight.

Stretch Mark Help

Joshua L. Fox, MD, a dermatologic laser surgeon in Fresh Meadows, New York.

Ask a dermatologist or dermatologic laser surgeon about having stretch marks treated with a pulsed-dye laser. The marks won't disappear altogether, but they should become less noticeable. Several laser treatments may be required.

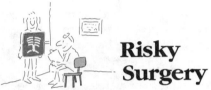

Risky Surgery

John M. Thorpe, Jr., MD, associate professor of obstetrics and gynecology, University of North Carolina at Chapel Hill School of Medicine.

Surgery to widen the vaginal opening during childbirth is rarely helpful. Called *episiotomy,* this common surgical procedure does not reduce the risk of vaginal or rectal tears. In fact, episiotomy increases the risk of tears. Yet episiotomies are still performed on the majority of first-time mothers in the United States. Many doctors who perform episiotomies routinely are unaware of the problems associated with the procedure. Episiotomy may be necessary in cases involving fetal distress or breech delivery.

Cervix-Sparing Hysterectomy

Ernst G. Bartsich, MD, associate attending obstetrician and gynecologist, New York Hospital–Cornell Medical Center, New York.

In an alternative to ordinary hysterectomy, only the top of the uterus is removed. *Supracervical* hysterectomy has been used to treat

139

fibroid tumors, pelvic pain, persistent bleeding and endometriosis. It's less likely than ordinary hysterectomy to injure the bowel and/or bladder...or to cause vaginal prolapse (a shift in the position of the vagina), sexual dysfunction or the "sense of loss" that is common following ordinary hysterectomy.

Vaginal Douching Danger

Donna Day Baird, PhD, epidemiologist, National Institute of Environmental Health Sciences, Research Triangle Park, NC.

After 12 months of trying to conceive, about 90% of women who had never douched became pregnant—compared with only 73% of the women who douched more than once a week.

Also: Douching may increase risk of pelvic inflammatory disease and other infections by spreading germs to the upper reaches of the uterus and fallopian tubes.

Unfaithful Husbands and Cancer Link

Keerti V. Shah, MD, professor, Johns Hopkins School of Hygiene & Public Health, Baltimore.

Women with unfaithful husbands are more likely to contract cervical cancer. A study of more than 1,200 men and women found that women whose husbands have other sexual partners are five to 11 times as likely to develop cervical cancer as those whose husbands do not stray. Incidence was eight times greater for women whose husbands frequented prostitutes. Researchers theorize that the husbands contract the human papilloma virus (HPV) during their extramarital liaisons and bring it home to their wives. Genital HPV infections are known to cause cervical cancer.

Sex and Urinary Tract Infections

Thomas M. Hooton, MD, associate professor of medicine, University of Washington, Seattle. His six-month study of 796 women was published in *The New England Journal of Medicine*, 10 Shattuck St., Boston 02115.

Frequent sex raises a woman's risk for urinary tract infection (UTI)...as does using a diaphragm with spermicide.

Study: Women who had sexual intercourse three times a week were three times more likely to have a UTI than women who abstained from sex. *Theory:* Intercourse introduces vaginal bacteria into the bladder. Spermicide kills beneficial bacteria but leaves infection-causing ones unharmed.

UTI Warning

Amee Manges, MPH, epidemiology researcher specializing in UTIs, School of Public Health, University of California, Berkeley. Her study of 302 women with drug-resistant UTIs was published in *The New England Journal of Medicine*, 10 Shattuck St., Boston 02115.

About 18% of urinary tract infections (UTIs) are now resistant to the most commonly prescribed antibiotic, *trimethoprim sulfamethoxazole* (Bactrim)—up from about 10% five years ago. UTI symptoms include abnormally colored or bloody urine...frequent or painful urination ... and pressure in the lower pelvis. If antibiotics do not clear up symptoms within two days, consult your physician about prescribing a different antibiotic. *To avoid UTIs:* Drink plenty of water ...urinate frequently—and immediately after sexual intercourse...and practice good hygiene.

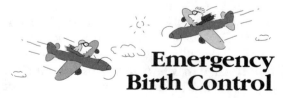

Emergency Birth Control

Roberto Rivera, MD, director, Family Health International, Box 13950, Research Triangle Park, NC 27709.

Taken shortly after "unprotected" sexual intercourse, oral contraceptives are a safe and reasonably effective way to prevent pregnancy. Emergency use of the Pill is roughly 75% effective at preventing pregnancy. Regular daily use of the Pill is 97% effective.

Caution: Emergency contraception should be initiated only under a doctor's supervision.

Safest Birth Control Pills

James McGregor, MD, professor of obstetrics and gynecology at University of Colorado Health Sciences Center, Denver.

Triphasic birth control pills are safest because they deliver *lower doses of estrogen* by weight to the body than earlier versions of the Pill. Pills that provide more than 35 micrograms of estrogen have been associated with increased probability of blood clots and stroke, particularly in older women.

Another benefit: The newer pills, which deliver varying hormone levels appropriate to the phases of the body's natural menstrual cycle, also cause less spotting in many women. Physicians prescribe an initial formulation that takes into account the patient's age and other factors—including susceptibility to acne. Physicians may vary the dosage after observing its side effects until the optimal formulation is determined.

Yeast Infection Relief

Study of 46 women with recurrent vaginosis by Eliezer Shalev, Central Emek Hospital, Afula, Israel, published in *Archives of Family Medicine.*

Yogurt relieves recurrent yeast infections. In a study, women who daily ate five ounces of yogurt containing live bacteria lactobacillus acidophilus had two-thirds fewer cases of recurrent vaginosis as before. This is the first study to demonstrate such positive effects from yogurt containing live cultures. *Theory:* Bacteria in the yogurt are believed to protect against infection either by maintaining an acidic environment in the vagina or by producing compounds such as hydrogen peroxide that kill harmful bacteria.

Ease Menstrual Cramps

Menstrual Cramps Self-Help Book by Susan Lark, MD, authority on women's health care in private practice in Los Altos, CA. Celestial Arts.

Avoid certain foods that can make menstrual cramping worse. Dairy products, fats, salt, alcohol, sugar and caffeine can all make cramping more severe.

Diaphragms and Cystitis Risk

Study of almost 800 sexually active women by researchers at University of Washington School of Medicine, Seattle, published in *The New England Journal of Medicine,* 10 Shattuck St., Boston 02115.

Women using diaphragms with spermicides for birth control change their bodies' internal environments in ways that allow the bacteria that cause cystitis to flourish. The more frequent the sex, the higher the risk.

If you have frequent bladder infections: Consider a different form of birth control.

More on Fertility Treatment

Zev Rosenwaks, MD, director, Center for Reproductive Medicine & Infertility, New York Hospital–Cornell Medical Center, New York.

The increasingly popular technique *intracytoplasmic sperm injection* (ICSI)—in which individual sperm are selected and injected directly into eggs—allows men with low-quality sperm to become fathers. Fertility experts had worried that sperm selected by lab technicians might be more likely to carry genetic defects than sperm "chosen" by nature.

Finding: Only 2.6% of ICSI babies suffered birth defects. That rate is comparable to that for children conceived normally.

Treatment for Ovarian Cancer

David Alberts, MD, professor of medicine and pharmacology, University of Arizona, Tucson.

Doctors have begun administering the anti-cancer drug *cisplatin* via an abdominal catheter instead of via an arm vein.

Benefit: Women who use the abdominal route have a 24% lower death rate. They're also less likely to experience hearing loss, nerve damage and other side effects.

This approach should be considered for ovarian cancer patients who have a small amount of tumor remaining after initial surgery.

Powder Risk

Linda Cook, PhD, epidemiologist, Fred Hutchinson Cancer Research Center, Seattle, leader of a study of 313 women with ovarian cancer and 422 without it.

Women who use talcum powder in the vaginal area right after bathing increase their risk of ovarian cancer by 60%. Women using powder deodorant sprays have a 90% increased risk. *Reason:* Unknown.

Self-defense: Avoid these products.

Fertility Drugs and Ovarian Cancer

David L. Healy, MD, PhD, chairman, department of obstetrics and gynecology, Monash Medical Center, Melbourne, Australia. His nine-year study of 10,358 infertile women was published in *The Lancet*, 42 Bedford Square, London, England WC1B 3SL.

Fertility drugs do not increase a woman's risk of ovarian cancer. Doctors have long thought that *clomiphene* (Clomid), *menotropins* (Pergonal) and other fertility drugs promote ovarian cancer. But a study found no evidence of increased risk. In fact, women who had taken fertility drugs had a slightly reduced cancer rate.

Theory: Infertile women pay more attention to their health. Thus, they're more likely to discover precancerous cysts earlier.

Ovary Removal Danger

Donna Kritz-Silverstein, PhD, associate adjunct professor of family and preventive medicine, University of California, San Diego. Her study of 1,150 women 50 to 89 years of age was published in *Circulation*, St. Luke's Hospital, Texas Heart Institute, MC1-267, 6720 Bertner St., Houston 77030.

Women whose ovaries have been surgically removed face an increased risk of heart disease, although the risk may not become apparent for 20 years. In a study, total cholesterol levels of women who had undergone a hysterectomy involving removal of *both* ovaries (bilateral oophorectomy) were seven points higher than women whose ovaries were intact.

Self-defense: Before undergoing a hysterectomy, discuss with your doctor whether removing your ovaries is necessary.

7

The Healthy Family

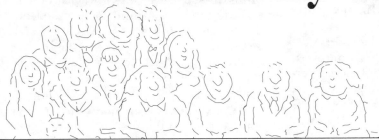

What You Need to Know About Your Child's Health Care

Charles B. Inlander

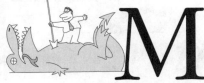

Many parents will find themselves seeking answers to the same old questions about their children's health...

●**How can I find a good doctor for my child?** While a pediatrician is the most obvious choice, family practitioners often make equally good doctors for children.

Carefully interview different types of doctors, then pick one that meets your requirements...one with a pleasant, caring attitude...a willingness to talk directly with your child as well as with you...a clean, orderly office...and a good system for fielding after-hours phone calls. Make sure your child gets along with the doctor and that the doctor accepts your health insurance plan.*

Caution: If the doctor belongs to a group practice, ask that you be allowed to make appointments specifically with him/her.

Ask if the doctor can provide you with educational materials regarding specific health issues. They're a big help when illness strikes —or during puberty.

●**Does my child need an X ray?** In addition to being costly, X rays, CT scans, magnetic resonance imaging and other diagnostic tests are typically frightening to children, risky and unnecessary.

They should be administered only if their findings will have a direct bearing on your

*To obtain a list of pediatricians in your community, send a self-addressed, stamped envelope to the American Academy of Pediatrics Pediatrician Referral, 141 Northwest Point Blvd., Box 927, Elk Grove Village, IL 60009.

Charles B. Inlander, president of People's Medical Society, a patient advocate organization, 462 Walnut St., Allentown, PA 18102. He is coauthor of several books on medical topics, including *Take This Book to the Pediatrician with You.* People's Medical Society.

child's treatment. If your child has a cough, for example, a chest X ray is generally unnecessary—unless the doctor has reason to suspect a serious lung ailment. Before agreeing to any test, question the doctor thoroughly to make sure it is necessary. *Key questions:*

- **What's the name of the test?**
- **Why is it necessary?**
- **What will it reveal that you don't already know?**
- **What will happen if the test is not performed?**
- **What are the possible side effects?**
- **Is a less-invasive test available?**
- **Will the test results change your method of treatment?**
- **Are childhood immunizations safe?** Most states require that all children be immunized against the following diseases—diphtheria, pertussis (whooping cough), tetanus, measles, mumps, rubella (German measles), poliomyelitis and Haemophilus influenza type B (bacterial meningitis). Experts are also now recommending varicella (chicken pox) and hepatitis B.

These vaccinations are typically administered between the ages of two months and 16 years. They are generally quite safe.

Exception: Pertussis. Half of all children who receive this five-dose vaccine develop fever, and, in rare cases, children have developed mental retardation or another permanent disability. However, because pertussis is such a serious disease, it is still prudent to have your child immunized.

To minimize risk: Insist that your child receive the *acellular* pertussis vaccine. It's less likely to cause dangerous reactions than the old vaccine, which remains in use.

The pertussis vaccine should never be given to any child who is over age six, who has a fever or has already had pertussis. Any child who experiences fever, shock, persistent crying, convulsions or neurological problems after the first pertussis shot should not receive any of the additional pertussis boosters.

- **My child has recurrent throat infections. Should his tonsils be removed?** Tonsillectomy is neither necessary nor particularly effective at curing recurrent ear or throat infections, even though doctors often urge surgery.

When it's appropriate: Only if the tonsils become so swollen that they interfere with the child's breathing, or if lab tests indicate the presence of abscesses behind the tonsils. In all other cases, it's best to treat such infections with antibiotics.

- **What about chronic ear infections?** Ear infections (otitis media) are common among children of smokers. If you smoke—stop. New mothers should avoid bottle-feeding their children. Research suggests that breast-feeding helps prevent earaches. Beyond this, there's no real consensus on treatment.

The American Academy of Pediatrics recommends use of oral antibiotics (usually amoxicillin), although some research casts doubt on their effectiveness. The surgical insertion of drainage tubes through the child's eardrums (tympanostomy) can cause serious complications, including severe infections and hearing loss.

Conservative approach—to discuss with your doctor: At the first sign of pain, give your child acetaminophen (Tylenol) or another non-aspirin painkiller. *Also helpful:* A heating pad held against the ear.

- **Do children's hospitals offer better pediatric care than general hospitals?** The standard of care in children's hospitals is no better than that in general hospitals with good pediatric sections. If your child requires inpatient surgery, pick a hospital that performs that surgery on a routine basis.

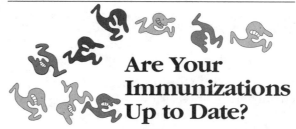

Are Your Immunizations Up to Date?

Timothy McCall, MD, a Boston internist, author of *Examining Your Doctor: A Patient's Guide to Avoiding Harmful Medical Care.* Citadel Press. He is a regular commentator on the public radio program Marketplace, and can be found on the Web at *www.drmccall.com.*

Most of us make sure our kids get immunized against infectious diseases like measles, mumps and polio. But we aren't so good at protecting ourselves. Each year, more than 60,000 adults in the US die of diseases that vaccines could have prevented. Compare that to fewer than 1,000 children a year.

About 20,000 adults die of influenza each year. Current guidelines call for everyone 65 or older to get a flu shot every fall, just before the influenza season starts. The guidelines also recommend flu shots for individuals with chronic diseases like heart or kidney disease, diabetes or HIV infection. Evidence suggests that flu shots may also benefit healthy individuals under age 65.

Flu shots don't always work in elderly or chronically ill people, whose immune systems tend to be weaker. If you have an elderly or chronically ill friend, coworker or family member, be sure to get vaccinated yourself. By doing so, you'll make sure they won't catch influenza from you.

One important vaccine that few people seem to know about is for the bacterium *pneumococcus*. Each year, 500,000 Americans get pneumococcal infections, primarily pneumonia. Forty thousand die from them.

I think everyone over 65 should get the pneumococcus vaccine. So should younger people with chronic heart or lung conditions, liver disease or diabetes—and people who have had their spleens removed.

People infected with the AIDS virus should get the pneumococcus vaccine as soon as they learn they're infected. As their immune system declines, the vaccine is less likely to be effective. Unlike the flu shot, the pneumonia vaccine usually needs to be given only once in a lifetime. Even so, only 14% of those at high risk have received it.

The other vaccine many adults overlook protects against two infections—tetanus and diphtheria. Current recommendations call for everyone to have a tetanus/diphtheria booster once every 10 years.

It used to be that people only got tetanus shots if they sustained a "dirty" cut and went to the emergency room. Recently, scientists discovered that many older people—some of whom haven't had a tetanus booster in decades—have lost protection against this potentially fatal disease.

Consequently, the recommendations have changed. Now all primary-care doctors should see to it that their patients are up to date with their tetanus shots, whether they cut themselves or not.

Some vaccines not recommended for the general public are appropriate for people at increased risk of particular infections. German measles (rubella) is of particular concern for women of childbearing age. It can cause severe birth defects.

Women who *might* become pregnant who have not had the rubella vaccine should have their blood tested for rubella antibodies. If no antibodies are present, they should have the vaccine right away—and avoid becoming pregnant for at least three months.

Hepatitis B causes fewer deaths than AIDS—around 5,000 a year in the US—but is almost 10 times easier to catch. Still, only about 10% of people at risk for hepatitis B have been vaccinated. IV drug users, sexually active gay men and anyone exposed to blood (health-care workers, dialysis patients, etc.) should get this safe and effective vaccine. The vaccine is also a good idea for sex partners of people with hepatitis B.

Vaccines are one of the great success stories of modern medicine. They only work, however, if you get them.

Healthy Toll-Free Calls

Matthew Lesko, coauthor, *Free Stuff for Seniors.* Information USA, Inc.

Many groups provide free health information by phone…

- **Eldercare Locator** gives referrals for home-delivered meals, transportation, legal assistance, housing options, more: 800-677-1116.

- **Patient assistance programs**—find out if your income makes you eligible for free prescription drugs from manufacturers: 800-762-4636.

- **Special services for veterans:** 800-827-1000.

- **Social Security questions**, duplicate cards, more: 800-772-1213.

- **Medicare information and problems:** 800-638-6833.

The Highest Life Expectancy

Study by Bruce Schobel, corporate vice president and actuary, New York Life Insurance Co., and Robert Myers, retired chief actuary, US Social Security Administration.

The world's highest life expectancy is in Japan. A Japanese boy born today can expect to live almost 76 years…a Japanese girl, almost 82 years. An American boy can expect to live 72 years…an American girl, 79 years. *Possible reasons:* Access to high-quality health care, low-fat diet, high standard of living.

Flu Self-Defense

Steven R. Mostow, MD, chairman, department of medicine, Rose Medical Center, Denver.

Get a flu shot. It is 70% effective at stopping each year's bug.

•**See your doctor immediately if you feel yourself coming down with the flu.** He/she can prescribe *amantadine* (Symmetrel) or *rimantadine* (Flumadine), or the newer drugs *oseltamivir* (Tamiflu) or *zanamivir* (Relenza), medications that minimize discomfort and prevent complications such as bronchitis, ear infection or pneumonia.

•**Keep a positive attitude.** Negative emotions depress the immune system, making you more susceptible to illness.

Remedy for Low Back Pain

Louis Kuritzky, MD, courtesy clinical professor of health and family medicine, University of Florida, Gainesville.

Most cases of low back pain are best treated with activity—walking, swimming, bicycling, etc.—*not* medication, rest or physical therapy. Nine out of 10 low back pain sufferers get better on their own, whether or not they receive treatment.

Preventing Back Injuries

University of California at Los Angeles study of 36,000 workers at The Home Depot in California from 1989–1994.

Back injuries can be prevented with the use of back-support belts (corsets). Despite earlier evidence to the contrary, the latest research concluded that use of the belts reduced low-back injuries by about a third. The biggest benefits were for men under age 25 and over age 35, and those doing material handling jobs.

Declaring War on Asthma

Richard N. Firshein, DO, assistant professor of family medicine at New York College of Osteopathic Medicine, and medical director of the Paul Sorvino Asthma Foundation, both in New York City. He is author of *Reversing Asthma: Reduce Your Medications with This Revolutionary New Program.* Warner.

The incidence of asthma has risen dramatically in recent years. In 1980, five million Americans were diagnosed with asthma. This year the number will be closer to 20 million—in part because of rising levels of ozone and other airborne pollutants.

What's the best way to prevent asthma? To treat it? For answers, we spoke with asthma specialist—and asthma patient—Dr. Richard N. Firshein.

CAUSES OF ASTHMA

Most doctors view asthma as simply a breathing problem caused by obstructed airways. To reduce this obstruction, doctors tend to rely on bronchodilators, adrenaline and other prescription drugs.

Trap: Drugs have severe side effects, including headache, nausea and rapid heartbeat… and they do *not* control the chronic inflammatory process that underlies asthma. Medication is one part of a comprehensive asthma program.

ASTHMA SELF-TEST

1. Are you breathing wrong? Proper breathing technique involves using the diaphragm to expand the belly. Asthmatics tend to breathe from the chest, lifting their shoulders as they inhale.

2. Do you need more than one breath to finish each sentence when speaking? Many asthmatics need to breathe in mid-sentence.

3. Do you have a rapid pulse? If so, you may be responding to a lack of oxygen or may have an underlying allergy.

4. Do you make a wheezing sound as you breathe? Wheezing is usually a sign of inflammation, narrowing of the airway or excess production of mucus.

5. Are you often anxious? Fear of suffocation gives many asthmatics chronic anxiety.

6. Are you in pain? Because they use the wrong muscles to breathe, asthmatics often have abdominal, back or chest pain...or tenderness in the ribs.

If you answered "yes" to three or more of these questions, see a doctor right away for a medical exam.

LIFESTYLE INVENTORY

As part of your medical exam, you and your doctor should review several key issues...

- **Allergies and intestinal complaints.**
- **Medication.** Discuss all prescription and over-the-counter drugs you take. Many drugs can exacerbate asthma, including hormones, antibiotics, antidepressants, antifungals, acid-blockers and antihypertensives.
- **Home environment.** Discuss where you notice symptoms most...how your home is heated and cooled...what sort of floor coverings you have...and what household cleaners you use.
- **Work environment.** Are you exposed to cigarette smoke, industrial chemicals, copier dust and other lung irritants? Is your office well-ventilated?
- **Dietary practices.** Deficiencies in magnesium, vitamins C and A and other antioxidant nutrients are contributing factors in many cases.
- **Immune status.** Do you suffer from frequent colds? Do you wake up tired after a full night's sleep? If so, your immune system may be compromised.

If this review finds a potential source of trouble, your doctor may want to test your blood or skin for allergies...evaluate nutrient levels in your body...test your immune response...and/or analyze your digestive tract.

Once the doctor understands the factors involved, he/she can help you plot a program to keep your symptoms in check.

ASTHMA-PROOFING YOUR HOME

Every asthmatic needs a "safe room"—someplace to go during an asthma attack. For most people, the best choice is the bedroom. *Here's how to prepare your safe room...*

- **Dust frequently** with a specially treated cloth that prevents dust from scattering.
- **Remove all carpeting.**
- **Encase your mattress, box spring and pillows in airtight vinyl covers.** This helps get rid of dust and dust mites, which can trigger an asthma attack.
- **Eliminate water leaks** and other sources of humidity.
- **Consider purchasing** a *high-efficiency particle-arresting* (HEPA) air filter. *Cost:* $200 to $400.
- **Consider getting rid of houseplants.** While plants themselves are not a problem, plant soil often contains mold, which can trigger an asthma attack.

AVOIDING TRIGGER FOODS

People are often surprised to learn that what they eat affects their breathing. For some, asthma is caused by unsuspected allergies or sensitivities to "trigger" foods—eggs, shellfish, nuts, seeds, soy, etc. For others, the culprit is pesticide residues or food additives.

Since no two people are alike in this respect, your doctor may order skin tests to identify specific triggers.

ANTIOXIDANTS TO THE RESCUE

Asthma is sometimes a result of lung damage caused by *free radicals.* These renegade molecules are found in polluted air and are produced by the body during vigorous exercise.

By consuming more antioxidants—which neutralize free radicals—many asthmatics notice a swift reduction in symptoms.

Antioxidant foods: Broccoli, cauliflower, squash, carrots, garlic and onions.

Many asthmatics are helped by taking a daily capsule of fish oil or—if they're sensitive to fish—flaxseed oil. Oils found in fresh salmon, tuna and mackerel have an anti-inflammatory effect on the lungs.

Ask your doctor about taking grape seed extract…and a daily supplement containing magnesium (250 mg)…vitamin A (4,000 IU)…vitamin C (1,000 mg)…and vitamin E (400 IU).

Magnesium reduces elevated levels of calcium, which can cause the breathing muscles to spasm.

Magnesium-rich foods: Tofu, spinach and beets.

For severe asthma, intravenous magnesium may be required.

THREE BREATHING STRATEGIES

●**Belly breathing.** Lie on your back on a mat, with knees bent and feet slightly apart. Place a hardcover book on your lower stomach, with the binding touching the bottom of your rib cage.

Breathe in through your nose. As you do, lift the book as high as possible using your stomach. Keep your chest relaxed and motionless.

As you exhale, use your abdominal muscles to squeeze every last bit of air from your lungs. Repeat slowly, taking about four breaths per minute.

●**Blowing out the candle.** Take a deep "belly" breath. Then exhale, pursing your lips firmly and blowing through them as forcefully as you can. Imagine that you're blowing out candles on a birthday cake.

●**"Breathing through."** If your breathing starts to accelerate because of emotional stress or an incipient asthma attack, shift over to belly breathing.

Notice any tension in your jaw, shoulders, chest or neck. Allow those body parts to relax.

Let your feelings "flow"—even if they're negative. Don't try to stop them with short, shallow breaths or clenched muscles.

Can't Stomach a Roller Coaster Ride?

Charles Kimmelman, MD, professor of otolaryngology, Manhattan Eye, Ear and Throat Hospital, New York, quoted in *Men's Health*, 33 E. Minor St., Emmaus, PA 18098.

Roller coasters are less fun as we age because the balance mechanism in the inner ear becomes less tolerant of excessive motion.

Solution: Take an over-the-counter motion-sickness medication before riding…eat a gram of powdered gingerroot—available at drugstores and natural-food shops…or wear a Sea Band, available at sporting-goods stores. This helps control nausea by stimulating an acupressure point on the inside of the wrist.

Easier Ways to Get Dressed

Richard B. Dewey, Jr., MD, assistant professor of neurology, University of Texas Southwestern Medical Center, Dallas.

Help for people with arthritis, Parkinson's disease or other disorders affecting coordination and flexibility…

●**Have a family member or tailor replace buttons and zippers** with Velcro fasteners wherever possible.

●**Have a shoemaker stick Velcro strips onto shoes** to make them easier to fasten.

●**Choose clothing that closes in front.**

●**Take off clothes from the more rigid side of the body first.**

●**If you must button clothes,** use a button hook.

●**Lower closet rods** to make clothes easier to reach.

GERD: A New Name For an Old Problem

Timothy McCall, MD, a Boston internist, author of *Examining Your Doctor: A Patient's Guide to Avoiding Harmful Medical Care*. Citadel Press. He is a regular commentator on the public radio program Marketplace, and can be found on the Web at *www.drmccall.com*.

In what may be a sign of the never-ending quest to give simple problems complex names, doctors are now regularly diagnosing *gastroesophageal reflux disease* (GERD). In the old days, we called this ailment hiatal hernia or esophageal reflux—or simply heartburn.

Whatever the name, GERD is what happens when stomach contents leak upstream into the esophagus, the muscular tube linking the mouth to the stomach. Typical symptoms include a burning sensation in the lower chest and an acid taste in the mouth.

The condition can be disabling, and severe cases can lead to esophageal cancer. Luckily, most cases can be controlled with lifestyle changes, drugs and—in extreme cases—surgery.

The first line of treatment for GERD is dietary modification. This involves avoiding foods known to trigger reflux. These include chocolate, coffee (including decaf), peppermints and other mints, citrus fruits and spicy or fatty foods. Drinking alcohol and smoking also promote reflux.

Certain medicines make GERD worse. These include the asthma drug *theophylline*, anti-inflammatory drugs like aspirin and ibuprofen, tricyclic antidepressants like *amitriptyline* (Elavil) and calcium-channel blockers, which are used for heart disease and high blood pressure. If you have GERD and are taking any of these drugs, ask your doctor about substituting another drug.

Anything that pushes on the belly encourages stomach acid to "backwash" into the esophagus. Tight clothing can do it. So can being overweight or even eating too much at a time.

When you're standing or sitting, gravity tends to keep stomach contents from moving upstream. For this reason, people prone to GERD should avoid lying down after eating, and should not eat or drink anything—even a glass of water—for a couple of hours before going to bed. Some people benefit by elevating the head of the mattress with a foam wedge or by placing the headboard on wooden blocks.

If lifestyle modification fails to bring relief, the first line of drug therapy for GERD is antacids. They bring quick relief by coating the esophagus and helping neutralize stomach acid. The next option is an over-the-counter (OTC) acid blocker, such as *Zantac 75* or *Pepcid AC*. If these drugs don't help, ask your doctor about prescription-strength versions. *Tagamet*, a similar drug, is no more effective than Zantac or Pepcid and is more likely to interact with other drugs.

Cisapride (Propulsid) and other prescription drugs that promote "motility" (movement of food through the gut) can also be helpful. These drugs can be used alone or in combination with other drugs.

The prescription drug called *omeprazole* (Prilosec) also appears to be very effective against GERD. Since this drug hasn't been on the market that long, some questions remain about its long-term safety.

The last resort for controlling GERD is usually surgery. In one procedure, called *fundoplication*, the surgeon wraps the upper portion of the stomach around the lower end of the esophagus. This operation can be very effective—although it isn't always and symptoms may recur years later.

If you go this route, be sure to ask your doctor about laparoscopic techniques. They require smaller incisions and afford faster recovery than conventional surgery. Check the surgeon's track record, too. Some have much better luck than others.

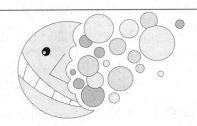

How to Extinguish Each Type of Heartburn

M. Michael Wolfe, MD, associate professor of medicine at Harvard Medical School, and a gastroenterologist at Brigham and Women's Hospital, both in Boston. He is coauthor of *The Fire Inside: Extinguishing Heartburn and Related Symptoms.* W. W. Norton.

It's all too familiar, that burning sensation spreading upward from the chest. Heartburn afflicts more than 100 million Americans, and we spend $3 billion each year on drugs to treat it.

Acid reflux, the condition that causes heartburn, can severely damage the esophagus—a condition that may necessitate surgery.

It can also cause asthma or chronic hoarseness…or send you to the emergency room with severe chest pain. And it increases your risk of esophageal cancer, which is often deadly.

Good news: Dietary strategies and minor lifestyle changes are often all that's needed to control heartburn. For more severe cases of acid reflux, new drugs are proving highly effective.

WHAT LIGHTS THE FIRE

For the first few minutes after you eat, food churns with stomach acid.

During this period, a valve-like muscle separating the stomach from the esophagus should constrict, preventing acid from splashing "upstream."

If this *lower esophageal sphincter* fails to close, acid seeps back (refluxes) into the esophagus. Doctors call this condition gastroesophageal reflux disease (GERD).

This is *hydrochloric* acid we're talking about here—as strong as the stuff that's in your car battery. The stomach is protected from injury by special cells in its lining—the esophagus is not.

THE GREAT MASQUERADER

The esophagus isn't the only organ vulnerable to acid reflux.

If even a little acid is inhaled into the lungs, you may develop a chronic cough.

If you have asthma, GERD can inflame the bronchial tubes, increasing the frequency and severity of attacks. In fact, GERD is an aggravating factor in 50% of all cases of asthma.

Acid in the voice box (larynx) causes chronic hoarseness. In severe cases of *acid laryngitis*, speaking becomes painful—even impossible.

Reflux can also cause a distressing "lump-in-the-throat" sensation…or a postnasal drip that forces you to clear your throat over and over again.

Problem: Fewer than half of all individuals with reflux-induced cough, asthma or hoarseness have noticeable heartburn. Consequently, even experienced doctors may fail to identify reflux as the cause of these conditions. That means these ailments go misdiagnosed—and *mistreated.*

Self-defense: If you experience any of these symptoms, ask your doctor about reflux. That advice holds true even if you do not have heartburn.

DIETARY STRATEGIES

Step one to beating GERD is to pinpoint the foods that relax the sphincter and/or boost production of stomach acid. *Usual culprits:* Fatty foods…dairy products…coffee (even decaf) and other caffeinated beverages…citrus fruits…red wine and other alcoholic beverages …chocolate…mint.

Mint? Despite its popularity as an after-dinner treat, *any* form of mint affects the esophageal sphincter.

Of course, when it comes to heartburn, the key is to find out what foods you should avoid.

BEHAVIORAL STRATEGIES

You may have heard that it helps to sleep with the head elevated—either by using an extra pillow or by standing the head of your bed on six-inch blocks.

Better: Using a foam wedge, such as the *Bedge. More information:* 800-525-4820.

Other helpful strategies:

- **Eat small meals.**

- **Don't lie down for at least three hours after a meal.** It's easy for acid to reflux into the esophagus when you're lying down.

- **Avoid tight clothing**, especially underwear. It forces acid into the esophagus.

- **When lifting a heavy object**, bend at the knees, not the waist. This puts less pressure on your stomach.

●**Avoid exercise for at least one hour after eating.** Even a brisk walk is enough to cause reflux.

●**Suck hard candy or chew sugarless gum.** Doing so stimulates the production of bicarbonate in the saliva, a natural antacid.

Over-the-counter (OTC) antacids are effective for mild, occasional heartburn. But they *don't* provide long-lasting relief.

H2 blockers like *cimetidine* (Tagamet HB), *famotidine* (Pepcid AC) and *ranitidine* (Zantac 75) can take up to an hour to start working. But they keep working for several hours and even at night—by blocking the effects of *histamine*, a chemical that induces the stomach to make acid.

To ensure prompt *and* long-lasting relief, I usually instruct my heartburn patients to take a liquid antacid and an H2 blocker. Remember, OTC drugs are for mild, occasional heartburn only. If you take a heartburn remedy more than three times a week—or if the pain is severe—see a doctor.

WHAT YOUR DOCTOR CAN DO

If you have chronic, severe heartburn, your doctor may want to perform an *endoscopy*. In this outpatient procedure, the doctor examines your esophagus using a thin fiber-optic viewing tube called an endoscope.

Endoscopy may reveal esophageal cancer or *esophagitis*—a potentially serious inflammation of the esophageal lining.

In especially severe cases of reflux, doctors prescribe very high doses of H2 blockers. This strategy may work wonders…or it may not be helpful at all.

If H2 blockers don't work, ask your doctor about proton-pump blockers like *omeprazole* (Prilosec) or *lansoprazole* (Prevasid). These drugs block acid secretion more effectively than H2 blockers. One dose usually works all day.

Omeprazole is often the best approach to reflux-induced asthma or laryngitis. In one study, it afforded relief for 73% of people who had reflux-induced asthma.

To keep symptoms from recurring, you'll probably have to take medication indefinitely.

Caution: Some of these drugs interact with other medications. Check with your doctor.

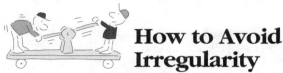

How to Avoid Irregularity

Adriane Fugh-Berman, MD, a Washington, DC–based medical researcher who specializes in women's health and alternative medicine. She is author of *Alternative Medicine: What Works.* Odonian Press.

How often should one have a bowel movement? In medical school, I was taught that "normal" people empty their bowels from several times a day to once a week.

I don't believe that anymore. Having a bowel movement more than once a day is okay. But having a bowel movement only once a week is definitely not normal—or healthful. Chronic constipation can lead to health problems.

First, chronic constipation promotes precancerous changes in colon cells. Presumably this is because these cells are exposed to bile acids and other toxins in intestinal waste for a longer-than-optimal period of time.

Constipation can also lead to hemorrhoids. People suffering from constipation often must strain to empty their bowels, and straining causes a buildup of pressure inside blood vessels lining the anal canal. Hemorrhoids are simply varicose veins in the anal canal.

What causes constipation? The most common causes are a lack of fiber in the diet… insufficient consumption of water…and a sedentary lifestyle.

Constipation is also a side effect of certain medications. These include codeine and other opiate painkillers…tricyclic antidepressants such as *amitriptyline* (Elavil)…*pseudoephedrine* (Sudafed) and other decongestants…and Maalox and other aluminum-based antacids.

Calcium can also be the constipation culprit. If you're taking calcium supplements, you should be taking magnesium supplements as well. Taken at about half the dosage of the calcium, magnesium helps counteract the constipating effect of the calcium.

Now for curing constipation. You've already heard that boosting your intake of dietary fiber can help make you regular. But I want to stress that you also need lots of water. In fact, eating more fiber without simultaneously increasing your intake of water can make constipation worse instead of better. I recommend drinking at least eight eight-ounce glasses of water each day.

Dietary fiber is found in fruits, vegetables and whole grains. If eating more high-fiber foods (and drinking more water) doesn't work for you, consider trying Metamucil or another over-the-counter psyllium seed product. Psyllium seed is a "bulking agent," and not a true (cathartic) laxative. Yet it's very effective against constipation.

Unlike laxatives, psyllium can safely be taken on a daily basis. Daily use of laxatives can lead to "lazy" bowels and to even worse constipation—not to mention dehydration and life-threatening imbalances in the body's sodium-potassium balance. Laxatives should be used only for occasional trouble.

One of the few laxatives recommended by conventional and alternative practitioners alike is tea made from the herb *senna*, which is available at health-food stores. Senna tea is quite effective, but I've found an even more potent remedy—*sennaed prunes*.

To make sennaed prunes, pour enough boiling water over a cup of prunes to cover them. Drop in a senna tea bag. Remove the tea bag after five to 20 minutes—the longer the bag stays in, the stronger the tea. Refrigerate the prune-senna mixture overnight before eating.

By the way, while caffeinated coffee has laxative properties, ordinary black tea contains *tannins*, compounds that cause constipation.

Mosquito Prevention

Bernice Lifton, a resident of Pasadena, CA, who has researched natural ways of eliminating pests. She is author of *Bug Busters*. Avery Publishing Group.

To mosquito-proof your property, eliminate any water-collecting places where they may breed.

Examples: Sagging gutters can accumulate water—so have them checked. Fix leaky outdoor faucets...put drainage by air conditioners so puddles do not gather underneath. Empty birdbaths every three days. If you put drinking water outside for pets, change it daily.

Also: Get rid of old tires and abandoned toys...and put away kids' wading pools that aren't being used.

Cuts and Scrapes

Alfred Lane, MD, professor of dermatology, Stanford University, Stanford, CA.

Many doctors advise patients to keep wounds dry to avoid infection. But in a study of premature babies, cuts treated with a petroleum-based ointment (*Aquaphor*) healed quicker and were less likely to become infected than those not treated. Researchers say the same treatment should also help adults' wounds.

No More Snoring

Gary Zammit, PhD, director of the Sleep Disorder Institute, New York.

Researchers believe snoring is caused by the vibration of soft tissues in response to turbulent air flow within the upper airway. Nasal strips, sold in drugstores, are narrow pieces of springy plastic encased in adhesive strips. When fastened to the outside of the nose so that the nostrils are opened up, the strip opens up the constricted passage, reducing the turbulence.

Caution: Their value for more serious disturbances, like sleep apnea, has not been demonstrated. If you suspect sleep apnea, seek expert evaluation. This condition can cause serious consequences.

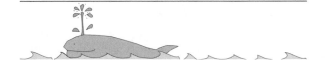

Children and Sex

Jan Faull, child development and behavior specialist, Seattle, writing online in *Family Planet*.

Talking to children about sex should not be a one-time talk—and not strictly anatomical. The topic will come up as a child grows older. When a child asks a straightforward question, answer directly and honestly in an age-appropriate way, using the correct names for body parts. Then respond to any follow-up questions.

Bottom line: Be glad your children come to you with questions—otherwise, they will go elsewhere to learn about sex. If you do not answer perfectly the first time, you can always restate your answer later.

No More Mumbling

Ann Mitchell, licensed speech pathologist with the Rehability Center, Falls Church, VA.

If you tend to mumble, take a deep breath and exhale slowly while counting out loud ...continue counting at a steady rhythm, leaving about half a second between the numbers. Most adults can reach between 15 and 20 before they need to inhale. If you can't get past 10, you need to practice taking deeper, more controlled breaths as you speak.

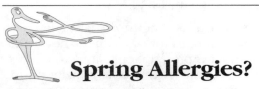

Spring Allergies?

Peter Boggs, MD, an allergist in private practice in Shreveport, LA, and former president of the American College of Allergy, Asthma and Immunology, Arlington Heights, IL. He is author of *Sneezing Your Head Off? How to Live with Your Allergic Nose*. Fireside.

If you suffer from seasonal allergies—as 22 million Americans do—both established and new treatments can relieve your allergy symptoms without putting you to sleep or forcing you to stay indoors.

HOW ALLERGIES START

Allergies occur when you inherit a genetic disposition to form allergic antibodies upon coming into contact with normally benign substances.

If one of your parents has an allergy, you have a 30% chance of being allergic, too. If both parents suffer from allergies, your risk jumps to 50% to 75%. If neither parent has allergies, your chance is only 13%.

You inherit and pass along only the propensity for allergies, not the specific allergies themselves.

Example: If your mother is allergic to cats, you may not develop the same allergy—but you may be allergic to pollen instead.

Still, having allergy-provoking genetic material isn't enough to prompt sniffling and sneezing. You must also be exposed to various allergens, such as dust mites...tree, grass or weed pollen ...animals...mold...feathers...insect stings...and certain foods. The allergens are so widespread that they're really impossible to avoid.

Example: The most common causes of hay fever during early spring are tree pollens. Later in the spring, grass pollens are typically to blame. And in the fall, weed pollens spur many people to suffer allergic reactions.

HOW YOUR BODY FIGHTS BACK

After you come into contact with an allergen, your body regards it as a foreign object. When your body next detects this substance, your immune system launches an all-out attack to get rid of it. During this offensive, chemicals such as histamine, leukotrienes and prostaglandin D2 are released.

These chemicals—and the ensuing nasal inflammation—are responsible for the allergy symptoms of congestion...runny nose and eyes ...sneezing...and itching in the nose, throat, eyes and ears.

TRADITIONAL TREATMENTS

•**Avoid allergy triggers.** This is the single most effective and inexpensive means at your disposal to ward off allergy symptoms. *Here's how to do it...*

•**Avoid outdoor activities between 5 a.m. and 10 a.m.** That's when pollen counts are highest.

●**Shower and change clothes when you come in** from working or playing outdoors. Pollen can cling to clothing and rub off on furniture.

●**Close windows and doors and run an air conditioner in the house and car** to filter pollen from the air you breathe. Avoid window and attic fans, which are notorious for drawing pollen into the house.

●**Antihistamines and decongestants** are the mainstays of seasonal allergy treatment. They're very effective for relieving symptoms quickly.

●**Antihistamines** don't prevent the allergic reaction, but they stop its symptoms, such as sneezing and watery eyes, by interfering with the action of histamine. A slew of nonprescription and prescription antihistamines is available today. They are generally effective but may cause drowsiness or dizziness. *Cautions...*

☐ **Don't take the antihistamine** *Hismanal* in combination with the antifungal drug *ketoconazole* or the antibiotic *erythromycin*. These combinations can lead to serious heart rhythm abnormalities.

☐ **Don't take antihistamines at all** if you have glaucoma, a persistent cough or an enlarged prostate.

●**Decongestants**—available with and without a prescription—relieve nasal stuffiness by constricting blood vessels in the nose. They can cause dizziness or nervousness and can make it hard to sleep. *Cautions...*

☐ **Don't use decongestants** if you have heart or thyroid disease, high blood pressure, diabetes or an enlarged prostate, without discussing it with your physician.

☐ **Don't use over-the-counter (OTC) decongestant sprays** for longer than five days. They may actually cause increased stuffiness.

●**Steroid nasal sprays.** Prescription steroid nasal sprays—such as Beconase, Flonase, Nasacort, Rhinocort and Vancenase—reverse swelling in the nose and block the allergic reaction.

When you spray these steroid nasal sprays into your nose once or twice a day, they also stop the twitchiness that plagues allergy sufferers—and makes the nose more likely to react to allergens and irritants such as cigarette smoke and other pollutants.

These steroid sprays work well when combined with antihistamines and decongestants. However, if you can't tolerate those drugs, they can also be used alone.

Important: Start using a steroid nasal spray one or two weeks prior to the allergy season to prevent the inflammatory process before it begins. Many sufferers use them daily for several months at a time. Steroid sprays cause few side effects if used at recommended doses.

●**Allergy shots.** If your allergy symptoms are severe...you have asthma...you get frequent ear infections...or you don't respond to oral or nasal allergy drugs—immunotherapy is another option.

Procedure: You'll be given a series of shots that contain progressively larger doses of allergen extracts.

You'll likely build up immunity to these allergens. You may, however, still need oral or nasal drugs to control your symptoms.

MEDICATIONS

●**Allegra** is a nonsedating prescription antihistamine.

●**Astelin** is a nasal antihistamine spray. It's available only by prescription. Astelin works within a few minutes after spraying, lasts 12 hours, doesn't cause drowsiness and has few side effects.

●**Claritin Reditabs** can be taken by children and adults who otherwise cannot take pills because they dissolve almost instantly when placed on the tongue.

●**Nasalcrom** is a nonsteroidal nasal spray that has been used for years and is now available without a prescription. Nasalcrom is extremely safe and effective at preventing the allergic reaction from taking place, reduces inflammation in the nose and doesn't cause drowsiness. Most sufferers use it three to four times a day, starting a week or two before the allergy season begins.

●**Zyrtec** is another prescription antihistamine. It may cause some drowsiness—though not as much as OTC antihistamines—and is safe and effective.

Hepatitis B Vaccine And Preteens

Ann M. Arvin, MD, professor of pediatrics and microbiology/immunology, Stanford University School of Medicine, Stanford, CA.

The hepatitis B virus (HBV), which can be transmitted sexually or via use of intravenous drugs, is 100 times more prevalent (and far more infectious) than the AIDS virus. All children 11 to 13 years of age should be vaccinated—whether or not their parents think they are sexually active or involved with drugs.

Kids Get Ulcers, Too

Mark A. Gilger, MD, assistant professor of pediatrics and gastroenterology, Baylor College of Medicine, Houston.

Causes include infection with the bacterium *Helicobactor pylori*...reaction to certain drugs...stress caused by serious injury, infection or disease.

Symptoms parents should look for: Recurrent abdominal pain...awakening in the night with abdominal pain...recurrent vomiting ...vomiting blood. Most ulcers are treatable with antacids...and curable with antibiotics.

Young Children Don't Need Pillows

Jay Berkelhamer, MD, chairman of pediatrics, Henry Ford Health System, Detroit.

Kids up to age two or three seem to sleep better without them. And pillows and other soft bedding can be dangerous to very young children—they may contribute to the suffocation of as many as 1,800 infants each year.

Music and Babies

Jayne M. Standley, PhD, professor of music therapy, Florida State University, Tallahassee. Her study of 20 premature infants was published in *Pediatric Nursing*, E. Holly Ave., Box 56, Pitman, NJ 08701.

Music helps premature babies grow stronger. When lullabies were played in a hospital neonatal unit, preemies' blood-oxygen levels (a key measure of health) went up. When the music stopped, their blood-oxygen levels fell.

Your Baby's Diet

Study by researchers at the University of Illinois, Urbana-Champaign, IL.

When your baby refuses new foods, try again tomorrow.

Reason: It's natural for a baby to reject unfamiliar tastes. But most babies will eventually learn to like most foods. In a study, when babies were offered pureed peas or green beans for 10 consecutive days, they ate twice as much on the tenth day as they had on the first.

What Never to Feed Young Children

Martha White, MD, director of pediatric allergy and research, Institute for Asthma & Allergy, Washington Hospital Center, Washington, DC.

Peanuts are easily aspirated into the lungs ...and peanuts are one of the most common—and dangerous—foods to which one may develop an allergy.

Most at risk: Those from high-risk families —where both parents or one parent and a sibling are food-allergic. Even trace quantities can trigger an attack in peanut-allergic individuals.

Example: A boy began wheezing when a jar of peanut butter was merely opened nearby.

Helpful: Alert teachers and other caregivers to the food allergy...have the child wear a

Medic-Alert bracelet (call 800-432-5378 for information)...older children should be taught to use spring-loaded syringes of epinephrine to ward off attacks after inadvertently ingesting a food to which they are allergic.

Exercise Benefits

James F. Clapp, MD, obstetrician, MetroHealth Medical Center, Case Western Reserve University, Cleveland, whose study of 65 newborn infants was published in the *American Journal of Obstetrics and Gynecology*.

Babies are more alert and less fussy if their mothers exercised regularly during pregnancy. *Note:* Always check with your doctor before starting any exercise program.

Prevent Infant Tooth Decay

Steven Grossman, DDS, co-chief of pediatric dentistry, Lenox Hill Hospital, New York.

Make sure your child's teeth are treated with fluoride...avoid sweet substances on pacifiers...use plain water in his/her bottle at bedtime...clean teeth and gums with a washcloth after feeding...brush his teeth once a day starting at age two or before...begin regular dental checkups as soon as the child's 20 baby teeth have erupted.

Lead and Obesity

Rokho Kim, MD, DrPH, instructor of medicine, Harvard Medical School, Boston. His study of 79 young adults was published in *Environmental Health Perspectives*, Mail Drop WC01 NIEHS, Box 12233, Research Triangle Park, NC 27709.

Exposure to lead during childhood can lead to obesity and shorter stature in adulthood. The greater the exposure between ages seven and 20, the greater the future weight gain.

SIDS Fact

E.A. Mitchell, MD, associate professor, department of pediatrics, University of Auckland, New Zealand, writing in *The Lancet*, 42 Bedford Square, London, England WC1B 3SL.

Sleeping with an infant can put the baby at increased risk of Sudden Infant Death Syndrome (SIDS). The reason isn't known—but may be related to airway obstruction or re-breathing air that a parent has exhaled.

At greatest risk: Infants whose mothers smoke. A mother who smokes may safely breast-feed and comfort her child in bed but should not let the baby sleep with her.

Getting Kids to Eat Fruits and Vegetables

Tufts University Diet & Nutrition Letter, 203 Harrison Ave., Boston 02111.

Kids eat more fruits and vegetables when healthful produce is part of meals instead of side dishes.

Helpful: Add pureed cooked vegetables to ground-meat dishes like meatloaf and hamburgers...substitute shredded carrots, zucchini or chopped spinach for some or all of the ground meat in lasagna or a casserole...add pureed or shredded vegetables and fruits to homemade muffins, cookies, cakes and quick breads...use pureed cooked apples or pears as a sauce for poultry, and whole pineapple chunks or rings to top baked or grilled chicken breast... mix unsweetened applesauce or fresh apples into hot cereal.

Kids and Sunglasses Safety

Stephen Miller, MD, director, clinical care center, American Optometric Association, St. Louis.

Children should wear sunglasses at the beach, pool or wherever sunlight will be reflected into their eyes.

Reason: A young child's eyes have less light-filtering pigment than an adult's eyes do, and are therefore especially vulnerable to cumulative eye damage from the sun's damaging UV rays.

Best: Lenses made of impact-resistant plastic or polycarbonate and that block 99% to 100% of both UVA and UVB rays.

The Value of Imaginary Friends

Jerome Singer, PhD, professor of psychology and child study, Yale University, New Haven, CT.

Imaginary playmates are the product of a child's needs and imagination. Two-thirds of preschoolers have them—and those who do tend to be more independent, cooperative with teachers and peers, happier and less aggressive than kids who do not have them. These playmates help children share ideas and feelings with adults that they might not otherwise feel comfortable expressing. Parents should accept imaginary companions—but not too enthusiastically. Kids need to feel that they retain complete control over imaginary friends.

Sleep and Behavior

Rafael Pelayo, MD, staff physician, Sleep Disorders Clinic, Stanford University, Stanford, CA.

Too little sleep can lead to behavioral problems in children. Sleepy children tend to subconsciously look for things to stimulate them. This can lead to disruptive behavior.

Bottom line: A hyperactive child may actually be suffering from sleep deprivation.

Guidelines: Eight to 12 hours of sleep a day from toddlerhood through adulthood.

Helpful: To get children to adjust to an earlier bedtime, move bedtime back by 15 minutes each day.

Poison Alert

Mark Wortman, *Yale Children's Health Letter*, Yale University School of Medicine, New Haven, CT.

Top causes of poisoning in kids: Household cleaning products...analgesics such as aspirin, acetaminophen and ibuprofen...cosmetics and personal-care products...household plants that are toxic if ingested.

Important: If you suspect poisoning or exposure, call your pediatrician or state Poison Control Center immediately.

Kids and Caffeine

Study of 400 New York City preschoolers, reported in *Eating Well*, Ferry Rd., Charlotte, VT 05445.

A study of 400 preschoolers found that 10% of them drink enough cola and iced tea every day to down an adult's caffeine equivalent of two cups of coffee.

Possible result: Jumpy and inattentive children.

Better: Drinks that are "caffeine-free."

Secondhand Smoke And Kids

Nancy J. Haley, MD, whose study was conducted while she was with the American Health Foundation, Valhalla, NY. Her study of more than 500 children, ages one to five, was published in *The New England Journal of Medicine*, 10 Shattuck St., Boston 02115.

Children who are exposed to tobacco smoke are three-and-a-half times more likely to develop respiratory illnesses—especially upper-respiratory problems—than ones who are not exposed. Children exposed to secondhand smoke have significant concentrations of a nicotine derivative in their urine. The more smokers in a child's home, the greater the concentration of nicotine by-products in the child's body and the greater the likelihood of respiratory problems.

Kids and Dehydration

Oded Bar-Or, MD, director, Children's Exercise and Nutrition Centre, McMaster University, Hamilton, Ontario.

Kids are more vulnerable to dehydration than adults. Youngsters don't sweat as much as adults, so they cannot cool their bodies as efficiently.

Problem: By the time a child feels thirsty, he/she is probably already at the beginning stages of dehydration.

Symptoms: Apathy...light-headedness... fatigue...nausea.

Helpful: To encourage kids to drink enough, offer them diluted fruit juice or sports drinks.

Avoid: Undiluted fruit juice and sweetened carbonated beverages, since their high sugar content can cause stomach cramps.

Skin Care for Kids in Puberty

Neal Schultz, MD, dermatologist in private practice in New York.

Eat plenty of fresh fruits and vegetables... drink lots of water...get regular exercise and fresh air...get plenty of sleep...keep skin clean by washing with gentle soap and water ...use sunscreen to protect against the sun's harmful rays.

Don't Forget This Person

How Was Your Day, Baby? A Childcare Journal for Working Parents by Melanie Goldish, a working mother in Hoffman Estates, IL. Tracer Publishing.

Take your caregiver to the pediatrician, too, when your baby has an appointment. He/she will have observed your baby closely and may have important information to tell the doctor. It can also be useful for the caregiver to hear what the doctor has to say.

Balloon Danger

Frank Rimell, MD, a pediatric otolaryngologist at the department of pediatric otolaryngology, University of Minnesota, Minneapolis. His study of more than 600 children who died or underwent endoscopy for removal of objects that were choking them was published in the *Journal of the American Medical Association,* 515 N. State St., Chicago 60610.

Children under the age of three are the most likely to choke on common objects—but balloons can be dangerous to kids of all ages.

Other dangerous items: Hot dogs, nuts, seeds, vegetable and fruit pieces.

Troubling: Some children can choke on objects that pass federal small-parts hazard tests aimed at keeping dangerously small items out of young children's hands.

Self-defense: Watch children carefully. Only allow young kids to play with items that are significantly bigger than the minimum size allowed under US rules, which is about the diameter of a toilet paper roll. And look for child-safety warning labels on toy packages.

Children and Choking

David Darrow, MD, DDS, assistant professor of otolaryngology and pediatrics, Eastern Virginia Medical School, Norfolk.

Most common objects that kill: Balloons and hot dogs.

Most common objects inhaled: Seeds... nuts, particularly peanuts.

Most common objects stuck in the throat: Coins. A child who inhales a foreign object into the bronchi and lungs will commonly have an episode of coughing, followed by wheezing. A child with an object stuck in his/her throat will complain of pain when swallowing and have severe vomiting. If you suspect your child has inhaled or swallowed an object, bring him to an emergency room for treatment.

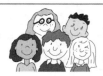

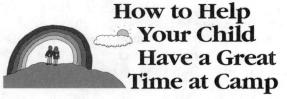

How to Help Your Child Have a Great Time at Camp

Bruce Muchnick, EdD, a licensed psychologist in private practice, Glenside, PA. His work includes psychotherapy with children and adults, management consulting and a "subspecialty" in camp psychology. Dr. Muchnick advises camp owners, directors, camping professionals and parents throughout the year and works with camp staffs during the summer.

Summer camp is more than a country vacation for children. At camp, kids learn to appreciate the outdoors, develop companionship and pick up skills that enhance self-reliance, cooperation and interdependence. These skills will remain with them throughout childhood and into adulthood.

Camp also serves as a kind of refuge where children can unburden themselves of the pressures at home. Camp frees them, gets their creative juices flowing and renews their sense of being kids.

To help your child have a successful time at camp this summer…

● **Learning to let go** allows children to develop autonomy and a stronger sense of self. It also gives parents a chance to take care of themselves and get to know each other again. When children return, parents can feel refreshed and be available and accessible to them again.

● **Prepare for camp together.** Decisions about camp—like where to go and what to pack—should be a joint venture, keeping in mind your child's level of maturity. If your child feels part of the decision-making process, his/her chances of having a positive experience will improve.

● **Don't buy a whole new wardrobe.** Camp is more rugged than life at home. A child doesn't need new clothes…and having well-worn clothes and familiar possessions will help ease the transition. This is especially important for first-time campers.

● **Talk about concerns.** As the first day of camp nears, some children experience uneasiness about going away. Children should be encouraged to talk about these feelings. Ask your child about his feelings rather than acting on what you think his feelings may be. Communicate confidence in his ability to handle being away from home and remind him about successes he has experienced in other situations.

● **Have realistic expectations.** Camp, like the rest of life, has high points and low ones. Not every moment will be filled with wonder and excitement. At times, your child will feel great while at other times he may feel unhappy or bored. And kids may not always get along well with each other.

Solution: Encourage your child to have a reasonable and realistic view of camp by discussing—in advance—both the ups and downs. Camp experiences will provide opportunities for problem solving, negotiating, increased self-awareness and greater sensitivity toward others. Don't send your child to camp feeling pressured to succeed. The main purposes of camp are to relax and have fun.

WHEN YOUR CHILD IS AT CAMP

● **Don't call within the first two weeks** if your child will be away at camp for the whole summer. It takes that long to adjust to being away…and a call from home may disrupt the process. It's hard to get an accurate sense of how a child is managing over the phone—this can be unsettling for you and your child, so it's best not to call at all.

● **Communicate in writing.** Summer camp offers kids and parents the chance to develop a rarely practiced skill—letter writing. Write as often as you want. Keep in mind that this is your child's connection to home and family.

Your letters should be upbeat. It's fine to write that you miss your child, but don't include things like *The house is so quiet without you.*

Better: Ask specific questions in your letters about your child's activities…bunk life…friends, etc. This will help him organize his letters home.

● **Packages are appreciated every now and then.** But don't send food—it's disruptive if some kids in the cabin receive food packages and others receive nothing. Receiving food packages may be contrary to camp policy. If your child asks you to sneak food packages, don't. Even if you think a rule is silly, breaking a camp rule might interfere with your child's sense of right and wrong.

Better: Send postcards, cartoons, newspaper and magazine articles, comics, game books, puzzles and other items that can be shared with friends.

Example: Tell your child...*I understand that you're hungry. That's why you have three great meals each day and snacks. I'll send you some comic books. Hope you enjoy them. Why don't you share them with your bunk?*

• **Don't make major changes at home.** This is not the time to redecorate his room or get rid of his pet snake. When kids return from camp, they like their rooms and their lives to be the same as when they left.

• **Help your child cope at camp.** Most kids need a few days to adjust to life at camp and being away from home. During this time, many experience homesickness. They miss familiar surroundings, parents, pets and friends.

Most kids cope with these concerns and—with the help of camp staff—build support systems. If your child's letters contain urgent pleas for you to bring him home, resist the temptation to rush to camp. Avoid making deals, such as *Give camp one more week. If you're still unhappy, we'll bring you home.*

Better: Support your child's efforts to work out problems with the help of the director and the camp's staff.

Communicate your love and confidence in your child's ability to work through problems. Remind him, if necessary, that he has made a commitment for the summer. Overcoming homesickness and upsets in the cabin and learning to care for oneself are important challenges faced at camp.

Important: If you sense legitimacy in your child's complaints, talk candidly with the camp director. Allow the director and staff an opportunity to apply their expertise in helping kids adapt to the routines of camp life. Follow up with another call a few days later. Most adjustment difficulties can be worked through.

• **Trust your instincts.** The occasional child who is truly not enjoying anything, having a miserable time and not adjusting to camp life

at all should be allowed to return home after a reasonable amount of time and effort.

Keep in mind that some kids feel guilty when an experience like camp does not work out for them. They may feel that they have let their parents down.

If your child leaves camp, let him know he has not failed and there will be other summers with other adventures.

WHEN YOUR CHILD COMES HOME

After a summer of fun, adventure and freedom, fitting back into the family and assuming responsibilities may be a challenge for some kids.

Strategy: Give him time and space for this reentry process. Support the positive changes you observe. Reintroduce "house rules" with patience and awareness that your child has done some maturing over the summer.

Safety Standards for Children's Camps

Reported in *Parents*, 685 Third Ave., New York 10017.

Is playground equipment well-maintained and age-appropriate? Are campers required to wear protective gear, such as helmets and pads, when playing sports? Are lifeguards certified by the YMCA or the Red Cross? Does the camp have a full-time health manager on-site who is certified in CPR and first aid and can administer medicines? Is there a nearby hospital for emergencies? Are camp vans and buses equipped with seat belts?

Warts and Children

Karl Beutner, MD, PhD, associate clinical professor of dermatology at the University of California at San Francisco.

About one in six school-age children will have warts at one time or another. While there are treatments, it isn't necessary to do anything. Often the warts will clear up by themselves. In children, 66% clear up in two years without treatment.

Treatments: Over-the-counter medications containing salicylic acid, which will get rid of warts within 12 weeks and is the least frightening treatment…or a dermatologist can freeze them with liquid nitrogen…lightly burn them with an electric probe…cut them off…or prescribe topical acids that are stronger than over-the-counter ones. The most effective treatment depends on the age of the patient, the number of warts and their locations.

Helping Your Kids Relax

Playwise: 365 Fun-Filled Activities for Building Character, Conscience and Emotional Intelligence in Children by Denise Chapman Weston, MSW, licensed play therapist, North Attleboro, MA. Tarcher.

Teach kids to breathe deeply—important to developing the relaxation habit. When blowing bubbles, have your child take deep breaths, then breathe slowly into the wand. Or tape a four-inch strip of crepe paper to the bridge of child-sized sunglasses so it hangs in front of your child's nose—have him/her blow on it to see how long he can keep it off his face. Or have him pick a short song to sing or hum in a single breath. Or have him inhale and exhale into a harmonica—and see how long he can keep it going.

Anxiety Disorders In the Family

Vanessa E. Cobham, PhD, lecturer, School of Psychology, University of Queensland, Brisbane, Australia.

More than 80% of anxious children have at least one parent who has a personal history of anxiety.

Good news: Cognitive-behavioral therapy is often helpful for such children—but only if the parent also undergoes therapy. For referral to a cognitive-behavioral therapist in your area, contact the American Psychological Association at 800-964-2000, *www.apa.org.*

How to Stop a Child's Bed-Wetting

Marla R. Ullom-Minnich, MD, a family physician in private practice in Moundridge, KS.

Reward the child for dry nights…have him change the sheets himself when he has an accident…have him practice holding his urine during the day for longer and longer periods of time.

Also helpful: A mattress pad that sounds an alarm when the child wets it. *Cost:* $60 to $90.

Bed-Wetting Prevention Alert

Rudi A. Janknegt, MD, head, department of urology, University Hospital, Maastricht, The Netherlands. His 24-week study of 66 bed wetters was published in the *Journal of Urology*, 1120 N. Charles St., Baltimore 21201.

Anti-bed-wetting nasal spray is often ineffective when the bed wetter has a cold or flu. Congestion keeps the medication, *desmopressin*, from being absorbed.

Good news: Desmopressin *pills* are 90% effective at stopping bed-wetting—even if the child or adult is congested.

ADHD Relief

Timothy Wilens, MD, associate professor of psychiatry, Harvard Medical School, Boston.

Attention deficit hyperactivity disorder (ADHD) can often be controlled with *desipramine* (Norpramin). In a study, 68% of adult ADHD sufferers treated with this

161

antidepressant experienced significant reduction in 12 of 14 symptoms (including short attention span). None of the ADHD sufferers given a placebo showed improvement. Desipramine is the only nonstimulant drug shown in controlled trials to be effective against adult ADHD. Stimulants, including *methylphenidate* (Ritalin) and *dextroamphetamine* (Dexedrine), remain the "first-line" drugs for ADHD.

Ear Infections

Matti Uhari, MD, associate professor of pediatrics, University of Oulu, Oulu, Finland.

Childhood ear infections can be prevented with sugarless gum sweetened with *xylitol.*

Study: Only 12% of kids who chewed the gum five times a day came down with ear infections. This compares with 21% who chewed gum sweetened with ordinary sugar (sucrose).

Theory: Xylitol blocks growth of *Streptococcus pneumoniae*, a bacterium thought to cause 30% of ear infections.

Childhood Ear Infection?

Elizabeth Barnett, MD, assistant professor of pediatrics, Boston City Hospital. Her study of ear infections in 484 children three months to three years of age was published in *Pediatrics*, 141 Northwest Point Rd., Elk Grove Village, IL 60009.

A single injection of the antibiotic *ceftriaxone* (Rocephin) works as well as 10 days of oral medication. Nearly two-thirds of all kids have at least one ear infection by their first birthday. Although oral antibiotics remain the first choice, an injection may be appropriate for children who are vomiting and can't keep medication down...children who refuse to take an oral medication...and children who are enrolled in a day care center that won't dispense medications. Parents should discuss with a pediatrician the best option for their child.

Restless Legs Syndrome... Almost Five Million Sufferers...How to Tell If You're One and What to Do About It

Arthur S. Walters, MD, associate professor of neurology at the University of Medicine and Dentistry of New Jersey–Robert Wood Johnson Medical School in New Brunswick. An expert on sleep disorders, he is the editor of *Sleep Thief, Restless Legs Syndrome* by Virginia N. Wilson. Galaxy Books.

If you have trouble sleeping because of a burning, tingling or "creepy-crawly" sensation in your legs, you may be suffering from *restless legs syndrome* (RLS).

This neurological disorder affects 2% of the population—some so severely that they're unable to sit still long enough to travel in an automobile or airplane or see a movie.

RLS isn't dangerous, but it can seriously disrupt your sleep and your quality of life.

TELLTALE SYMPTOMS

RLS sufferers generally have more leg discomfort when sitting or lying down than when standing. The leg discomfort is especially bad at night, making it hard to fall asleep.

Some sufferers kick during sleep. All have an almost uncontrollable desire to move their legs around.

RLS can strike at any age, but most cases occur after age 40. It often gets worse over time. There is no known way to prevent RLS.

One-third to one-half of all cases of RLS seem to be inherited. RLS can also be caused by nerve damage in the legs—typically the result of diabetes, kidney disease or a pinched nerve in the back...a deficiency of iron...or, theoretically, a deficiency of the neurotransmitter *dopamine*.

CONTROLLING SYMPTOMS

Some RLS sufferers derive relief from iron supplements. The typical dosage is 300 mg three times a day—but check with your doctor first to make sure supplements are right for you.

Others swear by supplements of vitamins E and B-12 and folate. My most severely affected patients, however, generally do *not* benefit from vitamin supplements.

What about nondrug therapies? *Two seem to be particularly helpful...*

● **Revise your sleep schedule.** Try to sleep when your RLS symptoms are least pronounced. You may be able to work out a flex-time arrangement with your employer to accommodate this schedule.

● **Avoid caffeine and alcohol.** They make RLS worse.

CONSULTING A DOCTOR

If symptoms persist, consult a doctor who has experience treating RLS patients. Unfortunately, RLS is often misdiagnosed as anxiety, stress, depression or garden-variety insomnia. Doctors often have a difficult time recognizing RLS, because patients seldom display the telltale leg symptoms in the doctor's office.

Once properly diagnosed, however—either by a primary-care doctor or a neurologist specializing in sleep or movement disorders—RLS can be effectively treated.

Well-controlled clinical trials indicate that 80% of RLS sufferers experience relief from long-term use of one or more of the following drugs...

● ***L-dopa, pergolide* (Permax) or *bromocriptine* (Parlodel).** These drugs boost dopamine levels. *Potential side effects:* Nausea, vomiting, light-headedness and fainting and "rebound" of symptoms into daylight hours.

● ***Clonazepam* (Klonopin) and other benzodiazepines.** *Potential side effects:* Drowsiness and mental dullness.

● **Acetaminophen with codeine, *oxycodone* (Percocet) and other opiates.** *Potential side effect:* Constipation.

Benzodiazepines and opiates can be addictive, but the risk is small if the drugs are used under close medical supervision.

FOR MORE INFORMATION

Send a 55-cent, self-addressed envelope to the Restless Legs Syndrome Foundation, Dept. WWW, Box 7050, Rochester, MN 55902.

Puberty Fact

Marcia E. Herman-Giddens, DrPH, associate professor of public health, University of North Carolina, Chapel Hill.

American girls reach puberty as early as eight years of age. At age eight, nearly half of African-American girls and 15% of white girls are starting to develop breasts and/or pubic hair.

Theory: Puberty may be partially triggered by estrogen-like compounds now found in everything from pesticides to plastic wrap.

Drawstring Danger

Dorothy A. Drago, MPH, product safety consultant, Gaithersburg, MD. Her study of drawstring accidents was published in *Archives of Pediatrics and Adolescent Medicine*, 535 N. Dearborn St., Chicago 60610.

To reduce children's risk of accidental strangulation, remove all drawstrings from the necklines and hoods of their jackets and other outerwear...and cut waist and bottom drawstrings to three inches. Between 1985 and 1995, eight American children suffocated when their drawstrings snagged on playground slides or school bus handrails or doors.

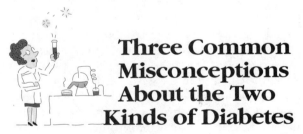

Three Common Misconceptions About the Two Kinds of Diabetes

David M. Nathan, MD, director of the Diabetes Center at Massachusetts General Hospital in Boston and author of *Diabetes*. Times Books. He is chairman of the Diabetes Prevention Program (DPP), a study examining whether type II diabetes can be prevented.

Diabetes is the most common chronic, serious ailment in the US. It's the leading cause of both blindness and kidney failure. It can cause nerve damage that requires amputations. And diabetes greatly raises the risk for heart disease and stroke.

Despite the wide swath diabetes cuts through our society, many people harbor misconceptions about the disease…

Misconception #1: Diabetes is a disease that *kids* get—and if you didn't get it then, you needn't worry about it now.

Misconception #2: Diabetes is an *old* person's disease—and middle-aged people needn't worry about it.

Misconception #3: When older people get diabetes, it's mild.

TWO TYPES OF TROUBLE

Both kinds of diabetes involve elevated blood sugar levels, along with abnormal metabolism of fat and protein.

Type I diabetes appears most often by young adulthood. But this type (once called *juvenile-onset* diabetes) accounts for only 5% to 10% of diabetic patients.

Type II diabetes strikes 8% to 10% of adults at some time in their lives. While type II usually develops after age 45, half of all people with the disease develop it before age 60.

Background: Blood sugar is normally regulated by insulin, an enzyme synthesized by beta cells in the pancreas.

In type I diabetes, an auto-immune reaction destroys the *beta cells*, leaving the body unable to make insulin. Without insulin injections, death may occur in a matter of days.

In type II diabetes—which is often associated with obesity—the beta cells fail to make enough insulin. Because type II diabetics may not need insulin shots, many people wrongly assume that the disease isn't serious.

The onset of type I diabetes is usually obvious. Common symptoms include extreme thirst, frequent urination, blurred vision or unexplained weight loss.

With type II, glucose levels rise so slowly that these symptoms take longer to show up… or develop so gradually that they're noticed only after complications start to occur.

Half of the people suffering from type II diabetes don't even know they have it. And—the longer diabetes goes untreated, the greater risk of complications.

TESTING GUIDELINES

The current testing guidelines issued by the American Diabetes Association urges all Americans age 45 or older to be screened for diabetes at least once every three years.

The screening test recommended by the guidelines is simpler and less unpleasant than the old oral *glucose-tolerance* test. That test—given after an overnight fast—required the patient to drink a sweet syrup, followed by a blood test two hours later.

The *fasting plasma glucose* test also requires an overnight fast. But the patient doesn't have to drink the sweet liquid or wait two hours.

With the old guidelines, anyone whose fasting blood sugar level was 140 or higher—or whose sugar level two hours after the drink was 200 or higher—was said to have diabetes.

With the current guidelines, the cutoff is 126. Research shows that complications start to develop when blood sugar rises above that level.

GETTING THE BEST TREATMENT

From diet and exercise to new drugs, there are now several ways to control type II diabetes and associated problems like high blood pressure, elevated triglycerides, low HDL (good) cholesterol, etc.

Caught early, type II diabetes can often be controlled with diet and exercise alone.

Eighty percent of type II diabetics are overweight. Once these patients lose weight—even as little as a few pounds—blood sugar level and metabolic state improve. So do blood pressure and cholesterol levels.

Unlike type I diabetics—who must carefully monitor the balance of carbohydrates to other foods at every meal—type II diabetics can mainly concentrate on cutting calories.

The best way to do this is to cut back on saturated fat…and to boost consumption of grains, fruits and vegetables.

What about eating less sugar? That's less important for type II than type I diabetics. However, since reducing sugar consumption can help keep blood sugar under control, it's worth doing.

Exercise reduces the body's insulin needs by boosting the cells' sensitivity to insulin. To get started, go for a 20-minute walk each evening

...or take the stairs instead of the elevator at work, while shopping, etc.

Caution: If you aren't used to physical activity, check with your doctor first.

When diet and exercise aren't enough to do the job, it's time for drug therapy. There are now a variety of medications that can help control type II diabetes...

●**Sulfonylureas** (SFUs) stimulate the pancreas to make insulin. Side effects can include *hypoglycemia* (low blood sugar) and weight gain.

●**Biguanides**, including *metformin* (Glucophage), reduce the amount of sugar released by the liver. This lowers blood sugar to levels similar to those achieved with SFUs—but without the side effects of hypoglycemia or weight gain.

●**Alpha-glucosidase inhibitors**, including *acarbose* (Precose), slow digestion of carbohydrates and block their absorption.

Because their effect on blood sugar isn't as powerful as that of SFUs and biguanides, these medications are generally better suited for mild diabetes.

INSULIN INJECTIONS

When oral drug therapy fails to control diabetes fully, insulin injections can dramatically lower glucose levels.

Most patients who learn to give themselves insulin injections are surprised at how simple and painless the process is.

Type II diabetes rarely requires the frequent injections needed to control type I—once or twice a day is often enough.

Cold Sore Relief

Spotswood Spruance, MD, professor of medicine, University of Utah School of Medicine, Salt Lake City.

People with cold sores used to have to wait for them to clear up.

The prescription antiviral agent *penciclovir* (Denavir) speeds healing of cold sores.

Bonus: Penciclovir ointment reduces the span of time during which the virus that causes cold sores is contagious.

Kegel Exercises Beat Incontinence in Women

Consumer Reports on Health, 101 Truman Ave., Yonkers, NY 10703.

Kegel exercises strengthen the pelvic-floor muscles surrounding the openings of the urethra, vagina and anus.

What to do: Contract pelvic muscles for five seconds, relax for five seconds. Repeat 12 times—eight times a day.

To identify your pelvic muscles: Practice interrupting urine flow during urination.

How to Stop Recurring Hemorrhoids

Bruce Yaffe, MD, a gastroenterologist and internist in private practice in New York City.

Stay regular by consuming about 30 grams of dietary fiber and at least 48 ounces of water per day.

Also helpful: Take an over-the-counter stool softener like *Colace* or a bulking agent laxative such as *Metamucil*...don't strain or hold your breath while defecating...clean the rectum with moistened wipes instead of dry toilet paper...and soothe the area with zinc oxide paste, petroleum jelly, cold compresses or an over-the-counter ointment such as *Balneol*.

If hemorrhoids are inflamed: Try warm baths, and wear cotton underwear and loose, nonbinding clothing.

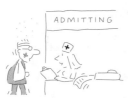

Keeping Wounds From Scarring

Alan Engler, MD, assistant clinical professor of plastic and reconstructive surgery, Albert Einstein College of Medicine, and a plastic surgeon in private practice, in New York City.

Don't wash the wound with hydrogen peroxide. Lubricate it with petroleum jelly or a topical ointment such as *bacitracin*.

•**Bandage the wound to minimize exposure to air.** Change the dressing once or twice daily.

•**Avoid exposure to sunlight.** It can cause skin to darken.

Pediatrician's Home Remedies

Norman Weinberger, MD, pediatrician in private practice in Norwalk, CT. He is a senior attending physician at Norwalk Hospital and on the faculty at Yale University School of Medicine. Dr. Weinberger is author of *You Just Don't Duct Tape a Baby: True Tales and Sensible Suggestions from a Veteran Pediatrician.* Warner Books.

Here are some of the problems my own adult kids ask me about their children—and what I suggest they do…

THE COMMON COLD

•**Make a cup of decaffeinated spice tea.** Add lemon and honey, and wait until it cools slightly. The tea is soothing and hot, which will combat stuffiness and open up the nasal passages. The honey in the tea can help soothe a sore throat as well. The lemon soothes and coats the throat with vitamin C.

•**Make old-fashioned chicken soup**—or use low-sodium canned soup. Not only will it make your child feel better, but making the soup keeps you too busy to worry.

•**Offer fun fluids.** The more fluids a sick child can drink, the better it is. The fluids help clean out the child's system.

Make colorful Jell-O water by doubling the amount of water in the Jell-O recipe…offer enticing flavored ices…or watered-down Gatorade.

FEVER

Fever is not usually as scary as most parents believe it to be. It is a sign that the body is fighting infection.

If you're concerned, take your child's temperature and make sure to tell the doctor how and when you obtained it.

If a high fever is not responding to acetaminophen (Tylenol), try a warm bath, which will dissipate body heat.

There is no reason for the water to be cold. Besides being unpleasant for the child, a cold bath can be dangerous. I have seen a really cold bath send a feverish child into shock. Alcohol rubs should also be avoided.

RASHES

Make sure you can tell your doctor…

•**When the rash began.**

•**Where on the body it began.**

•**How long it took to spread.**

•**Whether or not it itches.**

•**What color it is.**

•**Whether the bumps are flat,** raised or fluid-filled.

Do a little investigative work on your own, too. Did you just change laundry detergents? Often, it's a simple case of a reaction to a new food, lotion or sunscreen with PABA.

SUNBURN

For sunburn relief during winter vacations, try tea bags. Let the bags steep in boiled water for five minutes. Then, after they cool, remove from the water and apply the wet bags to the skin.

8

Reduce Stress, Lengthen Lives

You Can Make Stress Work for You

Kenneth Pelletier, MD, PhD
Stanford University School of Medicine

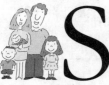Stress is an unfortunate fact of life. But possessing a healthy sense of control—a confidence in your ability to influence the course and destiny of your life —can help you influence stress by shortening its duration or avoiding it altogether.

How to reduce the different types of stress in your life…

STRESS AT WORK

Career demands cause a specific type of stress called *job strain*. It occurs when a job makes high psychological demands but allows little or no control, autonomy or discretion over tasks.

Strategy: Be more proactive, and try to divide your workload into blocks of manageable time. Schedule difficult tasks during your best hours. Set aside an hour or two each morning, if possible, when you don't take phone calls. Use that time to conquer your paperwork.

Examples: If you're constantly racing to meet deadlines, place a colored dot on one of the numbers on the clock in your office. Whenever the clock shows that hour, take deep breaths—in order to let go of cumulative stress and clear your mind. If you work at a computer all day, give your eyes and mind a break by periodically looking into the corner of the room—or out the window.

STRESS AT HOME

The time you spend with your family is the time for self-healing. But all too often, family members find that despite their physical closeness, they feel alone or isolated because there isn't any *positive interaction*.

Strategy: Enhancing family bonds is the key to managing stress and a happier, healthier life. Reduce external distractions by turning off the TV or radio *at least* once a week, and using

Kenneth Pelletier, MD, PhD, clinical associate professor of medicine at Stanford University School of Medicine in Stanford, CA. He is author of *Sound Mind, Sound Body.* Simon & Schuster.

167

that time for conversation or for an activity the entire family can enjoy.

Examples: Take a walk…go to the park… visit the library. Schedule weekly family councils to discuss problems and concerns or to celebrate family members' achievements.

STRESS AND PERSONAL OBLIGATIONS

Stress at home is not always caused by family problems, and in fact is often due to an overload of bills, errands and household chores.

Strategy: Ask yourself, *Is it worth dying for?* Often, we assign trivial tasks (such as getting to the cleaners before closing time) too much importance. The key is to prioritize what needs doing and focus on getting it done, instead of focusing on what can wait (which leads to more stress).

You may also want to consolidate errands and do the most important ones together.

To reduce accumulating bills, try to identify what you absolutely *need*, not what you *want*, relative to your level of income and debt.

STRESS AND YOUR PARTNER

Relationships take time, commitment and energy. Such efforts and demands can be particularly stressful when other areas of your life make similar demands. However, we can turn shortcomings or insecurities into assets and strengthen our ability to reach optimal health by acknowledging them to our partners and to ourselves.

Strategy: Isolate blocks of time to discuss issues of concern to both you and your partner. Instead of assuming one party is "right" and the other "wrong," place yourself in the other person's shoes and rehearse his/her perspective.

Most arguments occur during transitional periods of the day—when we get home from work, for instance. So take time to allow tensions to dissipate by changing clothes, taking a shower or walking outside before confronting or devoting attention to each other.

RELAXATION SECRETS

Truly successful people are not overburdened by stress. This is largely due to the fact that they perceive stress as an opportunity for learning…believe that they have control over their lives and destinies…and invest in altruism,

recognizing the need to see beyond their personal needs and devote time to helping others.

Research has shown that *attitude* toward oneself and the world is the key to managing stress. So, enjoying what is happening "now" can enable you to stay in the moment and release your mind from built-up concerns and tensions.

While stress-management skills are only part of a total lifestyle program to stay healthy, they can also allow the body and mind to relax and let go of accumulated tension.

EXERCISES THAT HELP TO MANAGE STRESS

Exercise I: While seated in a balanced, comfortable position, tense and then relax each muscle group. Focusing on your left arm and hand, silently say to yourself, three times, *My left arm is heavy and warm.*

Repeat with your right arm, and then move your attention to your head and face, imagining a cool breeze.

End the exercise by raising hands to chest while slowly inhaling and stretching your legs as you exhale.

Exercise II: Visualize a place, preferably outdoors, where you feel safe and undistracted. Allow that place to become as real as possible by paying close attention to details, such as the time of day, the colors, smells and sounds.

Imagine that whatever it is you want to change appears before you, and then transform the image in a positive way. Gradually allow the image to disappear and return back to your safe place.

Stress Avoidance Secrets: Proven Strategies

Robert M. Sapolsky, PhD, professor of biological sciences and neuroscience at Stanford University, Stanford, CA. He is author of *Why Zebras Don't Get Ulcers: A Guide to Stress, Stress-Related Diseases and Coping.* W.H. Freeman.

As the pace of American society continues to accelerate, the incidence of psychological stress keeps climbing. Stress is *not* just an annoyance. It has been linked to adult-onset diabetes, ulcerative colitis, atherosclerosis, high blood pressure and other serious ailments.

Yet we all know individuals who are *stress-resistant*—lucky folks who never seem "stressed out" despite the competing demands of career, family, etc.

To learn the secrets of stress resistance, we consulted Dr. Robert Sapolsky, a Stanford biologist and MacArthur "genius" grant recipient who has been studying stress for more than 15 years.

TWO SIDES OF STRESS

When confronted by a threat to its physical well-being, the body undergoes what is known as the *stress response*. It temporarily abandons its long-term "building projects"—growth, tissue repair, immune function, etc.

Instead, it floods the bloodstream with glucose, protein and fat from reserves in the liver and fat cells. Heart rate, blood pressure and breathing rate skyrocket. These physiological changes can save your life by giving you extra speed or strength…or a more focused mind.

Problem: The stress response occurs not only when we are confronted by *physical* danger, but also in situations that simply make us *feel* anxious—from getting stuck in traffic to having an argument with a spouse or coworker.

Research on both animals and humans suggests four effective strategies for limiting the toll taken by chronic stress…

A SENSE OF CONTROL

Having a sense of control over one's situation reduces the stress response. This has been shown in studies of humans exposed to a loud, intermittent noise.

Individuals who *believed* they could stop the noise by pressing a button felt less stress than subjects without this option—even though the sense of control was illusory.

But reducing stress is not as simple as saying, *Take as much control as possible.* In the case of an automobile accident, a diagnosis of a terminal disease or another uncontrollable event, suggesting that an individual can control the situation only adds feelings of guilt and inadequacy to stress.

In extreme situations it's usually better to *deny* personal responsibility for the problem—by identifying an *external* source of control.

Example: No one could have stopped the car in time.

Control is most helpful in coping with *moderate* stressors—traffic jams, supermarket lines, setbacks at work, etc.

If your boss gives you a tedious project, for example, look for areas in which you can exert control. Perhaps you could choose the members of your team, plot out a schedule for the project, etc.

PREDICTABILITY

Imagine asking your dentist, *How much longer will you have to drill?* It's much less stressful to hear, *Three minutes,* than it is to hear, *I don't know.*

Studies show that animals and humans given a warning signal before being subjected to a stressor experience less stress.

Caveat: This "early warning" must come far enough in advance to allow the subject to prepare…but not *too* far ahead.

With rats, flashing a warning light 10 seconds before the administration of an electrical shock reduces the stress response. A light that flashes one-half second before the shock has no effect.

When the light is flashed *five minutes* before the shock, rats experience more stress than if no light is flashed.

How can humans predict their stressors? By getting accurate, specific information.

Examples: Listening to the traffic report on the way to work…reading about treatment options for a serious illness…setting aside a specific time each day to speak with coworkers who otherwise might interrupt your workday.

HAVING AN OUTLET

A rat exposed to shock feels less stress if it's given an *outlet* for its nervous energy—the opportunity to run on an exercise wheel or gnaw on wood.

Humans benefit from outlets, too. Most people know what helps them relax—whether it's playing the clarinet, working out or practicing meditation. Each has been shown to lower blood pressure and adrenaline levels.

Most important: Create a change in tempo from the rest of the day. Pursuing your favorite activities three times a week has a greater effect on stress than saving all your outlets for the weekend.

CONTACT WITH OTHERS

As a threat to health and longevity, social isolation is second only to low socioeconomic status. Isolated people have a higher mortality rate than even smokers, obese people and hypertensives.

Implication: You can defuse stressful situations via physical contact with another person —holding hands, hugging, etc.

Exception: An Ohio State University study found that spouses in bad marriages had drastically suppressed immune systems.

People living alone needn't despair—health benefits can accrue from contact with a lover, close friends, fellow members of a church or synagogue, etc.

How to Turn Stress Into Strengths

Bruce Munro, PhD, director of behavioral medicine at the Institute of Stress Medicine–Jackson Hole, Box 279, Wilson, WY 83014. He is coauthor, with the late Dr. Robert Eliot, of *From Stress to Strength: How to Lighten Your Load and Save Your Life*. Bantam Books.

Feelings of stress are triggered by our natural survival mechanisms. Though few of us will encounter saber-toothed tigers in our daily routine, many of us are as stressed as our caveman ancestors when we're doing battle with the paper tigers of the modern workplace.

Much of our stress has to do with a mismatch between expectations and reality. As life's pressures mount and your burdens increase, the resulting pressures can have a catastrophic impact on your health. Cardiovascular damage is the most common result of stress—high blood pressure, heart attacks and strokes can be directly related to the amount of stress in your daily life.

Good news: There are steps you can take to diminish stress—even in the most difficult situations. How you react is your choice, far more than you realize.

Here are ways of identifying and controlling stress that can change your reaction pattern and lengthen your life…

HAVE A SOULMATE

We know that up to age 70, marriage reduces the risk of premature death and disability by about 50%. We don't have studies about living together, but presumably it works the same way. Having a friend, lover or companion to share your life and your feelings is one of the most important health insurance policies you can have.

Also helpful: Owning a pet, which enables you to interact emotionally. Caring for your pet will also distract you and prevent stress from building up.

MAKE FRIENDS

Do you have someone—other than your mate—who is genuinely interested in you… who will empathize with you…and listen to you and your troubles anytime?

Such strong friendships are especially important for men—because men aren't naturally as good at making friends as women are. Early training to be competitive hampers their efforts at friendship.

Example: When a group of women have lunch together, they all usually share in the conversation. At a table of men, however, what you normally see is one man talking at the others—and every man in the audience is just waiting for his turn to seize the floor.

Real friends are made one at a time, usually through shared activity. If you're a man, you may have to make a special effort to cultivate friendships—but it's worth the time and energy.

If you have friends who enjoy you as you are and with whom you can act naturally, you have a second ring of protection. They add more time and enjoyment to the length of your life.

RELIGIOUS CONNECTION

People who have religious connections that are *fulfilling* also have a health advantage.

Note that I said fulfilling. It's how you feel about your religious connections that counts, not how anybody else feels about them. Even if you go to religious services because you think you should—or if you're doing it for the sake of appearances or for your kids—that counts.

If your spiritual beliefs are a source of support to you—if your participation in prayer or meditation or religious services is nourishing—then you've reduced your odds of dying before 70.

AVOID PERFECTIONISM

Most successful people think they have to do everything perfectly. Perfectionists are hard on themselves and are horrible to work for. Because nothing they do is good enough, they project their dissatisfaction and put the blame on you. Nothing you do will ever be good enough, either.

How do you tell whether you're a perfectionist? If you find yourself frequently saying, *I should…I must…I have to.*

Solution: Prioritize your perfectionism. Pick two or three things in your job or your life, and focus your perfectionism on them. Constantly remind yourself that it is fine to do other things in a less-than-perfect manner.

BE ASSERTIVE

A person who is unassertive is a people-pleaser—someone who doesn't like to say "no" for fear others won't like him/her. If you feel you have to say "yes" to too many things, you'll get overloaded.

Unassertive people are usually angry *inside.* When overloaded, they blow their tops. Others feel this anger and become uncomfortable …then they push the unassertive person away.

Be assertive to make your work life go well. If there are problems at work, decide what needs to be changed and how. Then talk to your boss. Tell him you need feedback to do your best work.

THE VALUE OF VALUES

My definition of values is knowing just what you want to guide your life. A person who has no values and who doesn't know where he's going or doesn't care what he's doing will never make any progress.

Hans Selye, the physician who created the field of stress study, once said that *no wind blows in favor of a ship without direction.*

Being aware of what guides you can have a profound impact on every aspect of your life. Benjamin Franklin was a loser in his 30s. He simply couldn't get his life together. Finally, he hit on the strategy of writing what he wanted out of life. He referred to his list frequently. By means of this process he was able to make great advances and increased his contributions to American life.

Helpful: Write down 30 or 40 things you want on 3" x 5" cards, one item to each card. Go over the list, and choose the six items that are most important to you. Carry those cards around with you during the day, and refer to them at least twice a day to see how much you've been able to accomplish on each task.

DIVERSIFY YOUR LIFE

It's important not to focus only on one or two areas of intent. All of us need a variety of diversions, so that if one interest area becomes stressful or goes sour, there will be others that are doing well and can take up the slack.

People who lead stressful lives narrow the focus of their lives to just one or two areas. But if one of those areas develops a problem, there's a danger that they won't have other interests to fall back on. If a person has a range of interests, the others can sustain him through whatever reorganization is done.

Examples: Volunteer work is particularly life-enhancing. Not only does it distract you from dwelling on your own anxiety, but it also enables you to channel your energy in a positive way. Aerobic exercise conditions our bodies and creates a sense of well-being. It releases natural chemicals (hormones) that create optimism and improve our resilience and our resistance to stress and illness.

HUMOR LENGTHENS YOUR LIFE

We have to be able to laugh at ourselves and at humorous situations. If you've lost this ability, you're in trouble.

Helpful: Try watching comedies on TV or going to see funny movies. Laughter is very powerful medicine. I prescribe a daily dose until you've regained your sense of enjoyment in life.

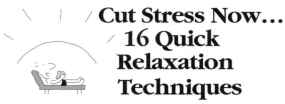

Cut Stress Now... 16 Quick Relaxation Techniques

Ed Boenisch, PhD, adjutant general of the Wyoming Military Department in Cheyenne. He is coauthor of *The Stress Owner's Manual*. Impact.

Practice the six-second release exercise. Anywhere, anytime you feel tense, inhale deeply for two seconds, then exhale for four seconds.

Say to yourself, "I'm relaxing." Let your shoulders and jaw drop. A wave of relaxation will flow downward.

●**Watch less TV.** Do not aimlessly channel surf. Do not watch violent or depressing shows.

Look through the television listings, and carefully select programs to watch. Emphasize uplifting, educational programs—those on the Discovery Channel and PBS, for example.

●**Don't take work home**...or take home to work. "Decompress" as you make the transition from one part of your life to another—so distress from one doesn't spill into the other.

Sing along with the radio...take a walk... nap...soak in a tub.

●**Look for humor in every situation.** Take yourself lightly and your work seriously. Read fun things—comics, cartoons, jokes—and share them with others.

●**Cultivate a "can-do" attitude.** As Norman Vincent Peale once said, "You are not what you think you are...but, what you think, you are."

●**Stop assuming the worst.** If someone cuts you off on the highway, don't automatically assume that the person is out to get you. Maybe he/she is rushing to the hospital to see a loved one who is desperately ill.

●**Take a 10-minute break.** At least once every hour, get up from your chair, stretch and move around. Doing so will help prevent stiffness and tension.

●**Listen to relaxing music.** Spend your day listening to instrumental classical or New Age music.

Good choices: George Winston, David Lanz, Enya, The Narada Collections.

●**"Box" your worries.** Categorize your worries into things you can/cannot control and things that are important/unimportant. If something is important and you can do something about it, take action. If it's unimportant and/or you can't do anything about it, let the worry go.

●**Take a one-minute vacation.** Pause to enjoy life's small, fleeting pleasures—the fragrance of a flower...the burbling of a brook... the tranquil beauty of freshly fallen snow...the cozy aroma of a wood fire. Notice and try to enjoy whatever is around you.

●**Practice "dot therapy."** Place adhesive dots wherever you need a cue to relax—on your car's rearview mirror...on your telephone handset...on your computer monitor.

Whenever you spy a dot, do the six-second release exercise.

●**Get an aromatic high.** Bring flowers to work. Spray perfume into the air. Light a scented candle. Floral fragrances reduce anxiety (even in the dentist's office)...cool, menthol-like scents boost energy...lavender is relaxing.

●**Boost your ego.** Carry a 3x5-inch card on which you've written all your good points. Whenever you start to feel overwhelmed, look at the card.

Ask those who care about you to contribute to your list.

●**Set realistic goals**—and envision yourself reaching them. If you're a salesperson, visualize yourself closing a deal with the client you're scheduled to see that day. You'll be less anxious when you go into the meeting.

●**Pet a dog or cat.** Doing so tends to lower heart rate and blood pressure—your own and those of the animal being petted.

●**Choose to be happy.** Abraham Lincoln once said, "Most folks are about as happy as they choose to be."

Each day, make a conscious effort to emphasize the positive and disregard the negative. Choose happiness day after day, and it soon becomes a habit.

Just Relax!

Janice Kiecolt-Glaser, PhD, professor of psychology at Ohio State University in Columbus, and a leading authority on mind–body medicine.

Dozens of studies have shown that emotional stress impairs the immune system. Relaxation reduces this stress, helping boost immunity. In one study, men and women who were taught relaxation techniques had a significant increase in the activity of natural killercells—a key marker in immune-system health.

Relaxation Can Control Seizures

Epilepsy: A New Approach by Adrienne Richard, an epileptic who uses mind–body techniques instead of anticonvulsants, and Joel Reiter, MD, neurologist, Santa Rosa, CA. Walker & Co.

An epileptic who practices deep diaphragmatic breathing daily in meditation may be able to stop a seizure from taking control.

Helpful: A partner can focus the epileptic on the relaxation techniques. If someone reminds him/her to relax and breathe deeply, the epileptic can switch into the relaxation technique and minimize the seizure's effects.

Quick Stress Buster

Jon Kabat-Zinn, PhD, director, Stress Reduction Clinic, University of Massachusetts Medical Center, Worcester, MA.

A five minute session lowers blood pressure, reduces levels of stress hormones and boosts feelings of well-being.

What to do: Sit comfortably, straight and tall …become aware of your breathing…visualize a mountain scene, noticing all the details… imagine changes taking place, the sun arcing across the sky, violent storms whipping up… focus on the mountain's stillness and calm throughout these events and carry this calm with you all day.

Sleep vs. Stress

Angela Clow, PhD, lecturer and coauthor of a study of 42 people at the University of Westminster, London.

Sleeping later reduces stress. In a study, people who woke up after 7:21 a.m. had lower blood levels of the stress hormone *cortisol* than those who woke up earlier. This was true even if they were woken suddenly at a later time…or went to bed later than usual. *Possible reason:* The body's natural "clock."

Cholesterol Levels Are Affected by Stress

Catherine M. Stoney, PhD, associate professor of psychology, Ohio State University, Columbus. Her studies of 127 airline pilots and 100 medical students were presented at the International Congress of Behavioral Medicine, Washington, DC.

In men, levels of LDL (bad) cholesterol rose 5% during periods of high stress. Women showed no stress-related rise in LDL. In another study, students who scored high on tests to measure conscientiousness had HDL (good) cholesterol levels about 4% higher than those who scored lower.

Good for Your Heart

James A. Blumenthal, PhD, professor of medical psychology at Duke University Medical School, Durham, NC.

Learning better responses to stress is good for your heart. This conclusion comes from experimental findings that people whose hearts are less able to pump blood in response to mental stress have three times more chance of a heart attack or heart surgery within five years than those whose hearts are better able to pump blood. Regular exercise and reacting to stress in a more relaxed way, perhaps by breathing deeply, are ways to head off the negative effects of stress.

Fight Stress Anytime, Anywhere

Alice Domar, PhD, researcher, Deaconess Hospital and Harvard Medical School, Boston, and author of *Healing Mind, Healthy Women*. Henry Holt.

I f you practice simple breathing exercises, you can fight stress anytime, anywhere. *Reason:* When people are upset they tend to take quick, shallow breaths.

Much better: Deep abdominal breathing. Make a conscious effort to relax your muscles and take deep breaths. Practice this form of breathing regularly, several times a day. Switch to it whenever you feel stressed or tense. It relieves anxiety and makes it easier for you to cope with whatever problem is causing your tension.

Plants and Stress

Ashley Craig, PhD, associate professor of health sciences, University of Technology, Sydney, Australia.

Houseplants help reduce psychological stress. In a study, brain wave activity was measured as 31 volunteers stared for two minutes at a plant, an abstract sculpture or a white panel.

Result: Those who stared at the plant experienced a 20% increase in alpha waves. These electrical signals are a sign of relaxation. Those who looked at the sculpture had no change in alpha wave activity.

Presumably, their inability to "figure out" the sculpture prevented relaxation. People who looked at the white panel also experienced a rise in alpha waves—but the effect of looking at the plant was far more powerful.

Top Stress Reducer

Karen Allen, PhD, research scientist, University of Buffalo School of Medicine, Buffalo, NY, leader of a study of 480 people under stressful conditions.

The top stress reducers are dogs. People who were facing stressful situations had the lowest heart rates and blood pressure if they were with their dogs—even lower than those of people who were with their spouses.

Possible reason: Dogs are perceived as completely nonjudgmental.

Music and Stress

Cheryl Dileo-Maranto, PhD, professor of music therapy, Temple University, Philadelphia, and president, World Federation of Music Therapy.

Music is a quick stress reliever. Listen to music for 10 to 20 minutes. *Helpful:* Sit in a comfortable chair, away from disturbances, with lights dimmed. Choose music you know well, instead of a new piece that might keep you alert …but avoid melodies that cause tension or remind you of anything unpleasant.

Instrumental music is preferable to songs with lyrics. *Reason:* The latter may distract you from relaxation and stimulate cognitive activity. If thoughts of the day's problems intrude, keep bringing your mind back to the music.

Writing Helps

Energy Secrets: For Tired Mothers on the Run by B. Kaye Olson, nurse and stress consultant, Lansing, MI. Health Communications.

Write down your nagging worries…make two columns on a sheet of paper, one labeled "Worries I can do something about" and the other "Worries I can't do anything about." Accept problems you can't change… and find solutions for those you can control.

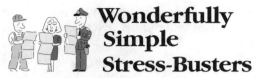

Wonderfully Simple Stress-Busters

Charles B. Inlander, president of People's Medical Society, a patient advocate organization, 462 Walnut St., Allentown, PA 18102. He is author of several books, including *63 Ways to Relieve Tension and Stay Healthy.* Walker.

The toll that stress takes on our nation's health and finances is daunting. Surveys by the National Institute of Mental Health and other groups reveal that...

● **Stress contributes to fully half of all illnesses in the US.**

● **At least 70% of all visits to the doctor** are for stress-related or stress-induced illness.

That's the bad news. The good news is that there are simple steps you can take to relieve and prevent stress...

● **Laugh more.** Laughter is one of the healthiest antidotes to stress. When we laugh, blood flow to the brain is increased, endorphins (hormones that give a sense of well-being) are released and levels of stress hormones drop dramatically.

Research at Loma Linda University showed that watching filmed comedy shows lowered blood pressure and reduced the risk of other cardiovascular problems.

The late author Norman Cousins put this research into practice to fight a crippling and irreversible form of arthritis. He rented funny movies each day, and laughed as much as possible. *Result:* His disease went into remission and he outlived all medical expectations.

● **Be more sociable.** When we're under stress, our instincts tell us to withdraw from the action and isolate ourselves. Nothing could be worse, according to stress experts.

Reason: Isolation allows us to concentrate more on our own problems, and perpetuates negative thinking—intensifying stress, rather than resolving it.

Research shows a clear link between isolation and failure to cope adequately with stress, along with a heightened vulnerability to illness.

When you feel stressed, respond by calling friends, or being around young children—they have a way of making you forget your worries.

Doing volunteer work is also a good stress-buster. A 10-year University of Michigan study found that men who did not do volunteer work had twice the death rate of men who volunteered once a week.

● **Be more decisive.** Indecision prevents you from taking action—reducing your sense of being in control, and thus intensifying stress.

How to overcome indecisiveness: First, write down the problem—and a list of your options. Include the option of doing nothing. Next, try *lateral thinking*—in which you consider unusual alternatives and their pros and cons.

Helpful: Be ready to compromise. There's hardly any decision that can't be modified at a later point.

● **Learn to be more assertive.** Many people incorrectly associate assertiveness with hostility or aggression. But assertiveness simply means expressing your feelings, letting others know your beliefs and opinions...and acting on your own behalf.

Psychologist James Mills, PhD, author of *Coping with Stress*, suggests these ways to become more assertive...

● **Speak up** when you feel it's warranted.

● **Initiate conversations** with others.

● **Concentrate on making your wishes and needs known to others.**

● **Make an effort to seek out and initiate friendships.**

● **Don't be afraid to disagree** with others.

● **Give out—and accept—compliments.**

● **Ask for information.**

● **Tell someone else about yourself.**

● **Break the stress–sleeplessness cycle.** On average, an adult needs between seven and eight hours of sleep a night. Lack of adequate sleep can make a person moody, angry and more vulnerable to illness and stress. *To beat sleeplessness...*

● **Develop a regular bedtime routine,** which will signal your mind that it's time to sleep.

• **Avoid alcohol, caffeine and tobacco**— all of which have negative effects on sleep.

• **Do something calming before going to bed.** And avoid doing things that may have an agitating effect. For example, don't watch a violent movie too soon before going to bed.

• **Don't use your bedroom for anything but sleeping and sex.**

• **Before retiring,** allot some extra time just to relax.

• **Give yourself pep talks.** If you're inclined to blame yourself for your problems, you may be guilty of negative self-talk, which causes stress.

Better: Talk positively to yourself. Tell yourself, "Good job" or "You handled that tough situation well." Practice in front of a mirror, if necessary. Eventually this positive talk will become an automatic response.

• **Reward yourself.** Rewards are a critical component of stress management. Those who reward themselves after completing a task by purposely engaging in something pleasurable, realize a boost in their immune systems that can last for several days.

Simple stress management technique: Schedule at least one pleasurable activity every day to reward yourself.

• **Write down pent-up emotions.** If you're under emotional stress, recording your feelings in a journal or diary can help relieve the problem—even when it involves marital or job difficulties.

This is especially true if you have trouble talking about worries or emotional issues, or if you have no readily available person to listen. The key may be the simple act of disclosure.

• **Slow down.** Try moving, talking and behaving in a more relaxed manner. You'll probably feel some of your stress start to ebb away. Stephan Rechtschaffen, MD, president of the Omega Institute for Holistic Studies, also offers these tips on slowing down...

• **Drive 10 miles per hour slower** than you usually do.

• **Pause at the table before you start eating.** When you eat, chew your food more slowly than usual.

• **When you get home in your car,** wait five minutes or so in your driveway before going inside. Listen to the radio, or just relax and ease into the transition.

• **Take a shower when you get home from work.** It will help relax you, and also signals a change from your work environment.

• **Let the phone ring a few times before you answer it.** Racing across the room to grab the phone triggers more stress.

9

Hospital and Surgery Awareness

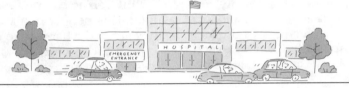

How to Have a Healthier, Happier Hospitalization

Theodore Tyberg, MD
Kenneth Rothaus, MD
New York Hospital–Cornell Medical Center

How can you be sure of receiving the best possible care during a hospital stay?

The first step is to become an informed patient. Being knowledgeable about your condition and treatment makes you more relaxed and confident—and therefore more likable.

Though it's not something they like to admit, doctors and nurses tend to provide better care to patients they like.

Of course, there's a fine line between being knowledgeable and being obnoxious. Try not to cross that line...but do not *let* yourself be ignored or mistreated.

Here are other strategies for ensuring you'll receive top-flight care...

BEFORE ADMISSION

• **Make sure hospitalization is necessary.** Schedule an appointment with your doctor to discuss your condition and the treatment options. Many procedures that once required hospitalization can now be done safely on an outpatient basis.

Examples: Hernia repair, cataract removal and breast biopsy.

• **Have your doctor explain the treatment you'll receive.** Find out how long the operation and recovery will take...and discuss scenarios that might unfold during your hospital stay.

A surgeon may decide *during* coronary angioplasty, for example, that you need bypass

Theodore Tyberg, MD, assistant professor of medicine, and Kenneth Rothaus, MD, assistant professor of surgery, both at New York Hospital–Cornell Medical Center. Dr. Tyberg and Dr. Rothaus are the authors of *Hospital Smarts: The Insider's Survival Guide to Your Hospital, Your Doctor, the Nursing Staff—and Your Bill!* William Morrow.

177

surgery. You and your surgeon should agree before you're wheeled into the operating room how the various scenarios are to be handled.

Do *not* expect your doctor to provide a detailed, step-by-step explanation of your treatment. If you'd like the details, ask him to steer you to relevant articles or books. The hospital's medical library may be open to patients.

●**Meet every doctor who will be involved in your care.** If you're scheduled for surgery, you'll want to meet the surgeon and the anesthesiologist. *Key questions to ask:*

●**Are you board-certified?**

●**How many cases like mine do you handle in a year?** If the number is 25 or fewer, ask your doctor why. Consider finding a new doctor or hospital.

●**Is this hospital appropriate for my condition?** For common medical problems and low-risk surgical procedures, a community hospital is fine. But teaching hospitals have more experience with serious conditions and complex, high-risk procedures.

Example: A woman was rushed to her community hospital emergency room with a severe headache...and was diagnosed with a brain aneurysm. The neurologist there had treated this life-threatening ailment only three times. After a couple of phone calls, the woman's husband had her transferred to a teaching hospital where 20 brain aneurysm repairs are done each year.

●**Learn hospital routines.** Call the hospital a week or so before your admission to inquire about admitting procedures, parking regulations, charges for telephones and televisions, etc.

Ask about the discharge routine. Will you be in a wheelchair? On crutches? Will you need an escort? Must you follow a special diet or other restrictions after you go home? Confirm details with your doctor.

●**Appoint a health-care advocate.** It's the job of this trusted friend or family member to speak on your behalf should you be unable to speak (during recovery from surgery, for example). Pick someone who is level-headed— *and assertive.*

To give your advocate more authority, sign a legally binding proxy. Obtain a proxy form from the hospital's patient services department —or from your lawyer.

If you have a living will, your advocate must make sure the doctor respects your wishes. Doctors tend to ignore living wills unless the patient advocate insists otherwise.

●**Pack wisely.** Take pertinent medical records, a list of allergies you have and a supply of the drugs you routinely take. Don't forget books and magazines and a list of telephone numbers of friends, family and doctors.

What about clothing? Bring slippers and a bathrobe. Pajamas aren't necessary—you'll receive a clean hospital gown at least daily. Leave jewelry and other valuables at home.

DURING YOUR STAY

●**Take an active interest in your care.** When unfamiliar people enter your room, ask who they are and what they're going to do. Consent to tests and procedures only *after* you've discussed them with your doctor.

Each time you see your doctor, ask what will happen next...and when to expect the next visit. Save questions about food, mail, etc., for a nurse or another nonphysician staff member.

●**Guard against mistakes involving drugs, food, etc.** Remind the staff of your condition and the treatment you expect. Have someone identify each drug before it's administered.

Examples: "Is this the blood thinner?" "Another IV bag! What's in that one?"

If your doctor tells you not to eat before surgery and housekeeping delivers a food tray, ask a nurse for an explanation.

A patient of ours who had surgery recently put a sticker on her leg that said, "Operate on this one." No one in the operating room thought this silly.

●**Insist that the staff wash their hands and don rubber gloves.** This is especially important if you have a fresh surgical incision. Don't be afraid to say, "I'd rather you wear gloves."

●**Don't suffer in silence.** Let the staff know about any discomfort—it might be symptomatic of a condition that needs attention.

Signs of a Good Hospital

John Connolly, EdD, former president, New York Medical College, Valhalla, and author of *How to Find the Best Doctors, Hospitals, HMOs for You and Your Family.* Castle Connolly Medical Ltd.

●**Accreditation**—by the Joint Commission on Accreditation of Healthcare Organizations.

●**Board-certified doctors.** At least 70% of staff doctors should be board certified.

●**Salaried "chiefs."** The chief of each medical department (medicine, surgery, pediatrics, etc.) should be paid for extra time spent overseeing the department.

●**Registered nurses.** At least 60% of the nursing staff should be RNs.

●**Well-maintained facilities.** Unclean and/or poorly maintained facilities may pose health and safety hazards.

●**Up-to-date equipment.** The best hospitals have the latest MRI machines, surgical lasers, mammography equipment, etc.

Hospital Rankings

Jesse Green, PhD, senior director, clinical evaluation and outcomes research, New York University Medical Center, New York City.

How reliable are the hospital rankings published each year by *U.S. News & World Report?*

Not very. The survey is based on three basic criteria—the hospital's human, physical and financial resources…the type of care it offers…and patient outcomes. But there are no objective data on these measurements.

Example: To rank hospitals by type of care, board-certified physicians are simply asked to name the top five hospitals in their various specialties. As you might expect, the doctors tend to pick hospitals they know.

Result: A small group of prominent hospitals—the "usual suspects"—get high scores.

Bottom line: Instead of revealing which hospitals are best, the survey reveals which hospitals are best regarded.

Shrewder Hospital Stays

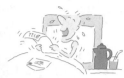

An Insider's Guide to Understanding Your Hospital Bill by Nancy Collins, RN, and Jan Sedoris, RN, hospital bill auditors. Eggman Publishing.

Keep a detailed log of treatments, drugs, services and supplies so you can later compare it with your itemized bill to ensure you're not being overcharged. If you're unable to maintain the log, ask a friend or family member to do it. *Also:* The log lets the staff know that you intend to keep informed of your situation.

Common mistakes found on hospital bills: Same supplies billed by more than one department, unrequested personal supplies—such as toothpaste—and charges for services not rendered, such as hours of physical therapy.

How to Win the Hospital Game

Charles Inlander, president of People's Medical Society, a patient advocate organization, 462 Walnut St., Allentown, PA 18102. He is author of several books, including *Take This Book to the Hospital with You: A Consumer Guide to Surviving Your Hospital Stay.* People's Medical Society.

Except for elective surgery, we usually cannot control when hospitalization for an ailment or operation will be necessary. But if a hospital stay is necessary, there are steps you can take to minimize the risk of injury and infection—and maximize your comfort and care.

BEFORE YOU GO

●**Be sure you need the treatment.** All procedures—and hospital stays—involve risk. Get a second opinion from another specialist before having any procedure. If the second doctor disagrees with the first doctor, get a third…or fourth opinion.

Example: If your first doctor urges you to have a bypass, but two or three other cardiac specialists feel your condition can be treated effectively with medication and diet, you would probably be wise to accept the recommendation of the majority.

●**Ask your surgeon how many such procedures he/she performs each year.** An adequate number depends on the procedure.

Example: If you need a bypass, look for a surgeon who has done 100 bypass operations within the last year.

●**Ask the doctor what his surgical success rate is.** Ask him how that compares with national figures for the same procedure. And confirm this with the medical director of the hospital.

●**Make sure the hospital your doctor chooses is the best one for your condition.** Different types of hospitals do different types of procedures well.

In general, local community hospitals are fine for uncomplicated procedures such as gallbladder removals, births, hysterectomies, etc.

But for a more serious procedure—such as open-heart surgery or a transplant—you're better off at a hospital that is affiliated with a major university *and* that has top specialists with extensive experience in the type of medical care you require.

●**Have all your preoperative tests done as an outpatient prior to admission**—preferably several days in advance. You don't want to be admitted to the hospital only to discover that a blood test or an X ray indicates your surgery should be postponed. This unnecessarily prolongs your hospital stay, which would also increase your costs.

●**Meet with your anesthesiologist or nurse-anesthetist *before* you are admitted.** Give him a list of all the prescription and over-the-counter drugs you are taking. Tell him about any medical conditions you may have.

IN THE HOSPITAL

●**Cut needless hospital costs by bringing everything you require**—including tissues, hand and body lotions, vitamins and medications for chronic conditions. Make sure these items do not appear on your bill.

If possible, have a friend or relative visit you each day for companionship and to speak up for you if you are not able to. Studies show that patients who ask the most questions—or who have family members who ask questions —get better care and have better outcomes than those who don't.

●**Understand that you can say *no* to anything.** One of your most important rights as a patient is your right to refuse services and treatment you don't want or understand.

Example: If you are getting a good night's rest without taking a sleeping pill, you can refuse the sedatives that are routinely administered to patients.

●**Question all tests.** Patients are sometimes given routine tests that are unnecessary, such as X rays or blood tests—or tests that are meant for other patients.

Key: Ask your doctor to tell you about every test in advance. If you were not advised of a test, ask the person who was sent to administer it whether your doctor ordered it…why the test is being done…and what the risks are.

●**Reduce your risk of medication mishaps.** Ask your doctor to show you the drugs he is prescribing for you while you're in the hospital. Note the shapes, colors and sizes.

If a nurse tries to give you an unfamiliar pill or liquid, refuse to take it until your doctor has been contacted and has identified and approved the medication.

Also ask your doctor what each pill is for and how often it should be administered. Keep a list so you don't forget.

●**Curb your risk of infection** by politely asking everyone who touches you—doctors, nurses, technicians—to wash their hands in the sink in your room. Unwashed hands are the leading cause of infections in hospitals, since doctors and nurses commonly move from room to room carrying germs.

If you must receive fluids intravenously, ask that the IV bag be mixed by the pharmacy staff —not by a nurse or technician. IV bags that are opened by nurses or technicians have higher risks of being contaminated with microorganisms circulating in the hospital.

●**Insist that your bathroom be cleaned and disinfected daily,** especially if you share a room.

NEGOTIATE YOUR RIGHTS

●**Ask the staff to rearrange their schedules to fit your needs.** If your doctor wants blood taken every eight hours, ask the technicians to draw your blood at 11 p.m., when you are just going to sleep, and again at 7 a.m., when you wake up, rather than at 8 p.m. and 4 a.m.

If the housekeeping staff routinely cleans your room at 2 a.m.—this is not uncommon—ask that they come back between 7 a.m. and 9 p.m.

●**If you don't want to be disturbed by interns and medical students** marching into your room during their rounds, tell the nurse or a patient representative (a hospital employee who acts as an arbitrator between you and the hospital) to note your wishes on your chart.

●**If your medication does not sufficiently control discomfort,** ask a nurse to call your physician and get approval to increase your medication.

Also helpful: Ask about less expensive, alternative methods of pain control that may be available at the hospital, including acupuncture, relaxation techniques and biofeedback.

How to Survive a Hospital Stay

Charles Inlander, president of People's Medical Society, a patient advocate organization, 462 Walnut St., Allentown, PA 18102. He is author of several books, including *Take This Book to the Hospital with You: A Consumer Guide to Surviving Your Hospital Stay.* People's Medical Society.

Some US hospitals are among the best in the world. Others are very, very good. But that doesn't mean that they are risk-free.

Better ways: You can greatly reduce the chance that something will go wrong in a hospital. To get special attention from doctors and nurses, take a few straightforward precautions and make use of inside information about the way hospitals operate. *Survival tactics...*

INFECTION SAFEGUARDS

Ten percent of hospital patients contract an infection after being admitted, adding $4,000 to $10,000 to a typical bill.

Examples: About 300,000 patients a year contract pneumonia in US hospitals. Other common hospital infections attack the urinary and respiratory systems. Staph infections are also a big problem.

Chief reason: Hospitals house a high percentage of infected people, many of whom have weakened immune systems. *Precautions:*

●**Make sure that all hospital staff members wash their hands before they touch you.** Don't be afraid to ask. It's your right.

●**Also ask personnel to put on a fresh pair of gloves** before touching you.

●**If you have a catheter, insist that hospital personnel monitor it at least three or four times a day.** A faulty catheter is an open door to infection.

THE TEAM APPROACH

Since you probably won't be at your most alert during a hospital stay, ask friends to help you monitor the treatment you receive.

Best: Ask three or more friends to stay with you in around-the-clock shifts.

Their very presence will help keep doctors and nurses on their toes, increasing chances that you'll receive above-average attention.

Myth: Guests are allowed to see you only during visiting hours.

Reality: Hospitals *hope* patients believe this, but visitors are *legally* allowed to see you at any time of day as long as they don't interfere with your treatment or that of any other patient in the room.

If your hospital stay is for more than a couple of days, consider making it more pleasant by decorating your room with some pictures from home or other familiar objects.

Leave valuables home. Many people have access to your room, so there's high risk of theft.

ATTENTION TO MEDICATION

With hundreds of patients receiving multiple medications each day, there's a great likelihood of a mistake in the type of medication you're given, in its dosage or in the frequency that it's administered.

The average error rate is 2% to 3%, meaning that in a 300-bed hospital there can be six medication errors an hour. *Precautions:*

●**Each time you receive medicine,** check to see if it's the same type you got on the last occasion. If it isn't, insist that hospital personnel check and double-check their instructions.

181

●**Similarly, ask staff members to justify any change** in the frequency of medication that you might notice.

●**Ask your doctor if the food you're served will have an adverse effect on your medication.** If it will, have him/her arrange for the appropriate diet.

REJECT THE UNKNOWN

If you don't understand a procedure or treatment, don't permit it until you *do*. Most hospitals will send in senior staff members to give you a proper explanation.

Myth: The release form you sign on entering a hospital means that you give up virtually all your rights.

Reality: You give up no rights whatsoever. You can accept or reject any type of treatment as well as any doctor who's assigned to you.

Exception: In life-or-death emergencies, hospitals are obligated to give you the appropriate treatment.

Above all, if you suspect that a doctor, nurse or other staff member is incompetent or negligent, call it to the attention of hospital authorities.

If hospital administrators don't correct the situation, ask for advice from an attorney who specializes in malpractice. If necessary, change doctors or even hospitals.

Many patients don't realize that they have the right to fire their doctor at any time and to leave the hospital whenever they wish.

SURGICAL SAFEGUARDS

If in the hospital for surgery…

●**Make sure that everyone involved in your surgery knows precisely what it's all about.** If you're having a cataract removed from your right eye, for instance, remind nurses, attendants, the anesthesiologist and the surgeon exactly which eye is to be operated on.

Some patients even use a marker to highlight the correct body part with an arrow or a circle. The measure might sound extreme, but it doesn't hurt to play it safe.

●**Choose a surgeon who frequently performs the operation.**

Rule of thumb: About 100 coronary bypasses a year and a higher frequency for more common operations, such as appendectomies. This is no guarantee of getting a competent surgeon, but it's an easy way to weed out those who lack experience.

●**Meet with your anesthesiologist before the operation.** The meeting alone can help you get better treatment because it makes you stand out as a real person. You'll no longer be the "gall bladder in room 305" but a person whom the anesthesiologist knows by name.

At the meeting, ask the anesthesiologist how many times he has performed your type of procedure. If he is inexperienced, ask for another anesthesiologist. Also tell him about all your medical conditions, including allergies —they can have an effect on anesthesia.

PURSUING DISPUTES

Not every mistake in a hospital is reason for a lawsuit. But if the error causes serious damage and you suspect negligence or (in rare cases) intent, check with an attorney.

Retain a lawyer who does nothing but malpractice work. Ask for recommendations from your regular attorney, the local bar association or from the Association of Trial Lawyers of America (202-965-3500).

Reputable malpractice attorneys can assess your chances of a successful lawsuit.

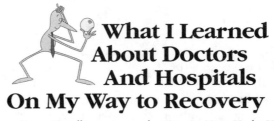

What I Learned About Doctors And Hospitals On My Way to Recovery

Evan Handler, actor and writer in New York. He is author of *Time on Fire: My Comedy of Terrors*. Little, Brown & Co.

By the time I was 24 years old, I had already played leading roles in five Broadway productions and three major movies. Then in 1985, just as I was up for a part in a film with Dustin Hoffman and Warren Beatty, I was diagnosed with leukemia…and told that my chances for survival were slim.

For the next five years, I learned a great deal about hospitals and doctors. I was in and out of four hospitals, and I saw more than 100 doctors as I underwent repeated courses of chemotherapy and a bone-marrow transplant.

Now I'm 35 years old and have been considered cured of the disease for more than seven years. I like to believe that part of the reason for my medical success was my intense curiosity and assertiveness during my treatment.

Here's what I learned about the medical system—and what anyone can do to ensure the best possible care for any serious illness...

●**Fight medical mediocrity and carelessness.** Someone dealing with a health crisis hopes to have a kindly doctor, like the ones shown on TV. But reality rarely lives up to that expectation.

Hospitals are large bureaucracies that are set up to care efficiently for many patients. Unfortunately, most are not designed to help individual patients flourish. The result is that any departure from conformity is often discouraged by administrators, doctors and staff—even when the standard procedure could *put your health at risk.*

Example: During my hospitalization, I had serious adverse reactions to several drugs routinely prescribed, including medications to combat the dangerous side effects of chemotherapy. So my doctors prescribed other drugs. Though this fact appeared on my bedside medical chart, *it was overlooked.* When nurses brought the standard medications to my room, I would have to remind them to check my chart—and request one of the alternative drugs that I could tolerate.

This meant delays while a doctor was summoned to write a new order...the pharmacy filled the prescription...and new tests were run. More than once, I was yelled at by nurses for the "trouble" I was causing—by insisting on medication that wouldn't make me sicker.

Don't be intimidated. It isn't easy to stand up for yourself when you're sick, vulnerable and dependent on others, so get support wherever you can.

When I was too weak to challenge the nurses' errors, my girlfriend did it for me. My refusal to conform may have made me unpopular—but it helped me survive.

●**If you have the time, it pays to shop for a doctor and a hospital.** My treatment began at one of the country's most renowned cancer centers. Yet I encountered conditions there that appalled me—ranging from a chronic shortage of bed linens to repeated examples of staff arrogance and insensitivity toward patients. There were even technicians who overlooked safe hygiene practices, such as properly sterilizing the catheters inserted into my body.

It doesn't have to be this way, as I realized only after visiting other, equally respected cancer centers. Many hospitals discourage comparison shopping—yet it's your right as a medical consumer to compare institutions and choose one you believe is right for you.

Self-defense: Get lists of medical centers and doctors from hotlines that specialize in your illness. Seek recommendations from everyone you know, especially people who work in the health care field. Call and visit medical centers. Interview doctors—dozens if necessary.

Consider not only the reputation of the person or facility, but the attitude with which you are treated as a potential patient. Are calls returned promptly? Are doctors and staff reluctant to answer questions...or are they generous with information?

Example: Be wary of any doctor or administrator who implies that, *Our facility is the only appropriate one for you. You would be foolish to accept any other. We are your only hope.*

Knowing what I now know, I would say to any doctor I was considering, *I want to work with someone who is willing to let me be a partner in the treatment. I don't want to be told what procedures may be "planned for" me. I want to know about the range of possible treatments, hear your recommendations and make my own decisions. I don't want interns and residents showing up every day to administer procedures and tests that I haven't been informed about.*

Look for the doctor who responds, *Of course —I wouldn't dream of anything else*—rather than the one who sputters...won't look you in the eye...or replies defensively, *Look, do you want to get well or not?*

●**Get the information you need about your illness and treatment.** The more you know about your condition and the treatment options, the easier it is to stand up for your rights.

While having faith in your doctor is important, you must always assume that there are other effective ways of dealing with your problem. You must be assertive.

Since accessibility to information about your illness is rare to nonexistent at most hospitals, it's up to you to do the research.

Strategy: Look for alternative treatments and medications by calling hotlines that specialize in your illness. Visit medical libraries and read journal articles yourself—or have a family member or friend do it for you. Call or visit a number of major medical centers known to treat your condition. You never know when you might discover information with which your doctor is not yet familiar.

There are also many medical professionals out there who would be willing to discuss options with you—even though they aren't personally treating you. Keep calling until you find them.

● **Choose your words carefully at hospitals.**
Midway through my treatment at the hospital, I decided to "fire" the cancer specialist with whom I had been working—and request another doctor. I didn't feel he was treating me with the respect and consideration I needed or allowing me to adequately participate in decision making. I also found his brusque manner and pessimistic outlook to be frightening and depressing.

Many patients don't realize that they have the right to change doctors—even when they're already in the hospital. The usual procedure is to make an appointment for a consultation with another doctor and explain to the new doctor that you are considering changing physicians. Then continue this approach while interviewing doctors until you find one with whom you feel most comfortable.

Important: When making the request, avoid specific criticisms about your first doctor. Instead, stick to the message, *We have trouble communicating.* Otherwise, you run the risk of creating a "political" mess that could affect your care, since most doctors are highly collegial and easily offended in this situation.

● **Explore alternative treatments.** I wouldn't recommend that people force themselves to try methods with which they're uncomfortable. But I'm glad I explored a variety of nontraditional therapies, from visualization and meditation to hypnotherapy and psychic healing.

I entered into this investigation in a receptive frame of mind—coupled with a healthy dose of skepticism. I viewed these techniques as tools to maximize my potential to heal, not as rigid formulas that guaranteed certain results.

To the rescue: With the help of family and friends, I sought out stories of unexpected healings. I read news accounts and books about alternative therapies, talked to people who had successful recoveries, attended a week-long retreat on guided imagery and other ways of coping with illness. I even had friends of friends recommend psychic healers.

I'm still a skeptic about many of these alternative therapies, but I believe that stimulating my emotions helped me cope with stress, which in turn affected my vulnerability to illness …and my ability to heal.

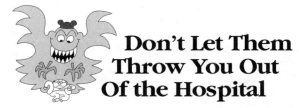

Don't Let Them Throw You Out Of the Hospital

Timothy McCall, MD, a Boston internist, author of *Examining Your Doctor: A Patient's Guide to Avoiding Harmful Medical Care.* Citadel Press. He is a regular commentator on the public radio program Marketplace, and can be found on the Web at *www.drmccall.com.*

In an effort to boost their bottom lines, HMOs and other managed-care plans are dramatically reducing the lengths of their patients' hospital stays. To remain competitive, many traditional insurers are adopting similar tactics.

From bypass surgery to cancer chemotherapy, the length of hospital stays has shortened dramatically. For bypasses, stays of two weeks were common just a few years ago. Now it's down to four days. Women having hysterectomies get as few as two days in the hospital.

This isn't all bad. There's good scientific evidence that hospital stays were *too long* in the past. Under the old system, doctors and hospitals had a financial incentive to keep patients hospitalized as long as possible. Under the new world of managed care, doctors can be penalized—or even fired—if their patients stay longer than the HMO deems necessary.

Unfortunately, the logic used by HMOs seems to be, "If cutting a little was good, then cutting more is better." Despite having already made dramatic reductions, HMOs continue to trim hospital stays.

Take the case of childbirth—the leading cause of hospitalization. In 1970, women having normal deliveries stayed an average of four days. By 1992, it was two days. A few years later, however, some California plans were hustling mothers out of the hospital after only eight hours.

In response, laws were passed mandating that insurers pay for two-day stays for normal deliveries and four days for C-sections. Unfortunately, these laws don't help people who are hospitalized for other reasons.

How can you prevent your loved ones or yourself from being thrown out of the hospital too early? *Be assertive.* Keep in mind that in calculating when to send you home, managed-care plans rely on best-case scenarios. Be prepared to explain why your case may not fit that definition.

If your specified number of days is up but you don't feel well enough to go home, tell your doctor (or have a family member do so for you). Though they don't always tell their patients, doctors have the ability to challenge the discharge decisions of insurance companies and hospital "utilization reviewers." If necessary, make your case to the hospital ombudsman.

The major determinant of whether it's okay to go home early is your medical condition. Any fever should be resolved. You should be able to take food by mouth. You shouldn't be so confused or lightheaded that you risk falling when you walk to the bathroom. If you've had surgery, you should be able to urinate on your own, and your pain must be controllable with oral medications.

The other important determinant is the situation at home. Is the environment conducive to healing? Will someone be there to take care of you? Will your insurer arrange for visiting nurses or other home care? Is there adequate backup if a problem arises? If these conditions aren't met, alert your doctor and insurance company.

Many people prefer to recover at home—if it's feasible. The surroundings are familiar, and there's more privacy. And given the risk of catching infections or developing other complications in the hospital, it makes sense to be discharged as soon as you can.

But the decision should be based on what makes sense *medically*—not on the HMO's bottom line. If you feel you're being taken advantage of, speak up. Tell whoever is trying to discharge you before you're ready that you'll hold them personally responsible if something goes wrong.

Cold Rooms and Heart Attacks

Steven Frank, MD, associate professor of anesthesiology, Johns Hopkins University School of Medicine, Baltimore.

Cold operating rooms can trigger heart attacks in surgical patients. Operating rooms are often kept cool for surgeons, whose scrubs can get hot.

Trap: The mix of anesthetic, low temperatures, cool intravenous (IV) fluids and an open incision can lower the patient's body temperature. In a study, patients given heated IV fluids and warmed with a forced-air heater suffered cardiac complications only 1% of the time. Patients who got the usual treatment suffered such complications 6% of the time.

Self-defense: Ask to be kept warm during surgery.

Common Hospital Billing Errors

John Connolly, EdD, former president, New York Medical College, Valhalla, and author of *How to Find the Best Doctors, Hospitals, HMOs for You and Your Family*. Castle Connolly Medical Ltd.

Up to 95% of hospital bills contain errors, and most of these errors favor the hospital. *Watch out for…*

•**Incorrect billing codes.** There are more than 7,000 five-digit codes for diagnostic tests, surgical procedures, etc. Don't trust the number. Look for the description of each procedure.

•**Duplicate billings.** These occur frequently with urine tests and other common tests.

•**Redundant or shoddy testing.** You should not pay for unclear X rays, blood tests ruined because of inadequate samples or any test that has to be repeated because of a mistake by the hospital lab.

•**Unauthorized charges.** Hospitals sometimes charge your credit card without your approval. Always insist on advance approval. Don't pay for anything you didn't approve— even if you received the treatment.

•**Phantom charges.** Hospitals often charge for procedures that—while not performed in *your* case—are usually a routine part of patient care. Watch out for charges for tests that were ordered and then canceled.

•**Unrequested items.** Often, these carry confusing names so they'll slip by uncontested. A $15 "thermal therapy kit" may be a bag of ice cubes. A $5 "urinal" may be a plastic cup.

•**Unbundling.** Routine procedures are sometimes billed separately, and the sum of these parts is often greater than the whole.

•**Arithmetic errors.** They may be honest mistakes, but the hospital won't correct them unless you bring them to its attention. Don't pay the bill immediately upon your discharge from the hospital. Take it home and look it over carefully.

The Truth About Hospitals and Medication Mistakes

Charles Inlander, president of People's Medical Society, a patient advocate organization, 462 Walnut St., Allentown, PA 18102. He is author of several books, including *Take This Book to the Hospital with You: A Consumer Guide to Surviving Your Hospital Stay*. People's Medical Society.

Medication mistakes can average 50 an hour in a medium-sized hospital.

Self-defense: Before taking medication at a hospital or having an IV started or changed, ask whether the doctor ordered it—and repeat your name to make sure that it is for you. If a loved one is unable to ask these questions—and friends or relatives aren't available 24 hours a day—pay for an attendant to do it. *Also:* If medication looks different or arrives at a different time, ask to see the doctor's order for the change.

Shorter Recovery Time

James A. Kulik, PhD, professor of psychology, University of California, San Diego. His study of 84 male bypass patients was published in the *Journal of Personality and Social Psychology*, 750 First St. NE, Washington, DC 20002.

Surgical patients go home faster when they're assigned to a semiprivate room.

Study: Bypass surgery patients were discharged an average of two days sooner when— before surgery—they shared a room with a postoperative bypass patient. This is compared with patients who had private rooms or who roomed with someone awaiting surgery.

Theory: Patients get better faster when they can talk with someone who has gone through the same experience.

Helpful: If you don't have a "post-op" roommate, seek out other patients in the hospital who have recently undergone the same surgical procedure.

Questions to Ask If Considering Heart Surgery

Julian Whitaker, MD, a trained surgeon who founded and runs the Whitaker Wellness Institute, which explores alternatives to surgery. Dr. Whitaker is author of *Is Heart Surgery Necessary? What Your Doctor Won't Tell You.* Regnery Publishing, Inc.

As far as I'm concerned, *90% of all heart surgery is unnecessary.* I recommend surgery to only 1% to 2% of patients with heart disease.

Opting for heart surgery isn't like taking vitamin C when you feel a cold coming on. You can't just "give it a try" and see what happens. You may sustain an enormous amount of unnecessary damage.

If heart surgery does not help you, it will harm you. Heart surgery hurts a lot, costs a lot and will weaken you for a long time.

Reality: Even necessary surgery can often be postponed while you try alternative therapies. The overwhelming majority of patients who are advised to undergo bypass surgery can afford to wait and are better off if they do.

Here are key questions that you should ask your doctor about heart surgery...and the answers I would give to my patients.

Why are you recommending surgery? Any of the following situations is a good reason for bypass surgery...

●**Significant blockage in the left main coronary artery.** Since this artery is only one inch long, blockage can cut off the blood supply to the entire left side of the heart.

●**Significant blockage in three or more arteries,** *plus* decreased left ventricular function (how well the left ventricle of the heart is working), *plus* an ejection fraction (percentage of blood ejected from the heart with each heartbeat) of less than 50%.

●**Incapacitating chest pain** that won't respond to medication and that limits your activities.

There are few other justifications for bypass surgery.

What is my real statistical risk of death or other serious harm (including new arterial blockages) from the surgery itself? How does that risk compare with the risks of other therapies? Heart surgery can kill you... whether you need the surgery or not. Ask your doctor to show you the results of the controlled trials in the US that are closest to your own situation.

In the two largest heart surgery studies to date, almost no group did better after surgery than groups treated in alternative ways. Furthermore, the death rate with nonsurgical techniques was lower.

What is the actual death rate? The death rate for bypass surgery varies in the US from 0% to 52%, depending on the hospital. The national average is 3% to 5%. After age 65, there is a *one in three* chance of heart attack, coma, stroke, kidney failure...or death.

Even the far-too-common procedure of angioplasty—in which a catheter is inserted into an artery in the groin and "snaked" through blockages—has a 2% to 4% death rate and leads to emergency bypass surgery 5% of the time.

How long will the effects of my surgery last? Heart surgery isn't always effective forever. Arteries treated with angioplasty reclose at a rate of 35% within six months. For about 70% of bypass patients, chest pain (angina) returns within five years.

Is there any way I can avoid surgery? If your doctor flatly says *no,* beware. Alternative options are *always* worth at least a discussion.

Obtain a copy of a groundbreaking article by Thomas B. Graboys, MD, a cardiologist on the staff of Harvard Medical School (*Journal of the American Medical Association* 1987, 258: 1611–1614). Take Dr. Graboys's five-step checklist to your doctor to discuss whether you meet the criteria defined by this group of researchers, called the Lown Group (from the Lown Cardiovascular Center in Boston).

If all of the following apply to you, you probably *don't* need surgery...

●**Your left ventricle isn't impaired or damaged** and your ejection fraction is more than 50%.

• **Your angina may be caused by something that could be remedied without surgery.**

• **An extensive treadmill exercise stress test doesn't show exercise-induced arrhythmias.**

• **It is possible to institute a nonsurgical therapy program.**

• **Your left main coronary artery is not blocked by more than 70%.**

What steps can I take to reduce my need for heart surgery? I call these measures the four pillars of therapy for reversing heart disease without surgery...

• **Diet.** Specialize in foods that are very low in fat. Fat should account for no more than 15% of your total daily calorie intake. This may be the most important step you can take. You'll lose weight, too, decreasing the stress on your heart.

• **Nutritional supplements.** Increase the amount of magnesium and potassium in your diet.

With your doctor's permission, take up to 1,000 milligrams of magnesium gluconate in pill form every day. Magnesium corrects heart irregularities, reduces cholesterol and helps control blood pressure. *Caution:* Dangerous for people with kidney failure.

Food sources of magnesium: Fresh fruits, deep green leafy vegetables, nuts, brown rice.

When potassium is depleted, the ratio of sodium to potassium rises—raising blood pressure. You can get enough potassium from foods. *Good sources:* Bananas, dried beans, lentils, oranges, tangerines.

• **Progressive exercise.** Exercise 20 minutes a day, three times a week. Little by little, increase the difficulty and the time spent. You'll lower your blood pressure, thin your blood and purge excess sodium by sweating. Ask your doctor to refer you to an exercise professional who can tailor a regimen to your situation.

• **Chelation therapy.** To reduce or eliminate angina pain, consider chelation therapy, which rids the body of harmful poisons. In each of 20 to 30 treatments—costing about $100 each—a synthetic protein called EDTA (ethylene diamine tetracidic acid) is administered intravenously. EDTA binds to the ions of toxic heavy metals and helps them dissolve in the blood.

Why this helps: Copper and iron are partially responsible for converting cholesterol into a damaging substance. Lead and mercury interfere with normal enzyme functions that help prevent plaque formation.

Many mainstream cardiologists disapprove of chelation therapy, an admittedly nontraditional technique. To explore the idea, contact the American College for Advancement in Medicine, 23121 Verdugo Dr., Suite 204, Laguna Hills, CA 92653, 949-583-7666 or 800-532-3688, *www.acam.org.*

Maybe I'm one of the small percentage who really does need heart surgery. How can I tell? People who really need surgery know they are very ill. They may have had a few heart attacks. Their symptoms may include severe chest pain that comes and goes, frequent shortness of breath, difficulty climbing stairs without resting, swollen feet and a host of other related warning signs.

I'd like a second opinion. Where can I get one? *Always* get a second opinion about proposed surgery, whether your health insurance requires it or not.

Don't consult a surgeon who is your doctor's colleague. Surgeons who operate all day tend to think cutting is a good idea. Instead, ask the American College for Advancement in Medicine or another reputable alternative medical organization for the name of a physician in your area who practices preventive medicine with a specialty in cardiac disease.

How to Prepare for Outpatient Surgery

Charles Inlander, president of People's Medical Society, a patient advocate organization, 462 Walnut St., Allentown, PA 18102. He is author of several books, including *Take This Book to the Hospital with You: A Consumer Guide to Surviving Your Hospital Stay.* People's Medical Society.

The night before outpatient surgery, note any illness and report it to your doctor. He/she may want to postpone the procedure.

• **Do not eat or drink anything after midnight** unless your doctor approves.

• **Wear comfortable clothes** to the hospital.

- **Do not wear makeup,** which makes it harder for anesthetists to monitor changes in skin tone.

- **Bring any medications you use** so the anesthetist and the surgeon know exactly what you are taking.

- **Arrange for transportation after the surgery** and for help at home for as long as your doctor recommends it.

Secrets of Rapid Healing After Surgery

Mehmet C. Oz, MD, a heart surgeon and cofounder and executive director of the Complementary Care Center at Columbia–Presbyterian Medical Center, New York.

A top-flight surgeon may be the most important ingredient for successful surgery, but the surgeon's skill is just one of many factors that affect the speed and ease with which a patient recovers after an operation. *To speed healing:*

- **Approach surgery as if it were an athletic contest.** The surgeon is your teammate. Make sure he/she is a member of the American College of Surgeons (312-202-5000)...and that he answers "yes" to these questions...

- **Do you encourage guest visits after surgery?**

- **Is it okay to wear headphones during surgery?**

- **Can my family bring in home-cooked meals?**

- **Would you mind if a massage therapist came in after the operation?**

- **Heed the surgeon's instructions about diet and medication.** Ask him about taking a daily vitamin supplement for seven to 14 days before an operation. This supplement should contain beta-carotene (up to 25,000 international units)...and vitamin C (2 to 3 grams).

For heart patients, I also recommend 1g a day of magnesium.

Caution: Stop taking vitamin E at least one week before surgery. It can cause the blood to thin.

- **Exercise regularly in the weeks prior to surgery.** I do *not* recommend vigorous exercise for someone about to undergo heart surgery. But gentle exercises like yoga or walking bring benefits without dangerously elevating the heart rate.

- **Lean on your loved ones.** Even before surgery, you may find it comforting to have family members present when treatment options are discussed.

Some family members prefer not to wait at the hospital during surgery. But they can find out ahead of time when you are expected to wake up—and plan to be there at that time.

- **Avoid hospital food, if possible.** When I'm ill, I don't want hospital food. I want my wife's cooking. Eating familiar food makes me feel better. When it's appropriate, I urge my patients to have some home-cooked meals brought in to the hospital.

Caution: Be sure home-cooked food does not violate any of your dietary restrictions.

- **Listen to tapes of soothing music during surgery.** Many surgical patients have at least some awareness even when under general anesthesia. The sound of surgical instruments at work or chitchat among the surgical team might be distressing—even though patients may not recall this distress afterward.

When I operate, I offer my patients tapes of soothing music to listen to through headphones...or let them bring in their own favorite music.

- **If you smoke, quit.** At the very least, stop smoking two weeks before surgery.

- **Practice stress management.** Several tried-and-true stress reducers can be adapted for use in the hospital...

- **Yoga.** Most patients can practice gentle yoga exercises within a few days after surgery. Yoga boosts strength and improves range of motion...and allows you to transcend your worries for a while.

- **Massage.** Some hospitals have massage therapists on staff. Others allow patients to make their own arrangements for in-room massage.

- **Hypnosis.** Self-hypnosis reduces not only presurgery anxiety but also postsurgical pain.

Ask your doctor or a hospital social worker to recommend a psychologist who is trained in hypnosis or other relaxation techniques.

Heart Surgery Recovery Fact

Thomas E. Oxman, MD, director of geriatric psychiatry, Dartmouth Medical School, Lebanon, NH.

Social support and religion help people survive heart surgery. Among people who had elective open-heart surgery, the risk of dying was four times greater for patients who did not participate in social groups, and three times greater for those without strong religious convictions. Patients with *neither* social support nor strong religious beliefs were 14 times more likely to die within six months of surgery as patients who had both.

Common Procedure May Be Unsafe

Alfred F. Connors, Jr., MD, director, Health Services Research and Outcomes Evaluation, University of Virginia School of Medicine, Charlottesville. His study of 5,700 critically ill patients was published in *The Journal of the American Medical Association*, 515 N. State St., Chicago 60610.

Called *pulmonary artery catheterization*, the procedure is used to diagnose and treat heart failure and other critical illnesses. It involves threading a catheter through a vein in the neck and into the heart.

Finding: Patients who underwent the procedure had a higher death rate and longer hospital stays than those who didn't receive it.

Self-defense: Before undergoing the procedure, patients should discuss its pros and cons with a doctor.

Shop Around First

Donald Palmisano, MD, JD, clinical professor of surgery and medical jurisprudence, Tulane University School of Medicine, New Orleans.

Shopping around for a hospital can result in better care and save you money on procedures that aren't covered or are only partially covered by insurance. Many doctors have admitting privileges at two or more hospitals. You can simply ask each hospital for a price estimate. If you are on a managed care plan and want to enter a hospital that is not in the plan, ask your doctor if he/she can help you negotiate for the hospital to accept whatever the managed care plan will pay. Because of increasing competition, some hospitals will agree.

Heel Surgery Danger

G. Andrew Murphy, MD, instructor of orthopedics, University of Tennessee, Memphis.

Surgery for chronic heel pain can cause fallen arches and a feeling of weakness in the foot. Called *plantar fascia release*, the operation involves cutting a band of tissue at the bottom of the heel.

Better: A conservative approach involving painkillers, stretching and, if necessary, injections of cortisone. Surgery should be considered only if the pain persists for more than a year.

Transfusion Trap

Karen Shoos Lipton, JD, CEO, American Association of Blood Banks, 8101 Glenbrook Rd., Bethesda, MD 20814.

Patients who donate blood for their own use during surgery—a process called *autologous donation*—don't always get to use it.

Self-defense: Your doctor should notify the hospital's transfusion service upon your admission to the hospital. Just prior to transfusion, a recheck of the patient's blood type is necessary.

Anesthesia and Operations

Norig Ellison, MD, professor of anesthesia, University of Pennsylvania School of Medicine, Philadelphia.

Many operations can be done with local or regional anesthesia. These include cesarean section, knee repair, appendectomy, hysterectomy and many other procedures that used to require general anesthesia.

Benefit: Local or regional anesthesia—in which the patient remains awake—usually offers the best opportunity for a swift, uneventful recovery.

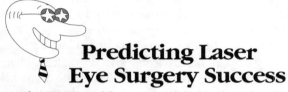

Predicting Laser Eye Surgery Success

Milton M. Hom, OD, an optometrist in private practice in Azusa, California.

Special contact lenses can help people who are considering vision-correcting laser eye surgery determine *in advance* whether the procedure will work for them. *Background:* Many ophthalmologists now use a 10-minute outpatient surgical procedure known as *laser in-situ keratomileusis* (LASIK) to correct aging-related vision trouble (presbyopia). Typically, LASIK is used to correct near vision in one eye, distance vision in the other. Some people can adapt to the resulting disparity between the eyes. Others can't. But by spending seven to 14 days wearing contacts that simulate the effects of LASIK, people can easily determine whether they would be able to adapt. The contacts can be fitted by an optometrist.

LASIK Surgery Warning

R. Doyle Stulting, MD, professor of ophthalmology at Emory University in Atlanta.

LASIK surgery to correct nearsightedness requires a highly experienced eye surgeon to minimize complications. LASIK corrects nearsightedness by using a laser beam to remove a thin layer of tissue from the cornea to flatten it. A study of 574 patients who had LASIK found that complications occurred about 5% of the time, and serious vision loss occurred in three cases. Complications were more frequent when the operation was performed by inexperienced surgeons.

Endoscopy...Is Your Doctor Competent?

Paul Jowell, MD, attending physician of gastroenterology, Duke University Medical Center, Durham, NC.

For years, gastroenterologists considered themselves competent at performing a given endoscopic procedure as long as they had performed it at least 50 times.

Now: Research suggests that adequate skill is achieved only when they've done the procedure at least 180 times.

Self-defense: If a doctor recommends endoscopy, ask about his/her experience level before agreeing to undergo the procedure.

To Reduce Blood Transfusion Risk

Neil Blumberg, MD, director, transfusion medicine, Strong Memorial Hospital, Rochester, New York.

Ask your surgeon if you're a candidate for *autologous donation* and/or *bloodless surgery.* Autologous donation involves donating your own blood for later use. That virtually eliminates your risk for blood-borne infection. Bloodless surgery involves the use of lasers and drugs to control bleeding during surgery. Since you lose less blood, you're less likely to need a transfusion.

All About the Latest Fat-Removal Technique

William P. Coleman III, MD, clinical professor of dermatology, Tulane University School of Medicine, New Orleans.

Ultrasound liposuction gets rid of even stubborn fat deposits—especially in the abdomen and in men's breasts. Like ordinary liposuction, the technique involves "vacuuming" fat out of the body using a long, thin tube (cannula) inserted through the skin. But ultrasound liposuction uses sound waves to *liquefy* fat cells before removal. *Cost:* $1,500 to $5,000—about the same as regular liposuction.

The Major Hospital Hazards and How to Avoid Them

Sheldon Blau, MD, clinical professor of medicine at the State University of New York at Stony Brook. He is coauthor of *How to Get Out of the Hospital Alive: A Guide to Patient Power.* Macmillan.

Most people make an assumption when they check into a hospital. "I'm safe here," they think. "I can trust these people to take good care of me."

But mistakes do happen—sometimes with serious or even fatal consequences.

I've been a doctor for more than 35 years, but I didn't grasp just how dangerous hospitals can be until I was hospitalized for an angioplasty three years ago.

An artery ruptured during the procedure, and I had to have emergency open-heart surgery to repair it. Then I caught a nasty staph infection from an unsanitary catheter. To top it all off, I developed phlebitis in my arm from repeated needle sticks. The swelling took months to heal.

My experience was not unique. Something similar could happen to you. But you can protect yourself if you know what to watch out for…

●*Trap #1:* **Being mistaken for another patient.** This occurs more often than you might imagine. Once you get your room assignment, ask if another patient on the ward has a last name that's the same as or similar to your own. If so, ask to be moved to another ward. Such a request might raise a few eyebrows—but your life may be at stake.

As soon as you move into your room, post a sign with your name and room number directly over your bed. Ask a friend or family member to spend as much time with you as possible throughout your hospital stay—asking questions, insisting that you get proper care, etc.

Your "patient advocate" should make it clear that he/she expects to be consulted on all treatment decisions. During my hospital stay, my wife was at my side 24 hours a day. Her persistence saved my life.

If you're having surgery: It's not unheard of for surgeons to operate on the wrong side of the body, take out the wrong organ, etc. To avoid such errors, meet with your surgeon the night before surgery. Discuss the procedure in detail, including the exact body part being operated on.

For absolute safety: A few hours before surgery, use a felt-tip pen to write CUT HERE on the incision site.

●*Trap #2:* **Catching an infection.** One in five people catch some sort of infection while hospitalized. Each year, 80,000 patients die as a result of such *nosocomial* infections.

Biggest threats: Staph infections and pneumonia. Staph can be deadly, especially if you come down with one of the new antibiotic-resistant strains.

What underlies the high incidence of hospital infections in the US? Dirty hands and medical equipment are the usual culprits.

Only one out of four doctors consistently washes his/her hands between patients. An even smaller proportion wash their stethoscopes between patients. The American

Medical Association has issued a warning about "killer stethoscopes."

Self-defense: Wash your own hands frequently, and insist that all doctors and nurses wash their hands before touching you. Be polite, but don't worry about offending anyone.

Alert the staff immediately if your room seems dirty or if you run out of soap or paper towels.

Make sure that any equipment that comes into contact with your skin has been swabbed with alcohol (or covered with a fresh disposable plastic shield). This goes for stethoscopes, thermometers, otoscopes (used to check the ears), infusion pumps, hemodialysis equipment and urinary catheters.

Special danger: Intensive care units (ICUs). Because ICU beds are so close to one another, infection risk is far greater in an ICU than in a private or semiprivate room.

●***Trap #3:*** **Getting the wrong medication.** A nurse might inadvertently give you the wrong drug...or give you the right medicine at the wrong dose, wrong time or through the wrong route.

Each year, tens of thousands of hospital patients die as a result of such medication errors.

Errors account for 40% of all adverse drug reactions in US hospitals, according to a Harvard study.

Self-defense: Learn the names, dosages and correct administration route of any drugs prescribed for you. Check this information with the nurse each time you're given a medication.

Learn the dosing schedule, too. Nurses sometimes fall behind schedule—and have to be reminded.

If you're given a pill or liquid (or intravenous fluid) that differs from what you've been getting, double-check with the nurse before taking it.

Alert the nurse *at once* if you experience any untoward reaction to a drug—pain or a burning sensation, shortness of breath, dizziness, confusion, tightness in your chest, numbness or itching. If you have any allergies, be sure they're listed on your medical chart.

Helpful resource: *The Johns Hopkins Handbook of Drugs* (Random House).

●***Trap #4:*** **Being robbed or assaulted.** With all the hospital staffers, patients, family members, delivery people, etc., roaming the hospital, it's difficult for hospital security to keep track of everyone.

Especially dangerous: Emergency rooms (ERs). More than half of all hospital violence occurs in the ER. One in three ER patients is armed. One in four is on some kind of illicit drug.

If you're going to the ER, bring a companion. While there, don't talk to or stare at anyone who is tense, loud or belligerent. Quietly alert a security guard or desk attendant instead.

Hospital parking lots can be dangerous, too. If you feel nervous, ask a hospital security guard to escort you to and from your car.

If you're staying in a hospital room, inquire ahead of time about security arrangements. Before going to sleep, make sure that the bathroom light is on and that the nurse call button is within easy reach.

Safer Surgery

Karen Allen, PhD, research scientist, University of Buffalo, New York. Her study of 40 cataract surgery patients who had local anesthesia was presented at a meeting of the American Psychosomatic Society.

Operations go better when the patient is allowed to select the music played in the operating room. In a study, surgical patients who picked the playlist had lower heart rates and blood pressure than patients who were not allowed to pick the playlist.

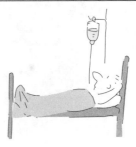

Best Hernia Surgery Option

Robert Kozol, MD, chief of surgery, Veterans Administration Medical Center, Detroit. His two-year study of 62 hernia patients was published in *Archives of Surgery*, 1411 E. 31 St., Oakland, CA 94602.

Old-fashioned hernia surgery may be better than the new laparoscopic (keyhole) surgery.

Pros of keyhole surgery: It requires only a tiny incision...it causes less pain...it permits faster recovery...and the surgeon can fix a bilateral (double) hernia in a single procedure.

Cons of keyhole surgery: It requires general anesthesia, while open-incision surgery allows local anesthesia...it's harder to perform than open-incision surgery...and it's more expensive.

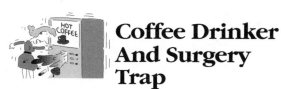

Coffee Drinker And Surgery Trap

Joseph Weber, MD, assistant professor of anesthesiology, Mayo Clinic, Scottsdale, AZ.

Coffee drinkers facing surgery can avoid postoperative headaches by having intravenous caffeine after surgery. Surgeons usually warn their patients to avoid coffee during the two hours prior to the operation. Consequently, these people are often experiencing caffeine-withdrawal headaches by the time they reach the recovery room.

Finding: Patients given intravenous caffeine after surgery had a lower risk for headache—10% versus 25% for those who didn't get caffeine.

Implication: Any coffee drinker scheduled for surgery should ask his/her doctor about postoperative intravenous caffeine.

Cataract Breakthrough

George Mintsioulis, MD, associate professor of ophthalmology, University of Ottawa Eye Institute, Ottawa, Canada.

A different type of cataract surgery makes for a faster recovery...reduces the risk of vision distortion...and improves eyesight right away instead of after the usual week to months.

Breakthrough: A *foldable* intraocular lens (IOL). Unlike conventional IOLs, which are made of a rigid plastic, the new lens can be slipped into place through an incision so small that no sutures are needed to close it. The patient generally does not even need an eye patch.

More information: Ask your ophthalmologist.

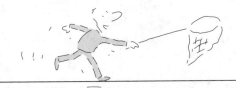

10

Health Secrets
For Men

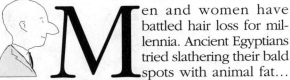

Hair Loss Prevention…
Replacement…Regrowth

David Orentreich, MD
Mount Sinai School of Medicine

Men and women have battled hair loss for millennia. Ancient Egyptians tried slathering their bald spots with animal fat… while Julius Caesar wore his famous laurel wreath low to hide a receding hairline.

These measures may sound silly to us now. But the methods tried since then—from prescription lotions to spray-on fake hair—aren't much better at growing hair.

Is there any truly effective way to stop hair loss? To find out, we spoke with hair specialist David Orentreich, MD…

●**What causes hair loss?** By age 50, hair loss affects more than 50% of men and 25% of women. Most of them have what's known as *androgenic alopecia.*

In men, this hereditary condition (also known as male pattern baldness) causes hair to recede from the forehead back to the crown. In women, it causes the hair to thin all over the head.

At the root of the problem—literally—are the male hormones *testosterone* and *dihydro-testosterone.* Present in both men and women, these androgens cause hair growth to "switch off."

●**What about other causes?** The second leading cause of hair loss is *alopecia areata.* This poorly understood autoimmune disorder inflames hair follicles and causes bald patches on the scalp—and sometimes on other parts of the body as well.

Hair loss can also be caused by thyroid trouble, pregnancy and other medical conditions that upset the balance of hormones in the body.

Some cases of hair loss are caused by "corn-rows" and other hairstyles that pull the hair too

David Orentreich, MD, assistant clinical professor of dermatology at Mount Sinai School of Medicine and a dermatologist in private practice, both in New York City.

tight. Such hairstyles cut off blood flow to the follicles, causing the hairline to recede.

●**Don't certain medications cause hair loss?** Yes. Some diuretics, antidepressants and cancer chemotherapy agents can cause temporary hair loss.

Sometimes even discontinuing birth-control pills causes sudden shedding of hair.

●**What's the best way to treat hair loss?** That depends on what's causing your hair loss. Sometimes all it takes is changing a prescription or hairstyle...or getting treatment for an underlying medical condition.

If the culprit is alopecia areata, injections of the anti-inflammatory drug *cortisone* often help.

A dermatologist simply injects tiny amounts of cortisone in a grid pattern on the scalp. This blocks the immune reaction underlying the hair loss, allowing hair to regrow.

If you're afraid of shots, cortisone lotion— 100 to 1,000 times more concentrated than what's sold over the counter—may work.

●**What about androgenic alopecia?** There is no cure for this form of baldness. Most of the time, however, aggressive treatment can keep the problem from getting worse.

I've learned that the hair loss drug *minoxidil* (Rogaine)—which boosts blood flow to the follicles—is not the miracle cure we had been hoping for.

Minoxidil lotion often works at first, but it soon loses its effectiveness. That's because poor blood flow to the follicles is only one piece of the puzzle.

The real problem is the presence of androgens. For that, you need an androgen-blocking drug. One such drug is *finasteride* (Proscar), a medication originally developed to treat prostate enlargement.

I've found that hair loss can often be stopped on a long-term basis by mixing minoxidil with finasteride and thyroid hormone or another drug that stimulates hair metabolism.

All the patient has to do is rub this three-drug "cocktail" into his/her scalp every day.

If a dermatologist has advised you to use minoxidil alone, ask about using it with these other drugs. Finasteride should not be used by men who are trying to father a child...or by women who are pregnant or trying to conceive.

●**What about growing new hair?** If hair loss is caught early enough, the three-drug cocktail may regrow enough hair that the problem is less noticeable.

This is especially true for women. Since their androgen levels are just 10% those of men, it's easier for finasteride to do its job.

When it comes to men who have been balding for more than 10 years or so, topical therapy is rarely enough. When my male patients tell me they want to regrow hair, I tell them that *oral* finasteride is their best bet.

Finasteride doesn't work in all cases, of course. When it does work, we still can't promise 100% regrowth. But since finasteride came on the market, I can do more for my patients now than ever before.

●**Are there any other options for regrowing hair?** You can always try hair transplants.

The basic hair-transplantation procedure was developed by my father, Norman Orentreich, MD, back in 1953. Although the surgery has been refined many times since then, the basic concept remains unchanged. We "harvest" healthy hairs from the back of the patient's head and transplant them to the bare areas up top or in front.

In the old days, the grafts were so large that they often left a sort of "clumpy" look. Now I use micro-grafts, which contain no more than two hairs each.

With micro-grafts, the appearance is so natural that after the transplant has grown in, the patient often can't tell exactly where it was. Several two- to four-hour procedures are required. *Cost:* $1,000 to $6,000 per procedure.

●**What about hair weaves?** A hair weave is really just a wig that's been sewn into your hair. Weaves often look good initially, but they are hard to maintain.

A transplant needs no special care. But a weave requires regular cleaning and tightening. That means frequent visits to the salon that installed the weave.

Make the Most of Less Hair

Anthony Palladino, barbershop owner, Beverly Hills, CA.

Have your barber help find a good style for you.

Surprising: If hair is cut shorter, it usually seems fuller. An all-around short cut makes hair look more evenly placed even if it is concentrated in the back and on the sides.

Other ideas: For a receding hairline, trim the forward part short while letting hair at your temples grow longer. For a bald spot, keep the back short and grow top-of-head hair long to cover the spot.

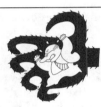

Domineering Men Die Sooner

Michael Babyak, PhD, researcher at Duke University Medical Center, Durham, NC, who conducted a study of 750 men over 22 years.

Men who exhibited such vocal characteristics as attempting to interrupt conversations and making quick responses were 60% more likely to die sooner than men who spoke quietly and were more laid back.

Theory: Socially dominating men need to be in control at all times. This increases levels of stress hormones in the blood, which can, over time, damage the heart and immune system.

Men and Their Metabolism

Susan Roberts, PhD, researcher at the Jean Mayer–USDA Human Nutrition Research Center on Aging at Tufts University, Boston.

As men age, their metabolism becomes less "flexible." A study comparing men in their 20s with those in their 60s and 70s found that when the men were fed an extra 1,000 calories a day, members of the younger group were able to naturally burn up some of the extra food, while the older group naturally burned up less and gained more weight. The research suggested that exercise may help older men burn off extra calories directly—and also indirectly—by improving the body's capability to speed up its metabolism.

Potbelly Risk

Eric B. Rimm, ScD, assistant professor of nutrition and epidemiology, Harvard School of Public Health, Boston. His five-year study of 28,643 men 40 to 75 years of age was published in the *American Journal of Epidemiology*, 111 Market Pl., Baltimore 21202.

Men with potbellies face a heightened risk of stroke.

Critical factor: The waist-to-hip ratio (WHR). In a study, men with the highest WHRs (above 0.98) suffered two to three times the number of strokes as men with the lowest WHRs (0.89). To calculate your WHR, divide your waist measurement by your hip measurement.

Almost All Men Can Become Fathers

Richard J. Sherins, MD, director, male infertility program, Genetic & IVF Institute, Fairfax, VA.

Men who have no viable sperm in their semen almost always have some unmoving sperm in their testicles. Those sperm can fertilize an egg if they are injected into it. This used to require expensive, painful surgery to obtain the sperm.

Now the sperm are aspirated through a thin needle in a procedure that is simple enough to be done in a doctor's office.

197

Infertility Factors

Emmett F. Branigan, MD, assistant professor of obstetrics and gynecology, University of Washington School of Medicine, Seattle. His one-year study of 95 couples with unexplained infertility was published in *The Journal of Reproductive Medicine*, 8342 Olive Blvd., St. Louis 63132.

Unexplained infertility is often the result of *leukocytospermia*, a condition in which the man's white blood cells adversely affect his sperm cells.

Good news: In a study, fertility rates increased *eightfold* when the man and the woman began taking the antibiotic *doxycycline*. Antibiotic therapy costs as little as $100, in vitro fertilization about $10,000.

Infertility and Infections

Harry Fisch, MD, director of the Male Reproductive Center at Columbia–Presbyterian Medical Center, 944 Park Ave., New York 10028.

Many male infertility problems come from infections. Bacteria or infection-fighting white blood cells present in the reproductive tract can severely affect both the production and motility of sperm, causing fertility problems. Many of these infections can be simply and effectively treated with antibiotics.

Also: A low sperm count may be a temporary condition caused by a current illness…or it may be a long-term holdover from a sexually transmitted disease contracted years ago but never completely cured. Antibiotics may rapidly clear up this problem, too.

Tight Underwear and Male Infertility

Carolina H. J. Tiemessen, MD, fertility specialist, St. Elizabeth Hospital, Tilburg, The Netherlands. Her study of sperm quality in nine men was published in *The Lancet*, 42 Bedford Sq., London WC1B 3SL, England.

Tight underwear can contribute to male infertility. For six months, men wore "boxers" and loose-fitting pants and avoided hot baths, saunas and electric blankets. During another six-month period, the men wore briefs and did not avoid these sources of heat.

Result: The men had lower sperm counts and reduced sperm mobility during the "brief" period.

Theory: The tight fit raises the temperature in the scrotum, impairing sperm formation.

Premature Ejaculation Help

Janet Lever, PhD, associate professor of sociology, California State University, Los Angeles, and Pepper Schwartz, PhD, professor of sociology, University of Washington, Seattle.

Premature ejaculation is the most common male sexual problem. Most cases can be easily fixed through a start–stop technique in which a man becomes more aware of his own arousal pattern and learns to change his technique.

More information: Consult your internist or urologist.

Safer Alternative to Vasectomy Reversals

Harry Fisch, MD, director of the Male Reproductive Center at Columbia–Presbyterian Medical Center, 944 Park Ave., New York 10028.

Men who have had vasectomies but now want children no longer need to have the surgery for vasectomy reversal. Instead, a small amount of sperm-containing tissue can be removed using local anesthesia—a procedure that takes only about a minute in the doctor's office, compared with about three hours in the operating room for a vasectomy reversal. The sperm is then injected into the wife's eggs through in vitro fertilization. About 500,000 men a year have vasectomies, and 1% to 2% have them reversed—a percentage that is increasing.

Impotence Drug News

Harin Padma-Nathan, MD, associate professor of urology at the University of Southern California and director of the Male Clinic in Santa Monica.

The impotence drug *alprostadil* can now be administered effectively at home *without* injections. Formerly, the drug had to be injected, which was often a painful process.

Now, a slender plunger device gently inserts the medicine—in the form of a tiny pellet—into the urethra.

About two-thirds of men for whom the technique works in the physician's office can also use it successfully at home. The effect typically occurs within about five minutes and lasts about one hour.

Snoring and Impotence

Karl Doghramji, MD, director, Sleep Disorders Center, Thomas Jefferson University, Philadelphia. His study of 250 subjects was published in *Sleep Research,* Brain Information Service, UCLA School of Medicine, Room 43-367, Box 951746, Los Angeles 90095.

Chronic poor sleep caused by snoring may disturb blood flow to the penis. A study found that about half of all impotent men also suffered from sleep apnea. Whether or not snoring causes impotence is unclear. However, there seems to be a clear association.

Self-defense: Impotent men should be checked for snoring and sleep apnea syndrome. If both are present, treatments are available—usually at sleep disorders centers. For referral to a sleep disorders center near you, contact the American Academy of Sleep Medicine, 6301 Bandel Rd. NW, Rochester, MN 55901. 507-287-6006, *www.aasmnet.org.*

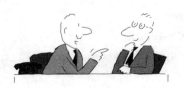

Curved Penis Help

Tom F. Lue, MD, professor of urology, University of California, San Francisco.

A curved penis can be fixed via surgery. The condition, called *Peyronie's disease*, occurs when erectile tissue on one side of the penis becomes scarred as a result of physical trauma —usually during intercourse—or a genetic disorder. In one procedure, erectile tissue on the opposite side is stitched together. The procedure, done under local anesthesia, takes about 30 minutes.

Strategies for Overcoming Impotence

Irwin Goldstein, MD, professor of urology at Boston University Medical Center. He is author of *The Potent Male*. Regenesis Cycle Publishing. The book is sold together with the video "Reversing Impotence."

Impotence can be a tough problem—but *not* because effective treatment is unavailable. A host of treatments introduced in recent years mean that most men can get help for this ailment.

The problem is that impotence is such a source of shame that many of the 30 million American men suffering from it are unwilling to seek help.

To tell a doctor a secret that's never been shared with anyone—maybe not even his spouse—is too much for some men.

The only advice I have for any man too proud to seek help for impotence is this—*get over it*. After all, would you rather endure a few minutes of embarrassment in the doctor's office...or forgo sexual satisfaction for the rest of your life?

GETTING HELP

Your first step should be to find a urologist who specializes in the treatment of impotence.

University-affiliated specialists are more likely to be up to date on impotence treatments than those without such an affiliation.

Any man suffering from impotence should be accompanied to the initial appointment by his sex partner.

Doctors used to think that nine out of 10 cases of impotence stemmed from purely psychological factors.

Now it's clear that while performance anxiety and other psychological problems often play a role, the vast majority of cases have physiological causes.

Examples: Injured blood vessels in the groin…atherosclerosis of arteries in the penis.

For this reason, diagnosing impotence requires a physical exam by a doctor *and* a psychological evaluation.

If your doctor cannot refer you to a sex therapist, get a referral by sending a self-addressed, stamped, business-sized envelope to the American Association of Sex Educators, Counselors and Therapists, Box 5488, Richmond, VA 23220.

A small percentage of men overcome impotence with the help of sex therapy…or following microvascular surgery to repair penile blood vessels damaged by groin injuries.

Treatments for Male Impotence

J. Francois Eid, MD, an assistant professor of urology at New York Hospital–Cornell Medical Center, and the director of the hospital's Sexual Function Center.

Male impotence—or erectile dysfunction, as doctors prefer to call it—is one of the most common untreated medical disorders in the world.

In the US, as many as 20 million men may have problems getting or maintaining an erection.

The disorder's prevalence increases with age. Only 5% of 40-year-olds experience erectile dysfunction. The rate among 70-year-olds is somewhere between 15% and 30%.

Of the men affected, however, only one out of 20 seeks medical help. That's unfortunate for two reasons…

- **Consistent loss of erection is not normal at any age**—and can actually be a symptom of an illness.

- **With many effective treatments now available** and many more on the way, erectile dysfunction can almost always be treated successfully.

More than 80% of all dysfunction can be traced to a physical (organic) cause—usually an inability to keep blood trapped in the penis after it becomes erect.

A much smaller percentage of cases is psychological in origin. These patients tend to be younger and usually report no erection at all with a partner, though they may be able to become erect when they're alone—watching an erotic movie, for example. (When the dysfunction is physical, the patient will usually have at least a partial erection.)

TREATING ERECTILE DYSFUNCTION

While its incidence is highest among older men, difficulty maintaining an erection is not a normal part of aging. A healthy male with a willing partner can expect to have one or two usable erections a week well into his 80s.

An occasional loss of erection is nothing to worry about. But if it happens consistently, see a physician who's very experienced at treating erectile dysfunction—either an internist specializing in erectile dysfunction (i.e., it makes up at least half of his/her practice) or a urologist.

Main difference: Only a urologist can surgically implant a prosthesis.

WHAT TO EXPECT

The first thing the doctor should do is take a medical history, including all psychological and sexual aspects of the dysfunction.

He should also give you a full physical checkup to identify any underlying illness that might be present. Difficulty in getting or maintaining an erection is often a predictor of vascular problems elsewhere in the body, including heart disease. *Other factors that can affect your erection include:*

- **High cholesterol.**

- **Cigarette smoking** (which constricts the blood vessels leading to the penis).

- **Excessive alcohol intake.**
- **Diabetes** (as many as 60% of diabetic men may have erection problems at some point).
- **Certain prescription drugs,** particularly blood pressure and cardiovascular medications, and some tranquilizers and antidepressants.
- **Radiation therapy.**
- **Pelvic surgery.**
- **Stroke or neurological disease,** including Parkinson's, Alzheimer's and multiple sclerosis.

Addressing these underlying causes can often solve the problem. If the dysfunction is psychological, you'll probably be referred to a certified sex therapist. If the problem turns out to be a simple issue of communication with your partner, a therapist could help you resolve it relatively quickly.

When the dysfunction involves more deeply ingrained issues—for example, inhibition or performance anxiety related to upbringing, religion and social background—it tends to be more difficult and time consuming to treat.

IT'S ALL IN YOUR MUSCLES

Most chronic erection problems aren't in a man's head, however, but in his muscle cells. Ninety percent of physical dysfunction occurs because the penis loses flexibility and elasticity over time, until its ability to trap and store blood becomes impaired. No matter how much blood flows into the penis, it leaks back out.

This happens because the muscle cells in your penis become thinner with age, while their supporting network of collagen (connective tissue) is no longer renewed as quickly as when you were younger, and becomes less elastic. As a result, the muscles in your penis are unable to fully relax—which is necessary for them to keep blood trapped in the penis.

FIVE TREATMENTS

Five types of treatment are now used to combat erectile dysfunction. Your choice of therapy should come only after discussing each option in detail with your doctor, and with your wife or sexual partner.

For a good outcome, it's vital to treat erectile dysfunction as a couple's problem, and include your mate in all aspects of treatment. I believe a supportive partner is the most important factor in regaining a full, healthy sex life.

- **Oral medications.** *Sildenafil* (Viagra) was approved by the FDA in 1998 and represents a new milestone in the field of erectile dysfunction. Viagra works by increasing blood flow to the penis, as well as causing penile muscles to relax. It does not initiate an erection, but helps store penile flow in response to sexual stimulation by counteracting the chemical in the body that diminishes an erection.

Viagra is effective regardless of the cause of the erectile dysfunction, including hypertension, coronary disease, prostate cancer, diabetes and depression.

Two other oral medications currently undergoing clinical trials—*apomorphine* and *Vasomax* —will probably not be as effective as Viagra. *Yohimbine* (a vasodilator), another popular oral medication, is worthless, in my opinion.

The antidepressant drug *Trazodone,* taken one hour before sexual activity, has been found to prolong erections in men who are able to obtain, but not maintain, an erection during intercourse. Trazodone, however, is much less effective than Viagra.

- **Topical cream.** *MUSE* (Medicated Urethral System for Erection), which contains a prostaglandin cream that's applied into the opening of the urethra just before intercourse, has also produced good results in clinical trials. This cream is a vasodilator, meaning that it causes blood vessels to widen—encouraging blood flow into the penis. However, patient response has been very disappointing. With the approval of Viagra, this method has become less popular.

- **Injection therapy.** Prior to FDA approval of Viagra, this was the newest form of treatment to emerge over the past 20 years, and is still the most effective treatment currently available. A drug is injected at the base of the penis 20 minutes before intercourse, using a very small needle. Like creams, the drug works by dilating the blood vessels. The result is usually a very natural, high-quality erection.

When it was first used in the 1980s, the injection of choice was a mixture of *papaverine* and *phentolamine.* The injections have some side effects, including scarring from repeated injections, and sometimes a painfully prolonged erection (solved by reducing the dosage).

Approved by the FDA in 1995, *prostaglandin E1* (Alprostadil), a substance that occurs naturally in penile tissue, is an injectable drug that can be self-administered at home. Tests show that scarring from prostaglandin E1 injections is minimal (occurring in only 1% of cases)—and the satisfaction rate is very high. This is currently the only FDA-approved method for penile injection.

Eight out of 10 men tested reported a usable erection and satisfactory intercourse. It also appears to work well for some cases of psychological dysfunction.

● **Vacuum device.** This is the least invasive method of all, involving no medication or surgery. A tube is placed over the end of the penis. The device creates a vacuum that encourages blood to flow in, creating an erection. A rubber ring is then snapped over the base of the penis.

While the success rate is very high with vacuum devices, only one-third of the men who buy them end up using them. *The complaints:* It's too cumbersome, while the erection that results can be a bit painful and is usually not quite as hard as normal.

● **Prosthetic device.** If injections, pills and creams don't do the job, you may want to think about having a prosthetic device implanted through a minor procedure in which a small opening in the skin is made between the testicles. This can be done using local anesthetic.

Currently the most popular device is an inflatable prosthesis, which includes a fluid reservoir and a small pump, which the patient activates to become erect. The prosthesis does not interfere with normal sensation or ejaculation. After implantation, the patient can't even feel it—or see it—and often his partner can't tell it's there. However, once the patient selects the prosthesis option, injection therapy or the vacuum device will no longer be appropriate. Fortunately, the prosthetic

device group of patients has an extremely high satisfaction rate.

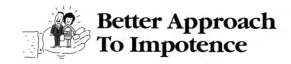

Better Approach To Impotence

J. Francois Eid, MD, an assistant professor of urology at New York Hospital–Cornell Medical Center, and the director of the hospital's Sexual Function Center.

A better approach to impotence is to treat the couple, not just the man. When partners are included in the process—from evaluation through treatment—the success rate increases dramatically over treating the man alone…no matter what treatment method is used.

Important: Solving the impotency problem does not miraculously solve any other problems in one's personal life. *Reality:* I see many couples who enjoy fabulous love lives even though the man is completely impotent… as well as many couples with awful personal lives for whom there is no impotence problem.

Impotence Predicts Heart Disease

Kenneth Goldberg, MD, director, Male Health Center, Lewisville, TX.

Twenty-five percent of men who see doctors for impotence caused by vascular problems have a heart attack or stroke within five years of the start of impotence. *Reason:* Sexual impotence is often caused by the same problems that cause heart trouble, including diabetes, smoking, high blood pressure and high cholesterol levels.

Hormones and Men's Health

Alvin C. Powers, MD, chief of endocrinology and diabetes at the Nashville Veterans Affairs Medical Center, and associate professor of medicine at Vanderbilt University Medical School, both in Nashville.

Four million American men suffer from low testosterone (*hypogonadism*), but only 200,000 receive treatment for the condition. Untreated, hypogonadism can cause impotence, depression, fatigue, excess body fat and osteoporosis. Many men fail to report these symptoms to their doctor.

Study: For six months, 227 men with low levels of testosterone were treated with the hormone. One group received it through a topical gel. The other used a patch, the most widely used form of supplemental testosterone.

Both groups had improvements in sexual desire and function as well as muscle strength. Bone loss slowed in both groups, too.

However, 66% of patch users reported skin irritation. Only 6% of gel users experienced such irritation.

The gel group also reported a greater increase in muscle mass and a decrease in body fat.

Implication: Testosterone gel is better tolerated and may be a more effective treatment than the patch.

Any man suffering from sexual dysfunction or depression should have his testosterone level measured. If the level is low, the doctor should consider prescribing testosterone.

FEWER PROSTATE SYMPTOMS

Many men over age 50 suffer from prostate enlargement. This noncancerous condition—*benign prostatic hyperplasia* (BPH)—causes frequent urination (particularly at night), often with decreased flow and dribbling.

Theory: Two contributing factors to BPH may be insufficient consumption of grains, beans and other isoflavone-containing foods... and excessive consumption of animal fat and protein.

Study: For three months, 29 men ages 50 to 75 took a daily supplement containing 40 milligrams (mg) of isoflavones (the amount in one cup of soy milk). The men experienced a 29% decrease in the frequency of nocturnal urination and a 10% increase in the rate of urinary flow.

More research is needed to compare this treatment with standard drug treatments and to determine its safety and effectiveness.

Saw Palmetto Benefits

Leonard S. Marks, MD, clinical associate professor of urology, University of California, Los Angeles, School of Medicine. His study of 44 men with benign prostatic hyperplasia was published in the *Journal of Urology,* 1120 N. Charles St., Baltimore 21201.

The effectiveness of saw palmetto against urinary problems associated with an enlarged prostate has been proven in numerous studies in other countries. But in the first US study of its kind, saw palmetto was shown to shrink swollen prostate tissue, thereby relieving the frequent urge to urinate...difficulty urinating...and the inability to empty the bladder fully.

More good news: Saw palmetto had *no* effect on testosterone levels. That suggests that the use of this herb does not reduce sex drive. Diminished libido is a common side effect of certain drugs used to treat prostate enlargement.

Treatment for Prostate Problems

Muta M. Issa, MD, clinical assistant professor of urology, Stanford University Medical School, Stanford, CA.

Benign prostate hyperplasia (BPH) is a common, age-related condition in which the prostate swells, impeding the flow of urine through the urethra. A treatment called *transurethral needle ablation* (TUNA) involves heating the prostate with radio waves emitted by a needle-like antenna inserted within the gland. TUNA requires only local anesthesia, and is up to 70% less costly and just as effective as conventional surgery.

Recovery time: One day (compared to three to four days for conventional surgery).

For the Enlarged Prostate

John Kabalin, MD, assistant professor of urology, Stanford University, Stanford, CA. His study of laser prostatectomy in 227 men was presented at a meeting of the American Urological Association, 1120 N. Charles St., Baltimore 21202.

Men with enlarged prostates find it easier to urinate following laser surgery. *Laser prostatectomy* clears away unwanted tissue just as effectively as standard surgery, in which the surgeon uses a wire loop or scalpel to remove prostate tissue…yet it causes virtually no bleeding and requires less anesthesia. The laser "cooks" the part of the prostate that encircles the urethra. This tissue disintegrates and is passed in the urine.

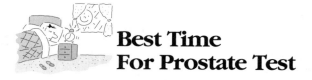

Best Time For Prostate Test

William J. Catalona, MD, chief, division of urology, Washington University School of Medicine, St. Louis.

A prostate-specific antigen (PSA) test is best performed at least 48 hours after having sex. Ejaculation can make a PSA reading jump. The test might then indicate possible prostate cancer. PSA readings return to normal 48 hours after ejaculation.

Prostate Test Schedule

H. Ballentine Carter, MD, associate professor of urology, Johns Hopkins University School of Medicine, Baltimore. His study was published in the *Journal of the American Medical Association*, 515 N. State St., Chicago 60610.

Men are typically advised to get their first annual *prostate-specific antigen* (PSA) test at age 50. But new evidence suggests that it's better to have the first test at age 40, followed by another at age 45 and then every other year starting at age 50. Experts believe this revised screening schedule should save lives by spotting tumors when they are still small and confined to the prostate gland, when treatment is most effective.

Best Treatments for Prostate Enlargement

Patrick C. Walsh, MD, urologist-in-chief at Johns Hopkins Hospital and director of the department of urology at Johns Hopkins University School of Medicine, both in Baltimore. Dr. Walsh developed the nerve-sparing radical prostatectomy procedure for treating prostate cancer. He is coauthor of *The Prostate: A Guide for Men and the Women Who Love Them*. Warner Books.

Prostate cancer gets lots of media coverage—but prostate enlargement is far more prevalent.

Technically known as *benign prostatic hyperplasia* (BPH), the condition affects more than half of men over age 50…and 80% of men by age 80.

The prostate is a walnut-sized gland that surrounds the urethra at the base of the bladder. It produces one component of seminal fluid and helps propel the fluid through the urethra during orgasm.

For unknown reasons, the prostate often begins to enlarge around age 40.

The enlarged tissue presses against the urethra, often leading to urinary problems…

Mild symptoms: Difficulty in starting the flow of urine…a weak urine stream…stopping and starting during urination…and dribbling afterward.

Severe symptoms: An urgent need to urinate up to several times an hour…a constant feeling of fullness in the bladder…and frequent awakening at night to go to the bathroom.

DIAGNOSING BPH

Although BPH is unrelated to a man's risk of developing prostate cancer, it's prudent to see a urologist if you're experiencing any urinary difficulties.

Reason: BPH and prostate cancer produce similar symptoms. Also, untreated BPH can lead to urinary tract infection or even bladder or kidney damage.

After reviewing your symptoms and medical history, the urologist should take a urine sample to check for infection. Then he/she should perform a digital rectal exam to feel for prostate enlargement.

The doctor should also test your blood level of *prostate-specific antigen* (PSA). A high level suggests prostate cancer.*

For mild BPH, the doctor will probably recommend *watchful waiting*. That involves simply keeping an eye on your symptoms, with checkups at least once a year to make sure no complications have developed.

Caution: Antihistamines and decongestants can worsen your symptoms. If you have BPH, ask your doctor about avoiding these drugs.

PROSTATE MEDICATION

More aggressive treatment may be called for if your BPH is clearly getting worse…if the symptoms are causing moderate discomfort… or if you're having to restrict your life to deal with them (such as always having to be near a toilet). Two classes of drugs are used to treat BPH…

•**Alpha-blockers** such as *terazosin* (Hytrin) and *doxazosin* (Cardura). These drugs—also used to treat high blood pressure—relax the prostate muscle.

*The American Cancer Society recommends an annual PSA test for all men starting at age 50 (age 45 for African-American men and men with a family history of prostate cancer). Caught early, prostate cancer may be curable via radiation and/or surgery.

•**5-alpha reductase inhibitors** such as *finasteride* (Proscar). It shrinks the prostate by blocking the prostate-stimulating effect of dihydrotestosterone.

In deciding which kind of drug is appropriate, it's important to understand that the prostate is made up of two types of tissue— *glandular tissue*, which enlarges, producing mechanical obstruction…and *smooth muscle tissue*, which squeezes the urethra shut.

Which drug is best for your BPH depends on which of the two kinds of tissue is the real culprit.

If your prostate is enlarged: Finasteride may help by shrinking it. It may need to be taken for six months to a year before symptoms begin to improve.

Side effects: Impotence occurs in fewer than 5% of men taking finasteride. Potency generally returns when medication is stopped.

If your prostate is of normal size: It doesn't help to shrink it. The treatment of choice is an alpha-blocker.

Side effects: Weakness, dizziness and drowsiness occur in up to 10% of men taking an alpha-blocker. To avoid these problems, ask your doctor about adjusting the dose and taking the drug at bedtime.

PROSTATE SURGERY

If drugs fail to bring relief, surgery can help. The "gold standard" for surgical treatment of BPH—the one considered most effective—is *transurethral resection of the prostate* (TURP).

In this procedure, the surgeon inserts a tiny lighted instrument called a *resectoscope* into the urethra. Excess tissue from the prostate's "inner ring" is chipped away bit by bit.

TURP is attractive to patients because it involves no incision…minimal postoperative pain …and a hospital stay of less than three days (followed by a week of rest at home).

If the prostate is of normal size, the surgical treatment of choice is *transurethral incision of the prostate* (TUIP).

As in TURP, a resectoscope is inserted through the urethra. But instead of chipping away tissue from the inner ring, the surgeon makes two tiny cuts in the muscular portion of the prostate. This relaxes its grip on the urethra.

Many men fear they'll become incontinent or impotent as a result of surgery. In fact, fewer than 4% of men who undergo TURP or TUIP experience such problems.

However, three out of four men who undergo TURP (and a slightly smaller proportion of those who undergo TUIP) experience retrograde ejaculation. In this condition, sperm liberated by orgasm go backward into the bladder instead of being ejected from the penis.

Retrograde ejaculation can render a man infertile. It is not dangerous, however, nor does it interfere with a man's enjoyment of sex.

MORE SURGICAL PROCEDURES

Two newer procedures destroy excess prostate tissue via heat administered via catheter...

• **Transurethral needle ablation** (TUNA) uses radio waves to produce heat.

• **Transurethral microwave thermal therapy** (TUMT) uses microwaves.

TUNA and TUMT have real advantages over TURP and TUIP. They can be done on an outpatient basis, for instance, and the risks of retrograde ejaculation, impotence and incontinence are smaller.

Prostate Cancer Drug

Glenn Gerber, MD, associate professor of surgery, University of Chicago School of Medicine.

The drug *mitoxantrone* (Novantrone) is highly effective at stopping pain caused by prostate cancer that has spread to the bones.

Study: Taken in combination with steroids, mitoxantrone significantly reduced pain in 38% of men with advanced cancer. This compared to 21% treated with steroids alone.

Also: The mitoxantrone group stayed pain-free for an average of eight months, compared to two months for the steroids-only group.

What's Better for Early-Stage Prostate Cancer— Radiation or Surgery?

Patrick Kupelian, MD, assistant staff, department of radiation oncology, Cleveland Clinic Foundation.

Early-stage prostate cancer responds just as well to radiation as to surgery—even though doctors often consider surgery the treatment of choice. In a study, 75% of patients given radiation were cancer-free after five years. That's roughly equivalent to the 76% who were cancer-free after surgical removal of the prostate. In choosing between the two therapies, men should consider the side effects associated with each—rectal bleeding from radiation...and incontinence from surgery.

Special consideration: Because of the potential for heart trouble, older men may be unable to have surgery.

More Prostate News

Glenn S. Gerber, MD, assistant professor of urology at the University of Chicago Medical School.

Surgery is extremely successful in treating early prostate cancer. A study of nearly 2,700 men between ages 48 and 79 with early prostate cancer who had their prostate glands removed surgically between 1970 and 1993 found that those with the least aggressive form of tumor had a 94% chance of surviving 10 years.

Those with *moderately aggressive* tumors had an 80% 10-year survival rate, while the comparable rate for men with the *most aggressive* tumors was 77%.

Researchers believe that in more recent years, the success rate has become even higher.

However, because surgery sometimes results in impotence and urinary incontinence, physicians say that for elderly men with slow-growing cancer, it may be better simply to wait and see how the cancer develops before deciding to operate.

Testicular Cancer Self-Defense

Mark Seal, MD, assistant clinical professor of urology at the Medical College of Ohio, and a urologist in private practice, both in Toledo. He is author of *The Patient's Guide to Urology.* High Oaks.

Although it does not get much publicity, testicular cancer is the most common malignancy among men 15 to 45 years of age.

Doctors don't know how to prevent the disease. Fortunately, however, it's now easy to detect—and cure.

Thirty years ago, testicular cancer proved fatal for 90% of its victims. Today the *cure* rate is 90%—and that includes advanced cases.

To reduce the threat of testicular cancer, all men should examine their testicles on a monthly basis. Monthly self-exams should start at puberty and continue until age 50. Testicular cancer is rare among older men.

In addition, any man in this age group should make sure his doctor performs a testicular exam with each checkup.

Testicular cancer is especially common in men who have had an undescended testicle (whether or not it was surgically corrected)… and in men with a personal or family history of testicular cancer.

HOW TO PERFORM A SELF-EXAM

The best time to do a self-exam is while showering. Gently anchor your right testicle with your right hand, and run your left index finger over the testicle's front and side surfaces.

Next, use both hands to check the back of the testicle. Gently squeeze the soft tubular structure (epididymis) that runs up into your lower abdomen.

Repeat this process on the left testicle, using your left hand and right index finger. The self-exam should take only 15 to 30 seconds per side.

If you find a lump or an area of tenderness, tell your doctor right away.

Helpful: Before starting a program of monthly self-exams, have your doctor check out your technique. This will also give you a "baseline" against which you can compare future self-exams.

If you're shy about touching yourself—many men are—consider asking your wife or sex partner to examine you.

One in three cases of testicular cancer are discovered by the patient's partner.

Good news: Most scrotal lumps are benign. *Non-cancerous causes of scrotal lumps include…*

●**Varicose veins of the scrotum** (varicocele). A varicocele feels a little like a bag of worms under the skin.

●**Sperm-filled cyst** (spermatocele). This consists of a pea-sized lump, clearly separate from the testicle.

●**Fluid buildup** in the scrotum (hydrocele).

●**Hernia.**

In examining a scrotal lump, your doctor will use his/her hands and check to see whether it can be "separated" from the testicle itself. If so, it's probably benign.

If the lump is intrinsic to the testicle, there's a good chance that it is cancerous. In such cases the doctor should perform blood tests to check for the presence of proteins associated with testicular cancer.

He may also do an ultrasound scan to see whether the lump is solid (possibly cancerous) or fluid-filled (probably benign).

TREATING TESTICULAR CANCER

Testicular cancer takes several forms. Treatment must be tailored to the particular form, although all cases necessitate surgical removal of the testicle, along with the attached structures (epididymis) and cord (blood vessels).

Chemotherapy and/or radiation therapy may also be appropriate, especially if the cancer has spread outside the testicle. One type of testicular tumor, called *seminoma*, is especially vulnerable to radiation.

Divorce and Men

David B. Larson, MD, MSPH, president, National Institute for Healthcare Research, Rockville, MD.

Divorce raises a man's risk of developing cancer.

Divorced men are 21 times more likely than married men to be admitted to a psychiatric hospital. Children of divorced parents are 30% more likely to die young than are kids whose parents stay married.

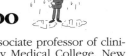

Breast Cancer Strikes Men, Too

Bonnie S. Reichman, MD, associate professor of clinical medicine, Cornell University Medical College, New York City.

Each year 1,400 American men develop the disease.

At greatest risk: Men with a family history of breast cancer—male or female.

Warning signs: A typically painless breast mass on one side…a swollen, sore breast…puckered, scaly or irritated skin patches on the breast…a firm lump or thickness in the breast …a crusty or retracted nipple…discharge from the nipple.

Low-Fat Diets and Men

William J. Kraemer, PhD, director of research, Center for Sports Medicine, and professor of applied physiology, Pennsylvania State University, University Park. His study of dietary and exercise routines of 12 men was published in the *Journal of Applied Physiology*, 9650 Rockville Pike, Bethesda, MD 20814.

Very low-fat diets can cause a drop in blood levels of testosterone, which is needed for muscle mass and strength.

At special risk: Wrestlers and other athletes who attempt to drastically reduce their fat intake.

Bottom line: The body needs a balance of nutrients—including fat.

11

Food and Nutrition Tips For a Healthier You

Dr. Dean Ornish's Secrets of Much Healthier Eating

Dean Ornish, MD
Preventive Medicine Research Institute and University of California at San Francisco

More and more information is emerging that documents the benefits of eating increased amounts of vegetables and substantially reducing consumption of red meat and other animal products.

Even the government has endorsed the healthfulness of a vegetarian diet for the first time in a new set of nutritional guidelines.

Here are the big health benefits of a vegetarian diet—and my strategies for making the switch...

WHY A VEGETARIAN DIET?

A plant-based diet is linked not only to lower rates of heart disease and stroke, but also to significantly lower rates of the most common cancers. These include breast and ovarian cancers in women, prostate cancer in men and colon and lung cancers.

Low-fat vegetarian diets also may reduce the incidence of osteoporosis, adult-onset diabetes, hypertension, obesity and many other illnesses.

In contrast, a meat-based diet is high in saturated fat, which your body converts to cholesterol. Such a diet is also high in iron, an *oxidant* that oxidizes cholesterol and makes it more likely to clog your arteries.

Iron also causes the formation of *free radicals*, which promote cancer and aging. A meat-based diet is low in the antioxidants that help prevent this from happening. *Also:* There

Dean Ornish, MD, who has proven the health advantages of a vegetarian diet in a series of studies during the past 20 years. He is president and director of the nonprofit Preventive Medicine Research Institute in Sausalito, CA and assistant clinical professor of medicine at the University of California at San Francisco. Dr. Ornish is author of several books, including *Everyday Cooking with Dr. Dean Ornish*. HarperCollins.

is no cholesterol in a plant-based diet, and with few exceptions (avocados, seeds, nuts and oils), a plant-based diet is low in both total fat and saturated fat.

A plant-based diet is also low in oxidants like iron (it has enough iron without having too much) and high in antioxidants like beta-carotene and vitamins A, C and E. Also, meat contains virtually no dietary fiber, which is high in a plant-based diet.

During the past few years, scientists have discovered and documented new classes of chemicals that help prevent illness and slow the aging process. These include bioflavonoids, carotenoids, phytochemicals and other substances that are high in a plant-based diet and low in a meat-based diet. In other words, there are more and more reasons to eat a plant-based diet.

The major reason for changing your diet and lifestyle, however, is not just to live longer or reduce the risk of illness or heart problems years later. It's to improve the quality of life *right now*.

To me, there's no point in giving up something that I enjoy unless I get something back in return that is even better.

MY EXPERIENCE

I began making changes in my own diet when I was 19 years old. My cholesterol and blood pressure were not a problem—they have always been low. I changed my diet and lifestyle because it helped me feel much better emotionally.

Today I have more energy and I think more clearly. I have an overall improved feeling of well-being. With a vegetarian diet, I can eat whenever I'm hungry until I'm full. I can eat delicious food—and I don't have to worry about my weight.

HOW TO SWITCH

●**Start by giving up meat *completely*.** Despite conventional wisdom, it is actually easier to make big changes in diet and lifestyle —all at once—than to make small, gradual changes.

First, you don't have to wait very long for the benefits. Most people find they feel so much better so quickly that the choices become clearer and worth making—not out of fear of dying but rather to increase the joy of living.

Second, your palate adjusts quickly when you make comprehensive changes in your diet so that you begin to *prefer* low-fat vegetarian foods.

●**Reduce fat in your diet.** Meat and fat are acquired tastes. Have you ever switched from drinking whole milk to low-fat or skim milk? At first, most people find that skim milk tastes like water and is not very good. After a week or two, it tastes fine. If you then go out to dinner and are served whole milk, it tastes too greasy and too rich.

The cow didn't change…your palate simply adapted. If you were always drinking some whole milk and some skim milk, the skim milk would never taste very good. It's easier if you just make a comprehensive shift and stop drinking whole milk altogether.

Similarly, while eating less meat is a step in the right direction, you may find it easier to give it up completely and consume more healthful foods. Otherwise, you get the worst of both worlds—you're eating enough to still have a taste for it, but you're not really getting all you want…and you don't feel much better.

Some people mistakenly assume that a vegetarian diet will automatically trim excess weight and prevent buildup of cholesterol in their arteries. But it is possible to eat a high-fat, high-cholesterol vegetarian diet, especially if you consume butter, whole milk, eggs, oils, avocados, seeds and nuts.

●**Center your diet on fruits, vegetables, grains and beans,** supplemented with moderate amounts of egg whites (which are high in protein and very low in fat and cholesterol) and nonfat dairy products, such as fat-free cheeses, yogurt and skim milk.

●**Eliminate *all* oils for optimal health and weight loss.** You have probably read that olive oil is good for your heart.

Reality: All kinds of oil are 100% fat—including olive oil. Olive oil is also 16% saturated fat…and your body converts saturated fat into cholesterol. Olive oil is *not* good for you, although it is less harmful than lard, butter or oils that contain even higher amounts of saturated fat.

Also, the more oil of any type you consume, the more weight you will gain. You will likely lose weight if you do nothing more than eliminate oils and products that contain oil from your diet.

Example: Instead of using oil to make pasta sauce, use vegetable-based soup stock, tomato sauce or the "juice" you get from sautéing fresh tomatoes in a nonstick pan.

●**Don't give up flavor.** A common misconception is that you have to choose between gourmet high-fat, meat-based foods that are delicious, beautifully presented and unhealthful…and low-fat vegetarian foods that are boring and bland and might make you live longer —or it just may *seem* longer.

You don't have to choose between good food and good health. High-fat meat-based meals can taste bad if they're prepared poorly …and low-fat vegetarian foods can taste great if they're prepared well.

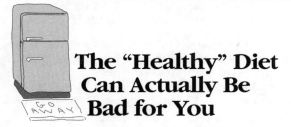

The "Healthy" Diet Can Actually Be Bad for You

Barry Sears, PhD, former staff scientist at the Massachusetts Institute of Technology, and president of Surfactant Technologies, a biotechnology firm in Marblehead, MA. He holds 12 patents for cancer treatments and dietary control of hormonal responses and is author of *The Zone.* HarperCollins.

Poor eating habits have led to an epidemic of obesity in the US. One in three adult Americans is now obese, as compared with one in four a little more than a decade ago.

Even people who follow the conventional wisdom for healthful eating—lots of carbohydrates, little fat and protein—often fail to lose weight. Why? Because, hormonally speaking, those guidelines are *dead wrong*.

When it comes to obesity, eating carbohydrates is a bigger problem than eating fat.

THE TROUBLE WITH CARBOHYDRATES

Modern humans are genetically identical to our Stone Age ancestors. Our digestive system, like theirs, evolved to handle a diet based on protein, fiber-rich vegetables and fruit.

Grains—the chief source of carbohydrates in modern diets—were unknown until the advent of agriculture, 10,000 years ago. That's only yesterday in evolutionary terms.

Problem: Carbohydrates cause a sharp rise in blood sugar levels. In response, the body makes more insulin, the hormone that lowers blood sugar levels and "tells" the body to store excess calories as *fat*.

Insulin also affects the body's synthesis of *eicosanoids*. These potent "superhormones" control virtually all physiological functions in the body—from the circulation of blood to digestion.

For optimum health, eicosanoids must be in balance. But high insulin levels cause the body to make more "bad" than "good" eicosanoids.

This can lead to platelet clumping, high blood pressure, reduced immunity and other potentially dangerous conditions.

A BETTER WAY TO EAT

Over the past 14 years, I have developed a simple yet precise eating plan that allows you to regulate levels of insulin and other hormones…and reach an ideal metabolic state.

Athletes call this state the "Zone," but in reality it is simply optimal control of hormonal function. You needn't be an athlete to realize the benefits. My program has been tested on heart patients, "ordinary" people and elite athletes, including professional football and basketball players.

All have reported greater mental focus and energy, better physical endurance, painless weight loss and improved cardiovascular function.

How do you reach the Zone? Treat food with the same respect you accord to prescription medications.

Specifically, you must regulate the *amount, proportion* and *rate of entry into the bloodstream* of all the nutrients you eat. And I mean *each time* you eat. Counting calories isn't necessary.

EATING IN THE ZONE

My eating plan has five major components…

●**Protein.** Besides serving as building blocks for every cell, dietary protein causes release of *glucagon*. This hormone works in opposition to insulin and works to maintain blood sugar levels.

To maintain proper glucagon levels, it's important to eat the right amount of protein.

Easy formula: At each meal, eat about as much protein as would fit in the palm of your hand. For most people, this translates into three to four ounces of low-fat protein.

Animal foods contain *arachidonic acid*, a fatty acid that the body uses to make "bad" eicosanoids. The fattier the meat, the higher the arachidonic acid content. That's why it's best to stick to chicken, fish, wild game (or range-fed meats), tofu and other low-fat protein sources …and to avoid organ meats entirely.

●**Carbohydrates.** For optimal hormonal balance, each meal should contain the proper ratio of carbohydrate to protein—4 grams (g) of carbohydrate for every 3 g of protein.

Emphasize "favorable" carbohydrates like fiber-rich fruits, vegetables and legumes. Since these are absorbed into the bloodstream slowly, blood sugar rises slowly…and insulin production is moderate.

Avoid "unfavorable" carbohydrates such as bread, rice, pasta, tropical fruits, dried fruits and fruit juices…and starchy or sweet vegetables, such as corn, potatoes, squash, carrots, peas and beets. These foods enter the bloodstream quickly, initiating a drastic insulin response.

If you do eat grains, stick with *whole* grains whenever possible. Their higher fiber content means slower absorption into the bloodstream.

What about dessert? An occasional treat is okay, as long as you balance your carbohydrate and fat intake by taking a "dose" of protein just beforehand—a few ounces of cottage cheese or sliced turkey, for instance.

●**Fat.** Though often treated as a dietary villain, fat in *moderate amounts* slows the rate of carbohydrate absorption, thus helping to moderate insulin response.

Fat also sends a satiety (satisfaction) signal to the brain, making you feel so full you'll *want* to stop eating.

Your ratio of grams of dietary fat to grams of dietary protein should be 1 to 3. Zone-favorable fats are largely monounsaturated—olive oil, canola oil, almonds, macadamia nuts, natural peanut butter and avocados.

Avoid butter, red meat and other sources of saturated fat.

●**Caloric restriction.** Have no more than 500 calories per meal. Too many calories from any source raises insulin levels.

●**Timing.** Except for the time you spend asleep, let no more than five hours pass between Zone-favorable meals or snacks.

This works out to three small meals and two snacks a day. If you eat breakfast at 7 a.m., have lunch no later than noon. If dinner isn't until 6:30 p.m., grab a mid-afternoon snack. Have a small snack at bedtime, too.

Vital: Snacks should respect the same 4 to 3 to 1 ratio of carbohydrate to protein to fat.

Examples: One ounce of hard cheese (or two ounces of cottage cheese) and half an apple… or one small muffin baked from a mix to which you added protein powder and substituted olive oil for butter.

Curative Curry?

Bandaru S. Reddy, PhD, chief, division of nutritional carcinogenesis, American Health Foundation, Valhalla, NY.

Rats exposed to a chemical that ordinarily causes colon cancer developed far fewer tumors when they were fed a diet high in *curcumin*. That's the ingredient that gives curry its bright orange color.

The tumors that did form in the curry-eating rats were less likely to grow and spread.

Fat-Free Food Trap

Walter Willett, MD, DrPH, professor of epidemiology and nutrition, Harvard University School of Public Health, Boston.

You can't eat a whole box of nonfat snacks and expect not to gain weight.

Reason: Whether it comes from fat or carbohydrates, a calorie is a calorie. Eat enough no-fat cookies, pretzels, etc., and your body will convert the excess calories into fat almost as efficiently as if you'd eaten the same number of high-fat snacks.

Surprising: If you eat 100 extra calories of fat, your body will store 97 of them. Eat 100 extra calories of carbohydrates, and your body stores between 80 and 90.

Better than Butter

Alice Lichtenstein, DSc, associate professor of nutrition, USDA Human Nutrition Research Center on Aging at Tufts University, Boston.

Although it's best to avoid butter entirely, a spread made of equal parts of butter and olive oil has about half the saturated fat of butter. It has lots of good-for-the-heart monounsaturated fats and few "bad" transaturated fats. Mix butter and oil in a food processor. Store in the refrigerator.

Eggs Can Be Part of A Healthful Diet

Barbara Retzlaff, MPH, RD, research dietitian, Northwest Lipid Research Clinic, University of Washington, Seattle.

Although they can be part of a healthful diet, eggs should be avoided by anyone with *combined hyperlipidemia* (elevated cholesterol and triglyceride levels). When patients with combined hyperlipidemia ate two eggs a day for three months, their total cholesterol levels climbed from 238 to 250...while LDL (bad) cholesterol levels rose from 149 to 162. In egg eaters who had elevated cholesterol

alone, levels were unchanged. *Note:* Cholesterol below 200 is considered desirable.

A Most Expensive Hamburger

Neal D. Barnard, MD, president, Physicians Committee for Responsible Medicine, 5100 Wisconsin Ave. NW, Suite 404, Washington, DC 20016.

America's appetite for meat causes an additional $29 billion to $61 billion a year in health-care costs. Individuals who eat beef, pork, poultry or fish face increased risk for high blood pressure...heart disease...diabetes...gallbladder disease...obesity and osteoarthritis... food poisoning...and cancer of the colon, lungs, ovaries and prostate.

Protein and Kidney Disease

Ping H. Wang, MD, assistant professor of medicine, University of California, Irvine.

Kidney patients have long been told to limit the amount of protein in their diet. An analysis of 10 studies involving 1,521 patients confirms that protein restriction does, in fact, significantly reduce risk of kidney failure or death in patients with nondiabetic kidney disease. It also slows progression of kidney disease in patients with insulin-dependent diabetes.

Two Are Better than One

Study of almost 6,000 adults, reported in *Tufts University Diet & Nutrition Letter,* 53 Park Pl., New York 10007.

People who live alone get fewer nutrients than those who live with others. People living alone are less likely to meet the recommended daily allowances of many nutrients.

213

But live-alones do better in limiting consumption of fat, cholesterol and sodium—probably because people tend to eat less when they eat alone.

Foods Can Change Your Moods

Judith Wurtman, PhD, nutrition researcher, Massachusetts Institute of Technology in Cambridge.

Sweet and starchy carbohydrates boost the level of a "stress-relief" chemical in your brain, serotonin, making you feel relaxed and in emotional control. *Examples:* Bagel, pasta, baked potato.

Foods high in protein can help increase mental alertness when you are running low on mental energy. *Examples:* Fish, poultry and dairy products.

Food Danger Zones

Stephen P. Gullo, PhD, president, Institute for Health and Weight Sciences, which offers one-on-one coaching to retrain eating habits and attitudes toward food, New York.

Food trouble spots are places where you're most likely to overeat—or eat the wrong foods. Some people are tempted in movie theaters, others have trouble at the office.

Self-defense: Understand your weaknesses and guard against them. If you cruise the vending machines at work every afternoon, break for a planned snack—eating healthful food like a banana.

Salt-Watchers

N. Nicole Spelhang, managing editor, *Mayo Clinic Health Letter*, 200 First St., Rochester, MN 55905.

If you're trying to cut back on sodium in your diet, be aware of these salt facts: Sparkling

bottled water has only 3 milligrams (mg) of sodium per 12 ounces, club soda has 75 mg... fresh turkey has less than 20 mg of sodium per ounce, but deli-variety turkey and ham each have more than 300 mg...even light soy sauce has more than 600 mg of sodium per tablespoon compared with 234 mg for a tablespoon of Worcestershire sauce.

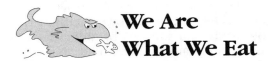

We Are What We Eat

Judith J. Wurtman, PhD, research scientist, department of brain and cognitive science, Massachusetts Institute of Technology, Cambridge. She is author of *Managing Your Mind & Mood Through Food* (HarperCollins) and *The Serotonin Solution*, a weight-loss book for people who overeat because of stress (Ballantine Books).

Folk wisdom has long held that our moods are influenced by the food we eat. That belief is gaining support from scientific research.

Food-mood strategies can't cure clinical depression or other serious psychological disorders. Such problems call for professional help. But they can be used to boost alertness at work...increase your sense of relaxation at home...and make it easier for you to tolerate life's ups and downs.

Mood-altering foods aren't unusual or hard to find. You don't have to follow a long, complex regimen before seeing results. They are ordinary, everyday foods...and in some cases, their effects are felt within as little as 30 minutes.

HOW FOOD ACTS ON OUR MOODS

Research suggests that food affects mood by altering the brain's production of chemical messengers called *neurotransmitters*...

The neurotransmitters *dopamine* and *norepinephrine* have an energizing effect. When your brain is producing these chemicals, you're alert, highly motivated and have fast reaction times.

The main building block of these "alertness chemicals" is the amino acid *tyrosine*. Eating protein—which contains lots of tyrosine—

raises tyrosine levels in the brain. This, in turn, boosts synthesis of dopamine and norepinephrine. *Result:* Greater mental energy.

The neurotransmitter *serotonin* has a calming effect. Its presence in the brain boosts concentration, relieves feelings of anxiety and—at night or if you're sleep-deprived—makes you feel drowsy.

To make serotonin, your brain needs a supply of the amino acid *tryptophan*. Like tyrosine, tryptophan is found in proteins. But eating more protein won't increase levels of tryptophan inside your brain. In fact, a high-protein diet *depletes* the brain's tryptophan supply.

Reason: Tryptophan must "compete" with tyrosine and other, more plentiful amino acids to enter the brain. It tends to be "crowded out" by them when you eat protein.

To increase the brain's supply of tryptophan, eat carbohydrates—*without protein*. Doing so triggers the release of insulin, which shunts some of the amino acids from the blood to other organs. Tryptophan, however, is left behind in the blood. With less competition from other amino acids, it can easily enter the brain.

BASIC FOOD-MOOD PRESCRIPTION

Because tyrosine and tryptophan can be dangerous when taken in pill form, it's best to use *food* to affect levels of these neurotransmitters.

Caution: The following principles are no substitute for eating a healthful, well-balanced diet. If you have diabetes, hypoglycemia or another diet-related condition, consult a doctor before changing your eating habits.

●**For greater alertness, motivation and mental energy...eat protein.** Just three to four ounces (less than half the size of a typical restaurant entrée) is enough to get tyrosine to the brain so it can be used to make dopamine and norepinephrine.

Best sources of protein: Fish, shellfish, skinless chicken, veal, lean beef and egg whites. Because these foods are essentially pure protein—with little or no fat or carbohydrates—they work especially quickly.

Other good sources: Low-fat dairy products, dried legumes, tofu and other soy products. These contain carbohydrates but are low in fat.

Avoid: Fatty foods, such as pork, lamb, fatty cuts of beef, most hard cheeses and other whole-milk products. High-fat foods divert blood from the brain to the digestive tract. They take a very long time to digest.

●**To relax and focus...eat carbohydrates.** As little as one to one-and-one-half ounces is all most people need. Overweight people and women during the two or three days just prior to menstruation may need up to two-and-one-half ounces.

Eating the carbohydrate without protein is crucial.

Reason: Protein will boost levels of amino acids that compete with tyrosine for entry to the brain. Instead of feeling calmer, you'll feel hyped-up. (If alertness is your goal, eating carbohydrates along with protein usually does not interfere with tyrosine's energizing effect.)

Best sources of carbohydrates: Gumdrops, licorice, marshmallows, jam and other sweets...grain-based foods such as bread, crackers, pasta, rice, popcorn and pretzels... and starchy vegetables such as potatoes.

Fruits and nonstarchy vegetables are not good materials for the brain's serotonin factory. A healthful diet includes plenty of both, but these are not the foods to eat when you need to feel calm or focused.

FOOD-MOOD STRATEGIES AND WEIGHT-LOSS DIET

Dieters often wonder whether these food-mood strategies lead to overeating—and to weight gain. In fact, these strategies are more likely to promote healthful eating...

Reason #1: Very small portions are needed to produce results.

Reason #2: The recommendations call for little or no fat. Not only is fat bad for you, but it also interferes with the food-mood effect.

MEALTIME POWER

For consistent results, use the food-mood principles to plan your meals and time your intake of proteins and carbohydrates...

●**Breakfast.** It should contain protein but little or no fat. *Options:* An orange, eight ounces of low-fat yogurt and a low-fat bran muffin...or cranberry juice and hot cereal with skim milk.

●**Morning snack.** A snack is OK for those who find it hard to eat even a light meal first thing in the morning…and those who eat breakfast so early that they feel hungry by midmorning. It will keep these individuals from coming to lunch so hungry that they overeat and feel sluggish all afternoon. *Good choice:* A small can of grapefruit juice, two rice cakes and one slice of skim-milk mozzarella.

●**Lunch.** It should be high in protein to keep you alert…and low in fat and calories, so you won't have to expend your energy digesting a heavy meal.

Don't *begin* lunch with a carbohydrate. If you have a roll or pasta before the entrée arrives, for example, you'll be sending tryptophan to the brain. That will dull your mental edge. *Instead:* Start your meal with a salad, juice or consommé.

●**Afternoon snack.** Few people need a snack after an energy-boosting lunch—unless they're carbohydrate cravers. For reasons we don't understand, these people start to feel irritable and scattered at midday. A handful of crackers or jelly beans will help them feel calmer and more focused.

●**Dinner.** Make sure it's high in carbohydrates if you want to relax. If you need to keep your energy up for classes or volunteer work, your dinner should be high in protein.

●**Bedtime snack.** If you have trouble unwinding at bedtime, eat one-and-one-half ounces of carbohydrates 30 minutes before retiring. (That's the equivalent of five or six graham crackers.) Make sure the snack is low in fat and protein.

Warm milk at bedtime is a *bad* idea. *Reason:* Milk contains quite a bit of protein, which most people find energizing.

POWER EATING AT CONFERENCES

To avoid the exhaustion that plagues many conference-goers, bring your own light breakfast—or skip breakfast altogether. Avoid heavy coffee-shop meals. Easy choices include a mini-box of fruit juice plus eight ounces of yogurt, or a single-serving box of cereal with low-fat milk and a banana.

If a buffet breakfast is part of the program, skip the hot table, where the high-fat foods are clustered. Instead, stick with fruit, cereals and low-fat muffins. During the coffee break, have coffee or tea, but skip the pastries.

At lunch, don't touch your roll until after you've eaten the protein part of the meal. If the entrée is a large serving, eat only half.

Pack a carbohydrate snack (such as graham crackers or fat-free cookies) in case you need to revive yourself during mid-afternoon presentations.

At dinner, emphasize protein if you need to be "on," carbohydrates if you're ready to unwind—just as you would at home.

Better Pasta Buying

Maggie Riechers, editor, *Healthy Decisions*, Georgetown University Medical Center, 3800 Reservoir Rd., Washington, DC 20007.

Buy pasta packaged in boxes, not in cellophane, and store it in a cupboard—not in glass containers on the counter. *Reason:* Exposure to light quickly robs pasta of much of its riboflavin.

Added Fiber Helps

Bruce Yaffe, MD, an internist and gastroenterologist in private practice, 121 E. 84 St., New York 10028.

Fiber supplements are effective for people who don't get enough fiber in their diets. They improve regularity, as well as firm up the movements of those who suffer from loose stools. People who don't eat enough natural sources of fiber such as fruits and vegetables should consider taking a fiber supplement like Metamucil. Other sources of supplementary fiber are oat bran and Citrucel.

Important: Supplements like Metamucil need to be accompanied by lots of fluid.

Tomatoes and Prostate Cancer Link

Edward Giovannucci, MD, assistant professor of medicine, department of nutrition, Harvard Medical School, Boston. The nine-year study of 47,000 men between the ages of 40 and 75 was published in *The Journal of the National Cancer Institute*.

Eating cooked tomatoes reduces the risk of prostate cancer by 50%.

A study of almost 50,000 men found that those who ate two or more servings of cooked tomato products a week had one-third less risk of developing prostate cancer than those who rarely ate cooked tomato products.

Fact: Approximately 10% of all men develop prostate cancer. Another study found that men who ate 10 or more servings of tomatoes each week benefited from the high content of *lycopene,* an antioxidant. Other antioxidants, such as beta-carotene and Vitamin A, had no effect on the risk of prostate cancer. And cooked tomato products seemed to bring out more lycopene than raw ones.

While tomatoes are the best food source of lycopene, there is a variety of other cancer-fighting foods to include in your diet, such as broccoli, cabbage, soybeans and carrots.

Red Meat and Non-Hodgkin's Lymphoma

Brian C.H. Chiu, MS, a researcher in the department of preventive medicine at the University of Iowa College of Medicine, Iowa City.

Eating red meat increases the risk of developing non-Hodgkin's lymphoma. A study of more than 35,000 women showed that those who ate the most red meat were almost twice as likely as those who ate the least to develop this cancer. Women who ate the most animal fat also had 1½ times the risk of developing the disease as those who ate the least.

Vegetarianism Can Mask Anorexia

David Herzog, MD, director, Harvard Eating Disorder Center, Massachusetts General Hospital, Boston.

People with eating disorders tend to spend a lot of time categorizing foods as "safe" and "unsafe." A vegetarian diet automatically rules out many unsafe foods—particularly the fatty, calorie-rich items.

Key question: Is your diet rigid and socially isolating? Most vegetarians can "get by" when eating in restaurants and at the homes of family and friends. However, eating disorder sufferers tend to withdraw from social situations in which food plays a central role.

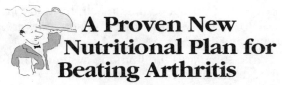 # A Proven New Nutritional Plan for Beating Arthritis

Stephen Sinatra, MD, director of education at Manchester Hospital and a cardiologist in private practice in Manchester, CT. He is author of *Optimum Health*. Lincoln Bradley.

As a cardiologist, I've long used a natural, nutritional approach for prevention and treatment of heart disease.

To my surprise, many of my heart patients have found that my nutritional therapy also helps reduce pain and swelling in their arthritic hands, knees and other joints. This observation led me to review the literature on nutrition and arthritis.

Ultimately, I developed a program of eating guidelines and nutritional supplementation designed specifically to ease the pain and inflammation of arthritic joints. (Of course, these same strategies help reduce the risk of heart disease.)

Follow these guidelines for at least eight weeks, and you'll see a significant reduction in pain and stiffness…

•**Raise your blood pH.** Each day, have a glass of carrot, apple or cherry juice. These juices have an "alkalyzing" effect on the blood.

Avoid orange juice, grapefruit juice and other citrus juices…as well as tomatoes, potatoes, eggplant and other foods from the nightshade family.

These "acidifying" foods lower blood pH. A lower pH promotes formation of crystals in your joints, which leads to arthritis.

●**Eat chlorophyll.** Be sure to drink a glass of green barley, chlorella or frozen wheat grass every day. Each of these is rich in this green pigment.

Chlorophyll helps remove excess heavy metals from the joints. Heavy metal atoms cause accumulation of *free radicals*, highly reactive compounds that damage the joints.

●**Eat cayenne and garlic.** Both herbs have an anti-inflammatory effect, helping to reduce swelling and pain.

I urge my patients to take a daily cayenne capsule. If it upsets your stomach, have it with bread or crackers. If stomach upset is severe, stop taking cayenne.

Garlic stimulates the immune system, which supports healing. Garlic also contains the antioxidant mineral selenium. It helps control free radical buildup.

●**Eat omega-3 oils.** Found primarily in flaxseed and fish oil, omega-3 oils stimulate the production of *leukotrienes*, natural compounds that inhibit inflammation.

I recommend taking one 1,000-milligram (mg) flaxseed oil capsule after each meal. The capsules can be found in any health-food store.

Another way to boost your omega-3 intake is to eat at least one—and preferably two—helpings of fresh fish per week.

●**Drink ginger tea.** In addition to being soothing to the stomach, ginger is a potent anti-inflammatory agent. I recommend one cup a day.

●**Eat Certo.** This pectin-containing gelatin powder, available in any supermarket, is very effective at reducing swelling in the joints.

Each day, consume one tablespoon (mixed with apple juice or another alkalyzing fruit juice to form a soupy gelatin). *Note:* It's unclear why Certo relieves arthritis.

●**Take multivitamin supplements.** A combination of antioxidant nutrients is the best way to fight free radicals.

Although fresh fruit and vegetables are rich in antioxidants, the best way to be sure that you get enough is to supplement your diet with multivitamins.

Be sure to select an iron-free supplement. Too much iron has been linked to an elevated risk of heart disease.

The supplement you select should contain no more than 1 mg copper (half the government's recommended daily allowance).

It should also contain folic acid, vitamin B-6, vitamin D, zinc and calcium—deficiencies in any of these nutrients can cause arthritis.

The supplement should also contain selenium and vitamin E. Both nutrients are especially good for morning stiffness.

●**Take coenzyme Q-10 and quercetin.** I recommend 30 mg of coenzyme Q-10 after each meal and 100 mg to 500 mg of quercetin once a day.

A remarkable substance, coenzyme Q-10 works to stabilize the membrane of every cell in your body. That prevents cell breakdown in your joints.

Quercetin blocks the release of *histamines* (inflammation-producing chemicals) into the bloodstream.

Both supplements are available in health-food stores.

●**Avoid caffeinated beverages**—coffee, tea and soda—as well as chocolate. A diuretic, caffeine washes nutrients out of your body, thereby undermining your efforts to eat a healthful, nutrient-rich diet.

Finish Your Cereal

Richard Wood, PhD, associate professor of nutrition, Tufts University Human Research Center, Boston.

Drink the leftover milk in your cereal bowl. *Reason:* Some of the vitamins and minerals in fortified cereals are dissolved into the milk while you eat.

Nonfat Pancake Recipe

Brand Name Fat-Fighter's Cookbook by Sandra Woodruff, RD, nutrition consultant, Tallahassee, FL. Avery Publishing Group.

Replace each tablespoon of oil in the batter with three-fourths as much nonfat buttermilk, nonfat yogurt, applesauce or mashed banana.

Example: If a recipe calls for two tablespoons of oil, use one-and-a-half tablespoons of your chosen fat substitute. *Also:* Replace each whole egg with three tablespoons of egg white or fat-free egg substitute.

Sparkling Waters May Be Sugary

Environmental Nutrition, 52 Riverside Dr., New York 10024.

Some clear beverages are really sugary soft drinks—but are placed on supermarket shelves near plain bottled waters and fruit-flavored waters.

Self-defense: Read the label to see the calorie content. Water has no calories. Soft drinks can contain 50 or more calories per six-to eight-ounce serving.

Lactose Intolerance

Michael D. Levitt, MD, associate chief of staff for research, Veterans Affairs Medical Center, Minneapolis.

A study suggests that only a fraction of those who think they are lactose intolerant actually are. The others have simply been swayed by widespread publicity about the condition. In a study of 30 people who thought they suffered from lactose intolerance, all were able to consume up to eight ounces of milk daily with negligible problems.

Antioxidants And Fewer Health Problems

Maureen Callahan, MS, RD, of Clearwater, FL, who writes frequently about nutrition and health. She is co-author of *The Miracle Nutrient Cookbook: 100 Delicious Antioxidant-Enriched Recipes and Menu Suggestions for Optimum Health.* Simon & Schuster.

The foods we eat have a big impact on our health—both positively *and* negatively.

Study after study shows that antioxidants—disease-fighting chemicals that occur naturally in many foods—have certain properties that may boost the immune system. They also reduce the risk of health problems—particularly heart disease and cancer.

While the antioxidants beta-carotene, vitamin C and vitamin E are available in supplement form, researchers recommend we try to obtain them naturally through the foods we eat.

ANTIOXIDANT-RICH FOODS

It is most prudent to build a proper diet through a diverse combination of foods. There are several foods that contain all three antioxidants. *They include...*

●**Mangoes.** Mangoes contain 57 milligrams (mg) of vitamin C—almost the full Recommended Daily Allowance (RDA)—as well as ample amounts of vitamin E and beta-carotene. No other tropical fruit provides all three.

●**Sweet potatoes.** They are low in calories and loaded with beta-carotene and vitamins C and E. One to two sweet potatoes—with or without the skin—almost meets the RDA for all three nutrients. Microwaving ensures that you don't lose these nutrients.

OTHER GREAT SOURCES

●**Beta-carotene is commonly found in leafy green plants.** Most health organizations recommend eating at least five fruits or vegetables a day, which amounts to a diet containing 6 mg of beta-carotene.

Beta-carotene is "fat soluble"—meaning that you need to eat a small amount of fat with the beta-carotene in order to absorb it. Scientists have not yet determined the exact amount of fat needed, but it is not a lot. This is one example of how fat in moderation is important to maintain good health.

• **Vitamin C.** The RDA for vitamin C is 60 mg. But researchers say that you need between 100 mg and 500 mg daily to fight off cataracts and other diseases such as cancer and heart disease. *Rich sources...*

• **One papaya** (188 mg).

• **Half a raw red, green or yellow pepper** (170 mg).

• **One cup of broccoli**—steamed or microwaved (98 mg).

• **10 to 12 strawberries** (85 mg).

• **8 ounces of orange juice** (124 mg).

Vitamin C is highly sensitive to heat and cooking. So when cooking vegetables, use a pressure steamer...or lightly steam or microwave.

• **Vitamin E** is one of the most potent antioxidants when it comes to fighting off disease. Studies show that the current RDA for vitamin E —10 mg for men and 8 mg for women—is probably too low to be able to offer much protection against disease. Preliminary studies show that anywhere between 100 mg and 400 mg of vitamin E daily might offer better protection.

Vitamin E is most commonly found in high-fat foods, such as vegetable oils and nuts. But —you don't have to eat a lot of them to reach the RDA.

Examples: One ounce of sunflower seeds (14.2 mg)...or one-quarter cup of wheat germ (4.1 mg)...or two tablespoons of peanut butter (3 mg).

Vitamin E can also be found in some leafy vegetables—and in sweet potatoes.

Although some experts recommend complementing dietary "E" with supplements (contrary to advice regarding other antioxidants), be aware that the synthetic "E" in supplements is not as potent as the form naturally occurring in foods.

A Good-for-You Frozen Treat

The Healthy Gourmet by Cherie Calbom, expert and speaker on diet and nutrition, Lake Ariel, PA. Clarkson Potter Publishers.

Freeze peeled bananas. Coat each in plain low-fat yogurt. Roll the coated bananas in chopped nuts and freeze again.

Cholesterol, Nutrition, Weight...and More

Andrew Weil, MD, director of the Program of Integrative Medicine at the University of Arizona College of Medicine in Tucson and a leading expert on alternative medicine, mind/body interactions and medical botany. Dr. Weil is author of several books, including *Spontaneous Healing* (Knopf) and *Natural Health, Natural Medicine* (Houghton Mifflin).

Our fascination with nutrition and how the foods we eat help or harm us continues to grow. Unfortunately, conventional nutritional science is quite primitive, resulting in considerable confusion even within the medical community.

This confusion exists because the general public and many physicians don't know how to interpret accurately the flood of new research on nutrition.

To help clear up some of the uncertainty, here are the answers to the big questions I'm frequently asked...

What is cholesterol—and what is the difference between "good" and "bad" cholesterol? Cholesterol is a waxlike substance that is needed for the body's normal metabolism. It travels through the blood system in little protein "packages" called *lipoproteins*.

One type of cholesterol is *low-density lipoprotein*—or *LDL*. It is commonly referred to as "bad" cholesterol because it damages the arterial walls. *High-density lipoprotein—or HDL—*is called "good" cholesterol because it appears to protect the arteries from damage.

Your body naturally produces all the cholesterol it needs. This is why you don't need any dietary cholesterol and should avoid foods that raise the cholesterol levels in your blood. If your cholesterol is too high, you are at greater risk of developing coronary artery disease.

What to do: Ask your doctor for your total cholesterol count and how it breaks down into LDL and HDL. Total cholesterol should be less than 180 milligrams per deciliter of blood—but a higher level may be fine if the ratio of HDL to LDL is high. If your total cholesterol level gets low enough—under 140, for example—you may not need to worry at all about the HDL/LDL level.

Exercise has been shown to boost HDL. Alcohol may also raise HDL, but since it has many adverse effects, I don't recommend you start drinking in order to boost your HDL level. If you do drink, opt for red wine and stick with one or two glasses per day.

How can I lower my level of bad cholesterol? Controlling cholesterol has more to do with what you *don't* eat than with what you *do* eat. While some foods help lower cholesterol, no one food will dramatically reduce cholesterol.

What to do: Cut back on saturated fats, which are found in meats, eggs, butter, whole milk and whole-milk products. They are also found in processed foods made with animal fats and in palm and coconut oils. The amount of saturated fat you consume has the most direct dietary influence on how much cholesterol circulates in your blood. Foods that contain cholesterol can boost your blood cholesterol level.

Don't assume that products labeled *cholesterol-free* are harmless. They may contain saturated fats, so read package labels carefully.

Oat bran can lower cholesterol slightly. Other foods and beverages that may be helpful if consumed each day include fruits and vegetables, onions, raw garlic, chili peppers, shiitake mushrooms and Japanese green tea.

How important is fiber…and how much do I need to eat? Fiber is a term for the *indigestible* components of the plant foods we eat. The intestines of people who eat a lot of fiber function better, since fiber increases the bulk and frequency of bowel movements. Constipation is often caused by a lack of fiber.

Studies have shown that adequate fiber intake may also lower the risk of colon cancer and prevent the incidence of irritable bowel syndrome and diverticulitis (inflammation of the intestines).

What to do: The average adult should eat 40 grams of fiber each day—about twice as much as most people consume. You can increase your fiber intake by eating cereals that contain bran. Read labels carefully to make sure the product contains between four and five grams of bran per one-ounce serving. You can also increase your fiber intake by including hearty amounts of fruits, vegetables and whole grains in your diet.

Should I be concerned about the pesticide residues on fruits and vegetables? Yes. Most produce carries traces of pesticides. And the waxes that coat fruits and vegetables (apples, cucumbers, peppers) often contain fungicides, which are toxic and cannot be removed, except by peeling.

What to do: Look for foods labeled *organic* or *pesticide-free.*

Be aware, though, that the term *organic produce* may or may not have any meaning, depending on local laws. In California, Oregon and some other states, produce cannot be labeled organic unless it meets strict criteria. But not all states have stringent guidelines. Ask your store's produce manager if you're unsure. Since pesticide-free produce is more costly, you should know which fruits and vegetables are most likely to be contaminated.

Produce that worries me most: Apples, carrots, celery, grapes (and raisins), green beans, lettuce, oranges, white mushrooms, peaches, peanuts, potatoes, strawberries and wheat flour.

What's the best way to cook vegetables? I prefer steaming or microwaving, which does the least damage to nutrients. Steaming can be used for many foods, including breads, vegetables and fish. Microwave ovens are convenient for thawing and heating as well as for making simple, individual servings. But there's some evidence that microwaving proteins for 10 minutes or more creates new, unnatural forms of proteins that may be harmful.

How can I better control my weight? My advice can be summed up in two words—*eat less*. Since fat is the densest source of calories—nine calories per gram compared with four calories per gram of carbohydrate or protein—the easiest way to consume fewer calories is to cut down on fat and eat more fruits, vegetables and grains.

At the same time, increase your aerobic activity to help burn off calories. As long as you stay on a low-fat diet and exercise for 30 minutes, five days a week, you should not regain the weight you lose.

Better Breakfasts

Brand Name Fat-Fighter's Cookbook by Sandra Woodruff, RD, nutrition consultant, Tallahassee, FL. Avery Publishing Group.

The healthiest breakfast cereals have whole grain listed as the first—and therefore main—ingredient. *Reason:* Whole grains contain essential fatty acids, vitamin E and other important nutrients. Also check the nutrition label for sugar content. A prudent daily sugar limit is 50 grams (four grams equals one teaspoon). Look for low-fat cereals—not necessarily *no-fat* ones.

Creamy Dishes Without Cream

Brand Name Fat-Fighter's Cookbook by Sandra Woodruff, RD, nutrition consultant, Tallahassee, FL. Avery Publishing Group.

Replace the cream called for in the recipe with an equal amount of evaporated skim milk.

Alternative: Replace one cup of heavy cream with one cup of regular skim milk plus one-third cup of instant nonfat dry milk powder. These substitutions work in quiches, sauces, casseroles, custards, puddings and other traditionally high-fat dishes.

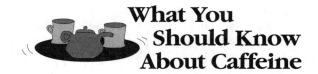

What You Should Know About Caffeine

Timothy McCall, MD, a Boston internist, author of *Examining Your Doctor: A Patient's Guide to Avoiding Harmful Medical Care.* Citadel Press. He is a regular commentator on the public radio program Marketplace, and can be found on the Web at *www.drmccall.com.*

Over the years, conflicting information has been written about the risks of caffeine. Studies have shown that drinking coffee has been tied to pancreatic cancer …high cholesterol…heart attacks…and birth defects.

Reality: The results of these studies have been called into question by health experts. That's because people who drink a lot of coffee tend to have other bad habits as well, such as smoking or not exercising—which may be the culprits.

CAFFEINE AND OSTEOPOROSIS

While caffeine in coffee, tea, cola, chocolate and some medications can cause jitteriness, trembling, irritability and insomnia, studies have not substantiated most of the claims about caffeine's negative *long-term effects.*

Exception: There appears to be a connection between consuming high levels of caffeine and osteoporosis—the thinning of bones that can lead to hip fractures, especially in older women. Risk factors for osteoporosis include being female, thin, white—particularly of Northern European ancestry—or Asian…not exercising…smoking…and having a family history of the disease.

Self-defense: If you are at high risk for developing osteoporosis, you should significantly reduce your caffeine intake and be sure to include enough calcium in your diet. In one study, women who drank at least one glass of milk per day were protected from the bone-thinning consequences of caffeine.

If you can't drink milk, take a calcium supplement. Calcium carbonate, sold in supermarkets, drugstores and health food stores, is an inexpensive and effective source.

Premenopausal women should take 1,200 mg/day…postmenopausal women, 1,500 mg/day. For best absorption, take no more than 500 mg at one time.

CAFFEINE WITHDRAWAL

People who are accustomed to drinking several cups of coffee a day may find that they develop headaches, difficulty concentrating, fatigue and depression if they eliminate caffeine from their diets.

If you decide you want to cut down on caffeine, it's best to do so slowly. Cut back by about 20% a week over a month—or more.

Slowly reducing the amount of caffeine in your system prevents withdrawal reactions. If headaches or other symptoms develop, increase your consumption slightly, then continue to slowly lower it over time.

Liquid Nutritional Supplements Are No Substitute for Real Food

Bonnie Liebman, MS, director of nutrition, Center for Science in the Public Interest, Washington, DC.

Liquid nutritional supplements, including brands such as Boost, Ensure, Resource and Sustacal, were originally created for the infirm and elderly. Today they're being promoted with slick commercials to active seniors as well as healthier, younger people who don't have the time to eat three square meals a day.

Reality: Most supplements contain a mixture of water, oil, sugar, soy, milk protein and added vitamins and minerals. *Better choices:* Fruits and vegetables, whole grain breads, yogurt. These old favorites also contain fiber as well as substances such as phytochemicals, which are believed to help prevent cancer and heart disease.

Distilled Water Is Safe to Drink

Richard P. Maas, PhD, associate professor of environmental studies, University of North Carolina, Asheville.

Distilled water provides an even higher degree of protection than other bottled waters for people with weakened immune systems who need to make extra efforts to avoid the Cryptosporidium parasite.

All About Food Allergies

Thomas Brunoski, MD, a physician in private practice in Westport, CT. Dr. Brunoski specializes in the treatment of medical problems with nutritional and allergy therapy rather than medication.

Every year, hundreds of people suffering from chronic health conditions—headaches, anxiety, asthma, heart disease, arthritis, mood swings and more—come to me for help.

One of the first questions I ask them is, *What do you eat?*

Reason: The most basic fact of our health is food, since every cell of our body comes from what we eat. Many people I see are making efforts to eat well, but their diets seem to betray them.

For many people, unsuspected allergies are present that can cause or aggravate a wide range of problems. If this seems likely, then I run a series of allergy tests to see what foods may be triggering their individual symptoms. Since it is almost impossible for a person to identify offending foods on his/her own, the findings are often surprising—not only to my patients but to me as well.

Once I discover which foods are making a patient sick—or worsening his condition—I'm able to prescribe a diet that can significantly improve that person's health.

The following are stories of just a few patients who have been helped by simply changing their diets.

ASTHMA AND ALLERGIES

A 30-year-old woman with a history of asthma told me her condition was getting worse, even though her doctor had prescribed four strong asthma medications. She had no energy, wheezed all the time and couldn't sleep because her coughing kept her awake. Her doctor told her that she might have to take oral steroid pills, which have unpleasant and harmful side effects.

Solution: First, I urged this woman to cut out all processed sugar. She could eat fruits since they contain fiber. Fiber binds sugar, releasing it over a longer period of time so that the body can digest it more slowly.

I explained that studies done in the 1930s at the Mayo Clinic suggested a link between sugar intake and asthma. These same studies found that a sugar-free diet helped control or even cure asthma in many children. (I also advised her to cut out caffeine, which seems to worsen asthma attacks.)

Because asthma is an allergic condition, I tested her for food allergies and found that she was sensitive to a variety of foods, including beef, milk, eggs, corn, tomatoes, wheat and peanuts.

Result: Within two weeks, the patient had stopped consuming sugar, caffeine and her specific "allergy foods," and she reported that she felt great. She had more energy…her sleeping had improved…and her husband was getting more sleep, too, since she wasn't waking him with her constant coughing.

During the past year, she has stopped using all asthma medications and hasn't had a single attack.

OSTEOARTHRITIS AND ALLERGIES

A middle-aged man came to me six years ago after being diagnosed with osteoarthritis. He suffered from pain in many joints and was taking over-the-counter and prescription pain medications, but his condition was worsening.

Solution: I advised him to cut out all junk food and start eating healthful meals, including salads. If there's such a thing as "miracle food," I'm convinced it is dark green salads—romaine, arugula and red leaf lettuce. These are loaded with vitamins, minerals and disease-fighting nutrients—flavonoids and retinoids.

I also tested him for food allergies and found he was strongly allergic to many things, including soybeans, oranges, potatoes, corn and onions. After following a diet devoid of these items for two months, the patient returned complaining that he felt better but still had pain.

I asked what he had been eating, and he replied, *Lots of chicken and broccoli.* So I did more tests and found that he was highly allergic to both of these foods. Broccoli was quite a surprise to me since I had never heard of anyone who was allergic to it.

Result: He stopped eating broccoli and chicken and started feeling better immediately. He also reported that he had little or no swelling in his joints. If he indulged his passion for these two foods, he felt achy the next day.

Eventually, I treated this man with oral immunotherapy (liquid allergy treatment that is administered under the tongue and that "desensitizes" people to particular foods or other allergens). Now he can eat both chicken and broccoli without trouble.

MIGRAINES AND ALLERGIES

A 27-year-old woman had migraine headaches once or twice a month. The symptoms were severe—extreme pain, nausea, vomiting and visual disturbances. She also felt fatigued much of the time. She mentioned that she had a childhood history of allergies, which is common in migraine patients. But she couldn't pinpoint any headache triggers—such as particular foods that might set off an attack.

Solution: Since sugar and caffeine are well-known migraine triggers, I advised that she eliminate them immediately. She also cut out processed foods since additives, including artificial dyes and preservatives—nitrites and sulfites—can cause a migraine attack. Testing revealed that my patient was allergic to a wide variety of foods. I suggested that she stop eating them as well.

Result: Within four weeks of starting her new diet, she hadn't experienced a single headache. One year later she remains headache-free. And with allergy desensitization, she is now eating the allergy-causing foods again—but no junk.

Spinach Pasta Contains Very Little Spinach

Reported in *University of California at Berkeley Wellness Letter*, Box 412, Prince St. Station, New York 10012.

One cup of cooked spinach pasta contains less than one tablespoon of spinach—which is just enough for color and a hint of flavor. The same is also true for other types of vegetable pastas.

Power Eating... Foods to Make You More Productive

Judith Wurtman, PhD, a research scientist in the department of brain and cognitive science at the Massachusetts Institute of Technology, Cambridge. She is author of *The Serotonin Solution* (Ballantine) and *Managing Your Mind and Mood Through Food* (Rawson Associates).

Whether you're an early bird or a night owl, you can maintain a high level of energy all day by eating the right foods at the right times.

HOW POWER EATING WORKS

Protein foods, such as meats, fish, poultry, dairy products, beans and eggs, contain the amino acid *tyrosine*. This stimulates the brain to produce *norepinephrine* and *dopamine*, two alertness chemicals. When eaten alone or with carbohydrates, such as breads, cereal products, fruits and vegetables, protein foods boost mental alertness and energy.

Never *start* a meal with a carbohydrate if you plan to work after the meal, because it may trigger drowsiness.

Reason: Carbohydrates contain the amino acid *tryptophan*, which triggers production of *serotonin*, a calming chemical.

FOODS THAT ENERGIZE

All low-fat protein foods produce quick mood-modifying and energy-boosting results. For most people, three to four ounces of the following work well...

Low-fat, low-carbohydrate foods, such as shellfish, fish, chicken (without the skin), veal, extra-lean beef, beans and legumes. *Also good:* Low-fat cottage cheese, yogurt, milk or tofu.

WHAT TO EAT

The body's "biological clock" plays a big part in how food energizes us. This clock causes us to feel the most energetic and the least stressed during the first six hours after awakening.

From then on, our energy level slowly decreases until the end of the day—usually within one hour of normal bedtime—when we shut down mentally.

The key to maintaining high performance levels is to eat foods that are energizing when your biological rhythms are beginning to slow down. *Meal guidelines:*

● *Breakfast:* A nutritious breakfast or a snack before noon keeps you from overeating at lunchtime. For maximum results, eat within three hours of awakening.

Best: A breakfast rich in protein foods, high in vitamins and minerals and low in fat.

Example: One piece of fresh fruit sliced (or one-half to three-quarters cup of berries) mixed into eight ounces of plain yogurt...a bran muffin with one or two teaspoonfuls of jelly or diet margarine ...one cup of coffee (black or with skim milk).

● *Lunch:* Your midday meal will either sustain your morning alertness or accelerate the drop in your energy level.

Best for you: A high-protein, low-fat, alcohol-free meal.

Examples: Three to five ounces of meat, poultry, seafood or fish...or eight ounces of low-fat yogurt or cottage cheese...or two ounces of low-fat cheese, such as mozzarella, ricotta or feta...or two eggs. *In addition:* One piece of sliced fruit (or one-half to three-quarters cup of berries) and two slices of whole-grain bread.

Myth: Pasta at lunch increases your mental and physical energy.

Reality: Most athletes load up on pasta before a prolonged endurance event because the body converts it to *glycogen*, which fuels the muscles...not the brain.

● *Dinner:* Your evening meal comes at a time when your biological rhythms are telling your body to shut down. To stay alert for evening projects, eat high-protein, low-carbohydrate foods.

Example: Four to five ounces of skinned, boneless, broiled chicken…one cup stir-fried mixed vegetables (broccoli, water chestnuts, onions, etc.) …three-quarters cup of steamed rice and one fresh orange. Never begin with a carbohydrate—breads, crackers, deep-fried vegetables, etc.

Caffeine alert: Your brain cells are most sensitive to caffeine first thing in the morning. *Recommended:* Limit your daily intake to one or two cups of coffee or tea when you get up (the effects will last up to six hours) and another cup in the middle of the afternoon.

Important: Avoid caffeine after 4:30 pm if it keeps you awake at night. However, if you have to work late or are fighting jet lag, a cup of coffee with dinner may keep you going a little longer.

PREPERFORMANCE EATING

The foods you eat before giving a speech, presentation or other public performance can make or break it…

• **Never perform on an empty stomach.**

• **Eat sparingly**—if possible, two hours before your performance.

• **Choose low-calorie**, low-fat foods.

• **Drink enough coffee or tea** to maintain your body's usual level of caffeine during your performance. *Caution:* If you rarely drink coffee or tea, don't start now. It will only make you more nervous.

• **Drink little or no alcohol**…and do not drink any alcohol in the three hours before your presentation.

Cancer Self-Defense

Ronald Estabrook, PhD, O'Hara professor of biochemistry, University of Texas Southwestern Medical Center, Dallas, who led a study of more than 200 cancer-causing substances found in the diet.

The biggest cancer threats are eating too much fat…and too many calories…and drinking too much alcohol—far greater cancer threats than consuming "cancer-causing" foods.

Reason: Most carcinogens, whether natural or synthetic, are present at levels so low that they pose an insignificant cancer risk.

Self-defense: Eat a varied and balanced diet that includes plenty of fruits and vegetables. This type of diet is not only better for your body but also helps protect against natural carcinogens. And, of course, don't smoke.

Wasted Food Statistics

William Rathje, PhD, professor of anthropology and archeology, University of Arizona, and director of the Garbage Project, which studies landfills, quoted in *The ULS Report*, Box 130116, Ann Arbor, MI.

Households that buy the highest proportion of processed foods also waste the highest percentage of fresh foods…

• **Vegetables make up one-third** of all wasted food.

• **22% are baked goods** and 18% are fruits.

Little-Known Blood Clot Buster

John Folts, PhD, professor of medicine, University of Wisconsin Medical School, Madison. His study of 15 people was published in the *Journal of the American College of Cardiology*, 415 Judah St., San Francisco 94122.

Purple grape juice prevents dangerous blood clots even more effectively than aspirin. *Flavonoids* in the juice reduce platelet "stickiness" by about 40%.

Researchers believe the same benefits can be derived from red wine and other kinds of grape juice—but not from grapes or "grape drink," which isn't 100% juice. The clot-fighting properties of grape juice are especially beneficial for certain heart patients.

Counting Calories

Soren Toubro, MD, associate professor of human nutrition, Royal Veterinary and Agricultural University, Copenhagen.

Counting calories is less effective at keeping weight off than eating a low-fat, high-carbohydrate diet.

Finding: Formerly overweight people who ate such a diet for one year regained less than one pound on average. Similar people who counted calories gained eight pounds. After two years, the calorie-counting group had regained 23 pounds each, those in the low-fat, high-carb group 11 pounds.

The Ultimate Summer Barbecue

Chris Schlesinger, head chef and co-owner of the East Coast Grill in Cambridge, MA. He is coauthor of *The Thrill of the Grill* and *License to Grill.* Morrow.

Come summer, everyone wants to cook out. But with steaks and burgers banned from many barbecues because of their high fat content, is there anything left that's really worth grilling?

Absolutely, says Chris Schlesinger, a Boston-based chef who is noted for his grilling recipes. Poultry, seafood, vegetables and even fruit make great alternatives.

Here are Schlesinger's six rules for healthful grilling. Together, they make for a great cookout.

AVOID CHARCOAL BRIQUETTES

Briquettes contain petroleum-based compounds that can wind up in your food. Lump hardwood charcoal—sold in supermarkets and hardware stores—makes a better choice.

These irregular lumps of pure charcoal are easier to light than briquettes…and they're free of petroleum products.

Gas grills are easy to use, but food cooked over gas just doesn't taste as good as food cooked over hardwood charcoal.

BUILD A TWO-LEVEL FIRE

If you're not careful, grilled food can end up getting burned on the outside and still be raw on the inside. To avoid this, build a fire with a high-heat area for searing…and a low-heat area to continue cooking food through.

Build your fire on one side of the grill. Once the coals are red-hot, use tongs to move a *few* over to the other side. Let food get well-seared before moving it to the "cool" side.

USE A CHIMNEY STARTER

Lighter fluid certainly does the job, but a chimney starter costs less and is just as convenient.

Fill the base of the starter with crumpled newspaper, then place it on the grill's fire grate. That's the *lower* grate, not the one the food touches. Fill the top with charcoal and light the newspaper.

Once the coals are red-hot, spill them onto the fire grate. Use long, fireproof mitts when handling the starter. Reattach the grill (cooking surface). Wait until the coals are covered with gray ash before grilling. Chimney starters can be purchased at hardware stores.

AVOID OIL-BASED MARINADES

Easy-to-make spice "rubs" are tastier than traditional oil-based marinades, and they're fat-free.

All purpose barbecue rub: Mix one-third cup each of freshly cracked black pepper, kosher salt, lightly packed brown sugar, paprika and cumin. Add two tablespoons each of cayenne pepper, ground allspice and ground ginger. Using your hands, rub it onto poultry or seafood before grilling.

USE STEAK SPARINGLY

If you love steak but fear its high fat content, use it as an accompaniment rather than an entrée. For example, add small bits of steak to a salad. Throw in some grilled portobello mushrooms for a texture and flavor so meaty, even confirmed steak lovers find them satisfying.

TOP FOOD WITH SALSA

Salsas are just as tasty as traditional barbecue sauces—*and* much better for you. Try topping grilled chicken or swordfish with a mixture of chopped tomatoes, fresh cilantro and lime juice.

Dangerous Diets

Stephen P. Gullo, PhD, president, Center for Healthful Living, 16 E. 65 St., New York 10021.

Beware of diets that do one or more of the following…

●**Claim weight losses of more than one to two pounds per week.**

●**Promote *miracle* foods** or supplements.

●**Restrict or recommend large quantities of specific foods** to the detriment of a balanced diet.

●**Imply that you can lose weight—and keep it off—without making any lifestyle changes or exercising.**

● **Rely heavily on case histories, testimonials and anecdotes**—but offer no scientific research to back up those claims.

●**Typically promise a "money-back guarantee."**

Simple Dieting Trick

Charles Attwood, MD, a physician in private practice in Crowley, LA, and author of *Dr. Attwood's Low-Fat Prescription for Kids*. Penguin.

Trim fat from your diet by remembering the simple acronym MEDICS.

●**M** is for meat…

●**E** is for eggs…and

●**D** is for dairy products.

Avoid or limit the first two and eat only non-fat versions of the third. And minimize consumption of I, C and S…

●**I** stands for *invisible fat* in nuts, soybeans, olives and vegetable oils.

●**C** is for condiments like ketchup, salad dressings, sauces and gravies.

●**S** is for cookies, candy, chips and other fatty snacks.

If You Need to Use Eggs…

Franca B. Alphin, MPH, RD, LDN, nutrition director, Duke University Diet and Fitness Center, Durham, NC.

To cut cholesterol and fat in recipes calling for eggs, use two egg whites instead of one whole egg. That cuts out all the cholesterol and 5 grams of fat—yet the dish should taste basically the same. If the recipe calls for more than one egg, substitute two egg whites for the first egg and only one egg white for each additional egg.

More About Flavonoids

Paul Knekt, PhD, head of laboratory, National Public Health Institute, Helsinki. His 26-year study of 2,748 men and 2,385 women 30 to 69 years of age was published in the *British Medical Journal*, Tavistock Square, London WCIH 9JR, England.

Fruits, vegetables, red wine and tea are all good sources of these potent antioxidants. Recently, researchers suggested that flavonoid-rich diets cut the risk of heart disease.

Now: Flavonoid-rich diets appear to reduce the death rate from *all* causes. In a study, individuals who ate the most flavonoids had a 25% to 30% lower risk of premature death than those who ate the least.

Arthritic Knee?

Timothy E. McAlindon, MD, MPH, assistant professor of medicine, The Arthritis Center, Boston University Medical Center. His eight-year study of knee pain in 556 participants in the Framingham Study was published in *Annals of Internal Medicine,* Independence Mall West, Sixth St. at Race, Philadelphia 19106.

In a study, individuals who consumed little vitamin D were three times more likely to have worsening of osteoarthritis of the knee than those who ingested high levels of vitamin D. The recommended daily allowance for D is 400 international units. Dairy products, cod liver oil, salmon and sardines are good sources of vitamin D.

Cut Kidney Stone Recurrence

Robert A. Hiatt, MD, PhD, assistant director, division of research, Kaiser Permanente, Oakland, CA. His five-year study of 99 kidney stone patients was published in the *American Journal of Epidemiology,* 2007 E. Monument St., Baltimore 21205.

Doctors have long urged kidney stone patients to adopt a low-protein, high-fiber, high-fluid diet. But a study suggests that the most important thing to do is to drink lots of water—six to 10 eight-ounce glasses a day.

Safer Meat Marinating

Reported in *University of California at Berkeley Wellness Letter,* Box 412, Prince St. Station, New York 10012.

Always marinate meat in the refrigerator rather than at room temperature.

Reason: Leaving the meat out allows bacteria to grow.

Do not put cooked meat back into an uncooked marinade or use it as a sauce unless you heat the marinade to a boil for at least one minute.

Reason: The used marinade could be contaminated by bacteria from the raw meat.

Cut the Fat

Cut the Fat! More than 500 Easy and Enjoyable Ways to Reduce Fat from Every Meal by the American Dietetic Association. HarperPerennial.

Put soups, broths, stews and baked beans in the refrigerator for 30 minutes before opening. Remove the lid, and skim off the solidified fat. This also works with *homemade* soups and stews—chill them and take out the fat that rises to the top.

Proven Diet for Arthritis Pain Relief

James Scala, PhD, a nutrition and health researcher for more than 30 years. Based in Lafayette, CA, he has taught nutrition at universities and medical schools in the US and abroad. He is author of several books, including *The Arthritis Relief Diet.* Plume.

If you have arthritis and think drugs are your only hope, think again. When scrupulously followed, a surprisingly simple diet plan has reduced arthritis symptoms for people all over the world. At least 15 major clinical studies have shown that this dietary approach works effectively.

THROW AWAY YOUR NSAIDS

The study's subjects—most of whom had had arthritis for many years—reduced their use of nonsteroidal anti-inflammatory drugs (NSAIDs), common arthritis medications. That means many, if not most, could stop taking them completely…and all of the subjects could get along with less.

That's pretty spectacular because NSAIDs have potentially severe side effects that get more serious over time. For example, they raise blood pressure and increase the risk of ulcers by about 15%. With long-term use, they can cause harm.

If you go on this diet, your arthritis discomfort should begin to abate within a couple of weeks.

Important: It will be three months before the diet has its full impact.

REBALANCING YOUR BODY'S CHEMICALS

Your goal is to create a better balance between two *prostaglandins* (hormone-like substances that your body cells make) so that you favor the one that reduces inflammation instead of the one that increases it.

The best way to decrease the harmful prostaglandin is with *eicosapentaenoic acid* (EPA). EPA is an omega-3 fatty acid found almost exclusively in the oils of fish and sea animals. Fish is good for you. It provides the most protein for the least number of calories and possesses the most healthful form of fat.

Caution: Most fast-food and frozen cooked fish contain ingredients that counteract the healthful effect by burying it beneath unhealthful deep-fried breading.

In restaurants, order baked, poached or broiled fish. Lemon juice is a tasty butter substitute.

Consume all the omega-3 oils you can. In addition to their inflammation-reducing properties, they also inhibit the development of arterial plaque that leads to heart disease and stroke. *Good sources of omega-3 oils...*

●**Fish...**especially deep-sea cold-water fish. *Excellent:* Salmon, herring, mackerel. *Good:* Bluefish, smelt, tuna and whitefish. If fresh fish are unavailable, eat frozen, canned or farmed fish (catfish, farm-raised rainbow trout, perch, cod and pike).

●**Fish oil supplements...**sold in health food stores and drugstores.

●**Flaxseed oil...**sold at health food stores and grocery stores. This powerhouse oil, which your body converts to EPA, is tasteless, golden yellow and easily added to foods such as hot or cold cereal, salad dressing, tuna salad or juice. One tablespoon or three capsules of flaxseed oil is equivalent to a one-gram EPA capsule.

Goal: Get at least three grams of EPA every day (five is better) in protein-rich fish and in capsules as food supplements.

EATING STRATEGY

●**Eat like a vegetarian—**but without limiting the amount of fish.

●**Chicken (skin removed)** is acceptable in moderation.

●**Venison and rabbit** are OK, but avoid all other meat. If you must indulge—eat low-fat red meat no more than once a month.

●**Cut back on milk and eggs** except for skim milk and egg whites.

●**Seek low-fat protein** from vegetable products such as tofu.

A salmon a day: If you eat just one meal of salmon each day and no meat or animal products, you'll feel better.

Caution: The nightshade plants—tomatoes, potatoes, eggplant and red and green peppers—cause inflammation for many, but not all, people with arthritis. To find out whether nightshades affect you, note in a food diary whenever you eat one nightshade, then don't eat it for three or four days. If you get a reaction in your joints within eight hours, try the food again. Same result? Avoid that food indefinitely.

THE WEIGHT GAME

Losing weight isn't the whole antiarthritis pain story, but it's definitely an issue. Extra body weight makes arthritis worse...not only in weight-bearing body areas, like the hips and knees, but also in common sites like the hands. No one is sure why.

The same is true for inflammatory disease in general, including migraine headaches, Crohn's disease and multiple sclerosis.

VITAMINS, MINERALS, FIBER AND MORE

Take a multivitamin and up to 500 milligrams of vitamin C daily.

Every day, put color on your plate—in the form of red, orange and yellow vegetables.

Certain substances that occur in some foods or are produced by the body, are capable of stimulating an immune response against the membranes in the joints, exacerbating arthritis. To help your body excrete these substances, eat enough fiber to have a bowel movement every 24 to 36 hours.

Excellent sources of fiber: Whole grains, such as bran cereal and whole wheat bread... fruits and vegetables. In addition, it helps to take a powdered fiber supplement, usually made from psyllium seed husks. Be sure to drink a lot of water when taking fiber supplements.

Don't deep-fry...stir-fry instead. When you cook with oil, use olive oil or canola oil. Peanut and soybean oils are acceptable—but not as good. Avoid corn oil—it helps the body make the bad prostaglandin.

TRACKING EVERYTHING YOU EAT

Help your health care practitioner—someone with interest and expertise in nutrition—treat your arthritis with diet. Present the facts in a food diary. Record everything you eat and drink, the amount, the time and why you ate it (main meal, snacking, felt faint, social occasion).

Each morning and evening, describe how your arthritis feels.

Examples: Inflammation, pain, stiff hands, inability to open an applesauce jar.

At night, evaluate whether your diet was balanced that day…whether you ate enough of the right stuff, too little or too much.

Bottom line: We eat an enormous amount of food in our lifetime—one bite at a time. Make each bite work for you, not against you.

Fruit Juice Trap

Barbara A. Dennison, MD, associate professor of clinical pediatrics, College of Physicians and Surgeons, Columbia University, New York City. Her study of 116 two-year-olds and 107 five-year-olds was published in *Pediatrics*, 141 NW Point Rd., Elk Grove Village, IL 60009.

Too much fruit juice can make kids fat. Children who drank more than 12 ounces of fruit juice a day were likely to be fatter and/or shorter than those who drank less.

Theory: Fruit juice is rich in calorie-dense simple sugars like fructose and glucose. Kids should consume no more than two six-ounce glasses of juice per day.

Eat Less Fat… Easy Ways

Men's Health, 33 E. Minor St., Emmaus, PA 18098.

Blot the grease on the top of pizza with a napkin. That will get rid of at least one teaspoon of fat.

●**Leave the last half-inch of take-out Chinese food in the container** so that you'll eat less sauce.

●**Make mashed potatoes with buttermilk**— or skim milk and butter-flavored seasoning— instead of using butter and whole milk.

●**Sauté meat and vegetables in fruit juice** or Worcestershire sauce instead of oil.

●**Do not drink alcohol on an empty stomach.** Alcohol increases food cravings and can trigger a high-calorie binge.

Other Calcium Sources

Barbara S. Levine, RD, PhD, director, Calcium Information Center, New York Hospital–Cornell Medical Center, New York City.

Broccoli, kale, bok choy and other leafy greens are calcium-rich…as are canned sardines and calcium-fortified orange juice, tofu and soy milk. If you worry about your calcium intake, ask your doctor about taking a daily calcium supplement.

Heartburn or Not?

M. Michael Wolfe, MD, chief of gastroenterology at Boston University and Boston Medical Center, and author of *The Fire Inside*. W.W. Norton.

Occasional mild heartburn in response to spicy foods is normal. But if you continuously suffer from heartburn more than two or three times a week or if it causes acute discomfort, you should consult a physician. This burning sensation, caused by acid that flows back from the stomach, can be associated with other symptoms, such as difficulty swallowing, crushing chest pain or hoarseness. These symptoms can indicate more serious medical problems such as asthma…or even esophageal cancer.

Ales, Beer and Alcohol

Nick Funnell, head brewer, Great American Restaurants, Centreville, VA.

Mild ales have less alcohol than normal beer, but more beer taste than nonalcoholic beers. Mild ales contain about 3% alcohol. Regular beer contains nearly 5%. Labels do not always point the way to less alcohol. Light beer is usually lower in calories but not much lower in alcohol content. Dark-colored beers may have stronger flavor than regular beers but not necessarily more alcohol.

Healthy Cheese Cooking

Skinny Italian Cooking by Ruth Glick, recipe developer and member of the International Association of Cooking Professionals, Columbia, MD. Surrey Books.

For healthier cooking with cheese, substitute low-fat varieties—and cut back the amount used. Use shredded mozzarella instead of sliced—it goes further—or sprinkle cheese on top of a dish instead of mixing it in. *Fresh-grated* Parmesan has a distinctive taste, so a little goes a long way—one-quarter cup has only seven grams of fat.

Medication Trap

Jerry Avorn, MD, associate professor of medicine, Harvard Medical School, Boston. His study of 3,500 New Jersey Medicaid recipients was published in the *American Journal of Medicine*, 105 Raiders Ln., Belle Mead, NJ 08502.

Stiffness, tremors and other symptoms attributed to Parkinson's disease may actually be side effects of drugs used to treat dementia, psychiatric problems or gastrointestinal complaints.

Danger: Doctors who fail to recognize this may prescribe *additional* medication to control the symptoms. The new drug may exacerbate tremors—and produce hallucinations and/or psychosis.

Self-defense: Before a new drug is prescribed for anyone with Parkinson's-type symptoms, the doctor should take him/her off the initial drug to see if the symptoms subside.

More Fat-Free Food Traps

Martin Katahn, PhD, professor emeritus, Vanderbilt University, and Lee Fleshod, PhD, former director of Nutritional Services, Tennessee Department of Public Health.

Makers of fat-free foods often compensate for the lack of flavor by adding extra sugar—boosting total calories significantly.

The extra calories from sugar can both add to your weight and increase the level of triglycerides in your blood, which raise the risk of heart disease.

Also: Independent analyses of "fat-free" foods often find fat content far in excess of what can legally be labeled "fat free."

Treatments for Nail Fungus

Mary Ellen Brademas, MD, clinical professor of dermatology, New York University Medical Center, New York.

Infected fingernails and toenails can be cleared up faster and better with two types of oral medication. Much more effective than creams, these prescription drugs—*Lamisil* and *Sporanox*—are incorporated into the nail bed and kill the fungus as the nail grows out.

Reducing Heart Attack Risk

Martha L. Daviglus, MD, PhD, assistant professor of preventive medicine at Northwestern University Medical School, Chicago. Her study was published in *The New England Journal of Medicine,* 10 Shattuck St., Boston 02115.

Eating just a small amount of fish may significantly reduce your chance of having a heart attack. A 30-year study of more than 1,800 men found that those who ate as little as seven ounces of fish a week had a 40% lower risk of fatal heart attack than those who ate no fish. Researchers believe that all kinds of fish are beneficial, including canned tuna and salmon. They advise people who wish to avoid heart disease to have at least two servings of fish a week in their diets.

Hidden Allergies...
How to Identify
The Causes

Janice M. Joneja, PhD, director of the allergy nutrition program at Vancouver Hospital and Health Sciences Centre in Vancouver, British Columbia. She is author of the medical textbook *Managing Food Allergy & Intolerance: A Practical Guide* (McQuaid) and coauthor of *Understanding Allergy, Sensitivity and Immunity* (Rutgers).

Ever had a rash, stomach problem or respiratory ailment that defied diagnosis? You might have been suffering from a hidden food reaction.

Up to 1% of adults and 7% of children under age five have at least one food *allergy*—an abnormal immune system response triggered by exposure to "foreign" proteins.

Food allergies can produce severe symptoms. Severe cases can lead to anaphylactic shock.*

Leading causes of food allergy: Fish (including shellfish)...cow's milk...eggs...wheat (including bread and pasta)...peanuts...tomatoes...spinach...strawberries...raspberries... oranges...mangoes.

It's estimated that 5% to 50% of all adults suffer from a related problem called food *intolerance*. This adverse reaction does *not* involve the immune system—but it produces similar symptoms.

Many cases of food intolerance are caused by a lack of one or more digestive enzymes. This deficiency impairs the body's ability to break down certain proteins in food.

Leading causes of food intolerance: Lactose ...sulfites...artificial colors...food additives like *monosodium glutamate*...histamines (compounds in fermented foods like cheese, sauerkraut, alcoholic beverages and vinegar)... *tyramine* (an amino acid in aged cheeses, yeast extract, wine, beer, raspberries and bananas) ...and food preservatives like *benzoic acid* and *sodium benzoate*.

*A potentially deadly condition marked by a drop in blood pressure, anxiety, reddening and swelling of the face, sometimes hives, tightness in chest and throat, difficulty breathing. Anyone experiencing these symptoms needs immediate medical attention.

PINPOINTING FOOD REACTION

Food allergies and intolerances manifest themselves differently in different people. A food that might give one person a rash might give another stomach pain.

Predictably, doctors often have a hard time pinpointing the trouble. Misdiagnoses are very common.

If you suspect certain foods are making you ill, ask your doctor to refer you to a food-allergy specialist—someone experienced in the use of the "elimination and challenge diet."

This diet—the only surefire way to pinpoint food reactions—has two phases. During the four-week *elimination* phase, all suspect foods are off limits. Symptoms often begin to clear up during this phase.

During the ensuing *challenge* phase, lasting a few weeks to a few months, suspect foods are reintroduced one at a time. The patient watches carefully to see if symptoms return.

Here are four case histories illustrating the most common—and commonly overlooked— food allergies and intolerances...

CASE HISTORY #1

Jack, a 48-year-old salesman, had a long history of headaches, bloating, gas and abdominal pain. His symptoms usually began an hour or so after breakfast and lasted all day. He also complained of constant fatigue and was having difficulty concentrating.

Jack exhibited no signs of gastrointestinal disease and had regular bowel movements. He went on a diet that excluded wheat, rye, oats, barley, corn and milk products. (He took an 800-mg calcium supplement to make up for the lost calcium.) In addition, he ate no raw fruit or vegetables—only cooked or canned were permitted—and no whole nuts or seeds.

After four weeks, Jack was "challenged" with each of the above foods. It turned out he was allergic to wheat, raw fruits and vegetables and highly fermented foods (cheese, wines, beer).

Now that Jack avoids these foods, his symptoms have abated. His energy has increased threefold, he says.

CASE HISTORY #2

Mary, a 50-year-old nurse, was troubled by constipation, mood swings and leg cramps. She was also concerned about the poor condition of her nails and teeth.

She was taking a variety of medications—including herbal supplements and an anti-depressant. Nothing seemed to help.

Mary's symptoms suggested an intolerance or allergy to several *different* foods. Indeed, an elimination diet revealed allergies to food additives, wheat and dairy products.

After giving up these foods for three months, her physical and emotional health improved. Within six months Mary was no longer constipated. She felt better than she had in 10 years.

CASE HISTORY #3

A 62-year-old telephone company employee named Virginia had a history of asthma and hay fever dating back to childhood. She was also bothered by stomach upset, flaky skin on her hands and feet...and a dangerously elevated cholesterol level.

Though she had been on a restricted diet, Virginia couldn't shake her symptoms. Then a series of elimination and challenge tests revealed sensitivity to certain nuts and seeds, wheat and and dairy products.

Within months of giving up these foods, Virginia's symptoms had disappeared, and her cholesterol level had fallen to normal.

CASE HISTORY #4

Rita, a 56-year-old computer worker, was plagued by diarrhea, gas and abdominal pain. She'd had these problems since childhood, but they had intensified over the past year.

When a thorough exam revealed no underlying illness, Rita was put on a diet that excluded grains, starches and sugar.

In the next four weeks, she reported only two episodes of diarrhea—and each occurred after she cheated on her diet. Subsequent challenges showed that she was affected adversely by foods containing refined sugar.

Having given up these foods permanently, Rita is now completely free of symptoms.

Diet and Alzheimer's Connection

William B. Grant, PhD, senior research scientist, NASA Langley Research Center, Hampton, Virginia.

High-fat diets may increase the risk of developing Alzheimer's disease. While this form of dementia has long been blamed on genetic factors, an analysis of dietary patterns around the world suggests that dietary fat may also play a role. *What the analysis found:* 5% of Americans over age 65 develop Alzheimer's. But Alzheimer's strikes only 1% of people over age 65 in China and Nigeria, where typical diets contain much less fat.

 # Social Drinking Facts

Jeff Cameron, MEd, an alcohol counselor with the early-intervention program DrinkWise, 157 Delhi St., Guelph, Ontario, Canada N1E 4J3.

Social drinkers average no more than 12 drinks a week...and no more than four drinks a day for men, three for women. Drinking more than that increases your risk of trouble. One drink equals one 12-ounce beer, five ounces of wine, 1½ ounces of spirits or three ounces of fortified wine.

To moderate your drinking: Abstain for at least two days each week. Doing so helps you think about your drinking and avoid habitual patterns. *Pace yourself.* Having more than one drink an hour raises your risk of becoming drunk. *Trace cause and effect.* What triggers your drinking? A visit from a friend? Watching sports? Plan strategies to drink less or not at all.

The Rest of the Story About Diet and Cancer…Fat vs. Fiber… And the Best Sources Of Cancer-Fighting Phytonutrients

Keith I. Block, MD, research assistant professor of medical dietetics and nutrition at the University of Illinois, and medical director of The Cancer Institute at Edgewater Medical Center, both in Chicago.

Despite our nation's 30-year "war" on cancer, the US cancer rate keeps rising. Overall, the odds that you'll die of cancer are 6% *higher* today than they were in 1970, according to one estimate published in *The New England Journal of Medicine.*

Good news: Eating the right foods sharply lowers your cancer risk. That's true if you are cancer-free…or if you have had cancer and are trying to avoid a recurrence.

Consider people in China and other countries whose typical eating habits are healthier than ours. They have *far* less breast, ovarian, prostate and colon cancers.

DIETARY FAT AND CANCER

If you're like the average American, roughly 40% of your daily caloric intake is in the form of fat.

But your risk of developing cancer (or having a recurrence) climbs four- to eightfold for each additional 10 percentage points of calories that come from fat.

Example: If you eat a 30% fat diet, your cancer risk is up to eight times higher than if you were to consume a 20% fat diet.

To keep your cancer risk low, fat should account for no more than 15% of your calories. The fats you do consume should be monounsaturated or polyunsaturated. Good sources of such fats include salmon, cod, canola oil, olive oil and flaxseed oil.

Saturated fats—like those found in meats, whole milk products and palm kernel oils—should be avoided. Saturated fats weaken the immune system, letting tumors flourish.

THE IMPORTANCE OF FIBER

A diet high in fiber—the indigestible part of grains, fruits and vegetables—reduces your risk of developing cancer, especially colon cancer.

In Sweden, cancer rates are low despite the fact that most Swedes eat a high-fat diet. Researchers theorize that their consumption of rye bread, which is rich in fiber, protects them.

How much fiber should you eat? Twenty-five grams a day is good, but 40 grams is ideal. Be sure to eat both *insoluble* fiber (the kind in whole wheat products) as well as *soluble* fiber (like that found in oat bran).

To make sure that you get enough fiber, your daily diet should include…

• **Two to three cups of whole-grain foods** —breads, brown rice, oat products, high-fiber cereal, etc.

• **One-and-one-half cups of beans and other legumes.**

• **Four to five cups of fresh vegetables**, including leafy greens, cruciferous vegetables, root vegetables and fruits.

Avoid candy, cakes and other sweets that contain refined sugar. Refined sugar can suppress the immune system, leaving you vulnerable to cancer.

CANCER-FIGHTING FOODS

Virtually all forms of produce are good for you, but certain fruits, vegetables and grains have special cancer-prevention powers. They're rich in *phytonutrients*, compounds that have been shown to deactivate carcinogens and even shrink tumors.

Your diet should stress these phytonutrient-dense foods…

• **Cruciferous vegetables.** Broccoli, cauliflower, cabbage and brussels sprouts contain *indole-3 carbinol* and *sulforaphane*, compounds that regulate hormone levels in such a way as to lower the risk for breast cancer.

These compounds also help protect cellular DNA against attack by carcinogens, including those in tobacco smoke.

• **Citrus fruits.** Oranges, grapefruit, lemons and limes contain more than 50 different phytonutrients. These include *flavonoids*, which block carcinogens from getting inside cells.

• **Currants, blackberries, apples, grapes and plums.** These fruits contain *saponins* and *quercetin*. These flavonoids help neutralize carcinogens, inhibit tumor growth and protect cells against attack by *free radicals*—renegade molecules produced during normal metabolism that can turn cells malignant.

• **Yellow, red and dark-green vegetables.** They contain *carotenoids*, which protect cells against oxidation and break down cancer-causing chemicals.

Tomatoes are an especially rich source of phytonutrients, including *lycopene*, *glutamic acid* and *turmeric acid*. These compounds block the formation of cancer-causing *nitrosamines*, protecting against stomach cancer and prostate cancer.

• **Garlic, onions, leeks and shallots.** By increasing the activity of immune system cells called *natural-killer cells*, these foods help destroy tumor cells.

One-two punch: After carotenoid-rich vegetables break down carcinogens, garlic, onions, etc., flush them from the body.

• **Soy foods.** In addition to saponins, foods made from soybeans contain the isoflavone *genistein*, a phytochemical that tempers cells' response to cancer-promoting hormones.

Soy consumption has been linked to reduced rates of breast, colon and prostate cancer.

Substitute soy milk and soy cheese for dairy products. A fermented soy product called *tempeh* is high in protein and particularly rich in genistein. Its meaty texture makes it great for casseroles and vegetable stir-frys.

• **Mushrooms.** Shiitakes and reishis, popular in Chinese cooking, contain *beta-glucan* and other immunity-boosting phytochemicals.

• **Sea vegetables.** Dark-green seaweeds like *kombu* and *wakame* are chockablock with trace elements that keep the immune system strong. They also contain "chelating agents," which remove toxins from the body.

• **Green tea.** This traditional Japanese beverage inhibits formation of nitrosamines, prevents genetic mutations and blocks the creation of tumors.

• **Turmeric.** This spice, found in curries, contains a powerful antioxidant called *curcumin*. It has been linked to lower rates of colon cancer.

Best Low-Fat Nut

Leslie Bonci, RD, nutritionist, Allegheny General Hospital, Pittsburgh.

Chestnuts have less fat than any other kind of nut. One ounce of dry-roasted chestnuts contains less than 1 gram (g) of total fat, less than 1 g of saturated fat and 70 calories (8% of which are from fat). An ounce of dry-roasted cashews—the second least-fatty nut—has 13 g of total fat, 3 g of saturated fat and 163 calories (72% of those from fat). *Other nuts, in order of increasing fat content:* Peanuts, almonds, pistachios, walnuts, pecans, hazelnuts (filberts), brazil nuts and macadamias.

Your Diet and Your Immune System

Elinor Levy, PhD, associate professor of microbiology at Boston University School of Medicine. She is coauthor of *The 10 Best Tools to Boost Your Immune System.* Houghton Mifflin.

For you to stay healthy—and to recover quickly from illness—your immune system must be healthy, too.

What can you do to optimize immune function? Exercise and stress reduction help. But evidence suggests that the most important contributor to immune function is what you eat.

THE ANTIOXIDANT SHIELD

By now, you have probably heard about free radicals. These ubiquitous molecules cause cells to break down, speeding the aging process, promoting heart disease and cancer and weakening the immune system.

There's no way to avoid free radicals. They're produced within the body as a result of normal metabolic processes. *But certain antioxidant compounds destroy free radicals…*

●**Vitamin E.** This potent antioxidant forestalls the gradual decline in immune function brought on by aging. It boosts synthesis of antibodies and encourages reproduction of key infection-fighting cells called *lymphocytes.*

People who take vitamin E supplements mount a stronger immune reaction against invading viruses and bacteria. They also enjoy a reduced risk for cancer.

Good sources of vitamin E include whole grains, seeds and vegetable oils. Since it's impossible to get enough E for full protection against free radicals from dietary sources, I tell my patients to take a daily supplement containing 200 international units (IU) of vitamin E.

●**Carotenoids.** These antioxidants increase the numbers of lymphocytes and natural-killer cells. Supplements are available, but the best sources are fruits and vegetables—especially carrots, kale, tomatoes and cantaloupes.

●**Vitamin C.** It energizes the immune system to react more vigorously to cancer cells and microbes. Diets rich in vitamin C have been linked to reduced risk for breast, colorectal and prostate cancer.

The optimal intake of vitamin C is 200 milligrams (mg) a day. You can get more than enough through your diet. Good sources of vitamin C include citrus fruits, cantaloupes and green peppers.

Caution: Larger doses can cause stomach trouble, kidney stones and—in some people—problems with iron metabolism.

MINERALS

Minerals are needed for the synthesis of proteins, which are key components of all cells and enzymes in the body…

●**Zinc.** The most important mineral for immune function, zinc boosts the number of lymphocytes and helps natural-killer cells attack cancer cells.

The average person needs 15 mg of zinc a day. Higher dosages seem to impair immune function.

One serving of fortified cereal (check labels) provides all the zinc you need. Meats (especially cooked oysters) and whole grains are also good sources. Zinc supplements generally are *not* necessary.

●**Iron.** An iron *deficiency* increases infection risk by weakening many different types of immune cells. Too *much* iron impairs immune function, too.

Women of childbearing age need 15 mg of iron a day. Men need 10 mg. Meats, beans and tofu are good sources.

Iron pills are a good idea *only* if a doctor has found you to be iron-deficient.

●**Selenium.** This mineral encourages growth of immune cells and stimulates production of antibodies.

Grains, nuts, seeds and fish are good sources of selenium. Because too much selenium can cause digestive and neurological problems, supplements generally are *not* a good idea.

LOW-FAT DIET

Excess dietary fat impairs your cells' ability to recognize viruses and bacteria, crippling your immune response. Even a diet that's *moderately* high in fat (41% of calories) *halves* the cancer-killing ability of immune cells.

Self-defense: Limit your intake of all fats to 25% of your total caloric intake. For most people, this means 44 grams (g) to 55 g of fat a day.

Avoid whole milk (8 g fat per eight ounces) …margarine (11 g per tablespoon)…fatty meat (14 g in three ounces of lean ground beef)… and nuts (18 g per ounce of pecans).

IMMUNITY BOOSTERS

Research is beginning to confirm what traditional healers have long known—that certain foods and herbs boost immune function…

●**Shiitake mushrooms.** Studies in Japan show that these mushrooms boost immune function and inhibit viral multiplication. In Japan, a shiitake derivative called lentinan is used as a cancer-fighting drug.

Shiitakes are tasty in soups, stews and vegetable dishes. Eat two to six shiitakes a week.

●**Reishi mushrooms.** These Chinese mushrooms boost reproduction of lymphocytes and trigger production of chemical "messengers" that coordinate immune system activity. Eat two to four reishis per week.

237

●**Garlic.** Garlic is a good source of selenium and of certain compounds with anti-infection and anticancer properties.

Season food with garlic at least three times a week.

●**Echinacea.** This popular herb boosts the ability of immune cells to swallow up cells infected with viruses...and stimulates production of compounds that coordinate the immune system's response against yeast infections.

Echinacea extract should be taken for no more than three days in a row—when you have a cold or flu, or feel one coming on. The usual dose is 30 drops of echinacea tincture, twice a day.

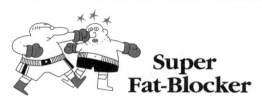

Super Fat-Blocker

Arnold Fox, MD, an internist and cardiologist in private practice in Beverly Hills, CA. He is coauthor of *The Fat Blocker Diet: The Revolutionary Discovery that Lowers Cholesterol, Reduces Fat, and Controls Weight Naturally.* St. Martin's.

In my 40 years of practicing medicine, I've seen every kind of diet aid you can imagine. But when it comes to producing lasting weight loss, I've never seen anything like *chitosan* (KITE-o-san).

This natural food supplement—made from the shells of lobsters—forms a gel in the stomach. This gel bonds with any fats that are present, forming fatty "clumps" that are indigestible. These clumps pass out of the body in the feces.

Animal studies have shown that chitosan taken before a meal blocks absorption of up to 50% of consumed fat.

One double-blind study in Italy found that people who ate a low-fat diet and used chitosan lost an average of 16 pounds ...compared with seven pounds for those who followed a low-fat diet without chitosan.

I usually tell my overweight patients to set a target weight, then take 1,000 milligrams (mg) of chitosan 30 minutes before eating lunch and dinner. Once the goal is reached, they can stop taking the chitosan.

Taking chitosan does *not* give you permission to eat whatever you want. But it will give you an extra push in the right direction.

There's no evidence that chitosan causes any side effects—but consult your doctor before trying it just to be safe, especially if you're taking any other medications.

Caution: Avoid chitosan if you're allergic to shellfish, or are pregnant or breast-feeding. Don't take vitamins A, D or E within four hours of taking chitosan. If you do, the health benefits of these vitamins will be lost.

Chitosan pills are available at most drugstores.

Anticholesterol Supplement

James W. Anderson, MD, professor of medicine and clinical nutrition, University of Kentucky, Lexington. His study of cholesterol levels in 248 men and women was reported at a meeting of the American Academy of Family Physicians.

Anyone with elevated cholesterol levels should ask a doctor about taking Metamucil or another supplement containing the bulking agent *psyllium*. *Finding:* Total cholesterol levels of volunteers who added 5 grams (g) (one heaping teaspoon twice daily) of psyllium to their daily diets fell 4.7% after 24 to 26 weeks. LDL (bad) cholesterol levels fell 6.7%. *Bonus:* Psyllium fights constipation. *Caution:* Psyllium should not be considered a substitute for cholesterol-lowering medication.

Which Fruit Contains The Most Antioxidants?

Ronald L. Prior, PhD, scientific program officer, US Department of Agriculture Human Nutrition Research Center on Aging at Tufts University, Boston.

Ounce for ounce, blueberries contain more of these disease-fighting compounds than any other fruit or vegetable.

Other rich sources of antioxidants: Concord grape juice, kale, strawberries and spinach.

12

Vitamins and Minerals Savvy

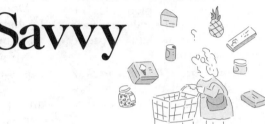

All You Ever Really Wanted to Know…Almost…About Vitamins and Minerals

Jeffrey Blumberg, PhD
Tufts University

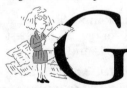

Given the many conflicting vitamin studies, it's easy to see why so many people are confused about which supplements to take and, of course, which ones to avoid.

To clear up the confusion, we spoke with Dr. Jeffrey Blumberg of Tufts University…

Does beta-carotene prevent cancer…or cause it? The body converts beta-carotene into vitamin A. But beta-carotene is also an antioxidant—which neutralizes "free radicals" in your blood. Left unchecked, these highly reactive compounds can damage tissues and cells and possibly lead to diseases such as cancer.

More than 200 studies suggest that beta-carotene does indeed play a role in *preventing cancer*. A Chinese study of 30,000 people showed a significant decrease in the incidence of cancer and mortality in those who took a combination of beta-carotene, vitamin E and selenium.

Conflict arose with the release of three major studies that contradicted established results…

● **Two widely reported studies** found that taking supplements of beta-carotene in the 30-to-50-milligram (mg) range may increase the risk of lung cancer. What wasn't mentioned in detail by the media was that those who developed cancer were heavy smokers, heavy drinkers and/or asbestos workers.

● **The other major trial** tracked 22,000 doctors and found that those taking 50 mg of

Jeffrey Blumberg, PhD, professor and chief of the Antioxidants Research Laboratory at Tufts University, Boston, one of the country's most prestigious schools for the study of health and nutrition. Dr. Blumberg is a leading vitamin supplement expert and has served on several national health advisory committees.

beta-carotene every other day for 12 years had no increased risk of cancer—but no decrease either.

However, this study tracked men in the highest socioeconomic group in the US—physicians who had full access to health care and were more likely than the average person to have healthy lifestyles. Evidence suggests a potentially modest effect of beta-carotene, which is unlikely to be readily found in a low-risk group.

Strategy: Because we are not certain whether large doses of beta-carotene increase the risk of lung cancer in smokers or heavy drinkers (those who have more than two drinks per day), people who smoke and/or drink heavily should avoid beta-carotene supplements. But nonsmokers who do not drink heavily can take between 10 mg and 20 mg of beta-carotene daily to reduce their risk of cancer.

Do iron supplements cause heart attacks?
One Finnish study showed a correlation between iron intake and increased risk of cardiovascular disease in older adults.

Reality: Several subsequent studies—most of which were conducted in the US—found absolutely no link between iron intake and heart disease.

Strategy: People age 50 or older who take a vitamin/mineral supplement containing the Recommended Daily Allowance (RDA) of iron —10 mg—need not worry that this minimal amount will trigger a heart attack.

Because people over age 50 do not need large amounts of iron anyway, it is best to steer clear of high-dose iron supplements—such as those containing more than 25 mg, which are wrongly promoted as "energizers" for the 50-plus crowd.

Women who are premenopausal should take 15 mg of iron per day…adult men should take 10 mg of iron per day.

Is folic acid only a must for pregnant women?
When taken during the weeks before conception and the first two months of pregnancy, folic acid helps prevent neural tube problems and other birth defects.

But folic acid is an important supplement for everyone. A major study suggested that folic acid might prevent more than 50,000 deaths from cardiovascular disease each year in adults.

Folic acid lowers blood levels of a toxic amino acid called *homocysteine*, which is produced in the normal course of cell metabolism. High levels of homocysteine significantly raise the risk of heart attack and stroke.

Folic acid may also protect against colon cancer.

Strategy: All adults need to consume 400 micrograms (mcg) of folic acid daily. Spinach and dark leafy lettuces, such as romaine, are good sources…but you would have to eat about two cups of spinach a day to get your 400 mcg.

Alternative: A multivitamin supplement containing 400 mcg of folic acid.

Does vitamin E prevent serious diseases?
Probably not at the current US RDA level—which is 30 international units (IU).

Numerous studies link considerably higher doses of vitamin E to a decreased risk of cardiovascular disease…some forms of cancer…and cataracts and macular degeneration.

Preliminary research also indicates that vitamin E may slow the progression of neurological diseases, such as Parkinson's and Alzheimer's.

A British study of 2,000 people who had suffered heart attacks found that those who took 400 IU or 800 IU of vitamin E daily for a two-year period had a 77% reduction in the incidence of a second attack.

Strategy: There is little risk in taking vitamin E—and there is much evidence that it prevents disease. Supplements between 100 IU and 400 IU daily are advisable.

Why supplements? It's almost impossible to get enough vitamin E from a low-fat diet. The richest dietary sources are vegetable oils and nuts.

Is it true that calcium is the most important dietary factor in preventing osteoporosis?
Almost every major health organization recommends that people get their RDAs of calcium. This mineral helps prevent osteoporosis and may reduce the risk of colon cancer and hypertension.

The problem is that calcium absorption depends on adequate levels of vitamin D in the body. The body manufactures vitamin D when it is exposed to sunlight. Vitamin D is also found in fortified milk and multivitamins.

As you age, your body becomes less able to manufacture vitamin D. About 80% of women over age 60—and almost as many older men—get less than two-thirds of the RDA of this nutrient.

Strategy: Make sure you get your daily dietary requirement of calcium—1,200 mg to 1,500 mg per day.

For those age 60 or older, a 400-IU vitamin D supplement daily is advisable.

Does vitamin C prevent colds? While there is no sound evidence that vitamin C *prevents* colds, some studies show that daily 1,000-mg to 2,000-mg supplements can *lessen* the severity and duration of colds. That's because vitamin C has an antihistamine effect.

In addition, numerous studies link a lower daily intake of vitamin C to a decreased risk of some forms of cancer and heart and eye disease.

Strategy: A National Institutes of Health study suggests the current RDA of 60 mg of vitamin C is far too low—and that doses of 200 mg may be closer to our actual daily requirement for optimal health.

To lower your risk of serious diseases, consume between 250 mg and 1,000 mg daily in food or supplement form.

Do chromium supplements aid in weight loss? Health food manufacturers claim that this trace mineral helps body-builders bulk up and the overweight shed pounds. The evidence for both claims, however, is weak.

Emerging research suggests that chromium may be an important player in the prevention of one of this nation's top killers—adult-onset or Type II diabetes—since chromium helps regulate glucose (sugar) levels.

Strategy: For people who are at risk for adult-onset diabetes because it runs in their families, studies suggest a 200-mcg chromium supplement daily. The average adult consumes only 25 mcg to 30 mcg a day, which may not be enough to ward off diabetes if you're at risk.

Important: Taking nutritional supplements can have health benefits, but too much of any nutrient can be dangerous to your health. Be sure not to exceed suggested dosages and to discuss any supplements with your doctor.

Which Mineral Supplements Should You Take?

Timothy McCall, MD, a Boston internist, author of *Examining Your Doctor: A Patient's Guide to Avoiding Harmful Medical Care.* Citadel Press. He is a regular commentator on the public radio program Marketplace, and can be found on the Web at *www.drmccall.com.*

Minerals—iron, calcium, chromium, zinc, etc.—are vital components of a healthful diet. But claims made about their health benefits extend far beyond the evidence. As with vitamins, it's important to remember the distinction between taking mineral supplements to prevent or treat dietary deficiencies and taking them in higher doses in an effort to improve health in other ways.

There's been a great deal of controversy over *chromium picolinate*. This dietary supplement has become very popular with body-builders and with people involved in weight-loss programs. But despite all the hoopla, there is little evidence that chromium picolinate is effective for these uses.

A study has raised questions about chromium picolinate's *safety*. When scientists exposed cells taken from the ovary of a hamster to high concentrations of chromium picolinate, they found that it caused severe chromosomal damage. This raised the possibility that the mineral supplement might be carcinogenic.

The industry that manufactures the supplement responded to this study within days, criticizing how the study was done and claiming that, when taken at the recommended dose, chromium supplements are completely safe. You have to wonder, though, if these critics might be more concerned with protecting their profit margins than your health.

There is less controversy about calcium, iron and zinc. Calcium supplements, especially when combined with vitamin D, exercise and/or hormone supplements, help prevent some of the normal bone loss that occurs as women enter menopause. It's even more important, however, to build strong bones in the first place by getting enough calcium when you're younger.

Adolescents and young adults—particularly women—should get 1,200 mg of calcium a day. Most get less than half of that amount. Elderly women should consume 1,500 mg a day. There is about 300 mg of calcium in a glass of milk or a cup of yogurt.

Those who don't get enough calcium in their diet should take a supplement. It's usually less expensive to buy a separate supplement like calcium carbonate than to try to get the full amount of calcium in a multivitamin.

Women of childbearing age, especially those who donate blood or have heavy periods, often need supplemental iron. Your doctor can give you a simple blood test that determines whether you are iron-deficient. It's best to have this test before you start taking iron. Too much iron in your system can pose a hazard to your health.

The average American gets only 80% of the recommended daily allowance of zinc, according to a study. If you suspect you're not getting enough zinc from your diet (good sources include shellfish, beef, beans and nuts), take a multivitamin that contains the recommended daily allowance.

Whenever you hear fantastic claims about the curative powers of mineral supplements, keep in mind that the multibillion dollar industry that manufactures them is behind a lot of the hype. As with vitamins, a balanced diet is the best way to ensure that you're getting the minerals you need. A simple multivitamin containing the *recommended daily allowances* of vitamins and minerals is safe, however, and provides insurance against dietary deficiencies.

Beware of higher doses. Until further studies sort out questions of effectiveness—and safety—their risks and benefits simply aren't known yet. In the meantime, it's your choice whether you want to be a guinea pig. Personally, though, I think I'll stay in the control group.

The Value of Herbal Ingredients

David Roll, PhD, professor of medicinal chemistry, University of Utah, College of Pharmacy, 201 Skaggs Hall, Salt Lake City 84112.

Don't pay extra for vitamin supplements with herbal ingredients. Herbal substances are of questionable value, and may interfere with vitamins in a manner that *blocks* your body from absorbing them. So you may wind up paying more for less.

Nutritional Supplements: What You Really Need For Optimal Health

Jeffrey Blumberg, PhD, professor of nutrition at Tufts University and chief of the Tufts University Antioxidants Research Laboratory, both in Boston.

Venture into any health-food store or pharmacy these days and you'll find yourself surrounded by nutritional supplements—from vitamins to bee pollen.

Is there any health benefit to taking supplements? Absolutely, says Tufts University nutritionist Dr. Jeffrey Blumberg.

Even if you aren't sick, says Blumberg, a few well-chosen supplements can make you much, much healthier…

Item #1: Few Americans get the Recommended Daily Allowance (RDA) for all nutrients. Only 9% adhere to the Agriculture Department's dietary guidelines.

Item #2: The RDA is based on the amount of each nutrient *needed* to prevent deficiency-related diseases—scurvy, beriberi, rickets, etc. Yet hundreds of studies confirm that risk of chronic diseases like cancer and heart disease can be minimized only by taking these nutrients at levels *in excess* of the RDA.

Item #3: It's virtually impossible to get sufficient quantities of some key nutrients from food alone—even with the most healthful diets.

KEY NUTRIENTS

•**Folic acid.** This B vitamin (also called folate) reduces blood levels of *homocysteine*. Research has linked high levels of this amino acid (a by-product of cell metabolism) to both heart attack and stroke.

Folic acid also guards against colon cancer and birth defects.

Since these defects occur in the first two months of pregnancy, any woman who even *thinks* she might become pregnant should take a daily supplement containing 400 micrograms (mcg) of folate.

Sources: Green leafy vegetables, whole-wheat bread, nuts, peas and beans. *RDA:* 400 mcg.

•**Vitamin B-6.** This vitamin works with folic acid to break down homocysteine. If all Americans upped their daily intake of folic acid and B-6, 50,000 fewer people would die annually of heart attack and stroke.

Sources: Meat, poultry, fish, liver, whole-grain products, most fruits and vegetables. *RDA:* 2 milligrams (mg).

•**Vitamin D.** This vitamin facilitates the body's absorption of dietary calcium. It's essential for healthy bones.

Sources: Fortified dairy products, fortified cereals and breads, liver, eggs and cod liver oil. Also synthesized in the skin during exposure to sunlight. *RDA:* 400 international units (IU).

•**Vitamin E.** Along with vitamin C and beta-carotene, vitamin E is a potent antioxidant. It neutralizes "free radicals," cell-damaging molecular fragments that circulate through the body.

Daily doses of vitamin E reduce the risk of heart disease…cancer of the esophagus, stomach and lung…and cataracts and other eye diseases.

Research also suggests that vitamin E can slow the progression of neurological diseases like Parkinson's and Alzheimer's.

Unfortunately, it's hard to get sufficient vitamin E from a healthful low-fat diet—so supplements are necessary.

Sources: Vegetable oil, wheat germ and nuts. *RDA:* 30 International Units (IU).

•**Beta-carotene.** More than 200 studies have shown that this antioxidant plays a key role in preventing cancer.

Sources: Broccoli, cantaloupe, carrots. *RDA:* There is no RDA for beta-carotene.

•**Selenium** is another cancer-fighting antioxidant. A study in China involving 30,000 people found a dramatically reduced risk of cancer among individuals who took supplemental vitamin E, beta-carotene and selenium.

Sources: Fish, shellfish, meat, whole-grain cereals, dairy products. *RDA:* There is no RDA for selenium.

•**Vitamin C.** Studies have linked this antioxidant to reduced risk of lung, colon and gastrointestinal cancers. It may also help prevent heart and eye disease.

The typical American diet provides 120 mg a day of vitamin C. That's twice the RDA, but a National Institutes of Health study suggested that the RDA is *too low*. A daily intake of 250 mg is better.

Sources: Citrus fruits, green peppers, broccoli, cabbage, cauliflower, potatoes, tomatoes. *RDA:* 60 mg.

•**Calcium.** This mineral is crucial for preventing osteoporosis—and it's *not* just for older women. A high calcium intake—along with sufficient vitamin D—is important for all ages, to build bone tissue and retain it.

Adults need 1,200 to 1,500 mg of calcium a day. To get this much from food, you'd need to drink about five glasses of milk…or eat several servings of yogurt, cheese or broccoli. For most people, it's easier to take a daily calcium supplement.

Sources: Dairy products, leafy green vegetables and beans. *RDA:* 800 mg.

THE THREE-PILL STRATEGY

All adults should take daily nutritional supplements with breakfast. This simple three-pill-a-day regimen provides high levels of the most critical nutrients—with minimal hassle.

Pill #1: **Multivitamin/multimineral.** It should contain 100% to 200% of the RDA for all vitamins mentioned above.

Check the expiration date on the bottle—pills lose potency as they age.

Pill #2: **Vitamin E.** Take a pill that contains 100 to 400 IU. If you prefer, take a combination pill containing vitamins E and C, beta-carotene and selenium.

***Pill #3:* Calcium.** The average person gets only about 750 mg a day in calcium from food sources. Since this is about half the amount you need for healthy bones, take one 600- to 700-mg calcium pill each day.

Which Vitamins? Which Minerals? Here's What I Do

Timothy McCall, MD, a Boston internist, author of *Examining Your Doctor: A Patient's Guide to Avoiding Harmful Medical Care.* Citadel Press. He is a regular commentator on the public radio program Marketplace, and can be found on the Web at *www.drmccall.com.*

When speaking with patients, I try to base my recommendations on the scientific data. There aren't any definitive studies about the benefits of vitamin supplements yet, but I'm going to tell you what I do based upon the evidence there is.

Each month, dozens of reports come out on the subject of vitamins and minerals. Despite all the information, many gaps in our knowledge remain. We know, for example, that people who eat diets high in certain nutrients like beta-carotene and vitamin C have lower rates of some cancers. Does that mean that taking a dietary supplement containing these vitamins will reduce your risk for cancer? No one really can say for sure.

Many medical experts say it's wrong for doctors to recommend something to their patients before there's scientific proof of its effectiveness. The problem is, people can't wait. In the "real world," we often have to make choices based on incomplete information. Even if the hard science isn't in yet, people want to know what makes the most sense now.

Many experts fail to recognize that there can be serious consequences to *withholding* recommendations until the proof is in. *Consider this:* As a first-year med student in 1979, I asked a professor who had just given us a lecture on

heart disease whether he would recommend a low-fat diet to people at risk for heart attack. No, he replied, there wasn't enough evidence yet.

I thought to myself that maybe there wasn't enough evidence for him, but there was for me. By that point I'd already been eating a low-fat diet for a couple of years. I had been doing so based on the theory that dietary fat contributes to the buildup of cholesterol in coronary arteries—a theory that seemed to have been confirmed by several preliminary studies.

Think of all the heart patients who might have benefited if doctors back then had been willing to recommend a low-fat diet. After all, the risk of cutting down on fat is pretty small.

The situation is similar with vitamin supplements today. There are theoretical reasons to take antioxidants (including vitamins C and E, beta-carotene and the mineral selenium). They gobble up free radicals, ubiquitous molecules that are thought to contribute to the development of both cancer and heart disease. And the evidence is that the risk of taking moderate doses of these vitamins is pretty small.

In that spirit, here are my educated guesses. Every morning, in addition to a multivitamin with minerals, I take 500 milligrams (mg) of vitamin C, 400 international units of vitamin E, 100 micrograms of selenium and 15 mg of beta-carotene. Whenever possible, I buy inexpensive store brands.

Even though I take these supplements, I firmly believe that a healthful diet is more important. If you eat poorly, I doubt you can undo all the damage by popping a few vitamins. Accordingly, I've been a not-too-strict vegetarian for years, consuming mostly whole grains, fruits, legumes, vegetables, a little fish and some low-fat dairy products like yogurt. To me, the vitamins are like a little added insurance.

My educated guesses could turn out to be wrong, so by all means stay tuned. New evidence might suggest the benefits of some vitamins not previously understood—while discrediting others.

Like me, plenty of doctors take dietary supplements, even if they don't recommend them to their patients. In this case, you may want to do what we do—and not what we say.

Timed-Release Vitamin Alert

The Vitamin Revolution in Health Care by Michael Janson, MD, American College for Advancement in Medicine. Arcadia Press.

Avoid "timed-release" vitamin and mineral supplements.

Reason: They cost more but may actually be less effective than the plain variety. Many vitamins, such as vitamin C, work best when they're present in the blood in high levels. This can be difficult to achieve with timed-release pills because they dissolve too slowly. *Also:* Some vitamins may not dissolve in time or in the right place to be well absorbed by the intestinal tract.

Exceptions: Both vitamin B3, or niacin, which can cause a temporary flushing of the skin, and iron, which can cause constipation and indigestion, should be taken as timed-release versions.

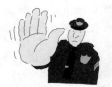

Where Never To Store Your Vitamins

Michael Janson, MD, American College for Advancement in Medicine, and author of *The Vitamin Revolution in Health Care.* Arcadia Press.

Never store vitamins in the refrigerator. Each time you open the bottle, warm air from the outside will mix with the cold vitamins, causing condensation. Over time the pills will become sticky and may actually begin to dissolve. *Also:* Don't store them in the bathroom, where heat and humidity can shorten their shelf life.

Better: Store vitamins in a pantry or on the kitchen counter where they'll stay dry and at room temperature.

Exceptions: Supplements of intestinal flora, such as *lactobacilli* or *bifidobacteria.* These should be kept in the refrigerator.

Depression and Vitamin B Connection

Maurizio Fava, MD, associate professor of psychiatry, Harvard Medical School, and director, depression clinical and research program, Massachusetts General Hospital, both in Boston.

Depression that fails to respond to antidepressants may indicate a deficiency of the B vitamin *folic acid* (folate). In a study of 213 depressed people, the antidepressant *fluoxetine* (Prozac) was less effective in those with low folate than in those with normal folate.

Self-defense: If you don't respond to an antidepressant, ask your doctor to check your folate level.

Calcium Is Inexpensive

Timothy McCall, MD, a Boston internist, author of *Examining Your Doctor: A Patient's Guide to Avoiding Harmful Medical Care.* Citadel Press. He is a regular commentator on the public radio program Marketplace, and can be found on the Web at *www.drmccall.com.*

You can get the medically recommended dosages of calcium, multivitamins and vitamins C and E for as little as 12 to 21 cents a day.

Key: Buy store brands, which are often made by the very same companies that manufacture the more expensive, best-selling supplement brands.

Vitamin B-12 Alert

Victor Herbert, MD, director of the hematology and nutrition laboratory at Mt. Sinai School of Medicine, New York, and editor of *Total Nutrition: The Only Guide You'll Ever Need.* St. Martin's Press.

Individuals over 50 years of age need to supplement their diets with at least 25 micrograms a day of vitamin B-12.

Take vitamin B-12 in tablets by itself—or combined with folic acid.

Don't take it in tablets that include other vitamins or minerals. *Reason:* When the pills dissolve in your stomach, the vitamin B-12 is destroyed.

Important: Do not take other vitamins prescribed for you by a health professional within one hour of taking vitamin B-12.

Vitamin C to the Rescue

Scott T. Weiss, MD, associate professor of medicine at Harvard Medical School, Boston.

Vitamin C may help prevent asthma, bronchitis and other lung problems. When researchers studied the diets and lung functions of over 2,500 people, they found that the people who consumed the most vitamin C had the best-functioning lungs. The difference in lung function between those whose daily diet contained an amount of vitamin C equivalent to that contained in 10 ounces of orange juice (99 milligrams) and those who had almost none was as great as that between nonsmokers and people who smoked a pack of cigarettes every day for five years.

Vitamin C and Arthritis

Tim McAlindon, MD, an associate professor of medicine at Boston University School of Medicine.

The progression of arthritis of the knee can be significantly slowed by vitamin C. An eight-year study of 640 people found that knee osteoarthritis progressed three times more slowly in those who consumed the most vitamin C than in those who ate the least.

Scientists offer two possible theories to explain this effect. One is that vitamin C's antioxidant properties mop up harmful free radicals that are released by the inflamed knee joint. The second theory is that vitamin C helps the body synthesize proteins that repair the arthritis caused damage. But either way—you win.

Vitamin C for the Heart

Joseph A. Vita, MD, associate professor of medicine at Boston University School of Medicine, Boston.

A study of 26 people with severely blocked arteries found that high doses of vitamin C helped their arteries open normally within two hours. Blocked arteries limit blood flow to the heart, causing angina and heart attacks.

Researchers theorize that vitamin C helps by suppressing superoxide, a substance that interferes with the body's natural way of opening arteries. Enough research has not yet been done to know how useful vitamin C supplements are as a treatment for artery problems.

Relief from Colds

Michael L. Macknin, MD, chairman, department of general pediatrics, The Cleveland Clinic Foundation.

Relieve symptoms and reduce the duration of colds by sucking zinc lozenges. They are available over the counter in drugstores.

Study: Cold sufferers were divided into two groups, one of which received zinc lozenges. This group reported that colds lasted an average of 4.4 days, compared with 7.6 days for the group receiving placebo lozenges. The group receiving zinc lozenges also reported suffering milder symptoms.

Dosage: The group took an average of five 13.3 mg zinc lozenges, totaling about 65 mg of zinc daily. The lozenges studied were zinc gluconate glycine (*Brand name:* Cold-eeze).

Vitamin C Danger

Sheldon Nadler, DMD, a dentist in private practice in New York City.

Chewable forms of vitamin C (ascorbic acid) may be bad for your teeth. Breath mints, chewing gum, etc., fortified with C are now being sold as easy ways to get your daily dose of this key nutrient.

Danger: Repeated exposure to any acid—including ascorbic acid—can corrode your tooth enamel. *Most damaging:* Habitual use of products containing more than 500 milligrams (mg) of C per piece.

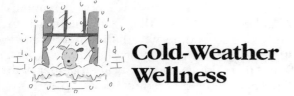

Cold-Weather Wellness

John H. Weisburger, PhD, senior scientist at the American Health Foundation, Valhalla, NY.

To get the vitamin C you need for winter, keep up your fruit and vegetable consumption—preferably at the same high level you would over the summer months. Vitamin C, along with other vitamins, is necessary for optimal health…and studies show that it lowers the risk of heart disease and some types of cancer.

Best: A minimum of five servings—fresh or canned—per day.

Alternative: Two 250-milligram tablets of vitamin C every day—one with a high-fiber breakfast and one at dinner. But these dietary supplements don't give you the extra nutrients or fiber that fruits and vegetables do.

Bladder Cancer and Vitamin C

Barbara Bruemmer, PhD, nutrition analyst, division of clinical research, Fred Hutchinson Cancer Research Center, Seattle. Her study of 667 men and women ages 45 to 55 was published in the *American Journal of Epidemiology*, 111 Market Pl., Baltimore 21202.

Bladder cancer risk can be cut by up to one-third by consuming lots of vitamin C, fruit and a daily multivitamin supplement.

What raises risk: Eating fried foods and smoking.

Vitamin C and Artery Link

Haruo Tomoda, MD, clinical professor of cardiology, Tokai University Hospital, Kanagawa, Japan. His study of restenosis in 101 angioplasty patients was published in the *Journal of the American College of Cardiology*, 655 Avenue of the Americas, New York 10010.

Vitamin C helps keep coronary arteries from clogging. Only 25% of angioplasty patients who took 500 mg of vitamin C a day suffered reclogging (a process called *restenosis*). But restenosis affected 43% of angioplasty patients who didn't take vitamin C. *Theory:* Vitamin C blocks restenosis by keeping oxidation of LDL (bad) cholesterol low. LDL cholesterol must be oxidized before it can attach to artery walls. Anyone who undergoes angioplasty should ask his/her doctor about vitamin C.

Vitamin D and Diabetes

Stanley Mirsky, MD, associate clinical professor at Mount Sinai School of Medicine, New York City.

Vitamin D may play a part in preventing diabetes. A Swedish study found that men with lower levels of vitamin D had higher blood pressure, higher triglyceride fat levels and higher insulin resistance, all factors associated with type II or adult onset diabetes. Four eight-ounce glasses of milk have enough vitamin D to provide the RDA of 400 international units.

Adults and Vitamin D

Study of 250 women in their 50s and 60s by Bess Dawson-Hughes, MD, chief, calcium and bone metabolism lab, Human Nutrition Research Center, Tufts University, Boston.

Adults need more than the recommended allowance of vitamin D. In a two-year study, women who received the Recommended Daily Allowance (RDA) of vitamin D —from both diet and supplements—lost twice as much bone from their hips as did women who received 800 International Units (IU) per day. Consider taking vitamin D supplements if you don't think you're getting enough of the nutrient from your diet, or if you don't get enough exposure to the sun, which allows the body to manufacture vitamin D on its own.

Vitamin E Protects the Lungs

Lindsey Dow, MD, consultant senior lecturer in care of the elderly, University of Bristol, Bristol, England. Her study of 178 people 70 years of age or older was published in the *American Journal of Respiratory and Critical Care Medicine*, 1740 Broadway, New York 10019.

Does vitamin E protect the lungs? In a study, the more of this antioxidant vitamin elderly people consumed, the better their lung function.

Caution: Researchers don't yet know exactly how much vitamin E is needed to improve lung function or if it is more beneficial when consumed in supplement form or in foods. Good sources include nuts, fresh vegetables and vegetable oil.

Vitamins vs. Birth Defects

Quanhe Yang, PhD, division of birth defects and developmental disabilities, National Center for Environmental Study, Centers for Disease Control and Prevention, Atlanta. His study of mothers of 117 babies was published in *Epidemiology*, One Newtown Executive Park, Newtown Lower Falls, MA 02162.

Doctors have long urged pregnant women to take a daily multivitamin—to prevent limb deformities in their unborn children. *Study:* Taking vitamins during the month before conception cut the risk of such defects by even more. *Self-defense:* Any woman who *might* become pregnant should take a daily multivitamin containing folic acid.

Vitamin E, Aspirin and Stroke Connection

Manfred Steiner, MD, PhD, a professor of medicine at East Carolina University School of Medicine, Greenville, NC.

Aspirin's proven antistroke power is multiplied when it is taken with vitamin E. A study of 100 people who had suffered *mini*-strokes, often a precursor of *major* strokes, found that taking vitamin E daily together with aspirin produced a reduction of up to 80%, compared with aspirin alone, in the number of anchor strands that enable dangerous clots to form in blood vessels.

Vitamin E and Cuts

James M. Spencer, MD, MS, director, Mohs surgery, University of Miami (FL) Sylvester Comprehensive Cancer Center. His three-month study was presented at a meeting of the American Society for Dermatologic Surgery.

Vitamin E *doesn't* help cuts and bruises heal faster—despite the common belief that it does.

Study: Fifteen volunteers applied vitamin E ointment to one-half of a wound twice daily. After three months, there was no difference in the rate of healing between the treated and untreated halves. And six of the volunteers dropped out, complaining of redness, swelling and skin irritation on the vitamin E side.

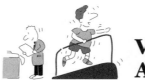

Vitamin E And Exercise

Kenneth Cooper, MD, MPH, inventor of aerobics and founder of the Cooper Clinic in Dallas. He is author of *Advanced Nutritional Therapies*. Thomas Nelson Publishers.

Vitamin E can reduce muscle soreness and damage from vigorous exercise. Studies found the benefit when people took large doses of vitamin E during the 24 hours before—*and* after—they engaged in vigorous exercise.

Recommended dosage: 400 International Units (IU) daily for adults. Physicians believe this effect comes from the ability of vitamin E to combat DNA-damaging free radicals released by exercise. Other researchers are studying the relationship between exercise and other vitamins, including riboflavin (vitamin B2) and vitamin C.

Beta-Carotene Update

Bruce Yaffe, MD, internist in private practice, 121 E. 84 St., New York 10028.

Don't discount beta-carotene—despite reports to the contrary.

Reason: Two of the three studies reported were flawed.

Problem: They used only high-risk people …and the higher death rate was not statistically significant. In nonsmokers and nondrinkers, other studies have shown beta-carotene helps prevent stroke and heart disease.

Best: Get 15 milligrams (mg) of beta-carotene daily from vegetables and fruits—particularly sweet potatoes, carrots, spinach, cantaloupe and mangoes.

Folic Acid Danger

Mark Dykewicz, MD, associate professor of internal medicine, St. Louis University Health Sciences Center.

Synthetic forms of this vitamin can cause hives, breathing problems, cramps and itching.

Problem: The FDA is urging food producers to fortify bread, flour and pasta with folic acid…and many vitamin supplements now contain folic acid.

Self-defense: Consult a doctor if you develop these symptoms after a meal—or while taking vitamins containing folic acid. (Stop taking the vitamins.)

Good news: You can get plenty of natural folic acid by eating dark green leafy vegetables, liver, nuts and wheat germ.

Folic Acid Benefits

Meir J. Stampfer, MD, a physician at Brigham and Women's Hospital, Boston, and the leader of one of the studies.

Folic acid may offer significant protection against heart attack and stroke. An inadequate intake of folic acid is associated with high blood levels of homocysteine, an amino acid which more than 20 studies have found increases the risk of stroke and heart disease.

Folic acid, a B vitamin, is found in dried beans, enriched whole-grain cereals, green leafy vegetables, peanuts, liver and orange juice. Researchers say that people eating five daily servings of fruits and vegetables receive enough folic acid (400 micrograms) to keep their homocysteine level down.

Magnesium Fights Migraines

Andreas Peikert, MD, neurologist, Munich–Harlaching Clinic, Munich, Germany. His 16-week study of 81 migraine patients was published in *Cephalalgia,* Henry Ford Hospital, 2799 W. Grand Blvd., Detroit 48202.

In a study, one group of migraine sufferers was given magnesium supplements, while a second group got placebos.

Result: 56% of the magnesium group reported fewer migraines, compared with 31% of the placebo group.

Caution: Magnesium supplements should not be taken by anyone who has kidney trouble.

Selenium vs. Cancer Facts

Larry C. Clark, MPH, PhD, associate professor of epidemiology, Arizona Cancer Center, Tucson. His eight-year study of 1,312 skin cancer patients 18 to 80 years of age was published in the *Journal of the American Medical Association*, 515 N. State St., Chicago 60610.

Selenium may help prevent cancer. A 10-year study of more than 1,300 people found that those who took 200 micrograms (mcg) of selenium supplements daily reduced their rates of colorectal, prostate and lung cancer by about half, compared with those who did not take the supplement.

Selenium is found in chicken, meat, seafood, grains, egg yolks, mushrooms, onions and garlic.

The average intake for US adults is only 108 mcg, so the supplement brings the total to approximately 350 mcg a day—considered a safe maximum. Don't overdo it, however—a daily intake of 1,000 mcg can cause side effects including hair loss and fragile nails.

Researchers conducted a study to determine whether selenium supplements prevent skin cancer.

What they found: Selenium did *not* affect skin cancer risk, but it *did* reduce deaths from cancers of the lung, colon, rectum and prostate. Skin cancer patients who took selenium developed 63% fewer prostate cancers, 58% fewer colorectal cancers and 46% fewer lung cancers. Ask your doctor about taking selenium supplements.

More Good Things About Selenium

Li Li, MD, PhD, Division of Cancer Prevention and Control, National Cancer Institute, Bethesda, MD.

Selenium may help protect the body against heart disease and cancer.

A study of 2,600 people in Finland found that the rates of both those diseases dropped by 60% as blood selenium levels rose from 60 to 103 micrograms per liter. The best sources of the mineral are seafoods, grains, muscle meats and Brazil nuts.

However, *don't* use selenium supplements without consulting your doctor first—it's easy to take too much, which is dangerous.

Chromium Picolinate Danger

Walter G. Wasser, MD, chief, division of nephrology, North General Hospital, New York City.

This popular weight-loss aid can cause kidney failure. *Case:* A 49-year-old nurse developed kidney failure after taking three times the recommended level of chromium picolinate for six weeks. *Bottom line:* Since the risk of chromium deficiency is small and the ideal dose is uncertain, there's no reason to take chromium supplements.

13

For a Healthy Sex Life

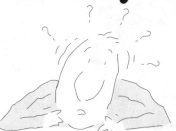

The Healing Power of Good Sex

Paul Pearsall, PhD
Henry Ford Community College

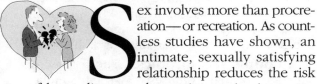

Sex involves more than procreation—or recreation. As countless studies have shown, an intimate, sexually satisfying relationship reduces the risk of heart disease…depression…migraine…premenstrual syndrome…and arthritis. It also boosts the immune system.

But sex is genuinely healing *only* if it transcends the mechanical, self-pleasure variety promoted by sex experts.

Indeed, the central goal of sexual healing should not be orgasm—but *connection with your partner.*

PHYSIOLOGY OF HEALING SEX

Healing sex brings a marked decline in bloodstream levels of *adrenaline* and *cortisol.*

These stress hormones provoke anxiety and reduce immune function.

In a study, women who were happily married had higher levels of natural killer cells and helper T cells than those in unhappy unions.

Healing sex is also a potent antidote for social isolation, which has been linked to serious illness and premature death.

A Yale study of 194 heart patients found that those without a spouse at home were twice as likely to die prematurely as those with a spouse.

HEALING SEX IS RARE

Most couples never experience sexual healing—because they're too quick to give up on their relationship. It takes at least *four years* to achieve the intimacy needed for sexual healing. Most couples split after only three years. Why do so many couples split? Because of lack

Paul Pearsall, PhD, professor of psychology at Henry Ford Community College in Dearborn, MI, and former director of education at the Kinsey Institute at Indiana University, Bloomington. He is author of *A Healing Intimacy* (Crown) and *The Pleasure Prescription* (Hunter House).

251

of intimacy. Intimacy doesn't just happen. You *make* it happen by treating your partner with care and genuine affection...and by taking the time to really connect, both in casual conversation and via sex.

Three factors are central to a sexually healing relationship...

•**Commitment.** Affairs and on-again-off-again sexual relationships are *not* healing because the two people never form a meaningful bond.

•**Consideration.** The bond between a couple must extend beyond the bedroom. Each partner must continually express tenderness and caring toward the other—by smiling...touching...being polite...giving compliments ...and showing respect.

•**Honesty.** There must be no secrets within the relationship—only total connection and total confidence.

HOW TO FORGE A SEXUALLY HEALING RELATIONSHIP

•**Spend time together.** For at least five minutes a day, sit or lie together—just the two of you. Cuddle. Talk. Let your bodies synchronize.

•**Listen more, talk less.** Ironically, good relationships involve little talk. Partners communicate via their own private language—subtle body movements, gestures, expressions and a sense of connection that arises only between lovers who grow ever closer as a result of sharing crises.

•**Do something special for your partner.** If you spend your days apart, call periodically during the day and say something like, "Honey, I've been thinking about you. I can't wait to see you."

If necessary, set an alarm clock to go off periodically to remind you to place the call.

You come to feel love by behaving lovingly, so even the simplest acts of connection can translate to intense sexual feelings.

•**Have sex only when it feels "right."** Trust your senses. If you rely on your "sex sense" for a month, you'll soon see that when you do have sex, it is more fulfilling and sensual.

•**Seduce your partner.** Instead of dressing up in a sexy costume—as sex therapists often recommend—use "brain power."

Send your partner mental "messages" all day long. At night, lie still in bed and send him/her more "sex waves." You'll be surprised at how seductive your own brain can be.

•**Fantasize about your partner.** Put on some sensual music and lie in bed with your eyes closed. Use your brain—not a vibrator or your hand—and envision yourself making love to your partner.

You may become aroused—even experience orgasm—but mental sex can be surprisingly fulfilling even if you don't.

50-MINUTE SEXUAL FITNESS PLAN

My sexual fitness plan—which you can add to your weekly exercise regimen—contains three components...

1. Shared laughter. Twenty seconds of laughter produces the same cardiovascular benefits as three minutes of aerobic exercise, studies indicate.

Studies also indicate that a good laugh strengthens the immune system by lowering cortisol levels and raising endorphin levels. And—couples who laugh together become closer and more in tune with one another.

2. Shared crying. Watching a good tear-jerker enhances intimacy—and sometimes leads to sexual arousal. Tears, which contain stress hormones and other chemicals, may be nature's way of washing toxins out of the body.

3. Couple "erotorobics." The following suggested sexual exercises may seem strange, but they increase your ability to respond to intimate physical contact...

•**Simulated sex.** Go through the motions of intercourse—with your clothes on.

•**Genital massage.** This stimulates blood flow in that area.

•**Dancing to erotic music.** Use the muscles you would if you were having intercourse.

•**Flirting.** Arch your back, sway your hips and stick out your chest. And practice sexual gazing and sexual smiling. Both can make you feel more sensuous.

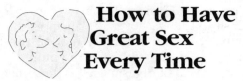

How to Have Great Sex Every Time

Edward W. Eichel, MA, a psychotherapist in private practice in New York City and the originator of the coital alignment technique. CAT is described in greater detail—and, yes, illustrated—in his book, *The Perfect Fit*. Signet. For more information on a CAT self-help videotape, call 212-989-1826.

O f all the concerns voiced by women undergoing sex therapy, none is more common—or emotionally distressing—than an inability to achieve orgasm during intercourse.

Only about 30% of women achieve orgasm regularly during intercourse (coitus).

Some women endure years of sex without a single coital orgasm. Typically, a woman relies upon a partner who "jumps through hoops" to bring her there, but never achieves the ideal.

Result: Sexuality, robbed of its playfulness and spontaneity, becomes more a chore than a pleasure.

TO THE RESCUE

A variant of the standard missionary position—known as the coital alignment technique (CAT)—not only helps the woman have an orgasm during coitus, but also boosts the odds that she and her partner will climax simultaneously.

Men who have long considered themselves sexually inadequate, as well as women who have worried they were frigid, can begin to experience sex with all its physical pleasure and emotional intimacy.

Bonus: Because good sex is usually synonymous with good communication, this improvement in a couple's sex life often carries over into other aspects of their relationship, bringing new levels of intimacy, contentment, and—important in this age of AIDS—commitment.

Unlike some other alternative lovemaking techniques, CAT is relatively straightforward. Couples have differed in the time necessary to master the technique, but with persistence, most have succeeded. Once mastered, it is remarkably effective—and quite reliable.

Study: Sexual response was measured in couples involved in committed relationships—before and after receiving CAT training. Prior to learning CAT, only 23% of the women reported achieving orgasm during intercourse on a regular basis. After CAT, that figure jumped to 77%. Before CAT, no women reported having regular simultaneous orgasms with their partners. Afterward, one-third of the women reported doing so.

Almost all participants reported at least some improvement in their sex lives following CAT training. In fact, the only participants who failed to benefit were those whose relationships were already jeopardized by nonsexual factors.

CAT BASICS

CAT encompasses five distinct elements, each designed to maximize contact between the penis and the clitoris, thus maximizing sexual response in both partners...

1. Positioning. The woman lies on her back. The man lies atop her, facing her much as in the conventional missionary position, but with his pelvis overriding hers in a "riding high" orientation.

His penis should be inserted into her vagina, with its shaft pressed firmly against her mons veneris—the soft fleshy mound covering the pubic bone above the vagina. She wraps her legs around his thighs, with her legs bent at an angle not exceeding 45 degrees and her ankles resting on his calves.

Important: He must let his full weight fall on her and must avoid using his hands or elbows to support his weight. While she may find this weight uncomfortable initially, it is essential to keep his pelvis from sliding back down off of hers.

2. Limited movement. Conventional intercourse involves a great deal of pushing, pulling and bracing of the arms and legs. CAT coitus focuses narrowly on the couple's pelvic movement. In fact, little additional movement is possible during CAT, given the partners' positioning. If additional movement is possible, the positioning is faulty.

3. Pressure-counterpressure. During ordinary intercourse, the man sets the rhythm while the woman moves little, if at all. In contrast, CAT calls for a rhythmic movement that is virtually identical for both partners.

Procedure: She performs an upward stroke, forcing his pelvis backward. He allows his pelvis to move, yet maintains a continuous counterpressure against her pelvis (and her clitoris).

In the downward movement, the pattern of movement is reversed, with the man pushing downward and the woman maintaining the counterpressure against his penis. As her pelvis moves backward and downward, the penis shaft rocks forward against her mons veneris, sliding to a shallow position in the vagina.

Note: Although the force of pressure and counterpressure is quite intense during CAT, the partners' actual movement is surprisingly slight.

4. Full genital contact. Repeated thrusting of the penis into and out of the vaginal "barrel," typical of conventional missionary intercourse, affords little direct stimulation of either the clitoris or the penis.

Typical result: His orgasm, even if perceived as pleasurable, is far less powerful than it might be...and she, having gotten little if any clitoral stimulation, fails to climax at all. In CAT, the penis and clitoris are held tightly together by pressure and counterpressure...and the penile-clitoral "connection" is rocked up and down in an evenly paced, lever-like fashion. This vibratory motion all but guarantees orgasms for both partners.

Bonus: Orgasms produced by CAT differ significantly from those produced by conventional in-and-out sex. Whereas a conventional orgasm is limited to a pulsating sensation, a CAT orgasm combines this with a "melting" sensation.

Among participants of the study, 90% of all subjects said that CAT intensified their orgasms ...and 60% said that it increased their desire for more frequent sex.

5. "Passive" orgasm. In ordinary coitus, the man thrusts faster and more deeply as he becomes increasingly aroused, while the woman typically slows down or even stops moving altogether. At the moment of climax, the partners' movements often become disconnected and may fall completely out of sync.

Result: The orgasm is incomplete, almost "spoiled."

Better: CAT prescribes complete coordination of movement by the partners, up to and beyond the moment of climax. In other words,

both partners make no effort to "grab" for orgasm, instead letting it "overtake" them.

The transition from voluntary motion preceding orgasm to the reflexive, involuntary movements typical of orgasm itself is thus fully coordinated. The possibility of incomplete orgasm is drastically limited.

Crucial: A conscious effort by both partners not to hold their breath or suppress natural sounds. Breathing freely and giving full rein to grunts, moans, spoken words and other vocalizations greatly facilitate orgasm—for the noise-maker and the listener alike.

Some couples report that the "reversed" CAT is an effective variation of CAT—if the man is much heavier than his partner.

Herpes Update

Anna Wald, MD, MPH, acting instructor, Virology Research Clinic, University of Washington, Seattle.

Genital herpes can be spread even without the presence of genital sores. In a study of 110 women with genital herpes, 65% of women "shed" virus particles at some point, both with and without accompanying lesions.

To reduce risk: Use condoms unless you're sure your partner is uninfected. *Also:* Viral shedding can be reduced by taking the prescription drug *acyclovir* (Zovirax), *valacyclovir* (Valtrex) and *famciclovir* (Famir).

How to Perk Up Your Sex Life

Judith Seifer, PhD, RN, president of the American Association of Sex Educators, Counselors and Therapists, Box 238, Mount Vernon, IA 52314. She is the host and co-creator of the *Better Sex* Video Series.

Remember the days when you had sex every other day—or even *daily?* Most couples make love less frequently as their relationships progress.

But your sex life needn't be dull—no matter how old you are or how long your relationship has lasted.

Here are the common problems that rob sex of its joy and satisfaction—and how to make things right…

LOSS OF DESIRE

Periods of low desire are usually linked to use of antidepressants or tranquilizers…depression…fatigue…or to disappointment, anger and other negative emotions that affect all relationships from time to time.

How can you boost your libido? First, make sure your partner doesn't think the problem lies with him. Admit that you have lost *your* desire.

If it's your partner whose sex drive has ebbed, gently encourage him/her to talk about it.

Good news: Talking about the problem usually leads to its resolution. If not, ask your doctor to rule out physical causes, such as the loss of estrogen during and after menopause.

Many menopausal women find their desire returns if they go on hormone-replacement therapy (HRT)…and researchers are evaluating testosterone-replacement therapy for men *and* women suffering from low libido.

IMBALANCE IN DESIRE

The old clichés are true. Women view intimacy in terms of acceptance, support and affection, whereas men think in terms of sexual intercourse. Many couples spend years struggling with this imbalance.

Mistake: Trying to get your partner to think the way you think.

Instead, look for ways to satisfy both the masculine need for intercourse *and* the feminine need to cuddle and talk. Embrace variety in your intimate encounters. Sometimes go for a quickie, sometimes go for a long, leisurely session. At other times, limit your touching to mutual massage.

IMPOTENCE*

Men who have persistent erection troubles —and their partners—come to view sex with anxiety and overwhelming seriousness. That makes good sex almost impossible.

*Impotence is defined as a "consistent inability to obtain or maintain an erection of sufficient rigidity to achieve satisfactory sexual intercourse." If a couple enjoys sex despite the man's inability to achieve an erection—that's not impotence.

Any man who is impotent in more than half of his sexual encounters should have a complete medical workup. He may have diabetes or heart disease.

Other common causes: Exhaustion, overeating, drinking, smoking, having high blood pressure and taking certain medications—such as antidepressants, antihypertensives and anti-anxiety agents.

Happily, most erectile problems are curable —thanks in part to an oral drug called *sildenafil* (Viagra)…the injectable drugs *papaverine* (Regitine) and *alprostadil* (Caverject)…and penile implants.

In many cases, a woman can give her partner an erection simply by performing oral sex …or by gently pressing the fatty pad of her thumb on his perineum. That's the firm area beneath the scrotum. These techniques stimulate the prostate gland, which is intimately linked to sexual function.

Most important: Take sex less seriously. Over a lifetime, you'll probably be able to count earth-moving sexual encounters on one hand. Even the most passionate couples wind up having mediocre sex about 20% of the time.

VAGINAL DRYNESS

Women of all ages can experience inadequate vaginal lubrication. This problem can lead to pain during intercourse and—eventually—the desire to avoid sex altogether.

Usual causes: Hormonal imbalances brought on by pregnancy, breast-feeding, menopause or infrequent sex.

To boost lubrication, couples should devote more time to foreplay…and use a lubricated condom or a water-soluble vaginal lubricant like Erogel or Slip.

Any menopausal woman who is experiencing vaginal dryness should ask her doctor about HRT. Estrogen usually restores vaginal moisture. For women who do not want to go on HRT, topical preparations are available.

SEXUAL BOREDOM

If you've been having sex on the same day, at the same time, in the same room, in the same position for years, the real question is, "How could you not be bored?"

Don't blame your partner for your boredom. Find ways to put the zest back into your sexual encounters. *What to do:*

●**Have sex in an unusual place**—your car, another room in the house, the shower, etc.

●**Schedule sex for a different time of day.** If you ordinarily have sex at night, try getting romantic in the morning. Or—make a date for an afternoon tryst at a local hotel.

●**Look for ways to expand your sexual repertoire.** If you don't practice oral sex already, you might want to give it a try.

Couples over age 55 are 50% less likely to engage in oral sex than younger couples. That's too bad. *Fellatio* and *cunnilingus* can increase intimacy and enjoyment for *both* partners.

Fellatio can help a man to have an erection. And most women find that stimulation of the clitoris—with the tongue, fingers or a vibrator—is the most reliable way to reach orgasm.

Cunnilingus can prime older women for intercourse by helping them to lubricate. It can even be a sexually satisfying substitute for intercourse if impotence or another problem renders that impossible.

Other ways to expand your sexual repertoire…

●**Fantasy.** Sexual fantasies spice up your sex life by giving you—and your partner, if you feel comfortable sharing them—new ideas. If you fantasize about being tied up and tickled with a feather, tell your partner. It just might lead to a sensual, exciting experience for both of you.

It's okay to imagine you're having sex with someone else while you're making love with your partner. That's normal and healthy.

●**Aphrodisiacs.** The best aphrodisiac around today is *green oat straw*. Taken daily, this oral homeopathic remedy boosts desire by increasing levels of circulating testosterone in both men and women. It's available at health-food stores.

Oysters, ginseng, chocolate and alcohol and other recreational drugs do *not* boost sex drive.

●**Erotic videos.** Men aren't alone in their enjoyment of watching others have sex. According to the Video Retailer's Association, 40% of adult videos are rented by women.

A woman who is turned off by hard-core porn may want to explore soft-core porn, women's erotica or instructional sex tapes.

●**Sex toys.** Vibrators, dildos, massage oils, etc., can dramatically enhance your sexual pleasure. *Important:* To keep the man from feeling "replaced" by a vibrator, couples should use it to stimulate both partners.

Discreet sources for sex toys: Eve's Garden, *www.evesgarden.com,* 800-848-3837 or Good Vibrations, *www.goodvibes.com,* 800-289-8423. Request their mail-order catalogs or order online.

●**Masturbation.** Both men and women often find it highly pleasurable to touch themselves during sex with a partner—or to watch their partners touch themselves.

Masturbation is also a powerful tool for teaching yourself to achieve orgasm—so you can better guide your partner.

RENEWING YOUR COMMITMENT

For the next week or month, treat your partner in a romantic way—just like you would like to be treated.

Example: Call your partner at the office just to say, *I love you.* Leave love notes in his briefcase, or her lingerie drawer. Bring home flowers. Start touching one another often in an affectionate way.

For nine out of 10 couples, these simple gestures make a dramatic difference in psychological and sexual satisfaction.

Love and Sex After 60

Robert N. Butler, MD, professor of geriatrics at Mount Sinai School of Medicine, New York. Dr. Butler is a former head of the National Institute on Aging. He is coauthor of *Love and Sex After 60.* Ballantine Books.

While the myth persists that the joys of sex are just a memory for folks in their 60s, 70s and beyond, the truth is far different. As long as you and your partner are healthy and willing, *there's no age limit to sexual fulfillment.* We've seen 90-year-olds who lead active, satisfying sex lives.

Too many older people, however, are deprived of this vital pleasure by correctable physical problems, poor lifestyle and self-defeating attitudes.

Sidestep these obstacles and you're likely to find that sex is as good as—or better than—ever.

HOW SEX IS DIFFERENT

At age 75, you're not the man or woman you were at age 25—not physically, emotionally… or sexually.

For men, in particular, the sexual difference is largely a matter of *time*. It takes longer to become aroused…longer to reach a climax…and the refractory phase (time interval between arousals) is longer.

But the good news is that your lifetime of experience—and maturity—will enrich the quality of your sexual encounters. Where sex in young adulthood is athletic, even explosive, it's often self-centered.

Couples who have weathered the storms of life (or those who fall in love in their later years) have often become more sensitive to each other's needs. Sex becomes a matter of mutual giving and sharing.

Important: Don't judge yourself by a youthful standard. Appreciate what you have today—it's different, but not inferior to yesterday.

CLEAR AWAY OBSTACLES

If your sex life isn't satisfactory, illness, not age, may be responsible. Diabetes, depression or an underactive thyroid can rob you of sexual desire.

Inflammation of the prostate may make sex uncomfortable. These conditions are treatable.

Heart disease can have an *indirect* impact on sex. People who suffer from angina (chest pain) or have had heart attacks are often anxious about sex, or avoid it altogether. But the risk of harm is actually very low…less than 0.3% of heart attack deaths occur during sex. Check with your doctor.

After menopause, vaginal tissues grow thinner and natural secretions dry up. This makes sex painful for some older women. Estrogen replacement can correct the problem, but recent studies have called into question the safety of the long-term use of estrogen.

If you'd rather forgo hormones, an over-the-counter vaginal lubricant like Replens will also help restore the pleasure of sex.

Some medications may reduce sexual drive and impair performance (especially for men). Blood pressure drugs, antidepressants, tranquilizers and diuretics (water pills) are the most common culprits.

Almost always, your doctor will be able to prescribe an alternative medication that will work just as effectively and spare your sex life.

IMPROVE YOUR LIFESTYLE

• **Exercise.** If your stamina is limited, you can't bring much vigor to sex—yet another good reason to exercise regularly. Try to exercise for at least 20 to 30 minutes, three to five times a week.

Brisk walking is the best exercise for most older people. Start by walking rapidly until tired, then rest and return at a leisurely pace to the starting point. Gradually increase the distance and pace. *Good goal:* Two to three miles in 45 minutes.

If you've been inactive for years, or have heart disease, consult your doctor before starting any exercise program.

• **Get enough rest.** A well-rested body is more eager and able to perform sexually. Try for seven or more hours of sleep a day. Take naps or rest breaks in the afternoon if you need them. Get medical help for persistent sleeping problems.

• **Avoid alcohol.** Several drinks may relax you and put you in the mood for sex, but can diminish your ability to perform. Even small amounts of alcohol affect you more than when you were younger.

Better: Avoid alcohol altogether, or limit yourself to a single drink for several hours before having sex.

• **Don't smoke.** The sexual organs—both male and female—fill with blood when arousal occurs, and nicotine interferes with this process by constricting vital blood vessels. Men who smoke may also have lower levels of testosterone.

• **Stay sexually active.** If you don't have sex regularly, desire and ability will dwindle. Stay in shape without a partner by masturbating.

If it has been years since you've been sexually active, pay special attention to lifestyle factors, be patient (and ask the same of your partner)...and expect that it may take several months to get back in practice.

SET THE SCENE

You're never too old for a richer, more romantic, more exciting sex life. Habit tends to make sex dull and routine. *The antidote:* Flexibility, creativity and caring.

●**Create a romantic setting.** One couple has "dates" at home—they dress nicely, have a candlelit dinner and then retire to the bedroom, which they've made inviting with fresh flowers and soft lights.

A vacation to a new, exciting place is also a great way to recharge your sexual batteries.

●**Be willing to change and explore.** Try new positions and techniques. If you've never read about sexuality, this is a good time to start.

●**Be stimulating and stimulated.** As most men grow older, they need direct physical stimulation of the penis to attain an erection. For women, leisurely, loving foreplay, which includes stimulation of the clitoris, increases pleasure and promotes orgasm.

Watching erotic videos and sharing your fantasies can make sex more exciting for both of you.

Important: Communicate. Tell your partner what feels good—and what doesn't feel so good.

●**Timing is key.** Sex doesn't have to be just a bedtime activity—particularly if you're retired and have more time.

Feel free to have sex when you're both energetic and in the mood. Many people are most rested and relaxed in the morning (and men are generally most potent then). Or unplug the phone, lower the shades and treat yourselves to a matinee.

WORK ON YOUR RELATIONSHIP

Sex is just part of a mature relationship. Tender, generous feelings increase the pleasure, while anger and resentment get in the way.

Desire and sexual performance are especially sensitive to the emotional climate.

Strive to be responsive to each other's feelings and needs—and not just in bed. Bring resentments and disappointments into the open, and do your best to resolve them.

Don't take each other for granted, but make a sustained effort to be interesting and interested. If boredom has crept into your relationship, look within for the deeper feelings you have for one another...and express those feelings sexually.

Exercises May Relieve Impotence

E. Douglas Whitehead, MD, urologist and director, Association for Male Sexual Dysfunction, 24 E. 12 St., New York 10003.

Simple pelvic-muscle exercises called Kegel exercises—long known to control urinary incontinence in men and women—may also relieve impotence in some men. The most common cause of impotence is impaired circulation, which leads to inability to retain sufficient blood within the penis. Researchers say Kegel exercises may work as well as surgery.

Prescription Drugs That Affect Sex

Deborah Carson, PharmD, associate professor of pharmacy practice, Medical University of South Carolina, Charleston.

Many people don't realize that medication can affect their sex lives. *Some common drugs and their side effects...*

●**Antidepressants.** Tricyclics like Elavil and serotonin reuptake inhibitors like Prozac and Zoloft can dampen sexual desire and interfere with orgasm and/or ejaculation.

●**Ulcer drugs.** Tagamet and Zantac in large doses can cause impotence, loss of libido and breast pain or enlargement.

●**Diuretics.** Thiazides like Anhydron and Lasix can interfere with ejaculation…dampen sexual desire…and cause impotence.

●**Anti-anxiety drugs.** Tranquilizers like Valium and Xanax can cause impotence and reduced libido and can interfere with orgasm and/or ejaculation.

●**Beta-blockers.** Inderal and Tenormin can cause impotence and decreased sexual desire.

Caution: It can be hard to distinguish a drug's side effects from the underlying medical condition. Never stop taking a drug without first consulting your physician.

Medicines affect different people in different ways. Often a different medicine for the same condition will be less likely to inhibit desire.

Better Sex, Better Sleep

The Doctor's Guide for Sleep Without Pills by Peter Tanzer, MD, in private practice, Pittsburgh, and clinical assistant professor of medicine, University of Pittsburgh School of Medicine. Tresco Publishers.

Improved sexual relations bring relaxation and reduced stress—two keys to better sleep. For many people, regular nighttime sexual relations seem to create a sense of satisfaction, calm and well-being, reduce anxiety and depression and let the participants sleep better.

Warning: Some people find that sex causes insomnia instead of relieving it…and they should avoid sex near bedtime.

Women Are Just as Likely as Men to Initiate Sexual Contact

Monica Moore, PhD, associate professor, department of behavioral and social sciences, Webster University, St. Louis.

According to cultural myths, it is the male who is the sexual aggressor in male–female relationships. But because a woman's ways of flirting—like standing close to her target or using seductive glances—are more subtle, it is the man who is seen as initiating contact…even in situations when he is simply responding to an invitation.

Saying No to Sex

Shirley Zussman, EdD, sex therapist, New York, and editor of *Sex Over Forty*, Box 1600, Chapel Hill, NC 27515.

To say *no* to sex gently, start by telling your partner why you are not in the mood. Assure him/her you find him desirable and he is not the reason for your lack of desire. Consider nonsexual intimacy instead—snuggling, doing some activity together—so you can still be close without being sexual…and set a date to make love in the near future.

Example: On the weekend, if you are too tired during the week.

If your lack of desire is caused by a relationship problem, say so and try to work it out. Talk at a neutral time and place—not in bed.

Sex and Heart Attacks

James E. Muller, MD, associate professor of medicine, Harvard Medical School, Boston. His study of 858 men and women who survived heart attacks was published in *The Journal of the American Medical Association*, 515 N. State St., Chicago 60610.

A study found that the risk of heart attack from sexual activity is only about two in one million. This compares with one in one million if the person did not engage in sexual activity during the prior hour. Heart patients who exercise regularly—meaning they simply walked briskly up a slight hill for 30 minutes a day—had no increased risk from sexual activity.

Sex Can Relieve Arthritis Pain

Warren Katz, MD, chief, division of rheumatology, Presbyterian Medical Center, Philadelphia.

Seventy percent of people in one study said their arthritis pain was relieved for up to six hours after intercourse.

Possible explanation: Sex triggers the release of natural cortisone and betaendorphins —two chemicals that relieve pain naturally.

Helpful: A warm bath or shower before sexual activity to relieve any initial stiffness.

Premature Ejaculation Drug

Stanley E. Althof, PhD, associate professor of psychology, Case Western Reserve University School of Medicine, Cleveland. His two-month study of premature ejaculation in 15 couples was published in the *Journal of Clinical Psychiatry*, Box 752870, Memphis 38175.

Delay premature ejaculation with the prescription drug *clomipramine* (Anafranil). Taken six hours before sex, clomipramine delayed ejaculation from an average of only 81 seconds after vaginal penetration to as long as 419 seconds. Couples reported greater sexual satisfaction while the man was on the drug.

Lovemaking Is More than Sex

Real Moments for Lovers by Barbara DeAngelis, PhD, a specialist in human relations and personal growth, Los Angeles. Delacorte Press.

Limiting lovemaking to sexual times puts tremendous pressure on sex lives and misidentifies the type of connection that true lovers want. The physical connection of sex is only a part of true lovers' intimacy. *Better:* Seek real moments of love with your partner—

moments to feel your love fully and rejoice in your relationship. Really making love means stirring up the feelings that constantly flow between you.

Drug for Genital Herpes

Bruce Yaffe, MD, internist and gastroenterologist in private practice, 121 E. 84 St., New York 10028.

Patients who have recurring episodes of these painful sores will get relief within six hours from *famciclovir* (Famvir)—a medicine that needs to be taken only twice a day when symptoms develop. Another drug— *acyclovir*—will also stop outbreaks, but must be used five times a day—and doesn't relieve the pain.

Dr. Ruth's Secrets of Great Sex

Sex therapist Ruth Westheimer, PhD, interviewed in *Investor's Business Daily*, 12655 Beatrice St., Los Angeles 90066.

Genuinely liking your partner…communicating well…being able to ask for what you want.

Sex Isn't Only for The Healthy

Robert Butler, MD, director, International Leadership Center on Longevity and Society, Mount Sinai Medical Center, New York, and author of *Love and Sex After 60*. Ballantine Books.

Generally, there is no medical reason why someone who is ill should abstain from sexual contact.

Example: Heart attack patients, after an initial recovery period, can usually safely have intercourse, and most actually benefit from it.

Helpful: Take preventive measures before making love, such as finding a comfortable position for both partners and taking nitroglycerin. Check with your doctor about appropriate precautions for your condition.

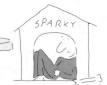

Better Communication

Sexual Healing: How Good Loving Is Good for You—and Your Relationship by Barbara Keesling, PhD, sex therapist, Los Angeles. Hunter House.

For greater intimacy, set aside a particular time for you and your spouse to practice asking *explicitly* what each other wants. Half the time, you do the asking...the other half, your spouse.

Benefit: No more second-guessing about what you or your partner wants.

Sex and Headaches

Fred Freitag, DO, associate director, Diamond Headache Clinic, Chicago.

Headaches associated with sex afflict about 3% of women occasionally.

Usual cause: Muscle strain of the neck and shoulders or rapid blood pressure increases from hormonal surges.

Self-defense: Stay in shape—sex requires stamina...take your time—extending foreplay lets hormone levels and heart rate rise gradually, not surge...change positions—certain positions cause more muscle strain and exertion than others.

Hysterectomies and Sex

Kristen H. Kjerulff, PhD, associate professor of epidemiology, University of Maryland, Baltimore, leader of a two-year study of 1,100 women, published in *The Journal of the American Medical Association*.

Hysterectomies don't diminish women's sexuality. Most women who have hysterectomies report more sexual activity and greater pleasure after the operation than before it.

Probable reason: The symptoms that usually lead to hysterectomies—including pain and heavy bleeding—keep women from enjoying sex fully *before* the operation.

Sexual Frequency

Domeena Renshaw, MD, founder/director, Loyola University sexual dysfunction clinic, Maywood, IL.

Married couples today have sex less frequently than couples 60 years ago. Then, married men and women in their 30s had sex about three times a week. Now the average is about twice a week.

Possible reasons: Dual-career marriages and other elements of a high-pressure modern lifestyle.

Home HIV Test Kits

Frederick Hecht, MD, assistant professor of medicine at the AIDS Program, University of California at San Francisco.

Home HIV test kits give results virtually as accurate as blood tests done at doctors' offices. After purchasing the kit, the buyer pricks his/her finger to take a blood sample and sends it to the company's lab. A code is given so that only the person with the code can obtain the results—which are available by phone within about a week. If the result is positive, the call is automatically directed to a company-provided counselor. *Cost of kit and lab work:* About $40.

Sensual Massage Made Easy

A Lover's Guide to Massage by Victoria Day, massage therapist and registered midwife, Bristol, England. Ward Lock, distributed by Sterling Publishing Co.

Start a sensual massage by putting oil on your hands and applying it to your partner with broad, easy strokes. Be very gentle at first, then feel through your fingers where to press harder. Keep your fingers relaxed. Use your whole palm and fingers for the massage. Keep strokes reliable and rhythmic, so the massage feels like a continuous sequence even though you move from one body part to another.

All About In Vitro Fertilization

Jonathan Scher, MD, obstetrician and gynecologist in private practice in New York, and coauthor of *Preventing Miscarriage: The Good News.* HarperPerennial.

Infertile couples seeking an egg or sperm donor should first contact an in vitro fertilization program or support group. These programs explain exactly how to proceed and what you need to find out about the donor. Trying to locate a donor by advertising is risky because of the unknown genetic background of the respondents. It may also cause future legal problems. The programs screen donors so you can specify factors such as preferred age, ethnic background and education. *Cost per attempt:* For sperm, about $200…for donated eggs, $1,000 to $3,000. Additional costs range from $6,000 to $10,000.

Questions that Keep Love Alive

Instant Insight: 200 Ways to Create the Life You Really Want by Jonathan Robinson, psychotherapist and seminar leader, Santa Barbara, CA. Health Communications.

Ask your partner: What helps you feel most loved by me?…Do you know what you do that makes me feel most loved?

Ask yourself: What act of love or kindness can I do for my partner this week?…What problems are we having that we are not talking about?…How can we talk about them?

Helpful: Plan to spend quality time together at least twice a week. Think about what you really love about your partner…and what fun things you can do together. Then work together to plan them.

Eminent Sex Therapist Reveals Her Secret Weapon Against Sexual Problems

Barbara Bartlik, MD, psychiatrist and medical sex therapist with the human sexuality program at New York Hospital–Cornell Medical Center in New York City. She studied with the late Dr. Helen Singer Kaplan, the renowned sex therapist, and was an associate in Dr. Kaplan's practice.

For most of us, erotica has long been taboo—an embarrassing vice. But as leading sex therapists have found, a new generation of "tasteful" videos and literature can be a powerful ally for couples struggling with sexual problems…or seeking to enrich their sexual relationship.

Even couples who find ordinary "porn" offensive often find that they enjoy—and benefit from—the new, sensitive erotica.

These materials—featuring interesting plots and caring, realistic relationships—are designed to excite *and* educate. They have proven helpful in resolving several common sexual problems…

SEXUAL ENNUI

The most obvious use of erotica is to spice up sex for couples who have fallen into a rut.

The late pioneering sex therapist Helen Singer Kaplan, MD, coined the term "hot monogamy" to describe couples who seek sexual adventure *within* marriage. This is done by using erotic toys, sexy lingerie, play-acting, reading and viewing erotica together.

PERFORMANCE ANXIETY

Old-style porn focuses exclusively on the sex act, emphasizing sexual prowess and anatomies of improbable proportions. That can exacerbate feelings of inadequacy in men (and women), contributing to impotence and performance anxiety.

Several more recent videos depict ordinary-looking people enjoying sex in the context of their broader lives. This gives viewers a more realistic standard against which to compare themselves, helping them overcome fears of inadequacy.

Some erotica depicts couples expressing passion *without* progressing to intercourse. Learning about noncoital ways to satisfy each other can remove pressure, rebuild confidence and curb anxiety—lessening performance concerns.

POOR COMMUNICATION

Many individuals find it hard to ask for what they want in bed—oral sex, anal stimulation, etc. They're simply unassertive...or they fear their partner will feel put down.

Erotica provides ways around this problem. One partner can say to the other, "Let's try what they did" or "I'd love it if we could do that."

In some videos, such as those in the *Femme* series (described on the next page), partners are shown giving each other suggestions and feedback in a sensitive, lighthearted way. Watching these "role models" can make talking about sex more comfortable.

SEXUAL INHIBITION

Even in our sexually liberated age, many adults come from restrictive upbringings that taught them sex is dirty and good people don't enjoy it. Many of these people never learned effective ways to give and receive sexual pleasure.

Erotica demonstrates a variety of ways to enhance foreplay and intercourse. And newer, plot-oriented tapes show people of all ages and from many walks of life enjoying sex. This can help viewers feel more comfortable with their own sexuality.

RELATIONSHIP CONFLICT

Pent-up anger or other conflicts with a partner can lead to loss of desire. This initiates a downward spiral in the relationship, since unsatisfying sex can lead to even more frustration.

To halt this spiral, couples must confront these conflicts directly—via honest conversation and perhaps counseling.

While couples are working out their difficulties, erotica can help reignite sexual interest, strengthening the bond between them.

LACK OF FOCUS

Some individuals have trouble focusing on their partners and find that they are unable to reach orgasm.

Typically, they're distracted by work pressures, concerns about body image or privacy, etc.

Erotica compensates for these distractions by "turning up the volume" of sexual excitement.

PROBLEMS THAT DON'T RESPOND TO EROTICA

Erotica is not helpful for...

- **Premature ejaculation.** Men with this problem need to focus on their own physical sensations, not images of others.

- **Sexual aversion.** For this problem, in which sex is extremely anxiety-provoking or distasteful, the partner or partners need to be exposed gradually to sexual activity.

- **Some individuals with a history of sexual abuse.**

Even minor problems sometimes require professional sex therapy. If the problem does not get better, seek professional guidance.

Helpful resource: American Association of Sex Educators, Counselors and Therapists, 804-644-3288.

WHERE TO GET EROTICA

Rent erotic videos at a neighborhood video store...or watch cable television.

Or browse through the classics of erotic literature in a bookstore's "sexuality" section. I recommend Anaïs Nin's *A Spy in the House of*

Love...Henry Miller's *Tropic of Cancer*...and D.H. Lawrence's *Lady Chatterley's Lover*.

If privacy is essential, consider using one of the following mail-order companies...

●**Critic's Choice Video**, 800-544-9852. Carries a selection of erotic videos, including the Playboy and Playgirl series.

●**Femme,** 800-456-5683. This video production company, started by former adult film star Candida Royale, features "female-friendly" erotic videos.

●**Sinclair Intimacy Institute**, 800-955-0888. Carries the Better Sex Video series, featuring realistic couples in tasteful settings.

  # Get in Sync

Al Cooper, PhD, clinical director, San Jose Marital and Sexuality Centre, San Jose, CA, writing online in *Self-Help & Psychology, http://cybertowers.com/selfhelp.*

Synchronize your sexual desire with your partner's by finding out what is knocking you out of sync—an overcrowded schedule, pent-up resentments, concerns about your attractiveness or your partner's—or anything else. Make decisions that will allow you to plan when to get together.

Examples: Go to bed earlier or later...or take turns setting up lovemaking sessions, so each of you gets a chance to do it your way.

Sleep Positions and Relationships

David Fogel, MD, medical director, Human Sexuality Institute, Washington, DC.

The way partners sleep may provide a window into the state of their relationship. Changes in a couple's sleep position may signal anger, vulnerability, longing, forgiveness, worry or other feelings.

Caution: Not all sleep-position changes are meaningful. Some may simply be a result of a change in the room's temperature.

14

Growing Older— Healthier

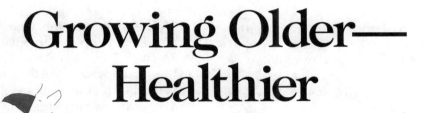

The Key to Successful Aging

Joseph A. James, MD
Beth Israel Medical Center

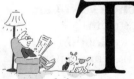

The best news about staying in good physical health as you age is not the break-throughs in medical tech-nology, but in the way good doctors now treat their older patients.

Changed goals: For years, patients would go to a doctor to get treated for a specific problem. But if you visit an experienced physician today, he/she is much more likely to check on a full range of physical and mental functions, with the idea of preventing disease or illness from taking hold by nipping any health problem in the bud as soon as it's spotted.

SUCCESSFUL AGING STRATEGY

•**It's now recommended** that doctors see their older patients (generally 59 years old… and above) at least *three times a year*—and once a year make a full assessment of the patient's physical and mental status.

•**This assessment employs a multidisci-plinary approach**—the doctor quickly refers the patient to an appropriate specialist if any preliminary test suggests a problem.

•**Preventive medicine is stressed**, including vaccinations and diagnostic tests.

•**The doctor is an active adviser on diet and exercise.**

•**If any medical problem *does* occur**—even a seemingly minor one—doctors will now treat it much more aggressively than in the past, when older patients were "expected" to become ill.

FINDING A GOOD DOCTOR

Many primary care physicians now have the equipment to make a full assessment right in their offices.

If you're looking for a doctor, seek out someone who treats a large number of older

Joseph A. James, MD, head of the Yarmon Division of Geriatric Medicine at Beth Israel Medical Center in New York City.

patients. For those who are age 70 or older and have several ongoing medical problems, I recommend seeing a geriatrician (a primary care doctor who specializes in age-related health issues).

FULL ANNUAL ASSESSMENT

Studies have shown that older people are significantly healthier from year to year if they have annual comprehensive assessments. This can be done by a doctor or a geriatric nurse practitioner. The health assessment should include...

●**An evaluation of your daily living activities.** How easy is it for you to dress, cook and shop for yourself? Are there any mobility or balance problems that need to be addressed?

●**Cognitive and psychological exam** that checks for any hint of early dementia, alcoholism (which may affect as many as one out of three people age 75 and older), side effects of medication or infection (both of which can cause delirium) and signs of depression, a common—and often undiagnosed—problem among seniors, and one that can be treated very effectively.

●**Nutritional risk evaluation.** This is very important. Many seniors don't eat the way they should, for a variety of reasons. Money can be an issue, or good shopping facilities might not be easily accessible. A physical disability such as arthritis could also make the act of cooking difficult.

The same is true of depression, or some other underlying medical problem. If there is a nutritional deficiency, nutritional supplements and more careful menu planning can help correct the problem.

●**Vision evaluation.** If a problem is diagnosed, the doctor should refer you to an ophthalmologist.

●**Hearing test**, using an audiometer. If any deficiency is spotted, you should be referred to an audiologist.

●**Urinary and bowel continence evaluation.** If there's even a slight problem, it's good to know about it. There are many things that can be done, either by your doctor or a urologist, to treat incontinence.

●**Basic dental evaluation.**

●**Full social evaluation**—including a look at how your support system of family and friends is holding up, what your general financial situation is, as well as key life decisions you'll be making—such as drafting a living will.

AGGRESSIVE SCREENING AND PREVENTIVE CARE

"Prevent it...or catch it early" is now the motto of doctors who cater to older patients. Your doctor should be making sure you are up to date on all important diagnostic tests and vaccinations, including...

●**Pneumovax vaccine.** Pneumonia can be fatal in older people, particularly those who live in cities. This vaccine is good protection against pneumoccocal pneumonia.

●**Tetanus vaccine.** This should be renewed every 10 years—something many adults forget.

●**A regular tuberculosis test.**

●**Annual mammogram**, to test for signs of breast cancer in women.

●**Annual prostate-specific antigen (PSA) blood test** to check for the signs of prostate cancer in men.

●**Flexible sigmoidoscopy.** This procedure checks for polyps in the colon, and should be done every three years.

●**Annual pelvic exam**, to check for signs of cervical or ovarian cancer in women.

●**Test for thyroid function.**

●**Annual evaluation of cholesterol** and triglyceride levels in the bloodstream.

●**Vitamin B-12 and folate evaluation**—for deficiencies that can lead to a decline in mental functioning.

●**Influenza vaccine shot** every autumn. This is important for all adults. Studies show that the flu vaccine curbs serious illness in all adult age groups.

AGGRESSIVE TREATMENT

While the tests listed above may seem expensive in the short term, they actually cost much, much less than the price of treating a serious illness further down the line.

This is why more and more HMOs and insurance companies are beginning to embrace the "whole-person" preventive philosophy—it saves them money.

Another part of this approach is to treat any illness, even a minor one, in an aggressive fashion.

Chronic problems like high blood pressure, diabetes, osteoporosis or mobility problems now get close attention from informed doctors. A wider range of treatments is now being used as well, including physical therapy and exercise and nutrition programs.

In the same way, swift aggressive treatment is now the rule for acute problems like respiratory infections or muscle or bone ailments. The view is that anything that takes away from your overall ability to live your daily life is a threat.

Finally, if you have any questionable health test results, expect your doctor to refer you to a specialist immediately. The older we get, the more important it is to get a qualified specialist's opinion—quickly.

Alzheimer's Self-Defense

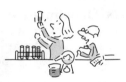

Peter V. Rabins, MD, MPH, professor of psychiatry at Johns Hopkins University School of Medicine, Baltimore. He is coauthor of *The 36-Hour Day,* a guide for Alzheimer's caregivers. Warner Books. Contact the National Alzheimer's Association (800-272-3900) for more information.

Alzheimer's disease—the most common cause of progressive deterioration of mental function—now afflicts four million Americans.

For the latest on this devastating illness, we interviewed Dr. Peter V. Rabins, a leader in the field...

● **What causes Alzheimer's?** There are several theories. *Two of the most widely circulated ones, however, have been largely debunked...*

● **Aluminum.** Though high levels of aluminum are often found in the brains of Alzheimer's patients, there is no evidence that this metal causes the disease. It is safe to use aluminum pans and to drink from aluminum cans.

● **Zinc.** As with aluminum, there is insufficient evidence to indicate that an excess of dietary zinc causes Alzheimer's. But one study did find a link between zinc and the clumping of proteins in the brain, a condition associated with Alzheimer's.

In light of this study, I think it's prudent to stick to federal guidelines for daily zinc consumption—15 milligrams (mg) for men and 12 mg for women.

● **If aluminum and zinc aren't the problem, what is?** Heredity may be to blame. Researchers have identified several different genes for Alzheimer's, including three that cause the form that strikes before age 65.

Researchers have also found a gene that produces a protein called APOE4. A study published in *The Lancet* suggests that if you inherit a copy of this gene from one parent, you have a 35% chance of developing Alzheimer's by age 90.

● **Is heredity the sole cause of Alzheimer's?** No. Studies suggest that some cases of Alzheimer's are associated with...

● **Head trauma.** A history of head injury doubles the chance that you'll get Alzheimer's. Thus it's vitally important to use seat belts, purchase a car with airbags and wear a helmet when riding a motorcycle (or—better—avoid motorcycles entirely). It's also a good idea to avoid boxing and other sports that can lead to head trauma.

● **Head circumference.** Researchers found that people who get Alzheimer's tend to have smaller heads than those who don't. If this provocative finding is confirmed, doctors may someday be able to assess a patient's risk by measuring his/her head circumference and other risk factors.

● **Education.** Alzheimer's patients tend to have less formal education than those without the disease. Formal education may delay the onset of the disease by four to five years.

● **How is Alzheimer's diagnosed?** No single test can diagnose Alzheimer's with absolute certainty. Doctors make a probable diagnosis on the basis of physical, psychological and neurological exams.

First, we perform lab tests to rule out other possible causes of dementia. The list of dementia-causing ailments includes stroke, thyroid disease, liver and kidney disease, vitamin deficiency, depression and long-term use of tranquilizers, antiulcer agents, antihypertensives and heart medications.

If you must take one or more of these drugs, make sure your doctor has prescribed the lowest effective dose.

Next, we observe the patient for signs that the dementia is progressing slowly. Rapidly progressing dementia usually suggests a problem other than Alzheimer's.

Finally, we look for memory loss plus impairment in one or more areas of mental functioning, such as language, visual perception and the performance of everyday tasks. Alzheimer's involves a *combination* of deficits.

●**How can I assess my risk of developing Alzheimer's?** *Two experimental tests that have been in the news recently are the...*

●**Eyedrop test.** The patient's eyes are dilated with eyedrops. In individuals with Alzheimer's (or a predisposition to Alzheimer's), the drops cause the pupils to dilate significantly wider than in people who face little risk of the disease.

Problem: Not everyone with Alzheimer's has dilated pupils after getting the drops...and many people without Alzheimer's do.

●**APOE4 test.** Using this blood test, doctors can determine if you have inherited one or more copies of the Alzheimer's gene.

I'm not recommending this test for my patients—even those with symptoms or a family history of Alzheimer's. All it can tell you is that if you inherit two copies of the gene, you're 2.5 times more likely to get Alzheimer's than someone who has not inherited this gene.

The real question, of course, is why anyone would *want* to know his risk of Alzheimer's—since there remains no effective means of preventing the disease.

●**What can I do to lower my risk?** Alzheimer's risk appears to be lower among people who take aspirin, ibuprofen or another nonsteroidal anti-inflammatory drug on a regular basis.

For postmenopausal women, estrogen-replacement therapy (ERT) may reduce the risk

of the disease—or at least delay its onset, though the evidence is conflicting.

●**I read that mental activity helps prevent Alzheimer's. Is that true?** We don't know that for sure, but I encourage my friends, family and patients to stay mentally—and physically—active, just in case.

Reading, doing crossword puzzles or engaging in other mentally demanding activities stimulates your brain cells. This may enhance connections between the cells, slowing the rate of age-associated memory loss.

●**What about "smart foods" and "smart drugs?"** Some people have started taking so-called *cognition-enhancers*—drugs and nutrients such as deprenyl, DHEA, ginkgo biloba and acetyl-l-carnitine. Unfortunately, there is no substantial evidence that these agents prevent Alzheimer's.

●**Is Alzheimer's ever reversible?** Despite media reports of miraculous cures, there hasn't been a single documented case in which someone with Alzheimer's got better.

Of course, patients *mis*diagnosed as having Alzheimer's disease can experience a restoration of memory when the underlying cause—typically depression or another medical disorder or drug effect—has been controlled.

On Healthy Aging

Peg Krach, PhD, associate professor of nursing, Purdue University School of Nursing, West Lafayette, IN.

People who remain healthy past age 85 share several attributes. They remain socially active ...are able to adapt to change and rebound from bad situations...rely less on medication than their less-healthy peers...view themselves positively, both physically and mentally...and have frequent contact with friends and family.

Also: They accept age-related ailments gracefully and with few complaints.

A Game Plan for Life Extension

Roy L. Walford, MD, professor of pathology at the University of California, Los Angeles, School of Medicine. He is author of *The Anti-Aging Plan*. Four Walls Eight Windows.

From Bulgarian yogurt to goat testicle implants, countless life-extension programs have been promoted. But only *caloric restriction* has been validated by scientific evidence.

More than 50 studies have shown that animals fed a calorie-restricted diet live 30% to 50% longer than animals allowed unrestricted eating. Calorie-restricted rats live about 55 months, compared with about 38 months for rats fed a "normal" diet.

No life-extension studies have been performed on humans. But my experience with Biosphere 2, the research habitat where I served as resident physician, supports the animal data.

Biosphere 2 was a self-contained habitat built under a massive dome in the Arizona desert. I lived there with seven colleagues from September 26, 1991, to September 26, 1993.

Since we could eat only what we could grow inside the dome, we often had to get by with less than we had been accustomed to.

Most of us consumed 1,800 to 2,200 calories a day. The average adult eats 2,400 to 3,000 calories a day.

BIOMARKERS AND AGING

During our time in the Biosphere, all team members experienced significant improvements in various "biomarkers" for aging.

Blood pressure, cholesterol levels, fasting blood sugar levels and white blood cell counts all declined. Meanwhile, our general health, disease resistance and overall vitality improved.

Blood samples taken during our stint in Biosphere indicated that insulin levels also declined. The hormonal changes were exactly like those seen in calorie-restricted animals.

HOW CALORIC RESTRICTION WORKS

Studies suggest that calorie restriction retards the aging process by...

● **Boosting the body's ability to repair damage** to its own genetic material (DNA).

● **Keeping the immune system "younger"** for a longer time.

● **Increasing the body's production of antioxidants.** These natural compounds help control levels of "corrosive" body molecules known as *free radicals.*

HOW TO CUT BACK ON CALORIES

If you are interested in extending the quality and quantity of your life, discuss caloric restriction with your doctor. Caloric restriction is not recommended for children, adolescents or pregnant women.

How many calories should you eat? It's hard to give one number that is appropriate for everyone. However, I suggest you start your antiaging plan by eating 1,800 calories a day.

On such a diet, weight loss is inevitable. But don't lose weight too fast. *Best:* In your first year on a calorie-restricted diet, lose no more than 25% of your weight.

If you lose weight more quickly than that, or your weight fails to stabilize after several months, up your calorie intake. In animal studies, too-rapid weight loss shortened life spans.

MOST HELPFUL STRATEGIES

● **Focus on foods with maximum nutritional value**—vegetables, fruits, grains and fish. You can eat more of them without exceeding your caloric guidelines.

● **Avoid sugar and alcohol.** They represent empty calories. You can, however, occasionally eat cookies, ice cream or other treats—so you don't feel deprived.

● **Eat less fat.** Try to get no more than 20% of your daily calories from fat.

● **Exercise.** While regular activity may not extend your life span, it will extend your *health span*. That's the period during which you remain active and healthy.

Ideal: Moderate exercise most days of the week, alternating between aerobic and muscle-building activities.

Mistakes Doctors Make When Treating Older Patients

Robert Butler, MD, professor of geriatrics and director of the International Longevity Center at Mount Sinai School of Medicine, New York City. He is the former director of the National Institute on Aging. In 1976, Dr. Butler won a Pulitzer Prize for his book *Why Survive? Being Old in America.* HarperCollins.

The older you are, the more likely you are to have health problems that require first-rate medical care. As many seniors have learned, however, it can be hard to find a doctor suited to care for *their* special needs.

How can older people be sure to get good medical care? We put that question to Dr. Robert Butler, a well-known crusader for elder rights. *He explained how important it is to watch out for the common mistakes doctors make when treating elderly patients...*

•*Mistake:* **Failing to appreciate the physical changes that come with age.** Most doctors now practicing know little about the aging body and its ills.

When we launched the geriatrics program at Mount Sinai in 1982, it was the nation's first.

A disease that causes one set of symptoms in a young person may manifest itself quite differently in an older person. Not all doctors realize that. And an unwary doctor can easily miss the diagnosis.

Example I: If a 30-year-old man suffers a heart attack, he is likely to experience severe chest pain. But chest pain is present in less than 20% of older heart attack victims. Instead, older victims may simply seem weak or confused.

Example II: An older person suffering from an overactive thyroid may exhibit apathy instead of hyperactivity, the classic symptom.

•*Mistake:* **Urging older people to "take it easy."** This is awful advice. Even if you've been disabled by a stroke or another medical problem, leading an active lifestyle helps keep you healthy and happy.

Researchers at Tufts University have shown that even people in their 80s and 90s can develop big, powerful muscles with a program of weight lifting. Such a program can literally put a bedridden patient back on his/her feet.

•*Mistake:* **Being too quick to blame health problems on old age.** Doctors often assume that health problems are inevitable in the elderly, exhibiting a defeatist "What can you expect at your age?" attitude.

They order fewer diagnostic tests and generally treat disease less aggressively in old people than in young people.

Example: An elderly woman seems confused and disoriented. *Assuming* that she has Alzheimer's disease, her doctor neglects to order tests that might show the real culprit to be an easily correctable drug reaction.

•*Mistake:* **Not giving the patient enough time.** A good physician will take the time to ask about your work status and lifestyle as well as your medical problems...and, in general, make you *feel* taken care of.

At each office visit, the doctor should ask about the symptoms you have reported in the past. He should also review your response to medications...and ask about new problems.

If you have a *hearing problem*, don't be afraid to ask your doctor to speak up.

Your first visit to a new doctor should be devoted to taking a thorough medical history, and conducting a physical exam and lab tests. This can take more than an hour.

Once this comprehensive exam is completed, you won't need another exam for a year—unless there's a health crisis.

•*Mistake:* **Failing to advocate preventive measures.** Some doctors seem to think, "Why bother trying to lower an elderly patient's cholesterol level. He's just going to decline anyway."

In fact, we now know that heart patients of *any* age can benefit from a program of dietary modification, lifestyle change and—if necessary—drugs or surgery.

•*Mistake:* **Giving inappropriate prescriptions.** Doctors are too quick to order tranquilizers and antidepressants for their older patients, thinking—incorrectly—that psychotherapy is of no use. And they often fail to realize that older bodies respond differently to drugs.

Example I: It can take an elderly person twice as long to "clear" *diazepam* (Valium) from his body as a young person. A dose appropriate for a young person could make an older person drowsy.

Example II: Older people often must take several different drugs at the same time. If the doctor fails to consider all the drugs, dangerous interactions could result.

If you're not sure your doctor knows all the drugs *you're* taking, put all your medications (including nonprescription drugs) in a paper bag and bring them to your next office visit.

Treatments for Parkinson's Disease

Abraham N. Lieberman, MD, chief of movement disorders at Barrow Neurological Institute in Phoenix, and clinical director, National Parkinson Foundation, 1501 NW Ninth Ave., Miami 33136. He is coauthor of *Parkinson's Disease: The Complete Guide for Patients and Caregivers*. Fireside Books.

More than one million Americans have been diagnosed with Parkinson's disease—the progressive, degenerative brain disorder. An equal number are thought to have the condition—but don't know it.

One percent of people over 60 have Parkinson's, as do 2% of those over 70. But the condition can strike at any age.

There's no cure for Parkinson's. Drugs remain the mainstay of treatment, although surgery has become an option.

THE SYMPTOMS

Most people are first alerted to the possibility that they have Parkinson's by friends or family members who notice…

- **Tremor.** It's most apparent when the hand or foot is relaxed. Most Parkinson's-related tremors are more pronounced on one side of the body.

- **Slow movement** (*bradykinesia*). People with Parkinson's swing their arms less when walking and take longer to wash dishes, take out the garbage, etc.

- **Rigidity.** Muscles become stiff and resistant to movement.

- **Poor balance.** Because they have trouble telling when they're standing straight, people with Parkinson's are likely to fall.

WHAT CAUSES PARKINSON'S

Parkinson's disease stems from damage to the *substantia nigra*. This region of the brain produces the neurotransmitter *dopamine*, which is vital to the function of a second brain area called the *striatum*—which controls movement.

Just what destroys the substantia nigra is unclear. Heredity is apparently a factor. Recent studies suggest that pesticides may play a role as well.

The existence of clusters of Parkinson's disease—as on the island of Guam—suggests that environmental factors may also be involved. But which agents might be involved is unknown.

Bottom line: There is no known way to prevent the disease.

THE FASTEST TREATMENT

The principal treatment is with a drug called *L-dopa* (Sinemet).

L-dopa is quite effective at controlling symptoms of Parkinson's. But there is a problem—fluctuating levels of the drug within the brain. When levels are low, Parkinson's symptoms return. High levels can cause tics, spasms and other side effects.

To maintain the right level, many Parkinson's patients take time-release L-dopa.

The drug *selegiline* (Eldepryl) helps maintain proper dopamine levels by blocking the action of an enzyme that ordinarily breaks dopamine down.

With or without selegiline, L-dopa works well for just so long. After five to 10 years, most patients have increased side effects and poorer response.

Doctors now have another drug in their anti-Parkinson's arsenal—*tolcapone* (Tasmar), though its usefulness may be limited by liver toxicity.

If you or someone you know is interested in participating in a clinical trial of these drugs, contact the National Parkinson Foundation (800-327-4545, *www.parkinson.org*).

SURGERY

Surgery has been used to treat Parkinson's since the 1930s. But techniques have vastly improved since then.

The most common form of surgery is *pallidotomy*. In this procedure, the surgeon inserts a tiny probe through the skull, then applies electrical current to destroy a region of the brain called the *globus pallidum.*

Pallidotomy does not cure Parkinson's disease. But properly performed, the surgery dramatically reduces tremor and improves the ability to move. It can be extremely helpful for patients who respond poorly to medication.

Because the globus pallidum lies deep within the brain, pallidotomy is risky. Even with a good surgeon, there is a 1% to 2% chance of hemorrhagic stroke.

The procedure can also cause temporary or even permanent confusion and disorientation.

If you are thinking about pallidotomy, ask your neurologist for a referral to an expert neurosurgeon.

FETAL TRANSPLANT

Some surgeons have begun taking tissue from the brains of 9- to 12-week-old aborted fetuses and implanting it into the brains of Parkinson's patients.

This transplanted tissue starts producing its own dopamine, making up for the lack of dopamine in the patients' brains.

As with pallidotomy, fetal transplantation carries a small but significant risk of stroke. But fetal transplants are often extremely effective—especially in people under 60. (The older you are, the less likely the transplants will take hold and flourish.) Following surgery, some patients find that they no longer need medication.

Problem: Because fetal transplantation is considered experimental, the cost of the procedure—about $50,000—isn't covered by most health insurance.

And because of political objections to the use of fetal tissue, the operation is available only in certain states.

Good Samaritan Hospital in Los Angeles and the University of Colorado Health Sciences Center in Denver have the most experience with fetal transplants.

Vitamin Deficiency And Memory

Robert M. Russell, MD, associate director, Jean Mayer US Department of Agriculture Human Nutrition Research Center on Aging at Tufts University, Boston.

Memory loss in elderly people is sometimes caused by a vitamin B-12 deficiency.

Self-defense: If you're over age 60, have your B-12 level checked by a doctor. If it falls below 300, taking a B-12 supplement should fix the problem. Some people need an injectable form of the vitamin. Check with your doctor.

Vitamins Do Help

Study by National Research Foundations and Memorial University of Newfoundland reported in *Money*, 1271 Avenue of the Americas, New York 10020.

People over age 65 who take multivitamins daily were found to be sick with infection-related illnesses only *half* as often as people who did not take vitamins.

Colon Cancer Detection

Marion Nadel, PhD, an epidemiologist in the Division of Cancer Prevention and Control, the Centers for Disease Control and Prevention, Atlanta.

Everyone 50 and older should be screened for colorectal cancer. According to the advisory panel to the US Public Health Service, effective methods include fecal-occult blood testing and sigmoidoscopy (or both).

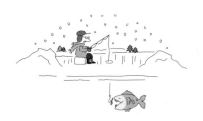

Stronger Seniors

Study of nursing home residents, ages 72 to 98—more than 80% of whom required a cane, walker or wheelchair—led by Maria Fiatarone, MD, chief, nutrition and exercise physiology laboratory, the Jean Mayer US Department of Agriculture Human Nutrition Research Center on Aging at Tufts University, Boston.

Strength training for seniors improves mobility and counteracts muscle weakness and frailty—at any age. A study of 100 nursing-home residents, average age 87, found muscle strength more than doubled after 10 weeks of a progressive resistance training program for hip and knee muscles. Exercise had substantial benefits even for people using canes, walkers or wheelchairs.

Bottom line: Exercise helps people of any age become stronger and more mobile.

Owning a Dog Can Extend Your Life

Erika Friedmann, PhD, a professor in the Department of Health & Nutrition Sciences at Brooklyn College, Brooklyn, NY.

A study of 369 heart attack sufferers found that those who owned dogs were far less likely to die within the first year than those who did not own dogs. Dogs make their owners feel wanted and needed. Dog owners also have to walk their pets regularly, and so are forced to get exercise, too.

Safer Lifting Now

Elizabeth Myers, PhD, assistant professor, Department of Orthopedic Surgery, Beth Israel Hospital, Boston.

People with brittle bones should be very careful about lifting.

Everyday activities like picking up grandchildren or lifting groceries out of the car can lead to painful compression fractures of the spine.

Researchers advise women with osteoporosis or others with fragile bones never to lift with outstretched arms or to bend from the waist while lifting.

Best way to lift: Keep arms as close as possible to the body and try not to bend at the waist.

How to Maintain Peak Mental Ability As You Get Older

Richard M. Restak, MD, clinical professor of neurology at George Washington University School of Medicine and Health Sciences in Washington, DC. He is author of *Older & Wiser* (Simon & Schuster) and *The Brain* (Bantam), which was the companion to the 1984 PBS television series of the same name.

Almost everyone experiences some decline in memory and reaction time after age 40. But a rich network of *neural connections*—links between brain cells that allow them to communicate—can help compensate for these losses.

A rich neural network may even help keep people from being incapacitated by Alzheimer's disease.

Extensive neural connections seem to act as a kind of *cognitive reserve*—allowing a person to function longer with the disease than someone whose mental resources were less extensive.

Good news: Brain cells can form new connections at *any* age. I'm 55 years old, and I'm taking steps *now* to preserve mental function *later*…

DEVELOP A CONSUMING PASSION

When your brain is involved in a wide range of activities, more neural circuits are created and maintained.

Helpful: Cultivating an interest in something totally different from your customary pursuits. A lawyer might take up bridge…or an accountant might learn to play the clarinet.

It's also a good idea to take classes in unfamiliar subjects. Studies have shown that higher education early in life helps ensure proper brain functioning in old age. It seems likely that intellectual activity *later* in life builds cognitive reserves as well.

GET REGULAR EXERCISE

Every day, I walk a few miles at a moderate pace. In addition to keeping the heart and lungs healthy, exercise boosts blood flow to the brain, fueling it with oxygen and glucose.

Another excellent form of exercise is the gentle Chinese martial art *tai chi*.

TAKE SUPPLEMENTS—SENSIBLY

Cellular damage caused by *free radicals*—renegade molecules formed in the body as a by-product of normal metabolism—is thought to be a major cause of age-related mental decline.

To neutralize free radicals, I make sure to get enough of the antioxidant vitamins A, C and E.

I eat lots of fruits and vegetables…and take a supplement containing 10,000 international units (IU) of beta-carotene (the precursor of vitamin A)…1,000 milligrams (mg) of vitamin C…and 400 IU of vitamin E (in the form *d-alpha tocopherol*, which has the highest "biopotency").

Since we tend to become deficient in zinc as we age, I also take a pill containing about 20 mg of this mineral every day. Zinc plays a key role in preserving the sense of smell.

●**Estrogen.** The Baltimore Longitudinal Study of Aging found that postmenopausal women who take estrogen are less likely to suffer from dementia than other women…and that women who already have dementia show improvement when they take estrogen.

Caution: Estrogen increases the risk for breast, uterine and ovarian cancer. Recent studies have refuted earlier findings that it protects against heart disease. Further studies are underway to investigate estrogen's role in the prevention and treatment of dementia. Women with a family history of any of these diseases generally should *not* take estrogen.

In men, estrogen promotes breast enlargement—so it's not a good idea for them to take it. Researchers hope to develop a drug that will stimulate men's estrogen receptors without "feminizing" side effects.

●**Anti-inflammatory drugs.** The Baltimore study also found preliminary evidence that taking nonsteroidal anti-inflammatory drugs (NSAIDs) such as *ibuprofen* might be protective against Alzheimer's.

Caution: Since NSAIDs can cause stomach trouble, they should be taken under a doctor's supervision.

●**DHEA.** Studies suggest that this hormone improves memory. But it increases men's risk for prostate cancer. We don't know if it poses any danger to women. More research is needed.

PREVENT STROKES

A stroke occurs when a blood clot or ruptured artery cuts off blood flow to the brain. New research links stroke-induced brain damage with Alzheimer's.

To minimize your risk: Exercise regularly, eat a healthful diet, avoid smoking and keep your blood pressure under control.

If a stroke does occur, new drugs can help arrest the damage. They must be administered *within hours*, however, so seek medical attention *immediately* at the first sign of stroke.

The signs of stroke include numbness on one side of the body…difficulty speaking or understanding speech…sudden headache…dizziness or loss of balance…and blurred or decreased vision.

CONTROL STRESS

Chronic psychological stress causes the body to make excess *cortisol*. Over time, high levels of this adrenal hormone can cause deterioration of the *hippocampus*, a part of the brain that plays a critical role in memory.

We can't always control events, but we *can* control our response to these events. One strategy I use is to reframe *frustrations* as *challenges*. I ask myself, "What's the best course of action to follow at this time?" I also use words that have a calming rather than tension-producing effect—for example, *concern* rather than *worry*.

MAINTAIN FINGER DEXTERITY

French researchers found recently that older women who knit retain normal mental function longer than their nonknitting counterparts.

I don't knit, but I always carry a crossword dice game with me. Whenever I have a few minutes to spare, I play it.

MAKE PRACTICAL ADAPTATIONS

Memory aids—from making lists to carrying a palmtop computer—are great for helping offset age-related memory loss. But do *not* become so dependent on these helpers that you allow your own natural abilities to atrophy.

Example: If I'm carrying a list of things to do, I'll check it only *after* I've called up as many items as I can from my own memory.

Vitamin E and Aging

Marguerite M.B. Kay, MD, Regents Professor of Microbiology and Immunology and Medicine at the University of Arizona, Tucson, and a geriatrician with The Veteran's Administration.

Vitamin E may help slow the effects of aging on the brain and immune system.

A study on mice found that when middle-aged and old mice were fed diets supplemented with vitamin E, normal age-related damage to vital proteins in their brain and immune system cells was delayed or prevented. Researchers believe that vitamin E, taken at the onset of middle age, will also slow damage due to aging in human brains and immune systems. The equivalent human dosage of vitamin E that was found effective in mice is about 400 International Units (IU) a day.

Caution: More than 1,000 IU a day of vitamin E may be dangerous.

Consider Nursing Home Transfer Policies

Joseph Matthews, author of *Beat the Nursing Home Trap*. Nolo Press.

On occasion, nursing homes try to send residents to hospitals or other nursing facilities to deal with temporary medical problems that can be handled at the nursing home itself.

Note: Transfers to other facilities for medical reasons cannot legally be made without the consent of the patient or legal proxy. The consent of the patient's attending physician should also be obtained.

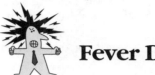

Fever Danger

Catherine Marco, MD, interim chairman of emergency medicine, Johns Hopkins Bayview Medical Center, Baltimore. Her study of 470 patients was published in *Annals of Emergency Medicine*, 11830 Westline Industrial Dr., St. Louis 63146.

Fever in an older person signals the need for hospitalization. In a study of patients 65 or older who went to the emergency room with a fever of 100 degrees or more, 76% were found to be seriously ill. Almost half showed no other outward sign of illness.

ERT to the Rescue

Sally Shumacher, PhD, professor of social sciences and health policy at the Bowman Gray School of Medicine, Winston-Salem, NC.

Estrogen replacement therapy (ERT) may help to delay—or prevent—Alzheimer's disease. Studies suggest that postmenopausal women taking estrogen supplements develop Alzheimer's at a lower rate than others. And—those who have Alzheimer's exhibit less severe symptoms. Estrogen may help the brain withstand Alzheimer's by fostering the growth and branching of nerve cells in the brain and by improving blood circulation there.

Exercise Improves Hearing

Helaine M. Alessio, PhD, associate professor of physical education, Miami University, Oxford, OH.

Research indicates that persons who are not physically fit improve their hearing when they begin regular aerobic exercise—and that persons who are fit are less susceptible to suffer a hearing loss as a result of exposure to loud noise.

Estrogen and Alzheimer's

Sanjay Asthana, MD, physician with the VA Puget Sound Health Care System in Tacoma, WA.

Estrogen treatment improves the memory and concentration of elderly women with Alzheimer's. An eight-week study of women in their 70s suffering from moderate Alzheimer's disease found that within one week those who were given estrogen via skin patches showed a significant improvement in their scores on standard tests of memory and attention. Those women given placebo drug patches showed no improvement. More research is needed to confirm these findings.

The Mind–Body Approach to Arthritis

Margaret A. Caudill, MD, PhD, codirector of the Arnold Pain Center at Deaconess Hospital in Boston, and pain management director of the Lahey Hitchcock Clinic in Nashua, NH. She is author of *Managing Pain Before It Manages You.* Guilford Press.

If you suffer from arthritis, you probably already know that medication provides only partial relief.

Fortunately, arthritis—as well as headaches, back pain and most other forms of chronic pain —can be managed via a set of mind-body techniques. These techniques cost nothing and can be self-administered. They are effective whether your pain is caused by a clearly identifiable disease or is of mysterious origin.

ACUTE VS. CHRONIC PAIN

Acute pain is the body's way of warning us that something is wrong. When we get this "warning signal," we take immediate action to protect ourselves.

Example: We drop a plate that's too hot to hold. Doing so helps us avoid additional injury and gives the injury time to heal.

With *chronic* pain, there is no hot plate to drop. With no obvious way to protect ourselves, we respond emotionally. We slip into depression…become unable to work…experience trouble with our relationships, etc.

The key to coping with chronic pain is to live well *despite* the pain.

KEEP A PAIN DIARY

Keeping a pain diary will help you look at your pain objectively.

What to do: Three times a day, rate the intensity of your pain, from zero (no pain) to 10 (the worst pain ever). Also—describe the sensation. Is it an ache? Burning sensation? Tightness?

Note what you are doing when pain strikes. Rate your distress—the frustration, anger, anxiety or sadness you feel in response to the pain.

Record what you did to alleviate the pain— took an aspirin, went for a walk, applied heat or cold, etc.

Your diary will help you pinpoint things that ease or exacerbate your pain…and clearly show the difference between the pain itself and your emotional response to it.

USE THE RELAXATION RESPONSE

In many cases, the psychological stress caused by pain is worse than the pain itself.

Stress causes muscular tension that can lead to new ills—headache or upset stomach, for instance. Stress also aggravates the fatigue that often comes with chronic pain.

By eliciting your natural "Relaxation Response," you can alleviate this emotional stress.

Technique: Pick a time when your pain is relatively mild, and find a peaceful place where you won't be disturbed. Sit comfortably or lie down. Use a heating pad, ice pack or pillows to make yourself comfortable, if necessary.

Focus on your breathing. With each exhalation, silently repeat a word or phrase of your own choosing. This can be something neutral, like "one"...or something uplifting, such as "God."

Or, count each inhalation and exhalation, starting over when you reach 10. When your mind wanders, gently bring it back to your focus word or phrase. Elicit the Relaxation Response for at least 20 minutes a day.

If you like, elicit the Relaxation Response while exercising. Just make sure your breathing and thoughts are synchronized with your movements.

PERFORM SELF-HYPNOSIS

Once you have mastered the Relaxation Response, add self-hypnosis. While deeply relaxed, close your eyes and imagine that your right hand is becoming pleasantly warm and heavy. Each time you exhale, imagine the pleasant sensation intensifying.

Now imagine a pleasant numbness that begins in your thumb, then moves to each finger with each exhalation. Feel it spread to your palm and the back of your hand, stopping at the wrist.

Place that numb hand on the painful area of your body, or imagine the numbness moving to that spot. When all the numbness has been "absorbed" by the painful area, return to your focus word.

End each session by returning the numbness to your right hand. Feel the normal sensations return to that hand, breath by breath.

PACE YOURSELF

Some chronic pain sufferers try to ignore their bodies—pushing on until the pain becomes unbearable. Others simply shut down, withdrawing from social and/or professional activities.

Better: Pace yourself. Learn to complete your daily activities and live as normally as possible.

To do this, you must...

• **Tune in to your body.** Use your pain diary and the Relaxation Response to become aware of subtle sensations that signal a flare-up.

• **Switch to a less demanding activity** when you feel pain building. If you're washing dishes when your pain worsens, sit down and use the time to pay bills. Go back to the dishes later.

CHANGE YOUR SELF-TALK

The meaning you ascribe to your pain makes an enormous difference in its effect on your life and your mood.

What does your pain mean to you? To find out, listen to your *self-talk.* That's the voice in your head that continually comments on and interprets your pain.

In individuals with chronic pain, self-talk is quite distorted. They tend to *catastrophize*— making a bad situation worse by engaging in exaggerated self-talk.

Example I: Instead of telling yourself you can bear a flare-up, you think, "This pain is unbearable."

Example II: Instead of acknowledging the many things you can still do despite your pain, you say, "My whole life is ruined."

Don't give in to such negative self-talk. Make a conscious choice to change it. Say your pain is too severe to keep a lunch date. You think, "My whole day is ruined."

Substitute a realistic interpretation. "This is unfortunate, but I can make other arrangements. I'll invite my friend to come here, and we'll send out for pizza."

PLAN FOR FLARE-UPS

No matter how well you manage your pain, there will be times when it becomes intense. To be ready for these episodes, keep a written list of strategies that make you feel better— things you can do to reduce the pain and ease your emotional distress.

Examples: Lying down...applying heat or ice...performing self-hypnosis...calling a friend ...or distracting yourself with a funny video.

HIGH-TECH HELP

Though medication can't stop chronic pain entirely, it can make your self-help program more effective. *Four drugs are especially effective...*

• **Gabapentin (Neurontin).** It seems effective for nerve pain caused by diabetes and post-herpetic neuropathy.

●**Mexiletine (Mexitil).** This is an oral form of the anesthetic lidocaine.

●**Fentanyl (Duragesic).** A new skin patch system delivers this potent painkiller continuously for three days.

●**Morphine (Duramorph).** The intrathecal pump constantly delivers morphine to the area around the spinal cord.

Risk Reducers

JoAnn Manson, MD, codirector of women's health at Brigham and Women's Hospital, Harvard Medical School, Boston.

The older a woman is at menopause, the less likely she is to die from heart disease —the leading cause of death in women. Studies show that the risk declines by about 2% for every year that menopause is delayed.

Other risk reducers: Cutting out cigarettes —smokers go through menopause earlier…regular exercise…maintaining a healthy weight…a low-fat diet.

Fainting Danger

J. King White, MD, cardiologist in private practice in Lake Charles, LA.

A fainting spell could signal a serious medical problem. One in five people faints at least once in his/her life.

Usual causes: Emotional stress, anxiety, the sight of blood, etc. But the older a person is, the greater the odds that a serious ailment is to blame—such as a heart disorder or a drug reaction.

To be safe: If you faint, see a doctor.

Best Shoes for Senior Citizens…

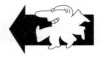

Steven Robbins, MD, associate professor of geriatric medicine, Center for Studies in Aging, McGill University, Montreal.

Those with hard, thin soles. Compared with going barefoot or wearing soft-soled tennis or running shoes, hard-soled shoes provide better "foot-position awareness," a sense that improves posture and helps maintain balance.

How to Guard Against Macular Degeneration

Neil M. Bressler, MD, associate professor of ophthalmology at The Wilmer Ophthalmological Institute of Johns Hopkins University School of Medicine in Baltimore.

Most people already know that diabetes and glaucoma can cause blindness. But one of the leading causes of vision loss is a breakdown of cells in the retina known as *age-related macular degeneration* (AMD).

This condition, which can be detected via a simple eye exam, causes four times more blindness in older adults than glaucoma or diabetes. One-quarter of people over age 65— and one-third of those over age 80—have early signs of the disease.

Scariest of all, AMD can rapidly progress from a minor vision problem to near total loss of "central" vision.

There's no way to restore vision loss caused by macular degeneration. But prompt treatment can often stop the disease in its tracks.

RETINAL BREAKDOWN

Macular degeneration gets its name from the *macula.* That's the exquisitely sensitive central region of the retina, the light-sensitive membrane at the back of the eye. The macula is what we rely upon for reading, driving, recognizing faces and other tasks that demand sharp vision.

Macular degeneration occurs when yellowish patches of material produced in the back of the eye called *drusen* begin to form behind a layer of cells in the macula.

In some cases, drusen cause no symptoms for 10 or even 20 years. But in some unfortunate individuals, drusen quickly give way to an abnormal proliferation of blood vessels and scar tissue within the macula itself.

WAVY LINES

It's at this point that symptoms often start to appear. Straight lines look wavy...or tiny blank spots appear in the center of your field of vision.

The course of the disease can vary. Some people with AMD lose the ability to read or drive within one year of the onset of symptoms. Others suffer comparatively minor vision loss—even after five or 10 years.

PREVENTION

Doctors have not yet found any way to eliminate the risk of developing AMD. *Preliminary research suggests, however, that the following two strategies may offer at least some degree of protection...*

•**Don't smoke.** Smokers seem to be more likely to develop the abnormal proliferation of blood vessels and scar tissue than nonsmokers. If you haven't yet kicked the habit, here's one more reason to do so.

•**Avoid heart disease risk factors.** The same factors that heighten the risk of cardiovascular disease—especially high blood pressure—seem to heighten the risk of losing vision from macular degeneration.

Let this reinforce your determination to cut your intake of saturated fat...control your blood pressure...get regular exercise...and avoid obesity.

EARLY DETECTION

Until doctors know more about prevention, the best way to protect your eyesight from AMD is via annual eye exams. The more conscientious you are about getting exams, the more likely you will be to catch AMD early—while it's still treatable.

Using a device called an ophthalmoscope, an ophthalmologist can easily see drusen and other retinal abnormalities that are the hallmarks of early macular degeneration.

There's no treatment for early AMD. But if the signs are there, it's vitally important to stay alert for the subtle changes in vision that suggest the disease is worsening.

Helpful: Check the vision of each eye separately every day. Some ophthalmologists suggest using an Amsler grid. Ask your eye doctor for one.

LASER SURGERY

Laser surgery is the only procedure proven to halt the progression of AMD.

This 15-minute outpatient procedure should help confine the troublesome blood vessels and scar tissue, thereby decreasing the risk of additional visual loss and protecting your remaining vision.

Laser surgery cannot restore the macula to its original state. Even if the operation goes well, odds are you'll find it impossible to read without low-vision aids that provide increased light and magnification.

After surgery, you'll need checkups—at one and three months later, and then every three or four months—for at least one year and possibly two. In about half of all cases, surgery must be repeated to take care of new areas of damage.

Important: Laser surgery is beneficial only when macular damage is limited to a tiny area—1.5 to 3 millimeters in diameter. That's why it's so crucial to see the eye doctor as soon as you notice symptoms. If you wait even a few weeks, it may be too late for effective treatment.

There's no good way to stabilize vision affected by larger areas of abnormal blood vessels and scar tissue. But two ongoing clinical trials may change that.

•**Study #1.** Doctors are evaluating the use of nonlaser surgical techniques to remove the damaged area and thus limit vision loss.

•**Study #2.** Doctors are trying to limit damage using *photodynamic therapy.* Dye injected into a vein in the patient's arm finds its way to the eye, where it concentrates in the abnormal blood vessels and scar tissue. Shining a harmless light into the eye causes a chemical change in the dye, rendering it toxic to only the diseased part of the retina.

For results of the study of photodynamic therapy with Visudyne, contact Novartis Ophthalmics at *www.visudyne.com.*

LOW-VISION AIDS

From high-power reading glasses and closed-circuit video systems to illuminated magnifying glasses, there are numerous visual aids to help you make the most of what vision you have remaining. These aids can make the difference in whether or not you can read or get around outdoors.

If your ophthalmologist isn't familiar with these devices, ask him/her to refer you to a low-vision specialist.

For more information on macular degeneration, send a self-addressed, stamped, business-sized envelope to the American Academy of Ophthalmology, 655 Beach St., San Francisco 94109.

Congestive Heart Failure And Blood Pressure Link

Daniel Levy, MD, director, Framingham Heart Study, Framingham, MA.

Controlling blood pressure is the best way to avoid congestive heart failure (CHF).

Trap: Doctors often overlook *isolated systolic high blood pressure*, the type most likely to cause CHF. In this form of high blood pressure, the first (systolic) number is 140 or higher…while the second (diastolic) number is 90 or below.

Implication: Patients with such blood pressure need close surveillance and may require treatment.

Alzheimer's Relief

Rachelle Doody, MD, PhD, associate professor of neurology, and codirector, Alzheimer's Disease Research Center, Baylor College of Medicine, Houston.

While not a cure, *donepezil* (Aricept) may benefit up to 80% of Alzheimer's patients. The drug slows breakdown of the brain chemical *acetylcholine*, which is vital for transmission of nerve signals. Donepezil is the second Alzheimer's drug to receive FDA approval. Unlike the first, *tacrine* (Cognex), it cannot harm the liver. And it must be taken only once a day. Tacrine is usually taken four times daily.

PSA Testing: More Harm than Good?

Timothy McCall, MD, a Boston internist, author of *Examining Your Doctor: A Patient's Guide to Avoiding Harmful Medical Care.* Citadel Press. He is a regular commentator on the public radio program Marketplace, and can be found on the Web at *www.drmccall.com.*

One of the most common questions I get from my male patients is whether they should have the *prostate specific antigen* (PSA) test. This simple blood test, I tell them, can detect prostate cancer at an early stage. What isn't known is whether getting a PSA test will benefit *you.*

In 1996, there were 317,000 newly diagnosed cases of prostate cancer in the US. With more than 40,000 deaths per year, it's become the number two cause of cancer death in men. Lung cancer remains number one.

Prostate cancer is very common. It has been estimated that 40% of all men over age 50 have it. But only about 8% of men ever get symptoms, and only 3% die of the disease. In other words, four out of five men with prostate cancer never get symptoms and nine out of 10 will die of something else. In the past, most of these men never found out they had cancer.

The PSA test changed all that. Before the test went into widespread use—beginning in the mid-1980s—there were only about one-third as many cases diagnosed per year. Even so, the number of prostate cancer deaths was about the same as it is today.

This points out one of the biggest problems with PSA testing. We now have the ability to detect cancer not just in those destined to die of the disease but also in the majority who will never get symptoms. Unfortunately, it's impossible to differentiate between the two groups —at least so far.

The second big problem with PSA testing is that it's not clear that the standard treatments for prostate cancer—radical prostate surgery and X-ray therapy—save lives. Many doctors and patients assume that they do. But no good studies have ever demonstrated their effectiveness. Such studies are now under way, but results won't be available for several years. In the meantime, the number of men undergoing prostate surgery has skyrocketed.

The side effects of radical prostate surgery, such as impotence and incontinence, are significant. Though surgeons in top prostate cancer centers report better results, a survey of men two to four years after the operation found that only 11% had had an erection sufficient for intercourse in the prior month. Almost a third wore adult diapers or clamps on their penises to control their urine. Radiation therapy also has significant side effects.

There are major disagreements among medical authorities about PSA testing. The American Cancer Society says men should have one every year starting at age 50 (earlier if they're African-American or have a family history of prostate cancer). The US Preventive Services Task Force does not recommend routine screening.

For my male patients over age 70 and for those whose life expectancy (due to other illnesses) is less than 10 years, I advise against PSA tests. The side effects of treatment simply outweigh the benefits. I tell younger men that a PSA test could save their lives—or it could cause them a lot of needless grief. Right now no one can tell you which.

I encourage my patients to learn as much as possible about prostate cancer. You might visit your local library. Remember, anything more than a couple of years old is outdated. If you (or the library) have access to the Internet, Oncolink (*http://oncolink.upenn.edu/disease/prostate*) is a great place to start.

Given the uncertainties, whether to have the PSA test is a highly personal decision—one each man must make in consultation with his doctor. As with any medical decision that hinges mostly on value judgments, however, it should be your values—not your doctor's—that dictate what you do.

Avoiding Disabling Falls

Steven L. Wolf, PhD, professor and director of research, department of rehabilitation medicine, Emory University School of Medicine, Atlanta. For a good introduction to tai chi, order the videotape *Tai Chi: A Gift for Balance*, Dr. Tingsen Xu, Box 98426, Atlanta 30359.

Elderly people may be less likely to suffer disabling falls if they take up *tai chi*, the ancient martial art that blends meditation with slow, rhythmic movements. Tai chi improves balance by teaching better control of the body.

Caution: Elderly people should begin tai chi training only after a doctor has ruled out neurological problems.

Free Eldercare

Free eldercare services hotline can refer you to any of more than 4,000 local agencies that may help meet your needs. Help is available for problems involving medical care, taxes, the law, investments, housing, transportation and much more. The Eldercare Locator Service in Beltsville, MD, is funded by the US Administration on Aging. Call 800-677-1116.

Dentist May Hold Key to Stroke Risk

Laurie Carter, DDS, PhD, director, oral and maxillofacial radiology, Virginia Commonwealth University School of Dentistry, Richmond.

Dental X rays may identify people at high risk for heart attack and stroke. Hardening of the carotid arteries, which lead to the brain, can often be seen in a panoramic dental X ray. This hardening of the carotids doubles risk of death from heart attack or stroke. *When X rays are taken:* Ask your dentist to look for calcifications in the carotid arteries.

Stroke Sufferer Fact

David J. Ballard, MD, PhD, professor of medicine, Emory University School of Medicine, Atlanta. His study of 38,612 patients age 65 or older was published in *Stroke*, American Heart Association, 7272 Greenville Ave., Dallas 75231.

Stroke victims live longer when they're cared for by a neurologist. Ninety days after suffering a stroke, patients who had been treated by a neurologist had a 36% higher survival rate than those under the care of a family physician.

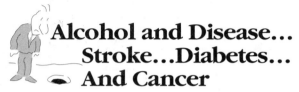

Alcohol and Disease... Stroke...Diabetes... And Cancer

Eric Rimm, ScD, a noted alcohol researcher and assistant professor of epidemiology and nutrition at Harvard School of Public Health in Boston.

The heavy toll of excessive drinking is all too obvious—from car accidents to liver disease, immune system problems and depression.

But the upside of alcohol is just as real. Drinking in moderation reduces the risk of developing serious illness.

Key: Knowing the level of drinking that is right for you.

HEART DISEASE AND STROKE

The evidence that moderate alcohol consumption cuts heart disease risk is very strong. More than 35 studies have shown that people who have one to two drinks a day are 25% to 40% less likely than nondrinkers to have a heart attack.

Moderate drinking seems to protect the heart by boosting blood levels of HDL (good) cholesterol...and by reducing concentrations of *fibrinogen*. That's a natural compound involved in blood clotting.

Alcohol's effect on the risk of stroke is more complex. *Ischemic* strokes (the most common kind) are caused by blood clots in the brain. One to two drinks a day protect against ischemic stroke the same way that they protect against heart attack.

Unfortunately, alcohol's anticlotting action may raise the risk for *hemorrhagic* stroke. This kind of stroke is caused by bleeding in the brain. Research has shown that people who consume three or more drinks a day are more likely than nondrinkers to suffer a hemorrhagic stroke.

Alcohol can raise or lower blood pressure, depending on how *much* you drink. If you're taking medication for high blood pressure, ask your doctor whether you should drink—and, if so, how much.

IS RED WINE SPECIAL?

You may have heard that red wine has special heart-protective powers. Red wine *does* contain antioxidants and other beneficial compounds not found in other alcoholic beverages. But an analysis of data from alcohol research around the world found that *all* forms of alcohol are equally effective at lowering the risk of heart disease.

To your heart, a drink is a drink. One drink equals four to six ounces of wine...12 ounces of beer...or 1.5 ounces of whiskey, gin or another "hard" liquor.

DIABETES

Moderate drinkers are 30% to 40% less likely than nondrinkers to develop adult-onset (Type II) diabetes. This common condition is associated with blindness, kidney failure and heart disease.

Researchers don't yet have an explanation for this antidiabetes effect. One theory is that drinking with meals slows food absorption, which keeps insulin levels steady. Another is that alcohol makes cells throughout the body more sensitive to insulin.

CANCER—A DIFFERENT STORY

There's simply no question about it—drinking *raises* the risk for cancer.

Malignancies of the mouth and throat are especially common among drinkers. But these cancers are rare, and the increase in risk is negligible if you have fewer than four drinks a day.

There is evidence that as little as two drinks per day raise the risk for colon cancer. That's a *very* common malignancy.

Good news: A common B-vitamin called folic acid, or folate, can neutralize this extra danger.

For people who consume at least the recommended daily allowance (RDA) of folate, moderate drinking does *not* appear to raise colon cancer risk. The RDA for folate is 400 micrograms (mcg) per day.

Folate sources: Fresh vegetables, cereals, orange juice, vitamin supplements.

The link between alcohol and breast cancer is stark. Studies consistently show that two to three drinks a day increase a woman's risk for breast cancer by 30% to 40%. Whether lighter drinking has any effect is unclear.

Epidemiologists advise women to have no more than one drink a day. At this level, the benefits to the heart outweigh the increased cancer risk.

Exception: If you are at high risk for breast cancer (your mother or sister developed the disease, for example), it's probably prudent to limit your alcohol consumption to two drinks per week.

The media has reported research showing that red wine reduces the risk for cancer.

Lab studies did show that *resveratrol,* an antioxidant found in red wine, blocks DNA damage that leads to cancer, detoxifies carcinogens and prevents tumors from progressing. But there's no evidence that resveratrol has any effect on humans. Not one population study has linked red wine consumption to reduced cancer rates.

Implication: Taking grape extract, eating grapes or drinking grape juice for resveratrol is unlikely to cause you any harm. But there's no evidence it will help you.

THE BOTTOM LINE

There's compelling evidence that moderate drinking—up to two drinks a day for men, one a day for women—is better for health than abstaining. This level of drinking reduces deaths from all causes by 15%—in men and women alike.

If you already drink moderately, feel reassured.

If you're currently a nondrinker, should you start drinking? Not necessarily. You may be among the minority who cannot keep their drinking at a beneficial level. Once you exceed three drinks a day, your risk of disease and death becomes higher—not lower.

Concentrated bouts of drinking are a bad idea, too. Having all of your weekly quota of drinks on the weekend won't help your cholesterol…and it might raise your risk of suffering a stroke or a lethal heart rhythm disturbance.

And a healthy heart won't help you much if you wrap your car around a telephone pole.

How Effective Is Colon Cancer Drug?

Leonard Saltz, MD, assistant attending physician, division of gastrointestinal oncology, Memorial Sloan-Kettering Cancer Center, New York City.

Patients with advanced colorectal cancer may benefit from *irinotecan* (Camptosar). In a study, this injectable drug shrank tumor size by 50% or more in 23% of cancer patients who had failed to respond to other drugs. In patients with no prior chemotherapy, the response rate was 32%.

Smoking Kills 400,000 Americans Each Year… Here's How Not to Be One of Them

Harlan M. Krumholz, MD, assistant professor of cardiology at Yale University School of Medicine in New Haven, CT. He is author of *No Ifs, Ands or Butts.* Avery.

If you're trying to quit smoking—or know someone who is—here are eight strategies that will maximize your odds of success:

1. Forget about switching to "light" cigarettes. Some smokers switch to low-tar, low-nicotine brands, thinking that doing so will cut the levels of these toxins in their bodies. Or they switch to a light brand as a prelude to quitting altogether.

Switching does *not* help. Studies show that people who switch unwittingly compensate by inhaling smoke more deeply or frequently. Tar and nicotine consumption remain at the same levels as before.

2. Develop a concrete plan. Only about 2% of smokers who try to stop are successful on any given try. Most people fail several times before succeeding.

You must approach smoking cessation as you'd approach running a marathon or tackling any other major project.

Set a firm date for quitting. Plan what you will do *every day* when the inevitable cravings hit. If you backslide, try again.

3. Try nicotine-replacement therapy. Nicotine patches (Habitrol, Nicoderm, etc.) and nicotine gum (Nicorette) can double your odds of quitting successfully.

Both patches and gum are effective. Some people enjoy the oral sensation of chewing gum. Others find chewing a chore, and prefer to use the patch. It administers nicotine continuously throughout the day.

Do *not* smoke while wearing a patch or chewing nicotine gum.

Pregnant women should probably not use the patch or gum, though continued smoking is likely to be more harmful than nicotine-replacement therapy.

Some people find that the patch irritates their skin. If you're among them, alert your doctor.

4. Enlist friends and family. Many smokers try to stop in secret—because they want to avoid embarrassment if they fail. That's the opposite of what should be done.

Tell friends and family—even your doctor—exactly what you intend to do. Ask them to check up on you periodically to see how you're doing. Apologize in advance for how irritable you'll be as you go through nicotine withdrawal.

5. Join a support group. Meeting with fellow quitters for as little as 20 minutes a week can dramatically improve your chances of success.

To locate a support group in your area, call your local hospital, the American Cancer Society (800-227-2345) or the American Lung Association (800-586-4872).

6. Find ways to motivate yourself. Think how much healthier you'll be after quitting… how you'll live longer…or how much money you'll save. Over a 10-year period, a two-pack-a-day habit costs roughly $30,000.

7. Consider alternative techniques. There's scant scientific evidence that acupuncture, acupressure, hypnosis and other alternative therapies help people stop smoking. Yet many former smokers swear by them. If you do decide to give an alternative therapy a try, be sure to find a practitioner with legitimate training.

8. Ask your doctor about antidepressant therapy. There's some evidence that *fluoxetine* (Prozac) and other antidepressants make it easier to quit for certain patients. Yet doctors are often reluctant to prescribe these drugs for smoking cessation. They fear that smokers will shake their addiction to tobacco only to become dependent on the antidepressants.

If you've tried quitting several times without success, however, the risk of becoming dependent on an antidepressant may be outweighed by the dangers posed by continuing to smoke.

Another potentially useful medication is *bupropion* (Zyban). It's been used to treat depression for several years under the name Wellbutrin. Exactly how it works isn't known, but the drug is thought to affect the neurotransmitter *dopamine* that may play a role in nicotine addiction. Studies have found that the combination of nicotine replacement and Zyban is more likely to result in smoking cessation than either drug alone. Side effects include dry mouth and insomnia. People who have epilepsy shouldn't use Zyban as it can cause seizures.

Getting the Right Treatment

Stephen B. Soumerai, ScD, associate professor of ambulatory care and prevention, Harvard Medical School, Boston.

Elderly heart attack patients rarely get the right treatment. Heart attack survivors who receive beta-blockers are 43% less likely to die and 22% less likely to be readmitted to the hospital than similar patients who receive other treatments. Yet in a study of 5,332 elderly heart attack patients, only 21% of those who *should* have been prescribed beta-blockers actually got them.

Problem: Many doctors have exaggerated concerns about the side effects of beta-blockers, including depression, loss of libido and fatigue. These concerns are based on old studies that have since been refuted.

Rural Living and Longevity Link

Mark D. Hayward, PhD, professor of sociology, Pennsylvania State University, University Park. His study, based on the National Longitudinal Study of Older Men, from 1966 to 1990, was presented at a meeting of the Population Association of America.

Men living in rural areas outlive their urban and suburban peers.

Theory: The rural way of life fosters tight relationships with family members, friends and neighbors. These social networks provide men with emotional support and assistance. There are no data on rural women.

Medical Care Self-Defense

Timothy McCall, MD, a Boston internist, author of Examining Your Doctor: A Patient's Guide to Avoiding Harmful Medical Care. *Citadel Press. He is a regular commentator on the public radio program Marketplace, and can be found on the Web at* www.drmccall.com.

To get the best medical care, you need to be informed and assertive. As a doctor, I'm in the unique position of hearing about and seeing the errors other doctors make most often during exams.

Here are some of the big mistakes doctors make and what you can do to prevent them...

***Mistake:* Prescribing drugs but not adequately explaining how to take them.** If medicine isn't taken properly, it may not work —or it may have unexpected effects.

Helpful: After your doctor writes out a prescription, ask how much of the drug to take... how often...if you should take it on an empty stomach...what to do if you miss a dose...and what to do if you develop side effects. Then have the doctor write out a schedule for the drug so you'll know exactly when to take it each day and for how long.

***Mistake:* Recommending treatment without involving you in the thinking process or diagnosis.** Urge your doctor to speak openly about what he/she thinks about your condition and the pros and cons of each treatment available. Be sure to take notes.

Important: When your condition requires elective surgery—or can lead to more serious complications—insist that you want time to think about the recommended treatment. This will give you time to research your ailment, seek a second or third opinion and consider alternatives.

***Mistake:* Coming to conclusions without considering the psychological factors in your life.** The mind can have a profound effect on your immune system, yet many doctors overlook its impact.

Helpful: If there are important changes going on in your life that your doctor should know about, such as marital problems or job issues, be sure to mention them—even if your doctor forgets to ask.

***Mistake:* Prescribing the "latest" drug.** Drug companies spend millions to influence the prescribing habits of doctors. Typically they try to get doctors to recommend brand-new drugs with high price tags and profit margins. What you want, however, is the best drug for your condition.

Helpful: Ask your doctor if there are any drugs that have been on the market longer than the one he is prescribing—and ask whether it would be acceptable to take those drugs instead. In general, older drugs have longer track records of safety and are usually cheaper.

***Mistake:* Giving you free samples of drugs that he normally would not prescribe.** Most patients love getting free samples. But drug companies give most of these samples for the newer drugs that they're trying to promote. These are often drugs with which doctors aren't too familiar yet.

Helpful: Before accepting a sample, ask your doctor how good the new drug is and whether there is another drug that is established —or cheaper—in prescription form.

Antiaging Supplements: Dr. Ken Cooper Explains What Works... And What Doesn't

Kenneth Cooper, MD, MPH, the inventor of aerobics and head of the Cooper Aerobics Center and the Cooper Clinic in Dallas. He is author of *Advanced Nutritional Therapies*. Thomas Nelson.

From DHEA (dehydroepiandrosterone) to melatonin, the market is now glutted with supplements purported to have antiaging properties.

Do these pills do what their proponents say they do? Are they safe? For answers, we went to Dr. Kenneth Cooper, the renowned exercise researcher and one of the earliest proponents of antioxidant supplements.

●**Of all the antiaging supplements, melatonin gets the most hype. Is it effective?** For occasional use to treat jet lag or insomnia, melatonin does seem to be safe and effective.

Melatonin has also shown promise against multiple sclerosis and certain forms of cancer, although research in these areas is in preliminary stages.

However, I am *against* the use of melatonin as an antiaging supplement. Most of the studies suggesting that it has antiaging effects have been done on animals. We just don't know if melatonin has the same effects on humans.

The safety of melatonin has never been fully established. Already there have been reports of troublesome side effects, including hangover and memory loss.

Since melatonin is a hormone, its long-term use might cause cancer—just as the long-term use of estrogen can raise women's risk for breast cancer. It's too early to know whether melatonin raises the risk for cancer. In the meantime, I'm not recommending it to my patients.

●**What about DHEA?** Short-term studies suggest that DHEA boosts the immune system, as its proponents claim.

But since DHEA stimulates the synthesis of sex hormones (testosterone in men and estrogen in women), it's only logical to think that it might also be promoting prostate and/or breast cancer.

Folks who take DHEA today might be inadvertently creating a time bomb with a 20-year fuse.

●**Is that also true for other hormones, like human growth hormone (HGH)?** Yes. A normal, healthy man who takes HGH and/or testosterone for their supposed antiaging properties may be upping his risk for prostate or testicular cancer and heart disease.

In my opinion, anyone who takes HGH or testosterone is playing with dynamite.

●**What about Pycnogenol, the pine bark derivative?** There's no doubt that this mixture of bioflavonoids has promise.

Some studies show that its antioxidant properties are 60 times stronger than those of vitamin E. But until we know for sure that it's safe, I don't recommend pycnogenol supplements to my patients.

●**Are there any antiaging supplements worth taking?** I'm a firm believer in supplements containing vitamins C and E and beta-carotene.

Although these antioxidants are not usually thought of as antiaging supplements, they do slow the aging process by helping to prevent the diseases associated with aging.

These three antioxidants work by neutralizing *free radicals,* renegade molecules that cause the cellular damage that underlies aging.

Vitamin E is especially beneficial. It blocks oxidation of LDL (bad) cholesterol, thereby preventing formation of the arterial deposits that underlie heart attack. Vitamin E also prevents DNA damage, which is thought to be the first step in the development of cancer.

Since it's almost impossible to get sufficient levels of vitamin E from food sources, I tell my patients to take a daily supplement containing 400 international units (IU) of *natural* vitamin E (*d-alpha tocopherol*).

Natural vitamin E is absorbed more efficiently than synthetic vitamin E.

If you smoke and/or have heart disease, ask your doctor about boosting this level to 800 IU a day. That might lower your risk of lung cancer —though it is still better to give up smoking.

●**What do vitamin C and beta-carotene do?** In addition to fighting free radicals, vitamin C now appears to be an effective remedy for mild arthritis pain. It's hard to get enough vitamin C from food, so I tell my patients to take a 500-milligram (mg) supplement twice daily.

Beta-carotene helps protect against heart disease, cataracts and certain cancers, including skin cancer.

I urge all nonsmokers to consume 25,000 IU of beta-carotene each day. You can get this amount in the form of a supplement...or from eating one and one-half average-sized carrots.

●**Anything else?** The mineral selenium seems to fight free radicals and help prevent cancer of the lung, colon, prostate and rectum. I would add 200 micrograms (mcg) a day of selenium to your vitamin/mineral "cocktail."

Finally, folic acid is now known to be critical for good health. It lowers bloodstream levels of *homocysteine,* a breakdown product of *methionine.* That's an amino acid that we get mostly from eating red meat and milk products.

Studies show a clear link between homocysteine levels and heart attack risk—even when cholesterol levels are low.

I tell my patients to take 400 mcg of folic acid a day in supplement form (800 to 1,000 mcg if heart disease is present).*

People over age 50 should take 50 mg of vitamin B-6 and 500 mcg of B-12 daily along with folic acid. Otherwise, vitamin B-12 deficiency can be masked.

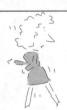

Osteoporosis Risk Indicator

Michael Holick, MD, PhD, chief of endocrinology, Boston Medical Center, 80 E. Concord St., M-1013, Boston 02118.

Prematurely gray hair is a risk factor for osteoporosis—loss of bone mass—in one's latter years.

*High homocysteine levels are also thought to cause neural tube birth defects. That's why obstetricians recommend folic acid supplements for pregnant women—even women who *might* become pregnant.

Persons who have hair that went more than half gray by age 40 have been found to be *four times* as likely to develop osteoporosis as other persons without prematurely gray hair. The reason for this is not known.

Safety: If your hair went gray early in life, consult with your physician and consider increasing your calcium intake.

To Minimize Osteoporosis Risk

Barbara S. Levine, RD, PhD, director, Calcium Information Center, New York Hospital–Cornell Medical Center, New York City.

Most women *and* men need to boost their calcium intake. New federal guidelines call for adults over age 50 to get 1,200 milligrams (mg) of the mineral per day. That's the equivalent of four daily servings of low-fat milk, yogurt, fortified orange juice or other calcium-rich food. Adults under age 50 should get 1,000 mg per day...adolescents, 1,300 mg. Old guidelines recommended 800 mg a day for most adults. *Danger:* The average adult consumes only 500 mg to 700 mg a day.

How to Stay Safe in This Crazy, Crazy World

Louis R. Mizell, Jr., an expert on criminal tactics. He is author of *Street Sense for Seniors.* The Putnam Berkley Publishing Group.

More than 4,000 Americans 55 years of age and older become crime victims in their homes every day.

Criminals target older people, expecting them to be less able to protect themselves and more likely to be poor witnesses.

Eighty percent of these crimes could be prevented if seniors learned more about criminal tactics and took a few simple steps to improve security. *Here are the facts about some of the most prevalent crimes and how to avoid them...*

HOME SECURITY

The idea that criminals will not enter an occupied house is a dangerous myth. Using force or trickery, crooks enter the homes of more than 500,000 people each year with at least one family member inside. *Most of these crimes would not occur if people took the following precautions...*

●**Don't open the door** unless you know who is on the other side. Every year, 15,000 seniors are victimized by the "push in" tactic when the criminal forces his/her way in. If you do not know the person, use a peephole and talk through the closed door.

Be aware that a determined criminal can push hard enough on a partially opened door to rip off most door chains that have not been professionally installed.

●**Don't trust people** just because they look respectable.

Example: In Miami, three little girls (one 10-year-old and two 14-year-olds) knocked at the doors of older people and melted their hearts with bright eyes and sweet smiles. After they were let in, one would slip into the bedroom and take cash and jewelry, while the other two distracted the victim. Before they were arrested, they had robbed 26 senior citizens.

●**Be wary of impostors.** More than 230,000 crimes per year are committed by criminals impersonating plumbers, gas and water inspectors, police officers, etc. Check the credentials of everyone who comes to your door *before* you open it. If you feel suspicious, call the organization he claims sent him.

●**Lock your door** whenever you leave your home, even if it's just to take out the garbage ...bring in the groceries...get the mail. Of the 3.2 million home invasions, 800,000 were the result of an unlocked door or window.

●**Keep your keys secure.** Someone who has your door keys has 24-hour access to your home, your family, your property and, of course, you.

●**Do not give your keys to anyone...** workers...home-care attendants...realtors...

unless you know you can trust them and all their relatives and friends who may also gain access to your keys. Three hundred thousand crimes are committed by criminals who surreptitiously obtain our keys.

●**Don't keep your car ignition key** on the same key ring with your house keys.

●**Don't leave your garage-door opener in your unlocked car.**

CAR-JACKING AND DRIVEWAY CRIMES

In today's mobile world, criminals have learned a variety of ways to exploit vulnerable people in and out of their cars. Driveway crime is rampant.

Example: A top Exxon executive was kidnapped from his 200-foot-long driveway on his estate in northern New Jersey.

Do not drop your guard when you get to your driveway. Check the rearview mirror as you approach your home and as you drive onto your driveway. If someone is following, keep your doors locked and circle the block. If they are still behind, drive to the closest police station.

If you see anyone suspicious by your house, keep your doors locked and blow the horn. If an unfamiliar vehicle is in your driveway, get a description, take down the license plate number and call the local police department from a neighbor's house before you go home. Keep your car doors locked and your engine running until you are certain there are no suspicious characters around.

Be aware of common ruses used by criminals to get you out of your car. *Two of the most common include...*

●**Bump and rob.** The criminal crashes into the victim's rear bumper...and robs her (victims are usually older women) when she gets out to inspect the damage.

●**Good Samaritan.** The criminal approaches his victim and points out that she has a flat tire (for which the crook is responsible). He then offers the victim a ride, and either robs or assaults her.

ATMS AND PAY TELEPHONES

Automatic Teller Machines (ATMs) and pay telephones provide *many* opportunities for criminals. At least 27,000 crimes, including kidnapping, murder, rape, car theft and robbery occur at pay phones each year. *To maximize security...*

●**Use machines and telephones that are in public view and well lit.**

●**Take along a companion** who can watch you from inside your locked car. If you do not have a car, have him stand 10 or 15 feet away to deter criminals.

●**Do not leave your car unlocked** or the keys in the ignition if you must go alone.

●**Face the street** when using the telephone.

●**Do your business quickly.**

●**Do not make withdrawals or deposits at the same place** or time every day.

●**Keep your PIN confidential.**

●**Be aware of your surroundings** and watch to see if you are being followed.

WISDOM

However safe you try to make your home, it will never be as secure as a bank. Do not keep large amounts of cash in your house. Word gets around.

Every year, thousands of seniors are the victims of robberies, losing hundreds of thousands of dollars.

Harry Lorayne's Cures For Absentmindedness

Harry Lorayne, who can memorize every person's name in a room of 200 people and recite from memory random pages of the latest issue of *Time* magazine. He is author of several best-selling books on memory, including the *Memory Power* package (book, audio and video cassettes), as seen on TV.

It is no longer necessary to accept loss of memory or a poor memory as an inevitable part of growing older. Absentmindedness is caused by a lessening of interest in humdrum activities like making and keeping appointments, performing daily rituals and keeping track of affairs and possessions. It can happen to anybody, at any age.

The good news is that there are simple techniques you can use to sharpen your memory and remember where you put things, people's names...even errands you have to run.

WHERE DID I PUT THAT...

You'll never misplace anything again if you clearly focus on the *present* for the moment it takes to set something down or put it away.

Do this by creating a picture in your mind that connects the object to its new home in a silly or absurd way. It's the outlandishness of what you imagine that makes it interesting to your mind, which in turn makes you *aware*.

Example: On your way to mail a letter before the post office closes, you mindlessly toss your reading glasses on top of the TV. When you get back home, you can't remember where you put your glasses.

Better way: At the moment you put your glasses down on the TV, form a cockeyed mental picture. For instance, imagine the TV antenna poking through the lens of the glasses and into your eye. When you need your glasses, you'll automatically recall the unusual image, shudder and quickly retrieve them.

Why it works: This mind-jogging system, and others like it, cures absentmindedness and forgetfulness by grabbing the mind by the "scruff of its neck"—forcing it to pay attention for a split second.

The reminder principle: Such memory games exercise your mind the way walking exercises your body. You become more creative and imaginative while simultaneously improving your memory. Some other mind-jogging techniques...

DID I TURN OFF THE...

Last week, as you headed down the sidewalk, you couldn't remember if you'd turned off the stove.

The week before, it was the iron.

Tonight, you're lying in bed wondering if you remembered to set the alarm.

Memory joggers: To be sure later that you've actually done these things, visualize a silly picture in your mind as you do them.

Example: As you unplug the iron, imagine that you're pulling your iron-shaped head out of the electrical socket. As you set the alarm in the evening, imagine that the button is piercing your finger or that you're using the clock radio to sleep on instead of a pillow.

Later, when you begin to wonder if you've remembered to do these ordinary, mundane tasks, the extraordinary images that come to mind will assure you that they have been taken care of.

And don't worry—your mind won't incorrectly "remember" that you've done these things, even if you use the same silly image each day. "True memory" will ensure that you remember the truth about what you have and haven't done.

WHAT'S HIS NAME...

An easy way to remember names is to think of familiar words that sound like the name you're trying to remember. You have probably heard about all this before. But—it really works. *Try it...*

When you're introduced to a person, really *listen* to his/her name.

If you don't hear it the first time, ask to have it repeated. That will not only help you remember the name, it will also make the person feel good and let them know that you care about meeting him/her.

To remember a person's name, use your imagination.

What does the name sound like? What does it remind you of?

It's best to come up with your own words or mental picture, since your originally created image is more likely to remind you of the person's name than would an image or word suggested by someone else.

Example: The name "Dr. Carruthers" sounds like "car udders." One way to remember this person's name, then, would be to imagine a car with udders.

HIS FACE IS FAMILIAR, BUT...

Now take your mental picture to the next step. Look again at Dr. Carruthers's face. Which of his features jumps out at you? Does he have a high forehead? An unruly mop of hair? Crooked or capped teeth?

Whatever feature seems most prominent to you today is likely to stand out for you in the future. Once you've identified Dr. Carruthers's

dominant feature, connect it to your substitute words—in this case, "car udders," and your mental picture of a car being milked.

Example: You might picture Dr. Carruthers's long white sideburns being cars (or having cars driving out of them)—and picture the udders on the car. To remember Carruthers is a doctor, picture stethoscopes attached to those udders. Now you've connected Dr. Carruthers's name to his face in a way you're not likely to forget! You've forced yourself to listen to the name...and really look at the face—and one will remind you of the other.

FIRST THE DENTIST, THEN...

Let's say you have a bunch of errands to run. Instead of writing them down and bypassing your memory altogether (and possibly forgetting the list), link them to each other in this silly way...

Example: You have to see the dentist, mail a letter, pick up a gallon of milk and stop to get new tires for your car. One possible way to link these errands together would be to imagine the dentist pulling stamped envelopes out of your mouth. You're pouring millions of stamped envelopes out of a milk carton instead of milk...a car is drinking milk out of a gigantic milk carton—or a gigantic milk carton is driving a car.

Replay these silly pictures in your mind. Then, as you leave the dentist's office, replay them again. Almost without effort, you'll remember each and every one of your errands—because one must remind you of the other.

Feeling Sad Can Kill

Susan Everson, PhD, MPH, associate research scientist, Human Population Laboratory, Berkeley, CA, who led a 10-year study of 2,428 men ages 42 to 60.

Feelings of hopelessness can make you ill. A study reported extreme pessimism is more hazardous to your health than depression. Men who reported moderate-to-high levels of hopelessness died at rates two to three times higher than those who were not so pessimistic. They also suffered cancer and heart attacks more frequently.

Curing Aggression

Helen H. Kyomen, MD, assistant attending psychiatrist, geriatric psychiatry program, McLean Hospital, Belmont, MA.

Estrogen therapy helps curb aggression in women *and men* suffering from severe dementia.

Background: Because they tend to take drugs for other medical problems, many dementia patients cannot tolerate the drugs ordinarily used to calm physical and sexual aggression. But in a four-week study, all patients given estrogen pills were less disruptive. Estrogen can cause some men to develop enlarged breasts (*gynecomastia*), but the benefits of estrogen therapy often outweigh this risk.

Hip Fracture Reduction

Dennis Black, PhD, associate professor of epidemiology and biostatistics at the University of California, San Francisco.

Alendronate, an osteoporosis drug, cuts the risk of hip fracture by half. The drug is sold under the brand name Fosamax. A three-year study of 2,027 osteoporosis patients who took the drug daily found that it reduced their chance of a hip fracture by 51% compared with those who took placebos. Fosamax is an alternative to estrogen, which is thought to also be effective in reducing fracture risk.

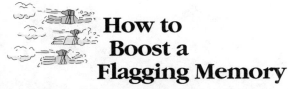

How to Boost a Flagging Memory

Adriane Fugh-Berman, MD, a Washington, DC–based medical researcher who specializes in women's health and alternative medicine. She is author of *Alternative Medicine: What Works.* Williams & Wilkins.

Do you—or does someone you love—keep losing keys, forgetting names or having other memory lapses? If so, you may be worried that the culprit is Alzheimer's disease or another incurable form of dementia. While it's a good idea to consult a doctor, the odds are that it is simple forgetfulness—which can be treated.

In some cases, memory problems—especially those associated with aging—stem simply from a lack of mental activity. If your job isn't particularly stimulating—or if you're retired—you might consider keeping a journal, joining a book discussion group, playing chess or Scrabble, doing crossword puzzles, etc.

Physical exercise is also a memory-enhancer. Aerobic exercise boosts circulation throughout the body—and that includes the brain. Increased blood flow to the brain has been shown to increase mental function.

Another way to ensure adequate blood flow to the brain is to eat a low-fat diet. The arteries that feed the brain are tiny to begin with, and any narrowing that occurs as a result of eating a fatty or cholesterol-rich diet drastically reduces oxygen flow. Blood flow problems can lead to tiny strokes, which are now believed to be the cause of much age-related memory loss.

These strokes—which generally produce no obvious symptoms—are typically caused by chronic high blood pressure and/or high cholesterol. So be sure your blood pressure and cholesterol are under control.

While there's no magic memory pill, the following supplements are safe…and beneficial for many people. They can be taken individually or in combination. For absolute safety, use them under a doctor's supervision.

• **Antioxidants.** Vitamins C and E and the mineral selenium all may help prevent memory loss. I usually tell my patients to take 400 international units (IU) of vitamin E a day, along with 1,000 mg of vitamin C and 100 micrograms of selenium. It's also a good idea to eat lots of fruits and vegetables. They contain lots of other antioxidants.

• **Phosphatidylserine.** This fatty substance was found to be helpful in preventing further deterioration in people with memory problems. In some cases, memory *improved* after several months of phosphatidylserine therapy. I usually recommend 200 to 300 mg per day.

Be patient—it may take three months before you notice any improvement.

Some alternative practitioners recommend a related substance called *choline* (or *lecithin*, which contains 10% to 20% choline). Neither choline nor lecithin looks anywhere near as good as phosphatidylserine, and they can cause unpleasant side effects.

●**L-acetyl carnitine.** This form of the amino acid carnitine plays a key role in energy production within the body. It seems to help both Alzheimer's patients and those with mild men-tal deterioration. The usual dose is 500 milli-grams (mg) to 1,000 mg three times a day.

●**Ginkgo biloba.** Like vitamin E, ginkgo helps thin the blood, boosting circulation inside even the tiniest capillaries—including those that feed the brain. Ginkgo also acts as an antioxidant, protecting the brain against attack by free radicals.

Ginkgo has been found to be effective in slowing the progression of Alzheimer's disease.

_____

15

Taking Care of the Outer You—Your Skin

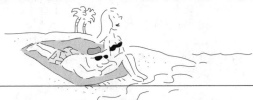

Make Your Skin Look Young Again Without Surgery

Joseph P. Bark, MD

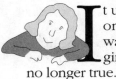It used to be that a face-lift was the only way to deal with skin that was wrinkled, sun-damaged, sagging or scarred. However, this is no longer true.

Today, while surgery is still required for serious problems, there are numerous safe, inexpensive *nonsurgical* techniques for rejuvenating your skin. *Here's a look at your options...*

ALPHA HYDROXY ACIDS

Glycolic, lactic, citric and other *alpha hydroxy acids* (AHAs) are found in a growing number of cosmetics. Excellent moisturizers, they also seem to minimize wrinkling, sun damage and acne—if used on a daily basis.

Even more effective: *Prescription* AHA products, which contain higher concentra-

tions of the acid. They're available from your dermatologist.

SUNSCREENS AND MOISTURIZERS

Sunscreens don't just prevent skin damage. They also help fade *existing* fine wrinkles.

Moisturizers keep skin soft and supple and *temporarily* improve its appearance. But they neither prevent nor reverse wrinkles. In fact, wearing moisturizer without sunscreen can raise your skin's vulnerability to sun damage.

VITAMIN A DERIVATIVE

Tretinoin (Retin-A) is a potent drug originally developed as a treatment for acne. Doctors may prescribe this vitamin A derivative to fade fine lines around the eyes...and to get rid of stretch marks and liver spots.

It's surprisingly effective when used on a regular basis, although it can take a year or more for the effects to become apparent.

Joseph P. Bark, MD, a dermatologist in private practice and a staff physician at St. Joseph Hospital in Lexington, KY. He is author of *Your Skin: An Owner's Guide.* Prentice Hall.

Tretinoin makes the skin appear smoother by thickening its outermost layer and "compacting" the layer of dead skin cells.

Caution: Tretinoin can cause redness and dryness...and can raise your susceptibility to sunburn. Because of the possible risk of birth defects, it's inappropriate for pregnant women.

Another formulation of tretinoin, Renova, is the first drug developed specifically for wrinkle removal. It reduces fine facial lines, brown spots and surface roughness just as effectively as ordinary tretinoin—and it's less likely to irritate the skin.

CHEMICAL PEELS

Chemical peels involve the application of concentrated AHAs (40% to 70% acid vs. 0.5% to 10% acid for over-the-counter AHA products). Peels are administered in a doctor's office.

A series of light *glycolic acid* peels helps remove damaged skin and improves the appearance of crow's feet and minor acne scars. The peel may cause stinging, as well as slight pinkness for a day.

Deeper peels, using *trichloracetic acid* (TCA) or *phenol*, are needed to obliterate wrinkles around the mouth, eyes and forehead, to correct irregular pigmentation and to eliminate liver spots.

The effects of a peel last for several years. However, peels may cause considerable pain, as well as persistent redness, skin tightness and scarring. Phenol peels are inappropriate for people with heart or kidney disease...or with dark skin.

Warning: Recovery from a TCA or phenol peel isn't pretty. Crust-like scabs that appear immediately after the peel can take up to two weeks to heal. During this period, it's essential to avoid the sun.

DERMABRASION

This procedure involves use of a rotating wire brush to "sand" off the upper two layers of skin, smoothing its appearance. Results last for several years.

Dermabrasion is good for removing acne scars, pockmarks and small wrinkles around the lips. For severe blemishes, two procedures, six to 12 months apart, may be necessary.

Caution: Dermabrasion can cause infection, scarring, variations in skin tone and extreme sun sensitivity. As with peels, the skin crusts over. Full recovery can take several months.

Also as with peels, dermabrasion works best for people with light complexions.

LASER PEEL

In this procedure—a new alternative to dermabrasion and chemical peels—the doctor uses a laser to "shear off" the epidermis. Laser peels are less likely than chemical peels to cause scarring and overlightening. They are also more precise.

Although crusting and redness still occur with a laser peel, recovery is usually faster. Laser peels are particularly effective against wrinkles around the eyes, age spots, scars and facial discoloration.

COLLAGEN INJECTIONS

Doctors can inject you with a natural protein called *collagen* to plump up facial skin and help fill in severe (cystic) acne scars and deep wrinkles.

Effects are immediate and last for four to eight months, until the collagen is resorbed. Then a new round of injections must be administered.

Infection and sun sensitivity at the injection site can occur following the injections. And allergies to collagen can cause excessive firmness and purple discoloration. This can last up to six weeks.

To make sure you're not allergic: Have two collagen allergy tests prior to receiving the injections. Do *not* have the injections if you have rheumatoid arthritis, Graves' disease, lupus or another autoimmune disorder.

Instead of collagen, some doctors have begun injecting fat "harvested" from elsewhere in the body (buttocks, back, etc.). Because the injected material is part of the body, there's no danger of allergic reaction. Unfortunately, it's not clear just how long fat injections last.

Low-Fat Diets May Reduce Skin Cancer Risk

Homer S. Black, PhD, professor of dermatology, Baylor College of Medicine, Houston. His two-year study of 76 patients was published in *The New England Journal of Medicine*, 10 Shattuck St., Boston 02115.

Skin cancer patients who were put on a diet that derived no more than 20% of calories from fat developed 70% fewer precancerous skin lesions (actinic keratoses) than similar patients whose diet remained above 36% fat. *Implication:* If you've had one skin cancer, adopting a low-fat diet can help you prevent a recurrence.

Help for Unsightly Scars

Tina S. Alster, MD, assistant professor of dermatology and pediatrics, Georgetown University Medical Center, Washington, DC. Her study of laser therapy on 16 heart surgery patients was published in *The Lancet*, 42 Bedford Square, London WC1B 3SL, England.

Red, raised scars (*keloids*) left on the chest following heart surgery can be made less visible—and less itchy—when treated with light from a pulsed-dye laser. The results from laser treatment appear to be long lasting, with no scar recurrence within the first year following treatment.

Does Your Hair Protect You from the Sun?

Zoe Diana Draelos, MD, clinical assistant professor of dermatology, Bowman Gray School of Medicine, Winston-Salem, NC.

A full head of hair does *not* offer full protection against skin cancer of the scalp. Scalp skin is just as vulnerable to sun damage as skin elsewhere on the body. When cancer does occur on the scalp, it's often very aggressive.

Self-defense: If you are bald or have thinning hair, rub SPF-15 sunscreen on your scalp… and wear a hat with a four-inch brim that goes all around the head. Even if you have a full head of hair, it's best to use conditioner or hair spray that contains a sunscreen.

Vitamin C vs. Wrinkles

Sheldon Pinnell, MD, professor of medicine and chief, division of dermatology, Duke University Medical Center, Durham, NC.

A prescription skin cream containing 10% vitamin C significantly reduced wrinkling and age spots in patients who used it for eight months. The vitamin "instructs" skin cells to produce new collagen, plumping the skin slightly. Called *Cellex*, the cream delivers 20 to 40 times the amount of the vitamin than can be absorbed from pills.

Skin Cancer— How to Protect Yourself

Perry Robins, MD, associate professor of dermatology at New York University and president of The Skin Cancer Foundation, 245 Fifth Ave., Suite 2402, New York 10016. He is author of *Sun Sense*, which can be ordered through this foundation.

The US is facing a growing epidemic of malignant melanoma, the deadliest form of skin cancer.

In the past 20 years, there has been a dramatic increase in the number of new cases reported.

Why the increase? We don't know exactly to what degree sunscreen really protects us, and not enough people are using it.

These are the most common questions I'm asked about skin protection and skin cancer…

•**Do you continue to recommend that people wear sunscreen?** Absolutely. Over the past 20 years, countless studies have shown sunscreen to be effective at preventing both sunburn *and* skin cancer.

Of course, sunscreen is *not* 100% effective. And wearing it does not give you complete freedom to bask in the sun all day.

●**What type of sunscreen is best?** Look for a sunscreen that offers protection against *both* forms of ultraviolet light—UVA and UVB.

UVB rays pose a greater threat of sunburn and skin cancer than UVA rays do. However, UVA rays can still be harmful if you are in the sun for prolonged periods of time.

Your sunscreen should have a sun protection factor (SPF) of at least 15...and if you plan to go swimming, it should also be water-resistant. With an SPF-15 sunscreen, you can remain burn-free for 15 times longer than you would with unprotected skin.

In regions where the sun's rays are particularly strong—such as in the South—use *sunblock* in addition to sunscreen.

Problem: Sunblock, which uses zinc oxide, talc or another opaque material to create a physical barrier to keep out rays, is messy and unattractive. Consequently, it is not appropriate for covering large areas of skin. I recommend using it only on two high-risk spots—the nose and the rims of the ears.

Avoid lotions containing mineral oil, cooking oil or cocoa butter. These products merely lubricate the skin. They do not block out harmful rays.

●**How should I apply a sunscreen?** Apply it liberally to all areas of skin that will be exposed to the sun. Do so at least 15 minutes before heading outdoors, so that it has a chance to be absorbed.

Pay special attention to easily overlooked areas—feet, earlobes, a bald spot, the backs of your hands, the tops of your ears, the nape of your neck and the tip of your nose.

Reapply at least once every three hours for as long as you're in the sun. Even with water-resistant sunscreen, it's prudent to reapply after going into the water or perspiring heavily.

●**I stopped sunbathing years ago. Do I still need sunscreen?** Yes. Your skin is at risk anytime you venture into sunlight—whether on the beach, in your backyard or on a brief walk. Sunscreens are *not* just for the beach!

In spring, fall and summer, applying sunscreen should become part of your daily routine. Rub it on just after your morning shower.

For office workers, a single morning application will suffice. If you work outdoors, reapply sunscreen frequently during the day. Even in winter, it's a good idea to wear sunscreen if you plan on being outdoors for more than a few minutes.

●**What else can I do to protect myself?** First of all, don't get too much sun too soon. On your first day in the sun, limit your exposure to just a few minutes. On each successive day, increase the length of exposure by a few minutes. If repeated exposure to the sun is inevitable, your goal should be to tan gradually rather than burn. A tan offers some protection by absorbing UV rays. *Other helpful strategies...*

●**Wear UV-blocking sunglasses.** Look for lenses that block at least 95% of UVB rays, 60% of UVA and 92% of visible light. Check the manufacturer's label...or look for the words "Z-80-3 Standard." A good pair of sunglasses will help protect your eyes from sunlight-induced cataracts.

●**Avoid sun exposure between the hours of 10 a.m. and 3 p.m.** The sun's rays are strongest during this period.

●**Always wear a wide-brimmed hat.** It should provide shade for your ears, forehead and neck.

●**At the beach, use an umbrella.**

●**What if I burn easily?** People who are fair-haired, light-skinned and blue- or green-eyed are *twice* as likely to develop skin cancer as dark-haired, dark-skinned, brown-eyed people are.

And—people who have a family history of skin cancer are at increased risk.

There are no special rules for these people to follow, except to be *extra* diligent in protecting their skin. For fair-skinned people, wearing a hat and using sunscreen every day are not just good ideas—they are absolutely *essential.*

●**What if I develop skin cancer?** Malignant melanoma is generally curable—if caught in its early stages, when it's very shallow. The deeper a melanoma gets, the more lethal.

To improve your chances of spotting a skin cancer in its earliest stages, give yourself a *total-body skin exam* at least once every three months. Look for any new growth or change in your skin. *Start today.*

•How do I perform this examination? You will need a hand mirror, a full-length mirror and a blow-dryer.

Begin with your head and neck, where 80% of all skin cancers occur. Examine your face, nose, lips and mouth, and your ears—especially the rims and lobes.

Use a blow-dryer to part your hair section by section. Standing with your back to the full-length mirror, use the hand mirror to examine the back of your scalp and neck. It may be better to ask a friend or family member for help.

Then continue downward, examining your back, hands, fingers, buttocks, genitals, thighs, ankles—right down to your toes.

The exam should take no more than 10 minutes.

Consult a dermatologist right away if you notice...

•A skin growth that increases in size and/or appears pearly, translucent, tan, brown, black or multicolored.

•A mole, birthmark or beauty mark that changes color, grows in size or thickness, changes in texture or becomes irregular in outline.

•A spot or growth that itches, hurts, crusts, scabs over, erodes or bleeds.

•An open sore or wound that persists for more than four weeks—or which heals and then reopens.

A Day Without Sunshine?

Wilma Bergfeld, MD, director of clinical research in dermatology, Cleveland Clinic Foundation, Cleveland.

Total sun avoidance is not healthful for you. The human body needs some sun exposure to synthesize vitamin D—merely five to 10 minutes a day is enough. And only a little skin need be exposed—even just a toe is enough.

Sunscreens Are Effective For Three Years After Purchase

Barbara A. Gilchrest, MD, Boston University School of Medicine, 80 E. Concord St., Boston 02118.

After that, some chemists say they may still be effective for another year—but there is no way for you to safely test them.

Self-defense: Discard unused sunscreen after three years. *Important:* Discard sunscreen immediately if it appears runny or starts to smell strange. This can happen if it's left in a hot car for too long.

Our Skin Would Change Very Little Over Time

Joseph P. Bark, MD, a dermatologist in Lexington, KY, and author of several books, including *Your Skin...An Owner's Guide.* Prentice Hall.

The most exposed areas of the body—particularly the face, scalp and arms—are the most likely to develop spots, dryness, wrinkles and skin cancer.

THE BEST GENERAL PROTECTION

•Use sunscreen. It's cheap and available without a prescription. If men used sunscreen instead of aftershave, they'd prevent many skin problems. Use a sun protection factor (SPF) of 30 or 50 (preferably 50) whenever you go out in the sun.

•Don't smoke. Smoking yellows the skin, dries it out and greatly increases wrinkling, especially around the mouth.

DRY, ITCHY SKIN

Complaints of dry skin are extremely common after age 50—for good reasons…

●**Less oil.** Some oil glands in the skin stop producing the oil needed for lubrication.

●**Winter itch.** In low-humidity areas such as the desert Southwest, and during the winter months elsewhere, water evaporates from the skin very quickly.

●**Overwashing.** We are a nation of clean freaks. We routinely wash away the oil layer that normally acts like plastic wrap, sealing in moisture. *Better:* Bathe every other day and don't scrub too hard. *Recommendations:*

●**Bathe, don't shower.** A shower equals an infinite number of rinsings. Sloshing around in the tub removes less oil.

●**Don't use bath oil.** Most goes down the drain. The residue will make the tub slippery, encouraging a fall. Instead, step out onto an absorbent mat and apply moisturizer while your skin is still wet, sealing in water. Pat dry.

Good moisturizers: Domol, Lubriderm, Hermal, Moisturel, mineral oil and the cheapest of all—Crisco solid. Crisco is great for itching, too. Rub it on gently with your fingertips.

●**Use tepid water.** Just as hot water flushes grease from dirty dishes, it flushes protective oils from your skin.

●**Choose a mild soap.** A major cause of dry skin is the daily use of harsh soap. *Good mild soaps:* Basis…Lowila…unscented Dove.

HARMLESS SPOTS

●**Liver spots.** The only connection between the liver and flat, dark brown "liver spots" (usually on the backs of the hands) is their color—although the liver was once wrongly considered their cause. "Age spots" is a more accurate term. I prefer to call them "birthday presents." These brown flat spots (called *lentigines*—the singular is *lentigo*) don't darken in the sun, as freckles do.

If you don't like the way your age spots or lentigines look, a dermatologist can freeze them individually with a quick spray of liquid nitrogen (it stings briefly) and they peel off over a week or two.

●**Seborrheic keratoses** look like drops of tannish to deep brown candle wax with superficial cracks ("splits"). They're hereditary, genetically timed to appear in later life. Seborrheic keratoses, which are extremely common, start small but can quadruple in size. *Prime sites:* The chest, back and temples.

If you have seborrheic keratoses that are flaky, itchy or unsightly, don't scratch or cut them off. A dermatologist can freeze them with liquid nitrogen. The crust that forms will fall off in two to three weeks.

WRINKLES

Wrinkles are harmless but can be reduced if they bother you. Sleep creases run vertically from scalp to chin and become more prominent on the sleeping side. To minimize sleep creases, vary your sleeping position. *Other ways to de-wrinkle:*

●**Retin-A** (tretinoin). This superb prescription cream is a good bet for keeping your skin fine and smooth as you age. *Caution:* Retin-A makes the skin much more sensitive to sunlight. Use sunscreen.

Caution: Many drugs besides Retin-A—most commonly the diuretics (water pills) taken for high blood pressure, heart problems and swollen legs—cause skin rashes or increase the burning effects of the sun. Results may be immediate or delayed for months—or years. If your skin gets red, a drug you're taking might be the culprit.

●**Collagen treatments.** Leather from cattle is chemically processed, broken into its component parts until it forms a thick gel and is then injected into the skin. The injections act like bricks that reassemble a "wall" under the skin to replace the collagen lost with age, especially in postmenopausal women.

Typical site: The upper lip. Lacking the support of a fat layer, the mouth folds in on itself.

The collagen treatment: Your dermatologist first tests a patch of skin on one arm. Thirty days later he tests near your hairline…to test for an allergic reaction. If no redness or itching results in two weeks, you'll have one collagen treatment (or possibly two, a few weeks apart). Benefits last for six to eight months. *Cost:* Several hundred dollars.

Mad cow disease isn't an issue with collagen, which is made from select herds.

●**Laser treatments.** These one-time treatments, done in the doctor's office, are especially effective for wrinkles above the lip and crinkly lines around the eyes. Treatment involves an extremely well-controlled quick burnoff of the outer layer of skin (epidermis) in a precisely defined area. The skin contracts and looks smoother.

What to expect: Some pain...weeks of healing...months of redness. Be aware that in some cases there may be permanent loss of skin color in the treated area, which will be more obvious the darker your natural skin color. The lighter your skin, the more pleasing the results. *Cost:* About $3,000 to $6,000.

BEWARE OF SUN SPOTS

For many types of skin cancer, having one spot or lesion increases the risk of recurrence. If you have ever had skin cancer, report faithfully to your dermatologist for follow-up visits.

"Sun spots," or actinic keratoses, are scaly red spots on exposed areas of the skin. They're generally harmless—but if left alone, up to 20% eventually turn into squamous cell skin cancers. Although this typically takes three to 10 or even 20 years, the potential for a malignancy makes it crucial to have them removed promptly.

Most common sites: The nose...face...tops of the ears...backs of the hands and arms.

How to tell if you have one: Close your eyes and run your fingers gently over your face. If you feel a scaly bump under the skin but can't see it, have it checked out. Actinic keratoses don't become visible for a while. They usually start out smaller than a pencil eraser (less than six millimeters in diameter) and get wider and more elevated over time, evolving to a button-like texture with a hard (indurated) base.

MELANOMA

This sometimes lethal form of skin cancer is dangerous at any age, but becomes increasingly likely over time, since its presence is closely related to accumulated exposure to the sun. Melanomas are flat to bumpy in texture, usually without cracks on the surface, and brown to black in color.

Bottom line: Any unrecognizable bump on your face—especially if it has any pigmentation at all—should be checked out by a dermatologist. If a biopsy reveals that it's a melanoma, or the doctor can definitely identify it as such, it must be removed immediately.

Melanoma Watch

Marianne Berwick, PhD, an epidemiologist at the Memorial Sloan-Kettering Cancer Center, New York City.

Inspecting your skin thoroughly can significantly reduce your risk from melanoma. A study of 1,200 people found that those who closely examined the skin over their entire bodies had a 63% lower rate of dying from melanoma. Dermatologists use the *ABCD* rule to identify suspicious moles and freckles—asymmetric shape, irregular borders, unusual color, diameter bigger than a pencil eraser's.

Sunlight Is Not the Only Threat to Skin

Pearon G. Lang, Jr., MD, professor of dermatology, Medical University of South Carolina, Charleston.

Skin cancer has also been linked to birthmarks, old scars and skin ulcers...immunosuppression caused by illness or chemotherapy ...human papilloma virus (the cause of warts) ...exposure to petroleum derivatives and other carcinogens.

Self-defense: Have birthmarks removed or checked annually...seek advice if a skin ulcer fails to heal or if a scar develops a growth or sore. If a wart doesn't respond to routine therapy, you may need a biopsy. A patient who is immunosuppressed or who has been exposed to carcinogens should seek advice if he/she develops a new growth or sore.

Rosacea Sufferers

Jonathan Weiss, MD, assistant clinical professor of dermatology, Emory University, Atlanta.

Ask your doctor about *MetroCream*. In a study of 128 patients, this prescription metronidazole *cream* resulted in a 58% reduction in redness and dry skin, compared with a 22% reduction with metronidazole *gel*. Improvements were noted within three weeks and continued throughout the study's 12 weeks. Rosacea, an acne-like condition that causes facial redness, usually appears after age 30.

Dandruff Shampoo Delay

John Reeves, MD, professor of medicine, University of Vermont, Burlington.

Dandruff shampoo can take up to a month to produce results—so don't give up too soon. The shampoos work by removing skin flakes…slowing production of flake-forming skin cells…minimizing scalp inflammation… and/or killing yeast that contributes to the problem. Various antidandruff shampoos appear to be equally effective, but which one is best varies from person to person.

The Big Mistake Shingles Sufferers Make

Michael N. Oxman, MD, professor of medicine and pathology at the University of California, and staff physician at the Veterans Administration Medical Center, both in San Diego. He is a member of the Scientific Advisory Board for the VZV Research Foundation, 40 E. 72 St., New York 10021.

If you have ever had chicken pox—and 95% of Americans have—you are at risk for the blistering rash and severe pain of *shingles*.

People who get shingles are often tempted to wait for the problem to clear up on its own. But waiting is the worst thing you can do.

Without prompt treatment with antiviral medication, shingles pain may become chronic.

We asked University of California virologist Dr. Michael N. Oxman all about shingles…

●**What is shingles, and who gets it?** Shingles is a disease of skin and nerves caused by reactivation of the *varicella zoster virus* (VZV) —the same virus that causes chicken pox.

After a bout of chicken pox, the virus doesn't leave the body. It travels up sensory nerve fibers from the skin and establishes latent (dormant) infections in sensory ganglia that last for the rest of an individual's life.

We don't yet know what causes reactivation. We do know that shingles occurs most frequently in people with reduced immunity—individuals taking corticosteroids or immunosuppressant drugs…undergoing chemotherapy…or suffering from HIV infection.

In some cases, shingles may even be triggered by psychological stress.

Shingles is especially common among people over 50—presumably because immunity declines with age. Among people who live to 85, half will get the disease.

●**Is shingles contagious?** You can't get shingles unless you've had chicken pox—and you can't catch shingles from someone who has shingles. However, if you've never had chicken pox, you can catch *chicken pox* from a *shingles* sufferer.

The shingles virus is similar to *herpes simplex virus*, which causes genital herpes. Unlike herpes simplex virus, however, VZV is *not* transmitted through sexual contact.

●**What are the symptoms?** Shingles usually begins with pain on one side of the body —typically on the trunk or around the eye.

The pain—often quite intense—is caused by inflammation created as the virus reproduces within nerve tissue. Pain is generally followed by a rash in the same area one to three days later.

Until the telltale rash appears, shingles is notoriously hard to diagnose. Depending on where the pain is, shingles can resemble a heart attack…gall bladder attack…appendicitis …kidney stone…or a ruptured spinal disk. Shingles can even be mistaken for glaucoma, if the eye is affected.

Once your doctor has ruled out these ailments, keep a close watch for the rash. It's essential to begin treatment as soon as the rash appears.

If treatment isn't started quickly, the virus may spread to other nerve cells. This can cause muscle weakness, hearing loss or other complications.

Most common complication: Chronic pain. Some patients with this disorder—called *post-herpetic neuralgia* (PHN)—are so sensitive that even the pressure of clothing on the skin can cause excruciating pain.

●**How is shingles treated?** Until a few years ago, there was no treatment. Then it was found that the antiviral drug *acyclovir* (Zovirax) was effective. But acyclovir must be taken in very high oral doses—or injected.

Some doctors used to prescribe steroids along with acyclovir. The thinking was that by reducing inflammation, steroids might prevent PHN.

Studies have shown that steroids do *not* prevent PHN. Moreover, they can lead to stomach ulcers and raise blood pressure.

Better: Two new antivirals, *famciclovir* (Famvir) and *valacyclovir* (Valtrex), are more easily absorbed than acyclovir...and these are far more effective.

●**What about controlling the pain?** Aspirin, ibuprofen or acetaminophen may be enough in some cases. For severe acute pain, doctors should prescribe codeine or another narcotic.

●**What if the pain becomes chronic?** Consult a doctor who specializes in pain management. Tricyclic antidepressants—prescribed at lower doses than for depression—are effective in 60% to 70% of patients with PHN.

Some patients appear to get relief from alternative treatments such as acupuncture or electrical stimulation.

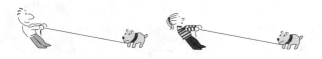

An Itch May Be More than Skin Deep

Neal Schultz, MD, a dermatologist in private practice, 1040 Park Ave., New York 10028.

When troubled by itching, focus on the cause. *Trap:* Severe, prolonged itching can indicate disease of the thyroid, kidney or liver...lymphoma...or other problems, so consult a doctor.

To be more comfortable in the meantime: Cool the skin with compresses or nonprescription lotions like *Sarna Lotion*. Oral antihistamines help itching from allergic reactions—and can be used for sedation if itching keeps you awake. Topical cortisone cream helps inflamed skin. If those don't help, ask your doctor about prescriptions. Ultraviolet light helps eczema and itching that has no obvious cause.

How to Tell When the Sun Is Dangerous

Joseph Bark, MD, a dermatologist in private practice in Lexington, KY. He is author of *Your Skin: An Owner's Guide*. Prentice Hall.

Here are some little-known facts about the summer sun and ways to protect yourself...

●**Shadow's length and sharpness.** If your shadow is shorter than you are—or there is no shadow—the sun is overhead and at its most powerful strength.

The same is true about the sun's intensity when your shadow—or the shade made by trees and other objects—is very sharp, deep and dark.

●**Altitude.** The higher you are in elevation, the thinner the ozone layer and atmosphere, and less protection against the sun's ultraviolet (UV) rays.

●**Sand/grass traps.** They reflect nearly 100% of the sun's rays. If you're at the beach or on a lawn when the sun is overhead, you get double the radiation.

• **Color.** The deeper the color blue of the sky, the less of a barrier there is between you and the sun's rays.

PROTECTING YOURSELF

• **Always wear the highest SPF sunscreen possible**—at least SPF 15—and be sure the sunscreen is waterproof.

Helpful: Men—use sunscreen in place of aftershave lotion. Women—use cosmetics that contain sunscreen.

• **Wear a hat with a wide brim** made from a tightly woven fabric that won't let much light pass through. Avoid baseball caps and sun visors…they don't protect the sides or back of the neck.

• **Wear large sunglasses** that fit close to your eyes and the bridge of your nose. Sunglasses stop you from squinting, protect against wrinkle formation and prevent cataracts and other eye disorders.

Caution: Avoid the small, John Lennon–style sunglasses. The dark lenses cause corneas to dilate, so they are exposed to light that slips in around the glasses. Instead, wear sunglasses at least as large as the eye's orbit—the hollow "cave" that houses the eyeball.

All-Year Sun Defense

Perry Robins, MD, associate professor of dermatology at New York University School of Medicine, New York, and president, Skin Cancer Foundation, 245 Fifth Ave., Suite 2402, New York 10016.

Always use sunscreen if you will be in the sun for any amount of time. Also use sunscreen that blocks UVA rays when spending a lot of time near glass.

Reason: Glass does not effectively block damaging UVA rays.

Women should use moisturizers that contain a broad-spectrum sunscreen (which blocks out both UVA and UVB rays) under makeup.

Much…Much Younger Looking Skin in 15 Minutes a Day

Rachel Perry, founder and chief executive of Rachel Perry, Inc., a natural skin care and makeup company based in Chatsworth, CA. She is author of *Reverse the Aging Process of Your Face: A Simple Technique That Works.* Avery Publishing Group.

You can actually reverse the aging process of your face. How? By using good quality facial cleansers and scrubs along with a few simple isometric facial exercises and self-massage. It takes only 15 minutes a day—and those minutes can be in the shower. My regimen works for men and women.

The general idea is to speed up the process of removing and replacing dead facial skin tissue. It's the dead tissue that leaves the skin tired and muddy looking.

Men don't get those fine lines above the upper lip that many women get because most men shave daily, automatically epidermabrading or exfoliating—i.e., removing dead skin tissue.

CLEANSE AND SCRUB

Daily cleansing and scrubbing is the key to removing dead skin cells.

For a *cleanser*, use either a creamy cleanser or foaming facial cleansing gel. Look for a spreadable consistency. A cleanser should not soak into your skin too easily. The cleanser removes oil and dirt.

A *scrub**—which is used for an abrasive scrub-massage—should have as many natural ingredients as possible. The word "scrub" or "cleanser" should be clearly marked on the container you buy.

For a scrub, I find that two ingredients—sea kelp and sea salt—have the necessary abrasive action, are antibacterial and give a smooth, refined texture to the skin. If you can't find a product with these ingredients, buy them in bulk and add ¼ teaspoon each of sea salt and sea kelp for each ounce of purchased product.

*Facial scrubs made from natural ingredients are available in varying degrees of abrasiveness and can be found in your local health food store or the health food section of your supermarket.

When you use a scrub, dampen your fingers first with water—the additional moisture gives the scrub more spreadability. Always look for products that are pH-balanced.

Caution: Use the scrub gently at first, until you get used to its abrasive action. You don't want to overdo it and leave red patches, or worse, break blood vessels in your face.

You'll also want a supply of small, rough, white cotton terry-cloth towels. Hand towels are a good size. I have seven—enough to last a week.

NOW, THE EXERCISES

It's a good idea to do these exercises whenever you apply cleanser and facial scrub.

Women may also want to do them whenever they apply moisturizer, night cream or even makeup base. This allows your fingers to move smoothly over your face.

Men might find it easiest to do them in the shower. Once you learn the exercises, they will quickly become automatic. After all, you work out to keep your body in good shape. You exercise your arms, legs, abdomen—why not exercise your face?

THE ETERNAL "O"

This exercise firms up the mouth, cheeks, nose and eye area…

First, form a large oval "O" with your mouth, pulling your upper lip downward over your teeth. Smile slightly, but don't move your mouth from the O-shape.

At the same time, squeeze your eyelids shut. The purpose of this phase is to stretch the skin tightly across your face, so you can massage it without worrying about damaging the elasticity of your skin.

The massage: Holding the O position with your eyes closed, use the fingertips of each hand to trace a complete circle around each eye.

●**Starting from the corners**, move over the eyebrows, then under the eyes (including the upper cheeks), for a complete circle.

●**Do this quickly**, a minimum of 10 times. Eventually, you work up to 50 times or more.

Nose: Next, massage your nose with downward strokes, five times.

Mouth: Then massage in a full circle around your mouth, five times in one direction, five in the other.

Forehead: Finally, put your fingertips at the bridge of your nose, and massage upward and outward over your forehead to your hairline, using five to 10 long strokes.

THE FIRMING SMILE

Now, for the bottom half of your face, to help prevent jowls and a double chin…

●**Roll your lips inward over your upper and lower teeth**, leaving a space of about ½ inch between your lips.

●**Smile as widely as you can**—with your *lower* jaw only.

●**Holding the exercise position**, and using your fingertips, massage the entire lower part of your face in small outward circular motions.

●**Start at the tip of your chin**, move up to your ears and then back down again, to a slow count of 10. With practice, work up to 20.

THE NECK REJUVENATOR

To keep your neck muscles firm, and your neck tissue smooth and supple…

●**Place your thumb under your chin**, and curl your tongue back in your throat until you feel the muscle directly under your chin protrude.

●**Now you can take your thumb away**—but continue to keep your tongue curled back.

●**Next, with your chin pointing upward**, stretch your neck as far to the left as possible, to a slow count of 10.

●**Repeat, rotating to the right.** At the same time, massage upward from the base of the neck with the fingertips of both hands, in long, vigorous upward strokes, up to the jawbone.

THE UPPER-LIP SMOOTHER AND AROUND-THE-MOUTH STRENGTHENER

To prevent those upper-lip lines, smooth the furrows that run from the corners of the mouth to the chin, strengthen the muscles around the mouth and firm the lips…

●**Press your lips together in a straight line**, smiling slightly.

●**Using the index fingers of both hands**, massage in tiny outward circular motions around the mouth, to a slow count of 10.

• **Squeeze your lips together harder and harder**, until you feel a tingling sensation.

• **Then immediately make a small "O" with your mouth**, to a slow count of 10.

• **Pucker harder and harder while massaging** in tiny outward circular motions around the mouth, to a slow count of 10. Release.

Do this exercise with the massage at least twice a day. And also do it whenever you can without the massage—while driving, cooking, cleaning, reading. It's a truly portable exercise.

Acne Drug

Diane Berson, MD, assistant clinical professor of dermatology, New York University School of Medicine, New York City.

The prescription lotion *sulfacetamide* (Klaron) clears blemishes by inhibiting the bacterial growth that causes acne—without drying the skin like other acne lotions.

In studies, acne sufferers who used sulfacetamide saw improvement within two weeks. It's effective in adults and adolescents.

UVB Rays Are Everywhere

Richard H. Grant, PhD, associate professor of agronomy, Purdue University, West Lafayette, IN.

Dangerous ultraviolet B (UVB) rays exist in shade as well as in direct sunlight. UVB exposure more closely correlates to how much *open sky* you can see than to whether you're in direct sunlight.

Example: If you're in a grove of trees with direct sunlight hitting you but with a limited view of the sky, you're probably getting *less* UVB exposure than you would get while standing in the shade of a lone tree where your view of the sky is less obstructed.

Helpful: Sunscreen, long sleeves, long pants and a broad-brimmed hat.

Skin Cancer Sufferer Risk

Morten Frisch, MD, PhD, senior epidemiologist, Danish Epidemiology Science Centre, Copenhagen. His study of 37,674 skin cancer patients was published in *Annals of Internal Medicine*, Independence Mall West, Sixth St. at Race, Philadelphia 19106.

People with skin cancer face an increased risk of developing other kinds of cancer. Compared with the general population, patients who had at least one basal cell carcinoma before age 60 had a 37% higher risk of developing breast cancer and a two- to three-fold higher risk of developing testicular cancer or non-Hodgkin's lymphoma.

Repairing Skin Damage

Joseph P. Bark, MD, a dermatologist in private practice and a staff physician at St. Joseph Hospital in Lexington, KY. He is author of *Your Skin: An Owner's Guide.* Prentice Hall.

Cosmetic surgery is the best option for repairing significant skin damage—deep wrinkles, severely sagging skin, pock marks and surgical or wound scars (including the red, raised scars known as *keloids*). Consult two cosmetic or dermatologic surgeons to get a balanced picture of the potential benefits and risks of any recommended procedure (including chemical peels and dermabrasion). Ask to see before-and-after photos of previous patients. *Also:* Ask for the names and phone numbers of those patients, and contact them before proceeding.

Sunscreen Danger

Brian L. Diffey, PhD, professor of photobiology, Dryburn Hospital, Durham, England.

Applying sunscreen incorrectly can raise your risk of skin cancer. To get the full sun protection factor (SPF), adults of average size must use about 1.2 ounces per application to cover their bodies.

Problem: Most people apply far less. Though they're wearing too little sunscreen, sunbathers assume they're protected and therefore stay out in the sun too long.

Self-defense: Apply sunscreen liberally and uniformly. Let it dry before going into the sun.

Sun Protection

Vincent DeLeo, MD, vice chairman of dermatology, Columbia University, New York City.

When it comes to blocking sunlight, a fabric's *weave* is more important than its color, thickness or any special coating.

Test: Hold clothing up to a light. If you can see through it, it won't provide adequate protection.

What Keeps Skin Young… And What Doesn't

Gerald Imber, MD, clinical assistant professor of surgery at New York Hospital–Cornell Medical Center, and a plastic surgeon in private practice, both in New York City. He is author of *The Youth Corridor: A Renowned Plastic Surgeon's Revolutionary Program for Maintenance, Rejuvenation, and Timeless Beauty.* William Morrow.

Although I've been a cosmetic surgeon for more than 20 years, I'm quick to point out that surgery is *not* the only way to keep your face looking youthful.

Proper skin care is more effective than you might imagine at keeping wrinkles at bay. The earlier you start taking care of your skin, the better the results.

Begin in your 20s, and your skin should keep its youthful appearance into your 50s and beyond.

Even if you're over 60, you can undo much of the damage caused by the combined effects of time and environmental stress, such as extremes of temperature, dryness, pollution and sunlight. You can also slow the skin's aging process.

That does *not* mean you should stock up on costly lotions. Cosmetic counters and drugstore shelves sag under the weight of products that claim to work miracles. None do.

But here are five products that really will have a noticeable effect on your skin…

ALPHA-HYDROXY ACID

Creams containing *alpha-hydroxy acids* (AHAs) are the first over-the-counter antiaging preparations that really work.

Derived from natural sources including sugarcane, grapes and milk, AHAs act as exfoliants, encouraging new cell growth, fading discoloration and reducing or eliminating fine lines.

There are now dozens of AHA creams on the market, each with its own "special" acid (lactic, citric, glycolic, etc.). All work equally well. Just be sure the label specifies an AHA concentration of 10% or so. That's the minimum strength capable of really smoothing the skin.

AHA creams yield noticeable results only after several months of daily use—so you must be patient.

Caution: Since once-a-day application of AHA gets such good results, some people assume that they might as well slather it on morning and night. *Bad idea.* Overuse of AHA cream can cause severe skin irritation.

For faster results: Ask a plastic surgeon or dermatologist about getting a light chemical peel. Such peels use a solution containing 30% to 70% AHA. They're performed in the doctor's office with no anesthesia.

In most cases the only side effect is a slight tingling and redness for an hour afterwards.

SUNSCREEN

Used properly, virtually any sunscreen on the market filters out ultraviolet A (UVA) and ultraviolet B (UVB) light. Those are the rays that cause premature aging.

Best: A sun protection factor (SPF) of at least 15. Do not assume that sunscreen with an SPF 30 allows you to stay in the sun twice as long as a sunscreen with an SPF 15.

Sunscreen gets sweated off quickly. I recommend reapplying it liberally at least once an hour. If you go into the water, reapply it as soon as you come out. I also recommend wearing a hat when venturing outdoors in sunlight.

ANTIOXIDANT VITAMINS

Vitamins C and E are the only vitamins proven to be beneficial to the skin. These antioxidant vitamins work by preventing the breakdown of collagen. That's the structural protein that keeps skin strong, smooth and elastic.

There's even some evidence that C and E help the body build more collagen.

I recommend taking 1,000 milligrams (mg) of vitamin C and 800 international units (IU) of vitamin E daily.

These vitamins must be taken *internally* to have any effect. Though it's a popular practice, there's no evidence that rubbing vitamin E oil or lotion onto your skin does any good. The vitamin molecules are far too big to penetrate the skin.

TRETINOIN

This vitamin A derivative (sold as *Retin-A*) smooths skin and erases fine wrinkles. It does so by speeding cellular turnover and stimulating the skin to produce collagen.

It's effective, but Retin-A can cause red, scaly patches. Luckily, there's a moisturizer-like formulation of tretinoin called *Renova*. It's not quite as effective as Retin-A but is less likely to cause irritation.

For visible results, tretinoin must be used for at least four months. To minimize the risk of skin irritation, I tell my patients to stop treatment periodically to allow the skin to recover. When and for how long you use tretinoin should be discussed with your doctor.

Retin-A and Renova are available only by prescription. AHAs and tretinoin can be used at the same time.

MOISTURIZER

Moisturized skin isn't any healthier than dry skin, but it certainly looks and feels as if it is.

Moisturizer hydrates dead cells on the skin's surface, temporarily preventing them from flaking off.

Any water- or oil-based formula will do the job, as will Vaseline or even Crisco. There's no medical reason to pay extra for fancy brands—no matter what "special ingredients" they contain.

The Dangers of Ultraviolet Light

Johanna Adami, MD, MPH, researcher, department of cancer epidemiology, University Hospital, Uppsala, Sweden. Her study of medical records of 113,000 cancer patients was published in the *British Medical Journal*, Tavistock Square, London WCIH 9JR, England.

Skin cancer may not be the only malignancy caused by sunlight. In a study, the lymph system cancer *non-Hodgkin's lymphoma* was 1.4 times more common among malignant melanoma patients than among healthy people ...and twice as common among patients with another common skin cancer, squamous cell carcinoma.

Theory: Ultraviolet light suppresses the immune system, crippling its ability to kill cancer cells.

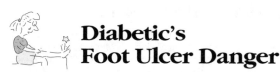

Diabetic's Foot Ulcer Danger

Lawrence O. Kollenberg, DPM, a podiatrist in private practice in Hot Springs, AR.

Diabetic foot ulcers that fail to heal sometimes necessitate the amputation of the toes, the foot or even the entire lower leg.

Now: Dressings containing freeze-dried bovine collagen help heal both infected and noninfected ulcers, helping to save the limb. In one study, all 24 diabetic foot ulcers treated with the collagen treatment healed within five months.

Also helpful: Don't walk barefoot...don't wear tight shoes...wash your feet every day with a mild, nondrying cleanser...and see a podiatrist on a regular basis.

Foot Pain Relief

Suzanne M. Levine, DPM, podiatrist and clinical instructor, New York Hospital–Cornell Medical Center, New York City.

People who suffer from chronic pain in the soles of the feet should avoid going barefoot.

Going barefoot—especially first thing in the morning—can rupture the scar tissue that forms overnight, forcing the healing process to begin anew the next night.

Self-defense: Until the foot has fully healed, always wear shoes or sandals.

Melanoma: What Your Doctor Isn't Telling You

Timothy McCall, MD, a Boston internist, author of *Examining Your Doctor: A Patient's Guide to Avoiding Harmful Medical Care.* Citadel Press. He is a regular commentator on the public radio program Marketplace, and can be found on the Web at *www.drmccall.com.*

The incidence of malignant melanoma, the deadliest form of skin cancer, has soared in recent years—probably because of the thinning of the ozone layer and our more active, outdoor lifestyles.

As you may know, your chance of surviving melanoma hinges almost entirely on how early it is detected. Found early, melanoma has a cure rate approaching 100%. Once the cancer has burrowed deep into the skin, however, the odds of long-term survival are slim.

Unfortunately, recent trends in the way doctors practice medicine may be making early detection of melanoma *less* likely. Because of their desire to reduce costs, health maintenance organizations (HMOs) are encouraging doctors to spend less time with patients. Yet the only effective way to check for skin cancer —and for precancerous conditions that might turn cancerous—is to examine the entire surface of your skin. That takes time.

Another factor interfering with early detection of skin cancer is that HMOs and other managed-care plans discourage primary-care doctors from referring patients to specialists. And *dermatologists* are the doctors most skilled at telling which moles are questionable.

Since you cannot count on your doctor to educate you about melanoma or do a careful screening of your skin, your best defense is to learn these things yourself. *Here are the basics...*

Fair-skinned people are at greatest risk. Blondes and redheads are two to four times more likely to develop melanoma than brunettes. Melanoma in blacks is uncommon, though it does occur. Melanoma tends to run in families. Be especially vigilant at checking your skin if a close relative had it. Any mole can become cancerous, but those present from birth are riskier.

The best way to prevent skin cancer is to avoid exposure to sunlight. That's especially important at midday, when ultraviolet (UV) radiation is peaking.

To reduce sun exposure, consider wearing a broad-brimmed hat, UV-blocking sunglasses and long pants and long sleeves. Cover all exposed areas with a sunscreen that has a sun protection factor (SPF) of 15 or greater. And don't assume cloudy days are safe. About 80% of UV rays make their way through the clouds. UV gets reflected into shady areas, too.

If you're at risk, examine your skin at least once every three months (or have a family member do it for you). *Look for these warning signs...*

- **Diameter larger than a pencil eraser.**

- **Irregular color**, sometimes with areas of red, white, gray or purple mixed in.

- **Irregular borders**, sometimes notched, with the color "bleeding" outward.

Melanomas are most likely to develop on parts of the body that get lots of sun exposure —especially the back and legs. But they can pop up anywhere, including such unlikely areas as the soles of the feet.

If there is any doubt whether a mole could be a melanoma, have it checked. If your primary-care doctor cannot rule out melanoma, have the mole biopsied by a dermatologist.

The poster on the wall of my office says it best. In a takeoff on the old school readers, it proclaims: "See Spot. See Spot Change. See a Doctor."

Periodic self-exam:

1. Examine body front and back in mirror, then right and left sides, arms raised.

2. Bend elbows, look at forearms, back of upper arms and palms.

3. Look at backs of legs and feet, spaces between toes and soles.

4. Examine back of neck and scalp with a hand mirror. Part hair to lift.

5. Check back and buttocks with a hand mirror.

More Skin Cancer Facts

Hensin Tsao, MD, PhD, melanoma researcher, department of dermatology, Massachusetts General Hospital, Boston.

Deadly skin cancer can lie dormant for more than a decade. Not too long ago, any patient who had a melanoma removed and then stayed cancer-free for 10 years was considered cured.

Finding: Melanoma can recur even after 15 years. Since treatments are now available for certain recurrences, melanoma survivors should have their skin and lymph nodes checked annually.

A Word About Surgery

Gerald Imber, MD, clinical assistant professor of surgery at New York Hospital–Cornell Medical Center, and a plastic surgeon in private practice, both in New York City. He is author of *The Youth Corridor: A Renowned Plastic Surgeon's Revolutionary Program for Maintenance, Rejuvenation, and Timeless Beauty.* William Morrow.

If you think you might decide to have cosmetic surgery, don't wait until you need a full face-lift.

Instead, start earlier and get several less invasive procedures (microsuction of the jowls, eye-lift, etc.). That way, you'll look great all along.

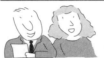

What Causes Tiny Red Lines on the Cheeks?

Thomas N. Helm, MD, assistant clinical professor of dermatology, State University of New York, Buffalo.

These tiny lines are usually nothing more than dilated blood vessels under the skin. Called *telangiectasia,* they're caused by sun exposure and by age-related thinning of the skin.

Good news: Dermatologists can remove them using an electric probe...or via laser therapy.

16

Health Alerts

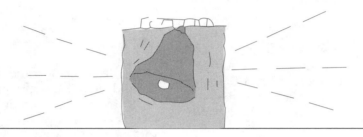

All About Leg Cramps

Norman Marcus, MD
Lenox Hill Hospital
International Foundation for Pain Relief

If you've been experiencing leg cramps but have neglected to do anything about them, you may be placing your life in jeopardy. *Reason:* While two of the three main types of leg cramps are benign, a walking-related cramp known as intermittent claudication can be a sign of heart disease.

•**Nighttime leg cramps** typically involve a spasm in the calf muscle that wakes you up. *To stop the pain:* Gently massage the knot while alternately flexing and extending your toes.

Also helpful: Ask your doctor about taking the prescription medication quinine sulfate…and about taking a daily supplement that contains 500 to 1,000 milligrams (mg) of calcium…1,000 mg of magnesium…and 400 international units (IU) of vitamin D.

The minerals are critical to proper muscle contraction. Vitamin D assures proper absorption of the minerals.

•**Post-exercise leg cramps** are usually caused by electrolyte imbalances brought on by heavy perspiration. These imbalances cause muscle and nerve cells to malfunction.

Helpful: Rest…drink water or a sports drink like Gatorade before and during exercise …and massage after exercise.

•**Intermittent claudication.** If walking gives you a cramp in one of your calves, see a doctor right away. Unlike other types of leg cramps, intermittent claudication is caused by reduced blood flow in one of the legs. In most cases, this reduction in blood flow is caused by the buildup of fatty deposits in leg arteries (atherosclerosis).

Danger: People who have fatty deposits in their leg arteries often have similar deposits in

Norman Marcus, MD, chief of pain medicine at Lenox Hill Hospital and president of the International Foundation for Pain Relief, both in New York City. Dr. Marcus is author of *Freedom from Pain*. Simon & Schuster.

their coronary arteries. In fact, if someone has claudication, there is a 50% chance that he/she also has heart disease.

Claudication causes bad cramps in one leg after walking even a short distance. Typically, the cramp disappears after a minute or two of rest…and recurs when you resume walking.

Other symptoms: Having one foot that has thicker toenails, is bluish in color, has less hair or is colder than the other foot.

Treatment for intermittent claudication is similar to that for coronary artery disease. In most cases, patients are urged to take long walks or get other regular aerobic exercise… quit smoking…and adopt a low-fat, low-cholesterol diet.

Some cases of intermittent claudication require leg surgery to clear away the blockages. In some cases, doctors are able to push aside the fatty deposits by snaking a balloon-tipped catheter through the skin and into the clogged artery. This procedure is called *balloon angioplasty.*

For severe cases, bypass surgery may be required. In this procedure the surgeon creates a "detour" around the blocked arteries by grafting a blood vessel from a large artery in the groin to an artery behind the knee.

In some cases, individuals who experience walking-related leg cramps are suffering not from claudication but from *pseudo*claudication.

This comparatively benign condition is caused by abnormal growth of bone tissue in the spine. As the bone grows, the bony sheath encasing the lower spinal nerves narrows. That compresses the nerves, causing them to register pain.

How can you tell pseudoclaudication from true claudication? Pain from claudication goes away within two minutes when you stop walking. Pain from pseudoclaudication persists for five to 10 minutes.

If pseudoclaudication is accompanied by leg weakness and loss of sensation, surgery may be needed. Injections of cortisone and local anesthetic into the spinal cord region may decrease the pain.

Diabetes Alert

John F. Amos, OD, chairman, department of optometry, School of Optometry, University of Alabama at Birmingham.

Annual eye exams are essential for all diabetics. See an eye doctor *right away* if you experience vision changes—blurred, fluctuating or double vision.

Disinfectant Danger

David Lewis, PhD, research microbiologist, University of Georgia, Athens. His study was published in *Nature Medicine*, 1234 National Press Bldg., Washington, DC 20045.

The disinfectant commonly used on medical and dental instruments does *not* kill the AIDS virus. Even when drill pieces and viewing scopes (endoscopes) used in the respiratory and gastrointestinal tracts spent two hours soaking in the disinfectant *glutaraldehyde*, the virus survived in blood-tainted lubricants used in these devices. While there's no evidence that contaminated lubricants have ever led to AIDS, occasional infections may go undetected.

Self-defense: Ask your doctor to sterilize endoscopes with ethylene oxide gas or peracetic acid, not simply disinfect them.

Rodent Danger

Bruno Chomel, DVM, PhD, assistant professor of population health and reproduction, School of Veterinary Medicine, University of California, Davis.

Hantavirus, which causes a respiratory illness that can be deadly, is thought to spread via inhalation of tiny particles of rodent droppings.

Self-defense: If you see signs of rodent infestation in storage rooms, cabins, etc., don't vacuum or sweep the floor. That can stir up feces-laden dust. *Better:* Don work gloves and a filter mask, then sprinkle or spray the floor with a mixture of bleach and water. Sweep the mess into a plastic bag, then dispose.

Another Danger In the Kitchen

Charles Gerba, PhD, professor of microbiology, University of Arizona, Tucson.

Dishcloths and kitchen sponges are often infected with *salmonella, staphylococcus* and other disease-causing germs.

Self-defense: Replace rags and sponges with paper towels. Or use a germ-resistant sponge such as Cell-O brand and wash it in hot water after each use. And be sure to wash your hands with an antibacterial soap after handling uncooked meat.

Good news: Adopting these simple strategies could prevent 90% of all food-borne illnesses.

The Scary Truth About Blood Transfusions

Edgar G. Engleman, MD, professor of pathology and medicine at Stanford University Medical School and director of the University's Blood Center, both in Palo Alto, CA. In 1983, under Dr. Engleman's direction, Stanford's blood center was the first in the world to test donated blood for the AIDS virus.

Although the nation's blood supply is safer today than ever before, many people remain fearful of catching AIDS or another disease from a transfusion.

For an update on transfusion safety, we spoke with Dr. Edgar G. Engleman, who pioneered the testing of donated blood for the AIDS virus in the early 1980s.

According to Dr. Engleman, the blood supply is now remarkably safe, especially when compared with 10 years ago. Risk of catching a serious infection is roughly one in 5,000. *There are several explanations for this increased level of safety...*

WIDESPREAD SCREENING

In the early 1980s, donated blood was screened only for hepatitis B and syphilis. Not until 1985 was testing for the AIDS virus (HIV) implemented on a nationwide basis.

Most blood banks did not launch efforts to screen for AIDS prior to the availability of a specific test, arguing that the risk of catching AIDS from a transfusion was tiny and the cost high. In fact, up to 2% of the units of blood transfused in some cities in the early 1980s harbored HIV. Thousands were needlessly infected, including Arthur Ashe and Ryan White.

Today, the Food and Drug Administration keeps close watch over blood banks. It doesn't hesitate to close down those that don't follow regulations.

MORE ACCURATE HIV TESTING

At one time, blood banks tested only for the presence of *antibodies* to HIV (not the virus itself). *Problem:* It can take a while after infection for antibodies to form. There is a window of time when a person's blood is infectious even though the virus isn't detectable via conventional antibody testing.

To offset this problem, more sensitive antibody tests have been developed.

Result: The window has shrunk from 24 weeks to about four weeks. In addition, the FDA has licensed a test for HIV itself. This test, which is mandated for use by all blood banks, shrinks the window even further.

And prospective blood donors are thoroughly questioned about possible risk factors for AIDS (homosexuality, intravenous drug abuse, etc.) before they are allowed to donate blood.

Bottom line: Roughly one in 400,000 transfusions now results in transmission of HIV. The new test should reduce the incidence to one in 700,000.

FEWER TRANSFUSIONS ARE GIVEN

A generation ago, doctors recommended transfusions even in cases that weren't life-threatening—to help people feel less tired after surgery, for example.

Today, doctors order transfusions only to save lives—not to make patients feel better.

BEYOND AIDS SCREENING

Blood banks now screen donated blood for the two strains of HIV, syphilis, hepatitis B and C, plus two other potentially deadly pathogens...

●**Human T-lymphotropic virus** (HTLV-1 and HTLV-2). Close relatives of HIV, these viruses cause cancer and other illnesses.

●**Cytomegalovirus** (CMV). It can cause a life-threatening infection in premature infants, chemotherapy patients, AIDS patients, transplant recipients taking immunosuppressant drugs and other individuals with poor immunity.

Diseases for which we are not yet testing, but which may be cause for concern, include...

●**Hepatitis G.** This newly discovered strain of hepatitis is less virulent than other strains—but more persistent.

●**Chagas.** This one-celled organism (protozoan) causes chronic infection, which can lead to heart failure.

As more people enter the US from areas where Chagas is endemic (chiefly Central and South America) the incidence of the disease in the US will increase. Even so, the number of cases spread by transfusion will probably remain low.

HOW TO AVOID BAD BLOOD

What can individuals do to protect themselves from tainted blood? First, it's important to remember that *blood transfusions save lives* ...and that people have died because they *refused* transfusions. Having said that, there *are* ways to minimize your risk...

●**Predeposit your own blood.** Autologous donation—banking your own blood—is the single most significant precaution you can take. Barring human error in the handling of your blood (extremely unlikely), your risk of contracting a transfusion-related illness is essentially zero.

●**Recycle your blood.** Many operating rooms are now equipped with "cell-saving" devices that collect blood draining from the surgical incision and reintroduce it into the body.

Called *intraoperative autologous transfusion* (IAT), this technique is often effective in emergency surgery—so it's definitely worth asking for. It cannot be used for intestinal surgery, tumor removal or any other operation in which blood could be contaminated with bacteria or cancer cells.

●**Know your options.** In California, surgeons are required to inform patients of their transfusion options. This is *not* the case in all states.

If your surgeon doesn't explain your options, ask him to do so. Alternatives should be discussed at least six weeks before surgery.

If significant blood loss is expected, a *series* of autologous donations may be required over several weeks. Blood cells can be stored for up to 42 days, frozen plasma for up to one year.

The surgeon isn't necessarily to blame if you should need a transfusion. However, you're likely to lose *less* blood under the hands of a good surgeon. Ask how many times he/she has done this procedure.

Some hospitals can provide plasma or platelets taken from one person. "Single donor" blood is generally less likely than "pooled" blood to carry disease. However, this isn't always practical. Given today's careful screening practices, the increase in safety is marginal at best.

Some patients scheduled for surgery ask friends and relatives to donate blood. The assumption is that blood from someone you know is safer than blood from anonymous donors.

In fact, friends and relatives are likely to be *first-time* donors (whereas the community supply consists mostly of blood from repeat donors), so their blood hasn't been subjected to repeated testing. Ironically, it may be less safe.

●**Ask about blood-boosting drugs.** Over the last decade, researchers have identified hormone-like substances that spur production of red blood cells, white blood cells or platelets. In many cases, these factors can be synthesized using recombinant DNA technology —and used as drugs.

Erythropoietin (EPO), one of the first of these to become commercially available, helps the body make more red cells. It's helpful for some patients with kidney failure and other chronic conditions that used to require repeated transfusions.

However, since the body takes up to a few weeks to manufacture blood cells in response to the EPO, its value in surgery is limited.

Lead Danger

Charles V. Shorten, PhD, associate professor of health, West Chester University, West Chester, PA.

Salad dressing stored in a crystal cruet can quickly become contaminated with lead. It's long been known that crystal goblets can leach lead into beverages. But this hasn't been considered a threat to children because so few drink from crystal. *However:* A study found that lead rapidly leaches into salad dressing. After one hour in a crystal cruet, lead levels hit 162 micrograms per liter (mcg/L). After 42 days, levels hit 665 mcg/L, eight times the level in distilled water.

Drinking Danger

Nedra Wilson, MS, RD, coordinator, Nutrition Information Service, University of Alabama, Birmingham.

Every glass of alcohol causes your body to lose water. If the water isn't replaced, you could become dehydrated.

Self-defense: Never use beer or any other alcoholic beverage as a thirst quencher. Remember to sip water whenever you're drinking beer, wine or any other alcoholic beverage.

Underwear Danger

Alan Matarasso, MD, a New York City–based plastic and reconstructive surgeon. His remarks were reported in *Archives of Internal Medicine*, 515 N. State St., Chicago 60610.

Tight garments may contribute to *deep vein thrombosis* (DVT), a potentially deadly ailment involving formation of a blood clot in the legs. Should the clot break away and travel to the lungs, this pulmonary embolism can kill within minutes.

Self-defense: Avoid restrictive clothing if you're at high risk for DVT. At-risk individuals include postsurgical patients, pregnant women and those who are bedridden.

Boating Danger

Neil Hampson, MD, medical director, hyperbaric department, Virginia Mason Medical Center, Seattle. His study of 27 poisonings was published in the *Journal of the American Medical Association*, 515 N. State St., Chicago 60610.

Pleasure boaters are vulnerable to carbon monoxide poisoning.

Danger: Air currents created behind a moving boat can draw carbon monoxide— colorless and odorless—from the engine exhaust into the boat. In a study of 27 on-board carbon monoxide poisonings, 21 involved engine exhaust...four involved emissions from onboard water heaters...and two involved emissions from gas generators. Many carbon monoxide poisoning cases go unreported because boaters blame their symptoms—headaches, nausea, dizziness and vomiting—on sea sickness.

Self-defense: Install a carbon monoxide warning sensor with an alarm in all gasoline-fueled cabin cruisers.

Allergy Attacks And Food

Stephen F. Kemp, MD, advanced subspecialty resident, clinical and laboratory immunology, University of South Florida College of Medicine, Tampa.

In a survey of 266 cases of the life-threatening allergic response *anaphylaxis*, 34% were caused by food, spices or food additives. *Usual culprits:* Shellfish and peanuts. Aspirin and non-steroidal anti-inflammatory drugs caused the most drug-related attacks. Anyone at risk for anaphylaxis should keep the drug *epinephrine* on hand.

Ear Thermometer Danger

Michael Yaron, MD, associate professor of surgery, University of Colorado Health Sciences Center, Denver. His study of 100 patients was published in the *Journal of Emergency Medicine*, University of California Medical Center, 200 W. Arbor Dr., San Diego 92103-8676.

In-the-ear thermometers are often unreliable. Only six of 10 adults with fever detected by an electronic rectal thermometer—considered the most accurate method for fever measurement—were found to have a fever with an ear thermometer. Oral thermometers are generally accurate.

Get a Tetanus Booster Shot Every 10 Years

Timothy McCall, MD, a Boston internist, author of *Examining Your Doctor: A Patient's Guide to Avoiding Harmful Medical Care*. Citadel Press. He is a regular commentator on the public radio program Marketplace, and can be found on the Web at *www.drmccall.com*.

The protection generated by a tetanus shot deteriorates over time. Older people, in particular, who have not had a booster shot in decades lose immunity to this completely preventable but potentially fatal disease.

Drinking Unfiltered Coffee May Raise Your Blood Cholesterol Level

Michael J. Klag, MD, an associate professor at Johns Hopkins University School of Medicine, Baltimore.

When Dutch researchers measured cholesterol levels of people who switched to unfiltered coffee brewed in French-press plunger coffee pots, they found that they rose by up to 20 points compared with those who stayed with filtered coffee. Scientists theorize that the jump was caused by two compounds that are trapped by coffee filters and have been shown to raise cholesterol levels and affect the function of the liver, which metabolizes cholesterol.

Another Secondhand-Smoke Danger

George Howard, DrPH, epidemiologist, Bowman Gray School of Medicine, Winston-Salem, NC, and leader of a seven-year study of 8,400 people.

Atherosclerosis—a thickening of the arteries that can lead to heart attack and stroke is another danger of inhaling secondhand smoke. Over time, the effects are cumulative. Regular inhalation significantly interferes with the ability of arteries to carry blood—increasing the risk of serious disease.

Yikes! Another Measles Shot?

Barbara Reynolds, Centers for Disease Control and Prevention, Atlanta.

If you were born after 1956 and received only one measles vaccination, a second may be needed to protect you. More than three million Americans between the ages of 20 and 37 are at risk of contracting measles despite inoculation. A single vaccination fails to provide immunity 5% of the time. That failure rate was only determined in 1989, and children up to age 12 then got second shots. You may not be protected if you were older than 12 in 1989.

Self-defense: Check your medical records. Have a second vaccination if necessary.

In-Line Skating Injuries On the Rise

Rodney M. Friedman, editor and publisher, *University of California at Berkeley Wellness Letter*, Health Letter Associates, Box 412, Prince St. Station, New York 10012.

In-line skating injuries will send more than 100,000 Americans to hospital emergency rooms this year. About two-thirds of these injured skaters will not be wearing a helmet, elbow and knee pads or wrist guards when they fall.

Stroke Diagnosis Danger

Louis R. Caplan, MD, professor of neurology and medicine, Tufts University School of Medicine, Boston.

Headaches, confusion, temporary blindness, seizures and other stroke-like symptoms are sometimes caused by a less serious neurological disorder called *reversible predominantly posterior leukoencephalopathy* (RPPL).

Danger: Some doctors begin treatment for stroke when the patient really needs adjustment of his/her blood pressure or immunosuppressant medication.

Good news: With proper treatment, patients with RPPL usually recover within days. RPPL is common among patients with high blood pressure and those taking immunosuppressant drugs after transplant surgery. It occurs when capillaries leak fluid into the brain.

Don't Cut Back on Caffeine Suddenly

Johanna Dwyer, RD, professor of medicine and community health, Tufts Medical School and School of Nutrition, Boston.

You may suffer withdrawal symptoms if you cut back on caffeine suddenly. *Better:* Lower your intake gradually. Try cutting half a cup of coffee from your diet every few days… or mixing regular with decaffeinated and gradually increasing the proportion of decaf. Also ease up on consumption of other caffeine-containing beverages, like some teas and soft drinks.

Hidden Dangers in Household Products… In Everyday Foods, Too

Samuel S. Epstein, MD, professor of occupational and environmental medicine at the University of Illinois School of Public Health in Chicago, and chairman of the Cancer Prevention Coalition, 520 N. Michigan Ave., Suite 410, Chicago 60611. He is coauthor of *The Safe Shopper's Bible: A Consumer's Guide to Nontoxic Household Products, Cosmetics and Food.* Macmillan.

Everyone seems to worry about smog and other sources of pollution *outside* the home.

But many everyday foods are tainted with toxic chemicals…and an EPA study of air in six US cities found that certain airborne toxins can be up to 500 times more concentrated indoors than outdoors.

Where do these dangerous airborne toxins come from? From cleansers, paints, cosmetics and other household products.

Problem: Federal regulations that govern the labeling of consumer products are woefully inadequate. Consequently, it's difficult for consumers to find out precisely which products contain dangerous ingredients or contaminants —and which are safe.

To find out how consumers can protect themselves, we spoke with Dr. Samuel S. Epstein, a noted toxicologist and chairman of the Chicago-based Cancer Prevention Coalition…

DANGEROUS PRODUCT AND SAFER ALTERNATIVES

●**Beef frankfurters.** The nitrite preservatives in beef frankfurters interact with *amines*, which occur naturally in meat and fish, to form potent cancer-causing compounds called nitrosamines.

Franks also may be contaminated with the carcinogenic pesticides *benzene hexachloride, Dacthal, dieldrin, DDT* and *heptachlor*…and with residues of powerful hormones.

Safer: "Nitrite-free" franks or—better still—tofu franks.

●**Bug killer.** Many household pesticides contain *propoxur*, a compound that is both carcinogenic and neurotoxic.

Safer: Brands that substitute *pyrethrum* or another natural, herbal pesticide for propoxur.

●**Cat litter.** Many brands contain *crystalline silica*, an eye and lung irritant and suspected carcinogen.

Safer: Litter made of a natural ingredient such as pulverized paper.

●**Flea collar.** Many flea collars contain the pesticide propoxur.

Safer: Flea collars made with natural, herbal pesticides.

●**Air freshener.** Some aerosol brands contain *orthophenylphenol*, a skin irritant and carcinogen. This is particularly dangerous because tiny aerosol droplets are readily inhaled deep into the lungs.

Safer: Solid air fresheners made with plant-based scents. It's best to avoid all aerosol spray products, including air fresheners, cosmetics and household cleaners.

●**Hair conditioner.** Some brands contain *formaldehyde* and the carcinogenic dye *FD&C Red #4.*

Safer: Natural, plant-based conditioners.

●**Hair dye.** Black and dark brown hair dyes have been linked to several kinds of cancer, including non-Hodgkin's lymphoma, multiple myeloma and leukemia.

Safer: Hair dyes that substitute plant-based substances like *henna* for the synthetic dyes.

Warning: Never buy hair dye that contains *phenylenediamine.*

●**Laundry detergent.** Brands that contain washing soda are highly caustic. Some brands may also be contaminated with a carcinogen called *1,4 dioxane.*

Safer: Vegetable-based detergents or laundry soap.

●**Makeup.** Cosmetics often contain talc, *titanium dioxide* and/or the preservative *BHA*—all of which are carcinogenic. In addition, *lanolin* found in many brands is often tainted with DDT.

Safer: Natural, plant-based cosmetics.

●**Moth repellent.** These often contain *naphthalene*, a neurotoxin, or *dichlorobenzene*, a highly volatile compound that is a potent carcinogen.

Safer: Cedar blocks, chips and sachets.

●**Paint stripper.** Aerosol strippers often contain *methanol*, a neurotoxin that is also a potent skin and eye irritant…along with *methylene chloride*, a carcinogen.

Safer: Get rid of old paint by sanding or scraping it off. To avoid inhalation of dust, wear a respirator mask.

●**Shaving cream.** Some brands contain the carcinogenic preservative BHA…along with *triethanolamine* and/or *diethanolamine*, which are nitrosamine precursors.

Others contain *Blue #1* and other cancer-causing dyes.

Safer: Natural brands—especially those that are applied with a brush.

●**Talcum powder.** Talc irritates the lungs and has been linked to ovarian cancer.

Safer: Products made with cornstarch.

●**Toothpaste.** Many popular brands of toothpaste contain Blue #1, which is a carcinogen.

Fluoride is also a suspected carcinogen.

Safer: Natural toothpaste without fluoride.

●**Weed killer.** Some brands contain sodium 2,4-*dichlorophenoxyacetate* (2,4-D), a carcinogen and neurotoxin.

Safer: "Weed whackers" or other tools for cutting rather than poisoning weeds.

•**Whole milk**—including whole-milk products like cheese and milk chocolate.

Milk fat is often laced with the carcinogenic compounds DDT, dieldrin, heptachlor and/or *hexachlorobenzene.*

In addition, milk products are sometimes tainted with antibiotic residues. Some of these residues cause allergic reactions. Others are suspected of causing cancer.

Ingestion of these antibiotic residues also promotes growth of potentially dangerous antibiotic-resistant bacteria inside the body.

Safer: Organic skim milk, especially brands labeled "bovine hormone-free."

Meningitis Warning

Ronald Ruden, MD, internist in private practice in New York.

acterial meningitis—the less common, *potentially deadly* type—is most prevalent in late winter/early spring. *Viral* meningitis is most prevalent in late summer/early autumn. Symptoms are the same—severe headache, fever, stiff neck. If you experience symptoms, see your doctor *immediately.* Bacterial meningitis requires antibiotics. Viral is treated simply with bed rest.

Prevention: Good hygiene—wash hands after using the bathroom…don't share food.

Even the Best Medical Labs Can Make Mistakes…

Charles Inlander, president of The People's Medical Society, a patient advocate organization, 462 Walnut St., Allentown, PA 18102. He is author of several books, including *The People's Medical Society Health Desk Reference.* Hyperion.

nd they can be dangerous—even deadly. The biggest errors occur on routine tests—especially Pap smears and PSA tests (for prostate cancer). If a test comes back negative and you still think something could be wrong—*get retested.* Ask your doctor to send the test to a different lab…or to send it to the same lab but under a different name. *Never* use the doctor's *in-office* lab—their error rates are much higher than commercial lab rates.

Also: Always make sure the lab your doctor uses is certified by the College of American Pathologists. If you don't trust the lab that your doctor uses, ask him/her to use a properly accredited one.

Asthma Attacks Can Be Triggered by Thunderstorms

A. Craig Davidson, MD, consultant physician, Guy's and St. Thomas's Hospital, London.

ulprit: Grass pollen and other airborne allergens stirred up by wind and rain.

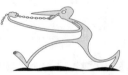

Nose Piercing Is Dangerous

William Castelli, MD, medical director, Framingham Heart Study, Boston.

ecause the nose is designed to trap airborne bacteria, it is one of the dirtiest places in the body. Many virulent bacteria, such as *staphylococcus aureus,* are harmless as long as they stay in the nose. But should the piercing needle force them into the bloodstream, they can cause serious illness—even death.

Glucose Level Alert

Linda J. Rhodes, MD, assistant professor of psychiatry, University of Texas Health Science Center, San Antonio.

levated glucose levels can trigger depression, fatigue, apathy and malaise. Diabetics should monitor feelings as well as glucose levels—and report problems to their doctor.

Cigar Dangers

Harlan Krumholz, MD, assistant professor of cardiology at Yale University School of Medicine, New Haven, CT, and author of *No Ifs, Ands or Butts: The Smoker's Guide to Quitting.* Avery Publishing Group.

Cigars have all of the health risks of cigarettes—including lung cancer, heart disease and stroke.

Trap I: Thinking that smoking cigars is safe because you don't inhale.

Reality: Cigar smoke contains more tar, nicotine and carbon monoxide than filtered cigarettes. You may not inhale as you puff, but you still breathe in the "secondhand" smoke.

Trap II: Giving in to the "George Burns phenomenon."

Reality: Just because someone else lived a long life despite an unhealthy habit doesn't mean you will, too.

Reality: Any amount of smoking puts your health—and others'—at risk.

Even Moderately High Blood Pressure Can Damage Kidneys

Michael Klag, MD, MPH, associate professor of medicine, Johns Hopkins University, Baltimore. His study of 332,544 men over 16 years was published in *The New England Journal of Medicine,* 10 Shattuck St., Boston 02115.

It has long been known that severely high blood pressure can cause kidney failure, but researchers have been unsure of what, if any, danger moderately high blood pressure poses to the kidneys.

In a study, men with mildly elevated blood pressure—140 to 159 over 90 to 99—were three times as likely to suffer kidney failure as were men with optimal blood pressure of below 120 over 80. Those with moderate hypertension—up to 179 over 109—had six times the kidney damage risk.

To the rescue: Your doctor will probably prescribe a pressure-lowering regimen.

Smokers' Sleep Trap

David Wetter, PhD, assistant professor, behavioral science, University of Texas, M.D. Anderson Cancer Center, Houston, and Terry Young, PhD, associate professor, preventive medicine, University of Wisconsin at Madison.

Smokers are more likely to have difficulty falling asleep, difficulty waking up, daytime sleepiness and nightmares. *Possible causes:* The stimulative effect of nicotine…nightly nicotine withdrawal…breathing difficulties associated with smoking. Over time, such sleep disturbances can result in fatigue, depression and impaired ability to think.

Shoveling Snow Stresses the Heart

Barry Franklin, PhD, director of cardiac rehabilitation, William Beaumont Hospital, Royal Oak, MI.

After two minutes of shoveling wet snow, heart rates of nine out of 10 men soared far above the zone recommended for aerobic exercise (70% to 85% of maximum heart rate). After 10 minutes of shoveling, heart rates reached 97% of maximum…and blood pressure was higher than when the men ran to the point of exhaustion.

Asthma Warning

Thomas Plaut, MD, asthma specialist and medical consultant to *Asthma Update,* 123 Monticello Ave., Annapolis, MD 21401.

Asthma patients cannot measure the ailment's severity by how they feel. A peak-flow meter is needed to determine lung function and ways to keep the disease under control. If you have asthma, make sure your doctor uses a peak-flow meter as the basis for determining therapy. And be sure the doctor teaches you how to use it at home between visits.

Lead Alert

Howard Hu, MD, ScD, associate professor of occupational and environmental medicine, Harvard School of Public Health, Boston.

Very low levels of lead are dangerous to adults, too. Adults who pick up traces of lead from environmental sources—like food cans, water pipes and lead paint dust—can develop high blood pressure and reduced kidney function.

Self-defense: Take the same precautions for yourself that you would for a child. *Start here:* Have your water tested to ensure lead levels are safe. The danger posed by lead-based paint should be evaluated and possibly removed by professionals—don't do it yourself. Take extra care with hobbies that expose you to lead, such as staining glass and shooting.

Lead Poisoning Alert

Study of 23 types of pool cue chalk, led by Mary Beth Miller, DO, department of medical toxicology, Good Samaritan Regional Medical Center, Phoenix, reported in *Pediatrics*, 141 NW Point Rd., Elk Grove Village, IL 60009.

Surprising source of lead danger: Pool cue chalk. Lead compounds are sometimes used to color chalk for pool cues. In one case, a 28-month-old girl who often put the chalk in her mouth developed elevated lead levels.

Self-defense: Buy pool cue chalk that does not contain lead. If unsure, take extra precautions to keep it away from children.

Toxic Chemicals Self-Defense

Robert G. Lewis, PhD, senior scientist, National Exposure Research Laboratory, Environmental Protection Agency, Research Triangle Park, NC.

To keep toxic chemicals out of your home, remove your shoes before coming inside, especially after working with insecticides or herbicides.

Also: Use a doormat...have carpets steam-cleaned...replace any carpet that is more than 20 years old. Traces of banned pesticides, such as DDT, can be found in some old carpets.

Who Should Be Vaccinated For Hepatitis B?

Mary Ann Littell, information specialist, American Liver Foundation, 1425 Pompton Ave., Cedar Grove, NJ 07009.

The vaccine is a good idea for international travelers...infants and adolescents...doctors, nurses, paramedics, firefighters and police officers...people on hemodialysis...members of the military...morticians and embalmers...patients and staff members at institutions for the mentally handicapped...members of ethnic or racial groups with high rates of hepatitis B infection—African-American, Native American, Hispanic, Chinese, Korean, Indo-Chinese, Filipino, Alaskan Eskimo or Haitian...people with multiple sex partners...intravenous drug users...recipients of clotting factor and certain other blood products...people living with or having sex with a hepatitis B carrier.

Weight-Lifting Danger

John D. Cantwell, MD, team physician for the Atlanta Braves, and a cardiologist in private practice in Atlanta.

Intense weight-lifting can be dangerous for individuals with high blood pressure. Anyone with hypertension or another risk factor for heart disease (cigarette smoking, high cholesterol, diabetes, etc.) should do strenuous exercise only with a doctor's permission.

Drowning Fact

Centers for Disease Control & Prevention, 1600 Clifton Rd. NE, Atlanta 30333.

Avoid alcohol before swimming—or while boating. From 25% to 50% of all adult drowning victims were exposed to alcohol at time of death.

Plastic vs. Wood Cutting Boards

Don Schaffner, PhD, extension specialist, food science, Rutgers University, New Brunswick, NJ.

When it comes to preventing bacterial contamination, food safety experts now favor plastic. But the best solution may be to have a plastic board for meat and poultry *and* a wooden board for fruit, vegetables and bread. Keep the boards separate to avoid cross-contamination. Clean them after each use with a solution of two teaspoons bleach in a quart of water. Plastic boards can be put in a dishwasher.

Caution: Sanitizing a wooden board in the microwave can cause a fire.

To Beat the Heat...

Stuart R. Rose, MD, head of the International Travel Clinic at Noble Hospital, Westfield, MA, and president, Travel Medicine, Inc., Northampton, MA.

Drink two to three quarts of water a day, even if you do not feel thirsty.

●**Drink two glasses two hours before any exercise.** Keep drinking cool water—not cold—during exertion.

●**Review medications with your doctor—** some can restrict sweat or increase production of body heat.

●**If you take prescription diuretics,** ask your doctor if you should change the dosage while traveling.

●**Replace salt lost through sweating** by drinking a sports drink or eating salty foods. If you have salt restrictions, consult your doctor.

Milk and Diabetes Connection

Hans-Michael Dosch, MD, professor of pediatrics and immunology, Hospital for Sick Children, Toronto. His study of diabetes in 140 infants was published in *The New England Journal of Medicine*, 10 Shattuck St., Boston 02115.

Infants given cow's milk formula during their first three months face an increased risk of diabetes later in life.

Theory: A protein in cow's milk—*bovine serum albumin*—is similar to proteins found in insulin-producing cells in the pancreas. In infants genetically predisposed to diabetes, antibodies that form to attack bovine serum albumin wind up attacking the pancreas cells as well.

Lesson: If possible, mothers should breast-feed their infants for the first three months of life.

Have a Foot Problem?

John T. Langloh, MD, staff orthopedist, National Hospital Medical Center, Arlington, VA.

Diagnose foot problems by checking your footprints. Dip your feet in water, then walk along a piece of brown paper. If you have a "light" footprint—little or no link between the ball of your foot and the heel— you may have a high arch.

Helpful: "Stability" shoes with extra arch cushioning...high-top sneakers.

If you have a "heavy" footprint, you may have flat feet. This can lead to arch or knee pain.

Helpful: Molded arch supports...shoes with "control" features...orthotic inserts.

Who's Reading Your Medical Records?

Timothy McCall, MD, a Boston internist, author of *Examining Your Doctor: A Patient's Guide to Avoiding Harmful Medical Care.* Citadel Press. He is a regular commentator on the public radio program Marketplace, and can be found on the Web at *www.drmccall.com.*

Patients discuss private matters with their doctors with the implicit understanding that the information exchanged is private. In reality, more and more people are gaining access to these confidential medical records and using the information in ways you never intended.

These days, insurance companies, credit bureaus and the like have assembled sophisticated databases that contain loads of private information. Unbeknownst to you, this information may be shared with other insurers, potential employers, marketing firms—and sometimes sold to anyone who will pay for it.

Worst of all, information you divulged to help your doctor help you may be used with just the opposite result. *Here are four true horror stories...*

●**A company changes its insurance policy to limit coverage** for AIDS-related problems after learning that an employee has tested HIV-positive.

●**A man is denied life insurance** after telling his doctor he was feeling "down" because he feared his company might be the victim of a hostile takeover.

●**A woman is fired** after her employer learns she needs a kidney transplant.

●**A hospital employee uses a computer to access the phone numbers of teenage female patients**, then calls them up and sexually harasses them.

To provide top-notch medical care, doctors need complete access to the most sensitive matters—drug use, sexual habits, etc. We need our patients to trust that their secrets will remain secret. If a young man doesn't feel comfortable telling a doctor he's gay, for example, then the doctor may misjudge the significance of a symptom, order the wrong tests, miss diagnoses and the opportunity to treat.

Until legal loopholes that allow unauthorized dissemination of medical information are closed, how can you minimize your risk? I recommend several strategies:

●**Never sign a blanket disclosure form.** Before agreeing to the release of your medical records, make sure you know who will be allowed to see them, which information they'll be given access to and what they need the information for.

●**Remind your doctor that your information must not be shared with anyone without your consent.**

●**Consider asking your doctor not to include especially sensitive information in your record.** You might say, "If I tell you something very personal that may be relevant to my care but that I don't want to be written in my chart, would you respect my wishes?" If your doctor is unwilling to honor your request, you'll have to decide whether you still want to reveal the information.

Keep in mind that keeping important information out of your chart could compromise your care down the road—especially if you see another doctor or if your doctor fails to remember what you said. Keep information out of your record only if you feel doing so is absolutely essential.

●**Be wary of any medical information you give out**, no matter how innocent it seems. A TV ad once offered free information on pollen counts to anyone who called an 800 number. The names of those who called were then used by the drug company that had sponsored the ad to market an allergy medication.

●**Get a copy of your medical records** to make sure all information is factually correct. An error in your chart could lead to the loss of employment or future insurance coverage.

In most states, you have a legal right to your medical records. In the rest, you can ask your doctor for a copy of your chart. If your doctor won't provide it, you've got to wonder whether your doctor views health care as a democracy or a dictatorship.

Fibromyalgia... New Strategies for Controlling Mysterious Pain and Fatigue

Robert M. Bennett, MD, professor of medicine and chairman of the division of arthritis and rheumatic diseases at Oregon Health Sciences University in Portland and a member of the medical advisory board of the National Fibromyalgia Research Foundation. For a free information packet on fibromyalgia, write the association at Box 500, Salem, OR 97308.

Fibromyalgia is a mysterious pain syndrome which afflicts four million Americans and is characterized by...

- **Chronic flu-like pain** in the muscles, tendons and/or ligaments.

- **"Tender points"**—areas of great sensitivity to touch.

- **Restlessness, numbness and/or tingling** in the arms and legs.

- **Sleep problems**—thought to be caused by pain and/or persistent leg twitching that makes deep, restful sleep impossible.

- **Chronic fatigue.** Many fibromyalgia sufferers feel tired even after a full night's sleep.

Some patients also report headaches, abdominal bloating and/or irritable bowel syndrome.

To learn more, we spoke with the nation's leading fibromyalgia researcher, Dr. Robert M. Bennett.

AN EMOTIONAL PROBLEM

For decades, doctors considered fibromyalgia an emotional problem. The consensus was that anxious or depressed individuals unwittingly "created" their symptoms.

Since the mid-1970s, several studies have proved this theory false. As it turns out, most fibromyalgia patients do *not* have emotional problems. In those who do, the problems are now believed to be the *result* of having to live with chronic pain—not the cause of the pain.

Fibromyalgia seems to be associated with chronic fatigue syndrome (CFS)—another disorder that has at least some connection with emotional problems. Up to 80% of CFS patients also have fibromyalgia.

Some researchers speculate that CFS and fibromyalgia are simply different terms for the same condition. Since neither syndrome is well understood, however, it's hard to know for sure.

HOW FIBROMYALGIA STARTS

While some cases begin with a flu-like infection, most start with lower back pain, whiplash or another localized pain. This pain then spreads to other parts of the body.

Why does the pain persist? What makes it spread? The culprit seems to be subtle changes in the central nervous system—possibly the result of abnormally high levels of certain neurotransmitters—that make people more sensitive to pain.

Because the disorder tends to run in families, researchers also suspect that there is a hereditary component.

THE GOOD NEWS...AND THE BAD

The good news is that fibromyalgia is neither crippling nor degenerative. It certainly isn't fatal.

Unfortunately, there is no cure. Most patients learn to manage their symptoms, but the pain may continue to flare up in response to injury, infection or stress.

Even worse, few doctors know much about the syndrome. That means it can be hard to get an accurate diagnosis.

If you think you have fibromyalgia, your best bet is probably a rheumatologist. To find one in your area, contact the Arthritis Foundation (800-283-7800).

DRUG THERAPY

Conventional arthritis drugs, including aspirin, do *not* seem to be particularly effective against fibromyalgia. Drugs that *do* seem effective include...

- **Amitriptyline** (Elavil) and other tricyclic antidepressants. Taken at low doses (10 to 25 milligrams [mg] instead of the 100 to 200 mg prescribed for depression), tricyclics help to reduce pain and promote sleep.

- **Zolpidem** (Ambien). This short-acting sedative can help fibromyalgia sufferers get much-needed sleep. However, because of the danger of dependency, zolpidem should be taken no more than twice a week.

•*L-dopa and carbidopa* (Sinemet). Very low doses of this drug—used mainly to treat Parkinson's disease—relieve restless-leg syndrome, a common problem for fibromyalgia patients.

•*Procaine or lidocaine.* These local anesthetics are injected into tender points. Injected properly, these drugs bring relief lasting several months.

•*Tramadol* (Ultram). A relatively new non-narcotic drug.

LIFESTYLE ISSUES

Since emotional stress can trigger pain, fibromyalgia patients must learn to pace themselves. Physical and occupational therapists can demonstrate less stressful ways to move... and suggest job modifications to make your work environment more comfortable.

It's particularly important to avoid long stretches of typing or other repetitive motions.

•**Exercise.** Although too much or too little exercise exacerbates fibromyalgia symptoms, gentle stretching or massage (including acupressure) and moderate exercise are essential. Shoot for 20 minutes of aerobic exercise three times a week.

•**Relaxation.** Since fibromyalgia pain isn't caused by muscle tension, deep breathing and other relaxation techniques aren't likely to reduce symptoms.

But learning to relax can keep tension from *exacerbating* the pain. Patients who know how to relax—via relaxation tapes, rhythmic breathing, hot baths, etc.—are better able to keep the problem in perspective.

•**Support groups.** As with many chronic diseases, fibromyalgia seems to be helped by active participation in a support group.

To find a group in your area—or to obtain more information on fibromyalgia—contact the Arthritis Foundation.

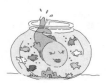

Aneurysm Alert

Harold Wilkinson, MD, chairman of neurosurgery at the University of Massachusetts, Worcester, MA.

When it comes to headaches, I consider myself lucky. I get them rarely, and I can always pinpoint the cause—most recently, giving up a three-cup-a-day coffee habit.

Though usually benign, headaches can be a sign of serious trouble—tumor, meningitis, etc. One cause that often gets overlooked is brain aneurysm—a weak, bulging portion of an artery—inside the skull. Left untreated, an aneurysm can rupture, causing a fatal "brain attack."

Each year, 25,000 Americans are stricken by ruptured aneurysms. Recently, a friend—just 36 years old—died after suffering a ruptured aneurysm.

What causes aneurysms? The risk factors include age (30 to 60 are the riskiest years), high blood pressure, atherosclerosis...and a family history of aneurysms.

The good news about brain aneurysms is that surgery is usually curative—if done within 24 hours of the rupture. Tragically, too many people shrug off their symptoms until it's too late.

If you suddenly get "the worst headache of your life"—especially if you have any of the risk factors—see a doctor right away.

Avoiding Drug Errors

David W. Freeman, editorial director, *Bottom Line/Health*, 281 Tresser Blvd., Stamford, CT 06901.

Doctors are notorious for having bad handwriting. Making matters worse, many common medications have similar names—Accupril and Accutane, Lovastatin and Lotensin, Prilosec and Prozac...to name but a few.

Bad handwriting plus confusing drug names can cause big trouble. *Real-life example:* A doctor wrote an order for 2 milligrams (mg) of the blood pressure drug *Cardura* on a patient's hospital chart. But the pharmacist read the doctor's scrawl as 2 mg of the anticoagulant *Coumadin.*

Luckily for this patient, a nurse caught this potentially lethal error and called the doctor, who cleared things up. Of course, not every nurse is as vigilant.

How does one guard against such errors? I put that question to Diane D. Cousins, RPh, a prescribing error expert with the US Pharmacopeia, the nonprofit organization that sets national drug standards. She said that each time a doctor writes a prescription for you, insist that he/she write legibly *and...*

● **Avoid use of Latin words and abbreviations** for drug names and directions for use.

● **Include a brief notation of the drug's purpose.**

● **Include your age and weight.**

● **Specify dosages using metric values** (grams, milligrams, etc.) or international units (IU) instead of the old-fashioned apothecary terms (drams, minims, etc.).

● **Write a zero** *before* **a decimal point (for fractional doses)**...but not a zero *after* a decimal point. For example, 0.5 mg instead of .5 mg, but 3 mg instead of 3.0 mg.

Please take the time to see that your doctor complies. It just might save your life.

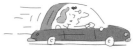

Gas Fumes Danger

Victoria Strand, MD, consulting physician, department of respiratory and allergic disease, Karolinska Institute, Huddinge University Hospital, Stockholm.

Fumes from gas appliances and heavy traffic can render the respiratory tract unusually sensitive to pollen.

Study: Adult asthmatics experienced an average 52% decrease in lung function when exposed to airborne pollen if they had breathed such fumes a few hours earlier.

Self-defense: Have gas appliances inspected annually...equip gas stoves with exhaust fans (or open a window when cooking)...open a window when operating a gas dryer...avoid jogging on busy streets.

Important: If sufficient household ventilation cannot be arranged, asthmatics should consider switching to electrical appliances.

Checking Up on Your Thyroid Could Save Your Life

Lawrence Wood, MD, a member of the thyroid unit at Massachusetts General Hospital in Boston, and coauthor of *Your Thyroid: A Home Reference Ballantine.* For more information, contact the Thyroid Foundation of America, 350 Ruth Sleeper Hall–RSL 350, 40 Parkman St., Boston 02114. 800-832-8321.

If you've been feeling run down, the problem could be your thyroid gland. Research suggests that *hypothyroidism* (thyroid deficiency) is far more common than previously believed. One study found signs of the disorder in 8% of women and 3% of men.

Hypothyroidism is especially common among older people. Over age 60, up to 17% of women and 8% of men have it.

The thyroid gland, located just below the Adam's apple, is responsible for regulating body metabolism. Besides reducing your energy level, hypothyroidism can cause elevated cholesterol levels, weight gain, depression, constipation and/or brittle hair and nails.

CAUSES OF THYROID TROUBLE

The leading cause of hypothyroidism is scarring of the gland caused by inflammation. This condition is known as Hashimoto's disease.

Other causes include viral infection, certain drugs (including lithium and iodine) and radiation therapy delivered to the neck for cancer.

Mild cases of hypothyroidism often go undetected—because the symptoms are too subtle to be detected by the individual.

Doctors at Massachusetts General Hospital in Boston studied a group of patients with mild hypothyroidism. Most of these patients *thought* they were well. In a double-blind study, each was treated, in turn, with thyroid and placebo tablets.

Result: Most patients felt better when taking the thyroid tablets. Some felt more energy, others were less depressed or less constipated.

These findings suggest that low-dose thyroid treatment may be beneficial even for people who don't know they have thyroid trouble.

CHECKING THYROID LEVELS

The easiest way to detect hypothyroidism is via a blood test for a pituitary hormone called *thyroid-stimulating hormone* (TSH). Ordinarily, TSH stimulates the thyroid gland to make *triiodothyronine* (T3), *thyroxine* (T4) and other thyroid hormones.

If levels of these thyroid hormones fall too low, the pituitary automatically makes more TSH. So, abnormally *high* levels of TSH are a clear sign of hypothyroidism.

If your thyroid is producing too much hormone (a condition called *hyperthyroidism*), TSH levels in your blood will be abnormally low. If your TSH levels are abnormal, your doctor may order other tests.

The TSH test can be obtained by your primary-care physician during a routine checkup.

Cost: $40 to $80.

WHO SHOULD GET TESTED?

Everyone age 50 or older should have his/her TSH levels checked at least once every five years. Start at age 35 if you have...

- **A parent, sibling or child who has had thyroid trouble.**

- **A visibly swollen thyroid gland** (goiter). If you think you have a goiter, see a doctor. The condition can be the first sign of thyroid cancer.

- **Prematurely gray hair.** Even a single gray hair before age 30 is a sign that you may have an overactive or underactive thyroid.

- **Insulin-dependent diabetes.**

- **A tendency toward left-handedness.** For unknown reasons, left-handed people seem to be predisposed to thyroid trouble.

- **Pernicious anemia.**

- **White spots on the skin known as vitiligo,** a thyroid-related immune disorder.

Important: A diagnosis of hypothyroidism should always be confirmed by a TSH test.

TREATING HYPOTHYROIDISM

Hypothyroidism is easily corrected by taking a daily tablet of T4 (from which the body can make T3). This treatment, taken indefinitely, can be prescribed by your regular doctor.

Most people with hypothyroidism feel well after two to three months of taking the pills.

Your doctor will probably start you on a low dose of thyroid hormone and check your TSH levels every few weeks until the proper dosage is found.

Dosing requirements can change, so have your TSH levels checked about once a year.

Caution: Thyroid pills should not be taken with iron supplements. Iron blocks the absorption of thyroid hormone.

OVERACTIVE THYROID

Low levels of TSH generally mean hyperthyroidism. This condition can occasionally be caused by inflammation of the gland or too much iodine in the diet. But the most common cause is a hereditary condition known as Graves' disease.

Graves' usually strikes between age 20 and 40. Signs include swelling of the thyroid, weight loss, anxiety, hair loss, muscle weakness and a rapid heartbeat.

If you're diagnosed with Graves', your doctor will probably refer you to an endocrinologist for additional testing and treatment.

THYROID LUMPS AND TUMORS

About one of every 25 people has one or more small nodules in their thyroid gland.

If a nodule is detected, your doctor should evaluate it further. Tests may include a TSH level, imaging studies (an ultrasound or a radioactive thyroid scan) and a thyroid biopsy.

Nodules that prove to be cancerous should be surgically removed. Surgery is often combined with radioactive iodine, thyroid supplements and X rays or chemotherapy. Most cases of thyroid cancer can be cured via these means.

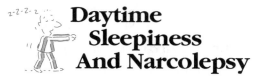

Daytime Sleepiness And Narcolepsy

Michael Thorpy, MD, director of the Sleep–Wake Disorders Center at Montefiore Medical Center, Bronx, NY, and director of the National Narcolepsy Registry.

Do you find yourself nodding off several times a day? If so, you may be one of the hundreds of thousands of Americans who suffer from narcolepsy.

Narcolepsy usually starts around puberty. It's thought to be largely hereditary, although in many cases it shows up only after it's been triggered by a head injury, an intensely emotional experience or another event.

Narcolepsy symptoms start subtly and become more pronounced with time. The disorder is typically diagnosed about 10 years after symptoms first appear.

Telltale symptoms: Excessive daytime sleepiness and an uncontrollable urge to sleep.

Narcoleptics *know* they're about to fall asleep—they don't typically black out in midsentence—but can do nothing to keep from doing so.

THREE RELATED DISORDERS

Many people who suffer from narcolepsy also suffer from one or more related disorders...

●**Cataplexy.** This form of sudden muscle weakness is brought on by strong emotions. You might begin to argue with your spouse, for instance, only to have your head droop uncontrollably and your knees weaken.

●**Sleep paralysis.** This frightening phenomenon is marked by an inability to move the body after awakening in the morning.

Episodes of sleep paralysis can last anywhere from a few seconds to several minutes.

●**Hypnagogic hallucinations.** These unusually vivid dreams occur at the very onset of sleep.

Hypnagogic hallucinations come about when a person goes immediately from wakefulness to *rapid eye movement* (REM) sleep without first progressing through lighter stages of sleep.

GETTING HELP

If you think you have narcolepsy, organize your day so that you can take short, frequent naps (less than 20 minutes). To avoid accidents, always take a brief rest before driving or operating dangerous equipment.

Avoid alcohol and caffeine. Alcohol won't prevent sleepiness, and it can cause you to wake up late at night. Caffeine is simply not potent enough to keep you awake.

If these simple remedies don't help, consult a board-certified sleep specialist. He/she may ask that you spend a night in a sleep disorders center, where the type, depth and quality of your sleep can be measured.

For referral to sleep specialists in your area, contact the American Academy of Sleep Medicine at 507-287-6006, *www.aasmnet.org.*

HELPFUL MEDICATIONS

●**Stimulants.** *Pemoline* (Cylert), *methylphenidate* (Ritalin), *dextroamphetamine* (Dexedrine) and related drugs simply help you stay awake.

Although stimulants are quite effective at controlling drowsiness, they can have side effects, such as anxiety, headaches, insomnia and increases in heart rate and blood pressure.

●**Antidepressants.** Drugs like *protriptyline* (Vivactil) and *fluoxetine* (Prozac) fight cataplexy. Protriptyline can cause dizziness, dry mouth and sexual dysfunction. Fluoxetine can cause insomnia and sexual dysfunction.

●**Sleeping medications.** *Clonazepam* (Klonopin) and *zolpidem* (Ambien) improve nighttime sleep. However, clonazepam is addicting and can cause daytime drowsiness.

Zolpidem is nonaddicting, but it can cause daytime sleepiness, nausea and headache.

NATIONAL NARCOLEPSY REGISTRY

To learn more about narcolepsy and/or to add your name to the National Narcolepsy Registry, contact the National Sleep Foundation, 1522 K St. NW, Suite 500, Washington, DC 20005, 202-347-3471.

Web site: www.sleepfoundation.org

E-mail: nsf@sleepfoundation.org

17
Weight Success

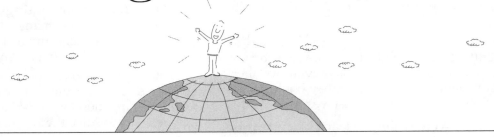

The 10 Secrets of Successful Weight Loss

Anne M. Fletcher, MS, RD

If you're trying to lose weight, it's easy to be discouraged by the experts. Doctors and dietitians routinely cite pessimistic figures like the notorious "95% failure rate." According to this statistic, 95% of all dieters gain their weight back—and then some.

The truth about weight loss may not be nearly so dire. A survey by *Consumer Reports* found that one in four readers who used commercial diet programs had kept off at least two-thirds of the weight they had lost.

Twenty-five percent is still a lower success rate than most of us would like. But instead of focusing on dieting failures, I decided to look at what's different about people who *don't* gain weight back.

I consulted the experts who *really* matter—160 people, each of whom had lost at least 20 pounds (average weight loss for this group turned out to be 63 pounds) and who had kept the weight off for at least three years.

It turned out that there were 10 common threads among these "successful losers"...

1. They believed they could do it. Most of the people I surveyed had lost and regained their weight at least five times before successfully keeping it off. But they didn't give up.

The turning point for many of them came when they realized they were sick and tired of the weight-loss battle. Instead of using this feeling as an excuse to stop trying to lose weight, however, the successful dieters somehow felt empowered by it. The feeling made them resolve to take control.

2. They lost weight for themselves—not someone else. All her life, one young woman I interviewed had been told by her mother

---

Anne M. Fletcher, MS, RD, a registered dietitian who has counseled hundreds of overweight people. A leading writer on nutrition, she is the former executive editor of the *Tufts University Diet & Nutrition Letter* and author of *Thin for Life*. Chapters Publishing, Ltd.

327

(and everyone else), "You have such a pretty face—if only you'd lose some weight!"

She lost and gained weight repeatedly. Inside, she was angry that people didn't accept her the way she was. By the time she entered college, she weighed more than 200 pounds. But it was there that she met a man who loved her that way.

Ironically, because she finally felt accepted, she was able to lose weight once and for all—for her own sake.

3. They found out what worked for them. About half the people I talked to lost weight on their own. Others used a commercial diet center or a self-help group...or consulted privately with a dietitian.

In addition, successful people learned to accept a target weight that was realistic for them. This goal might be slightly above their ideal weight, but they knew they could go no lower without starving themselves.

4. They were willing to learn a new way of eating—for life. Many dieters go back to their old eating habits once they lose weight. That's why most dieters regain weight.

The weight-control masters accepted low-fat eating as a *way of life*. They learned to enjoy fruits, vegetables and grains. They found ways to add low-calorie flavor by using spices, lemon or lime juice and low-fat products. Gradually, they noticed that they didn't feel good when they ate high-fat foods.

5. They deal with slipups immediately. While they aren't obsessed with the scale, most weigh themselves once a week to once every few days. They have a narrow window of acceptable weight regain (typically five to 10 pounds). When their weight exceeds this "buffer zone," they do what's necessary to lose it.

Some people exercise more. Others cut back on sweets...pay closer attention to portion sizes...or keep a food diary to increase their awareness of what they eat. But each person I talked to had a plan of action—and used it before the weight gain could get out of hand.

6. They say nice things to themselves. Negative self-talk can be self-fulfilling. An

example is the "now-I've-blown-it" phenomenon that's familiar to many of us: *I ate one cookie. I'm a pig. I might as well eat the whole bag.*

The weight-loss masters give themselves positive and encouraging messages even when they make mistakes: *I resolved not to eat two helpings, but I slipped. I'll be more careful the rest of the day.*

7. They exercise. Nine out of 10 of the successful people I interviewed exercise regularly. They aren't fanatics, and few of them work out every day. But they've managed to find simple activities like walking that they can work into their daily routine.

8. They face their feelings. Back when they were overweight, many of the people I spoke to automatically turned to food whenever they felt upset, bored, lonely or anxious.

What they learned to do instead was get to the source of the negative emotion—by noticing the feeling, identifying the cause and figuring out a way to solve the problem.

Many of their solutions are quite simple. When bored, they leave the house and do something fun. When lonely, they call a friend. When angry, they confront the person who's mistreating them.

9. They enjoy life. A number of the now-successful people used to spend so much energy taking care of others that they neglected their own needs. Eating was their only reward.

Some people who kept weight off have developed what I call a "healthy selfishness." They're still considerate of others, but they take care of themselves, too.

As one woman put it, *I found that when my own needs were met, I was better at meeting the needs of others.*

They've also found ways to reward themselves without food—from pursuing a hobby to seeking more satisfying relationships.

10. They get support. They ask their families not to leave junk food laying around...call a buddy when they're tempted to overeat... and request encouragement and pep talks from friends and family.

Beer Drinkers Really Do Have Bigger Bellies

Bruce B. Duncan, MD, PhD, an epidemiologist at the Federal University of Rio Grande do Sul, Porto Alegre, Brazil. His study of the drinking habits of more than 12,000 adults was published in the *American Journal of Epidemiology*, 2007 E. Monument St., Baltimore 21205.

Compared with both nondrinkers and those who drink an equivalent amount of alcohol in wine, adults who drink six beers a week are rounder around the middle. *Danger:* Potbellies have been linked to increased risk of heart disease.

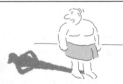

Why Diets Fail

Steven A. Lamm, MD, clinical assistant professor of medicine at New York University School of Medicine in New York. He is author of *Thinner at Last*. Simon & Schuster.

One out of three Americans is overweight, ranging from a few pounds to obese. Most of these people have been on numerous types of diets—many of which have failed.

Here's why dieting no longer makes sense—and new thinking about effective weight loss…

WHY DIETING FAILS

When you diet, your brain—in an act of self-defense against perceived starvation—signals your body that you need more food…and lowers your metabolism so you store more fat. Both actions make it harder to reach your dieting goals.

With each repeated cycle of dieting, it takes longer to lose weight and it comes back quicker. What's more, you are likely to accumulate extra pounds each time.

Important: Taking off weight isn't the main problem—keeping it off is. Despite the best nutrition, exercise regimens and diet plans in the world, 90% of dieters regain one- to two-thirds of lost weight within one year and almost all of it within five years.

Getting out of the diet mode requires that you accept that obesity is a complex medical problem that requires a multipronged solution, including possible drug intervention. Being very overweight is not a result of a lack of willpower or discipline, so stop blaming yourself for your size and deluding yourself that you won't wake up hungry tomorrow. You will, because your brain sabotages your best efforts at psychological control and makes it impossible to resist cravings.

Also recognize that constant dieting can perpetuate your weight problem by adversely affecting your metabolism.

Important: A chronic overweight problem can only be managed, never cured. To keep your weight in "remission," you must be constantly vigilant, eating healthfully and exercising regularly.

A HEALTHY EATING PLAN

Here's how to start on a healthy eating plan for life…

● **Stop obsessing over your weight and your appetite.** Rather than keeping you "in control," mental preoccupation with dieting is practically guaranteed to keep you overweight because you're constantly thinking of food.

● **Adhere to the following eating guidelines** developed by the Department of Agriculture…

● **Eat 20% of your calories from protein sources, 20% from fat and 60% from carbohydrates.** People with a weight problem should reduce their carbohydrate intake to about 40% and increase protein intake to 40%.

● **Cut back on foods that are high in saturated fats,** including potato chips, ice cream and red meat. They aren't good for you and seem to spark primitive hunger urges.

● **Decrease your intake of simple carbohydrates**—sugars. Instead, concentrate on eating more complex carbohydrates—breads, rice, pasta, potatoes, fruits and vegetables—which will give you energy and make you feel full.

● **Don't skip meals.** Not eating at regular intervals is a foolproof way to get fat—it convinces your body you're starving and need to conserve fat.

●**Don't eat less than 1,200 calories a day.** When you go on such a low-calorie diet, your body starts to break down muscle tissue to use for energy so it doesn't have to dip into its fat stores. You lose weight, but you lose muscle as well as fat, which means that after your diet you'll end up with a higher percentage of body fat to muscle mass. That will make your metabolism work even slower.

●**Start or continue an exercise program.** *Ideal:* Engage in aerobic activity—walking, running, swimming or bicycling—for an hour three times a week. *Second best:* Exercise moderately for 30 minutes five times a week.

To build muscle and offset muscle loss brought on by dieting, also engage in resistance training—using free weights or weight machines—twice a week. Weight training can speed your loss of fat, help you ward off osteoporosis as you age and enhance your endurance.

Important: Unless you are willing to exercise regularly, you will not succeed in keeping weight off.

FINDING A PHYSICIAN

Discuss drug treatment for obesity with your primary care doctor. If your doctor won't prescribe drugs for you, ask for a referral to an obesity specialist. Or contact the American Society of Bariatric Physicians (303-779-4833) for the name of a doctor who prescribes medication as part of a comprehensive weight-control program. Approximately 60% of physicians today offer such a program.

Wonderful Ways to Keep Weight Off Once You've Lost It

Joyce Nash, PhD, a clinical psychologist in San Francisco and Palo Alto, CA. She is author of several books on behavioral medicine, including *Now That You've Lost It*. Bull Publishing Co.

It's a lot easier to lose weight than it is to keep off the excess pounds. When you are trying to lose weight, you're singularly focused on the task at hand. But once you're down to your target weight, you have to balance weight maintenance with other factors in your life.

On a daily basis, that requires you to continually correct yourself and bring yourself back on course.

Weight management is a journey rather than a destination.

PSYCHOLOGY OF WEIGHT MAINTENANCE

Positive thinking patterns are crucial to successful, long-term weight management. *People who are not successful at managing their weight tend to…*

●**Make excuses** that let them overeat or not exercise.

●**Focus narrowly on the pleasure of eating** and forget their weight-management goals.

●**Doubt their ability to change.**

●**Set unrealistic expectations** for themselves or others.

●**Judge themselves—and other people—harshly.**

In contrast, those who are successful tend to…

●**Remind themselves of their long-range goals.**

●**Notice even small successes** in weight management.

●**Use positive self-talk** to keep themselves on the right track.

STRATEGIES FOR WEIGHT MAINTENANCE

●**Make exercise a regular part of your life.** Without regular exercise, weight maintenance is exceedingly difficult.

Of course, making exercise a part of your daily routine is easier said than done. I recommend you choose a range of activities that you enjoy and can turn to when you're in different moods—or confronted by bad weather.

Example: I walk outside for an hour a day. On days when it rains, I cycle on a stationary bicycle indoors.

●**Reduce fat calories to 30% of your daily intake.** Most Americans eat more fat than they need. We're exposed to a lot of fatty, highly palatable foods, so we develop a taste for foods that are readily available. However, you can change your taste buds and actually learn to prefer low-fat foods.

Strategy: Start small. Eat bread without butter, salad with little or no dressing and chicken without its skin.

Bonus: After consuming low-fat foods for a while, you'll find that eating fatty foods makes you feel physically and psychologically uncomfortable...bloated, sluggish, even nauseous.

● **Control binges.** Between 25% and 50% of all people who attend weight-management programs are bingers. The biggest trigger for binges is negative emotions—anger...depression...anxiety.

Strategy: Keep a two-week journal to record your eating behaviors—meals, snacks, binges. Also record the circumstances—how you feel, what you are doing and your thoughts when you are eating. This will help you identify triggers for eating and develop strategies to avoid them.

Example: I recently treated a female patient who often felt angry and responded to her negative emotions by bingeing. Once she identified her anger as a trigger for excessive eating, she was able to examine her anger cycle and pick and choose which battles to fight and when to let the anger pass away. She also learned to express her anger—by confronting the person who had precipitated the anger in her, for instance—in ways other than eating.

● **Eat moderately.** To successfully maintain a low weight level, you must keep your caloric intake under control.

Strategy: Eat anything you want, but keep your calories in a moderate range. The government recommends between 1,600 and 2,800 calories each day to maintain weight for most adult men and women. However, your best range for maintaining weight will depend on your age, sex, lifestyle, activity level and other factors. Experiment with adding on and taking off calories to find the range that's best for you.

● **Think smart.** Focus on your long-term goal of weight maintenance, give yourself instructional thoughts and pat yourself on the back for positive behaviors.

Mistake: At the office, a coworker is passing around slices of cake. As a slice comes your way, you see only the cake, not your goal. You rationalize, telling yourself that you've been good for weeks and you shouldn't be deprived when everyone else is eating it.

Better: As a slice comes your way, remind yourself that you've worked hard to lose weight, you feel great and you want to keep the weight off. You tell yourself that the momentary pleasure of the cake isn't in your best interest. You decline the cake. As your coworker moves on to someone else, you feel good about yourself and congratulate yourself for forgoing temptation.

● **Handle lapses.** Everyone backslides on occasion.

Strategy: Avoid turning a lapse into a relapse. Instead of having a second donut, go to the gym to burn off the calories or cut back on calorie intake tomorrow.

● **Create a lifestyle that is satisfying to you.** The last thing you want to say at the end of your life is that you devoted the majority of your life to watching your weight. While weight maintenance is important to health and psychological well-being, your life should be about something more meaningful.

Create a mission that makes you feel your life is worth living. Find a way to be creative, contribute to society or do something that's important to you.

Maximize Your Gardening "Workout"

Jeffrey Restuccio, author of *Fitness the Dynamic Gardening Way.* Balance of Nature Publishing.

Heavy digging, raking, laying sod, turning compost and other garden chores burn 300 to 400 calories an hour.

To burn even more: Use hand tools, such as an old-fashioned push mower instead of a power mower, a rake instead of a leaf blower ...wear wrist and ankle weights to increase calories burned...split tasks into 30-minute segments so you'll get a good workout each day.

Caution: Don't overdo it.

Metabolism Slows With Age

Johanna Dwyer, DSc, RD, director, Frances Stern Nutrition Center, New England Medical Center, Boston.

Metabolism slows with age—beginning as early as age 35.

Result: Weight gain simply from continuing to eat as you did when you were younger.

Self-defense: Weight training and regular aerobic exercise to increase muscle mass and keep your metabolism running more quickly. *Also:* Consume foods that are full of nutrients but low in calories—drink vegetable juice instead of soda, eat multigrain bread instead of white. You can continue eating most of your favorite foods—just reduce the portion sizes.

Dieting for People Who Have Trouble Dieting

Louis Aronne, MD, director of New York Hospital's Comprehensive Weight Control Center. He is author of *Weigh Less, Eat More.* John Wiley & Sons.

If you're like most people, you have probably tried all the weight-control approaches—but haven't been successful in losing all the weight you want...or keeping it off.

WHY WE OVEREAT

One of the major reasons you're overweight may be that you can't control your urge to eat. Food cravings are a result of a chemical imbalance in the brain. They start in the hypothalamus, the brain's hunger center, which sends out chemical messengers—*neurotransmitters*—to tell you when, how much and what to eat.

Although it sounds very simple—some neurotransmitters say eat...others say stop eating—the delicate balance between messengers can easily be disturbed.

Add to that the unlimited amounts of food available everywhere today and the fact that you don't have to physically exert yourself to get food, and you've got a setup for out-of-control eating.

HOW TO CONTROL FOOD URGES

To fight your cravings, you must learn how to curb the levels of neurotransmitters the brain sends out. The only way to stifle your urge to eat now is to change your exercise and eating patterns. *Here's how...*

● **Keep a weight-control journal for one month.** Research has shown we don't know how much we really eat in a day—sometimes we underestimate by as much as 75%.

Helpful: Buy a small notebook that you can carry with you everywhere. Each time you eat or drink something, write down what it was, how much you consumed, when and where, what you were doing before and how you felt while eating.

Reason: If you use the journal every day—all day—you'll identify hidden food traps in your routine...determine if stress prompts you to eat...discover the types of foods that trigger you to overeat...learn how exercise affects your appetite.

● **Start an exercise program.** You've heard it over and over again, but exercise is truly the key to weight-control success.

Build exercise into your everyday life—climb the stairs instead of taking the escalator...walk to the corner store instead of taking the car...park far away from the mall so you'll have farther to walk.

Engage in up to an hour of aerobic exercise—walking, running, biking—and resistance exercise—calisthenics or weight training—at least three times a week.

Example: Do 10 minutes of aerobic activity mixed in with resistance training three times a day...or 30 minutes once a day. Studies show that both ways are equally beneficial for people who are just starting to exercise.

If you're already someone who works out regularly but wants to burn more calories, vary the intensity of your workout.

Example: Set the treadmill so that you walk up hills of different heights, followed by flat surfaces.

●**Learn about the components of a nutritionally balanced diet.** The government recommends that adults eat the following daily…

●**Six to 11 servings of pasta, cereal, rice and bread.** *Example:* One serving equals a half cup of pasta.

●**Three to five servings of vegetables.** *Example:* One serving equals a half cup.

●**Two to four servings of fruits.** *Example:* One serving equals one banana.

●**Two to three servings of dairy products.** *Example:* One serving equals eight ounces of milk.

●**Two to three servings of meat, poultry, fish and eggs.** *Example:* One serving equals two to three ounces.

●**Sparing amounts of fats, oils and sweets.**

Exception: If you suffer from i*nsulin resistance*—a condition where the body must produce increasingly large amounts of insulin to maintain blood-sugar levels—moderate your intake of cereal, bread, pasta and other carbohydrates. Instead, follow a slightly higher-protein, lower-carbohydrate diet than the government recommends.

Reason: You actually crave carbohydrates, but carbohydrates make you eat more because they quickly raise and then lower your insulin levels. Your body thinks your blood-sugar level will drop too much and sends out a signal requesting more food.

You can find out if you are insulin-resistant —a quarter of the population is—by keeping your weight journal and tracking your response to carbohydrates. Or you can talk to your doctor about it.

●**Don't skip meals or severely limit your food intake.** This prompts your brain to produce more *neuropeptides*, which trigger a gnawing desire for carbohydrates.

If you ignore the urge, your brain dispatches another chemical, called *galanin*, which instructs your body to eat and store fat. Together, the two produce irresistible cravings.

●**Be prepared for cravings as you change to a healthier diet.** The good news is that the cravings will fade.

Helpful: Satisfy cravings for carbohydrates by eating small amounts of food—a small piece of fruit, a pretzel.

Manage your cravings for sweets by eating a small portion of a nonfat product, such as a graham cracker or a hard candy. Large portions may have lots of calories, so beware. If you must have chocolate, eat a few chocolate kisses.

●**Control stress.** When you are under pressure, your body produces *cortisol*—a hormone that tells your body to put out more neuropeptides and galanin. As a result, you crave carbohydrates and fats.

Helpful: While you can't eliminate stress entirely, you can learn to control it. Find the best stress-buster for you—exercise…practice deep-breathing or meditation…perform muscle relax-and-release exercises…take a warm bath…read a book…or listen to music.

For some people, stress reduction actually suppresses the appetite by decreasing levels of certain compounds in the body that can spur weight gain.

Surprising Calorie-Burner

Harold Bloomfield, MD, psychiatrist in private practice in Del Mar, CA, and coauthor of *The Power of 5.* Rodale.

Sipping ice water burns calories. Whenever you drink something cold, your body raises your metabolism to keep your body temperature from falling. That process burns calories— eight 16-ounce glasses of ice water will burn an extra 200 calories per day.

The Fat Bank

50 Essential Things to Do When the Doctor Says It's Heart Disease by Fredric Pashkow, MD, medical director of cardiac rehabilitation, Cleveland Clinic Foundation. Plume Books.

Use "fat banking" to maintain a healthful diet without feeling as if you can never have fatty foods. Look at calorie and fat allotments as balances in a bank account. You can draw on them as you would from a bank. If you know you will want a high-fat food on a certain day, you can "build up your bank balance" by cutting your fat intake for some days before…or reducing fat intake afterward to bring your account back into balance.

Also helpful: When eating a meal containing high-fat food, eat a small amount of that food and balance it with low-fat choices—lots of vegetables, or fruit for dessert.

Simple Secrets of Permanent Weight Loss

Kathleen Thompson, coauthor of *Feeding on Dreams: Why America's Diet Industry Doesn't Work & What Will Work for You.* Avon.

Each year, Americans spend $33 billion on commercial diet programs—and much of that sum is essentially wasted.

Reason: The premise on which these programs are based—cut calories and lose weight—is at least 20 years out of date. In study after study, it has been thoroughly discredited.

Weight loss isn't that simple. The hard part isn't losing weight, but keeping it off. Unless you're willing to eat frozen dinners and drink low-cal shakes for the rest of your life, that is almost impossible on most of the commercial weight-loss programs.

Not surprising, then, that many dieters shuffle unsuccessfully from one diet plan to the next—losing weight on one program, putting it back on and then moving on to another plan.

In fact, counselors working for the leading commercial diet plans freely admit that perhaps nine of 10 people who try one commercial diet program wind up trying two or three…or more.

WEIGHT-LOSS PRINCIPLES

How do you take weight off and keep it off —once and for all? *There are three fundamental principles for effective and lasting weight loss…*

Principle #1: Take control of your life and your weight. Turning responsibility for what you eat and what you do over to anyone else is deadly. You must design a program for yourself. You also must open your life to self-inspection.

Often, eating is a survival skill. It's a way of coping with frustrations and disappointments. Life can be very difficult. Eating can get you through it.

Overeating becomes a way to maintain emotional health—although physical health is jeopardized as a result.

To overcome this self-destructive approach to food, you must learn to separate food itself from its emotional symbolism. You may need the help of a psychologist specializing in weight problems.

For referrals to a psychologist in your area, contact the National Association of Anorexia Nervosa and Associated Disorders, Box 7, Highland Park, IL 60035, 847-831-3438, *www.anad.org.*

Principle #2: Accept your body. Focus not on how your body looks, but on what it enables you to do. Don't compare yourself with the ideal body put forth in sexy movies or magazine ads. After all, body shape is determined largely by heredity. We tend to look like our mothers and fathers—and that persists even if we're successful at losing weight.

Principle #3: Make food a pleasure. Avoid thinking of food as a moral issue. "Good" foods are those you think you should be eating— fruits, vegetables, beans, pasta, etc. "Bad" foods taste good but are fattening—cakes, candy, sugary soft drinks, etc.

Substituting good foods for bad *sounds* like a good idea, but odds are it's just setting you up for failure. *Problem:* Even if you could steer clear of "bad" foods for several months, you'd give in to temptation—possibly by going on an eating binge.

Better way: If you like cheesecake, allow yourself the freedom to eat it on occasion. By removing this cheesecake "taboo," you reduce your obsession with it.

DIETING VS. YOUR SET POINT

The only way to ensure lasting weight loss is to lower your set point—the weight your body "thinks" it should weigh. When people overeat, they generally gain weight only temporarily, returning to their usual weight, or "set point" when they resume their previous eating habits.

Similarly, when you go on a low-calorie diet, your body wants to keep you from starving. As a result, your metabolism slows to maintain your set point. *Result:* Weight loss occurs very slowly. When you resume your normal eating patterns, your weight quickly rises to its former level.

To lower your set point, reduce your intake of dietary fat and increase your lean muscle mass. In other words, lighten up your eating habits and exercise enough to build muscle.

CUTTING OUT DIETARY FAT

●**Start small.** You're not going on a diet, you're changing the way you eat for the rest of your life. So there's no need to cut out dietary fat all at once.

You might start by switching to milk instead of cream in your coffee, then switching to low-fat mayonnaise on your sandwiches, etc.

●**Eat what you like.** If you already enjoy certain low-fat foods, make them staples of your diet. Make a list of your favorite high-fat foods, and find a way to substitute low-fat versions for some of them.

●**Keep track of your fat intake.** Buy a nutritional guide that lists the fat content of each food. Use it to calculate how many grams of fat you consume each day.

The maximum number of grams of fat you can eat each day and still lose weight is determined by your age, sex and medical condition, among other things.

A woman over 30 should probably consume no more than 20% of her calories in the form of fat. A man over 30 can probably get away with up to 25%. (One gram of fat equals about nine calories.)

●**Make sure the whole family adopts healthful eating habits.** If your spouse has an ice cream sundae for dessert, you probably won't feel satisfied with a pear. But if everyone in the family starts eating healthfully, there's less temptation.

THE IMPORTANCE OF EXERCISE

The more you exercise, the more muscle you build. And because muscle cells burn dietary fat more efficiently than fat cells do, gaining muscle mass speeds your metabolism. *Payoff:* A thin person can eat much more fat than a fat person without gaining weight.

If you've been inactive for a long time, begin by exercising just five or 10 minutes a day. Gradually build until you're exercising at least 20 minutes a day, three to four days a week.

The point is to do what you like. Otherwise, you'll quickly give up exercising. If you used to play a lot of volleyball or softball, for example, try to work these activities back into your schedule. If you're joining a gym, look for one where you feel comfortable. One reason people stop going to the gym is that they feel they don't measure up. If you feel intimidated by a fancy club, try the local "Y" instead.

Consider hiring a personal trainer. If you can't afford one, pool your money with a few friends and hire a trainer to come to one of your homes. Invest in headphones and a few good exercise tapes.

Free Yourself from Food Cravings

Elizabeth Somer, MA, RD, author of *Food and Mood.* Henry Holt. She is editor-in-chief of *Nutrition Alert*, Nutrition Communications, 4742 Liberty Rd. S., Suite 148, Salem, OR 97302.

Here are some simple ways to rid yourself of food cravings...

●**If you crave something sweet,** eat a bagel with low-sugar jam instead of candy.

●**Make gradual changes in your diet**—not abrupt ones, which can upset mood-altering brain chemicals.

●**Eat regularly**—not skipping breakfast. *Helpful:* Eat smaller amounts more often.

●**Take a daily multivitamin** containing minerals, too.

●**Drink at least six glasses of water** every day.

Body Shape and Health Risk

Stephen P. Gullo, PhD, president, Institute for Health and Weight Sciences, New York City, and author of *Thin Tastes Better*. Carol Southern Books.

Extra weight at your waist increases risk of heart attack, high blood pressure, stroke and diabetes—but extra weight centered on the hips and thighs may not.

To check out your "body shape risk," measure your waist at its narrowest point, and your hips (over your buttocks) at their widest point. Divide the inches measured at your waist by those measured at your hips.

An increase in health risks are related to a ratio that's greater than 1.0 for men, and 0.8 for women.

A Diet for Life

James Merker, MPA, CAE, executive director, American Society of Bariatric Physicians, Englewood, CO.

Don't start a diet simply to meet some short-term weight goal.

Example: Trying to drop a few dress sizes in time for a special party.

Problem: Pounds that are shed quickly are likely to return just as fast—if not faster.

Better: Focus on long-term, permanent weight control, which requires a similar long-term, permanent change in lifestyle.

Vegetarian Diets: Results Last Longer

Neal Barnard, MD, president, Physician's Committee for Responsible Medicine, 5100 Wisconsin Ave. NW, Suite 404, Washington, DC 20016. A physician and psychiatrist, he is also author of *Eat Right, Live Longer*. Harmony Books.

Totally vegetarian diets are best at successfully modifying eating habits in a way that produces lasting results.

Mistake: Many doctors recommend moderate diets because they believe patients will cheat on strict diets or give up on them entirely. But research shows dieters are *more* likely to follow strict diets than moderate ones.

Reasons: The diet regime is clear-cut, so cheating can't be rationalized. And...strict diets bring faster results—and with them the vital positive reinforcement of visible success.

Do Your Feet Hurt?

Carol Frey, MD, orthopedic surgeon, University of Southern California Foot & Ankle Clinic, Los Angeles, and author of a five-year study of 580 women.

As weight increases, feet grow larger and a person is more likely to have foot and ankle trouble.

Example: Overweight women were three times as likely to have ankle pain as women of normal weight.

Lose Weight—Even While You're Sleeping

Keli Roberts, a personal trainer in Los Angeles and author of *Fitness Hollywood*. Summit Group.

To lose weight...lift weights. The number of calories burned in any one weight-lifting workout is not very high—but a person with more muscle mass uses up more calories *all the time*, even while sleeping.

In one study, one group of people exercised aerobically three times a week for 30 minutes, while another split the sessions between aerobics and strength training. The aerobics group members lost four pounds during the study, but people who added strength training lost 10 pounds...*and* gained muscle mass.

Diet Doctors' Weight-Loss Secrets...and How They Keep Weight Off

Mary Dan Eades, MD, an internist specializing in weight loss and metabolic medicine. She is in private practice, with her husband, Michael Eades, MD, in Little Rock, AR; Stephen Gullo, PhD, president of the Institute for Health and Weight Sciences in New York, which offers one-on-one coaching to retrain eating habits and attitudes toward food; John McDougall, MD, founder and director of The McDougall Program at St. Helena Hospital in Deer Park, CA.

The secret to looking and feeling younger than your years is following a nutritious diet and exercising regularly. But there are many different strategies for battling everyday temptation and staying slim—so we asked three top diet doctors how they do it...

MARY DAN EADES, MD

My diet is focused on getting the correct balance of foods so that metabolic hormones, particularly insulin, help the body use nutrients as they should. As a result, I consume moderate amounts of protein and fat, and I'm selective about the carbohydrates I eat.

Today, at age 43, I weigh 135 pounds and stand 5'5" tall—with less than 24% body fat.

● **I eat adequate amounts of protein.** Protein is the most essential food that the body needs to survive. I eat at least 10 to 12 ounces of protein each day when I am trying to lose or maintain my weight.

I get the protein in the form of lean red meat, fish, poultry, low-fat cheese, eggs and tofu. By eating protein in correct proportion to other dietary components, I am able to burn the incoming fat as fuel for energy rather than store it—as would be the case if I were eating a lot of protein-rich foods and not enough of the other types.

● **I select my carbohydrates carefully.** I keep my carbohydrate intake to a minimum—about 60 to 80 grams daily because of their adverse impact on insulin—especially starchier

sources and refined carbohydrates. I primarily get those carbohydrates from a wide variety of fruits and vegetables that pack a big vitamin punch.

● **I take a daily multivitamin supplement** to ensure I'm getting all of the nutrients I might otherwise miss.

● **I exercise regularly.** I practice kung fu—a high-impact aerobic and resistance training regimen—four times a week for one hour. Or, if I can't get to kung fu class, I run and work out with weights.

STEPHEN GULLO, PhD

Living a very busy lifestyle surrounded by fine foods, I frequently find myself tempted to overeat. Obesity runs in my family, and I have the same weight-control problems as my patients. If I'm not careful about what I eat, I can easily add eight to 10 pounds to my 5'11", 168-pound frame. I'm especially prone to weight gain around the abdomen. And that is particularly unhealthful.

Pizza is my downfall. Just one slice can cause me to experience continuing cravings for more pizza, bread and other flour products for weeks. *To cap my craving for pizza, I try to minimize my trigger-food problem by "boxing it in"...*

● **Limiting** the quantity I eat.
● **Controlling** how often I eat it.
● **Avoiding** all the locations at which I usually am inclined to eat this particular food.

If self-control doesn't work, I "box it out"—temporarily banish pizza from my diet. It's hard at first, but eventually I stop craving the food. If I find myself thinking about it, I use diversion. Some activity that diverts the mind usually turns off the craving almost instantly.

To avoid temptation, I follow a few guidelines...

● **Shop carefully at the supermarket,** since that's where most weight problems begin. I avoid shopping in the late afternoon or right after work, when blood sugar plummets and we're prone to impulsive food purchases. Before I put any product in my shopping cart, I ask myself, *Is this a food I have* *a history of abusing?* If it is, I put it back on the shelf.

• **When traveling, I don't accept hotel mini-bar keys.** I also ask the maid not to leave cookies or candy on my pillow. Availability creates craving.

• **Never show up at a restaurant hungry.** It is easy to attack the bread basket. Instead, I eat sugar-free Jell-O, nonfat yogurt, nonfat soup or fruit before dining out. Sometimes before a meal I have cold tomato juice, which is a natural appetite suppressant.

• **Exercise regularly.** I jog or put in time on the "strength trainer" NordicTrack for 45 minutes two to three times a week and do additional strength training. This helps me burn 10% to 15% more calories than I would normally.

• **Take supplements.** I believe in the importance of vitamins and antioxidants. Every day, I take vitamin E (400 International Units [IU]), vitamin C (500 milligrams [mg] in the morning and 500 mg at night), folate (400 mg), selenium (100 mg) and a baby aspirin.

• **Use cognitive-switching techniques.** This involves replacing negative food thoughts with healthy ones.

Example: Instead of saying, *I'll have just one slice of pizza* (which is not true to my history with this particular food), I tell myself that the craving I'm feeling is only temporary...the desire will pass...and that as much as I want a slice of pizza at that instant, I want to be healthy and in control of my life.

JOHN McDOUGALL, MD

At age 22, I weighed 220 pounds and stood 6'1" tall. Today, I'm 49 and I weigh 175 pounds. I'm a vegetarian who relies on the starch-based diet followed by the people from China, Japan and the Middle East.

In these cultures, people have lower levels of obesity, heart disease, breast cancer and other health problems than do those who follow the typical high-fat American diet. *Here's what I do...*

• **I eat minimal amounts of protein and fat.** As a vegetarian, I don't eat meat, fish, poultry or dairy products. I believe they lead to medical problems. I get all the protein I need from vegetable sources. I also avoid vegetable oils, margarine and shortenings as well as refined and simple sugars.

• **I eat mostly carbohydrates.** My diet consists largely of whole grains (such as breads, pasta and rice)...root vegetables (potatoes, sweet potatoes, yams, turnips, parsnips)... beans, peas and lentils...and green and yellow vegetables. I can eat these foods until I've satisfied my hunger. I eat limited amounts of fruits (because they can be high in sugar and calories) and limited amounts of low-fat dressings and sauces.

• **I don't take vitamin supplements** because I get all the nutrients I need from my diet. While I don't eat dairy products, I get sufficient calcium from potatoes, rice, corn and other vegetables that contain the mineral.

• **I exercise moderately.** Luckily, my low-fat diet doesn't call for intensive activity to maintain my weight. I try to be physically active in my routine. I downhill ski in winter and swim, windsurf and walk in summer. I also work out with weights with a personal trainer one hour each week year-round... although I wish I had time to do more.

Calorie Buster

Pietro Tonino, MD, chief of sports medicine, Loyola University Medical Center, Maywood, IL.

Running on a treadmill burns more calories than using any of five other common exercise machines. Exercisers who ran on a treadmill burned about 700 calories per hour, compared with those who used a stair machine (627 calories per hour)...rower (606)... cross-country ski machine (595)...stationary bike with arm motion (509)...and standard stationary bike (498).

The Real Reason It's So Hard to Lose Weight

Albert Ellis, PhD, creator of rational emotive behavior therapy and author or coauthor of more than 700 papers and books, including *The Art & Science of Rational Eating*. Barricade. He is the president of the Institute for Rational Emotive Behavior Therapy, 45 E. 65 St., New York 10021.

Why is it so hard to lose weight? It is not because we don't know which foods to eat (and which to avoid).

In most cases, persistent obesity is the result of *irrational beliefs*.

These are the things we tell ourselves—consciously or unconsciously—about the events in our lives and our reactions to them.

They're why so many of us wind up using food to satisfy *emotional,* not physical, hunger.

By replacing these beliefs with sound self-statements, it's possible to change your eating behavior—and your weight.

START WITH SELF-ACCEPTANCE

Few people recognize the incredible irony that underlies most cases of obesity—that is, if you're serious about losing weight, you must first learn to accept yourself. You must do so *unconditionally,* with all your eating and weight problems.

Putting yourself down—for being fat, for falling short of your eating goals or for any other reason—may *feel* like a powerful motivational tool. In fact, it hampers your efforts to change your eating habits.

Trap: If you habitually put yourself down, you'll eventually come to view yourself as weak and unable to change—and, perhaps, not *worth changing.*

Self-flagellation also makes you feel bad. And people regularly use overeating to soothe bad feelings.

How does one move toward greater self-acceptance? *There are two key strategies...*

●**Focus on behavior.** Don't confuse what you *do* with who you *are*. Just because you overeat (behavior) does not mean you're a bad person (character).

Each of us does millions of things during a lifetime. Some are good. Some are bad. Learn to say, "*Overeating* is bad" rather than, "*I* am bad."

●**Change "shoulds" and "musts" to preferences.** Shoulds and musts are among the most common—and most destructive—irrational beliefs. *If you think that...*

●**Life *should* be less stressful...**

●**You *should* be able to eat whatever you want...**

●**You *must* become thinner...**

●**Other people *must* treat you fairly...**

...then you'll feel angry and miserable when these demands aren't met.

Let's face it. Life *isn't* fair, and others don't always treat us the way we'd like them to. Yet insisting that things be otherwise doesn't change things. It just wastes time and energy—and makes us chronically upset.

When we recast these demands as *preferences,* they lose their power to make us miserable.

Example: Don't tell yourself, "I *must* be thin." Tell yourself, "I *prefer* to be thin."

THE ABCD METHOD

Each time you catch yourself overeating, analyze the situation using the following simple technique. Some people find it helpful to do this in writing. *Pause for a moment, and...*

●**Identify the *Activating* event.** This is the situation that preceded your distress.

Examples: Your boss gave you a poor performance evaluation...you had an argument with your spouse...you stepped on the scale only to see that you'd gained five pounds.

●**Notice your irrational *Beliefs* about the negative event.** In addition to using *should* and *must* and putting yourself down, irrational beliefs can stem from *awfulizing* (blowing events out of proportion)...and *low frustration tolerance* (viewing frustration and discomfort as *intolerable* rather than *inconvenient*).

Examples: "My boss *should* appreciate me more, and it's *awful* that he/she doesn't"..."My spouse *must* always be supportive and good-natured"..."Dieting is *too hard* and I cannot *stand* it."

There's nothing wrong with feeling frustrated, depressed or angry occasionally. But when you convince yourself that these feelings are to be avoided at all costs, you subject yourself to needless pain.

• **Consider the *Consequences* of your irrational thinking.** The greater your awareness of your irrational beliefs, the easier it will be to see that they lead to undesirable consequences—emotional *and* behavioral.

Example: If you believe life should not include problems and challenges, you're likely to spend much of your time feeling resentful and discouraged. You're also likely to avoid taking responsibility for choosing what to eat.

When you accept that restricting your eating may be difficult but not *horrible* or *impossible*, you can focus on pleasures other than eating.

• ***Dispute* your irrational beliefs.** Simply identifying problematic events, beliefs and their consequences isn't enough. You must vigorously *challenge* your ineffective self-statements. *Ways to dispute irrational beliefs...*

• **Evidence.** Is it *proven* that fat people are worthless? That you should always get what you want?

• **Logic.** How does it follow that going off your diet once or twice means you'll never lose weight?

• **Pragmatism.** Is this belief really helping you to reach your goal? Would a different belief be more helpful?

• **Role-playing.** Have a friend repeat your own irrational beliefs one at a time—while you forcefully argue against them.

Proven Ways to Lose Weight Wisely

Anne M. Fletcher, a registered dietitian and author of *Eating Thin for Life: Food Secrets & Recipes from People Who Have Lost Weight & Kept It Off.* Chapters Publishing.

Based on interviews with more than 200 people—each of whom successfully lost an average of 64 pounds and kept off the excess weight for at least three years—I've found that it isn't necessary to spend a lot of money to lose weight.

Most of these people accomplished their goals without spending thousands on a gym membership or spa vacation. They didn't buy a $3,000 treadmill...have surgery to reduce their stomachs' capacity to hold food...or go on an expensive diet-drug regimen.

Instead, they made reasonable changes to both their eating and exercise habits—changes that last a lifetime.

Lessons from the people I interviewed who lost weight without going broke...

• **Write down what you eat.** Some of us underestimate by up to half what we eat when we don't record each morsel. It's the little snacks—the handful of peanuts or the bite of your spouse's dessert—that can trip you up.

Helpful: Many people find it helpful to keep track—in a notebook—of everything they eat while they are losing weight. And—most of those I surveyed continued to record what they ate on a weekly or occasional basis to maintain weight loss. Just the act of keeping track of what is consumed helps many people to cut back.

• **Buy a digital food scale, measuring cups and spoons and a fat and calorie counter.** Many people are unaware of what constitutes an accurate food portion. We're all used to "supersizing" our meals, so our servings often are much larger than those listed on food labels.

Example: Some calorie counters list a bagel as weighing two ounces. Yet the plump, fresh bagels we get at the bakery typically weigh four ounces—doubling their calorie count to more than 300.

Total cost: Less than $100.

Once you get a handle on *real* portion sizes, you will be able to put away the scale and books. But don't discard them.

Reason: It's a good idea to periodically check to make sure you are still eyeballing portions correctly and that your calorie and fat counts are on target.

• **If you need help losing weight, shop around for a value-conscious program.** Half of the people I studied lost weight on their own. The other half needed help from professionals or programs. There's nothing wrong with signing up for commercial programs, but they don't have to cost an arm and a leg.

Nonprofit support groups like TOPS (Take Off Pounds Sensibly, 800-932-8677) and Overeaters Anonymous (505-891-2664) are inexpensive, costing just a few dollars a week. Some programs don't charge at all.

Weight Watchers (800-651-6000) is affordable, costing about $20 to join and $10 a week to attend meetings.

●**Walk it off.** By far, walking was the top exercise choice of the people whom I surveyed.

Reasons: It doesn't cost anything…you can do it outdoors or indoors at a mall…with a dog or friends…near your home or at a local university or school…at a low, moderate or high intensity—whatever you are comfortable with.

Important: More than half of the people I surveyed did more than one kind of exercise to break the monotony of a daily workout.

●**Take advantage of community adult education exercise programs.** At night, many local schools open their doors to adults for physical education classes such as aerobics, calisthenics, swimming or country line dancing. These classes are typically inexpensive (less than $50), last for several weeks and are taught by experts.

●**Borrow low-fat cookbooks from the library.** Test the recipes, and if you like one book especially well, buy it…and use it.

Or, since most of us tend to eat the same 10 dinners over and over again, select five to 10 low-fat recipes and copy them from the book onto recipe cards.

●**See a registered dietitian (RD) at the local hospital.** Not only can RDs assess where your eating habits are falling short, they can devise a personalized plan for you that will help you to control your food intake and get the nutrition you need.

Cost: A visit to an RD costs about $40. If you have a weight-related medical illness, such as diabetes or high blood pressure, the cost may be covered by your health insurance.

●**Spend your snack money on fruits and vegetables.** The people I interviewed told me that this was their biggest secret of weight loss and weight maintenance.

More on How to Control Food Cravings

Leslie Bonci, RD, nutritionist, University of Pittsburgh Medical Center.

Distract yourself by taking a short walk or doing something else for five minutes, until the craving passes…set limits on your consumption—two cookies instead of half the bag…find a healthful substitute for what you're craving—an apple instead of a brownie, for example.

Scent Therapy Can Help You Lose Weight

Alan R. Hirsch, MD, assistant professor of neurology and psychiatry at Rush–Presbyterian–St. Luke's Medical Center in Chicago. He is also neurological director of The Smell & Taste Treatment and Research Foundation, Water Tower Place, Suite 990W, 845 N. Michigan Ave., Chicago 60611. He is author of *Dr. Hirsch's Guide to Scentsational Weight Loss.* Element.

Physicians have long been aware that people who lose their sense of smell (a condition known as *anosmia*) often wind up gaining weight.

My research shows that overweight people who sniff food aromas do just the opposite—they *lose* weight.

Study: More than 3,000 overweight people were given a pen-like inhaler containing the scent of apple, peppermint or banana. They were asked to sniff the scent whenever they felt hungry.

Over the course of the six-month investigation, participants took from 18 to 288 whiffs a day…and lost an average of 30 pounds apiece.

The more frequently the subjects sniffed, the less hungry they felt—and the more weight they lost. Some people wound up losing even more weight than they intended to lose.

It's not yet clear whether these individuals will be able to keep the weight off. My hunch, however, is that scent-induced weight loss will prove to be no easier or harder to maintain than weight loss brought about via more conventional means—special diets, exercise regimens, appetite suppressants, etc. Follow-up studies may provide an answer to this important question.

WHY SNIFFING WORKS

What explains the connection between sniffing food and losing weight?

One likely possibility is that *sniffing* food somehow tricks the brain into *thinking* that the body is actually consuming food.

Another theory: Inhaling a pleasant food aroma helps eliminate the subtle anxiety that often causes people to overeat.

Whatever the explanation, it's clear that food scents do help curb overeating.

PRACTICING SCENT THERAPY

If you'd like to lose weight via "scent therapy," try these simple strategies...

•**Take time to sniff your food before eating.** Inhale as deeply as possible to make sure the aroma-causing molecules reach the olfactory bulb. That's the part of the body responsible for the sense of smell.

•**Chew your food thoroughly.** The more thoroughly you chew, the more scent is liberated.

If you're eating alone—or can do so without offending your dining partner—you might even try "blowing bubbles" into each mouthful of food before swallowing.

By doing so, you maximize the mixing of food molecules with air molecules.

•**Opt for fresh foods whenever possible** ...and eat them hot. Fresh, unprocessed foods tend to have stronger scents than packaged or canned foods. Hot food is more aromatic than cold food.

•**Add a pungent herb, spice or condiment to bland foods.** If you're eating rice, for example, you might top it with steak sauce. You might sprinkle chopped garlic on your salad ...or add a splash of ketchup on cottage cheese.

USING AN INHALER

If you prefer, you can use a scent inhaler. For information on where to purchase one, contact The Smell & Taste Treatment and Research Foundation at 312-938-1047.

Keep the inhaler with you at all times. When you find yourself feeling hungry, inhale the scent three times into each nostril.

Vary scents you inhale, and stick to food odors you like. If you don't find an odor pleasant, it *won't* help you lose weight.

Caution: Do not use an odor inhaler if you suffer from asthma or migraine headaches. These conditions may worsen if you do.

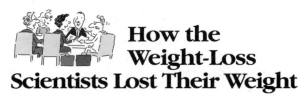

How the Weight-Loss Scientists Lost Their Weight

Richard Heller, PhD, and Rachael Heller, PhD. He is adjunct professor of pathology at Mount Sinai Medical School in New York and professor of biomedical sciences at City University of New York (CUNY). She is assistant clinical professor of pathology at Mount Sinai and assistant professor of biomedical sciences at CUNY. They are coauthors of several books, including *The Carbohydrate Addict's Lifespan Program*. Dutton.

A s scientists who have been overweight, we know firsthand that food cravings and weight gain don't always result from lack of willpower.

Instead, they may be caused by biological addiction to carbohydrates and an overabundant production of the hormone insulin.

CARBOHYDRATES AND INSULIN

Our research shows that as many as 75% of overweight people—and 40% of normal-weight people—suffer from a biological imbalance involving insulin.

Insulin is a hormone that helps your body use and conserve food energy in three ways...

•**Insulin *tells* your body when to eat.**

•**Insulin *delivers* food energy** to wherever the body needs it.

•**Insulin *commands* the body to save food energy** stored in fat cells for a time when no food is available.

Many people produce so much insulin that their bodies are unable to absorb it all. As a result, they wind up with an excess of insulin in their bloodstreams. This imbalance leads to a cycle in which they experience overpowering cravings for carbohydrates, such as breads, pastas, snack foods and cakes. When they eat carbohydrates, the body releases even more insulin.

The result is constant hunger pangs, intense and recurrent cravings for carbohydrates, easy weight gain and difficulty losing weight.

Fortunately, carbohydrate addiction and insulin imbalance can be corrected so that you can lose weight and be healthy for the rest of your life—without feeling deprived or struggling to manage your eating patterns and your weight.

ARE YOU A CARBOHYDRATE ADDICT?

Ask yourself the following six questions. *They will help you find out if your body has trouble managing carbohydrates...*

●**After eating a full breakfast, do you get hungrier** before it is time for lunch than you would if you had skipped breakfast altogether?

●**Do you get tired after eating a large meal** or find that you get sluggish and/or hungry in the afternoon?

●**Have you been on diet after diet,** only to regain all the weight that you lost and more?

●**Does stress, boredom or tiredness make you want to eat?**

●**Do you sometimes feel that you aren't satisfied,** even though you have just finished a meal?

●**Do you find it harder to take off weight**—and keep it off—than when you were younger?

If you answered "yes" to *two* of these six questions, you are probably mildly carbohydrate-addicted.

If you answered "yes" to *three* or *four* questions, you are likely to be moderately carbohydrate-addicted.

If you answered "yes" to *five* or *six* questions, you probably have a severe carbohydrate addiction that may be greatly affecting your life.

MANAGING YOUR CARBO INTAKE

We have created a simple plan to help restore the carbohydrate addict's body to its natural balance.

This regimen has worked for both of us—Rachael lost 165 pounds and Richard lost 45 pounds, and we have maintained that weight loss for more than 12 years. It has also worked for 80% of the 1,000 carbohydrate-addicted patients we counseled at Mount Sinai Hospital in New York.

The plan does not require you to deprive yourself of carbohydrates, only that you limit them to one meal a day to prevent the release of excessive amounts of insulin.

TWO CATEGORIES OF FOOD

●**Carbohydrate-rich foods,** including breads…grains…cereals…ice cream…milk…yogurt…fruit and juices…luncheon meats…pasta…noodles…rice…snack foods…sweets…and starchy vegetables—beets, squash, carrots, zucchini, corn, tomatoes, peas and potatoes.

●**Craving-reducing foods,** including red meat…poultry…fish…cheese…tofu…oils…fats…dressings…nonstarchy vegetables—brussels sprouts, green beans, peppers, lettuce, asparagus, broccoli and mushrooms.

OUR BASIC PLAN

●**Eat one balanced Reward Meal® every day for breakfast, lunch or dinner.** This is a balanced wholesome meal—not a binge—that includes all of the foods you need for good nutrition and health. Start with two cups of fresh salad. The rest of the meal should consist of…

●**One-third craving-reducing protein,** such as meat, poultry, fish, cheese, eggs or tofu.

●**One-third nonstarchy vegetables.**

●**One-third carbohydrate-rich foods** such as starches, starchy vegetables and snack foods, fruits, juices or sweets.

We don't believe that you need to weigh your food or count calories or fat grams when following the plan. Simply use good sense and listen to your body when sizing up portions.

●**Complete your Reward Meal® within one hour.** If the meal lasts longer, your body will continue to release insulin in response to the carbohydrate-rich foods, and you'll be hungry all over again.

●**Eat only craving-reducing foods at all other meals and snacks.**

We're not saying our plan will work for everyone. All programs must be individualized to suit particular lifestyles and needs. But we believe that carbohydrate addiction is so pervasive that, for most people, our plan is worth trying.

Working with your physician, follow the program for two weeks. You should immediately notice a lessening of your cravings.

If you don't, try adjusting the program until you notice a difference—for example, you may need to eat between-meal snacks…adjust the proportions of your meals…or adjust your intake of nutritional and other dietary supplements.

Another Benefit of Losing Weight

Gary Zammit, PhD, director, Sleep Disorder Institute, New York.

It is possible to cure snoring by losing weight.

Study: Males who snore heavily were placed on a six-month weight loss program. *Result:* Among the men who lost six pounds, the amount of snoring dropped 50%. Among those who lost 13 pounds or more, snoring was virtually eliminated.

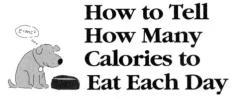

How to Tell How Many Calories to Eat Each Day

Ellen Coleman, MPH, nutrition consultant, The Sport Clinic, Riverside, CA.

Use the *Harris-Benedict equations* to determine your *basal energy expenditure (BEE)*.

For men: BEE = 66 + 13.7W + 5H − 6.8A.

For women: BEE = 665 + 9.6W + 1.7H − 4.7A. In each equation, W equals weight in kilograms (kg), H equals height in centimeters (cm) and A equals age. To make metric conversions, multiply your height in inches by 2.54 and divide your weight in pounds by 2.2.

Example: A 40-year-old man who is 5 feet 10 inches (178 cm) tall and who weighs 195 pounds (88.6 kg) needs 1,897 calories a day. 66 + (13.7 x 88.6) + (5 x 178) − (6.8 x 40).

Note: The BEE is based upon how many calories are needed each day by a *sedentary* person. Add *another* 100 calories for every 15 to 20 minutes of light exercise (walking, gardening, etc.). Add 150 to 200 calories per 15 to 20 minutes of vigorous exercise (running, swimming, etc.).

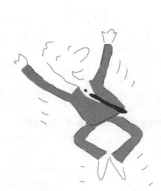

18

Healthy Attitudes for Your Work and Home Environment

Carpal Tunnel Syndrome: New Preventive Steps

George Piligian, MD
Irving J. Selikoff Center for Occupational and Environmental Medicine

The medical condition known as *carpal tunnel syndrome* (CTS)—and related disorders belonging to the category of *cumulative trauma disorders* (CTD)—are among the most widespread and most frequently discussed workplace disorders.

BACKGROUND TO THE PROBLEM

CTS results from the entrapment of one of three main nerves supplying the hand as it goes through the wrist. It can be diagnosed by a physical exam and an objective diagnostic test called nerve conduction velocity and EMG. Related ailments or CTDs as a group may be harder to diagnose because objective diagnostic tests are not yet available for all of them.

Common symptoms to train employees to watch for: An early sign of CTS is a change in the sensations in your hand—such as tingling—or just being aware that the hand doesn't feel right. Later on, pain, numbness or weakness may occur.

If ignored, CTS can progress to the loss of hand-muscle control and crippling.

COST THREAT

As if difficulty in diagnosing CTDs weren't bad enough, once a person has gotten to the advanced stages of a CTD, the symptoms are often impossible to reverse completely.

Implication for businesses: Prevention of such ailments is a company's best—and virtually only—defense. The next best defense is trying to help workers who do become affected as soon as the very first symptoms appear.

Risk of ignoring early signs: Once symptoms become severe, the employee will probably

George Piligian, MD, occupational medicine physician at the Irving J. Selikoff Center for Occupational and Environmental Medicine, Mount Sinai Medical Center, New York.

345

face disability leave and prolonged medical treatment—with surgery the most likely treatment for very severe cases.

Result: The cost of coping with an employee suffering from a CTD very often falls most heavily on the business through its health insurance and disability insurance policies. Difficulty of diagnosis notwithstanding, CTS and related conditions are a real and growing problem for business.

REDUCING THE RISK

Employees are most at risk when they do repetitive tasks, especially when they must work in an awkward manner, using poorly designed tools and equipment.

Increased use of computers is believed to be a leading cause—because of several factors involving work style and use of the body while at the computer.

Assume that complaints of CTS are real and justified. In fact, since symptoms are progressive, the more you can encourage workers to come forward at the first hint of possible trouble, the better for the worker and for the business.

Milder cases, caught early, may be stopped from progressing by making minor changes in the work function, coupled with physical therapy to ease the symptoms. Some people may be able to continue working at a fairly high level while getting treatment. But often, significant changes in work pace and work style are needed to arrest progression of the symptoms.

ADDITIONAL PREVENTIVE MEASURES

●**Listen to employee complaints** that certain jobs, especially repetitive jobs, are causing discomfort or pain. Worker complaints of headaches, neck or back pain, persisting fatigue of hand and arm muscles, and changes in sensation from these parts can all be early warning signs of CTDs.

●**Adjust workstations.** Watch out for employees who look uncomfortable at their tasks. Watch for jobs that seem to force workers into awkward postures. Are work desks and tables adjustable for the workers using them? Are there tools that workers seem to be having trouble using? Listen for complaints that certain tools "just don't feel right." Don't assume that "one size fits all" when it comes to office equipment. Some equipment may have to be redesigned to accommodate individual workers.

●**Redesign jobs to minimize repetitive motions.** Try to rotate jobs among several employees so no one worker must perform the same task over and over again. If repetitive work can't be reduced, at least provide frequent breaks and rest periods.

●**Reduce stress.** Since stress or workplace organizational factors are apparently contributing factors to some CTDs, do whatever is possible to reduce the stress level in the workplace. If frequent absences and irritability levels are increasing, it is likely that stress is too great.

●**Consider using outside expertise.** Seek the nearest university hospital center that has an occupational health clinic with experience in research in this relatively new field. Consult with people on the staff who have experience in spotting and eliminating workplace hazards.

Caution: Many entrepreneurs have begun to do business in ergonomics—claiming expertise in preventing CTDs. The quality of many of these so-called experts is hard to evaluate.

Stand Up Straight

Susanne Callan-Harris, MS, PT, physical therapist, department of sports medicine, University of Rochester, NY.

Surprising cause of carpal tunnel syndrome: Slouching. Poor posture while working at a computer weakens the shoulders and upper back due to lack of use. When the upper body is weak, the forearms and wrists have to do more work when typing. Repetitive-motion strain, such as carpal tunnel syndrome, may result.

Healthier Computer Use I

Study by Alan Hedge, PhD, director, Human Factors Laboratory, Cornell University, quoted in *Office Systems97*, 1111 Bethlehem Pike, Box 908, Springhouse, PA 19477.

Avoid computer eyestrain by occasionally shifting your focus to distant objects to relax eye muscles. Also, keep the monitor at or below your horizontal line of sight and 18 to 30 inches from your eyes. Symptoms of eye strain include blurred vision, dizziness and headaches.

Healthier Computer Use II

Steelcase Corp., office furniture and design specialists, Grand Rapids, MI.

Antiglare filters on computer screens reduce health and vision problems while increasing productivity among full-time computer users. In a study of optical glass antiglare filters, 80% of users said the filters made it easier for them to read computer screens, and 89% said filters increased the quality of the screen image. The percentage of computer users complaining of tired eyes dropped from 86% to 40%…lethargy from 78% to 36%…itching or watery eyes from 60% to 28%…focusing trouble from 60% to 33%…dry eyes from 52% to 24%…headaches from 53% to 32%.

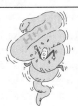

What HMOs Won't Tell You

Alan Mittermaier, president, HealthMetrix Research, Inc., a company that assists employers in evaluating HMOs and other managed-care providers, Box 30041, Columbus, OH 43230.

When a company contracts for any outside services, the customary procedure is to monitor the supplier to ensure that it consistently delivers what it committed itself to deliver. When it comes to health maintenance organizations (HMOs), however, many companies ignore that basic business practice.

The lapse could be especially expensive today. *Reason:* No matter what happens in Congress in regard to health insurance, health care costs are still expected to rise in the coming years.

CRUCIAL COMPARISON

The good news: It is easier to monitor the performance of an HMO than those at most companies might think.

Essential: At least once a year, compare the company's current HMO with nationwide HMO performance measures.

Advantages: By giving the HMO an annual checkup, the company can pick up early warning signals of potential trouble. Even if it remains in good shape, knowing how the HMO stacks up against competitors puts the company in a better bargaining position when the contract comes up for renewal.

How to do it: Use the *Health Plan Employer Data Information Set* (HEDIS), available from the National Committee on Quality Assurance (NCQA) in Washington, DC. The database establishes guidelines for comparing HMOs in approximately 60 key areas of performance.

Nearly all HMOs—especially those with superior performance—provide the HEDIS data to companies that request them.

When a company first compares its HMO against industry norms, it often hires a consultant. For $5,000 to $10,000, most health care consultants will steer a company through the initial procedure and also teach managers how to do it themselves in the future. *Several important performance criteria include:*

● **The medical-loss ratio.** The term refers to the ratio of an HMO's medical expenses to the revenue it collects in premiums. Most managed care industry observers agree that a medical-loss ratio of less than .80—where less than 80% of premium income is spent on medical coverage—is inappropriate.

On the other hand, a ratio of .80 to .85 is a reliable sign that the HMO is financially stable and not spending an excessive portion of its income on marketing or administrative overhead.

Caution: Be careful about renewing a contract with an HMO whose ratio fluctuates significantly from year to year. A severe downward dip might indicate that the organization has suddenly found a need to market itself more aggressively. That can occur if an HMO suddenly loses a large number of members.

An upward surge can be a bad omen, too. It could indicate, for instance, that an HMO has incurred unexpected medical expenses which could spell financial difficulty. This can result if the HMO finds itself with a large number of unexpectedly costly medical cases.

If trouble does occur, an HMO may try to cut corners on service or concentrate on attracting new members instead of servicing current ones.

Exceptions: New HMOs may have more fluctuations in their medical-loss ratio than HMOs that have been in business for many years.

●**Disenrollment rates.** This term refers to the percentage of employees who have dropped out of the HMO.

The statistics aren't as obvious as you might think, since meaningful figures can't include employees who drop out because they change employers or move away. The statistics to look at are those of workers who opt out of the plan and go into another.

Rule of thumb: Be leery of an HMO with a disenrollment rate of more than 10% a year or one with a steadily rising disenrollment rate.

●**Preventive care.** While there's no guarantee, companies can usually hold down health care premiums by using an HMO that stresses preventive care. For that reason, periodically check HEDIS statistics for the HMO's performance, compared with industry norms, in children's immunization, mammography and prenatal care.

A reduction of these services can point to higher costs in the future.

EVALUATING A NEW HMO

If the company decides to change HMOs, or if it is considering using one, the first step is, again, to get the HEDIS data for organizations the company is considering.

Next, check with current and past clients as you would with any other supplier. *But also take a hard look at...*

●**Prices.** The best HMO isn't necessarily the one with the lowest premium, but the one whose services match up closest with the company's benefits policy.

Example: If a company's current policy requires no employee copayment for office visits, it might look for a less expensive HMO than a business that currently recoups part of its health care outlay by requiring a $25 copayment.

●**Quality.** As a rule, try to contract with an HMO that's accredited by either the NCQA in Washington or the Joint Commission on Accreditation of Health Care Organizations in Oak Brook Terrace, Illinois.

Both organizations set rigorous standards. Information supplied by the NCQA is generally supplied in layman's terms and is therefore easier to understand. Nevertheless, it is prudent for companies that use managed care for the first time to hire a consultant to evaluate the data.

●**Access to primary-care physicians.** The key here is the number of physicians that an HMO lists that are actually accepting new patients. Often, an HMO's provider directory lists an impressive array of family physicians, internists and pediatricians, but many of them don't accept new patients. HEDIS tracks the percentage that do.

Rule of thumb: Select HMOs where at least 75% of the listed physicians accept new patients.

●**Patient satisfaction.** That's easy to overlook but critically important. *Reason:* The best health care plan in the country won't do a company much good if employees don't like it.

Recommended: In addition to talking with past and current clients, ask a prospective HMO for results of its latest patient satisfaction survey, preferably one conducted by an independent organization. If the HMO conducts its own survey, ask to see the questionnaire in order to spot any question-bias.

Rule of thumb: There's usually a trade-off between employee satisfaction and limiting choice of providers, a big factor in lowering costs.

Example: An HMO that limits employees to a small network of physicians may save a company money, but it is also likely to create dissatisfaction, especially if employees cannot continue to use their own personal physicians.

Are You Taking Advantage Of the Family and Medical Leave Act?

US Department of Labor Research, cited in *Benefits and Compensation Solutions*, 10 Valley Dr., Greenwich, CT 06831.

Only 2% to 4% of eligible employees are taking advantage of the Family and Medical Leave Act, despite fears that the Act would put a strain on business. Under the law, businesses with 50 or more employees must allow employees to take as much as 12 weeks a year of *unpaid* leave to handle family illnesses, births or adoptions.

Everyone Has Anxiety— More...or Less

Jerilyn Ross, MA, LICSW, director, The Ross Center for Anxiety and Related Disorders, 4545 42 St. NW, Suite 311, Washington, DC 20016. Ross is author of *Triumph Over Fear: A Book of Help and Hope for People with Anxiety, Panic Attacks, and Phobias*. Bantam Books.

You're suffering from anxiety when, stuck in traffic and late for an appointment, your heart starts pounding and your hands start sweating.

Or—an argument with your spouse makes your muscles tense up, and your knees feel weak.

An occasional bout of some anxiety is not only unavoidable, it's healthy. This emotion serves a constructive function—to prepare you to deal with stressful situations...to motivate you to avoid adversity and to solve problems.

But *frequent*, intense anxiety is not a healthy condition...

WHEN ANXIETY ITSELF IS THE PROBLEM

There is reason to be concerned about anxiety when the symptoms are out of proportion to the triggering event or situation...or the anxiety interferes with your ability to attend to everyday activities and responsibilities.

High-performing managers who live and work in a stressful environment of challenge and change usually can tell the difference between normal anxiety and anxiety that is out of control. *Typical:*

●**An executive has been a polished speaker for years**, experiencing a normal case of jitters before he/she begins each presentation but never afraid of the experience. Then during a particular presentation, for no apparent reason, he has a panic attack—his heart begins to race, he experiences shortness of breath and lightheadedness—and is sure he is going to pass out. As a result, the manager begins to be fearful that those jitters will overwhelm him in the *next* presentation—and so starts to make excuses and refuses invitations to speak.

●**A manager has made many business trips by plane**, experiencing the usual anxieties when planes hit turbulent air or landings are delayed because of bad weather. Then, for some reason, the anticipation of those fears becomes overwhelming. The manager begins to balk at taking business trips and declines a promotion that would require even more travel.

Problem: Fears caused by the anticipation of a panic attack can interfere with normal everyday living. These are fears of the actual feelings themselves.

These are not fears of flying or fears of talking before groups of people. They are fears that the feelings themselves will be overwhelming...turning talks and presentations into total disasters. A person fears he may lose control or make a fool of himself—that the racing heart and shortness of breath will kill him or that he may be losing his mind.

Caution: Competent managers very often self-diagnose these symptoms as "all in their heads"—to be conquered by self-discipline.

They often work in a business culture and environment that encourages people to be strong and tough it out.

They are embarrassed to reveal their fears. And even though many of these symptoms are overwhelming to the person experiencing them, their peers and subordinates may not see any outward signs of the terrors within.

Anxiety disorders are the most common mental health problem in America today. Between 13% and 25% of Americans suffer from these problems—which can manifest themselves as panic attacks, phobias or obsessive-compulsive disorder.

Fortunately, anxiety disorders are also among the most easily treatable mental disorders.

Like hypertension and diabetes, the symptoms generally respond favorably to medication and training in behavior modification by qualified psychotherapists.

Trap: While anxiety sufferers have no reason to be embarrassed about their feelings, or to believe that there is no remedy, fewer than 25% of the people who suffer these irrational fears actually receive treatment.

THE RIGHT MEDICINE

Anyone who went to a doctor over 10 years ago in search of relief from an anxiety problem and had a disappointing experience with prescribed medication should not be reluctant—if necessary—to try again now. Prior to the mid-1980s, doctors usually treated panic symptoms with drugs that were potentially habit-forming and not always very helpful. More effective treatments are now available.

No one pill will make all the symptoms of an anxiety disorder magically disappear. Even though many people do recover completely from their distressing symptoms, anxiety disorders are generally a chronic condition that can be greatly relieved though rarely eradicated by to the right medication and behavior therapy.

A psychiatrist trained in managing anxiety disorders may prescribe *Xanax* (alprazolam) ...or *Klonopin* (clonazepam)...or *Prozac* (fluoxetine hydrochloride)...or *Paxil* (paroxetine) ...or *Tofranil* (imipramine).

Many more medications specifically designed to treat panic disorders are undergoing Food and Drug Administration testing.

A psychotherapist who specializes in anxiety disorders can generally train patients in ways to modify their thoughts and behavior effectively and efficiently, and at far less cost than for other mental conditions. Consult your doctor for referrals to experienced psychotherapists in your area.

"OUTS"

In addition to using medication it is often possible to learn to manage irrational anxieties on your own.

Key: Use your creativity to give yourself an "out"—either actual or imaginary—from anxiety-provoking places or situations.

Example: If you start sweating due to anxiety related to a luncheon meeting to discuss renewal of a contract with a major customer, take note of the location of the restaurant's phone and restrooms—places you can easily retreat to for a needed emotional break—and then make a graceful retreat if you need to.

Important: An out—something that helps you to face the scary situation—is not a crutch. A crutch is something you use to keep yourself away from the activity. A crutch is having someone else do the shopping because you are afraid of stores...sticking to side streets while driving instead of using highways...walking up steps instead of using elevators. An out, on the other hand, is anything that gets you *in*.

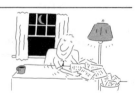

Workaholism Self-Defense

Joyce Kilmartin, president, Equilibrium, Inc., a company that provides seminars and workshops to help people balance their lives, Box 738, Barrington, RI 02806. The company also produces a *Personal Life Audit* and *Goal Planning Kit*.

A major problem with workaholism is that today many businesspeople wear it almost as a badge of honor. In their minds, being overworked is tantamount to success.

Reality: Truly successful people know how to keep their lives in balance. They know the importance of work but also of family and physical and emotional health. In the end, managers with balance in their lives are more creative, more productive...and more likable.

By contrast, a person who pursues work to the exclusion of all other activities is headed for trouble.

Example: Late in life, you begin to think back on your accomplishments and the first thing that comes to mind is a set of Italian luggage or a condo on Maui. Then you start wishing that you'd been closer to your children.

HOW MUCH IS TOO MUCH

The question, of course, is how to tell when commitment to work changes from a healthy drive to succeed—into a prescription for despair. There's no clear answer that applies to everyone, but there are some very reliable warning signs...

●**It's dark when you leave for work and dark when you return from the office**, even in summer.

●**No matter how hard you work**, it never seems to be enough.

●**You have no fun in your life**, but you do have fantasies of escaping.

●**You don't really know what's going on in the lives of your loved ones.**

●**You're plagued by aches and pains** and are too tired for sex.

LESS OBVIOUS SIGNALS OF WORKAHOLISM

●**Forgetting things that you've known for years**—such as your ATM password or a close relative's birthday. That kind of forgetfulness is a sign that professional concerns are monopolizing your mind.

●**Inability to get into the car without turning on the radio**—or getting on the phone. The habit is often a sign that you feel obliged to juggle facets of your life instead of focusing on the real task—in this case, driving.

●**Buying exercise equipment**—or a health club membership—but never using it. Successful people are purposeful. They understand the importance of following through, whether it's finishing a marketing report or losing five more pounds. Burnout candidates have good intentions, but can't get off the track toward exhaustion.

REGAINING BALANCE

It's rarely easy to change your behavior. *How to facilitate change:*

●**Take active steps to remain focused on the goal of leading a life that's balanced among work, family and your emotional well-being.** One of the most effective ways is to isolate yourself for an hour or two. A setting close to nature is especially helpful.

Ideal: By the ocean. In this environment, list the 10 people and things that are most important in your life. Almost always, family appears ahead of work.

●**Enlist the help of a friend.** Choose a person who has known you for a long time, both professionally and personally.

Be honest with this confidant about your desire to be successful and to enjoy life more fully. Listen to his/her feedback, and ask him to recommend specific actions you can take.

If you're married, bring your spouse into the change process. Nearly always, you'll discover that your spouse has been hoping that you'd achieve more balance.

●**Avoid major shifts in lifestyle.** Instead, make small, incremental changes, such as delegating someone to attend an unimportant meeting.

Monumental changes are nearly always impossible, but small ones are self-reinforcing. If your productivity rises once you start delegating, for instance, it's unlikely that you'll go back to the days of slavish attendance at every meeting.

Ask your confidant to encourage you to take a chance on small lifestyle changes. Surprisingly, many small changes will become part of your permanent regimen.

●**Learn something new that you've always wanted to know.** New knowledge isn't just satisfying for its own sake. It makes you a more interesting and creative person. And it serves the purpose of adding variety to your life, refreshing your spirit and thereby reducing the chances of filling all of your time with work.

But again, take it in small steps. Start lessons on a musical instrument you like, but don't bite off more than you can chew.

●**Improve your health.** Eat more healthfully, get more sleep, exercise more frequently and spend more time outdoors. *Also helpful:* Yoga and meditation.

Almost always, better health brings a higher level of confidence, and that too is self-reinforcing.

351

Highly confident people don't have to prove themselves by working 14 hours a day.

Most top achievers, consciously or otherwise, follow these steps. They know what their priorities are in life and never stop learning. They take care of their health. And with the help of a confidant, they work toward incremental improvements in the overall balance of life.

Hostility, Stress And Disease

Redford B. Williams, MD, professor of psychiatry, Duke University Medical Center, Durham, NC. He is also coauthor of *Anger Kills*. Harper Perennial.

Intense anger is nearly as likely as strenuous activity to cause a heart attack. People with stressful jobs also have a higher incidence of high blood pressure. After a heart attack, an optimistic outlook and supportive social ties can play a major role in successful recovery.

Simple Stress-Reducing Office Routine

Chicago Institute of Neurosurgery and Neuroresearch.

Millions of Americans who suffer from back and neck pain are unable to identify a specific incident as the root of their discomfort.

Surprisingly, it doesn't take bungee jumping or moving a piano to bring on a backache. In fact, one of the most common causes of back and neck problems is simply doing too much of nothing at all.

Sedentary jobs that necessitate sitting at a desk or computer terminal for extended lengths of time can be hard on your body. Maintaining the same position for hours on end can lead to constant muscle tension, joint strains, permanent muscle shortening, decreased circulation and other damaging conditions that contribute to back and neck pain.

Are those of us who make a living glued to an office chair hour after hour, day after day, destined for bad backs? Absolutely not. You can counteract the negative effects of prolonged sitting by breaking up your day with brief, frequent periods of activity.

Perform the following five-minute series of stretches twice a day and supplement this quick routine with hourly strolls around the office. Stretching, coupled with a minute or two of upright movement each hour, helps reduce stress, ease muscle tension and strain, improve circulation and relieve pain.

If you're experiencing severe or persistent pain, consult a doctor.

1. Reaching behind your back, clasp your fingers together with your palms facing in. Slowly raise and straighten your arms. Hold this position for several seconds, then slowly release. Repeat three times.

2. Raise your elbows while keeping your hips stationary. Twist your upper body at your waist to the right. Hold this position for several seconds, then repeat on your left side. Repeat this stretch on each side three times.

3. Place your fingers behind your head. Squeeze your shoulder blades together until you feel tension through your upper back, then slowly release. Repeat three times.

4. Stretch your right arm across your upper body. With your left arm, pull your right elbow toward your left shoulder. Hold this position for several seconds, then reverse arms. Repeat three times.

5. Clasp both your hands together above your head. While stretching your hands upward, slowly lean to the right side, then left. Do not arch your back. Keep your knees slightly bent. Repeat three times.

6. Lean against a support with your left leg forward and your right leg back. Your left leg should be bent and your right leg should be straight. With your right heel on the floor, slowly move your hips forward until you feel a stretch in your right calf. Hold for 30 seconds before releasing, then reverse legs. Repeat three times.

7. Extend and separate your fingers until you feel the stretch. Hold this position for five seconds. Relax, then gently bend your fingers.

8. Bring your left hand to your upper back from above while bringing your right hand to your upper back from below. Slowly move your hands as close together as possible and hold. Release after several seconds, then reverse arms. Repeat three times.

9. Tuck in your chin slowly. Hold this position for two seconds, then release. This exercise counteracts the effects of leaning forward to stare at a computer monitor.

10. Sit up straight and extend both of your legs out from your body. Hold this position for several seconds, then release. Repeat three times.

How to Reduce Job Stress

Valerie O'Hara, PhD, founder of the La Jolla Institute for Stress Management, and a psychotherapist in private practice in Grass Valley, CA. She is author of *Wellness at Work: Building Resilience to Job Stress* and *Five Weeks to Healing Stress: The Wellness Option.* New Harbinger.

It has gotten to the point where you can't sleep. Your body aches. You snap at your spouse…your kids…and your dog. These symptoms are common. So is the cause—*job stress.*

How can you get relief *without* quitting? Regular exercise, sound nutrition and some form of daily meditation are effective stressbusters. But there are some lesser-known antidotes to try…

TAKE A SICK DAY

Do so *before* you feel you can't stand the stress any longer. Temporarily removing yourself from the work environment gives you the time and the distance you need to reflect on the precise causes of your stress…and how to eliminate them.

If you don't call in sick now, your body may soon force you to. Epidemiologists say that more than 80% of all visits to primary-care physicians are for stress-related illnesses.

KEEP A JOURNAL

Use your time off from work to experiment with keeping a journal. The idea behind "journaling" is to create a stress diary, in which you detail the sources of your work stress…and list what you like about your job.

When it comes to psychological stress, the way you *perceive* your circumstances plays a big part in determining your response to them. Often, we exaggerate work problems in our own minds. Writing them down helps us recognize this exaggeration.

Example: Jenny, a registered nurse, came to me complaining bitterly about "never-ending paperwork." She insisted that she hated her job.

Journaling helped her realize that she spent only one-quarter of her time dealing with paperwork. The rest was devoted to caring for patients—something she truly loved.

By changing the way she perceived her job, Jenny learned to contain her stress—not exaggerate it.

MAKE A CHART

A thought-replacement chart is a tool that helps retrain your immediate responses to stressful situations.

What to do: Take a piece of paper, and divide it into three columns. Label the first column "Trigger Situations," the middle column "Negative Self-Talk" and the third column "Positive Thought Replacement."

In the first column, jot down the regular sources of your job stress. In the center column, describe your usual responses to these situations. In the third, write what a friend would say to make you feel better…or what you would tell yourself if you were in a good mood.

Next time you find yourself in one of these situations, use those statements from the third column to talk back to yourself. Doing so will change your perception and defuse your stress.

Example: Larry felt overwhelmed by the increased workload associated with his recent promotion. Whenever his boss gave him a new project, he thought, "I'll never get this done on time. I might as well give up. I don't deserve this promotion."

Larry's thought-replacement chart helped him change this self-talk to: "I can take it one step at a time. I can prioritize and delegate. I can do this job."

Larry still has just as much work. But his new, more positive perspective on the situation has helped him better deal with it.

SCHEDULE WORRY TIME

Sometimes talking to yourself about a problem isn't enough to solve it. In such cases, you must take action.

If you find yourself spending too much time agonizing over what action to take, schedule regular "worry focus" sessions.

Allot 30 minutes a day to focus on what's stressing you out. Brainstorm possible solutions on your own...or with the help of a coworker. When your time is up, banish any worries by telling yourself, "No, those thoughts are for the next worry focus."

DON'T FORGET TO RELAX

Balance your worry focus sessions with one or more daily "worry breaks"—predetermined times when you simply refuse to dwell on anything stressful.

If the idea of having to remember to take your break makes you anxious, tie it to a regular activity—a shower, jog, commute, meal or something else that's already been incorporated into your routine.

Many people would like to try deep breathing or another relaxation exercise—but they get so caught up in the workday that they forget to take a break.

In such cases, the solution is to set up a visual reminder.

Example: Vicki, a personnel manager, found that a few moments of deep breathing and visualizing herself sitting by a waterfall did much to calm her nerves. But she kept forgetting to take advantage of this technique—until she hung a picture of a waterfall in her office to prompt her.

THINK TWICE ABOUT CAFFEINE

The coffee, tea, soda, etc., that you depend on to get through a stressful morning may *cause* additional stress later in the day.

Two cups of coffee a day contribute to anxiety. More than two cups *creates* anxiety.

Find out how much caffeine is contained in the beverage you drink. To encourage yourself to have noncaffeinated alternatives, tape a note on your mug reminding you to have herbal tea instead.

Better still, keep a half-gallon bottle of water on your desk. Try to finish it by the end of the work day. It will keep hunger at bay, discouraging stress-related snacking. When your body is properly hydrated, it works better and produces more energy—energy you need to do your job well and fight stress.

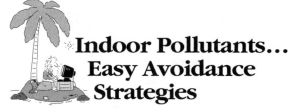

Indoor Pollutants... Easy Avoidance Strategies

Leo Galland, MD, director of the Foundation for Integrated Medicine and an internist in private practice, both in New York City. He is author of *The Four Pillars of Healing*. Random House.

Environmental pollution can cause all sorts of ailments, including asthma, allergies, immune system suppression and even cancer.

Smog, toxic-waste dumps, chemical-laden streams and other examples of *outdoor* pollution get lots of media attention. But for most of us, pollutants *inside the home* pose much bigger threats to our health.

Here's how to create an environmentally safe home...

PROHIBIT SMOKING

Establish a firm no-smoking policy. That goes for pipe and cigar smoking as well as for cigarette smoking.

If someone in the family smokes and is unable or unwilling to quit, make sure he/she smokes outside. To discourage smoking by guests, get rid of ashtrays...and consider posting a sign that reads NO SMOKING PLEASE.

In addition to raising your risk for cancer and heart disease, secondhand smoke aggravates asthma and raises children's susceptibility to sore throats and ear infections.

Cancer-causing tars in tobacco smoke cling to curtains and upholstered furniture long after cigarettes have been extinguished.

DON'T WEAR SHOES

If you wear shoes in your home, you track in pesticides, lead and other toxins each time you come home. These chemicals can be difficult to clean up—especially if they're deposited on carpets.

In Japan and many other countries, it's customary for house guests and occupants to leave their shoes at the door. Follow their example. Go barefoot...or wear slippers, if you prefer.

CONTROL MOLD

Household mold can cause everything from eczema and asthma to joint pain, fatigue and headaches. Some molds excrete *tricothecenes*, toxic compounds that suppress the immune system and cause leukemia.

Molds flourish in moist air. Use a dehumidifier to keep relative humidity indoors below 50%. Simple models are available for about $100 at hardware stores.

Make sure your basement and attic are well-ventilated. Install exhaust fans in your kitchen and bathrooms—to get rid of moisture that builds up during cooking and showering.

Do not install carpeting in bathrooms, basements or other areas where dampness or high humidity is a problem.

Check your refrigerator daily. Remove food with any signs of mold. Once a week, clean showers, tubs, cabinets under the sink and other mold-prone spots. Using gloves, apply an antiseptic solution made of 50% hydrogen peroxide and 50% water.

CHECK GAS APPLIANCES

Gas stoves, heaters and clothes dryers must be properly vented to avoid exposure to carbon monoxide (CO), nitrogen dioxide (NO2), formaldehyde and other toxic emissions.

Especially hazardous: Gas appliances with a pilot light. If your home has any such appliances, replace them with electric appliances...or with pilotless gas appliances, which have an electrical ignition system.

Even low-level exposure to CO—if prolonged—can cause memory impairment and hearing loss. Nitrogen dioxide can cause persistent cough and sore throat.

Self-defense: Install a CO monitor in your kitchen. *Cost:* About $50. For more information, call the Consumer Product Safety Commission at 800-638-2772.

WATCH OUT FOR FORMALDEHYDE

Formaldehyde is commonly found in particle board, plywood and other building materials. It can leach out of these materials into the air.

Breathing formaldehyde-laden air can cause dizziness, shortness of breath and a burning sensation in the eyes, nose and/or throat. Prolonged exposure has been linked to chronic headache, memory loss and cancer.

If you're planning to remodel your house, use formaldehyde-free building materials. If your home already contains materials made with formaldehyde, give them a coat of *Safe Seal* varnish or another hard lacquer.

Since new clothing, carpets and furniture can give off formaldehyde, too, it's a good idea to air them out for several days before using them. Put them in an unoccupied room with open windows.

GET AN AIR FILTER

Every home should have an air-filtration system. There are three major types of filters available...

- **Negative ion generator.** By giving particles of smoke and dust a small electrical charge, it makes them adhere to floors, walls and furniture, where they can be removed by sweeping or dusting.

- **HEPA (high-efficiency particulate arrestor) filter.** This is a folded paper element that filters out dust, pollen and smoke.

- **Activated charcoal filter.** It filters out formaldehyde and *volatile organic compounds* (VOCs), which can irritate the lungs and cause cancer.

For more information on air filters, call Allermed at 972-442-4898.

...AND A WATER FILTER

In most parts of the country, tap water has been treated with chlorine to kill bacteria. Unfortunately, chlorine reacts with organic matter (typically leaves that fall into the water system) to form *chloroform* and other *trihalomethanes*.

These compounds are known to cause bladder and rectal cancer.

Self-defense: Use an activated carbon water filter (such as those made by Brita and Water Pik) for any water used for drinking or food preparation. Such filters, which also remove lead, are inexpensive and widely available. *Cost:* About $20.

Since trihalomethanes can evaporate into the air while you shower, it's also a good idea to install a charcoal filter on your shower head. *Cost:* About $70.

What about bottled spring water? It's generally chlorine-free, but some brands are contaminated with bacteria. Call the manufacturer to make sure it comes from a protected spring, and request an analysis.

CONTROL DUST

House dust can contain lead (from lead paint and lead-tainted soil), as well as VOCs from paint, adhesives, carpeting and cleaning solutions.

Self-defense: Damp-mop all floors and other horizontal surfaces (windowsills, furniture, etc.) once a week. Vacuum carpets three times weekly.

CHOOSE PRODUCTS CAREFULLY

Paints, solvents, cleansers, furniture polishes, air fresheners and other common products can contain a wide range of toxins. To limit your exposure to these noxious chemicals, use nontoxic alternatives.

Helpful resource: Dr. Samuel Epstein's *The Safe Shopper's Bible* (Macmillan).

Caution: Never mix products containing ammonia and chlorine. These compounds react to form *chloramine*, a toxin that can cause severe lung damage.

MAKE YOUR HOME OFFICE SAFE

Computers, copiers, fax machines and especially laser printers often emit VOCs. Keep all such devices in one room—not a bedroom. Make sure the room is well-ventilated, and install an air filter.

If possible, leave the room each time you print out a document.

Environmental Control of Allergies

Harold Nelson, MD, senior staff physician and allergist, department of medicine, National Jewish Center for Immunology and Respiratory Medicine, Denver.

Often, the best defense against airborne allergens that trigger hay fever and other allergies is to control your environment. This means avoiding situations in which allergies are likely to strike and taking steps to minimize allergic reactions when avoidance isn't possible. *General strategies...*

• **Do not plan outdoor activities for the middle of the day or afternoon.** Ragweed pollen peaks between 11 a.m. and 1 p.m. Grass is the "safest" in the late afternoon and early morning.

• **Take "safe" vacations during the height of allergy season.** *Best destinations:* The mountains or the beach, which are often pollen free.

• **Avoid alcohol.** In some people with nasal allergies, alcohol swells blood vessels in nasal passages, causing increased nasal stuffiness.

• **Don't hang clothes and sheets outdoors to dry.** They'll catch windblown pollen and molds.

• **Stay away from smokers.** Cigarette, pipe and cigar smoke—as well as cooking smoke from grills and campfires—can trigger sinusitis.

ALLERGY-PROOF YOUR HOME

• **Rent an air-filtration system before buying one.** This will let you try it out first to see if it works. A filtration system is not all that useful for house dust mite allergy, but may help those allergic to animal dander.

• **Cover your mattress with plastic.** *Also:* Pillows need to be covered or washed...replace feather pillows with polyester—foam pillows can get moldy. *Helpful:* Wash bedding in hot water at least once every two weeks.

• **Consider removing carpeting from your bedroom.** Even when cleaned regularly, carpets and rugs can harbor mites. To limit animal dander problems, keep pets away from those areas that are carpeted.

19

Taking Care of Your Eyes, Ears and Teeth

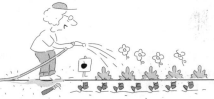

The Simple Secrets of Avoiding Serious Eye Troubles

James F. Collins, MD, FACS
Center for Eye Care

Everyone over 40—not just those who wear glasses or contact lenses—should see an ophthalmologist once every year or two…and then *annually* after age 65. Most eye problems develop slowly, but the major diseases increase sharply after age 65.

Tests for eye health cost approximately $50 to $125. A visual field test for peripheral vision costs another $75.

Downside: Medicare may not pay for preventive care, especially if the doctor doesn't find a problem.

The three most common eye diseases are cataracts, glaucoma and a disease that is less familiar to most…macular degeneration. A cataract is a human eye lens that has lost some of its clarity and become cloudy or opaque. Age-related cataracts, the most common type, can start as early as age 40.

Rarer causes: Eye injuries…certain drugs, including steroids (such as prednisone or cortisone)…diabetes. Many people have some degree of cataract formation by their 60s or 70s.

The extent of impairment depends on the location and extent of haziness in the lens—as well as to what the individual person is accustomed. A person who does crossword puzzles or fine sewing might be more bothered by cataracts than someone who doesn't do close work or much reading.

The most common types of cataracts progress slowly and symptoms can be treated as they develop. In early stages, cataracts are treated with new eyeglass prescriptions and the use of sunglasses. Relatively few people with cataracts

James F. Collins, MD, FACS, a practicing ophthalmologist and medical director of the Center for Eye Care in West Islip, NY. Dr. Collins is author of *Your Eyes…An Owner's Manual*. Prentice Hall.

require surgery. When surgery is necessary, however, it's nice to know that cataract surgery is one of the most consistently successful operations performed today. Unless an additional eye disease has intruded, the chance of restoring vision to its former level is more than 95%.

The surgeon removes the cloudy inner part of the human lens (cataract) and replaces it with an artificial lens. The outer part of the human lens (the capsule) is left in place. About one-third of the time, the capsule grows hazy and an opening must be cleared with painless laser treatment months or years later.

Previously, treatment techniques required waiting until a cataract was "mature" before it could be frozen and removed. Now the timing is based on individual need, such as a person's inability to drive a car or play golf. Cataract surgery enables many people to drive for the first time in many years.

GLAUCOMA

Glaucoma is a group of disorders that involves excessive pressure within the eye. Damage to the optic nerve causes partial vision loss. The degree of severity varies greatly.

Only an ophthalmologist can interpret the subtle tests required to make a diagnosis. Most cases of glaucoma can be controlled before loss of vision is significant.

Keys to success: Early detection…proper treatment…compliance with doctor's orders.

The most common type—*primary open angle glaucoma*—is an insidious disease that's treatable in early stages but can progress to permanent blindness.

The "angle," formed by the cornea and iris, contains the meshwork of the eye that permits fluid to drain out.

The incidence increases dramatically after age 40 (striking about 2% of people in that age group), and increases steadily after that.

Symptoms usually don't appear until loss of peripheral vision becomes noticeable. Only regular eye exams will catch this type of glaucoma early.

The slow loss of peripheral vision can creep up on you. *Tip-offs:* You trip over furniture… drive up on curbs…turn your head more broadly to see around you.

Treatment: Eye drops, pills, laser surgery and even conventional incisional surgery, if necessary.

Much rarer: Narrow angle and acute angle closure glaucoma. Drainage from the eye shuts down. This may cause sudden, severe pain (usually in one eye), blurred vision, redness and swelling in the eye, headache and nausea. Intense nausea with minimal eye pain may cause this form of glaucoma to be misdiagnosed as a severe digestive ailment and not treated properly as a result.

MACULAR DEGENERATION

A frequent cause of the loss of sharp vision is macular degeneration. The macula is the central portion of the retina, which is a thin, transparent tissue that serves as the nerve cell layer of the eye.

The most common type by far is dry (*atrophic*) macular degeneration, which often causes no symptoms. Only an ophthalmologist can properly diagnose it.

Rarer: Wet (*exudative*) macular degeneration, a hemorrhage into the macula, accounts for about one-tenth of cases but more than 90% of severe visual loss caused by age-related macular degeneration.

Main symptom: A gradual loss of central vision or, in the case of "wet" macular degeneration, a sudden drop-off of vision.

Other causes of sudden vision loss include acute glaucoma, blood clots and hemorrhages. Migraines can also cause sudden, temporary loss of vision, usually off to one side.

Photodynamic therapy, which uses a low-powered laser in concert with the drug *verteporfin*, has shown great promise in arresting the downward course of the "wet" variety.

RETINAL BREAKS…AND DETACHMENT

A retinal break is a round hole or horse-shoe-shaped tear in the retina. Fluid can pass through and accumulate under the retina, pulling it away from the layers of the eye underneath—leading to a retinal detachment. A tiny detachment may not be noticed but larger detachments can lead to profound vision loss and even blindness.

At risk: Anyone who has had an eye injury or blow on the head…is very nearsighted

...has a family history of retinal breaks or detachment...has severe diabetes. Some diabetics develop abnormal scar tissue in the vitreous gel (a thick, clear, jelly-like substance that fills the eyeball, cushioning and protecting it from within) that can contract, causing retinal tears and detachments.

Modern advances have made retinal tears and detachment much less common after cataract surgery than they used to be.

More rarely, a retinal tear can also cause a torn retinal blood vessel, resulting in bleeding into the vitreous gel. This in turn can cause sudden loss of vision.

Symptoms of a retinal break: You may see "flashers" or "floaters" or suddenly notice that a specific part of your vision is "missing," suggesting that a large section of the retina has become detached. Some retinal detachment can also cause few or no symptoms and only be discovered during a thorough eye examination.

Treatment for a retinal break: An ophthalmologist carefully tracks any retinal break for the development of retinal detachment. Laser treatment is often used as a preventive measure.

Treatment for retinal detachment: Surgical reattachment, sometimes involving multiple procedures. The prognosis for recovery is best when treatment is prompt.

PROTECT YOURSELF

• **Wear sunglasses** with ultraviolet-blocking lenses.

• **Keep your blood pressure at normal levels.**

• **Take supplements of vitamins A, C and E and minerals zinc and selenium.** The compounds made specifically for eyes are generally better than multivitamins because they contain larger amounts of zinc and selenium.

• **Eat a healthy diet.** A proper diet is better for your eyes than vitamin supplements. Favor dark green, leafy vegetables such as spinach and collard greens.

In one impressive study of people with early macular degeneration, those who ate a diet heavy in dark green vegetables were three to four times more likely to preserve good vision than those who did not.

• **Don't smoke.** Cigarette smoking robs the eyes of important nutrients and aggravates cataracts.

Follow the above recommendations even more closely if you have either of two risk factors that can't be controlled: A genetic predisposition—the condition tends to cluster in families—and eye color.

People with light-colored eyes, especially those with blue irises, have a much higher incidence of macular degeneration.

To be sure all's well, take a simple test with your glasses on. Cover one eye at a time. Do you see equally well through both?

A Sign of Diabetes?

Michael Yablonski, MD, chairman of ophthalmology, University of Nebraska, Omaha.

Bloodshot eyes can be a sign of diabetes. If your eyes are frequently red, consult a doctor.

Other causes: Allergies, eyelid infections, sickle-cell anemia.

Better Cure for Corneal Infections

Terrence P. O'Brien, MD, assistant professor of ophthalmology and director of ocular infectious diseases, Wilmer Eye Institute, Johns Hopkins Hospital, Baltimore. His four-month multicenter study of 140 ulcerative keratitis patients was published in *Archives of Ophthalmology*, 2870 University Ave., Madison, WI 53705.

The antibiotic eyedrops *ofloxacin* (Ocuflox) cure the potentially blinding eye infection *bacterial ulcerative keratitis* just as fast and with less irritation than the standard therapy (a mixture of two antibiotics that must be specially formulated by a pharmacist). After four weeks, corneal infections were cured in 90% of patients who used ofloxacin—compared with 86% who used the mixture.

Cataract Self-Defense...
Sunglasses...
Supplements...
Surgery

Julius Shulman, MD, assistant clinical professor of ophthalmology at Mount Sinai Medical Center, New York City. He is the author of *Cataracts: The Complete Guide from Diagnosis to Recovery for Patients and Their Families.* St. Martin's Press.

Like gray hair and wrinkles, a gradual clouding of the eye's crystalline lens—the transparent light-focusing structure just behind the iris—represents a normal part of aging.*

While removal of the cloudy lens remains the only cure for cataracts, modern surgical techniques make this operation far simpler and safer than it used to be.

We've also learned a great deal about the role that environmental factors play in cataract formation—and how to slow the process...

PREVENTING CATARACTS

Scientists now know that sunlight and other sources of ultraviolet (UV) light may hasten formation of cataracts—not to mention macular degeneration and other potentially blinding eye disorders.

Self-defense: Just as you use sunscreen to protect your skin from sunlight, you should use UV-blocking eyeglasses to limit your eyes' exposure.

Whenever you venture outdoors in bright sun, wear sunglasses that block UVA and UVB light. Both glass and plastic lenses are okay. There is no advantage to polarized lenses.

If you wear corrective lenses, be sure to choose lenses that screen UV. Other strategies for forestalling development of cataracts include avoiding smoking and limiting your exposure to air pollution.

Inside the body, toxins found in cigarette smoke and air pollution have an oxidizing effect, causing formation of highly corrosive compounds called *free radicals.* These

---

*Some people develop cataracts at 50, some at 90. Past age 65, about 30% have them, and by 75, more than 50%. Cataracts can also be caused by eye trauma—a ball or fist striking the eye, for instance.

compounds attack cells, including those in the crystalline lens.

A daily dose of antioxidants—especially vitamins E and C—will help limit production of free radicals. I tell my patients to take a daily supplement containing 400 international units (IU) of vitamin E and 500 milligrams (mg) of C.

Diabetics are at special risk for cataracts, apparently because of fluctuations in blood sugar levels. These fluctuations cause the lens to swell, which disturbs its delicate metabolism and causes clouding.

If you have diabetes, check your blood glucose levels often and take other measures to keep your blood sugar tightly controlled.

Long-term use of *prednisone* or another oral corticosteroid—prescribed for rheumatoid arthritis, ulcerative colitis, asthma, lupus, etc.—causes a steep increase in cataract risk. Ask your doctor about nonsteroidal anti-inflammatory drugs (NSAIDs) and other alternatives. *Inhaled* steroids, including those used in asthma inhalers, don't seem to promote cataracts.

Self-defense: Have your eyes examined every two years if you are under 60...every year if you are older or have diabetes...twice a year if you are taking corticosteroids.

WHEN TO TREAT CATARACTS

The first symptoms of cataracts are often unusual sensitivity to bright light (photophobia) and blurred vision—a problem that's especially noticeable while you're driving at night.

As lens transparency declines, you may develop nearsightedness (myopia), which makes reading glasses unnecessary. If you're already myopic, you may need a stronger prescription.

Anyone who experiences symptoms suggestive of cataracts should see an ophthalmologist right away. He/she can give you a stronger eyeglass prescription, if necessary...and conduct tests to rule out other causes of vision loss, such as glaucoma and macular degeneration. Without prompt treatment, these eye conditions can lead to blindness.

Good news: As long as eyeglasses can correct your vision to 20/50 or better—that's the point at which vision trouble begins to affect daily activities—cataract surgery is generally unnecessary.

Exceptions: Prompt surgery for cataracts is necessary if…

• **You drive and your corrected vision falls below 20/40**—the legal standard in most states.

• **You have chronic eye inflammation.**

• **Your cataracts threaten to cause glaucoma.**

Ultimately, when to have surgery is a *personal* decision. A passionate reader or stamp collector may want his cataracts removed sooner than someone whose leisure pursuits are hiking or movies.

If a doctor recommends cataract surgery, ask why. Do not agree to surgery unless you are having significant problems with your daily activities…or your symptoms are reducing your quality of life.

SURGICAL OPTIONS

The treatment of choice for most cataracts is an outpatient procedure known as *phacoemulsification*. In "phaco," the surgeon pulverizes the lens with sound waves from a tiny ultrasound probe inserted into the eye.

Phaco requires only one tiny ⅛-inch incision—and none or very few stitches. Healing takes two to three weeks.

An older technique—*extracapsular cataract extraction* (ECCE)—requires a ½-inch incision that must be closed with up to 10 sutures.

ECCE is also performed on an outpatient basis, but it's almost always less desirable than phaco because healing can take up to eight weeks.

Exception: ECCE is better than phaco for advanced cataracts, which are too hard to break up with sound waves.

Since phaco is usually preferable, be suspicious of any doctor who recommends ECCE.

Both phacoemulsification and ECCE are performed under local anesthesia (injected into the eyelids). Some surgeons now use *topical* anesthesia, in which anesthetic is delivered to the eye via eyedrops.

Cost of surgery: $1,500 to $2,000.

REPLACING THE LENS

Until the 1970s, people who underwent cataract surgery had to wear thick "Coke bottle" lenses afterward—to make up for the lost lens.

With modern surgery, thick eyeglasses are unnecessary. The surgeon simply replaces the lens with a plastic or silicone intraocular lens prosthesis.

Unlike a natural lens, the prosthesis has a fixed focal length—that is, it cannot change shape to accommodate both near and far vision.

In most cases, you must make a choice—do you want the lens primarily for reading and other close work…or for distance vision?

If you pick near vision, you'll need ordinary looking (not Coke-bottle) eyeglasses for distance vision—and vice versa.

If cataract surgery is to be performed on both eyes, ask the surgeon about placing a near-vision lens in one eye and a distance-vision lens in the other. That way, you may avoid the need for eyeglasses entirely.

Obesity and Cataracts

Robert J. Glynn, ScD, associate professor of medicine, Harvard Medical School, Boston. His five-year study of 17,764 male physicians 40 to 84 years of age was published in *Archives of Ophthalmology*, 600 Highland Ave., F4-334, Madison, WI 53792.

The fatter you are, the greater your risk of cataracts. In a study, the leanest men had the lowest risk. Smokers also face an increased risk of cataracts.

Protect Your Eyes with Good Nutrition

Studies quoted in *Health*, Box 56863, Boulder, CO 80322.

People who eat at least five servings of vegetables a week cut in half their risk of suffering *macular degeneration*—the most common cause of blindness in older Americans. Researchers believe that antioxidants in vegetables tie up oxygen molecules known as "free radicals," which otherwise damage the eyes over time. Also, the vitamin A in vegetables prevents loss of night vision.

361

Asthma Danger

Samy Suissa, PhD, director, division of clinical epidemiology, Royal Victoria Hospital, Montreal. His review of medical records of 48,118 asthma patients was published in the *Journal of the American Medical Association*, 515 N. State St., Chicago 60610.

Long-term use of high-dose steroid inhalers can cause glaucoma. Steroid inhaler use has increased sharply over the last 10 years. But in a study, asthmatics who used high-dose steroid inhalers eight times a day for three months or more were 44% more likely to develop glaucoma than were similar asthmatics who did not use inhaled steroids.

Self-defense: Asthmatics who use high-dose steroid inhalers should have their eyes checked by an ophthalmologist.

Glaucoma Busters

Sally Mellgren, MD, an ophthalmologist in private practice in Vista, CA. Her study was presented at a meeting of the American Academy of Ophthalmology.

Fight glaucoma with a low-fat diet and regular exercise. A common age-related eye disorder, glaucoma is caused by the buildup of pressure inside the eyeball. *Study:* Doctors put their glaucoma patients on a primarily vegetarian diet and a program of moderate exercise. After two weeks, fluid pressure in their eyes fell an average of 11.3%.

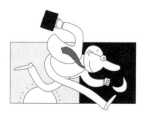

Glaucoma Treatment Without Side Effects

Joel S. Schuman, MD, associate professor of ophthalmology, Tufts University School of Medicine, and director of the glaucoma service, New England Eye Center, both in Boston.

The glaucoma eyedrops *brimonidine* (Alphagan) seem less likely than other glaucoma drugs to cause troublesome side effects. *Brimonidine* works by reducing production of *aqueous humor* (the clear, watery fluid in the eye). It's unlikely to cause heart rate and blood pressure disturbances, which prevent glaucoma patients with asthma and heart conditions from using other glaucoma drugs. Everyone age 40 or older should be checked for glaucoma every two years.

Better Glaucoma Testing

Richard Mills, MD, ophthalmologist, University of Washington in Seattle.

The standard glaucoma test, which measures pressure inside the eye, may not be the most effective way to diagnose the disease

Reasons: Eye pressure fluctuates, so any single measurement may be normal...and some people with glaucoma never develop above-normal eye pressure. *Better:* An inspection of the back of the eye to find damage to the optic nerve and measure any loss of peripheral vision.

Eye Exam Timetable

John Shoemaker, assistant vice president, Prevent Blindness America, 500 E. Remington Rd., Schaumburg, IL 60173.

Healthy adults 20 to 39 years of age should see an optometrist or ophthalmologist once every three to five years (every two to four years for African-Americans). Between ages 40 and 64, it's every two to four years for both Caucasians and African-Americans. For

Caucasians and African-Americans age 65 or older, it's every year or two.

Important: People with a family history of glaucoma or another eye ailment should have their eyes examined more frequently. Consult an eye doctor right away if you experience any vision problems.

Eye Exercise

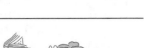

Paul Planer, OD, an Atlanta optometrist and author of *The Sports Vision Manual.* International Academy of Sports Vision.

Exercise your eyes while working at your computer by hanging a newspaper page on the wall about eight feet from where you sit …every 15 minutes, look away from the computer screen and focus on the newspaper…bring the headlines into focus and then shift your gaze back to the computer screen…repeat five times before returning to work.

Itchy Eyes?

George W. Fulk, OD, PhD, professor of optometry, Northeastern State University, Tahlequah, OK.

Your eyelashes might be infested with mites. These microscopic bugs are usually harmless—unless they become too numerous.

Self-defense: Ask your doctor or optometrist about using the topical gel *pilocarpine* (Pilopine) to treat the problem.

"Red Eye" Danger

Michael Yablonski, MD, chairman, department of ophthalmology, University of Nebraska, Omaha.

Though usually a minor condition caused by a bacterial or viral infection, red eye is sometimes symptomatic of *iritis*—a potentially blinding inflammation of the iris.

Other symptoms: Excessive tearing…pain in reaction to light…cloudy vision…headaches.

Good news: The problem usually clears up following a few days or weeks of treatment.

Treatment: Cortisone-like eyedrops to control inflammation. They are sometimes used in conjunction with a drug to dilate the pupils… and pain medication.

Does My 10-Year-Old Need Bifocals?

George Fulk, OD, PhD, professor of optometry, Northeastern State University College of Optometry, Tahlequah, OK.

Bifocals help keep certain children from becoming extremely nearsighted. They work by relieving eye stress when kids do "close work." Mildly nearsighted kids fitted with bifocals may be 50% less likely to become extremely nearsighted than kids fitted with regular eyeglasses.

Eyedrop Danger I

Douglas Koch, MD, associate professor of ophthalmology, Baylor College of Medicine, Houston. His study of 70 red-eye sufferers was published in *Archives of Ophthalmology*, 2870 University Ave., Madison, WI 53705.

Decongestant eyedrops used to clear redness can cause eyes to become even redder. In 70% of patients studied, increased redness was caused by the "rebound" effect. That is, patients using the nonprescription eyedrops developed even greater redness when the effects of the drops wore off. The other 30% were allergic or had a toxic reaction to *tetrahydrozoline* or another ingredient.

Good news: Rebound redness and inflammation usually clear up when sufferers stop using the drops.

Self-defense: Use nonprescription eyedrops for no longer than four days. Or try artificial tears—they contain no irritating ingredients. If redness persists, see an ophthalmologist.

Sunglasses Update

Stephen Miller, clinical care unit, American Optometric Association, 243 N. Lindbergh Blvd., St. Louis 63141.

Cheaper sunglasses may protect eyes as well as the more expensive ones. As long as the label promises UVA and UVB blockage of at least 99%, a $15 generic pair of sunglasses will give just as good protection from ultraviolet radiation as a $200 pair. With higher-priced sunglasses, you are paying for the frame design and a brand name.

Eyedrop Danger II

Douglas Koch, MD, associate professor of ophthalmology, Baylor College of Medicine, Houston, and coauthor of a study of 70 people with unexplained conjunctivitis, published in *Archives of Ophthalmology.*

Vasoconstrictor eyedrops—widely available without a prescription—can hurt eyes if used too frequently, by causing conjunctivitis (pinkeye).

Self-defense: If you develop inflammation, redness, discomfort or discharge while using drops, stop using them immediately. Be especially cautious about using drops containing *naphazoline* or *tetrahydrozoline hydrochloride.*

Examples: Clear Eyes, Murine Plus and Visine.

Eye Injury Reduction

Paul Vinger, MD, associate clinical professor of ophthalmology, Tufts University School of Medicine, Boston.

To reduce risk of eye injury, ask for *polycarbonate* lenses whenever you buy eye-

glasses. They resist shattering far better than glass or other plastics. *Test:* Lenses made of *high-index plastic* shattered when hit by a tennis ball going 40 miles per hour. Lenses of *allyl resin* shattered when struck by a tennis ball moving at 55 mph. Glass withstood impacts of up to 89 mph. *Polycarbonate* lenses did not shatter even when bombarded at speeds of up to 130 mph.

Wraparound Sunglasses Offer Best Protection

Safe in the Sun by Mary-Ellen Siegel, MSW, social worker and therapist, department of community medicine, Mount Sinai School of Medicine, New York. Walker & Co.

Any sunglasses that fit closely are also good. If sunglasses do not fit closely, almost three times as much UV radiation reaches eyes. Make sure sunglasses fit comfortably and snugly.

Ideal: Frame distributes weight evenly on your nose…hinges are sturdy…and ear pieces don't have too much play.

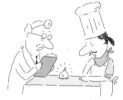

Food for Your Eyes

Johanna M. Seddon, MD, associate professor of ophthalmology, Harvard Medical School, Boston.

In a study, those who ate spinach or other dark, leafy green vegetables, such as collard and mustard greens, two to four times a week had healthier maculas (central part of the retinal layer) and better vision than those who did not. Eating greens five or six times a week resulted in greater benefits. Results combined vegetables of all types, canned or fresh, cooked or raw.

Possible explanation: These greens are rich in lutein and zeaxanthin, pigments that are vital to the visual process but that can become damaged or destroyed by light and with age.

Surprise: Carrots—usually considered good for vision—contain very little lutein and zeaxanthin.

Better Hearing

George A. Gates, MD, professor of otolaryngology–head and neck surgery, University of Washington, Seattle.

Profoundly deaf adults may benefit from a cochlear implant. This device—long recommended primarily for deaf *children*—is surgically implanted behind the ear. It transforms sounds into electrical impulses that the wearer can "hear."

The implants improved lip-reading ability in 90% of those who got them…and 10% to 20% of people who got them were able to communicate without lip-reading.

Free Hearing Test

George Biddle, executive director, DAHST (Dial A Hearing Screening Test), 300 S. Chester Rd., Swarthmore, PA 19081.

Free hearing test by phone can reassure you about a feared loss of hearing—or warn you of the need for medical attention. The call involves listening to four tones in each ear. Failure to hear a tone warns of a problem. Call 800-222-EARS between 9 a.m. and 5 p.m. Eastern time to obtain the phone number of a local hearing clinic through which the test will be administered.

Exercise May Improve Hearing

Study of 26 people by Helaine Alessio, PhD, associate professor of exercise physiology, Miami University, Oxford, OH.

Subjects were able to hear faint sounds twice as well after they had worked out for one-half hour two or three times a week for two months. *Possible explanation:* Improved circulation to the inner ear may improve hearing ability.

How to Prevent Hearing Loss

Christopher Linstrom, MD, chief of otology at New York Eye and Ear Infirmary in New York City, and assistant professor of otolaryngology at New York Medical College, Valhalla.

We tend to take our hearing for granted—until we start to lose it. And once hearing loss occurs, it's usually *irreversible*.

The gradual loss of hearing that occurs as we age is called *presbycusis*. It's very common. By age 60, most people have a slight weakness in their ability to hear sounds above 4,000 hertz (cycles a second). Unfortunately, that's the range in which speech falls.

The first sign of presbycusis is usually an inability to make out consonants—to distinguish between "sit" and "spit," for example, or "pants" and "dance."

Irreversible hearing loss can also be the result of high fever, measles, scarlet fever and certain other diseases…or, rarely, a side effect of surgical anesthesia.

A third form of hearing loss occurs when a small bone in the middle ear called the *stapes* loses its ability to transmit sound to the auditory nerve.

This hereditary condition, *otosclerosis*, afflicts 3% of the population, mostly women. It may start at puberty, but typically comes on in the 20s, 30s or 40s.

PROTECTING YOUR HEARING

You can't do much about your genes or your age, but you can protect yourself against the major enemy of hearing—exposure to loud noise.

Sustained noise above 85 decibels (the loudness of a shout or a crying infant) damages the nerve endings that transmit sound signals to the brain. As with presbycusis, the speech frequencies around 4,000 hertz are the first to go. Then higher and lower frequencies are affected.

A 30-year-old who has spent years in a noisy factory, or used a jackhammer without hearing protection, may have the hearing of someone 50 years older.

You run a similar risk if your nights are spent at a disco, club or bar where the music is deafening. Or if you keep the volume of your Walkman too high.

Self-defense: Do everything necessary to avoid prolonged exposure to loud noise. If the noise level at a club causes pain or ringing in the ears, *leave.*

If sustained noise is unavoidable—at work, for example—use a noise-blocking headset... or foam rubber or molded wax earplugs. For maximum protection, wear a headset *in addition* to earplugs.

When buying ear protection, look for a noise-reduction rating (NRR) of 15 or higher. Putting cotton in your ears is *not* very effective. Cotton has an NRR of only five to 10.

What about brief exposures to loud noise? You probably won't suffer any hearing loss from the occasional fire engine roaring past (though it is a good idea to plug your ears with your fingers). But even one *very* loud burst—a gunshot, for example—can cause permanent trouble.

If you experience ringing in the ears and your hearing seems less acute after a loud noise, *and it's not back to normal in a day or two,* consult a hearing specialist.

To find a good one, call a local hospital's ear, nose and throat department...or contact the American Academy of Otolaryngology–Head and Neck Surgery at 703-836-4444.

CHRONIC EAR INFECTIONS

A bad cold or flu often causes fluid to build up in the ear. If fluid accumulation becomes chronic, delicate structures in the middle ear can be permanently damaged.

If your stuffiness persists for longer than a month, or if ear infections recur frequently, your doctor may prescribe a powerful decongestant or insert a ventilation tube through your eardrum.

To prevent injury to your eardrum, avoid flying when you have fluid in your ears. If your trip can't be postponed, ask your doctor for a good decongestant. During the flight, gently pop your ears by swallowing hard.

COPING WITH HEARING LOSS

Your doctor will probably recommend a hearing test to pinpoint the extent and cause of your problem. It's rare, but hearing loss can stem from a tumor of the brain or cranial nerve. It's especially important to rule out a tumor if your hearing loss is more pronounced on one side.

A hearing test is conducted in a noiseless, insulated testing booth. It tests both the *level* (speech-reception threshold) and the *clarity* (word discrimination score) of hearing.

Some hospitals and hearing aid makers offer a "telephone hearing test," but such tests aren't very accurate.

Does your hearing loss stem from a problem in the transmission of sound through the inner ear? From damage to the auditory nerve? What frequencies are affected? The hearing test should answer these questions.

Some conditions can be corrected surgically. If you have otosclerosis, for example, a simple outpatient procedure to insert a tiny "piston" in the inner ear restores normal hearing 90% of the time.

If you need a hearing aid, get an audiologist's help in choosing the most appropriate model.

Today's devices—which must be painstakingly calibrated—are different from those of decades past. Most are small enough to fit inside or behind the ears or on eyeglass frames. And most have electronic filters and precise volume controls that let you amplify just the frequencies that give you trouble.

Some state-of-the-art devices are programmable. You can preset them for listening comfortably to conversation or music, indoors or outdoors. *Cost:* $400 to $2,000.

Caution: Never buy a hearing aid via mail-order or telephone.

COCHLEAR IMPLANTS

The latest treatment for hearing loss is the *cochlear implant.* Implanted in a bone next to the ear, this miniature computer turns sound into electromagnetic energy, which is fed into the inner ear to stimulate the auditory nerve.

Cochlear implants are appropriate only for individuals with profound hearing loss in both ears that cannot be helped by a hearing aid.

Though cochlear implants can boost the hearing of otherwise deaf people, they cannot provide the same sound quality of a good hearing aid.

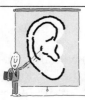

Earlobes...What They Can Tell You

William J. Elliott, MD, PhD, associate professor of preventive medicine and pharmacology, Rush-Presbyterian–St. Luke's Medical Center, Chicago. His study of 264 heart patients was published in the *American Journal of Medicine*, 105 Raiders Ln., Belle Mead, NJ 08502.

Creased earlobes are a better predictor of future heart trouble than diabetes, high blood pressure, smoking, high cholesterol, family history of coronary disease or obesity. In a study, having one creased earlobe raised the risk by 33%. Having both earlobes creased raised the risk by 77%. The link between earlobe creases and heart disease is not yet understood.

Self-defense: If your lobes are creased, ask your doctor about strategies to lower your risk.

No More Earaches When Flying

Jeffrey Jones, MD, director, department of emergency medicine, Butterworth Hospital, Grand Rapids, MI. His study of 190 fliers with recurrent ear pain was reported in *Annals of Emergency Medicine,* 11830 Westline Industrial Dr., St. Louis 63146.

Take one decongestant tablet containing *pseudoephedrine* at least 30 minutes before your flight leaves. A study found that following this regimen relieved discomfort in 68% of travelers with recurrent ear pain, compared with only 38% of those who took a placebo. One pill works all day, so there's no need to take more if your flight is delayed.

Important: Check with your doctor before trying this regimen to ensure that the pseudoephedrine does not conflict with other medications or health conditions.

Getting Help for Ringing in the Ears From Tinnitus Sufferer Dr. Stephen Nagler

Stephen M. Nagler, MD, director of the Southeastern Comprehensive Tinnitus Clinic in Atlanta. A tinnitus sufferer himself, he is a member of the board of directors of the American Tinnitus Association, Box 5, Portland, OR 97207.

Forty-four million Americans experience the hearing disorder *tinnitus*—ringing in the ears—on an occasional basis. Six million have chronic tinnitus.

Tinnitus makes it hard to concentrate and can disrupt sleep. It can lead to depression—or even suicide.

WHAT CAUSES THE NOISE?

Tinnitus is *not* a normal consequence of aging. It's usually caused by damage to the delicate "hair cells" lining the *cochlea*, a snail shell-shaped structure of the inner ear.

The most common causes of hair cell damage are...

• **Loud noise.** A single loud noise (such as an explosion) can permanently damage the hair cells. More often, tinnitus stems from years of exposure to loud music, factory noise, etc.

Self-defense: Avoid loud music. Wear sound-absorbing earplugs whenever you spend time around a noisy machine.

Inexpensive earplugs are available at hardware stores. If you anticipate repeated or prolonged exposure, custom-molded earplugs from an audiologist—or sound-absorbing earmuffs—offer better protection.

Ineffective: Stuffing your ears with cotton.

• **Drugs.** Transient tinnitus can be caused by many common drugs, including aspirin. Among the drugs that can cause *permanent* tinnitus are *cisplatin* and certain other chemotherapeutic agents...and aminoglycoside antibiotics like *streptomycin* or *gentamicin.*

Self-defense: Anytime your doctor prescribes a drug, ask about the risks—including the risk of tinnitus. Make sure the benefits outweigh the risk.

●**Diseases.** Tinnitus can be symptomatic of high blood pressure, arteriosclerosis, thyroid disorders, diabetes and certain other diseases.

Tinnitus can also stem from head and neck injuries...or from disorders of the middle or inner ear, including otosclerosis and Ménière's disease. In rare instances, tinnitus is caused by a tumor of the auditory nerve.

Self-defense: If you suffer from any of these ailments, be sure to get adequate treatment. If you develop tinnitus, consult a doctor right away.

SOUND MASKING

Most tinnitus sufferers crave silence. Ironically, the most effective treatment is often to "bathe" yourself in sound.

●**Music.** Try listening to different kinds of music. Notice if any helps mask the tinnitus or simply distracts your attention.

●**White noise generators.** These tabletop devices produce static noise or nature sounds (wind, surf, etc.). They're available from electronics stores. *Cost:* $100 or less.

●**Tinnitus maskers.** These are white noise generators worn in or behind the ear, like a hearing aid. Certain maskers function as both a white noise generator *and* a hearing aid.

Tinnitus maskers must be custom-fitted by an audiologist. *Cost:* $1,000 or more.

AUDITORY HABITUATION

Auditory habituation combines use of a tinnitus masker or hearing aid with educational sessions that help the tinnitus sufferer change the way he/she perceives the sound.

This technique—administered by an audiologist or physician—can be quite effective. Eighty percent of those who try it get significant relief. However, the process can take two years.

Ultimately, the tinnitus sufferer comes to have a *neutral* rather than a *negative* perception of the sound. It's like wearing pants—you can feel the cloth against your skin if you think about it. Most of the time, however, you're unaware of the sensation.

MIND/BODY TECHNIQUES

●**Cognitive-behavioral therapy.** It helps tinnitus sufferers avoid the distorted thinking that aggravates their suffering.

Example: "The noise is driving me crazy. I cannot get any work done."

For referral to a cognitive-behavioral therapist, call the American Psychological Association at 800-964-2000. Make sure the therapist has experience treating tinnitus.

●**Self-hypnosis.** Some unscrupulous hypnotherapists claim that tinnitus sufferers can be hypnotized to no longer hear the sound. Not true. But self-hypnosis can help them come to terms with their ailment.

More information: Contact the American Society of Clinical Hypnosis, 130 E. Elm Ct., Suite 201, Roselle, IL 60172, 630-980-4740.

●**Biofeedback.** This technique employs electronic gear that lets you monitor your brain waves and muscular contractions. Using this gear, tinnitus sufferers learn to control their own physiological reactions to the noise.

For a list of biofeedback practitioners in your area, send a self-addressed, stamped, business-sized envelope to the Association for Applied Psychophysiology and Biofeedback, 10200 W. 44 Ave., Suite 304, Wheat Ridge, CO 80033.

●**Guided imagery.** Simply imagining yourself in a tranquil setting can help eliminate the frustration caused by tinnitus.

What to do: A few times a day, close your eyes and spend a few minutes picturing yourself aboard a sailboat. Imagine the smell of the sea, the feel of the sun on your skin, the sound of spray, etc.

You're headed for an imaginary island where your tinnitus magically disappears.

TINNITUS MEDICATION

Some patients get relief from *alprazolam* (Xanax). If congestion or allergies seem to be compounding the problem, an antihistamine may be helpful.

The herb *ginkgo biloba* has been used with some success.

Caution: Ginkgo can interfere with blood clotting. If you take it on a regular basis, make sure your doctor checks your bleeding and clotting time at least twice a year.

For Healthy Gums

Andrew Weil, MD, director, program of integrative medicine, University of Arizona, Tucson.

Floss daily with *unwaxed* floss. It's better than waxed floss at getting under the gum line.

●**Massage gums** with your fingertips. Or— stimulate gums by *gently* running the end of a toothpick under the gum line.

●**Brush sore gums** with a paste made of hydrogen peroxide and baking soda. Leave it on for a few minutes, then rinse well.

●**Rinse with goldenseal**, an herbal disinfectant sold in health food stores. *Mix:* One cup warm water, one-quarter teaspoon salt, one-half teaspoon—or the contents of one capsule—goldenseal powder. Rinse two to three times a day.

●**Take coenzyme Q-10.** This natural supplement is thought to improve gum health.

●**Have teeth professionally cleaned** at least twice a year.

Cleaner Kids' Teeth

Eli Grossman, DDS, consultant, New Institutional Service Company, Northfield, NJ. His study of 32 children eight to 12 years of age was published in the *Journal of the American Dental Association*, 211 E. Chicago Ave., Chicago 60611.

Electric toothbrushes help children keep their teeth cleaner.

Study: Kids who used an electric toothbrush with a small head designed especially for children (Braun Oral B Plaque Remover for Kids) removed 65% of dental plaque.

Kids who used a regular manual toothbrush removed 42% of plaque.

Best Dental Floss

Peter L. Jacobsen, DDS, PhD, professor of diagnostic sciences, University of the Pacific Dental School, San Francisco.

If your teeth are tightly spaced, use Glide, Colgate Total or another low-friction floss. For widely spaced teeth (if you can see between your teeth at gum level), use a woven floss like Oral-B Ultra Floss or Super Floss. If you tend to shred floss, use dental tape instead.

Better Brushing

Academy of General Dentistry, 211 E. Chicago Ave., Suite 1200, Chicago 60611. Send for the Academy's free pamphlet *Brush Up on Your Dental Facts for Adults and Seniors.*

Three to four minutes of brushing are needed to get teeth really clean. The average person brushes for less than one minute.

Helpful: Listen to the radio or stereo while you brush. Most popular songs last three to four minutes.

Vegetarians Are at Higher Risk for Periodontal Disease

Holly Lucart, Academy of General Dentistry, 211 E. Chicago Ave., Suite 1200, Chicago 60611.

The diets of strict vegetarians may lack sufficient calcium, vitamins D, B2 and B12, and complete proteins.

Self-defense: Replace the calcium by eating green vegetables, grains and nuts. Replace other missing vitamins by taking a daily multi-vitamin. Vegans—who eat no animal products at all—are at greatest risk.

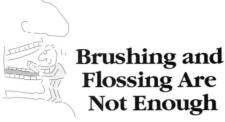

Brushing and Flossing Are Not Enough

Tom McGuire, DDS, president of Tooth Fitness, a Grass Valley, CA, firm that produces dental wellness programs for corporations. He is author of *Tooth Fitness, Your Guide to Healthy Teeth*. St. Michael's Press.

We all know the importance of brushing and flossing. But when it comes to other aspects of tooth care, there remains a great deal of confusion. *Here are the answers to the most common questions patients have about teeth...*

●**How often should I have my teeth professionally cleaned?** The usual advice—once every six months—is rather arbitrary. Go as often as your dentist or dental hygienist says is necessary. If you have advanced gum disease, or if you're bad about brushing, that might be as often as once a month.

●**My gums bleed when I brush. Should I be worried?** Many people think a little bleeding is normal. *Not true.* Bleeding gums are an early sign of gum disease (*gingivitis*). Untreated, it can lead to serious bacterial infection.

Gingivitis can usually be reversed in one to three weeks by daily flossing and by brushing after meals.

Helpful: After brushing, rinse with a mixture of one-quarter teaspoon salt and four ounces of water, to get rid of bacteria.

If bleeding persists for more than three weeks, see your dentist. You might have *periodontal* disease. An advanced form of gum disease, it won't respond to self-treatment.

Other danger signs: Sensitivity to heat or cold, sugar or acidic foods...sudden pain in the affected area...bleeding...the sensation that something is pressing on the root of a tooth.

Over time, periodontal disease can cause bone loss in the jaw. Left untreated, it may result in tooth loss.

Warning: Periodontal disease can increase the risk of heart disease. If you suspect you have gum disease, see your dentist at once—especially if you are predisposed to heart disease.

●**What causes gums to recede?** The likeliest cause is gum disease, although after age 50, gums naturally begin to pull away from the teeth. Though severe recession can lead to tooth decay, most cases of receding gums are a *cosmetic* problem.

●**What can I do to prevent gum disease?** Supplements of vitamins C, A and B-complex have been shown to help. So has eating less sugar. Sugar speeds formation of plaque (film made of food particles, bacteria and saliva), which causes decay and gum disease.

●**What kind of toothbrush is best?** A tear-drop-shaped model with soft bristles about one inch long. If your mouth is small, choose a "junior-size" brush.

The brush should have no more than four rows of clear (not colored) bristles. They make it easier to detect signs of bleeding from brushing.

Brushes with clear plastic handles stay cleaner longer—they allow bacteria-killing ultraviolet light to penetrate to the bristles.

After brushing, rinse your toothbrush in warm water. Stand it up to dry. Allowing a brush to lie flat permits the water to pool...and bacteria to grow. To help control bacteria, soak brushes once a week in mouthwash.

●**How often should I replace my toothbrush?** Every three months—sooner if the bristles become flattened or frayed.

It's also a good idea to replace your brush after each professional dental cleaning—to prevent exposing clean teeth to bacteria from the old brush.

●**Do electric toothbrushes do a better job?** Electric and ultrasonic brushes provide more brush strokes per second, but they're often less effective than manual brushes at reaching the back teeth and the inner surfaces of the lower front teeth.

Instead of an electric toothbrush, you might consider buying an *oral irrigating device.* Such devices send a jet of water deep below the gumline, where brushes and floss can't reach. They should be used *in addition to* brushing and flossing.

Best model: The Water Pik, with the Pik Pocket subgingival irrigation tip attachment.

When using an irrigator, keep the pressure low. For maximum benefit, fill the reservoir with antibacterial mouthwash or saline solution, instead of water.

●**What brand of toothpaste is best?** They are are all pretty much alike. It's the *brushing* action that cleans the teeth and keeps the gums healthy.

For adults, use the toothpaste that tastes best to you. If you hate the taste of your toothpaste, you're apt to avoid brushing.

People who have gum problems should avoid "whitening" toothpastes, which tend to be abrasive.

Important: Don't swallow toothpaste. Most brands contain artificial coloring, flavoring, sweeteners, etc., whose health risks aren't fully known.

Since children tend to swallow toothpaste when they brush, I recommend a natural toothpaste like Tom's of Maine for them. It's free of additives.

●**What about special flosses?** Unwaxed floss, which has a rough surface, is better than waxed, thin or "friction-free" floss at removing plaque and dislodging food.

Exception: If your teeth are closely spaced, or if unwaxed floss causes pain or becomes frayed, try a coated or ultrathin floss. Otherwise, you're likely to forgo flossing altogether.

Avoid *colored* flosses. They make it hard to detect bleeding.

Flossing technique is more important than what type of floss you use.

Proper way: After inserting a 12- to 18-inch piece of floss between two teeth, press it to one side, and guide it down using a back-and-forth, shimmying motion.

Caution: Pulling floss "up and out" can dislodge a filling. Instead, let go of one end of the floss and slide it through the space between the teeth.

Floss at least every night—after brushing but *before* spitting out all the toothpaste. If you have an area in which food gets trapped, floss every time you brush.

●**Should I be using a fluoride or anti-plaque rinse?** Yes. I recommend using these before brushing (or when you cannot brush following a meal). Fluoride is very good at fighting decay.

If your water isn't fluoridated, children should be given fluoride drops, from age one-and-a-half until age 16. Fluoride taken during that time is the best way to prevent tooth decay in adulthood.

●**What's the best way to whiten teeth?** For superficial stains caused by cola, coffee or cigarettes, try a whitening toothpaste. Follow instructions carefully. Overuse can strip protective enamel from your teeth.

For severe stains, ask your dentist about tooth-bleaching. Dentist-administered bleaches are faster, more effective and less likely to irritate your gums than do-it-yourself bleaches. *Cost:* $100 to $300 per bleaching.

●**How often should I have dental X rays?** When starting with a new dentist, have a set of *full-mouth, bitewing and periapical* (root) X rays. After that, have bitewing X rays annually (every six months if you're prone to decay). Depending on your checkups and your dentist's recommendations, you can go up to five years between full-mouth and periapical X rays.

●**Are amalgam (silver) fillings really dangerous?** Amalgam fillings, which contain the toxic metal mercury, can cause nausea, memory loss and neurological problems. If you're concerned about mercury toxicity, consider replacing them. Look for a dentist who advertises mercury-free or cosmetic dentistry.

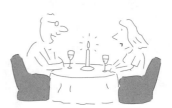

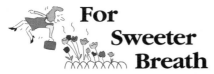

For Sweeter Breath

Alan Winter, DDS, associate clinical professor of dentistry, New York University School of Dentistry and partner, Park Avenue Periodontal Associates, 30 E. 60 St., Suite 302, New York 10022.

Rinse your mouth after eating. Rinse carefully after eating starchy or sugary foods.

●**Scrape the back of your tongue every day** with a toothbrush to remove bacteria. (The tendency to gag will decrease.)

●**Avoid coffee**, alcohol, tobacco and sulfur-containing foods like garlic and onions.

●**Drink water or chew sugarless gum** when your mouth is dry to produce more saliva.

●**Eat parsley**—a natural breath freshener.

●**Avoid over-the-counter mouthwashes.** Most just disguise bad breath briefly.

Important: Sucking on candy mints and cough drops is not a solution because they cause decay.

If the problem persists, see your dentist and doctor to see if you have an underlying dental or digestive problem.

Laser Whitening Procedure

Gary F. Alder, DDS, director, dental residency program, Rush–Presbyterian–St. Luke's Medical Center, Chicago.

Discolored teeth can now be whitened quickly and painlessly with a laser. In this procedure, teeth are painted with peroxide bleach, then zapped with a blue argon laser. The 90-minute treatment—performed in a dentist's office—works on coffee and tobacco stains as well as on the discoloration caused by the antibiotic tetracycline. Teeth are noticeably brighter immediately after treatment...and continue to whiten for several days. Laser whitening is better and faster than home bleaching.

What Causes a Burning, Itching Sensation Inside the Mouth?

Trey Petty, DDS, associate professor of medicine, University of Calgary Medical School, Calgary, Canada.

Several serious ailments can cause this sensation, so those experiencing the problem should be examined thoroughly by a dentist or doctor. However, you may be suffering from *burning mouth syndrome* (BMS), a mild but mysterious ailment that affects mostly post-menopausal women.

Helpful: Lozenges containing *capsaicin*—the substance that puts the kick in cayenne pepper. Capsaicin lozenges are not available commercially, but they can be made by a pharmacy—or even at home.

Recipe: Dissolve two cups of brown sugar, ¼ cup molasses, ½ cup butter, two tablespoons water and two tablespoons white vinegar in a heavy pan over low heat. Boil gently, stirring frequently until the mixture reaches 300°F. Stir in ½ teaspoon cayenne pepper. Drop by teaspoonfuls onto wax paper and let harden. Start with three lozenges per day. Taper back as pain subsides.

20

Keeping Fit Pays Off

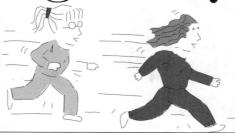

Jack LaLanne's
Fitness Magic

Jack LaLanne

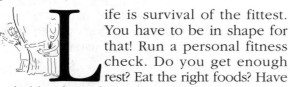

Life is survival of the fittest. You have to be in shape for that! Run a personal fitness check. Do you get enough rest? Eat the right foods? Have a hobby that relieves stress? Exercise to accumulate reserves of energy that will be like money in the bank for the day you need it?

The only way to increase your strength, energy and vitality is to stress your body beyond what it's accustomed to doing.

People up to 95 years old have *doubled* their strength and endurance in a short time with weight-training programs.

A 90-year-old person can't lift a weight as heavy as a 21-year-old person can. But each can work to his own capacity…and get results.

People rationalize about not exercising. Their main excuse—*I don't have the time.*

Would you sell your arm for $100 or your leg for $1 million? No, because your most priceless possession is your body. Shouldn't you spend a little time keeping it in good shape?

How you look is a billboard of the way you regard yourself. As you become fitter, and look and feel better, your self-esteem will rise…a good first step for improving your sex life as well.

If you're afraid you'll have a heart attack—be aware that the people who have heart attacks are the ones who *don't* exercise.

MAKE GOOD USE OF COMMERCIALS

When a commercial interrupts a TV show, don't get a snack—exercise instead. *Here's an easy one…*

●**Get up/get down.** Lower yourself gently to the floor and lie on your back. Stand up.

Jack LaLanne, fitness expert who opened his first gym in 1936 and has promoted physical culture for 65 years. Mr. LaLanne is author of several books, including *Revitalize Your Life After 50: Improve Your Looks, Your Health and Your Sex Life.* Hastings House.

373

Repeat slowly...then quickly. Practice until you can do it fast 15 times in a row. Invite your children or grandchildren to join in.

MAGIC FIVES

I devised these five simple exercises to trim and firm every part of the body. You can do Magic Fives almost anywhere. Your only gym equipment is a straight-backed chair and one or two books.

Start by doing each exercise slowly to a count of 10. Build stamina by exercising a little more vigorously each time, four or five times a week. Consider watching yourself in a mirror to see how well you're doing. Visualize yourself as you want to look. Breathe deeply to bring oxygen to your bloodstream and burn fat.

1. Swings. These work many muscles simultaneously. Hold a light book between your hands. Place your feet shoulder width apart. Bend your knees slightly.

Bend over at the waist. Breathing out, slowly swing the book down between your legs, trying to touch an imaginary wall behind you. Breathing in, swing the book back up again over your head. Keep your arms straight and try to touch the imaginary wall immediately behind you with the book.

2. Knees to chest. Excellent for the waistline, hip flexibility, abdominal muscles and lower back.

Sit at the very edge of a straight, hard chair. Holding both sides of the seat to keep your balance, lean back until your shoulders touch the back of the chair. Draw both knees as close to your chest as you can (or lift one knee at a time until you can lift both at once). When you become advanced, hold a book between your knees.

Lower your legs. Then make pedaling motions, pretending you're riding a bicycle. Progress from short movements to large ones. With each rotation, extend your leg down close to the floor before continuing.

For variation, do these exercises while lying on your back on the floor or on your bed.

3. Leg lunges. For sagging hips and flabby thighs.

Stand to one side of a chair. Hold on to the back of it. With your right leg, lunge forward as if you were fencing. Bring it back. Repeat with your left leg. As you get stronger, bend your knee more and step farther out. Keep your upper body erect throughout.

4. Leg extensions to the back. Tremendous for your back muscles all the way down from your neck to the bottoms of your feet. Firms the buttocks.

Facing a chair, bend at the waist and hold both sides of the seat. Keep your arms straight and back away from the chair until you feel comfortable.

Slowly lift your right leg backward as high as possible while pointing your toes, looking up, breathing in and tensing your hips tightly. You can bend your left knee a bit. As you lower your leg, breathe out...put your chin on your chest...and round your back, tensing your abdominal muscles. Repeat with your other leg.

5. Two-way punches. These cardiovascular exercises work most of the upper body muscles. They'll burn calories and trim your waistline.

● **Forward punches.** Helpful for your arms, shoulders, upper back and chest. Stand with your feet shoulder-width apart. Bend your knees a bit. Visualize a punching bag in front of you and punch it hard with one hand at a time. Imagine that your elbow is hitting a wall behind you as it comes back. Increase the pace.

● **Overhead punches.** Works the backs of your arms, the sides of your waist and your calves. Improves your posture.

Clench your fists, stand erect and punch your right arm overhead, pretending you're trying to hit the ceiling. Rise up on your toes as you go. Drop the opposite elbow down as low as you can. Alternate arms. Do this exercise rapidly.

● **Combination punches.** Assume the position for forward punches. Pull your waist in and punch forward rapidly, hitting your elbows against an imaginary wall behind you. Quickly switch to an overhead punch. As each arm comes down, push your elbow down as low as you can. The faster you punch, the more calories you'll burn. When you become more advanced, hold a book in each hand for extra resistance.

TRIM UPPER-ARM MUSCLES

The muscle on the back of the upper arm typically gets flabby as people age. That is because the triceps are not used very often. *To tone that muscle:*

• **Do overhead punches** (described above).

• **Push a weight**, such as a small barbell, above your head.

• **Stand with your back to the wall and your arms down**, with your palms against the wall. Push yourself away from the wall and back again. *Bonus:* You'll exercise the backs of your shoulders and improve your posture.

TAKE RESPONSIBILITY

I spend at least one hour a day lifting weights…and another hour swimming. Can't you find 20 minutes a few times a week to keep yourself in shape?

Caution: Always check with your doctor before starting an exercise regimen.

The Dangers Of Too Much Exercise

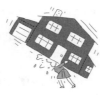

Kenneth H. Cooper, MD, MPH, president and founder of The Cooper Aerobics Center in Dallas and a leading exponent of exercise for almost three decades. He is author of numerous books on health and fitness, including *Dr. Kenneth H. Cooper's Antioxidant Revolution.* Thomas Nelson.

When I was writing my first fitness book, *Aerobics*, back in 1968, I believed that a regimen of sustained, strenuous exercise was necessary for health and longevity…and more was better.

In the decades since then, countless studies have helped to radically refine this basic "exercise prescription."

It's become clear that the health benefits of less exercise—less strenuous *and* less time-consuming—are almost as great as a very demanding workout program.

We've also learned that *excessive* exercise exacts a toll on our bodies—in the form of everything from musculoskeletal injuries to increased risk of cancer.

Finally, we've come to recognize the vital role that *antioxidants* can play in protecting exercisers against cancer, heart attack, arthritis and other diseases.

HOW MUCH EXERCISE IS BEST?

In 1989, Steven Blair, PhD, a researcher here at The Cooper Aerobics Center, shook the scientific world.

In measuring the fitness of more than 13,000 American men and women, Blair found that the 20% who were fittest were 65% less likely to die over the next eight years than the 20% who were least fit. No surprise there.

The shock was that the biggest reduction in mortality came from only a *slight* increase in exercise. Those who were just a tad fitter than their most sedentary peers enjoyed a 55% lower death rate.

Implication: Very moderate physical activity gives the biggest health return on your investment of time and energy.

A modest exercise regimen confers increased energy and endurance and a stronger, more resilient cardiovascular system. This "aerobic training effect" lowers your risk of disease…and raises your life expectancy by up to two-and-one-half years.

I now believe that there's no *health-related* reason to do anything more strenuous than take a brisk walk (two miles in less than 30 minutes) three times a week. Or three miles in 45 minutes, twice a week.

Next month I turn 65, and I follow a slightly more strenuous schedule. I walk or run two to three miles, four or five times a week. I want to stay at a higher level of fitness so I can safely engage in more strenuous activities like mountain climbing, skiing and an occasional five-kilometer running race.

WHY MORE ISN'T BETTER

People who exercise harder than this may be doing themselves more harm than good.

375

I'm talking especially about individuals who run 30 miles a week or more.

For starters, the risk of muscle injury rises *steeply* once you run much more than 15 miles a week. Most people I know who used to work out at this level have had to cut back sharply—because of chronic injuries. Many of those who kept running long distances eventually had to quit altogether. Some required hip or knee replacements.

But muscle and joint problems are just the beginning. It turns out that serious exercisers may be unusually vulnerable to life-threatening illnesses.

One of my friends, a 50-mile-a-week runner, died of a brain tumor at age 50. Another friend who loved to run marathons succumbed to cancer at age 60.

In my practice, I've seen many cases of cancer and heart disease among elite athletes.

Studies examining the relationship between exercise and health, like Dr. Blair's, indicate that the death rate goes up slightly for those at the peak of the fitness pyramid.

What's to blame? I'm now convinced that the most likely culprit is a class of highly unstable oxygen molecules.

HOW TO PROTECT YOURSELF

Oxygen is essential for life, as we all know. But when chemical reactions strip an oxygen molecule of one or more electrons, it becomes highly reactive. This so-called *free radical* launches an attack on the body's cells.

Result: Arteriosclerosis, cancer, immunity problems—even an increased risk of cataracts.

Free radicals are plentiful in polluted air (including air tainted with automobile exhaust and cigarette smoke). They're also generated during the normal energy-burning process of metabolism.

Fortunately, the body is equipped with special enzymes that neutralize free radicals. But while moderate exercise helps this self-defense system "gear up" for battle, *excessive* exercise floods the body with free radicals. This may overwhelm this system.

At special risk: People who run outdoors in an urban setting. They get an extra dose of free radicals from car exhaust, smog and other airborne toxins.

To protect yourself—especially if you exercise regularly—you need *antioxidants* to help the body neutralize free radicals. These include vitamins C and E and beta-carotene (a precursor of vitamin A).

Like many health experts, I think it's best to get these antioxidants by eating five to seven servings of fruits and vegetables each day.

Dark-green and yellow vegetables are rich in beta-carotene. One-and-a-half medium-sized carrots or one sweet potato a day provides enough to give you protection. Citrus fruits are good sources of vitamin C. Seeds, nuts and vegetable oils have vitamin E.

For an extra margin of protection, take supplements every day. Here's what I've found to be best for regular exercisers...

- **1,000 milligrams (mg) of vitamin C** (2,000 mg if you're over 50).

- **400 international units** (IU) of vitamin E (600 if you're over 50).

- **25,000 IU of beta-carotene** (50,000 if you're over 50).

- **200 to 240 micrograms** (mcg) of folic acid.

- **1 mg vitamin B-12.**

If you exercise strenuously (running more than 30 miles a week, for example), boost the doses to 3,000 mg of vitamin C...1,200 IU of vitamin E...and 50,000 IU of beta-carotene.

To keep vitamin costs under $5 a month, buy generic supplements in bulk (500 tablets at a time).

Just be sure the vitamin E is in its natural form (d-alpha tocopherol). It gets into cells and body fluids more efficiently than the synthetic form.

Walking Your Way to Better Health

Mort Malkin, DDS, attending surgeon at Brooklyn Hospital Center, New York. A noted authority on fitness and walking, he is author of *Aerobic Walking—The Weight-Loss Exercise*. John Wiley & Sons.

Walking may be *the* ultimate form of exercise. It can provide just as much of a workout as running—even cross-country skiing—without the inconvenience, expense or risk of injury associated with those activities.

With a few simple alterations to your stride, walking is also a great way to melt away pounds and strengthen muscles. And, of course, walking is a weight-bearing exercise (good for bone-building)…and it can be done anywhere. All you need is a decent pair of shoes.

OPTIMIZING YOUR STRIDE

Conventional walking is too easy to be much of a workout. That's because it uses only a small part of the body's muscle mass.

According to a Columbia University study, conventional walking is mostly momentum. Only in the final third of the stride do the muscles produce power for forward movement… and even then the power comes from only the modestly sized calf muscles—the *soleus* and *gastrocnemius*.

To boost the fitness value of walking, you must put more muscle to work. The larger the muscle mass you involve with each stride, the greater the health benefits, including weight loss.

Here are three ways to optimize your stride…

●**Make the muscles work earlier.** Most walkers apply power only to the *end* of each stride, as they push off with the ball of the foot and the toes.

Instead: Start extending a backward force against the ground the instant your heel touches down. Think of pulling the ground under your body with your leg. This action involves the back of the thigh (hamstrings) and the buttocks (*gluteals*). Together, these muscles are up to five times bigger than your calf muscles. End each stride with a push-off as you normally would.

●**Swing your hips.** Most people use only the legs to carry their feet forward.

Better: Reach forward with the hip of the leg that is coming forward for the new stride.

Picture a line through your hips, running from left to right. If you're strolling, this line stays perpendicular to the direction of travel. In aerobic walking, the line should be at a 45 degree angle to the direction you're headed.

Result: You work your abdominals, lower back muscles and even more of the gluteals.

●**Boost your speed.** Focus on acceleration as soon as your heel strikes the ground. Imagine your eyes on a level plane. As you walk, keep them level, with no bouncing.

Look at a lamppost, tree or another object that is relatively close to you. Walk so smoothly that the object does not jiggle.

BODY BENEFITS

Put more muscle mass to work, and you will more quickly derive the benefits of walking—better fat metabolism, improved glucose tolerance, a lower resting heart rate, reduced stress, etc.

The difference between plain walking and aerobic walking is dramatic.

Example: A woman with insulin-dependent (adult-onset) diabetes joined one of my walking classes. For several years, she had been walking five miles six days a week. She needed 20 units of insulin a day. Her blood sugar level averaged 135.

After trying the proper technique for one month, she found she needed less insulin—12 units daily. Her blood sugar level had declined to a more normal 99.

GETTING STARTED

To reduce your risk of injury, start your walking program gradually. You can begin by taking a 10- to 20-minute stroll, three or four days a week, even if you're already fit.

Add five minutes a week, working up to an average of 40 to 50 minutes a session. This is the ideal workout length for weight loss and health benefits.

As you increase workout time, also increase your speed. *You'll know you've reached the proper intensity if…*

• **You're *slightly* out of breath** throughout the workout.

• **You're a bit above the comfort zone** but are able to finish the workout. On a scale of 5 (resting) to 20 (all-out effort), your level of exertion should be about 14.

• **You're able to talk in phrases only,** not complete sentences. In fact, you won't feel like talking at all.

PICKING THE RIGHT SHOES

Try on a wide variety of walking and running shoes to find the pair that best fits your feet.

Look for: Moderate cushioning...a low, beveled heel...roominess in the toe box...flexibility...an "Achilles notch" at the back of the collar (to allow space for your Achilles tendon).

Have a salesperson check the wear pattern on your old shoes before he/she recommends a new pair.

Inexpensive Ways To Shape Up

Patrick Netter, home fitness expert and consultant, J.P. Netter Marketing, 11693 San Vincente Blvd., Los Angeles 90049.

Rent—or buy—workout videos from your local video store...contact an area high school about evening exercise classes for adults ...create your own home gym by buying a single well-made exercise machine—the cost will be less than joining a health club...exercise with friends to make it more difficult to put off working out.

Health Clubs Can Be Unhealthy

Rodney Basler, MD, dermatologist and past chairman of the American Academy of Dermatology's task force on sports medicine, Lincoln, NE.

Even the cleanest-looking health club can, in actuality, be full of hidden germs.

Self-defense: Grab a towel when you walk in and keep it between your body and the equipment...instead of wearing skin-baring tank tops and short shorts, exercise in T-shirts and thigh-length shorts...wear flip-flops in the shower. Pooled water on shower floors and damp carpeting can lead to athlete's foot...before using a hot tub, make sure the water is clear—cloudy water and deposits along the sides of the tub are signs of bacterial growth.

Beware of Health Club Scams

Stephen Isaacs, a lawyer and coauthor of *The Consumer's Legal Guide to Today's Health Care.* Houghton-Mifflin.

The costly lifetime memberships that health clubs advertise are a bad deal. *Reason:* They last for the club's lifetime, *not yours.* When you do join a health club, read the fine print in contracts *very carefully.* Some contracts contain a comprehensive liability waiver that relieves the health club of responsibility for all accidents...even those that are caused by its own negligence.

Exercise Beats Dieting

John Foreyt, professor of medicine and psychiatry at Baylor College of Medicine in Houston and director of its Nutrition Research Clinic.

Exercise is more important than dieting for weight loss. In a study, researchers followed three groups of people who wanted to lose weight. One group exercised and dieted, the second dieted without exercising, the third exercised without dieting. After two years, only the group that exercised without seriously dieting maintained their weight losses.

Reason: These people said that, after working out, they didn't want to fill up on high-calorie, high-fat foods and instead ate sensibly and lost weight.

The Right Time To Exercise

Tom Thomas, PhD, professor of nutritional sciences, University of Missouri, Columbia, quoted in *Runner's World,* 33 E. Minor St., Emmaus, PA 18098.

Exercise *before* a fatty meal to minimize the artery-clogging effects of the food. A one-hour exercise session about 12 hours before a high-fat meal significantly cuts the amount of fat circulating in the blood after the meal. Exercising after the meal has little effect. *Bottom line:* If you expect to eat a high-fat dinner at night, do a one-hour run, for example, first thing in the morning.

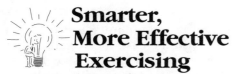

Smarter, More Effective Exercising

Mort Malkin, attending surgeon at Brooklyn Hospital Center, New York, and author of *Aerobic Walking—The Weight-Loss Exercise.* John Wiley & Sons.

Unless you take the proper precautions you should avoid using weights when walking for fitness.

Why: Hand weights can cause shoulder and back pain...ankle weights can strain knees and throw you off balance.

More effective than weights: Increase your walking pace.

Exercise and Longevity

Urho Kujala, MD, PhD, unit for sports and exercise medicine, University of Helsinki, Finland.

Exercise prolongs life regardless of heredity. A study of 16,000 adult twins who were tracked for 19 years found that the active twin had a substantially lower chance of dying prematurely.

General finding: Persons who jogged, walked briskly or performed equivalent exercise for 30 minutes at least six times a month had a 43% lower death rate than persons who were sedentary.

Dr. Kenneth Cooper's Exercise Plan

Kenneth H. Cooper, MD, MPH, president and founder of The Cooper Aerobics Center in Dallas and a leading exponent of exercise for almost three decades. He is author of numerous books on health and fitness, including *Dr. Kenneth H. Cooper's Antioxidant Revolution.* Thomas Nelson.

I've been a fitness enthusiast for several decades. But my ideas about exercise and health have changed with the times, as new medical data have emerged.

EXERCISING WISELY

For the average American, it is clear that moderate exercise is best. Moderate exercise minimizes the risk of musculoskeletal injury... it's a realistic level of exercise for most people...it's easy...and it doesn't take a lot of time.

At The Cooper Aerobics Center, we have shown that moderate activity reduces deaths from heart attack, stroke, diabetes and cancer by 55%—and increases longevity significantly.

The best exercises to perform to obtain health and longevity benefits, in no particular order, are cross-country skiing...swimming... running...cycling...and walking.

You can perform indoor or outdoor versions of these activities—and mix and match among them to keep up your interest.

A WEEKLY WORKOUT PLAN

Before you start an exercise program, consult a physician for a checkup and an exercise stress test if you're a healthy male over age 40 —or a healthy female over age 50.

Here's a great moderate-level weekly workout plan almost anyone can do...

Aerobic exercise: Perform an aerobic activity at least three times a week. Make sure each session includes...

●**A three- to four-minute stretching session.** Stretch your legs—hamstrings, quadriceps and Achilles tendons—and your back before and after exercising. Also stretch out your shoulders if you're preparing to do an activity with intensive arm movements, such as swimming or cross-country skiing.

Stretches should be gentle and continuous, not pulsing. Breathe evenly while stretching and stretch to the point of resistance, not to the point of pain.

●**A five- to 10-minute warm-up.** Do your chosen exercise at a slower pace to ready your musculoskeletal system for more intense activity.

Example: Walk at 75% of your usual speed until you break out in a light sweat.

●**A 20-minute aerobic segment** performed at a sustained low speed. After six to 10 weeks, gradually increase your speed and distance, and add arm movements to intensify the workout.

To become aerobically fit, walk up to 45 minutes, five times a week...or 60 minutes, two to three times a week.

●**Five-minute cool-down.** Exercise slowly again to bring your heart rate back down to normal.

●**Integrate muscle-toning exercises into your regimen.** Use weight machines or hand-held weights, or perform push-ups or stomach crunches at least twice a week for 20 minutes.

Reason: Toning exercises keep your muscles in shape—including your heart—improve strength, stamina and flexibility, and reduce the potential for injury.

You can perform muscle-toning exercises on the same days you perform aerobic activities or on alternate days.

KEEP IN MIND

●**Aging increases the risk of injury.** Therefore, the intensity of exercise becomes less important than the duration of exercise. You get as much cardiovascular aerobic benefit from walking a 12-minute mile as you do from running a nine-minute mile.

Important: Shoot for a 12- to 15-minute-per-mile pace when walking.

●**Stretching becomes more important.** It can reduce stiffness and risk of injury and improve athletic performance.

Important: If you feel pain, immediately stop what you're doing. If pain persists, have it evaluated by a physician.

●**You may gain some weight as you age**—but that's not unhealthy if you continue to exercise. Don't worry about extra pounds if you're within 20% of your ideal weight.

Better Weight-Lifting Workouts

Patrick Netter, exercise/fitness equipment consultant, 333 Bonhill Rd., Los Angeles 90049.

You'll develop better muscle tone and strength if you increase the weight rather than the number of repetitions. As soon as you can do three sets of 12 reps with moderate effort, add five to 10 pounds to the weight. *Also:* When doing reps, do them slowly. Fast and jerky repetitions build up momentum. That can cause strain or injury to your muscles and joints.

Short Exercise Sessions May Be Better

John Jakicic, PhD, assistant professor of behavioral medicine, University of Pittsburgh School of Medicine, and leader of the study of 56 women.

In a study, overweight women who exercised in three 10-minute sessions lost more weight than women who exercised in one 30-minute session.

Possible reason: The shorter-duration workouts seemed easier for the women to do—so they did them more diligently, and ended up doing more total exercise than the women who did longer workouts.

Do-It-Yourself Sports Drink

Nancy Clark, MS, RD, author of *Nancy Clark's Sports Nutrition Guidebook*. Human Kinetics.

During strenuous workouts lasting an hour or more, sports drinks such as Gatorade and Powerade are better than water for replacing carbohydrates depleted during exercise. But athletes can save money by making their own sports drinks.

Recipe: Dissolve one tablespoon sugar and a pinch of salt in a glass with one tablespoon of hot water. Add one tablespoon orange juice (or two tablespoons of lemon juice) and seven ounces of ice water.

Antiarthritis Exercise

Marian Minor, PhD, PT, an associate professor at the University of Missouri School of Medicine, Columbia.

Walking and cycling—dynamic exercise—are good for people with arthritis.

A study found that dynamic exercise produced greater improvement in muscle strength, physical conditioning and joint mobility than the isometric or range-of-motion exercises usually recommended for people with rheumatoid arthritis.

Improved joint mobility makes it easier to move around and perform everyday bending and stretching activities.

The best way to get into a suitable noncompetitive exercise program that does not overstress your capabilities—join a group with other people who know about arthritis. Local chapters of the Arthritis Foundation may be able to direct you.

Exercise Is Good for Asthmatics

Francois Haas, PhD, pulmonary physiologist, New York University Medical Center, Rusk Institute, 400 E. 34 St., New York 10016.

Aerobic conditioning helps increase lung capacity and strengthens the heart, making it easier to draw oxygen into the lungs and easier for the heart to pump oxygen-rich blood.

Helpful: Any exercise that raises the heart rate above normal limits...even walking.

Self-defense: Take medication to open the bronchial tubes at least 20 minutes before exercising. Warm up for 10 minutes before strenuous exercise. Avoid asthma-provoking situations like exercising in cold, dry weather or when the air is filled with pollution or allergens.

How to Stick With Your Exercise Regimen

Charles Roy Schroeder, PhD, professor of exercise physiology at the University of Memphis. He is author of *Taking the Work Out of Working Out*. Chronimed.

Have you ever committed yourself to an exercise routine—only to quickly abandon it?

If so, your commitment was probably based on the prospect of *future* goals—weight loss, lower cholesterol, firmer muscles, etc.

There's nothing wrong with these goals, but they are rarely enough to keep you motivated.

To stick with a routine, you must find ways to enjoy exercise itself. How do you do *that*? Dr. Charles Roy Schroeder, one of the country's leading exercise physiologists, recommends these strategies...

• **Consider your personality and lifestyle when picking an exercise routine.** If you have a demanding, people-oriented job, you might enjoy a repetitive, solitary workout like swimming or jogging.

If you thrive on competition, pick a competitive sport like tennis, basketball, etc.…or pepper your workouts with goal-oriented elements, such as timed sprints.

- **Be aware of bodily sensations.** It's easy to overlook the pleasurable feelings that accompany exercise. Make it a point to be aware of these *kinesthetic* sensations—the rhythm of your breathing…the motion of your joints… the ebb and flow of tension as your muscles contract and release.

- **Add music.** The right music can make your movements more graceful and rhythmic. It can also set a pace for you.

Avoid loud or insistent music—the kind favored by many aerobics instructors. Blaring music directs your attention away from the pleasurable kinesthetic sensations.

If you're running, bicycling or skating, it's best not to wear earphones. They can make it hard for you to hear traffic or other potential hazards.

- **Work out with a mirror.** Mirrors enable you to see your muscles at work at the same time you *feel* them working—and that helps focus your mind.

Mirrors also let you check for correct form… and let you enjoy the gradual improvement in your appearance as you get into shape. That helps keep you motivated.

- **Vary your exercise routine.** Make your workout interesting by varying…

- **Speed and intensity.** Alternate between light and heavy weights. Experiment with different resistance settings on the exercise bike. Vary your running pace.

- **Magnitude.** On a stair-climber, take one step at a time for several steps…then two steps at a time…then three…and then back to one.

- **Range of motion.** Instead of lifting a weight all the way up on each repetition, lift it one-quarter of the way and then lower it. Then lift it halfway and lower it…and then lift it three-quarters of the way.

Also: Add motions that spread the work over additional muscles.

In the arm curl, for example, standard form is to hold dumbbells with hands down at sides, then bend at the elbows to bring forearms up in front of chest.

As you raise your forearms, try moving your elbows forward at the same time. That works the shoulder muscles.

- **Form.** On a bicycle, move your hips from side to side as you pedal…or push harder on alternate sides (LEFT right left, RIGHT left right).

- **Get a workout partner**—someone who is open to the idea of exploring pleasure in movement. Motivate and inspire each other.

- **Be playful.** Throw in some skipping steps as you jog. In the pool, pretend you are a dolphin or a submarine. No one has to know what you're thinking.

Giving free rein to your imagination will make exercise more enjoyable.

Better Stationary Biking

Hold It! You're Exercising Wrong by Edward Jackowski, founder of Exude, a one-on-one motivational and fitness company based in New York. Fireside.

Unless you want to add bulk to your lower body, don't bike with much tension on the wheels. The more tension, or resistance, you ride with, the bigger your leg muscles will become. *To improve muscle tone without building size:* Pedal with little or no tension at a high speed—80 to 120 rotations per minute (RPM).

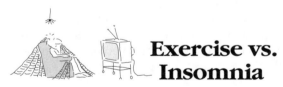

Exercise vs. Insomnia

Peter Tanzer, MD, in private practice in Pittsburgh, clinical assistant professor of medicine, University of Pittsburgh School of Medicine, and author of *The Doctor's Guide for Sleep Without Pills.* Tresco Publishers.

Exercise can help beat insomnia. Exercise *well before* bedtime. Later, as you cool down, you will begin to relax and be ready for sleep.

Exercise too near bedtime is stimulating, causing increased alertness that can interfere with falling asleep.

Caution: If an exercise routine helps you sleep better, keep it up. If you stop, insomnia may return in a few days.

Exercise Surprise

Kenneth Cooper, MD, MPH, president and founder, The Cooper Aerobics Center, 1220 Preston Rd., Dallas 75230.

Shorter exercise sessions held more frequently may be better for weight loss than fewer, longer sessions.

Reason: The body burns additional calories for several minutes after exercise ends.

In theory, the calories burned during one 30-minute session equal the ones burned in three 10-minute sessions of the same intensity. But the three-session approach means the body has three post-exercise calorie burns instead of one.

"Tubing" Your Way to Strong Muscles

Brian B. Cook, senior kinesiologist (exercise specialist) at Total Physio, a physiotherapy and rehabilitation clinic in Hamilton, Ontario. He is coauthor of *Strength Basics: Your Guide to Resistance Training for Health and Optimal Performance.* Human Kinetics.

If you'd like to boost your strength and muscular endurance but weight lifting isn't right for you, "tubing" is a safe, effective alternative.

Tubing—stretching a length of rubber hose—is perfect for older individuals and for anyone just beginning or resuming an exercise program after a sedentary period. It's also good for those who lack access to weights…who want a break from conventional weight training…or who wish to stay toned while traveling. (Rubber tubing takes up little room in a suitcase.)

Tubing is very inexpensive. The recommended 12-foot length of ⅜- to ½-inch diameter tubing costs about $20. It's available from sports/fitness stores and medical supply houses.

You can make handles on the tubing simply by tying a loop on each end. If you prefer, look for tubing made just for exercise—it comes with built-in handles.

Caution: Check the tubing before each use. If you find nicks and/or tears, replace the tubing.

TUBING SCHEDULE

Do at least three 30-minute tubing workouts each week. First, stretch for five to 10 minutes. Then do two sets of 10 repetitions of each of the following exercises. After three weeks, progress to three sets of 10 reps each.

Important: Unless otherwise indicated, the tubing should be lightly stretched when you are in the starting position.

CHEST PRESS

Lie on your back with your legs bent and feet flat on the floor. Anchor the tubing under your shoulders. Place your elbows on the floor at chest height and your hands above your elbows.

Exhale and stretch the tubing to arm's length. Inhale as you slowly return to the starting position.

HALF SQUAT

Stand on the tubing at its midpoint, with feet shoulder-width apart. Holding the tubing handles, extend your arms straight down at your sides. The tubing should be fully stretched. Look straight ahead, with your abdominals tight and chest up.

Inhale as you slowly squat until your knees are bent at a 90-degree angle. Exhale as you slowly return to the starting position.

BENT-OVER ONE-ARM ROW

Lean on a chair with your left hand. Slightly bend your knees and hips, keeping your back parallel to the floor. Stand on the tubing with your right foot. Place the left foot behind you to stabilize your body.

Hold the slightly stretched tubing in your right hand, letting your arm hang straight down from the shoulder. Inhale as you pull your hand up toward your shoulder, keeping your elbow snug against your body. Exhale as you lower your hand to the starting position. Repeat, then switch arms.

BICEP CURLS

Stand on the tubing with your feet shoulder-width apart, knees slightly bent. Keep your arms against your sides and palms pointed slightly forward, with the handles in your hands.

Exhale as you slowly curl your hands up to your shoulders, keeping your elbows next to your body. Inhale as you lower your hands to the starting position.

SEATED CALF PRESS

Sit on the floor. Straighten your right leg and loop the tubing around the arch of the right foot. Keep the left leg bent, with the foot flat on the floor.

Hold the handles in both hands at chest level. Exhale as you point the toes of the right leg. Inhale as you return to the starting position.

Repeat. Then do the exercise using the left leg.

How to Get the Most Out of Your Workouts

Miriam E. Nelson, PhD, associate chief of the Human Physiology Laboratory at the Jean Mayer US Department of Agriculture Human Nutrition Research Center on Aging at Tufts University in Boston. She is author of *Strong Women Stay Young*. Bantam.

Working out at a health club can be a great way to build strength and endurance. But only a fraction of the estimated 19 million Americans who now belong to health clubs are getting their money's worth.

Here's how to make sure *your* money—as well as your time and sweat—are well spent.

ASK FOR GUIDANCE

You may *think* you're exercising under the watchful eyes of the fitness trainers who are on duty at your health club.

But most trainers adopt a hands-off approach to interacting with club patrons. To avoid seeming rude, they'll correct your technique *only* if you're about to injure yourself.

Unless you take the initiative and ask for help, you may never know that you're leaning too heavily on the handrails of the stair climber…or that the short jerks you use to move the weight on the "lat pull-down" are less effective than slow, smooth movements.

Next time you work out at the gym, ask an instructor, "Am I using this piece of equipment correctly? Is there a way I could get more out of it?"

DO STRENGTH TRAINING FIRST

If you're just beginning an exercise program, don't start with aerobics classes or another cardiovascular workout. If you do, you'll probably find it hard to keep up. That's because your muscles, ligaments and bones aren't yet strong enough to take the punishment.

Instead, get a couple of weeks of strength training under your belt. Aerobic activity will then be more enjoyable.

CHALLENGE YOURSELF

It's definitely not true that you must experience pain to make fitness gains. But if you want to see noticeable improvements in strength, you must be willing to push yourself a little.

How much weight should you lift? In general, you should be able to lift a given weight only eight to 10 times before your muscles become so fatigued that you must rest.

Sharp pain is a signal to stop exercising immediately, since it could indicate a joint problem.

If you have any medical concerns, consult a doctor before beginning an exercise regimen.

BUILD BOTH SIDES OF YOUR BODY

Even if their bodies look perfectly symmetrical, most people are stronger on one side. They tend to favor that side when working out with leg-extension machines and other weight machines that involve use of both arms or legs at the same time. As a result, the stronger side always stays stronger.

When exercising both legs or arms at the same time, be conscious of challenging the weaker limb. Do not depend on the stronger one to lift the weight.

DON'T HOLD YOUR BREATH

Most people instinctively hold their breath while lifting heavy weights. But breath-holding during exertion is hazardous—especially for individuals suffering from heart disease, high blood pressure, diabetes or glaucoma. It causes excessive pressure in the chest and abdomen.

Safer: Exhale as you lift the weight...and inhale as you lower the weight. If you have trouble getting the rhythm right, count out loud as you lift.

PREVENT DEHYDRATION

You already know that it's important to drink water while working out. But it's just as important to down at least eight ounces of water *after* a workout—even if you're not thirsty.

Sports drinks such as Gatorade are appropriate only for long-distance runners and other endurance athletes.

MAKE YOUR WORKOUTS SOCIAL

Exercise with a friend. Good conversation makes those minutes on the treadmill zip by... and just being near someone you like can keep you going through a series of weight lifts.

Your workouts are also a good way to keep up with people you might otherwise be too busy to see. Finally, knowing that your workout buddy will be waiting for you at the gym makes it more likely that you'll stick to your exercise schedule.

RECORD YOUR PROGRESS

Motivate yourself by keeping an exercise log that charts your growing fitness. Such a log makes it easy to remember the proper seat adjustment, the resistance and the other settings for each machine.

Overrated Exercise Machines

Research led by William Whiting, biomechanics specialist, Los Angeles, reported in *Women's Health Letter*, Box 467939, Atlanta 31146.

Abdominal muscle exercise machines are highly overrated. They are no more effective than old-fashioned crunch exercises. Claims like losing 10 pounds in 10 days are based on using them with nutrition and aerobic exercise programs. Crunches—done with or without a device—do not burn enough calories

to achieve significant weight loss. And—they do not provide enough resistance to help users get a rippling, washboard-type abdomen.

Dance for Health and Fun

David Nieman, DrPH, professor of health and exercise science, Appalachian State University, Boone, NC 28608.

Dancing is better exercise than walking. Ballroom dancing burns 210 to 385 calories per hour. More vigorous Western or swing dancing burns up to 400 calories per hour. Walking 2.5 to 4.5 miles per hour burns about 210 to 315 calories per hour. In addition, dance classes are an excellent way to meet people—since you usually rotate partners throughout the lesson.

Better Sleeping

Donald Bliwise, PhD, director of the Sleep Disorders Clinic at Emory University School of Medicine, Atlanta.

Exercise during the day can help you sleep better at night. Researchers set up a program of moderate exercise four times a week for a group of people between age 50 and age 76 who had difficulty sleeping at night and they found that they were able to sleep more soundly. Experts say that to help sleep, exercise should be done earlier in the day, well before supper time. *Best:* Bike riding, brisk walking or other moderate aerobic exercise.

Finding the Fountain Of Youth

Research conducted by Gary Hunter, PhD, professor of human studies, School of Education, University of Alabama.

Strength training is the closest thing to a "fountain of youth."

Study: Women as old as age 77 who began training on weight machines increased their physical strength more than 50% within four months. Such strength is vital in preventing debilitating injuries often associated with aging—from gradual weakening and lessening of mobility, to osteoporosis and injuries from falls. The women in the study also increased their walking speed by 18% even though walking was not part of their training.

Important: Aerobic exercises such as walking and swimming, while excellent for general health, do not provide strength benefits. Resistance training with weights or machines is necessary to accomplish this.

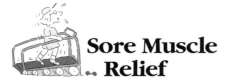

Sore Muscle Relief

Patrice Morency, MS, director, Innerweave Clinic, Portland, OR.

Soothe sore muscles with a hot/cold shower. Start with two minutes of hot water, then change to cold water for two minutes. Repeat this hot/cold cycle five times.

Why it works: The temperature changes cause alternating constriction and dilation of blood vessels. That helps flush lactic acid—the chemical that underlies soreness—from the muscles.

Hot Weather Jogging

Jeff Galloway, former Olympic runner who conducts fitness clinics in the US, writing in *Runner's World*, 33 E. Minor St., Emmaus, PA 18098.

Keep your head wet by pouring water over yourself at the start of your run and every 10 to 20 minutes...wear light, synthetic clothing so sweat will evaporate faster...after the run, cool down by pouring water over yourself or taking a cool swim or shower.

Best Swimming Exercise

Men's Fitness, 21100 Erwin St., Woodland Hills, CA 91367.

When swimming for exercise, use a basic crawl stroke. Cover as much water as possible with each stroke. Measure progress by how many strokes it takes to swim the length of the pool. Breathe every other stroke. Avoid holding your breath for several strokes. Keep power coming from your arms—two or three relaxed, shallow kicks per stroke are plenty. To sharpen strokes, swim as fast as possible with clenched fists.

Exercising to Lose Weight

Robert McMurray, PhD, professor of sports science and nutrition, University of North Carolina, Chapel Hill.

Exercising to lose weight works if you can do at least 45 minutes of aerobic and strength training five days a week. *Regimen:* Change your routine on a daily or weekly basis to lower the risk of muscle strain and reduce monotony.

Example: Switch between swimming and walking. Performing a variety of exercises will keep more muscles toned and may burn more calories.

Easy Rheumatoid Arthritis Relief

Mary J. Bell, MD, assistant professor of rheumatology and clinical epidemiology, Sunnybrook Health Science Center, University of Toronto. Her six-week study of 150 rheumatoid arthritis patients was presented at a meeting of the American College of Rheumatology.

Exercise helps ease joint stiffness caused by rheumatoid arthritis. Patients who did light exercise—walking and stretching—for as little as three hours over a six-week period reported a significant reduction in stiffness. Exercise is also effective against osteoarthritis.

Walking with Weights Works!

David Nieman, DrPH, professor of health and exercise science, Appalachian State University, Boone, NC.

Walking with weights burns more calories than walking without weights.

To avoid injury: Start with a one-pound weight in each hand. Gradually increase to five pounds. Keep stride length normal and consistent...and walk slowly until you've adjusted to the weights.

Caution: Swinging your arms excessively while carrying hand weights can cause elbow or shoulder injuries. If possible, alternate use of hand weights with ankle weights and weight vests.

How to Develop the Exercise Habit

Adele Pace, MD, an Ashland, KY, psychiatrist with a special interest in fitness. She is author of *The Busy Executive's Guide to Total Fitness.* Prentice Hall.

Everyone knows that exercise is good for you. That it reduces your risk for heart disease, diabetes and cancer. That it lowers your weight while raising your spirits. But for too many of us, the gap between couch and gym is just too great.

Many people embark on an ambitious exercise program only to lapse back into inactivity after a few workouts. These people fail to develop the *exercise habit* that keeps some people up and active through all kinds of moods and weather.

A POSITIVE ADDICTION

As with food and sex, we have an innate appetite for physical activity. Working out triggers production of *dopamine* and other pleasure-giving neurotransmitters, and the brain comes to crave this rewarding "bath" of neurotransmitters.

Consequently, people who work out regularly develop a sort of addiction to exercise.

For them, exercise is no longer a chore or obligation. It's a pleasurable habit.

How do you reach that point? The key is finding a way to *enjoy* your workouts. If you dread exercise—if you expect it to be painful and/or boring—it will be. Anticipate pleasure, and you'll find that instead.

SELF-EDUCATION IS KEY

Having a vague notion that exercise is beneficial does nothing for your attitude. You must read up on the specific, concrete rewards of exercise.

Good sources of information: *The American College of Sports Medicine Fitness Book* (Human Kinetics)...and Dr. Robert Cooper's *Health and Fitness Excellence* (Houghton Mifflin).

Find out exactly how exercise strengthens the muscles and boosts endurance. Learn how regular workouts cut your risk for heart disease as effectively as quitting smoking.

Talk to enthusiastic exercisers. Get them to tell you how they feel during and after working out. Ask them why they do it. Catch their excitement.

When I was a medical resident, I knew I should exercise. But I had no time—or so I thought. I asked a student—a 25-mile-a-week runner—why he wasted the time when his schedule was already jammed.

He explained vividly how running gave him extra energy and honed his concentration. He claimed that the 30 minutes a day he spent running actually made him a better student.

Guess what? He graduated first in his class.

REWARD YOURSELF

One good way to train yourself to become a habitual exerciser is to bolster your brain's natural reinforcement system with external rewards.

During your workouts, envision the cold drink you'll treat yourself to after it's over...or promise yourself a bagel or low-fat muffin.

Set up a system of short-term rewards for meeting your goals. If you've faithfully walked 30 minutes a day all week, indulge yourself with a good book or movie...a new article of clothing...or an afternoon off from work. Enjoy this special treat with a clear conscience.

To maintain your interest—and boost your fitness—continually revise your goals upward.

As your conditioning improves, shoot for a 20-minute-a-mile pace, then a 15-minute-a-mile pace (or whatever pace seems reasonable for you).

Record your progress in an exercise journal. Review it periodically to remind yourself of just how far you have come.

SECRETS OF EXERCISE SUCCESS

•**Exercise with a buddy.** Running, walking or weight-training with a like-minded individual is far more pleasurable than working out alone.

When you have an exercise buddy, each exercise period becomes a social occasion as well as a workout. You look forward to getting together. You can compare notes and encourage each other, too.

•**Help others with their exercise programs.** In addition to *seeking* help in forming an exercise habit, *give* help to a friend or family member who wants to get into shape. Doing so makes it harder to accept your own excuses for not working out.

If you have kids, exercising together certainly qualifies as "quality time." By encouraging your kids to exercise, you help them cultivate a life-long, life-giving habit.

Helping others works even if the other "person" is a dog. I became a committed runner as a result of taking my overweight Collie-Shepherd mix, Sam, on a daily two-mile run. No matter how tired I feel, I refuse to let the pup miss his exercise.

•**Combine exercise with another activity.** I exercise outdoors as much as possible, resorting to the gym only when bad weather hits (or for weight-lifting).

Like many people, I find stair-climbers and stationary bicycles boring. To make working out on them more palatable, I read magazines and medical journals as I step or pedal.

When I run on a treadmill, I listen to self-help audio tapes. One of my favorites is Dr. Denis Waitley's six-tape set *The Psychology of Winning* (Nightingale Conant).

•**Include several different kinds of exercise in your repertoire.** You might run one day, bike the next, swim the next, etc. "Cross-training" helps you achieve full-body fitness while staving off boredom.

EXERCISING ON THE ROAD

Before departing, call ahead to find out if health club facilities are available at your hotel (or nearby). If you return to the same city frequently, scout out the best exercise opportunities.

If you've been cross-training, you'll have no trouble getting in a good workout—whether the available facilities are geared to running, bicycling, swimming, etc.

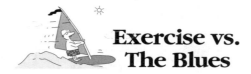

Exercise vs. The Blues

Kathleen Moore, PhD, research associate, department of psychiatry, Duke University Medical Center, Durham, NC. Her study of 57 depressed people 50 years of age or older was presented at a meeting of the Society of Behavioral Medicine.

Even short workouts—as brief as eight minutes—are enough to enhance mood.

Earlier studies showed the psychological benefits of *sustained* exercise. But this is the first to suggest that brief workouts reduce feelings of sadness, tension, fatigue, anger and confusion.

21

The Whole You—
The Mind/Body
Connection

Deepak Chopra's Secrets of Having Boundless Energy

Deepak Chopra, MD
Sharp Institute for Human Potential and Mind/Body Medicine

Fatigue is one of the most common problems doctors are asked to treat. Complaints about exhaustion are likely to continue, given our busy schedules and many demands on our lives.

Yet despite the large number of people who feel tired day after day, fatigue is an unnatural state. Such fatigue does not occur in animals or children. When children and animals are tired, they rest and awaken renewed.

But adults have the ability to maneuver around their biological needs. They drive themselves...resist the natural, biological cycle of alternating rest and activity...and become depleted.

To banish common fatigue, we need to rediscover our basic harmony with nature. The secret of recovering our harmony can be found in a mind/body system of health, which is based on the understanding that your own mind/body system is inseparably connected to the systems of nature.

WATCH WHAT YOU EAT

You can increase your energy by eating fresh, pure foods. By contrast, foods that lack freshness and are highly processed deplete the body of energy. *Foods especially rich in natural energy include...*

- **Fresh fruits and lightly cooked vegetables.**
- **Wheat, rice, barley and other whole grains.**
- **Nonmeat sources of protein**, such as dried beans. For those who balk at a vegetarian diet, fish and poultry are acceptable substitutes.

Deepak Chopra, MD, executive director of the Sharp Institute for Human Potential and Mind/Body Medicine, 1110 Camino Del Mar, Suite G, Del Mar, CA 92014. He is author of numerous books, including *Boundless Energy* (Harmony Books) and *The Seven Spiritual Laws of Success* (New World Library).

• **Honey as a substitute for refined sugar.**

Foods that deplete energy and should be avoided include red meat, aged cheese, alcohol, coffee and smoked and canned foods. This does not mean you must completely avoid anything but energy-boosting foods.

Any system that is too rigid will create further imbalance. Instead, experiment with these suggestions and notice what proportion makes a significant difference in your own energy level.

STRENGTHEN YOUR DIGESTION

Poor digestion can lead to fatigue in two ways...

• **Energy for the body is lost when food is not adequately metabolized.**

• **When food residue lingers undigested**, impurities and toxins may accumulate, placing stress on the body.

How to strengthen your digestion and boost your energy level...

• **Create a calm atmosphere for dining.** Instead of always working through lunch and watching TV during dinner, enjoy yourself and pay attention to your meal. Conversation is fine —but avoid controversial subjects.

When the body is accustomed to a routine, digestion will be automatic. So stick to regular mealtimes.

• **Eat your biggest meal at lunch.** Research indicates that this is the time when metabolism is most efficient.

• **Sip warm water or herbal tea throughout the day** to normalize the metabolic rate and eliminate toxins.

Helpful: Fill a thermos with warm water, which enhances digestion. Keep it nearby and take a few sips every half-hour.

REDUCE STRESS

Tension drains the body of energy, causing it to function less effectively.

Better: Make it a priority to spend time on relaxing activities. Everyone has favorite pastimes, and some of these can even take place during the work day.

Classic stress-relievers: Meditation, a massage, sex, a warm shower or bath, playing or listening to music...and a change of scenery.

EXERCISE IN MODERATION

Americans' obsession with strenuous exercise is creating an epidemic of exhaustion. Pushing ourselves past what our bodies are naturally designed to handle results in long-lasting fatigue.

Solution: For maximum energy, exercise seven days a week for 15 to 20 minutes at a time. Some fitness experts recommend taking a day off between workouts—but that's because our average workouts are too strenuous. Instead, exercise daily, but to only 50% of your capacity.

Example: If you are able to swim 20 laps, only swim 10. You'll feel energetic—and over time, your capacity will increase.

KEEPING NATURAL RHYTHMS

The body is most responsive to certain activities when they are performed at specific times of the day.

Before electric light was invented, our schedules were more in keeping with these natural rhythms under which our bodies evolved. Rediscovering them will help you feel energetic every day.

• **Awaken between 6 a.m. and 7 a.m.**

• **Exercise in the morning**—or, if this isn't possible, no later than three hours before bedtime.

• **Eat lunch between 12 p.m. and 1 p.m.**

• **Eat dinner between 6 p.m. and 7 p.m.** ...and wind down with restful activities afterward, such as going for a walk, reading, playing games with your family or listening to music.

• **Go to bed between 10 p.m. and 11 p.m. each night.**

Helpful: If you try going to bed at 10 p.m. but find you have trouble falling asleep, don't worry about it. Just rest quietly with your eyes closed. Clear your mind, and avoid dwelling on anything that is troubling you. Your body will get the rest it needs. Over time, you'll gradually notice an increase in energy in the morning, and you'll be able to fall asleep at the earlier hour.

TAKE PLEASURE IN LIFE

Joy is a natural energizer. If you're having a good time, you'll never be fatigued. In fact, studies have found that 80% of people suffering from chronic fatigue score higher than normal on measures of depression and anxiety.

Solution: Practice shifting your awareness to the positive. We can't avoid negative events, but we don't have to dwell on them.

Treat others with kindness, tolerance and love...refuse to entertain negativity...and pay attention to the joy and playfulness that can be found all around you. Learn to meditate to help you get in touch with nature and enable you to see these simple joys.

EXCEPTION TO THE RULE

If you are bothered by persistent fatigue, have a thorough medical checkup to rule out a treatable physical cause—such as anemia, thyroid problems or mononucleosis.

Nine Things You Can Do in Under Five Minutes to Improve Your Health

Harold H. Bloomfield, MD, a psychiatrist in private practice in Del Mar, CA. He is coauthor of *The Power of 5*. Rodale Press.

Split-second schedules don't leave much time for relaxation. So—here are nine ways to boost your happiness and limit stress in under five minutes.

1. Practice "one-breath" meditation. You don't have to spend years mastering meditation. This one-breath method is a powerful, straightforward relaxation technique that can be practiced anytime, anywhere. Try it whenever you feel fatigued or out of sorts.

What to do: Sit in a comfortable chair. Straighten your back, relax your shoulders and take a deep breath. Let the air "open" your chest. Imagine it filling every cell in your body. Hold the breath for a moment, then exhale, releasing every bit of tension.

Also helpful: One-touch relaxation. Place your fingertips just in front of your ears. Inhale and clench your teeth. Hold for five seconds. Exhale, and let your jaw muscles go loose.

Repeat this exercise three more times, using half the original tension, then one-fourth, then one-eighth. Then take a deep breath, press your fingertips against your jaw, let it go slack and say, *Ah-h-h-h.*

Imagine you are breathing out any tightness.

2. Inhale an energizing scent. Research suggests that lemon and peppermint scents are energizing.

Helpful: Have an occasional cup of lemon or peppermint tea...chew sugarless peppermint gum...keep a bottle of peppermint and/or lemon extract to sniff...add a couple of drops to a small scent dispenser...or experiment with potpourri containing other energizing scents such as pine, jasmine, lavender or orange.

3. Sip ice water. It keeps your cells hydrated and helps you burn calories.

Reason: Whenever you drink something cold, your body raises your metabolism to keep your body temperature from falling. That process burns calories—eight 16-ounce glasses of ice water will burn an extra 200 calories per day.

Strategy: Start the day with eight to 16 ounces of ice water. Sip a 16-ounce glass every hour or two, keeping one next to you at work and at home. All told, you should drink eight glasses by the end of the day.

4. Bask in bright light. Most people get a powerful surge of energy from sunlight or bright indoor light. Make use of this effect by moving your desk chair closer to a window...or take a five-minute outdoor walk every few hours.

Also helpful: Each day, get five minutes of nonpeak sun—before 10 a.m. or after 3 p.m.—without sunscreen or sunglasses and enjoy the full mood-lifting effects of sunlight.

5. Cook with "nutriceuticals"—vegetables, herbs and spices that have specific healing properties:

•**Garlic and onions** boost the immune system, helping prevent colds.

•**Basil, cumin and turmeric** help prevent cancer of the bladder and prostate.

•**Black pepper, jalapeños, mustard and hot red peppers** all boost your metabolism for several hours. That helps burn fat.

•**Cinnamon** helps metabolize sugar, keeping your blood sugar levels steady.

6. Check your reading posture. Poor posture—leaning over a desk, for instance—can cause tension headaches, vision problems and pain in the jaw and/or neck.

Self-defense: Bring reading material up to your field of vision or use a book stand to hold a book at the proper angle. If you tend to spend a lot of time on the telephone, invest in a headset. You should never cradle the telephone between your ear and shoulder.

7. Do trigger-point therapy. Wherever you feel tense, feel for a tight band of muscle tissue—a trigger point. Press or squeeze it with light to moderate pressure. Continue pressing for five to 10 seconds, then release.

8. Curb indoor pollution. Whenever possible, keep your windows open. Keep gas appliances properly maintained to limit their output of carbon monoxide. Use exhaust fans in the bathroom, kitchen and garage whenever you use these rooms. All gas appliances should be checked annually—and properly vented to the outside. Make your home and office smoke-free.

9. Do absolutely nothing. "Lyming" is the Caribbean art of doing nothing—without feeling guilty about it. Try lyming frequently to give your brain time to process all the information it receives over the course of a day.

Helpful: Take a five-minute "mental vacation" every few hours. Picture your favorite beach or other getaway place. The idea is to escape the rat race briefly—but completely.

20 Minutes a Day To a Much Happier, Much Healthier Life

Herbert Benson, MD, associate professor of medicine at Harvard Medical School, and president of the Mind/Body Medical Institute and coauthor of *Timeless Healing: The Power and Biology of Belief.* Scribner.

In more than 30 years of practicing medicine, I have found that the most impressive healing force—one that is universally accessible—is the power of the individual to cure himself/herself.

REMEMBERED WELLNESS

Doctors have long known that many patients will show improvement if they are given a placebo—a "dummy" pill—simply because they believe that the pill prescribed by the doctor will be effective. Most of the success physicians had before the modern era of scientific medicine probably came from this effect, because most of the medicines they used back then had little or no pharmaceutical value.

Example: During my college years, I spent one summer working as a seaman on a merchant ship. Knowing I was a premed student, my fellow sailors came to me after shore-leave carousing to cure their hangovers. I gave them vitamin tablets, the only pills I had to dispense, and was amazed to see how effectively they cured my shipmates' symptoms.

Most researchers dismiss this "placebo effect" as an unwanted complication that makes it difficult to carry out objective research into the effect of medical treatments. But, the placebo effect shows how powerful belief can be in enlisting the body's own curative powers.

When patients trust a physician, a treatment he recommends can be remarkably effective even though scientific medicine says it should not work. I think we should recognize the remarkable ability of the human mind to direct the body away from illness and toward health by dropping the expression "placebo effect" in favor of a positive term such as "remembered wellness."

Examples: In 1979, Harvard's Dr. David P. McCallie, Jr., and I studied a variety of treatments that had been used to relieve angina in the past—but that were revealed to have no physiological effect. We found that as long as the medical profession still believed in them, they worked 70% to 90% of the time. Later, when better-informed physicians began to doubt them, the effectiveness of these treatments dropped by more than half.

More recent studies have shown that remembered wellness helps patients obtain relief more than 70% of the time from chest pain, fatigue, dizziness, back pain and congestive heart failure.

MIND AND BODY

Remembered wellness is a powerful tool for restoring health. You can use it purposefully by training your body to enlist the mind's power of belief.

Brain researchers have found that thinking about a particular event produces the same pattern of activity in the brain as actually experiencing the event. The brain sends signals to the body that make it react the same way to the mental image as it would to the actual experience.

Example: When the old blockbuster movie *Lawrence of Arabia* was playing, movie theater concession stands experienced record demand for drinks. Moviegoers who had been watching desert action for two hours emerged during the intermission as thirsty as they would have been had they actually spent that time in the Arabian desert.

Our brains continuously produce images with powerful bodily effects. In particular, most of us today are continually exposed to stressful situations of one type or another, from heavy traffic...to work deadlines...to family problems.

The brain's natural response to stress, known as the fight-or-flight response, is to pump out adrenaline and other stress hormones. These substances increase blood pressure and produce harmful effects on the body, including blockage of blood vessels, disturbances in heart rhythm, anxiety, depression, anger and hostility.

Medications are not effective in the long run in dealing with the symptoms of stress.

A better way is to enlist the body's own recuperative power of remembered wellness.

One particularly effective method is to practice the *relaxation response*.

LET HEALING BEGIN

The *relaxation response* is the result of practicing mental focusing techniques that prevent an agitated mind from jumping from one stress-producing thought to another. When the mind calms down, the body follows suit. The relaxation response slows the body's metabolism and produces slow brain waves that are associated with pleasurable feelings.

To produce the relaxation response: Sit in a comfortable position, close your eyes, relax and breathe slowly and naturally while silently repeating a particular phrase you have chosen.

The focus phrase can be a religious word, phrase or prayer of particular significance to you, or a secular term that has a calming effect. *Examples:* "God, grant me the serenity"... "Peace".."Relax."

If your mind wanders, passively disregard the disturbing thoughts and return to your focus phrase.

Continue for 10 to 20 minutes, then allow other thoughts to return to your mind, open your eyes and sit for another minute before getting up.

Free of distraction, the body will be encouraged to use its own recuperative powers.

THE LIFESAVING POWER OF BELIEF

When people believe that life is meaningful and that they have a mission to accomplish, they are strongly motivated to commit all their inner mind/body resources to help them fight illness. That combination sometimes produces medical miracles.

Example: My patient, a deeply religious 71-year-old widow, having overcome diabetes and several heart attacks, was suffering from an advanced case of throat cancer. When her doctor recommended surgery to remove half her jaw, she refused, insisting that she would be able to survive with radiation therapy, another proven but less aggressive therapy.

As she suffered the devastating side effects of radiation, she never lost the belief that she would survive so she could continue helping other people. She bolstered her powers of resistance by practicing the relaxation response, and her many friends and relatives across the country complemented her fervent prayers with prayers of their own.

Five years later, the tumor has vanished, and my patient is fitter than she has been for a long time.

BOTTOM LINE

Modern medicine has many effective medications and procedures that target specific diseases. Both physicians and patients need to recognize that these techniques work best when they are used in combination with the patient's own inner beliefs.

How to Use Guided Imagery for Wellness

Mitchell L. Gaynor, MD, associate director of the Strang–Cornell Cancer Prevention Center, and assistant clinical professor of medicine at New York Hospital–Cornell Medical Center, both in New York City. He is author of *Healing Essence: A Cancer Doctor's Practical Program for Hope and Recovery.* Kodansha.

Can your imagination protect you from cancer and other serious ailments? Can it cure disease? Extend life? Can it make you less anxious and more fulfilled?

Although more research needs to be done, preliminary studies suggest that the answer to each of these questions is *yes.*

To harness the power of your imagination, you must practice guided imagery on a daily basis.

This easy mental exercise involves creating and then focusing on a tranquil mental picture —basking in the warm sun on a sandy, windswept beach, for instance. Psychologist Jeanne Achterberg has called *guided imagery* "thinking without words."

HOW THE MIND HEALS THE BODY

Over the last eight years, I've taught thousands of cancer patients to use guided imagery for healing and recovery...and the same technique can be used by *healthy* individuals to become happier, more relaxed—and less vulnerable to illness.

My imagery regimen, which I call *Essence*, is not a substitute for medical care. It's an adjunct to conventional cancer therapies like chemotherapy, radiation and bone marrow transplantation.

A scientific field called *psychoneuroimmunology* (PNI) has demonstrated clearly that the mind plays a key role in health and illness.

Specifically, negative psychological factors like stress, depression and pessimism impair the immune system...while joy, optimism and other positive emotions enhance it.

In one landmark study, breast cancer patients who practiced meditation and guided imagery in addition to receiving conventional medical care lived *twice* as long as a control group who got only conventional medical care.

In another study, conducted at Yale University, patients suffering from depression began to feel much better when they visualized scenes in which they were praised by people they admired.

By using my Essence program, you can cultivate positive, health-promoting emotions— and assist in your own healing.

ESSENCE AT WORK

One of my patients, a 28-year-old man, had experienced a complete remission from cancer after receiving a bone marrow transplant. But he hadn't slept in three months. He was afraid he would never wake up.

Guided imagery gave him a sense of peace that enabled him to release the fear. Soon, he was able to get the restorative sleep he needed to stay well.

Another patient was benefiting from chemotherapy, but the nausea caused her so much suffering that she was thinking about discontinuing it.

With my program, her anxiety and nausea dissipated. She was able to get on with her lifesaving treatment.

When another of my patients discovered that cancer had spread to his liver, he was sure that the disease was too advanced for chemotherapy to help.

My program helped him realize that he was a person, not a statistic...and that the outcome *in his case* was uncertain. He had a partial remission, and is back at work a year after his diagnosis.

Even if your illness cannot be cured—and not all can—my program can help eliminate *emotional* suffering.

THE ESSENCE OF ESSENCE

Most of us were brought up with a clear picture of how our lives were supposed to turn out. We suffer because our lives fall short of our expectations.

We struggle against the reality of disease. *It's not supposed to be this way,* we think…or *Life's not fair.*

But deep within each of us lies the true self —our "essence." It's the part of you that doesn't judge your life, but accepts it. It doesn't smother unpleasant feelings. It doesn't turn physical pain into emotional pain with thoughts such as, *I just can't stand this* and *Why must this happen to me?*

You experience your essence only when your mind becomes quiet and your thoughts recede. Meditation helps, but I've found that my program works faster.

I ask my patients to do this for 20 minutes, twice daily…

Sit in a quiet setting, breathing slowly. Let the breath come through your nose, into your upper abdomen and out through your mouth.

Focus on a positive thought, preceded by the word "infinite." *Examples:* Infinite peace… infinite love…infinite healing. *Next…*

- **Experience whatever negative emotion is troubling you.** Try to envision the emotion as a physical thing, endowed with shape, temperature, color, etc.

- **See your essence as a white light just above your head.**

- **Surrender your pain,** suffering or sadness. Imagine the negative emotion being swallowed by the white light.

- **Empower your healing.** Breathe deeply, and as you inhale, visualize white light going into the region of your body once occupied by suffering or pain.

- **Nurture the idea of a positive outcome.** Imagine a life free of pain, fear and suffering.

- **Create an imaginary channel** that lets the white light of your essence continuously flow into the place where you experience negative emotions.

- **Embody your own healing power.** Imagine each cell of your body being suffused with the white light.

While I developed this technique for cancer patients, it can also heal the suffering caused by any illness, including heart disease, arthritis, etc. It can even help people who are healthy.

We all suffer fears, painful memories and disappointments. We forget who we truly are as we struggle to meet unrealistic expectations …and condemn those around us who fail to meet our expectations of them. We push these feelings aside, but they take their toll.

Simply focus on whatever is bothering you —job stress, marital strife, etc. At the same time, visualize your essence. Let its healing power flow through your mind and body.

How to Use Your Mind to Improve Your Health

Steven Locke, MD, assistant professor of psychiatry, Harvard Medical School, Boston, and chief of behavioral medicine, Harvard Pilgrim Health Care, New England's largest health maintenance organization. Dr. Locke is coauthor of *The Healer Within.* Mentor.

While some doctors still caution against using creative visualization and other "mind–body" techniques to the exclusion of conventional medicine, studies make it increasingly clear that one's attitude and emotional state play key roles in the prevention of—and recovery from—illness.

We asked Harvard Medical School scientist Steven Locke, MD, about the relationship between the mind and the immune system…

What effects do positive emotions have on immunity?

Close relationships with friends and family members seem to have significant and highly beneficial effects on the immune system. Several studies have shown, for example, that married people live longer than those who are single or divorced. Other studies have linked happiness and positive emotions to longer survival among cancer patients.

Study I: Eighty-six women with advanced breast cancer were divided into two groups.

One group received standard medical care… the other received medical care *and* weekly group therapy sessions.

Result: The women who received group therapy lived nearly twice as long as those who received only medical care.

Study II: Melanoma patients were divided into two groups. The first group received medical care only…the second group received medical care as well as stress-management training.

Result: Those in the second group suffered far less distress over their cancer diagnoses than those in the first group…their immune functions were much stronger…and their rate of survival was greater. *Also:* There was a greater trend—though not statistically significant—for melanoma to recur in the first group.

How do negative emotions affect the immune system?

Stressful events, such as the death of a family member, marital separation, the loss of a job—even taking a college exam—cause marked deficits in the immune function, as measured by changes in the number and function of specialized blood cells.

Unknown: Whether or not these events increased susceptibility to illness. Also unknown is whether depression and other emotional problems cause cancer. While they can lead to self-destructive habits that cause cancer, there is no clear evidence that they themselves result in the illness.

Is there a cancer personality?

Some researchers suggest that there are behavior patterns—including suppression of hostility or a helpless/hopeless attitude—that place some people at greater risk for cancer.

In my opinion, the notion that your personality determines your cancer risk is simplistic and emotionally destructive. Cancer is bad enough without believing your illness is your fault.

Reality: People develop cancer not because of personality defects but because of hereditary predispositions to the disease…exposure to tobacco smoke or other carcinogens…a high-fat, low-fiber diet…or excessive alcohol use.

Is there any value in guided imagery, deep relaxation and other "alternative" techniques?

Such techniques certainly give those who are ill a psychological boost by engendering a sense of empowerment.

Less certain: Whether these techniques do what they are intended to do—marshal the immune defenses against pathogens.

In a study at Ohio State University, elderly people received training in progressive muscle relaxation.

Result: The subjects had significantly more natural killer-cells—a type of immunity that protects against viral illness and cancer—in their bloodstreams after the training than they did before.

Caution: These techniques are unproven for cancer or other terminal illnesses. Patients who wish to use them should not abandon their conventional treatments in the belief that these techniques will cure them.

Does laughter play a role in the battle against illness?

Norman Cousins, the late editor and essayist who wrote about his personal health battle in *Anatomy of an Illness*, was among the first to argue that laughter does *not* play a role. He felt misunderstood about the power of laughter. He believed what made the difference for him was the sense of empowerment from being an active participant in his treatment. Although he used comedies to induce positive emotions, he emphasized hope, a sense of control and loving support as critical factors in healing. Research, however, suggests laughter may affect immunity.

Study: Watching a humorous video (in this case a comedian) reduced levels of adrenaline and cortisol in the bloodstream—according to scientists at Loma Linda University in California. These and other substances that suppress immunity are produced by the body in great quantities during times of stress.

Is it true that hostile, angry people die younger?

Dr. Redford Williams and his associates at Duke University found that certain forms of hostility—cynicism and mistrust—are associated with higher mortality. Other studies suggest that people who are either too angry or who never express their anger may be at higher risk. At Harvard, my colleagues and I did a study of various psychosocial factors and immunity.

Among our findings: People who were deemed most hostile had lower natural killer-cell activity.

Possible explanation: Hostile and mistrustful individuals may have poor social networks. Many studies suggest that the support of friends and family plays a protective role in health.

Can mind power combat a common cold?

Stress increases the likelihood of developing colds. Since relaxation techniques have increased immune responses in other studies, deep breathing and meditation might be helpful in strengthening resistance to the cold virus. Although this hasn't been well researched, it seems worth a try.

Your Mind And Your Health

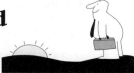

Elliott Dacher, MD, who practices internal medicine and conducts healing and wellness seminars nationwide, 11469 Washington Plaza W., Reston, VA 22090. He is author of *Whole Healing: A Step-by-Step Program to Reclaim Your Power to Heal.* Dutton.

When left unexpressed and unresolved, emotions such as anger, hostility and feelings of loss and stress are dangerous to your health. So are feelings of powerlessness.

Example: A study in *The Journal of the American Medical Association* showed that people who had little or no control over their jobs reported feeling "helpless and powerless"—and were more likely to develop heart problems and elevated blood pressure levels.

Though feelings of anxiety will arise, they can be managed so that your health is not compromised by them.

WHY PALMS SWEAT

Our minds have greater influence over our well-being than most of us realize. The human brain produces chemicals called *neuropeptides* —messengers that deliver information to various parts of the body. The medical world recently discovered that neuropeptides are also produced outside the brain—in tissues, organs and even in the immune system's white blood cells. Neuropeptides, nerves and other neurotransmitters link every part of the body, creating a kind of inner conversation. What happens in one area or organ can affect numerous other organs.

Example: If you are about to give a speech and are feeling nervous, your brain may send neuropeptides carrying an anxiety-provoking message to your stomach (creating butterflies). In turn, your stomach may send similar messages to the back of your neck (triggering stiffness), your heart (causing palpitations) and your hands (resulting in sweaty palms).

Medical researchers now recognize that it is impossible to separate the mind's health from the body's health. What you believe, think or feel will affect your body in the short and long term, and a growing number of experts strongly suspect that you can use your mind not only to ward off illness but also to heal yourself when you get sick.

USING YOUR MIND

● **Tap into your power of choice.** To combat feelings of helplessness and powerlessness— in the workplace, in personal relationships or in your health care—make informed, intelligent choices.

Example: In the area of health care, it's crucial to realize you can't allow yourself to be helpless, relying on practitioners or institutions to make the best choices for you or to ensure your long-term health. You need to take charge.

When you see your doctor, make sure you're armed with information about your condition. Visit your public or hospital library …read medical journal articles…check out online sources, such as HealthWorld (*www. healthy.net)*, which provides access to articles on medical conditions.

By making informed choices in every area of your life—and by acting rather than being acted upon—you will gain that important sense of control.

● **Listen to and trust your body.** Each day, I see patients who complain of sore throats or colds that just won't go away. When I ask them, *Have you taken time off work to get well?* the answer is almost always, *No.*

My message to them: *If you were any animal other than a human, you would listen and respond to your body telling you to rest. You would find a resting place somewhere, curl up and go to sleep until you felt better.*

Too often our "intelligent" mind tells us we absolutely must finish a project at work or we must devote a Saturday afternoon to coaching our child's soccer team, even though we're exhausted. We ignore the signals sent by our bodies and our more intuitive and wiser minds.

Symptoms of illness may be more than signs of a physical problem. Often, they are a signal that something is out of sync in your life, that some aspect of your approach to life needs changing.

If you're chronically tired or sluggish, your body may be telling you to exercise more or change your diet—or simply unplug your phone and crawl into bed for a healing rest.

When you learn to listen to and trust the messages your body sends, you will be taking an important step toward achieving optimal health.

• **Give your mind a rest.** Just as your body needs sleep for renewal and optimal health, your mind needs periods of quiet and solitude.

A quiet mind reveals important things about your life, changes you may need to make to create a healthier and richer lifestyle. Inner information such as this cannot break through constant mental chatter. A period of solitude "recharges" the brain and the body.

Helpful: I often tell people, especially working parents, to take a half day off from work …or spend a Saturday alone…or go to a retreat or spa for a weekend and reflect, read, walk or listen to music.

• **Confide in a friend and/or keep a journal.** When you think only about your problems, it's likely that you'll end up obsessing about them —and feeling even more stressed.

Helpful: Spend time with a trusted friend, sharing your innermost fears, your sadness over the loss of a loved one or your feelings of anger or bitterness about a problem at work. Research shows that something as simple as social support greatly enhances one's health.

Or spend 15 to 20 minutes every evening writing in a journal. Research shows that talking with a close friend about your feelings or writing them down greatly relieves stress. Writing also imposes order on a particular situation, so you are more able to resolve problems.

I've kept a journal for 20 years and when I look back on what I've written, I discover thought and behavior patterns—good ones and bad ones. I see decisions I've made and directions I've taken. Often I realize that I need to change certain patterns in order to achieve a more truly healthful life.

• **Look for meaning in every part of your life.** Finding meaning in one's life, studies show, is an essential part of good health. While it's easy to discover meaning in the positive aspects of your life, such as your loving relationship with your children and joy in your work, it is difficult to find meaning and purpose in life's difficulties and crises.

When you face a difficult situation at work or in a personal relationship, rather than feeling powerless or angry or resentful, ask, *Is there something I can learn from this situation?*

When you find positive meaning in every aspect of your life and start to realize that there is a greater force operating, you begin to develop the spirituality essential for true health.

• **View health as a lifelong process.** Most of us think of "health" as the absence of disease. But health is much more than being symptom-free and more than fixing what's broken. Everything we do, feel or experience plays a role—good or bad—in our health.

I like to think of health as an art—a lifelong process of developing, shaping and composing our lives.

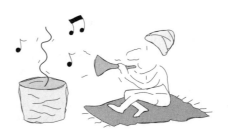

How to Make Your Mind Very Sharp

Harry Lorayne, who can memorize every person's name in a room of 500 people and recite from memory random pages of the latest issue of *Time* magazine. He is author of several books on memory, including *The Memory Power Package*, as seen on television.

I am over 70 years old. I can remember 500 names at a time or numerals consisting of an almost infinite number of digits. When I'm not applying my memory systems, then my memory isn't as good as when I was young. But, when I am using my memory systems, I remember better than anyone alive today!

You can use my systems to *regain* memory. Bob Norland did. He wrote to me when he was 75. Bob had had a stroke, and doctors told him he would never be able to remember again. His daughter brought him my systems. Now 80, Bob still works, but can't write with his right hand. So when he takes orders on the phone, he must rely on his memory for names, order numbers, prices and phone numbers.

When I was just starting out back in the 1950s, the big memory guru was David Roth. I first met him when he was 91. A few years later, he told me the Rotary Club was throwing him a party for his 94th birthday. He said, "I won't do much, just get everyone's name and telephone number...and repeat it back...person by person."

He died at age 96, with his full mental capacity. Applying these ideas keeps you young.

ONE-A-DAY MENTAL EXERCISES

Mental exercises are the key to keeping your memory sharp. I do crossword puzzles regularly. I also do "one-a-day" mental exercises. They force me to think. *Here are three examples (answers at end of article)...*

1. Take a pad and pencil. Draw a line, from left to right, about one inch long. How can you make it shorter without erasing, cutting or folding the paper?

2. Chickens are 50 cents each, ducks are three dollars each and turkeys are 10 dollars each. You want to spend exactly 100 dollars, but also take home 100 birds. How many of each bird should you buy?

3. Look at the Roman numeral IX. How can you add one symbol, and make the number 6?

WORKING THE "SYSTEMS"

All you need to do to use my systems effectively is stay alert and aware. They're based on ancient memory systems going back to Aristotle, with a few twists of my own. I use these systems constantly, whether walking down the street, driving or waiting in line. *Here's how to start...*

●**Original awareness.** You can't forget something if you never remembered it in the first place. *Turn that around, and you've got the solution to remembering:* If you remember something originally, how can you forget it?

●**Observation.** Essential to *original awareness*—anything you wish to remember must first be observed.

●**Association.** This is the best way to sharpen your observation, and thus your *original awareness.*

In order to remember any new piece of information, it must be associated to something you know or remember in a ridiculous way.

●**Linkage.** Once you *associate* an item by picturing it in a *ridiculous* way, you can *link* it to anything else. That's how you can remember long sequences.

Let's say you want to remember the following six words, in sequence—airplane, tree, envelope, earring, bucket, sing. *Here's how...*

Airplane: Picture an airplane. Now you want to link "airplane" to "tree." Think of a ridiculous image that connects, or associates, those two things in your mind's eye.

Examples: A gigantic tree flying instead of a plane...an airplane growing up out of the earth like a tree...airplanes growing on trees...millions of trees as passengers boarding an airplane. These are crazy, impossible pictures.

Envelope: Picture millions of envelopes growing on a tree. See it clearly, just for a second.

Earring: You open an envelope and millions of earrings fly out and hit you in the face. Or you're wearing envelopes on your ears instead of earrings.

Bucket: A gigantic bucket is wearing earrings.

Sing: The gigantic bucket is singing.

Putting it all together: Your first image is of an airplane. Then a gigantic tree is flying out of an airplane. When you think of tree, your next "link" is of millions of envelopes growing on a tree. You open an envelope and millions of earrings fly out. A gigantic bucket is wearing earrings. The gigantic bucket is singing. Practice thinking of those images, and you'll have the sequence. Using the same method, you can remember 10, 15, 20 or 30 or more items in sequence.

MAKING THE CONNECTION

Making your pictures ridiculous is key. *Four ways to do that are...*

●**Substitution.** Picture one item instead of the other. *For example,* imagine a tree flying instead of an airplane.

●**Change proportion.** Try to see items larger than life. That's why many of my suggestions are "gigantic."

●**Exaggeration.** That's why I often suggest you see "millions" of an item.

●**Action.** Action is always easy to remember. The *link,* tying ridiculous images to each item, can work with *anything.*

You can even do it with numbers. It's easy, once you learn how to associate each number with a specific image.

For names, even foreign words, you make your image by substitution.

Example: Let's say you want to remember the states in alphabetical order. After "Minnesota" comes "Mississippi." How to link them? Well, you can't picture Minnesota, but you can picture a "mini soda." Now, imagine a "Mrs. Sipping" a "mini soda." So, when you think of mini soda (Minnesota) you will automatically think of a Mrs. Sipping (Mississippi).

We all forget mundane things. It's the unusual, the obscene, the violent that we remember.

That's what makes the systems work.

The use of images in memory systems isn't new. Aristotle wrote, "We must speculate with images."

I added the ridiculous aspect. For kids it's not a problem. I asked a bunch of kids to visu-alize a piano coming out of their ears. Adults sometimes have a problem with that. But kids don't. One said, "I saw a piano coming out of my ear and a platypus was playing it!"

Society dulls your imagination. Don't let it!

Answers to one-a-day exercises: 1) Draw a line above it that is two inches long. The first line is shorter. 2) 94 chickens, one duck, five turkeys. 3) Add a capital S. Now you have: SIX.

How to Stimulate Your Cerebellum

Arthur Winter, MD, FICS, a neurosurgeon at the New Jersey Neurological Institute, Livingston, NJ. He is coauthor of *Build Your Brain Power—The Latest Techniques to Preserve, Restore and Improve Your Brain's Potential.* St. Martin's Press.

The cerebellum lies at the back of the skull, beneath the cerebrum. It is responsible for coordinating body movements, and is particularly vulnerable to age.

Helpful: Practice new motor skills to stimulate the region.

Cerebellum test: Stand with your hands at your sides and close your eyes. Touch your nose with one index finger then the other. Repeat four times.

Do this exercise and at least some of the ones listed below daily:

●**Charades** (which substitutes body control for speech).

●**Pat your head with one hand and rub your stomach with the other** for a count of 20—then reverse hands and repeat.

●**Use a pair of scissors to cut out a picture** from a newspaper or magazine, sticking as closely to the outline as possible.

●**Try to stack 100 pennies** or dimes as high as you can before they tumble.

●**Play tennis or go bowling**—both sports require coordinating body movements and vision.

●**Listen to dance music** (this actually stimulates the "dancing" areas of the brain).

Mind–Body Made Easy

David W. Freeman, editorial director, *Bottom Line/ Health*, 281 Tresser Blvd., Stamford, CT 06901.

We've all heard about the health benefits of meditation and other mind/body techniques. But who has time to practice these techniques?

We all do, says Gloria Keeling, president of the Mind/Body Fitness Training Institute in Maui, Hawaii. *Even if you can't always find time to meditate, the following strategies can easily be incorporated into your daily routine...*

●**Start each day with a positive thought.** Don't get out of bed until you've had one. *Example:* "I am a healthy, loving person." If you can do so without disturbing your bedmate, say the affirmation out loud.

●**When brushing your teeth, *only* brush your teeth.** Focus on the taste of the toothpaste, the feel of the foam, etc. Practice this type of "mindfulness" whenever you wash the dishes, make the bed, etc.

●**Practice "eating meditation."** Eat slowly. Savor the taste and texture of each bite. You'll enjoy food more...and make more healthful food choices.

●**When someone talks to you, focus all your attention on what he/she says.** Do not think about how you'll respond. Good listeners are good thinkers—and have better relationships.

●**Do "mini-checkups."** While driving or doing chores, notice how you feel. If you feel anxious or tired, spend a few minutes doing deep breathing.

●**Get outside.** Stargaze. Walk barefoot. Listen to birds singing, water flowing, etc. Affirm your connection to nature.

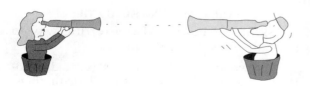

Empower Yourself

Jane Shuman, motivational speaker, Shuman & Associates, 2475 Boxwood Ln., Aurora, IL 60504.

Empower yourself by visualizing and affirming what you want to have happen—*as though it has happened already*. Pick a situation in which you want to have more control. Relax. Breathe deeply and quietly. Visualize the situation in as much detail as possible. Imagine yourself having a powerful, positive response to it. Focus on the image of your success daily until you actually meet the challenge.

The Healing Power of Friendship

Jacqueline Olds, MD, assistant clinical professor of psychiatry at Harvard Medical School in Boston, and a psychiatrist in private practice in Cambridge, MA. She is coauthor of *Overcoming Loneliness in Everyday Life*. Birch Lane Press.

America is in the midst of a loneliness epidemic—and the isolation is undermining our health. Yet because our culture esteems self-reliance and abhors dependency, many of us are ashamed to admit we're lonely...and too proud to reach out.

In American society, saying you're lonely suggests that you're weak—or unable to attract friends. Yet total self-reliance is a myth, and loneliness is *not* a sign of weakness. It's an alarm system—a signal that we need to bring people into our lives.

A HIDDEN PROBLEM

Because of the stigma of admitting to loneliness, many people don't even *know* they're lonely—much less what to do about it.

They may call the problem "low self-esteem" and look to the past for solutions. What they really need to do is get more involved with the people around them. Of course, those who are too depressed to do so need to have their depression treated first.

Our seeming obsession with the most intimate details of strangers' lives—as evidenced

401

by the rise of "tell-all" television talk shows—is another manifestation of our isolation.

When you lack a circle of people you know well, gossiping about strangers is a way to fill the gap. But it isn't very satisfying.

HEALTH RISKS OF LONELINESS

Evidence is growing that loneliness has serious health consequences...

James House, PhD, a University of Michigan sociologist, reviewed studies of 37,000 people in the US, Sweden and Finland.

What he found: People who had no serious medical problems but who lived alone and/or had few friends were twice as likely to die over a decade as people who had more social connections.

•**A Duke University study found** that heart attack survivors who were married or had confidants had an 82% five-year survival rate. Those who had neither had a 50% five-year survival rate.

•**Ohio State University researchers have shown** that having a close circle of friends helps block stress-related declines in immune function, as measured by natural-killer cell activity.

INCREASING ISOLATION

Harvard's Robert Putnam has reported a serious decline in the number of Americans involved in church groups, political clubs, the Red Cross and similar community organizations.

A 1992 survey bolsters Putnam's contention. It found that 39% of Americans said they socialized with neighbors no more than once a year ...compared with 28% in 1974. It doesn't look as though this trend is going to change anytime soon.

Several college students have told me that having a significant relationship will only hinder their careers. Their priorities are so skewed that they see such a relationship as a burden that will make it hard to reach their "real" goals.

CULTIVATING FRIENDSHIPS

No matter how busy our lives, it's essential that we make room for others. Even if you're married, you need close friends *other* than your spouse. It's unreasonable to expect one relationship to meet all your emotional needs.

Even if your spouse *could* meet all your needs, it's risky to depend solely on him/her. What would happen to you if something happened to him?

Many people assume that a friendship forms naturally when we meet people we like and invite them to get together once in a while.

But liking someone and intending to get to know that person aren't enough. To grow, friendships need a context—a shared endeavor that provides regular contact.

INTEREST GROUPS

Interest groups can provide this environment—but only if they have a long-term focus. Helping out on a one-time political campaign doesn't give you the same sense of connection that you would get from helping on the park cleanup crew every week.

If you're shy about approaching new groups, consider inviting someone you already know to go *with* you to a meeting.

In addition to a context, friendships need some degree of mutual dependency and mutual obligation.

Examples: Watering each other's plants when one of you is out of town...holding a joint garage sale...looking after each other's kids for the afternoon...sharing a vegetable garden that joins two yards.

One obvious way to start this kind of exchange is to *offer* your help. Ask if you can bring some groceries by for a coworker who's sick, or collect mail for a neighbor who's out of town.

Even better approach: Ask for a favor. For many of us, this goes against the grain. We worry that people will stop liking us if we impose. This is one of the first cultural values we acquire in America.

More often than not, though, people are delighted to be asked for their assistance. Because you were willing to go out on a limb by asking them for help, they'll be more likely to turn to you when they need a hand.

STRENGTHENING FAMILY TIES

Asking for help is also a terrific way to strengthen bonds *within* families.

Example: My husband's 98-year-old grandmother seemed depressed at family gatherings.

She's still an excellent seamstress, so on one of these occasions we asked if she'd mind trying her hand at a pile of mending that had stacked up. Suddenly, she felt happy and useful. She left the gathering more cheerful than we'd seen her in months.

Even if your family is spread out across the country, working on shared projects will bring you closer together.

Example I: Geographically dispersed siblings can help each other catalog old family photos or compile oral histories.

Example II: Families can take on charitable causes that hold particular meaning for them—such as contributing to the American Liver Foundation if a relative needed a liver transplant.

Once we acknowledge our need for other people, we open the door to a life that is healthier, more connected and more satisfying.

How the Great Self-Help Experts Help Themselves

Joan Borysenko, PhD, cofounder of the Mind/Body Clinic at New England Deaconess Hospital in Boston and president of Mind/Body Health Sciences in Boulder, CO. She is author of *Minding the Body, Mending the Mind* (Bantam) and *A Woman's Book of Life* (Riverhead).

Wayne Dyer, PhD, a reknown motivational speaker and author of numerous books, including *Your Erroneous Zones* (HarperCollins) and *A Promise Is a Promise* (Hay House).

Bernie Siegel, MD, founder of Exceptional Cancer Patients in Middletown, CT, which provides information and therapeutic support to people with life-threatening and chronic illnesses. He is author of several books, including *How to Live Between Office Visits.* HarperCollins.

The stress and tension that accompany the demands of work and family affect everyone today. Yet some of us handle the pressure better than others, by calmly dealing with the struggles we face.

To uncover the secrets of people who keep cool while pursuing excellence, three of the country's leading self-improvement experts share the techniques they use when tension strikes…

JOAN BORYSENKO, PhD

A demanding schedule that keeps me on the road about 200 days a year is a source of great pleasure and potential stress. Lectures and workshops for hospitals, corporations, churches and civic groups on topics ranging from medicine and psychology to spirituality, stress and women's health require constant research. There's a never-ending series of book-writing deadlines and production schedules for audiotapes, all of which make a busy life. And until five years ago, when my younger son left for college, I was also balancing family and career.

Research on stress hardiness reveals that when work is deeply meaningful—when we are committed and passionate about what we do—there is less stress. That is certainly true for me.

Self-defense: While attitude helps me manage stress, so do family, friends and health habits. Medical research shows that meaningful relationships are critical to health and well-being. Being in touch with friends and family is a priority for me—even if it means enormous phone bills when I call from abroad.

Health habits are important, too. But the busier and more stressed our lives become, the easier it is to make excuses for being couch potatoes.

Example: I live high in the Rocky Mountains, where I love to hike in the stark beauty and crystal-clear air. For me, hiking and yoga are priorities when I'm home. When I'm traveling, I have to be more creative. I specifically request hotel accommodations near hiking trails rather than in downtown areas…I take the stairs rather than the elevator…and I order take-out lunches and use the spare time to take walks.

Eating well is another challenge when life is hectic. I eat oatmeal and fruit for breakfast and adhere to a largely vegetarian, whole-foods diet to cut down on fat and junk.

Since I teach meditation and extol the benefits of prayer, I am fortunate that my work reinforces this great source of comfort and creativity.

Most mornings and evenings, I meditate, which reinforces my gratitude. During the day, I try to become aware of my breathing. Is it shallow stress breathing…or deep, energizing, relaxing breathing?

403

A few minutes of the latter makes a big physiological and psychological difference. And when I shift my breathing, it makes me more aware of what's on my mind. Am I complaining...or am I aware that life is the most precious gift?

When I remember to be grateful, it shifts me into the now. Stress is replaced by peace, and I realize that life—with all its joys and sorrows—is an incredible and awesome adventure.

WAYNE DYER, PhD

My life is full of stressful things—demanding writing deadlines, complex travel schedules and the special stress of canceled or delayed flights.

And...I'm a parent of eight children, ages six to 22—seven of whom live at home, which is where I work.

With a crush of obligations, it's important to realize that it is not *things* that make us upset. The events themselves are meaningless. It's how we react that counts. How we choose to process any event is entirely up to us. If we choose inner peace, we'll have peace.

Self-defense: To help change my thoughts and stress levels, meditation is the most important thing I do. Every day, I meditate for at least 20 minutes in the morning and again at night.

I also avoid a sedentary lifestyle, which can make me more susceptible to stress. To be in the natural flow of health, healing and love, we must move about.

Examples: Instead of driving to the store to buy milk, I walk. And when I went away for two months to write my latest book and my office was on the eighth floor, I made a commitment to use the steps, not the elevator. I also get up most days at 4:45 a.m. and run 12 to 15 miles.

When annoying things happen, I remind myself that the universe has a purpose and things happen for a reason.

If tensions or stress levels rise in a group situation, I excuse myself and find a quiet place to meditate for 10 minutes. By the time I come back, peace has usually returned.

And—I make sure to be inspired at all times. The word inspired comes from *in-spirit.* When you're inspired by what you do, you're removed from the stress of the physical realm and deep into what is called the *zone.* You have an overriding objective...and you are on track.

BERNIE SIEGEL, MD

As a doctor, I see many heartbreaking situations each day. To help me better understand and cope with them, I started keeping a journal years ago.

At first, I made notes to myself during the day. But after I got home, I did not always remember the details of the day. So I learned to write more elaborate notes to help my recollections. Despite my efforts, I was still unable to resolve my emotions. I knew the events were affecting me because I knew how my mind and body felt each evening.

To the rescue: Instead of viewing difficult events as stressful, I remembered what my mother had taught me—that difficulties are part of life...that they can be viewed as redirections...and that something good can come of them.

I began to realize that I have only one real problem—*me.* I found that I could refocus my thoughts by reminding myself that everything in life is fragile...that we are mortal and are here for just a limited period of time. By refocusing my thoughts, I am able to concentrate on what I truly love rather than be distracted by the details of everyday life. This is not about selfishness but about how we contribute our love to the world.

Another lesson that I have learned is that whatever happens in life will happen, regardless of what I think. I do not judge events as good or bad. Situations I might have shortchanged as "problems" or "failures" have redirected my life and led to things for which I am now grateful.

Helpful: Every morning, I go running for at least one hour and listen to my inner voice and any other voices that want to speak to me. I also leaf through inspirational books that I keep on a shelf in my office, reading a paragraph or two to keep refocusing on what is truly important. The *Hazelden Meditation Series* (Hazelden Publishing and Education) is particularly helpful.

Throughout the day, I meditate. My goal is to turn my entire day into a meditation. Once I can love enough and have enough faith, that will occur.

Several times a day, I stop to think about my behavior and how I am acting. I find that I'm never entirely happy with how I have behaved. But I forgive myself and continue to rehearse and practice—just as any athlete would do—to stay in touch with myself.

To stay in touch with my feelings, I keep a journal, and at least once a week, I write poetry or prose, paint pictures or construct something with my hands. These activities help me integrate what I'm experiencing rather than shut off events from my emotions.

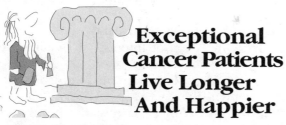

Exceptional Cancer Patients Live Longer And Happier

Bernie Siegel, MD, founder of Exceptional Cancer Patients in Middletown, CT, which provides information and therapeutic support to people with life-threatening and chronic illnesses. He is author of several books, including *How to Live Between Office Visits.* HarperCollins.

In more than 30 years as a surgeon, I treated thousands of cancer patients. Over the years, I noticed that while some of my patients denied their true feelings about their illnesses, others remained upbeat and insisted on taking responsibility for their lives.

These "exceptional" cancer patients managed to thrive emotionally despite being sick. In many cases, they fared better *physically* as well—outliving their less optimistic counterparts by months or years.

What's the secret of being an exceptional patient? Two factors are involved—*inspiration* and *information.* Even if you do not have cancer, pondering these eight questions—developed by George Solomon, MD—should inspire you and provide you with helpful information…

•Do I get a sense of meaning from my work, daily activities and relationships? People who dislike what they do often get sick as a result of the inevitable psychological stress

…or because sickness offers a convenient way out of an unpleasant situation. Each of us should work at something we see as contributing to the world.

I've seen many cancer patients suddenly quit their jobs and start doing what they always wanted to do. Many of these individuals lived longer, healthier lives.

Each of us must realize that despite the apparent constraints on our lives, we are free to do what we want to do.

•Am I able to express anger appropriately? When an infant isn't given what he/she wants, he bellows—for food, affection, a dry diaper, etc.

Like babies, adults deserve to be treated with respect and love. If we don't get treated that way, we must express our displeasure. We must tell others that we do not intend to let ourselves be stepped upon.

Sadly, most of us have been taught that expressing anger is wrong. We block our negative feelings instead, inhibiting our own healing powers and building up a reservoir of rage.

•Am I capable of asking friends and family (and my doctor) for help? You have an absolute right to ask for help whenever you need it. This goes for practical day-to-day items like food and transportation, as well as for emotional support when you're feeling sad or lonely.

Asking for help isn't a matter of selfishness. It's a matter of survival.

•Am I able to say "no" when asked for a favor I can't do—or do not feel like doing? Just as you have the right to ask others for favors, you have the right to decline requests from others.

Doing so doesn't mean you don't love the person asking the favor. It means you recognize that it's you alone who gets to choose how to spend your time.

Of course, your family and friends have every right to say no to your requests.

•Do I engage in health-promoting behaviors based on *my* needs? Others have no right to decide what you should or shouldn't do regarding exercise, diet, the treatments you seek (or don't seek), etc. You alone do.

Listen to others, but don't be afraid to follow your own path.

●**Do I spend enough time playing?** By play, I mean any activity so enjoyable that it causes you to lose track of time. If you can lose track of time, you won't feel as if you're ill for the duration of the play—no matter how dire your prognosis.

●**Do I frequently feel depressed and/or hopeless?** Many cancer patients fall into the trap of getting depressed *about* being depressed. Instead, you must confront your depression and learn from it.

You may need antidepressants and/or psychotherapy. No matter what, *learn* from the darkness—and accept that having cancer actually gives you a sense of freedom.

●**Am I dutifully playing a role while neglecting my own needs?** Many people identify themselves only by the roles they play—husband or wife, mother or father, valued employee, etc.

When these individuals are no longer able to play that role because of cancer, they lose all sense of identity.

I often ask cancer patients, "How would you introduce yourself to God?" If you introduced yourself as a lawyer or a teacher, I think God would say, "Come back when you've learned who you really are." Each of us is a unique creation. We are much more than the obvious roles we play.

Intentional Healing: The Do-It-Yourself Way to Perfect Health

Elliott S. Dacher, MD, a fellow of the Institute of Noetic Sciences, Sausalito, CA. He is author of *Intentional Healing: A Guide to the Mind/Body Healing System* (Marlowe & Co.) and *Whole Healing* (Dutton).

To most people the word "healing" means doctors and drugs—regaining health with the help of others.

But the most powerful kind of healing is what we do for ourselves, by our own thoughts and actions, by the way we live.

This *Intentional Healing* is based on a conscious decision to maximize well-being. *Instead of passively enduring the physical ravages of stress, suffering the consequences of bad health habits and allowing negative emotions to plague our days and nights, we...*

●**Tap into the powers** that are naturally within us.

●**Take control of our minds and bodies** to use these powers to the maximum.

If you're in good health, Intentional Healing will help you stay that way. If you're ill, it can combine with medical care (if needed) to make you well.

KEYS TO HEALING

The twin pillars of Intentional Healing are *mindfulness* and *self-regulation*.

Mindfulness is becoming aware of what your mind is doing.

Self-regulation is harnessing the mind's power to ease your body into a healthier state.

Most people go through life barely conscious of the thoughts and feelings that course through their minds. But many of these thoughts and feelings are destructive.

Examples: Worry, anger and fear all tighten muscles, tax the circulation and trigger the release of stress hormones that in time take their toll on every system of the body.

MEDITATION

Mindfulness involves *waking up* to what's going on in your mind, observing patterns of thought and patterns of feeling in order to change and control them.

The first step to mindfulness is a daily meditation exercise...setting time aside to stop, be still and listen to what's going on within your mind. *For 30 minutes each day...*

●**Sit in a quiet place, eyes closed,** hands comfortably on your thighs. Take a deep breath and then breathe normally, counting each cycle of inhalation and exhalation up to 10. Do this three times.

●**Now focus your attention on your abdomen,** how it rises and falls with each inhalation and exhalation.

●**When thoughts enter your mind, simply observe them** without getting caught up in them. Let them pass. Then turn your attention back to your breathing.

●**If you feel restless, bored or uncomfortable, observe these feelings, too.** Then, when your mind quiets, focus again on your breathing.

You may feel extremely relaxed and peaceful after a few minutes...or you may not. There's no right or wrong way to feel...the point of the exercise is simply learning *to experience the present*.

IN THE MOMENT

Everyday life offers constant opportunities to practice mindfulness. *Examples...*

●**When you eat,** slow down. Eat slowly and mindfully, to keep your digestive system in a relaxed condition. Be aware of the color and aroma of the food. Note the feeling of each mouthful, the changing subtleties of flavor and texture, the movement of your jaws, the sensation of swallowing.

●**When you wash the dishes,** be conscious of the way each plate and utensil feels, the sensation of water on your skin. Be aware of your thoughts in a detached way, then return your full attention to the task at hand.

●**When talking with others,** pay complete attention. Erase judgments and reactions from your mind...instead of planning your response, be silent and listen fully to what the other person has to say.

LEARNING TO REGULATE YOUR BODY

Health is a natural result when your body functions in a balanced way, neither too revved up nor too fatigued. We run into trouble when external pressures and events—or our own feelings (particularly anxiety) disrupt the balance. That creates stress...widely recognized as a villain in a host of illnesses, from eczema to backache to heart attack.

By learning to regulate your own body, you cease to be at the mercy of health-destroying stress. Whenever you wish, you can ease your body into a healthy balance.

●**Relaxation** is a critical skill. Many people find that regular practice of mindfulness makes them more relaxed and eases stress. Practice an exercise called complete breathing...

Sit in a straight-backed chair. Close your eyes and place both hands on your abdomen. Feel your hands rise as you inhale deep down into your abdomen, making it expand as if it were a balloon. Continue breathing in to fill your chest with air—feel your chest muscles expand. Draw in more air so your shoulders rise slightly.

Release the breath, allowing it to flow smoothly out of the chest, then slowly contract your abdomen to expel the rest of the air.

Repeat the cycle 10 times. Do three groups of 10 complete breaths.

●**Healthy lifestyle.** This is another important way to take control of your body. By exercising regularly, you reduce stress, strengthen your heart and circulatory system and enhance the activity of your immune system.

Brisk walking, at least 20 minutes, four times a week, is a sensible, healthy exercise schedule.

The foods you eat have a significant effect on how your body functions. Choose a diet that will promote the health of your heart, arteries and digestive system...

Build your diet around fresh fruits and vegetables, and unprocessed foods rich in carbohydrates and fiber.

●**Keep animal fats to a minimum.**

●**Reduce your intake of salt.**

●**Drink lots of water.**

●**Have modest-sized meals.**

CREATE A HEALTHY LIFE

Our *attitudes* have a constant impact on our bodies.

Greed, selfishness and contentiousness generate relentless stress. But when we resolve to live at peace with the world and other people, we create for ourselves an environment that promotes healing. *Strive for...*

●**Contentment.** This mental attitude finds satisfaction in what life gives you. This doesn't mean abandoning your goals, but being patient with the pace of progress, enjoying each day.

●**Simplicity.** This requires you to know the difference between what you want and what you need. The simpler you make your life, the less turmoil you will cause yourself.

●**Honesty.** Be honest with yourself and all around you.

●**Harmlessness.** Abstain from actions and words that injure others. Make a conscious choice to nurture feelings of goodwill toward everyone.

●**Solitude.** Only when outside noise quiets down can you listen to your mind and body. Spend a half hour a day alone in a quiet room or out in nature. Give yourself space for reflection…it's as necessary for healing as food or sleep.

For Deep Relaxation: Yoga Made Very Simple

Alice Christensen, president of the American Yoga Association, 513 S. Orange Ave., Sarasota, FL 34236. She is author of *20-Minute Yoga Workouts*. Ballantine.

If you're chronically anxious or simply feel "stressed out," consider giving yoga a try. This 5,000-year-old system of exercise, breathing and meditation is wonderfully effective at clearing the mind and easing muscular tension.

It also fosters a profound sense of self-confidence—a feeling that you can handle whatever comes your way.

BASIC YOGA PROGRAM

A basic program takes about 20 minutes each day. Some people prefer doing yoga in the morning. Others prefer early evening. Either way is okay. Just make sure you do it at the same time of day—every day.

The only "equipment" you'll need is a quiet room…loose, comfortable clothing…and a blanket, large towel or another pad on which to sit comfortably.*

YOGA BREATHING

To help focus your attention inward, start with two minutes of "complete breath" exercises.

Sit cross-legged on a firm cushion on the floor, or find another seated position in which your back is straight but relaxed.

*For more information on yoga, or to order videos or audiotapes, contact the American Yoga Association.

Begin inhaling slowly and deeply through the nose. Relax your belly so that it expands with each incoming breath, and let your chest and ribcage expand. At the very "top" of each inhalation, your shoulders will lift slightly. At this point, exhale by relaxing your shoulders and then your ribs. Then tighten your belly to squeeze the air out. Relax and repeat.

Important: When we breathe ordinarily, each inhalation lasts longer than each exhalation. With yoga breathing, inhalation and exhalation should take the same amount of time.

Breathe *in* for a count of five…then *out* for a count of five until you've established a rhythm. Then focus on the sound of your breath.

ARM AND SHOULDER STRETCHES

These three stretches—each done while standing—loosen the joints and ease muscular tension.

●**Arm roll.** Hold your arms out to the side, elbows straight, hands held up as if stopping traffic. Rotate your arms forward in three large circles, then backward in three large circles. Then do three *small* circles in each direction.

●**Head roll.** With arms at your sides, bend your head forward while relaxing the muscles in the back of your neck. Slowly tilt your head to one side, then back, then to the other side, then to the front.

Do this head rotation three times clockwise, then three times counterclockwise.

●**Side stretch.** Keep your feet slightly more than shoulder-width apart, with arms held out to the side. Inhale deeply. Then exhale as you bend to the right. Slide your right hand down your right thigh toward the knee, and bring your left arm overhead. Breathe in, and return to an upright position.

Do the same stretch on your left side. Repeat three times on each side.

SPINE STRETCHES

These poses are especially beneficial if you work at a desk.

●**Sun pose.** Stand with feet together. As you inhale, raise your arms from the side until they're overhead. Look upward. Exhale as you bend from the waist. Reach as far forward as you comfortably can, and grasp your ankles, calves or knees.

Hold for a moment, then inhale as you return to an upright position, raising arms to the side until they're overhead. Lower arms in a circle as you exhale. Repeat twice.

●**Baby pose.** Sit on your feet. Slowly bend forward until your head approaches the floor. Let your arms rest at your sides with elbows bent. Hold for at least one minute.

●**Corpse pose.** Lie on your back with feet slightly apart and arms at sides, palms up. Close your eyes. Relax your entire body, paying particular attention to the face and stomach. Rest for at least one minute.

YOGA MEDITATION

Meditation teaches us to *observe*—rather than worry about or act upon—the thoughts that constantly flit through our minds.

This lets us withdraw from the never-ending bombardment of desires, fears, regrets, etc.… and find peace by turning our attention solely to the present moment. Start by lying face up on your pad, with arms at sides, palms up. Remain as still as possible.

For the next two minutes or so, focus on each part of your body in turn. Envision each part separately…and relax it.

Start with your forehead, then your eyes, face, neck and shoulders. Move down your body, relaxing each in turn—arms and hands…chest and abdomen…hips, legs and feet…then back up the spine to the neck and head.

Gently bring your attention to your forehead. Silently repeat "om" several times.

Your aim is to think of nothing. If thoughts intrude, don't worry—and don't try to *force* them to stop. Gently return your attention to the experience of silence.

Trap: The more you fight to *control* your thoughts, the harder your thoughts will resist you. Instead, just observe the thoughts as if they were passing by in the distance.

After meditating for 10 minutes or so, open your eyes. Wiggle your fingers and toes, open and close your fists. Take a deep breath. Stretch your arms and legs. Your yoga session is over.

As you become more skilled at meditation, you should be able to *remember* and *reproduce* the feeling at will—to achieve instant relaxation anytime, anywhere.

Midlife Wisdom

Kathryn Cramer, PhD, psychologist and founder of The Cramer Institute, which helps individuals and organizations master transition and change, 10411 Clayton Rd., Suite 305, St. Louis, MO. She is author of *Roads Home: Seven Pathways to Midlife Wisdom*. William Morrow & Co.

Restlessness, boredom, physical and emotional changes, a lack of creativity and/or a sense of something looming on the horizon are often signs of a midlife crisis.

I call them the *readiness signals* that tell you to begin a journey to midlife wisdom—which happens by traveling seven important pathways.

MENTAL MASTERY

Mastery is your ability to capitalize on your accumulated knowledge and experience to solve problems.

Conscious attention to the details of your life will lead to better judgment in problem-solving. However, experts say that today we are bombarded with information at 1,000 times the rate our grandparents were.

We decide which of these bits of information to notice or ignore in the first place—but most of us don't realize that we've overdeveloped this skill because we've done a lot of selective *not noticing* by midlife.

Helpful: To become more aware of the details in your life, ask yourself these questions at the end of each day:

●**What did I learn today?** Be specific. Write down what you accomplished, what you thought and said. Recall any new skill or understanding you acquired.

●**How did I learn what I learned?** This will help you pinpoint how you learn best and most naturally.

●**How can I increase the use of this type of learning in my everyday life?** If you find yourself learning through reading, consider expanding your reading to other areas.

PHYSICAL VIGOR

There are two reasons that people who are between the ages of 35 and 65 must tune in to how they feel about their bodies…

●**The physical component of your journey** is intricately tied to all the other components. Your mind, emotions and relationships

409

cannot be at their peak if your body is not functioning at least near its best.

● **Much of what upsets midlifers can be fixed or improved upon.**

These simple habits can have a powerful impact on your physical and mental well-being…

● **Eat breakfast daily.**

● **Avoid snacking.**

● **Maintain your ideal weight.**

● **Exercise regularly.**

● **Sleep seven to eight hours a night.**

● **Don't smoke.**

● **If you drink, drink moderately.**

EMOTIONAL VITALITY

To remain emotionally healthy, you must be able to recover from past and present disturbing situations and enrich your connections to people and events.

I've found that during the first half of life, experiences of joy usually emanate from events that go your way.

During the second half of life, however, emotionally healthy adults are capable of experiencing true joy despite the bad things that might happen to them. We lose the grandiosity of youth that says we can and must be the force at the center of life.

Unfortunately, most of us have little emotional training before midlife, so we have trouble responding competently to anger, pain and fear.

Helpful: Write down what disturbs you about an experience for which you would like to have a different emotional response. Recall childhood experiences that triggered similar negative feelings. How did you react? Feel the pain of not expressing your feelings as a child. Feel compassion for the child you were.

INTERPERSONAL EFFECTIVENESS

Interacting well with others requires that we be able to establish caring relationships and unify the strong and sensitive aspects of our personalities.

Example: Are you happy when you give someone a gift? For mature adults, the satisfaction of giving a gift far outweighs the thrill of receiving one. In fact, experts call this altruism the hallmark of maturity and the foundation of satisfying relationships.

Many midlifers have problems stemming from a lack of this altruistic development. Some couples have lost their ability to reach out to each other in truly compassionate ways. Or parents don't know how to be compassionate toward their teenage children.

Helpful: Select a person you feel is an adversary. Write down traits you admire and traits you loathe. Then write a few sentences about your adversary as though you have no feelings toward him/her. Be objective and detached.

Reflect on the admirable, negative and neutral traits you assigned to your adversary. Pretend you're getting to know this person for the first time.

Watch for insights as a result of your more balanced view. Once you have achieved emotional distance from this person, try approaching him anew, emphasizing the attractive and neutral traits over the negative. You'll see your former opponent's viewpoint more clearly.

EXCEPTIONAL COMPETENCE

We need to perform complex tasks, assume leadership and mentor roles and contribute significantly to the world based upon our talents and desires.

By the time we hit midlife, we've become good at tasks we have performed for years. Use this competence to free your time and attention and get focused on the important goals of the second half of your life. It is a time to confirm or readjust priorities and develop a vision, as you did when you were young.

Important: Do not compare your successes and failures with those of others. This will deflate or inflate your view of yourself unnecessarily. You will underestimate the value of what you have done, or you may end up with a false sense of superiority that will squelch your motivation.

SPIRITUAL SERENITY

Midlife spiritual anxiety is exceedingly normal. If we don't struggle to find more satisfying answers to age-old questions about life and our mortality, we risk facing old age with fear and anger as our main companions. *Helpful…*

● **Come to terms with life.** Our mortality is less frightening when we feel we have made the most of our lives.

●**Give in to feelings about your mortality.** Crystallizing your feelings can lead to a clearer sense of life purpose and a greater degree of life satisfaction.

PERSONAL INTEGRITY

Being happy with yourself and your work requires personal integrity, an integration of the many parts of your personality working together as one cohesive whole. People with personal integrity don't act one way at work and another way at home. They have the same standards of honesty, behavior and emotional response wherever they are.

Strive to bring out the best in yourself and others. Remind yourself to help others who need help, and be generous with your time and energy. Your reputation and enthusiasm will soar.

Four-Step Plan for Beating Obsessions and Compulsions

Jeffrey M. Schwartz, MD, associate research professor of psychiatry at UCLA School of Medicine. He is author of *Brain Lock: Free Yourself from Obsessive-Compulsive Behavior*. HarperCollins

---

You're not sure you turned off the stove, so you go home to check. After you leave again, you're *still* unsure. What if the house burned down? So you check *again*. And *again*. This is classic *obsessive-compulsive* behavior. Dread arising from intrusive thoughts (obsessions) leads to repetitive behavior (compulsions).

One of my patients washed his hands 100 times a day. He knew they were clean but couldn't shake the feeling they were dirty...and scrubbed until his hands were cracked and raw.

Five million Americans suffer from *obsessive-compulsive disorder* (OCD), whose symptoms make daily life exceedingly difficult. Countless more have minor obsessions and compulsions they would like to get rid of.

Examples: Getting up at night to check and recheck a lock...rereading the same passage to make sure you got every word...having unspeakable thoughts of violence that you can't get out of your mind.

We've made great strides in pinpointing the cause of the maddening symptoms...and developing a therapy that really helps.

A GLITCH IN THE BRAIN

OCD is caused by a biochemical imbalance in the *caudate nucleus*, a region of the brain whose function is to control another part of the brain called the *orbital cortex*.

Ordinarily, the orbital cortex serves as a sort of "error-detection system." When the caudate nucleus malfunctions, the orbital cortex is left stuck in the "on" position. This "brain-lock" condition creates a "something-is-amiss" feeling that won't go away.

To the rescue: My four-step program can control OCD within a matter of weeks.

STEP 1: RELABEL

Since obsessions and compulsions won't go away of their own accord, your first step is to *relabel* them by making mental notes.

If you feel compelled to count all the blue cars you pass on the highway, for example, tell yourself, "I don't *need* to count the blue cars. I'm having a *compulsive* urge to do so."

This inner dialogue brings you back to reality. By *observing* your brain—neither giving in to the compulsion nor pretending it doesn't exist—you bolster your "Impartial Spectator." That's the innermost part of your personality...and what will allow you to conquer OCD.

STEP 2: REATTRIBUTE

The next step answers the question, "Why won't these terrifying thoughts, urges and behaviors go away?" *Reattribute* these symptoms to their true cause—a biochemical imbalance in the brain.

Think of OCD anxiety as a mental alarm system—with a hair-trigger. The siren may wail incessantly, but that *doesn't* mean you must pay attention to it.

Helpful: Silently reflect on the phrase, "It's not me, it's OCD." Doing so stresses the distinction between your thoughts and fears... and your real self.

Once you learn to separate yourself from your urges and anxieties, you can *choose* not to act on them.

STEP 3: REFOCUS

Each time your obsession or compulsion resurfaces, *refocus* your attention on a pleasurable, constructive activity—taking a walk... gardening...doing needlepoint...listening to music...playing a computer game.

Your goal is to pursue the activity for at least 15 minutes. At first, however, you may be able to go no longer than five minutes.

The longer you refrain from acting on a compulsive urge, the weaker it becomes. Even if you ultimately give in, you still come out ahead. You're learning to tolerate psychological discomfort...and building up your power to say "no." This is profoundly empowering.

STEP 4: REVALUE

The more diligently you practice relabeling, reattributing and refocusing, the more fully you'll recognize your obsessions and compulsions for what they are—worthless distractions having no value whatsoever.

This process will gradually become automatic. Without even thinking, you'll be able to devalue the thoughts and urges and fend them off until they fade.

BENEFITS OF THIS METHOD

Some people experience a profound sense of relief after using my four-step technique for only a single day. For most people, however, it takes about eight to 10 weeks.

Do *not* expect your urges to go away completely. Each incremental improvement—you put off checking the lock for five minutes—brings you closer to full control. Praise yourself for each step forward!

The four-step method is more than a behavioral technique—it has physiological effects. Studies using *positron emission tomography* (PET) show that in individuals who practice the four-step method, brain function returns to normal.

WHAT ABOUT MEDICATION?

Some recently developed drugs—including the antidepressants *fluoxetine* (Prozac) and *fluvoxamine* (Luvox) and the antianxiety drug *buspirone* (BuSpar)—greatly weaken the fear that makes OCD urges so hard to resist.

I think of these drugs as "training wheels"—a useful aid when you're just getting acquainted with the four-step method.

Once you master my program and your brain biology begins to change, you'll be able to reduce the dosage...or give up the drugs completely.

22

Natural Ways and Herbal Solutions

Herbal Teas...
How to Grow Them and
Brew Them, Too

Marietta Marshall Marcin

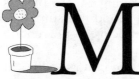

Many herbs can be used for tea. Although they won't reach the fullness or height they would outdoors, you can grow them indoors. Simply choose a spot where the plants will get plenty of sun—ideally a south-facing window that gets light all day.

HERBS THAT MAKE GREAT TEAS

Your gardening store likely stocks the seeds or will know a mail-order source. *Here are some of my favorites...*

•**Fennel seeds, leaves and root** are excellent stomach and intestinal remedies. When brewed, they also arouse appetite and expel mucus accumulations. The tea tastes like anise, peppermint and licorice.

•**Lemon balm tea** has been used for colic, cramps, bronchial catarrh, dyspepsia, some forms of asthma and headaches.

•**Mint tea** can be made from 30 different varieties. Mint teas relieve cramps, coughs, poor digestion, nausea, heartburn, abdominal pains, headaches and other ailments attributed to nerves.

•**Thyme tea** is ideal for calming nerves, alleviating indigestion and clearing the mucous membranes.

DRYING AND STORING

•**Using scissors**, cut leaves just before the flower forms for the fullest flavor and best leaf color when dried.

•**Wash leaves or branches quickly in cool water**...and lightly towel dry. Then spread on a mesh rack and place in a slow oven set at 100° to 125°. Leave the oven door open, and stand nearby, as the leaves dry in just a few minutes.

Marietta Marshall Marcin, a gardener in Winnetka, IL, who grows 34 herbs in her garden. She is author of several books, including *The Herbal Tea Garden: Planning, Planting, Harvesting & Brewing.* Storey Communications.

Or dry them in a microwave on a very low setting for one minute or less.

BREWING

Cover one teaspoon dried leaves—or three teaspoons fresh crushed herb—with one cup boiling water. Steep for 10 minutes and strain.

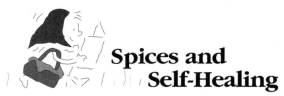

Spices and Self-Healing

James A. Duke, PhD, a botanist in Fulton, MD. He is now retired after spending 30 years at the US Department of Agriculture in Beltsville, MD. He is author of numerous books, including *The Green Pharmacy*. Rodale Press.

Did you know that celery seed fights gout? That bay leaves stop headache pain? We didn't know either—until noted botanist James A. Duke, PhD, shared with us his picks for the most useful medicinal spices*...

BAY LEAF

Good for: Migraines, diabetes.

Healing properties: Bay leaves are rich in pain-killing compounds called *parthenolides*.

They also contain a compound that boosts insulin's ability to control blood glucose.

Eating food seasoned with bay leaves helps prevent diabetes...and helps keep adult-onset (Type II) diabetics from worsening to the point that they need daily insulin shots.

How to use: Make a tea by steeping several bay leaves in hot water. Or add bay leaves to chicken or bean soup.

Caution: Bay leaves themselves should not be eaten.

CAYENNE

Good for: Chronic pain, arthritis, ulcers, bronchitis, colds, influenza.

Healing properties: Cayenne contains *capsaicin*, a compound proven to block Substance P. That's the brain chemical involved in transmission of pain impulses.

*Check with your doctor before using spices for medicinal purposes. Do *not* substitute "spice therapy" for medication prescribed by your physician.

Capsaicin also boosts the body's production of natural painkillers called *endorphins*...and destroys the ulcer-causing stomach bacterium *Helicobacter pylori*.

How to use: For pain relief, soak gauze in a hot pepper sauce containing cayenne, and apply it to the painful area. My wife has found this very effective for her back pain.

For ulcers or for blocked air passages, add one-half teaspoon hot pepper sauce or cayenne to hot lemonade, and drink.

CELERY SEED

Good for: Arthritis, gout.

Healing properties: Celery seed contains more than a dozen distinct anti-inflammatory compounds. The same compounds are found in celery stalks.

How to use: Take two capsules of celery seed extract (available in health-food stores). You can also eat four stalks of celery.

GARLIC

Good for: Heart disease, high blood pressure, impaired immunity.

Healing properties: One of nature's most potent antibiotics, garlic inhibits growth of fungi, yeast and bacteria—including strains that are becoming resistant to synthetic antibiotics.

Garlic also contains *allicin*, a compound that works like aspirin to thin the blood. Because of this blood-thinning effect—plus its proven cholesterol- and blood-pressure-lowering powers—garlic is effective at preventing atherosclerosis.

How to use: I add garlic cloves to almost every dish I cook. I also cook with chives, leeks and onions. All have properties similar to those of garlic.

Each time my grandchildren visit, I take garlic pills to ward off any infections they might have brought along with them.

Fearing bad breath, some people prefer "deodorized" garlic pills. But I'm convinced that the more a garlic pill stinks, the better it is for you.

Beware: If you take aspirin to prevent a heart attack, garlic may thin your blood too much. Discuss this with your doctor.

LICORICE

Good for: Enlarged prostate, ulcers.

Healing properties: *Glycyrrhizic acid*, the major active ingredient in licorice, prevents conversion of testosterone to dydrotestosterone. This reduces swelling of the prostate, thereby putting an end to frequent urination, the most common symptom of prostate enlargement.

Licorice also contains numerous antibacterial compounds, including some that kill ulcer-causing bacteria.

How to use: Munching on licorice candy will *not* work. That's because most licorice candy sold in the US is made with anise, not licorice.

Instead, use a piece of licorice root to stir your tea. The active ingredients will steep into the tea—and act as a natural sweetener, too.

You can also add licorice root extract to hot drinks. Licorice root and licorice root extract are available at health-food stores.

Caution: Too much licorice can raise blood pressure...and cause heart problems. If you have high blood pressure, consult a doctor before using licorice.

ROSEMARY

Good for: Alzheimer's disease.

Healing properties: Sometimes called the "herb of remembrance," rosemary contains five compounds that seem to prevent the breakdown of *acetylcholine*, a neurotransmitter that's deficient in patients with Alzheimer's.

I believe that rosemary works just as well as the Alzheimer's drug *tacrine* (Cognex). Tacrine works in only 25% of patients...and it can cause liver damage.

I also believe that eating rosemary can reduce one's risk of *developing* Alzheimer's.

How to use: Rosemary can be added to all sorts of recipes, including fish and chicken dishes.

Since there's evidence that rosemary can be absorbed through the skin, you might try tossing rosemary sprigs into your bath...using rosemary shampoo...and rubbing rosemary lotion into your skin.

Ginger for Upset Stomach...and More

Stephen Fulder, PhD, a biochemist and private research consultant in Galilee, Israel, and a former lecturer at London University. He is author of numerous books, including *The Ginger Book: The Ultimate Home Remedy*. Avery.

If you're like most Americans, the closest you get to ginger is an occasional glass of ginger ale.

But in many parts of Asia, ginger is highly valued as a medicine. It's part of daily life for billions of people—as a safe, effective home remedy for a variety of ailments, including stomach upset, the common cold and poor circulation.

Powdered ginger—the kind you find in the spice section at the supermarket—is potent enough. But fresh ginger is even more potent ...and organic fresh ginger more potent still. *Here's how to use ginger...*

•**Stomach upset.** A ginger "tea" made with one-third teaspoon of powdered ginger (or one teaspoon of grated ginger) in a cup of hot water with a squeeze of lemon provides fast relief for motion sickness, nausea, vomiting or simple indigestion.

You can also buy ginger capsules or tablets at health food stores. In that case, you'll want to take two 500-milligram (mg) capsules.

Ginger calms the stomach, stopping the sensation of nausea, and speeds the digestive process.

•**Common cold.** Take two cups of ginger tea (or two 500-mg capsules) three times a day.

•**Poor circulation.** For cold hands and/or feet, take one cup of ginger tea (or a 500-mg ginger capsule) once a day, preferably in the morning. You won't see results quickly—it's more of a preventive measure than a cure.

But don't wait for an illness to come along. I love to add a slice of fresh ginger to ordinary tea...or grate it into stir-fried vegetables. I take some every day. So should you.

Medicinal Herbs: Growing Your Own to Improve Physical and Emotional Health

Miranda Smith, horticultural writer and teacher at the New England Small Farm Institute, Box 180, Belchertown, MA 01007. She is author of *Your Backyard Herb Garden*. Rodale.

In recent years, we've come to appreciate anew the medicinal value of herbs. Used properly, herbs offer a safe, natural alternative to many drugs—to energize, relax, help wounds heal, etc.

Most people buy their herbs at a health food store. But many herbs are easy to grow, whether you've got a big backyard or just a few pots on a porch.

GARDENING IS GOOD FOR YOU

Gardening is a wonderful antidote for psychological stress...a source of solitude...a respite from everyday problems. And with all the digging, hoeing, etc., it gives a pretty good workout.

You might even discover that gardening is good for the spirit. It's one thing to *read* "all things are connected," quite another to *experience* it in your garden.

Tending your herbs every day, you see in concrete terms how sun, rain, soil and your own care affect your plants. You begin to feel as if you were an integral part of the rhythms of nature.

Herbs can be grown from seedlings or seeds. You can get them from a local nursery...or a mail-order company, such as Richters, 357 Hwy. 47, Goodwood, Ontario L0C 1A0. 905-640-6677, *www.richters.com*.

CHAMOMILE

This plant produces daisy-like flowers on stalks that grow up to three feet tall. Full sunlight is best, but it tolerates partial shade.

German chamomile grows erect and can be planted six to eight inches apart. *Roman* chamomile is low, with creeping stems. Allow 18 inches between plants.

Uses: Chamomile tea, prepared from freshly picked or dried chamomile flowers, is quite relaxing. Taken 15 minutes before bedtime, it induces sleep. Chamomile tea also calms cranky toddlers and eases teething pain.

Caution: If you're allergic to ragweed, avoid chamomile tea.

COMFREY

This bushy plant grows three to five feet high, with drooping tubular flowers that range in color from blue to yellow and cream. Comfrey prefers full sun but will grow in partial shade. Give each plant at least three square feet.

Uses: Comfrey is for *external* use only. A strong comfrey *decoction*—a tea-like solution used on the skin—promotes healing of cuts, burns and bruises.

FENNEL

This herb grows up to five feet tall, with tiny yellow flowers that appear at midsummer. Plant six inches apart, preferably in full sunlight.

Uses: Fennel tea aids digestion. It also reduces colic in infants...and flatulence in children and adults.

FEVERFEW

This hardy two-foot perennial bears white daisy-like flowers. Plant seedlings in full sun or partial shade, spacing them 12 inches apart. Feverfew thrives even indoors in a pot, as long as it gets direct sunlight.

Uses: A tea of feverfew leaves has been shown to reduce the severity *and* intensity of migraine headaches. It can be drunk up to three times a day, between meals. Or simply chew one to four fresh leaves a day.

Caution: Stop using if you develop mouth sores.

LAVENDER

This plant grows up to two feet tall. Its lovely flowers yield a sweet, clean fragrance. Plant in full sun or partial shade, one to three feet apart. It will grow in containers, too.

Uses: Lavender tea calms jangled nerves. A cold lavender tea compress relieves headaches.

LOVAGE

One lovage plant, which grows up to six feet tall, can supply your needs for a full year. It prefers partial shade.

Uses: Use lovage as you would use celery, in cheese and egg dishes, soups, stews, salads, etc. You can apply lovage tea to wounds as an antiseptic. Or—drink it to stimulate digestion.

MARJORAM

This plant grows one foot tall, with tiny white or pink blossoms. Space seedlings six to eight inches apart, in full sun if possible. It will grow in containers.

Uses: Marjoram tea helps settle an upset stomach. Use it lukewarm as a gargle for throat inflammation.

PENNYROYAL

This perennial grows up to one foot high, with bluish flowers. Set plants in full sun or partial shade, six to 10 inches apart.

Uses: Pennyroyal is a natural insect repellent. Rub the leaves on your skin…or put a bouquet of pennyroyal sprigs on your picnic table. Occasionally crush the leaves to release their bug-unfriendly fragrance.

Caution: Do not take pennyroyal internally. It is poisonous.

THYME

Thyme grows up to 15 inches high. Set groups of plants one foot apart, in full sun or partial shade.

Uses: Thyme tea settles the stomach. Also, add to bath water. Thyme's antiseptic qualities help raw, rough skin.

MAKING HERBAL TEA

Steep fresh or dried herbs for 20 minutes in a tightly stoppered container. Immediately refrigerate any unused portion.

Some herbs can cause stomach irritation, headache and other side effects. To start out, make an extremely weak tea. See how it affects you. Once you're confident that you can tolerate weak tea, increase the strength a bit to find what works best for you.

Flower Remedies

Jamison Starbuck, ND, a naturopathic physician in family practice and a lecturer at the University of Montana, both in Missoula. She is past president of the American Association of Naturopathic Physicians and a contributing editor to *The Alternative Advisor: The Complete Guide to Natural Therapies and Alternative Treatments.* Time Life.

Dried flowers of *calendula officinalis* are good for burns, cuts, scrapes, acne, tonsillitis and canker sores, vaginitis, rashes, athlete's foot and sunburn.

During the Civil War, these bright orange and yellow flowers provided the major line of defense against infection. Today you can buy dried calendula flowers, ointment, tincture or spray at most health food stores…or grow your own.

Calendula flourishes in almost any climate, whether it's planted in a pot or in the ground.

Most nurseries sell bedding plants in the springtime. Be sure to ask for *calendula officinalis*—not marigolds.

Flowers harvested between June and September are most potent. Dry them out of direct sun on a mesh screen for one to two weeks. Store in an airtight container.

Hot calendula tea helps soothe ulcers. Gargle with cool tea for inflamed tonsils or canker sores.

To make tea: Pour 10 ounces of boiling water over ⅔ cup of the flowers. Let it steep for 15 minutes. Or add five to 10 drops of calendula tincture to a cup of hot water.

Apply tincture or spray to rashes, cuts, scrapes or acne with a cotton ball. Spraying is good for sunburn, vaginitis and pinworms. Use ointment on scabs, eczema and psoriasis.

To make ointment: Melt ½ cup of petroleum jelly over low heat in a double boiler. Add a handful of dried calendula flowers. Heat on low for an hour. Strain out the herb and pour into a glass jar.

When to Consider Alternative Therapies

Timothy McCall, MD, a Boston internist, author of *Examining Your Doctor: A Patient's Guide to Avoiding Harmful Medical Care.* Citadel Press. He is a regular commentator on the public radio program Marketplace, and can be found on the Web at *www.drmccall.com.*

Consider alternative therapies if your ailments do not respond adequately to conventional medicine…and for stress-related problems like anxiety and insomnia. But do not abandon conventional medicine for unproven approaches marketed as homeopathic or natural. And—remember that even natural treatments have side effects. Some herbs and vitamins can cause problems if taken in large doses…in combination with certain other herbs and vitamins…or with conventional medicines.

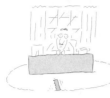

Treat Stress and Depression the Natural Way

Michael J. Norden, MD, clinical associate professor of psychiatry at the University of Washington, Seattle. He was among the first to publish medical accounts of the varied uses of Prozac and has been a pioneer in the integration of psychopharmacology and alternative treatments. Dr. Norden is author of *Beyond Prozac.* ReganBooks/HarperCollins.

The stress of modern life has given rise to a worldwide epidemic of depression. Mood disorders are more prevalent now than ever before, and they're occurring at younger ages.

What's causing this epidemic? Much of the blame may well rest with technology, and the sweeping lifestyle changes it has encouraged.

Our bodies and brains evolved for a Stone Age existence, when daily life was governed by the rising and setting of the sun and the changing of the seasons. Today, people seem to live at a breakneck pace, 24 hours a day, all year long.

Problem: Fast-paced living brings reduced levels of the neurotransmitter *serotonin*, a key buffer against depression.

On the advice of their doctors, many people have turned to antidepressants to relieve their malaise. For serious depression, that's prudent. However, it often makes more sense to find natural, nondrug ways to boost serotonin levels…

GET MORE LIGHT

Exposure to bright light has been shown to raise serotonin levels. Unfortunately, indoor lighting averages only 200 to 500 lux. That's too weak to do the trick. Outdoors, sunlight can climb above 100,000 lux.

Being exposed to artificial light *at night* (when our ancestors would have been asleep)

throws off the production cycle of *melatonin.* This key neurochemical affects a variety of bodily functions, including serotonin synthesis, making it another important buffer against depression.

Antidote: Get outdoors as much as possible during the day. If you live in a "gray" climate, consider buying a light box (10,000 lux). This device—available for $200 to $400—can be used while reading, exercising or watching TV.

Caution: Light boxes should not be used by people with retinal disease.

Best brands: Apollo Light Systems (800-545-9667), Hughes Lighting Technologies (800-544-4825) and The SunBox Company (800-548-3968).

Also helpful: Dawn simulators. These devices use light to awaken you naturally on dark winter mornings.

SEEK OUT NEGATIVE IONS

Air with high concentrations of negative ions—molecules with an extra electron—is clearly linked to positive moods. Unfortunately, city air contains 10 times fewer negative ions than air in the country or by the seashore. Ion concentrations are even lower inside air-conditioned offices.

Antidote: If you can't live in the country or near the ocean, buy a negative-ion generator. These devices boost serotonin levels, improving mood and promoting sleep.

Be sure the machine you buy generates *small* negative ions. That's the kind shown to yield psychological benefits.

Best brand: Bionic Products of America (800-634-4667).

GET MORE SLEEP

Adults today get 20% less sleep than before the invention of the electric light. Most of us need at least eight hours of sleep a night. Nearly 50% of Americans get less.

Sleep deprivation produces a sharp decrease in serotonin levels. It is strongly linked to depression.

Antidote: Make sleep a priority. If you feel sleepy during the day, or if you need an alarm clock to wake up, you probably need more shut-eye.

Strategies: Keep the bedroom cool and dark…avoid work or stimulating TV for at least one hour before bedtime…cut down on caffeine and alcohol…exercise late in the day (but at least five hours before bedtime)…rise at the same time each day. On days when you can't get the sleep you need, nap.

GET REGULAR EXERCISE

Exercise—an excellent serotonin booster—is linked not only with better moods, but also with better overall health. Yet despite the so-called "fitness revolution," Americans get less exercise today than even 10 years ago. We get far less exercise than our hunter-gatherer ancestors.

Antidote: Find an exercise you enjoy, and do it regularly. Aerobic exercise several times a week is ideal, but any kind of exercise is better than none.

RETHINK YOUR DIET

Our ancestors survived mostly on green plants and small game animals, which were low in fat but high in cholesterol.

Lesson: While some middle-aged men and others at high risk for heart attack should take steps to lower high cholesterol levels, cholesterol levels below 160 confer a heightened risk of depression, accidents and suicide. Apparently, low cholesterol levels interfere with the regulation of serotonin.

That doesn't mean we should binge on saturated fat. It does suggest that we should be wary of cholesterol levels that are too high *or* too low.

What about carbohydrates? They do appear to improve serotonin function *temporarily.* Over the long term, however, a high-carbohydrate diet diminishes your sense of well-being.

Reason: Carbohydrates quickly raise blood sugar and insulin levels. Elevated insulin signals the body to store food as fat—making it less available for energy. Insulin also boosts production of certain prostaglandins linked to depression.

Antidote: Eat a diet that's more in line with that of our hunter-gatherer ancestors…

•**Emphasize fruits and vegetables** while limiting consumption of grains and sweets. When you do eat grain, stick to whole grains. They have a less drastic effect on blood sugar than white bread or processed cereal.

•**At every meal, maintain a protein-fat-carbohydrate** calorie ratio of 30%-30%-40%.

•**Keep meals under 500 calories.** Don't let more than five hours pass between meals (except when you're asleep). Frequent, small meals keep insulin levels lower than a few large meals.

•**Do not eat red meat or egg yolks more than once a week.** These foods contain a chemical precursor to a brain chemical that is associated with depression.

WHAT ABOUT ANTIDEPRESSANTS?

Anyone who is so depressed that he/she has trouble functioning at work or at home should seek a medical diagnosis.

•**Fluoxetine** (Prozac) is the best known of a group of antidepressants called *selective serotonin reuptake inhibitors* (SSRIs). These drugs avoid many of the serious medical risks of older drugs.

But Prozac can cause decreased libido, delayed orgasm, insomnia and agitation…and may suppress melatonin levels.

Over the short term, this is probably not a concern. For patients who take the drug for a year or more, however, the effect on melatonin might have negative implications for long-term mood and health.

•**Sertraline** (Zoloft) and *paroxetine* (Paxil) are similar to Prozac but may be better or worse in a given individual.

•**Fluvoxamine** (Luvox) is another SSRI that appears to have fewer side effects than Prozac. Unlike Prozac, it raises melatonin levels.

•**Nefazodone** (Serzone)—the newest antidepressant on the US market—affects serotonin more subtly and seems free of Prozac's most objectionable side effects. It may be particularly helpful in treating depression accompanied by anxiety or insomnia.

•**Venlafaxine** (Effexor) acts on serotonin and boosts levels of *norepinephrine* (the neurochemical affected by earlier antidepressants called tricyclics). It has a good track record in treating cases that fail to respond to other medication.

•**Bupropion** (Wellbutrin) does *not* act on serotonin. In fact, we're not quite sure *how* it works. In a tiny percentage of cases, it has been associated with seizures. This risk can be minimized by lowering the dosage and spreading doses out throughout the day.

Effective Remedies from Your Kitchen Cabinet

Jamison Starbuck, ND, a naturopathic physician in family practice and a lecturer at the University of Montana, both in Missoula. She is past president of the American Association of Naturopathic Physicians and a contributing editor to *The Alternative Advisor: The Complete Guide to Natural Therapies and Alternative Treatments*. Time Life.

Next time you're searching for relief from an acute ailment, look in your kitchen. Chances are you'll find as many remedies there as in your medicine chest.

●**Cold.** Try ginger tea. Both an antiviral and anti-inflammatory remedy, it helps prevent chills and reduces the buildup of phlegm. *What to do:* Peel and thinly slice a two-inch piece of fresh gingerroot. Put it in a saucepan and cover with 12 ounces of water. Bring to a boil, then gently simmer for seven minutes. Strain, add honey and the juice of one-half fresh lemon. Sip six ounces every three hours.

●**Sinus congestion.** To clear your nasal and sinus passages, try a *steam inhalation with dried thyme leaves.* Thyme is a good antiseptic and decongestant. *What to do:* Pour a quart of boiling water into a bowl. Add a heaping teaspoon of dried thyme leaves. Drape a large, dry cotton towel over your head and hold your face about 12 inches above the bowl. Breathe in the thyme-laced steam for eight minutes. Then gently blow your nose.

●**Bladder infection.** If you experience early symptoms of a bladder infection—such as pain when urinating or increased frequency—try *parsley tea.* Parsley is a mild natural diuretic that contains virtually no calories and also flushes the bladder of pesky organisms that can cause infection. *What to do:* Bring one quart of water to a boil, turn off the heat and add one cup of fresh parsley, stems and leaves. Cover and steep for 15 minutes. Strain and drink one cup of cool tea over a two-hour period. Repeat the process four hours later. If your symptoms worsen or persist for more than 24 hours, see your health-care provider.

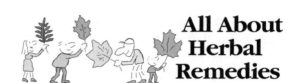

All About Herbal Remedies

Daniel B. Mowrey, PhD, president of the American Phytotherapy Research Laboratory, a nonprofit research facility in Lehi, UT. He is author of several books on herbal medicine, including *Herbal Tonic Therapies*. Keats Publishing.

Even if you eat right, exercise regularly and get plenty of sleep, herbal supplements can raise your health to a whole new level.

As explained here by one of the country's leading herbalists, Dr. Daniel B. Mowrey, so-called "tonic" herbs confer an impressive array of health benefits, including increased energy and stamina...heightened immunity...reduced risk of heart disease...improved liver function ...reduced joint inflammation.

If you'd like to add herbal remedies to *your* medicine chest, start with the following eight tonic herbs.* All are available at health food stores.

Unlike drugs, herbal preparations are not regulated by the FDA. Ask the store clerk to recommend a reputable brand.

The doses listed are based on capsules containing 850 milligrams (mg) to 900 mg of the herb.

Caution: Consult a doctor before starting any herbal regimen—especially if you have a heart ailment or another chronic illness and/or you are using prescription or over-the-counter medications. Herbal remedies can dangerously interact with certain drugs.

**Editor's note:* Certain remedies are inherently unsafe. *Comfrey, borage, chaparral* and *coltsfoot* can cause liver disease...*ma huang* can cause a rise in blood pressure that is particularly unsafe for those with heart or thyroid disease or diabetes...*yohimbe* can cause tremors, anxiety, high blood pressure and rapid heart rate.

If you develop a rash, nausea, hives, headaches or hay fever-like symptoms while taking an herb, stop using it immediately.

CAYENNE

Cayenne is good for the cardiovascular system. A mild stimulant, the herb also helps maintain muscle tone in the stomach and intestinal walls and enhances digestion. Cayenne is also an excellent "activator herb," amplifying the benefits of other herbs you take.

Daily dose: Two capsules. Or use ground cayenne as a spice.

ECHINACEA

Echinacea fights illness on two levels. First, it boosts levels of white blood cells, *B-* and *T-lymphocytes* and *phagocytes*—the key components of a healthy immune system. Second, it neutralizes invading microorganisms.

German researchers have shown that echinacea stops staph, strep and fungal infections, along with a variety of viruses.

Daily dose: Two capsules. Be sure the capsules contain the *whole* root in powdered form, not extract.

Used intermittently, liquid extract of echinacea makes a soothing balm for sore throats. Using an eyedropper, let a few drops fall against the back of your throat.

GARLIC

This spice helps prevent heart disease by lowering cholesterol levels and blocking formation of fatty deposits in the coronary arteries. It also boosts levels of T-cells, a critical component of the immune system.

Animal and human studies have shown that garlic also relieves arthritis. It contains sulfur compounds, which are known to have significant anti-inflammatory properties.

Daily dose: Two pills. Or use a garlic clove or garlic powder in your cooking.

GINGERROOT

Gingerroot is an excellent remedy for indigestion, constipation, diarrhea and nausea (including morning sickness). There's no good explanation for why it works. But my research suggests that ginger is even more effective than Dramamine at preventing motion sickness. It is also effective against the flu.

Be sure to buy capsules made from the *whole* gingerroot—not extract.

Daily dose: For mild motion sickness, two capsules 15 minutes before you depart (and two to four more every hour or whenever symptoms return). For serious gastrointestinal upset, take six to 12 capsules an hour.

LAPACHO

A South American herb, lapacho contains *napthoquinones* (N-factors), unique compounds that have antiviral and antibiotic properties. It's effective at preventing colds, flu and bacterial and fungal infections.

Taken in capsule or tea form, lapacho soothes painful joints...and boosts energy levels. Lapacho also stimulates activity of enzymes in the liver, enhancing its ability to remove toxins from the blood.

In Brazil, lapacho is used to treat leukemia and cervical cancer, and lapacho salve is used to treat skin cancer.

Studies suggest that the herb may also be effective against breast cancer.

Make tea by simmering the purplish paper-thin inner lining of the bark in hot water for 20 minutes, then strain and let cool. Leftover tea can be refrigerated.

Daily dose: To prevent illness, four capsules or two cups of tea. To treat an infection, six capsules or one to two quarts of tea.

MILK THISTLE

One of the world's most studied plants, milk thistle is very good for the liver. By stimulating protein synthesis, it boosts levels of key liver enzymes, speeding regeneration of damaged liver tissue. It also inhibits *lypoxygenase*, an enzyme that destroys liver cells.

Studies show that milk thistle can help reverse the effects of hepatitis and cirrhosis.

Daily dose: Two capsules.

PYGEUM EXTRACT

Derived from the bark of an African tree, pygeum has been shown to prevent—and even relieve—benign enlargement of the prostate. It contains *phytosterols*, which are potent anti-inflammatory compounds. Pygeum also contains *triterpenoids*, compounds that have an antiswelling effect.

Daily dose: To prevent prostate enlargement, two capsules. To shrink an enlarged prostate, four capsules.

YERBA MATE

This South American herb boosts energy and stamina without causing the jitters that caffeine can cause. Anecdotal reports suggest that yerba mate is also effective against asthma and allergies, though the mechanism is unknown.

Yerba mate is best taken as a daily tea. Pour boiling water over yerba mate leaves, let sit for 10 minutes, then strain and serve.

Daily dose: Two to four cups.

Fight Allergies with Stinging Nettle

Nancy L. Snyderman, MD, associate clinical professor of otolaryngology at the California Pacific Medical Center in San Francisco. A medical correspondent for ABC-TV's "Good Morning America," she is also author of *Dr. Nancy Snyderman's Guide to Good Health.* William Morrow.

As an ear, nose and throat doctor, I prescribe lots of allergy and cold preparations. I used to rely on conventional antihistamines and decongestants. Unfortunately, these drugs can cause drowsiness, dry mouth, nervousness and other side effects. They often do more harm than good.

While preparing an interview with alternative medicine advocate Andrew Weil, MD, he told me about *stinging nettle* (Urtica dioica). This herb is great for stuffy noses caused by allergies. It takes a little longer to work—up to 48 hours—but *doesn't* cause side effects.

Since then everyone in my family has used the herb. I recommend it to my patients, too, particularly those with seasonal allergies like hay fever.

Nettle is safe even when taken over an extended period. In fact, you can use it throughout allergy season. Or take it as soon as you feel a cold coming on. Be sure to follow the dosage directions listed on the bottle.

It's unclear how nettle works. It may constrict small blood vessels in the nose...or it may block the body's production of *histamines*, chemicals that stimulate production of mucus.

Stinging nettle is available in capsules or in tincture form. I prefer Eclectic Institute's freeze-dried nettle capsules because I believe they're especially potent. They are available at health-food stores or from the manufacturer at 800-332-4372.

Alternative Remedies for Hay Fever

Freeze-dried preparations of the herb *stinging nettle* (Urtica dioica) are often helpful... and unlike antihistamines and decongestants, they do *not* cause troublesome side effects.

Caution: *Nettle tea* and capsules containing air-dried stinging nettle are less effective.

Also helpful: *Quercetin*, a compound derived from citrus fruits and buckwheat. Quercetin supplements should be taken as a preventive measure starting several weeks before allergy season. Consult a doctor before taking stinging nettle or quercetin.

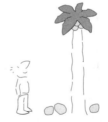

Healing Secrets From a Mayan Medicine Man

Rosita Arvigo, DN (doctor of naprapathy, a branch of chiropractic), director of the Ix Chel Tropical Research Foundation, Belize. She is coauthor of *Rain Forest Remedies: One Hundred Healing Herbs of Belize.* Lotus Press.

In the past decade, the National Cancer Institute has tested nearly 2,000 rain forest plants for anticancer and anti-AIDS activity. Hundreds of drugs have been developed this way, including *vincristine* (Oncovin) for leukemia and *paclitaxel* (Taxol) for ovarian cancer.

For the past 20 years, Dr. Rosita Arvigo of Chicago has lived in the rain forest of the tiny Central American nation of Belize. There, she and Michael Balick, PhD, associate director of the New York Botanical Garden, have studied medicinal plants, including those used by the late Don Elijio Panti, a 103-year-old "medicine man," who was legendary among the Maya of Belize.

Unlike modern drugs, these plants have been proven over thousands of years of use to be effective and safe. They are available at grocery stores, health food stores and garden centers…

Caution: Plant remedies should not be used by people with allergies to plants. Anyone who experiences heart palpitations or a skin rash from a medicinal plant should discontinue its use.

Recently, we asked Dr. Arvigo about these plants—and how we can put them to work in our own lives…

●**Basil.** Basil tea relieves fever, indigestion, anxiety and insomnia. Lab tests have found that basil oil has antibacterial and antifungal properties.

Boil a handful of fresh leaves (or two tablespoons of dried leaves) in two cups of water for five minutes, then strain. Drink hot before meals or at bedtime.

●**Lemon grass.** Among the Maya, lemon grass tea is widely used to reduce fever. It is also effective against coughs and colds.

Lemon grass causes perspiration and promotes the excretion of phlegm.

For treating fever in an adult, boil one mashed root and 10 leaves of the plant in three cups of water for 10 minutes. Drink hot, go to bed and wrap up warmly.

For fever in children, boil 10 leaves in three cups of water for 10 minutes. Give the child one-half cup of tea six times daily.

●**Marigold.** Taken as a hot tea, the larger, yellow varieties of marigold are great for treating colic. Marigold tea also relieves fever, stomach pain, flatulence and headaches.

To make tea, boil two or three flower heads in one cup of water for five minutes. Let the tea steep for 10 minutes. Give a baby spoonfuls of the warm tea.

Herbal bath: Boil a double handful of marigold flowers and leaves in a large pot of water for 20 minutes. Let the water cool, then pour it into a plastic baby tub. Bathe the infant for 10 minutes, then wrap him/her warmly and put him to bed.

●**Oregano.** This herb is widely used in Belize as a remedy for upper respiratory tract infections. It also relieves indigestion.

Oregano can be taken in tea form…or fresh or dried oregano leaves can be added to soups, stews and sauces.

To make tea, pour three cups of boiling water over one-half cup of fresh-picked leaves or three tablespoons of dried leaves. Let steep for 15 minutes, then strain. Drink one cup before each meal.

●**Periwinkle.** Although periwinkle contains potent anticancer compounds, it's best used as a remedy for sore throats.

Place nine pink flowers in a pint of water, and soak in sunlight for three hours. Sip the resulting tea all day long when you have a sore throat or cold.

●**Red rose.** This garden favorite makes a cooling tonic for hot, humid days. It also helps cool fevers and prevent diarrhea. *For children:* Boil one red rose and nine leaves in one cup of water for five minutes, then steep for 15 minutes. Strain and drink. *For adults:* Boil three roses and nine leaves per cup of water.

Safe, Simple Fix for Minor Injuries

William Pawluk, MD, MSc, director of clinical programs, Division of Complementary Medicine, University of Maryland School of Medicine, Baltimore.

From sprains and bruises to toothache, bone fracture and postsurgical discomfort, the homeopathic remedy *arnica* is good for just about any pain caused by physical trauma. Unlike aspirin and other over-the-counter painkillers, arnica pills have no side effects.

In a 1991 English study on patients hospitalized for acute injuries, arnica relieved stiffness and improved psychological well-being in 98% of patients, compared with 57% of patients given a placebo.

Arnica works *fast*. One of my coworkers fell and pulled a muscle. Ordinarily, it would take a week or two for pain from such an injury to subside. Yet within three days after he started taking arnica, his pain was gone.

It may even be beneficial to take arnica *before* sustaining an injury. Many marathoners use it before they race. In Canada, horse trainers have begun to use arnica to coax a little more speed out of their thoroughbreds.

Arnica is derived from a mountain plant called *leopard's bane*. It's sold in "potencies" ranging from 6x or 6c (low potency) to 200c (high potency).

In general, higher potencies are best for chronic conditions, low potencies for acute conditions. But speak with your doctor before taking a dose.

Arnica is safe in a wide range of dosages—from one pill every eight hours to four pills an hour. If pain persists, see a doctor.

Arnica is available in health-food stores, pharmacies and mail-order homeopathic pharmacies.

Two Herbs that Calm the Colon

David Edelberg, MD, clinical instructor at Northwestern University School of Medicine and chief of holistic and preventive medicine at Grant Hospital, both in Chicago. He is also chairman and medical director of American Holistic Centers, a group of clinics offering physician-supervised alternative medical care.

If you're plagued by diarrhea, cramping and intestinal gas, you may have *irritable bowel syndrome* (IBS).

What causes IBS? Emotional stress is often involved.

Whatever its cause, IBS can be controlled with two herbs...

•**Peppermint** relaxes smooth muscle surrounding the large intestine, curbing spasms.

During flare-ups of IBS, I tell my patients to take *enteric-coated* peppermint oil—one or two capsules three times a day between meals.

If this dosage causes a burning sensation during bowel movements, lower the dose.

•**St. John's wort** eases anxiety by acting as a mild tranquilizer and antidepressant. It lowers levels of the brain chemical *monoamine oxidase* (MAO). High levels of MAO have been linked to depression.

The usual approach to reducing MAO levels is to take an MAO inhibitor such as Marplan, Nardil or Parnate. But foods that contain *tyramine*, including aged cheese, bananas and pepperoni, can interact with MAO inhibitors—*perhaps lethally*.

There are no dietary restrictions with St. John's wort (though it can make fair-skinned individuals sensitive to sunlight). Take one capsule twice a day with meals.

Both herbs are available at health-food stores.

Mail-order source: Arrowroot Standard Direct (800-234-8879).

Food and Healing

Annemarie Colbin, founder of the Natural Gourmet Institute for Food and Health, 48 W. 21 St., New York 10010. A certified health education specialist and certified culinary professional, she is author of several books, including *Food and Healing*. Ballantine.

You are probably well aware that a low-fat, high-fiber diet can help prevent disease. But is there such a thing as food that heals?

The answer is *yes*.

For more than 30 years, I've been studying the effects of food on health. I have also tried out many remedies based on centuries-old folk wisdom.

Based on my observations and those of my students, I'm convinced that certain foods *do* help the body heal more quickly from a number of minor ailments...

COLDS AND FLU

The best natural remedy is garlic. By boosting the immune system and killing bacteria, it helps keep a mild viral illness from turning into a serious bacterial infection.

Swallow one small clove or several small pieces every four to six hours until symptoms subside. Wash this garlic "pill" down with a glass of orange juice or water.

Don't worry about bad breath. If you don't chew the garlic, no one will be able to smell it on your breath.

CONSTIPATION

You probably know that whole grains and fresh fruits and vegetables—especially prunes —help "normalize" colon function.

But these natural remedies won't do much good unless you wash them down with plenty of water. Vegetarians should have four to six glasses a day, meat-eaters at least eight.

Ironically, constipation is sometimes caused by consuming *too* much dietary fiber. If you suspect this is your problem, cut back on raw produce. Continue to eat whole grains—especially brown rice. It seems to be more easily digested than other high-fiber foods. And drink plenty of water.

COUGH

If you have a "wet" cough (one that produces phlegm), drink hot liquids—especially hot-and-sour soup or another spicy soup. Wet coughs should be encouraged—they are the body's way of expelling bacteria and other pathogens.

Also helpful: Hot apple or pear juice with cinnamon (from the Chinese medical tradition).

To stop a "dry" cough or a tickle in the throat, eat something salty—like *umeboshi plums.* These pickled plums are sold in health-food stores and Japanese groceries. Or—try licorice tea. It strengthens the lungs and is a traditional herbal remedy for asthma.

DIARRHEA

Mild diarrhea can often be controlled by eating small amounts of cooked white rice…or grated raw apple that is allowed to turn brown, so it develops the soluble fiber pectin.

Caution: Seek medical attention for severe, prolonged diarrhea or diarrhea accompanied by vomiting. That can signal dysentery, food poisoning or another life-threatening infection.

HEADACHE

Tension headaches are often triggered by insufficient food or insufficient fluids…or by prolonged exposure to summer heat.

Remedy: Two or more cups of cool juice. I've seen this "prescription" relieve headaches in as little as five minutes.

Fruit juice—especially apple or apricot juice —seems best. I don't know whether that's because of the pleasant flavor or because it gets carbohydrates and fluids into the system quickly.

For a headache caused by drinking too much alcohol or eating too much sugar, eat olives, anchovies or umeboshi plums.

You might also try steamed vegetables sprinkled with sesame salt. My father had an easy and delicious variation on this idea—eating a scallion that's been dipped in salt.

For a headache that stems from caffeine withdrawal, chew a piece of lemon. The strong, sour taste somehow counteracts the body's response to less caffeine. Drink plenty of water to prevent dehydration.

Over the years, I've noticed that migraines can be triggered by eating potato chips or another oily food on an empty stomach.

Remedy: "Spiked" lemon tea. Squeeze half a lemon into a cup. Dice the peel and simmer in 1¼ cups of water for 10 minutes. Strain into the cup. Add a pinch of cayenne or ½ teaspoon of grated fresh ginger—or ¼ teaspoon of powdered ginger. Sweeten with maple syrup or barley malt.

SORE THROAT

To soothe a sore throat, drink tea made from ginger or slippery elm (the latter can be found in health-food stores). Slippery elm lozenges are also effective.

Ginger tea is made by simmering three to four slices of fresh ginger in a cup of water for eight minutes. It is also good for coughs, chest congestion and motion sickness.

STOMACH UPSET

If you have heartburn or another form of *gastroesophageal reflux,* eat *cooked* food only —it's easier to digest.

Intestinal gas can often be relieved by an "antacid" made of *kudzu,* a starch made from the root of the kudzu plant. It's sold in health food stores.

425

Dissolve one tablespoon of kuzu in a cup of cold water. Cook, stirring until thick. Then add a tablespoon of soy sauce.

To make kuzu pudding, dissolve two tablespoons kuzu in a cup of apple juice. Add a teaspoon of vanilla if desired. Cook, stirring constantly, until thickened. Fold in a tablespoon of tahini (sesame paste). Eat hot or cold.

Soothing and very relaxing, kuzu pudding is an excellent remedy for stress or insomnia. Kuzu has also been shown to reduce cravings for alcohol.

RESPECT YOUR TASTE BUDS

Don't force yourself to eat foods you dislike. If you find a food distasteful, it probably isn't something that will help your body.

Fast Headache Relief Without Drugs

Art Ulene, MD, medical correspondent for the NBC-TV's "Today" show and clinical professor of obstetrics and gynecology, University of Southern California School of Medicine, Los Angeles.

If you frequently get headaches, you should know about my natural self-treatment program. The program combines dietary strategies (identifying and avoiding "trigger foods") …daily exercise and relaxation…plus visual imagery (creative visualization).

Imagery can be used anywhere, anytime. It's good both for warding off headaches…and for keeping them from getting worse.

My program is *very* effective. When I tested it with 19 headache sufferers, they reported 33% fewer headaches.

Their use of painkillers fell by 40%. That's important because while drugs do relieve pain, they can cause nausea and other side effects. In some cases, the side effects are worse than the headaches.

Caution: If you've just begun to get headaches, or if your pain is severe, consult a doctor. About 2% of headaches have an underlying cause that needs treatment—sinusitis, inflammation of a blood vessel or even a life-threatening problem like aneurysm or brain tumor.

But for tension-type and migraine headaches, imagery works very well.

What to do: Close your eyes and relax. Picture a red light attached to the part of your head that hurts. The light represents your pain.

Imagine slowly dimming and then extinguishing the light. This should take three to five minutes. As the light disappears, so should your headache.

If you're at home, use visualization along with a cold pack. A bag of frozen peas is good.

Natural Remedies For Fatigue

Adriane Fugh-Berman, MD, a Washington, DC–based medical researcher who specializes in women's health and alternative medicine. She is author of *Alternative Medicine: What Works.* Williams & Wilkins.

Do you feel tired all the time? Do you lack the energy you used to have? Join the club. Chronic fatigue is an extremely common complaint—and one with many different causes. *Here's what you need to know to get to the root of your problem…*

●**Lack of sleep.** Although sleeplessness seems an obvious reason to be tired, it's often overlooked. These days, people like to brag about how little sleep they need. But there are actually very few people who truly need only five or six hours a night. Most of us need eight. Some of us need nine or 10. Just because you can get by on six or seven hours a night does *not* mean that's all the sleep you need. If you suffer from persistent fatigue, see how much better you'll feel with an extra 30 or 60 minutes of sleep each night.

Maximize the *quality* of your sleep, too. Never work or worry in your bedroom. Make your bedroom as quiet as possible—use earplugs if you must. If street lamps or other sources of light outside your window bother you, try heavy drapes or an eye shade.

●**Lack of exercise.** Too little exercise can cause fatigue—or make it worse. Of course, overexercising can also cause fatigue, but moderate exercise is actually an energizer. What's moderate? Twenty to 60 minutes three times a week is ideal. Do *not* exercise within two hours of bedtime. Doing so may interfere with your sleep.

•**Medication.** Sleeping pills can cause a sort of fatigue "hangover" in many people. That goes for *melatonin* as well as prescription sedatives like *diazepam* (Valium). Fatigue can also be a side effect of many other over-the-counter and prescription medications, including blood pressure drugs like *propranolol* (Inderal) and *atenolol* (Tenormin)…as well as many antidepressants and antihistamines. If you suspect your medication is making you tired, ask your doctor about alternatives.

•**Diet.** Heavy meals, especially late in the day, or particularly starchy meals can cause fatigue. If you insist on a heavy meal, have it early in the day. A hearty breakfast is less likely to sap your energy than a hearty lunch or supper.

What else can you do to boost your energy? Consider taking vitamin and herbal supplements. *B-complex* is especially effective—take this supplement once a day. *Vitamin B-12* is good, too. Take 1,000 micrograms a day. Since B-12 is found almost exclusively in meat and dairy products, many strict vegetarians suffer from B-12 deficiency—and from chronic fatigue as a result.

Vitamin B-12 may be better absorbed when it's injected, and some people swear by injections for an energy boost. I generally prefer B-12 tablets. They're far less costly and, I think, just as effective.

Coenzyme Q-10 helps fight fatigue by maximizing the heart's pumping efficiency. Take 30 mg once or twice a day.

Ginseng tea, capsules or extract can be a potent source of energy. Be sure not to mix ginseng with caffeine or another stimulant. The combination can cause palpitations or irregular heartbeat.

Siberian "ginseng" isn't really ginseng at all, but another plant species called *Eleutherococcus*. It, too, has energizing qualities. Both herbs are *adaptogens*, meaning that they help the body to adapt to stress.

If these measures don't boost your energy, see a doctor. You may be suffering from depression, anemia, chronic fatigue syndrome or another disease that requires medical intervention.

Natural Alternatives to Common Medications

Michael T. Murray, ND, professor of botanical science at Bastyr University in Seattle. He is author of *Natural Alternatives to Over-the-Counter and Prescription Drugs.* Morrow.

Conventional medications can be quite effective at controlling symptoms…but they can also cause nasty side effects.

Fortunately, there are natural alternatives to many of the most common prescription and over-the-counter (OTC) drugs. Available in health-food stores, these herbs, plant extracts, vitamins, etc., are often as effective as the medications they replace—and less likely to cause side effects.

If the idea of using natural remedies seems "flaky" to you, it's probably because mainstream doctors in the US tend to be strongly biased against them.

This bias is *not* shared by doctors elsewhere. In Germany, for example, the herb *St. John's wort* (Hypericum perforatum) is prescribed for depression eight times more frequently than synthetic antidepressants like *fluoxetine* (Prozac).

Here's a list of drugs you may be better off without, along with the natural alternatives with which to replace them.

Important: Choose products with labels specifying the concentration of active ingredients …and use them only under medical supervision.

HEADACHE REMEDIES

It's no secret that people with recurrent headaches tend to use lots of aspirin, ibuprofen and acetaminophen. Few people realize, however, that these OTC painkillers cause "rebound" headaches in 70% of the people who use them. That is, painkillers taken to stop pain wind up causing *more* pain.

***Alternative I:* Magnesium.** Many tension-type and migraine headaches stem from a slight deficiency of this mineral. If your headaches do, magnesium oxide supplements should bring relief. Take 600 milligrams (mg) per day, divided into three 200-mg doses.

***Alternative II:* Feverfew.** This herb is particularly effective against migraines. Take 80 mg of an extract containing at least 0.2% of *parthenolide*, the active ingredient in feverfew. No side effects have been reported.

ACID BLOCKERS AND ANTACIDS

Acid blockers like Zantac, Tagamet and Axid fight stomach upset and ulcers by blocking the release of stomach acid. But in doing so, they disrupt the digestive process. This can lead to nutritional deficiencies.

Acid blockers have also been linked to liver and kidney problems, yeast infection (*candidiasis*) and breast enlargement in men (*gynecomastia*).

Antacids like Tums and Maalox can cause a rebound effect, in which the stomach generates more stomach acid as the antacids wear off. Many antacids contain aluminum, which some suspect may be a cause of Parkinson's and Alzheimer's disease.

***Alternative:* Deglycyrrhizinated licorice** (DGL). It promotes synthesis of the natural substances that line the intestinal tract, protecting it against acid irritation. In studies DGL has proven *more* effective than acid blockers and Maalox.

Typical dosage: Two 380-mg tablets, taken 20 minutes before meals.

Caution: If you have persistent stomach pain—especially pain that grows worse on an empty stomach—see a doctor. You may have a peptic ulcer.

ANTIHISTAMINES

Benadryl and other OTC antihistamines are effective at relieving nasal congestion, runny nose and other cold and hay fever symptoms. But they can cause dry mouth and drowsiness.

Nonsedating antihistamines are available by prescription only.

***Alternative:* Quercetin.** This derivative of fruits and flowers keeps the body from releasing histamine and other compounds that trigger cold and hay fever symptoms.

Typical dosage: 200 mg, taken five minutes before meals.

SLEEPING PILLS

As many people suffering from insomnia have learned, sleeping pills can impair mental and physical function…and make it hard to "get going" in the morning.

***Alternative:* Valerian.** This herbal sleeping aid works better than sleeping pills, without causing any morning "hangover."

Typical dosage: 150 mg, taken 45 minutes before bedtime. Look for a product that contains 0.8% *valerenic acid*, valerian's active ingredient.

ANTIDEPRESSANTS

All prescription antidepressants cause side effects. Almost half of all people who take fluoxetine or *sertraline* (Zoloft), for example, notice a decreased sex drive.

***Alternative:* St. John's wort.** Double-blind studies have proven this herb to be *more* effective than prescription antidepressants. St. John's wort appears to be safe, though it can cause sun sensitivity and stomach upset.

Typical dosage: 300 mg, three times a day. Buy a product containing 0.3% of the herb's active ingredient, *hypericin*.

FINASTERIDE (PROSCAR)

Enlarged prostate (also known as *benign prostatic hyperplasia*, or BPH) affects 50% of men over age 60. Symptoms include frequent urination and a weak or uneven urine stream.

Doctors usually treat BPH with *finasteride*. This drug blocks synthesis of testosterone, the hormone that fuels the growth of prostate tissue.

But finasteride can take up to six months to relieve symptoms. It can also cause depression and impotence.

***Alternative:* Saw palmetto.** This herb, widely used in Europe, has proven effective against BPH in many studies. It causes no major side effects.

Typical dosage: 160 mg, twice a day. Expect improvement within four weeks. Buy a *fat-soluble* extract that contains 85% to 95% fatty acids and sterols.

Caution: Any man who thinks he has BPH should have a full physical. Urinary difficulties can be symptomatic of prostate cancer.

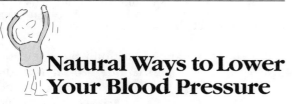

Natural Ways to Lower Your Blood Pressure

Stephen Fortmann, MD, associate professor of medicine at Stanford University School of Medicine, and deputy director of the Stanford Center for Research in Disease Prevention, both in Palo Alto, CA. He is coauthor of *The Blood Pressure Book: How to Get It Down and Keep It Down.* Bull Publishing.

If your blood pressure is in the "danger zone" (140/90 or above), you may already know that taking steps to lower it will reduce your risk for heart attack, stroke, kidney failure and other serious ailments.

You might *not* know that the same steps are beneficial if your pressure only *slightly* exceeds the upper limit of normal (120/80). Even if your pressure is below 120/80, you'll enjoy long-term health benefits if you make certain lifestyle changes...

LOSE WEIGHT

Not everyone with high blood pressure is obese, and not all obese people have high blood pressure. But for most people, losing weight reduces blood pressure.

Rule of thumb: A loss of one pound of body fat brings a one-point drop in systolic blood pressure (the upper number).

If you need to lose weight, set realistic goals. Plan to lose about one to three pounds a month.

EXERCISE REGULARLY

Exercise pumps up your metabolism, helping you burn more calories and preserve muscle tissue. Exercise seems to have a direct pressure-lowering effect, too.

Finding: When sedentary people began exercising regularly, their systolic pressure fell about 10 points.

Walking is an excellent form of exercise. Here's how to pack more walking into your everyday life...

● **Walk or bike to work, on errands, etc.** If it's too far to do so, consider parking your car a block away...or getting off one stop early on the bus or train.

● **Walk as much as possible while at work.** Take stairs instead of elevators. Walk to a coworker's office instead of telephoning. Take a brief walk at lunchtime...and during each work break.

● **At day's end, take a 15-minute walk** with a friend or family member. A late-afternoon walk helps you unwind...and takes the edge off your appetite.

REDUCE SODIUM INTAKE

The salt industry has been pushing the idea that only a minority of "salt-sensitive" people have to worry about the pressure-raising effects of sodium.

Reality: For most people, restricting sodium intake reduces blood pressure by two to three points.

Americans eat a great deal of salt without realizing it. Fast food—pizzas, hot dogs, hamburgers, etc.—are often loaded with sodium. So are canned foods, frozen dinners, prepared salad dressings and sauces, processed poultry and meat, pretzels, potato chips and smoked fish.

I tell my patients to avoid table salt and salty foods whenever possible. An adult needs only 200 mg of sodium a day. A single roast beef sandwich contains four times that amount.

In the supermarket, check labels for sodium content. When you cook, season with herbs instead of salt.

INCREASE POTASSIUM INTAKE

An analysis of 33 different studies by Paul K. Whelton, MD, of Tulane University, found that the systolic blood pressure of people who took potassium supplements dropped an average of five points.

Potassium supplements are okay, but it's better to get your potassium from foods. Potassium-rich foods include apples, melons, bananas, potatoes, tomatoes and nectarines.

Each day, have at least two servings of fruit and three servings of fresh vegetables. Juices are rich in potassium. Watch out for tomato juice, though. Most brands of tomato juice are sky-high in sodium.

REDUCE MEAT CONSUMPTION

Vegetarians tend to have lower blood pressure than nonvegetarians. Why? One possibility is that the antioxidants in fruit and vegetables help lower blood pressure.

Another is that the calcium in fruits and vegetables is easily absorbed. Calcium seems to help reduce blood pressure.

REDUCE ALCOHOL CONSUMPTION

In some individuals at least, regular drinking raises blood pressure. For these people, abstaining brings significant declines in blood pressure.

Example: A two-drink-per-day drinker who stops drinking might experience a 10-point decline in systolic pressure. Heavier drinkers who go on the wagon can experience a drop of up to 20 points.

Implication: Any hypertensive who regularly has more than two drinks a day should curb his/her alcohol intake.

DO RELAXATION EXERCISES

Psychological stress causes a transient rise in blood pressure, but doctors still don't know whether stress has any long-term effects.

It's clear, however, that relaxation exercises can bring lasting reductions in blood pressure. Many individuals who practice relaxation regularly experience as much as a five-point drop in systolic pressure.

What to do: Twice a week for 15 minutes—set an alarm clock so you won't have to keep track of time—sit on a comfortable chair in a quiet room.

Close your eyes. Relax your right arm until it feels warm and "floppy," then move on to your right thigh, calf, ankle and foot…left thigh, calf, ankle and foot…left arm…abdomen and buttocks…chest…neck…jaw and forehead.

Once your entire body is relaxed, envision ripples on a lake, soft breezes blowing through grass or another soothing scene.

SEVERE HIGH BLOOD PRESSURE

If your blood pressure is 140/90 or higher, your doctor will probably prescribe anti-hypertensive medication. Even so, lifestyle changes might enable you to get by on a lower dosage …or reduce your blood pressure to the point that drug therapy is no longer necessary.

Meditation Lowers Blood Pressure

Robert Schneider, MD, director of the Center for Health and Aging Studies, Maharishi University of Management, Fairfield, IA.

In a study, patients with mild hypertension who practiced *transcendental meditation* (TM) twice a day had a greater drop in blood pressure than those who learned progressive muscle relaxation—tensing and relaxing muscles one at a time. They also had a greater drop in blood pressure than those who reduced salt and calorie intake and exercised regularly.

Also: The TM users' blood pressure reduction was about the same as that in people who take blood pressure medication.

In TM, you sit with your eyes closed and repeat a word or sound—a *mantra*—until feeling restful.

Meditation and Pain Control

Amy Saltzman, MD, member of the board of trustees, American Holistic Medical Association, 4101 Lake Boone Trail, Suite 201, Raleigh, NC 27607.

Meditation helps control pain—and promotes general health. A series of studies published in prestigious medical journals over the past decade found that practitioners of meditation report significant decreases in pain, anxiety, depression, blood pressure and other physical symptoms—allowing doctors to decrease medication and doctors' visits.

The Benefits of Massage

Tiffany Field, PhD, director, University of Miami's Touch Research Institute, Dept. of Pediatrics, Box 016820 (D-820), 1601 NW 12 Ave., Miami 33101.

Massage promotes general good health, not just relaxation. Massage also strengthens the immune system by increasing the number of natural killer cells in the body.

Study: HIV patients who received regular massage showed reduced stress and improved immune function. Massage may soon be considered as basic a component of good health as diet and exercise.

Secrets of Self-Healing From Chinese Medicine

Roger Jahnke, OMD (doctor of Oriental medicine), an acupuncturist and Chinese medicine practitioner in private practice in Santa Barbara, CA. He is author of The Healer Within: The Four Essential Self-Care Methods for Creating Optimal Health. *HarperCollins.*

An avalanche of medical research shows that the human body is capable of remarkable feats of self-healing.

Self-healing happens automatically when you cultivate your body's innate self-healing powers.

How do you do that? *Chinese medicine makes use of four simple techniques...*

- **Deep breathing**
- **Gentle movement**
- **Self-massage**
- **Meditation**

Put these techniques to work for just 10 to 15 minutes a day, and you'll be more energetic and alert...and less vulnerable to illness and the negative effects of stress.

Although these techniques can be done as often as you like, it's a good idea to combine all four briefly first thing each morning.

DEEP BREATHING

Americans have forgotten how to breathe. We typically take very shallow breaths. This pattern of breathing constricts blood vessels, contributing to high blood pressure.

Shallow breathing also impairs immune function. It does so by slowing the circulation of antibodies and immune cells throughout the body.

By making a conscious effort to breathe slowly and deeply, you can counteract these physiological disturbances. *Try the following exercise right now...*

- **Take a slow, deep breath through your nose.** Allow the lower portions of your lungs to fill, then keep inhaling until your lungs are fully inflated.
- **Exhale slowly for 10 seconds.** You can exhale silently...or with an audible sigh of relief. Allow yourself to drift off into deep relaxation.

While even a single deep breath is beneficial, the accumulated effect of many such breaths is dramatic. Resolve to do two or three deep breathing sessions each day.

Do one session before getting out of bed in the morning, another just before you go to sleep at night.

Some people prefer to do deep breathing periodically throughout the day.

You might decide to take a deep breath each time the telephone rings...each time you stop at a red light...or each time you open the refrigerator. The point is to develop a habit of breathing deeply all day long.

GENTLE MOVEMENT

Research confirms that easy, low-intensity exercise provides virtually all the disease-fighting benefits of vigorous exercise—with far less risk of injury to both your muscles and joints. *The "flowing technique" is very popular in China...*

What to do: Stand with your feet shoulder-width apart and shoulders relaxed. Let your arms dangle at your sides. Bend your knees slightly...move your tailbone beneath your spine so as to "lengthen" your back...and lower your chin as if nodding "yes."

Rest briefly, begin to inhale slowly and turn your palms forward. Swing your arms forward and upward, slowly rising onto the balls of your feet as you do. Raise your hands (palms up) to shoulder height, keeping your elbows slightly bent. Turn your palms downward. Slowly lower your arms and exhale. Return your heels to the floor. As your hands pass your legs, allow them to swing back slightly while gently lifting your toes.

Repeat 10 to 15 times, developing a gentle rhythm.

SELF-MASSAGE

Self-massage has been a powerful healing tool in China for thousands of years...

•**Hand massage.** Using your left thumb, apply gentle pressure to the palm of your right hand. Place your remaining fingers on the back of the right hand for support.

Increase the pressure gradually until you're exerting about the same pressure needed to squeeze a new tennis ball.

Massage your hand all over, noting any areas of tenderness. Massage the fingers as well—all the way out to the tips. Finally, grasp each finger of your right hand on either side of the nail. Pinch gently.

Switch hands, and repeat. To conclude, return to any tender spots on either hand and knead them gently for a few additional minutes.

•**"Energizing" the internal organs.** Place your palms over the lower edge of your rib cage, near the sides of your body but still on the front. Rub your palms against your body in a circular motion, breathing easily and deeply as you do. Feel the warmth generated by your hands penetrating toward your organs.

Next, place one hand on your breastbone (sternum), the other on your navel. Rub in a circular motion with each hand.

Move both hands to your lower back, and repeat the process. The Chinese believe that sending warmth into the organs improves health and heals disease.

MEDITATION

Meditation reduces blood pressure, dilates blood vessels and stimulates the production of essential neurotransmitters and hormones.

One of the easiest and most powerful meditation techniques is *mindfulness*. Using this technique, you can free yourself of psychological and physical stress by focusing closely on a single bodily sensation.

Breath-awareness exercise: As you stand, sit or lie comfortably, focus all your concentration on the sensation of your breath as it passes through your nostrils. Your nostrils should feel cool as fresh air enters…and warm as you exhale.

You can do this mindfulness exercise for as briefly as a moment or as long as 20 minutes.

Notice that as long as you hold the focus on your breath, it's impossible to worry or think about stressful situations.

Ancient Chinese Secret For Relaxation and Better Health

Simon Wang, MD, PhD, professor of physiology at Guangxi Medical University in Guangxi, China. He is author of *Qi Gong for Health and Longevity.* East Health Development Group.

Qi gong is the ancient Chinese art of relaxing, rejuvenating and healing the body and the mind. It consists of exercises that boost the flow of *qi* (pronounced chee), the universal life force within the body.

According to the principles of Chinese medicine, qi flows through the body along channels called *meridians.* As long as this flow is smooth, the body remains healthy. But any blockage or imbalance of qi quickly results in illness.

To learn more about qi gong and how to use it in our own lives, we spoke to Dr. Simon Wang, who has received a standard Western medical education, but has spent years studying and using qi gong…

No one knows exactly how qi gong works. My own hunch is that it affects the release of hormones in the body.

I could relate countless anecdotes about the effectiveness of qi gong. My 66-year-old father, for instance, has practiced it for years…and he never even gets a cold. *But qi gong has also been shown to be effective in many clinical studies…*

•**In a controlled study at the Shanghai Hypertension Research Institute,** subjects showed improved cerebral blood flow after 12 months of qi gong training. Headaches, high blood pressure and several other ailments are associated with reduced blood flow in the brain.

The same study showed reduced levels of blood lactate after qi gong training—suggesting a beneficial reduction in metabolic rate.

•**Studies conducted at the Traditional Medical College in Beijing** showed that people taught qi gong experienced a marked rise in alpha brain waves. Alpha waves are associated with a calm, alert state.

•**A study of 68 AIDS patients in San Francisco** showed that two months of qi gong training brought a 13% to 22% rise in the number of infection-fighting white blood cells.

HOW TO PRACTICE QI GONG

There are many types of qi gong. All involve manipulating the flow of qi via meditation, breathing exercises and self-massage.

Qi gong can be practiced while standing, sitting or lying down. It can be done anywhere you can find a little peace and quiet—at home or at work...or even while traveling.

Weather permitting, it's best to do qi gong outdoors. The flow of qi is stimulated by fresh air and close proximity to plants.

Qi gong works best if done every day, on a life-long basis. Devote 20 minutes or so each morning to learning qi gong, and within two months you should feel calmer and more refreshed.

Here is my daily routine. I do it every morning, immediately upon waking...

RELAXING YOUR MIND

Lie in bed or sit cross-legged on a bed or the floor. Relax. Concentrate on breathing naturally for a minute or two.

Next, concentrate on "guiding" qi to an area deep within your brain, just behind your forehead. Imagine this "qi cavity" glowing with red or yellow light...or imagine that it's filled with ocean waves, a green meadow or another natural scene.

Concentrate on these images for five minutes. Gradually, a sense of calm will wash over you.

RUBBING YOUR HANDS

Now activate the qi cavities in your hands. Shift your focus from your head to your palms. Gently rub your palms together for a minute or two. Then use one palm to rub the back of the other hand for another couple of minutes.

Reverse hands and repeat, breathing naturally throughout.

RUBBING YOUR ARMS

Continue focusing on your palms. Close your eyes, and run your left palm up the outside of your right arm, from the wrist to the top of your right shoulder. Rotate your right arm outward, and run your left palm all the way down the inside of your right arm.

Do this 20 times, then switch arms and repeat.

BATHING YOUR FACE

Close your eyes. Gently press the tip of your tongue against the back of your upper teeth. Cover your face with your palms, with your fingers pointing upward.

Using both hands, rub your face from forehead to chin. Then rub it again from chin to forehead. Repeat 20 times, until your hands and face feel warm.

RUBBING YOUR CHEST

Use your right palm to rub from the top of the right side of your chest, down and across your body to the lower portion of the left side of your chest.

Then take your left palm and rub from your upper left chest down and across to your lower right chest.

Repeat 20 times, concentrating on the center of your palms.

RUBBING *DAN TIAN*

Close your eyes. Using your right palm, rub your abdomen, just below the navel, in a tight, circular pattern. Repeat 20 times.

The lower abdomen contains the *Dan Tian* point, one of the most important of all qi cavities.

RUBBING *YONG QUAN*

Yong Quan is a qi cavity in the center of the sole of each foot.

Place the fingers of your left hand against the bottom of your right foot—at the point where the arch meets the ball of the foot. Rub rapidly in a circular motion 20 times, concentrating on the Yong Quan point.

Then switch to your right hand and left foot, and repeat.

Some Medicinal Oils Are Very Good for You

Richard N. Podell, MD, clinical professor of family medicine at Robert Wood Johnson Medical School in New Brunswick, NJ, and a physician in private practice in New Providence, NJ. He is author of several books, including *Patient Power*. Fireside.

Conventional wisdom has it that oils are something to keep *out* of our diets. These liquid fats are just too laden with calories.

But there are certain oils that have great medicinal properties...

EVENING PRIMROSE OIL

Oil extracted from the seeds of the evening primrose plant *(Oenothera biennis)* is rich in *gamma-linolenic acid* (GLA).

Native Americans used the evening primrose as a medicine, and modern research has confirmed that its oil can help in a variety of conditions.

•**Diabetes.** Many people who have diabetes wind up with *neuropathy,* a form of nerve damage that causes pain and weakness. An impressive body of research shows that evening primrose oil can help diabetics guard against neuropathy.

In one 1993 study conducted in seven hospitals in England and Finland, 50 diabetic patients took 12 capsules of evening primrose oil daily for one year. Another 50 diabetic patients took an olive oil placebo for the same period of time.

Result: Those who took evening primrose oil experienced significant reductions in pain and weakness, and improvements in nerve function and reflexes. Those who got the olive oil experienced no such improvements.

BORAGE OIL

Borage *(Borago officinalis)* is a plant with blue star-shaped flowers. Oil extracted from its seeds contains an even higher concentration of GLA than evening primrose oil. Four standard capsules contain as much of the beneficial fatty acid as 12 evening primrose oil caps.

•**Psychological stress.** In a controlled study conducted at the University of Waterloo in Ontario, Canada, and reported in the *Journal of Human Hypertension,* 30 healthy college students were divided into two groups. The first group took nine borage oil capsules a day for 28 days. The second group took a placebo for the same time period. Before and after the supplement period, they were given a psychological test known to cause stress.

Result: The students in the borage oil group exhibited much less stress when they took the test the second time. Those in the placebo group exhibited no decline in stress the second time around.

FISH OIL

Salmon and other cold water fish are rich in *omega-3* fatty acids—substances the body uses to synthesize "good" prostaglandins.

A growing body of research suggests that fish oil is powerful medicine against a number of illnesses.

•**Crohn's disease.** This inflammatory bowel condition causes severe diarrhea and abdominal pain, and interferes with nutrient absorption. Crohn's disease often goes into remission only to flare up several weeks or months later.

One study done in Italy and published in *The New England Journal of Medicine* showed that fish oil supplements brought striking benefits to people with Crohn's.

In the study, 78 patients who were in remission took either nine fish oil capsules daily or a placebo.

Result: After one year, 74% of the control group had suffered relapses. Only 41% of those who took the fish oil relapsed.

USING MEDICINAL OILS

While there's little risk in taking a daily capsule of evening primrose oil, borage oil or fish oil on your own, be sure to check with your doctor first. He/she should be able to help you determine a dosage appropriate for you.

Certain risks are associated with use of natural oils.

Example: Fish oil can thin the blood enough to cause internal bleeding, especially when taken along with other "clot-busters" like garlic or aspirin. In some cases, it raises blood sugar and cholesterol.

Eat Away Arthritis

Lauri M. Aesoph, ND, a naturopathic physician in Sioux Falls, SD. She is author of *How to Eat Away Arthritis.* Prentice Hall.

Cayenne, ginger and turmeric can bring marked relief from arthritis pain. These spices work by blocking release of *substance P,* a brain chemical that transmits pain signals and activates inflammation in the joints.

Important: If you decide to begin "spice therapy," let your doctor know—so he/she can adjust your arthritis medication.

●**Cayenne.** Cayenne can be eaten as a spice …or applied in cream form to painful joints. In a study, up to 80% of arthritis patients were helped by an over-the-counter cream containing cayenne pepper extract *(capsaicin)*.

Capsaicin cream is sold in drugstores under the brand names Capzasin-P, Pain Free and Zostrix.

Caution: Applying the cream to broken skin can cause pain. Also—don't eat cayenne if you have an ulcer.

●**Ginger.** In a study, ginger eased pain and swelling in 75% of arthritis patients. You can add fresh gingerroot to your cooking. Or take one to three gingerroot capsules a day.

Caution: Consuming more than 3 g of ginger at a time can cause stomach upset.

●**Turmeric.** This spice contains *curcumin*, a compound that reduces swelling. In one study, arthritis patients took either 1,200 mg of curcumin or 300 mg of the arthritis drug *phenylbutazone*. Both groups showed comparable improvement in symptoms, but the drug caused side effects.

Cook with turmeric…or take two curcumin capsules three times daily.

Caution: Limit daily turmeric consumption to one meal…or six capsules.

Natural Remedies for Impotence

Adriane Fugh-Berman, MD, a Washington, DC–based medical researcher who specializes in women's health and alternative medicine. She is author of *Alternative Medicine: What Works*. Williams & Wilkins.

The first step in overcoming impotence is to find out which type you have. *Physical* impotence is caused by nerve damage (often as a result of injury or chronic conditions such as diabetes)…or poor circulation in the penis (often caused by fatty deposits in penile blood vessels). In addition, certain drugs can cause physical impotence. Nine out of 10 cases of impotence are of physical origin.

Psychological impotence stems from emotional stress, depression or strife within your personal relationship. If you have this form of impotence, your best bet is psychotherapy or couples counseling. About 10% of all cases of impotence have a psychological basis.

How can you tell physical from psychological impotence? Find out whether you have erections during sleep. There are fancy machines for measuring "nocturnal penile tumescence." But you don't need them. Here's a simple, inexpensive test you can do at home.

Just before going to bed, use tape to fasten a perforated strip of stamps around the base of your penis. Don't wrap your penis too tightly. You should be able to slip a coin between the stamps and your skin. In the morning, check to see if the strip of stamps has broken. Do this every night for a week.

If you're consistently breaking the stamps, odds are you have a psychological problem. Consider asking your doctor for referral to a therapist. If you're *not* breaking the stamps, your problem is probably physical. If so, your next step is to determine whether any medication you're taking is the culprit.

A variety of over-the-counter (OTC) and prescription drugs—and many herbal remedies—can cause impotence. These include the herb *ephedra* or decongestants containing the ephedra derivative pseudoephedrine…blood pressure medications, especially beta-blockers such as *propranolol* (Inderal) and *atenolol* (Tenormin)…and *selective serotonin reuptake inhibitor* (SSRI) antidepressants such as *fluoxetine* (Prozac) and *sertraline* (Zoloft).

If you suspect that your impotence is a side effect of a drug, ask your doctor about switching to another drug. If drugs *don't* seem to be causing your impotence, consider trying one of the natural remedies that are effective against impotence…

●**Ginkgo biloba.** Good circulation to the penis is essential for good erections, and this potent blood thinner helps boost circulation throughout the body. In a study by Alan

435

Cohen, MD, of the University of California at San Francisco, 32 of 37 patients with sexual problems (including impotence and inability to achieve orgasm) got better when they took 120 mg of ginkgo extract twice a day.

•**Ginseng.** Although it's best known as a mild stimulant, ginseng is also effective against impotence. Two varieties of ginseng are readily available—*Panax ginseng* and *Panax quinquifolius*. These can be taken as a tea, in capsule form (take one or two daily) or liquid extract (one or two dropperfuls a day). Be sure to take it in the morning. Taken in the evening, its stimulant properties can cause insomnia. Never combine ginseng with coffee or any other stimulant food or drug.

Made from the bark of a West African tree, *yohimbe* is often touted as a cure for impotence. Unfortunately, it can raise blood pressure and heart rate and cause anxiety, dizziness, headache and tremor. A pharmaceutical form of the herb, *yohimbine*, is available by prescription. However, I don't recommend either version of the herb because of these disturbing side effects.

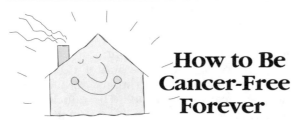

How to Be Cancer-Free Forever

Sidney Winawer, MD, chief of gastroenterology and nutrition service at the Memorial Sloan-Kettering Cancer Center and professor of clinical medicine at Cornell University Medical College, both in New York. He is author of *Cancer Free: The Comprehensive Cancer Prevention Program*. Fireside.

Cancer may soon surpass heart disease as America's number-one killer. That's the bad news.

The good news is that by making certain lifestyle changes now, most people can reduce their risk of developing cancer by 50%.

STAYING CANCER-FREE

•**Boost your fiber intake to 25 grams a day.** People who consume a lot of fiber have a lower incidence of colon cancer. Some experts feel that because fiber speeds the transit of waste products through the digestive system, carcinogens in the stool don't linger in the colon.

But because people who are chronically constipated have no higher risk of colon cancer than their more regular counterparts, we're beginning to think fiber fights cancer in other ways.

By filling up on fiber, you don't have room for a lot of cancer-friendly fats. You're also less likely to consume as many calories and more apt to maintain a healthier body weight. Excess weight may put you at risk for many types of cancer, including prostate, colorectal and breast cancers.

What I do: I consume 15 to 20 grams of fiber every morning by combining Bran Buds —a cereal with about 12 grams of fiber in a one-ounce serving—with one-half cup of raisin bran and one sliced banana.

Beans and lentils are also good sources of fiber. One cup of cooked beans or lentils contains about eight to 12 grams of fiber.

Important: Remember to drink at least six glasses of water a day when consuming large amounts of fiber.

•**Reduce your dietary fat intake to no more than 20% of your total daily calories.** High-fat diets are strongly related to the risk of colon cancer. A fatty diet may also increase your risk of prostate cancer or hasten its progression. And while there's no clear-cut evidence that fat triggers breast cancer, women who live in cultures where little fat is consumed have lower incidences of the disease.

•**Eat five or more servings of fruits and vegetables a day.** Both contain *antioxidants*—substances that counteract cancer-causing free radicals, which form in our bodies following exposure to sunlight, tobacco smoke, car exhaust and other pollutants.

Fruits and vegetables also are packed with cancer-fighters called *phytochemicals*. One of the most powerful anticancer phytochemicals is *sulforaphane*, found in broccoli, cabbage, brussels sprouts, bok choy and cauliflower. Sulforaphane appears to boost the body's natural defenses by activating an enzyme that removes carcinogens from cells.

Garlic and onions—especially raw—contain the phytochemical *allyl sulfide*, which neutralizes certain carcinogens.

And soybeans contain *genistein*. Genistein curbs uncontrolled cell proliferation and competes with estrogen, which has been linked to breast, ovarian and uterine cancers.

How to get five or more servings of fruits and vegetables a day: Fruit with cereal and orange juice in the morning...two vegetables at both lunch and dinner...fruit juices during the day...fruit for dessert.

●**Exercise aerobically for 30 minutes, three to five times a week.** A study by Harvard researcher I-Min Lee, MD, found that exercise helps reduce all types of cancer—possibly by enhancing immune system functions. Tests done on people who exercised even moderately showed that they had higher circulating levels of natural killer cells following their workouts.

A University of California at San Diego/Veterans Administration Medical Center study found that exercise more than tripled the participants' natural killer-cell counts. Regular exercise may reduce the risk of prostate cancer, possibly by lowering testosterone levels. Physical activity also reduces the risk of breast, uterine and ovarian cancers by reducing estrogen levels and improving body-fat distribution. (Studies suggest that women who carry their weight in the upper and mid-body may be especially cancer-prone.)

●**Limit alcohol to four drinks a week.** Excessive consumption of alcohol damages cells, activates certain carcinogens in the body, irritates the lining of the mouth, throat, esophagus and other places (making them more hospitable to cancer) and depresses the body's immune system.

Beer contains potent cancer-causing agents called *nitrosamines*. Another carcinogen, *urethane*, turns up in bourbon, sherry, fruit brandies and other alcoholic beverages.

●**Stay out of the sun.** Ultraviolet rays promote skin cancer and may lower the body's immunity in general.

Wear a *broad-spectrum* sunscreen with a sun protection factor (SPF) of 15—preferably higher—whenever you plan to be outdoors for more than 10 minutes. It is also beneficial to wear a broad-brim hat and tight-weave clothes to block the sun.

●**Teach yourself to relax.** Though we can't say that stress "causes" cancer, we know there's a link between high levels of stress and the disease. Chronic low-level stress may also play a role. Some experts theorize that intense or long-term stress reduces immunity.

Reduce stress, and you may lengthen your life. Regular exercise is a stress-buster. So are pleasurable activities such as dancing, listening to music, socializing with friends, enjoying hobbies, viewing humorous or uplifting movies, etc.

●**Consider taking one aspirin a day.** We're not sure why aspirin has an anticancer effect, but we think it may inhibit cell proliferation and thus reduce the likelihood of tumor formation.

Aspirin may promote cell death—so that precancerous cells die before they have a chance to settle in and reproduce.

No one knows how much aspirin a person needs a day to prevent cancer, but we think about 81 milligrams (mg) (a low-dose pill) may be as effective as higher doses. Check your pharmacy for low-dose aspirin.

Important: Consult your doctor before taking aspirin regularly.

●**Don't smoke.** Smoking increases the risk of colon and other cancers—in addition to heart and pulmonary disease.

For more information about cutting your risk of cancer, call the Cancer Information Service at the National Cancer Institute, 800-422-6237.

Good Things About Ginkgo Biloba

Varro Tyler, PhD, ScD, distinguished professor emeritus of pharmacognosy, Purdue University, West Lafayette, IN.

Ginkgo biloba has long been known as a natural memory booster. But this herbal remedy is also effective against dizziness...

ringing in the ears (*tinnitus*)...and the on-again, off-again leg pain called *intermittent claudication*. Each of these ailments can be caused by sluggish circulation.

How ginkgo works: It helps lower abnormally high levels of platelet activating factor (PAF), a natural body compound that promotes blood clotting, thus inhibiting circulation.

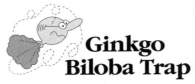

Ginkgo Biloba Trap

Marc Rosenblatt, MD, assistant professor of ophthalmology, Mount Sinai Hospital, New York City.

A 70-year-old man who had been taking 40 milligrams (mg) of the memory-boosting herb *ginkgo biloba* twice a day began experiencing blurred vision.

When doctors examined him, they found blood oozing down the iris of his eye.

Diagnosis: The bleeding was caused by the combination of *ginkgolide B*, a powerful

blood thinner found in ginkgo, and aspirin, another drug with blood-thinning properties. The man was taking both.

Self-defense: Do not take ginkgo with another blood thinner unless your doctor says it's okay. Avoid ginkgo if you have a bleeding disorder.

Lavender and Insomnia

Alan Hirsch, MD neurological director, The Smell & Taste Treatment and Research Foundation, Chicago.

Lavender oil is a safe and effective remedy for insomnia sufferers.

What to do: Place several drops of essential oil of lavender on a cloth and leave it on your nightstand, or fill an electric diffuser with oil to disperse fragrance throughout the room... grow your own lavender and keep a basket of flowers at your bedside...or make an herbal pillow filled with these leaves (fill with fresh leaves every three weeks).

23

Health Care Smarts

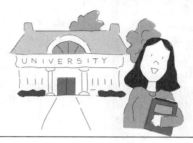

Why Personal Medical Research Is So Important

Fred D. Baldwin, PhD

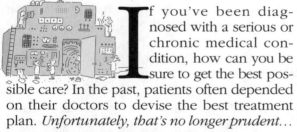

If you've been diagnosed with a serious or chronic medical condition, how can you be sure to get the best possible care? In the past, patients often depended on their doctors to devise the best treatment plan. *Unfortunately, that's no longer prudent...*

● **Medical knowledge is changing so rapidly** that few doctors can keep up. Each month, several hundred articles are published in medical journals—about cardiology alone.

● **Your doctor may be biased toward certain treatments** because of his/her training. Surgeons tend to favor surgery. Internists tend to recommend pills.

● **Your doctor may decide not to recommend a costly therapy** because of cost-cutting pressure from an HMO.

The truth is that you may never find out about a treatment that could cure you unless you do your own medical research.

Example I: A woman with a brain tumor was told by her doctor that her only option was surgery, which could leave her partially paralyzed. She contacted a support group and learned of a noninvasive alternative called the "gamma knife," a form of radiation therapy. Five years later, she's completely healthy.

Example II: Doctors told a woman with non-Hodgkin's lymphoma that her chances of survival were slim. Then her mother read about clinical trials of an extra-high-dosage form of chemotherapy known as *CHOP*. The woman has now been symptom-free for more than a year. Doctors say her prospects are excellent.

RESEARCH SERVICES

If you're low on time or energy—and don't mind paying for medical information—consider using a research service. For a fee of $125

Fred D. Baldwin, PhD, a Carlisle, PA, medical writer and coauthor, with Suzanne McInerney, of *Infomedicine: A Consumer's Guide to the Latest Medical Research*. Little, Brown.

to $400, such services will scan huge medical databases and assemble a bound report containing copies of relevant articles.

Reputable research services include…

•*The Health Resource,* 933 Faulkner, Conway, AR 72032. 800-949-0090.

•*Institute for Health and Healing Library,* 2040 Webster St., San Francisco 94115. 415-923-3681.

•*Schine Online,* 39 Brenton Ave., Providence, RI 02906. 800-346-3287.

DOING YOUR OWN RESEARCH

People are usually happy with the reports they obtain from these services. But by paying someone else to find out about their disease, they're missing out on self-education—a process many people find empowering.

Patients find that actively doing their own research helps allay their anxiety, making them feel hopeful instead of hopeless and helpless.

Good news: Doing sophisticated medical research has become easier than ever before. If you own a computer with a modem, you can do much of your work from home.

If you don't own a computer, see if you can use one at your local public or medical school library. To find a medical library near you, call the National Library of Medicine (NLM) at 888-346-3656.

•**Read about your ailment in consumer health guides.** Look it up in *Mayo Clinic Family Health Book* (William Morrow)…*The American Medical Association's Family Medical Guide* (Random House)…and *The Merck Manual* (Merck Publishing Co.).

If you have trouble deciphering medical terminology, pick up a copy of *Mosby's Medical Dictionary* (Mosby-Year Book).

•**Search out top specialists.** If you have a serious ailment, odds are your family doctor will urge you to see at least one specialist. But many doctors are obligated to refer you to a specialist whose name is on a list provided by an insurance company. This might not be the most highly skilled specialist.

Self-defense: Ask your doctor, "If this were your problem, whom would *you* consult?" As you contact the various experts, ask them the same question.

•**Put powerful databases to work for you.** Hundreds of health-oriented databases have been compiled by research facilities and libraries around the country.

The best is *Medlars,* the online database system of the NLM at *www.nlm.nih.gov.*

Medlars encompasses 40 separate databases —including *Medline*, with abstracts of more than 11 million journal articles. NLM offers PubMed and Internet Grateful Med, two free systems to search MEDLINE. PubMed's retrieval engine links over 700 journals for full text of articles.

Also on the NLM Web site, you'll find Medlineplus for information on hundreds of diseases, conditions and wellness issues. Drug information, online medical dictionaries, a medical encyclopedia and links to other government health resources are available.

Medline can be accessed through libraries… and via online services like America Online. To contact the NLM, call customer service at 888-346-3656 or visit *www.nlm.nih.gov.*

You can do a similar search using *Index Medicus.* This vast *printed* index lists the same journal articles as Medline. It's available at most medical libraries.

•**Focus on the latest research.** Pay special attention to *review* articles. These summarize state-of-the-art treatments. They give a great overview and are usually written by top experts.

Note where these experts are, and contact them. If you have trouble getting through on your own, ask your doctor to arrange a consultation for you.

Grateful Med can be set up to screen databases for review articles only. If you're using a print source like *Index Medicus*, look for articles whose titles contain the words "Current Trends," "Current Status" or "Review."

•**Look into clinical trials.** The National Institutes of Health (NIH) acts as a clearinghouse for information on clinical trials being conducted at research facilities around the country.

To find out if you're eligible to participate in a clinical trial at the NIH's Warren Grant Magnuson Clinical Center in Bethesda, Maryland, call 800-411-1222…or go to *www.cc.nih.gov.*

To find out about cancer trials, contact the National Cancer Institute at 800-422-6237. To find out about AIDS trials, contact the US Department of Health and Human Services at 800-874-2572.

● **Look into alternative treatments.** A good place to start is Dr. Marc Micozzi's *Fundamentals of Complementary and Alternative Medicine* (Churchill Livingstone).

You can also call the NIH National Center for Complementary and Alternative Medicine Clearinghouse (888-644-6226) to learn about alternative approaches for your ailment.

If you have computer access, check out alternative medicine resources at *www.healthfinder.gov, www.altmedicine.com* or *www.drweil.com.*

Beware: Some organizations listed on the Web are fronts for companies that sell rather dubious nutritional supplements.

● **Seek out others who have had your ailment.** They can be found via online discussion groups. Also, check out Medical Matrix at *www.medmatrix.org.* It lists medically oriented "newsgroups" on the Internet.

To find a support group: Contact the National Self-Help Clearinghouse (212-817-1822) or the National Organization for Rare Disorders (800-999-6673). Or—consult *The Self-Help Sourcebook* (American Self-Help Clearinghouse).

Making Sense of Medical News

Timothy McCall, MD, a Boston internist, author of *Examining Your Doctor: A Patient's Guide to Avoiding Harmful Medical Care.* Citadel Press. He is a regular commentator on the public radio program Marketplace, and can be found on the Web at *www.drmccall.com.*

Look beyond headlines. Media reports often exaggerate the importance of individual studies.

● **Consider the source.** Worry about ulterior motives if the study was sponsored by a pharmaceutical manufacturer or an industry association.

● **Were animals or humans studied?** Results from animal studies can't always be correlated to humans.

● **How many subjects were studied?** Too few means that the results are less likely to be valid.

● **Were the subjects like you?** A study of elderly men may mean little to you if you're a 35-year-old woman.

● **Don't overinterpret results.** Just because a study finds that garlic helps protect against some cancers, doesn't mean garlic is a cancer cure.

● **Don't change your lifestyle based on a single news report.** Stay with tried-and-true advice, such as sticking to a balanced, low-fat, high-fiber diet.

The Terrible Truth About Medical Misinformation

John Allen Paulos, PhD, professor of mathematics at Temple University, Philadelphia. Dr. Paulos is author of *A Mathematician Reads the Newspaper.* Basic Books.

It seems you can't open a newspaper or turn on the TV these days without a dose of medical information—the latest risk to health, the newest treatment breakthrough, etc.

Unfortunately, much of what we read and see is grossly misleading. That can cause needless worry—or give needless reassurance. It can also lead us to adopt unsound health practices.

To guard against medical misinformation, keep in mind some basic facts about science, reporting and human nature...

SCIENCE VERSUS JOURNALISM

Scientific knowledge progresses *slowly* and *tentatively.* Most new studies add only a small piece to a very large puzzle.

On the other hand, reporters get paid for being dramatic. Pressure to produce an exciting story leads them to make studies sound more conclusive than they actually are. And bad news is inherently more compelling than good news.

Example: Finnish researchers found a higher rate of lung cancer among smokers who took beta-carotene supplements. Because many other studies have suggested that beta-carotene helps prevent cancer, this made for some pretty frightening headlines.

But the study wasn't all it was cracked up to be. The people in the study had been smoking heavily for an average of 36 years...and they continued to smoke during the six years of the study. Their experience was not necessarily applicable to others.

The researchers themselves conceded that the slight increase in cancer they found could have been simply the result of chance. That fact was ignored in most media reports.

READING BEYOND THE HEADLINES

Newspaper headlines are designed to grab the attention of readers. TV spotlights sensational sound bites and eye-popping visuals. But in science, the truth usually lies in the details—which are presented later, if at all.

Our emotions affect our interpretation of information presented to us. Once we see a picture of a child who is bedridden with leukemia, we're unlikely to pay much attention to how or why he/she got there.

Remedy: Recognize your tendency to jump to conclusions. Read the whole story. As you do, ask yourself the same questions a good journalist would ask—who, what, where, when, why, how and how likely.

If details are lacking, don't make any judgment until you get all the facts.

WHAT DO THE NUMBERS MEAN?

Statistics lend an air of authority to any health-related story. But what do the numbers refer to? Where did they come from? Reporters often ignore these all-important questions.

Example: It has been widely reported that condoms have a "16% failure rate." The figure came from a 1990 survey in which people were asked whether their birth control method had ever failed. Though 16 in 100 condom users surveyed said that condoms had failed, that does not mean that condoms fail 16% of the time.

Be especially wary of surveys in which people "self-report" complex information. People don't always tell the whole truth.

WHAT'S THE REAL RISK?

To judge by the media, virtually everything puts us at risk of some dread disease.

First question to ask: Just how big is the risk? We tend to overreact to threatening, unfamiliar things, particularly when they lie outside our control.

Try to look at risk-related statistics rationally, not emotionally.

Example I: Illicit drugs can indeed be deadly. But even the scourge of heroin (6,000 deaths a year) and cocaine (8,000 deaths) pale in comparison to the toll taken by tobacco (400,000 deaths) and alcohol (90,000 deaths).

Example II: To sound dramatic, a reporter might emphasize that 2,500 people die each year from a particular disease...and drive home the point with heart-wrenching interviews with their families.

But 2,500 deaths out of the total US population is not very significant.

Example III: Most of us have heard that "one woman in eight will develop breast cancer." But this figure is for *lifetime incidence.* It fails to take into account the fact that a woman's risk rises with age. It also assumes that all women will live at least to age 85.

In fact, fewer than one 20-year-old woman in 200 will develop breast cancer by the time she reaches age 40...and only one 40-year-old in 25 will develop breast cancer by age 60.

The reported rise in breast cancer risk sounds even less terrifying when you consider that much of the rise can be attributed to widespread screening, which has brought more cases to light ...and that our ever-lengthening life spans are enabling more women to reach the age at which the disease usually strikes.

Bottom line: News reports often omit the context that gives meaning to statistics.

RESPECT THE POWER OF CHANCE

Ten people with advanced cancer receive a drug and have a dramatic remission? It *might* have been the drug...or they might have gotten better anyway.

When evaluating medical news, look for *statistical significance.* Statistically significant results are those that cannot be attributed to random chance.

The smaller the sample size (the number of people, animals, etc., participating in the study), the more likely that a dramatic result was due to chance.

When two things happen together, don't assume that one *causes* the other. A question that news reports often ignore is whether confounding variables may be responsible.

Example: A study found that people who drink wine have fewer heart attacks than those who drink beer or hard liquor. Does wine have a magic ingredient? Or is there another explanation?

One explanation researchers mentioned (but news summaries didn't) is that wine drinkers tend to be more educated and affluent than beer and whiskey drinkers. It's well known that wealth and education go hand in hand with greater health and longevity.

This is one reason why double-blind, controlled studies are more convincing than others.

In such studies, two matched groups are compared. One group receives a drug, for example, the other doesn't...and neither the experimenters nor the experimental subjects know which group is which. This makes it more likely that observed effects are due to the drug and not other factors.

On the other hand, be skeptical of anecdotal reports. Anyone can select a striking story. With no basis for comparison, however, even the most vivid event is meaningless.

Example: When a talk show guest blamed his wife's fatal brain cancer on her cellular phone, this caused panic among cellular phone users—and even sparked a decline in cellular phone stocks.

But about 10 million people now use cellular phones, and the overall brain cancer rate in this country remains at six per 100,000. By chance alone, you'd expect 600 phone users to develop the disease each year. Far fewer cases have been reported.

LOOK TO THE SOURCE

Any study appearing in a scientific journal like the *The New England Journal of Medicine*, the *Journal of the American Medical Association* or *The Lancet* has undergone a rigorous quality-control process known as peer-review.

Peer review means that experts in the field have judged the study to be of sufficient quality and importance to merit publication. An unpublished finding reported on TV has not been subjected to peer review—and is therefore less credible.

While "expert" commentary isn't foolproof, it's more reliable than a reporter's interpretation.

Of course, if you really want the details, you'll need to read the original journal article.

How Does Your HMO Stack Up?

The National Committee for Quality Assurance (NCQA) has begun rating and accrediting health-maintenance organizations.

Rated: The quality of an HMO's medical treatment...physicians' qualifications...preventive health services...medical record-keeping... the appropriateness of care...patients' rights.

While evaluations are paid for by participating HMOs, one in eight tested so far has received a failed rating. *www.ncqa.org.*

Picking an HMO

Susan Pisano, director of communications, American Association of Health Plans, 1129 20 St. NW, Suite 600, Washington, DC 20036.

Before enrolling in a health-maintenance organization, put these questions to the HMO representative...

●**Are there participating doctors near where I work or live?**

●**Where can I go for care at night or on weekends?**

●**Does the plan offer a choice of doctors?**

●**What percentage of participating doctors are board-certified?**

●**Does the member services department have useful information** about participating doctors?

Ask the HMO for references. Ask friends and family members about their experiences with HMOs, too.

The Value of Lab Tests

Marc Silverstein, MD, director, Center for Health Care Research, Medical University of South Carolina, Charleston. His study of lab tests in 531 patients, average age 63, was published in *The American Journal of Medicine*, 655 Avenue of the Americas, New York 10010.

Routine lab tests are of little value for apparently healthy individuals. Many doctors order urinalysis, complete blood count, thyroid studies and blood chemistry as part of physical exams. But besides being costly, these four tests are unlikely to uncover a health problem in such individuals. If your doctor recommends the four tests as part of a routine physical exam, ask him/her to explain the health benefits of the information derived from these tests...and how the results will change his recommendations.

Avoiding Anxiety During an MRI

Helen Wahba, RN, staff nurse, department of radiology, MetroHealth Medical Center, Cleveland.

One in 10 people scheduled to undergo magnetic resonance imaging (MRI) find it impossible to do so.

Reason: Claustrophobia. MRI scanning involves lying down for 25 to 60 minutes in a very narrow tunnel for a very noisy exam.

Here's how to make the process much more bearable...

●**Ask your doctor to explain MRI testing procedures** well before your scheduled test. Pamphlets are provided by most scanning sites.

●**Have a family member or friend stay in the room with you during the scan.** If possible, ask this person to hold your ankle during the exam.

●**Make sure you are in a comfortable position before the exam begins.** A pillow under the knees reduces the strain on your back.

●**Keep your eyes closed throughout the procedure.** Drape a cloth over your eyes...

Editor's note: Less-confining "open" MRI machines are now available, but they may produce less-detailed images.

and imagine sitting on a beach or in your favorite chair at home.

●**Ask that the air conditioning be turned up.** That way, you can avoid the "closed-in" feeling of a too-warm room.

●**Wear prism eyeglasses.** These glasses let you see out of the tunnel while you're lying on your back. Ask loved ones to sit at the end of the tunnel so you can see them.

Ulcer Testing

A. Mark Fendrick, MD, University of Michigan School of Public Health and School of Medicine, Ann Arbor, MI.

Delay invasive tests for ulcers until you have tried drug therapy. Research shows that nearly all people with ulcers are infected with bacteria that are associated with ulcer recurrence. Medical guidelines now recommend using antibiotics to kill the bacteria.

Trap: Doctors may routinely order an initial uncomfortable endoscopy for patients suspected of having ulcers. *Better:* Have a blood test done to detect the antibodies. Consider antibiotic therapy if the test is positive. Have an endoscopy only if symptoms fail to disappear.

Genetic Testing Can Save Your Life...or Ruin It

Ellen Matloff, MS, a genetic counselor at the Yale Cancer Center in New Haven, CT. She specializes in counseling patients at high risk for certain forms of cancer.

Over the past 20 years, hundreds of diseases have been linked to mutations in certain genes. A growing number of these mutant genes can now be detected via a simple blood test.

How much influence does your genetic makeup have over your health? What can you do if a hereditary ailment runs in your family? Who should undergo genetic testing?

For the answers to these and other questions, we spoke with Yale genetic counselor Ellen Matloff...

●**To what extent is illness determined by "bad" genes?** We shouldn't really call these genes "bad." We all have genetic mutations. Each of us is probably predisposed to at least one disease—whether it's cancer, heart disease, high cholesterol or a blood disorder.

Having a mutation that has been linked to a specific illness doesn't *guarantee* that you'll develop that illness. It just means you're at high risk.

In many cases, you can minimize the risk by adopting a healthy lifestyle...and by keeping an especially close watch on your health.

With some genetic defects, including those causing certain types of thyroid and colon cancer, risk of developing the disease in question can be close to 100%. That means anyone with the mutant gene who lives to age 85 is almost certain to develop the cancer unless the organ is removed—no matter what other preventive measures are taken.

With other mutant genes, the risk is less certain. If you have one of the recently identified genes linked to breast cancer, for example, you have an 85% chance of getting breast cancer by age 85. The general population of women face a 10% risk of breast cancer.

These mutations are also associated with a 50% to 60% lifetime risk of ovarian cancer (versus a 1% lifetime risk for the general population).

●**For which diseases is genetic testing available?** Testing is now available for literally hundreds of diseases, including some hereditary forms of cancer of the breast and colon. That number is growing every year.

●**Who should undergo genetic testing?** For mutations associated with Huntington disease, muscular dystrophy and other *rare* illnesses, genetic testing is appropriate if the individual has already begun to show symptoms of the illness...or if he has a family history of the disease. The test results help the doctor confirm a suspected diagnosis.

Presymptomatic testing: Available for some forms of hereditary breast, ovarian, colon, thyroid and skin cancer—is appropriate only if...

●**One or more close family members** (parent, sibling, grandparent, aunt or uncle) has had the cancer in question.

●**A close family member had the cancer at an early age.** For breast cancer, early is considered to be age 40 or younger. Or, if the family member had the cancer more than once—in both breasts, for example. Consult your doctor.

●**What's involved in genetic testing?** Typically, a sample of blood or skin (cells scraped from the inside of the cheek) is required for testing.

The sample may be tested at the hospital—or sent out to an independent lab. Results are available within one to three months. Be sure to find a hospital that offers genetic counseling services along with testing. To find one, contact the National Society of Genetic Counselors (610-872-7608) or the information desk of your local hospital.

●**What if I test positive?** For some diseases, there's nothing you can do to alter your fate. Take Huntington disease. Even if you find out that you have the mutation linked to this fatal neurological disease, there's no way to prevent the nerve degeneration or slow its progress.

In such cases, one benefit to screening is the *elimination of uncertainty*.

Someone who tests positive for the gene for Huntington might opt not to have children—for fear of passing on the mutation to them...or of being too ill to raise them.

Another person might choose to begin his family at a younger age, to use donor sperm or eggs or to do prenatal testing.

That person can now make meaningful plans for the future—make out a will, settle finances, even choose a nursing home. This may also be a time to consider spending more time with friends and family and to enjoy life to the fullest.

Many people find the reduced uncertainty to be positive—even if the news is bad.

With cancer-related mutations, the outlook is more positive.

Say you test positive for a mutation linked to breast or ovarian cancer. Your doctor may recommend that you have a mammogram or ultrasound scan more frequently than is ordinarily recommended. That way, you'll be able to detect any tumor at its earliest possible stage.

If you have the gene for colon cancer, you might have colonoscopies more frequently.

A more aggressive approach would be to take out the organ before it develops disease.

If you have your thyroid removed and take thyroid supplements, for example, your risk of thyroid cancer is almost zero.

A woman with a family history of breast cancer might opt to have her breasts removed. This approach, known as "prophylactic mastectomy," is an extreme step. But it can be a lifesaver.

Knowing you're at risk for a certain ailment can motivate you to stick to a healthy lifestyle —eating a low-fat, high-fiber diet, avoiding smoking, etc.

●**How should I go about deciding whether or not to get tested?** Discuss testing with a genetic counselor, your doctor—and your entire family. Consider what would happen if you were to test positive—or negative. Take time to think this over.

Many individuals who initially clamor to be tested ultimately decide not to—once they realize just what's involved.

In most cases, we recommend waiting until at least age 18 before getting tested for adult-onset disorders. Children should be tested only if there's a family history of a treatable childhood disease.

Easily Overlooked Medical Deductions

Nadine Gordon Lee, tax partner, Ernst & Young, LLP, 787 Seventh Ave., New York 10019.

Use this list as a reminder of some of the medical deductions you can easily overlook when you prepare your tax return...*

●**Alcoholism and drug abuse treatment.**

●**Contact lenses.**

*These expenses are deductible only to the extent that their total exceeds 7.5% of Adjusted Gross Income.

●**Contraceptives**, if bought with a prescription.

●**Hearing devices.**

●**Hospital services fees** (laboratory work, therapy, nursing services, and surgery).

●**Impairment-related work expenses** for a disabled individual.

●**Lead paint removal.**

●**Medical transportation**, including the standard mileage deduction.

●**Orthopedic shoes.**

●**Seeing-eye dog.**

●**Special equipment for the disabled.**

●**Special diet foods** prescribed by a physician and taken in addition to your normal diet.

●**Special schools for a handicapped child.**

●**Tuition fees** charged by a school for medical care.

●**Wigs** essential to mental health.

Refund Break for the Ill

Nicholas T. Scott, CA-9, No. 94-15321.

The statute of limitations for filing a return is temporarily suspended during a period when a person is incapacitated and unable to file a return. So when alcoholism rendered a person incapable of filing a return, the statute of limitations was *extended* and he could later file for a refund after the date on which the refund deadline normally would have expired.

Health Benefits Alert

Study by the Institute for Clinical Outcomes, 2681 Parleys Way, Suite 201, Salt Lake City 84109.

Be wary of insurance plans that severely limit the list of drugs for which they will reimburse you.

Reason: Forcing doctors to use a second-choice medication often leads to longer recovery times and may increase the cost of treating a particular illness.

Prostate Cancer Fact

American Institute for Cancer Research, Washington, DC.

About 90% of men who are diagnosed with prostate cancer before it has spread beyond the prostate gland—and who are then treated surgically—can expect to live at least another 15 years.

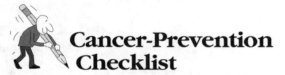

Cancer-Prevention Checklist

Hugh Shingleton, MD, national vice president for cancer detection and treatment, American Cancer Society, 1599 Clifton Rd., Atlanta 30329.

●**Colorectal.** Men and women age 50 and older should have a sigmoidoscopy every three to five years and a fecal occult blood test every year.

●**Rectal/prostate.** Men and women age 40 and older should have a digital rectal exam every year, and men age 50 and older should have a prostate-specific antigen (PSA) test every year.

●**Cervical.** Women age 18 and older (or whenever sexual activity begins) should have a pap test every year until age 39.

Exception for women 18-39: After three or more consecutive annual pap tests with normal findings, the test may be done less often at the doctor's discretion.

Women age 40 and older should have a pap test every year.

●**Uterine/ovarian.** Women between age 18 and 39 should follow the above recommendations for a Pap test. Women age 40 and older should have a pelvic exam every year.

●**Breast.** Women age 20 and older should self-examine their breasts at least once every month. Women between age 20 and 39 should have a manual clinical examination by a health professional every three years and a clinical exam every year once they reach age 40. Women between age 40 and 49 should have a mammogram every one to two years and every year once they reach age 50.

●**Other.** Both men and women between age 20 and 39 should receive health counseling and a cancer checkup every three years, and every year once they reach age 40.

Cellular Phones and Cancer Risk

Kenneth J. Rothman, DrPH, senior scientist, Epidemiology Resources, an epidemiology research and education company in Newton, MA.

In a study of 250,000 cellular phone users, there was no increase in overall mortality. The study included "flip phones," which have antennas that must be held close to the head. It did *not* specifically address the question of whether these phones cause cancer.

You Can Catch Up On Sleep

Allan Pack, MD, PhD, director, Center for Sleep and Respiratory Neurobiology at the University of Pennsylvania, Philadelphia.

Recovery sleep need not be hour-for-hour, because sleep-deprived people go into deeper sleep more quickly and may need less recovery sleep than the sleep they lost.

Best Ways to Protect Your Lower Back

Natural Medicine for Back Pain: The Best Alternative Methods for Banishing Backache by Glenn S. Rothfeld, MD, founder and medical director of Spectrum Medical Arts in Arlington, MA. Rodale Press.

Anyone who sits for long periods of time each day is at high risk for developing lower back pain.

To reduce the risk: Cross your legs at the ankles, not the knees…stand up and walk around at least once every half hour.

Important: Your office chair should have a straight back…armrests…enough width and depth for you to move around…a back bulge that curves into the small of your back…seat padding that does not give more than half an inch.

If you do overstress your back and experience pain, apply cold as soon as possible. Continue the cold treatment periodically for one or two days.

Reason: Cooling the back helps prevent minute tears in the muscles from bleeding and reduces painful fluid accumulation.

After one or two days, switch over to heat treatments—two or three times a day, for 15 minutes at a time. This relaxes the muscles and reduces the pain. Moist heat—a hot water bottle wrapped in a wet towel—is better than dry heat from a heating pad.

Back Injury Study

Ann Myers, ScD, associate professor of nursing, Alfred State College, Alfred, New York, and leader of a study of 600 city employees.

A study found that back injuries are twice as common among workers who have little control over their jobs as they are among workers who have a greater say in how they do the same kind of work.

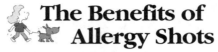

The Benefits of Allergy Shots

Peter Creticos, MD, associate professor of medicine, Johns Hopkins University School of Medicine, Baltimore. His three-year study of 77 patients was published in *The New England Journal of Medicine*, 10 Shattuck St., Boston 02115.

Asthma attacks caused by exposure to pollen respond better to allergy shots than to oral allergy medication. The shots have long been used to control sneezing, runny nose and other *nonrespiratory* symptoms of ragweed allergic rhinitis (hay fever). But it's been unclear whether these shots are helpful to patients with ragweed-induced asthma.

Finding: Patients treated with allergy shots needed less medication, could breathe easier and were less sensitive to ragweed.

How to Tell if You Are Allergic to Nickel

James Marks, MD, professor of medicine, Pennsylvania State University College of Medicine, Hershey.

Nickel is often overlooked as a cause of allergic reactions. The silver-white metal is found in everything from pierced earrings and keys to tools, zippers and, of course, nickel coins.

Symptom: An itchy, crusty and blistery rash.

Helpful test: Tape a nickel to your skin on a hot day. If your skin turns red, consult a dermatologist.

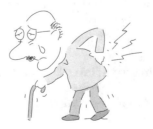

Lyme Disease Update

Charlene C. DeMarco, DO, a tick-borne disease specialist in private practice in Egg Harbor, NJ. Her study of 89 patients with late-stage Lyme disease was presented at the International Conference on Macrolides in Lisbon, Portugal.

Lyme disease responds well to the antibiotic *clarithromycin*. Of 28 patients who took 250 mg twice daily, 20 had moderate relief of the arthritis that's characteristic of the late stages of Lyme. Results were less dramatic in those who got once-a-day medication. Other antibiotics for late-stage Lyme disease must be injected. Late-stage Lyme disease occurs within 24 months of being bitten by an infected tick.

Lyme Disease Self-Defense

Allen C. Steere, MD, director of rheumatology and immunology, New England Medical Center, Tufts University School of Medicine, Boston.

Remove the tick and save it in a vial…label the container with the date and location where you were likely to have been bitten…at the first signs of infection—rash, joint pain, fever, other flulike symptoms—take the tick to your doctor.

Reason: Knowing what kind of tick bit you helps the physician with diagnosis and treatment. It is not generally of value to analyze the tick itself for infectious agents.

Illness Can Be Good for You

Randolph M. Nesse, MD, professor of psychiatry, University of Michigan Medical School, Ann Arbor, and author of *Why We Get Sick: The New Science of Darwinian Medicine.* Times Books.

Some disease symptoms show that the body's natural defenses are working properly. Nausea and vomiting remove potentially fatal toxins from the body. Fever is a defense against infection. Coughing also removes toxins. Disease and health are more closely related than most people realize. The human body repairs damage by having cells divide—but the same mechanism gone awry can lead to cancer.

To Avoid Spreading Cold Sores…

Rodney Basler, MD, assistant professor of internal medicine and dermatology, University of Nebraska Medical Center, Omaha.

Always use sunscreen on your lips when outdoors…keep blisters clean and dry…coat them with petroleum jelly or a similar substance to prevent cracking…do not share cups, straws, toothbrushes or towels during an outbreak. For people with frequent outbreaks, ask your doctor about taking low doses of the antiviral drug *acyclovir* to prevent outbreaks or lessen their severity. The medicine is sold by prescription under the name *Zovirax.*

Hooray!! Lower Cost Prescription Drugs

Charles Inlander, president of The People's Medical Society, a patient advocate organization, 462 Walnut St., Allentown, PA 18102. He is author of several books, including *The People's Medical Society Health Desk Reference.* Hyperion.

To save money on medications that your doctor prescribes, you can…

●**Buy generics**—they can cost 70% less than virtually identical name brands.

●**Buy in bulk**—ask for a six-month prescription instead of a one-month supply that's renewable five times.

●**Play it safe with new medicines** by buying just a one-week supply until you find out about any possible side effects.

●**Shop around**—different drugstores price the same medicine differently.

•**Use mail order**—check with your employer or other services to find a good place to send for mail-order prescription drugs. Ordering through the mail will generally get you the lowest prices.

Help for Ex-Ex-Smokers

John Hughes, MD, professor, department of psychiatry, University of Vermont, Burlington.

Quitting smoking takes most smokers five or six tries. Very few people quit for good after the first time...but too many get discouraged when they can't quit and then don't try again.

Bottom line: Don't stop trying to quit smoking. Eventually you will be successful.

Heavy Smokers and the Nicotine Patch

Study of 522 smokers by Jorn Olsen, MD, PhD, University of Aarhus, Denmark, published in *The American Journal of Epidemiology.*

Heavy smokers using nicotine patches to kick the cigarette habit should start out with the highest-strength patches and gradually taper off.

Reason: If the initial dose doesn't deliver enough nicotine, smokers may quickly stop the treatment. Over-the-counter patches currently available deliver from 21 milligrams (mg) to 7 mg of nicotine a day.

Cost: About $30 for one week's worth of patches.

24

Emotional Health Means a Happier You

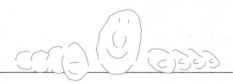

How Your Emotions Affect Your Health... Proven Ways to Stay Well

John Travis, MD, and Regina Sara Ryan
Wellness Associates

The flood of news about health and fitness these days can be more confusing than helpful. If you've been exercising or eating "right" for years but still feel frustrated and unfulfilled, you are not alone.

There are ways to take charge of your health by tapping your inner resources effectively. The changes that we support are simple and are designed to increase self-awareness, since all aspects of life are interdependent.

Example: When you're worried about something, you're also likely to have an upset stomach.

What may appear to be individual events are really interconnected aspects of a larger, more complex system.

When you master small changes, you build a fortified base from which to take further steps on your healing journey toward wellness.

Although many people associate wellness only with fitness, nutrition or stress reduction, wellness is really much more. Wellness brings people into a domain of self-responsibility and self-empowerment.

SET GOALS FOR WELLNESS

Goals keep you on course. And more than that, goals are like magnets—they tend to attract people and resources that help get them accomplished. It's almost magical how this happens.

Often people set their sights too high and then quit completely when they don't make the grade. Approach these "impossible" goals by breaking them down into manageable parts.

BREATHING REDUCES STRESS

Stress is inevitable—you need it to warn you about the negative forces of life. But there are

John Travis, MD, and Regina Sara Ryan, coauthors of *Wellness: Small Changes You Can Use to Make a Big Difference.* Ten Speed Press. Dr. Travis is director of Wellness Associates, 21489 Orr Springs Rd., Ukiah, CA 95482.

many forms of stress that wear you down and cause a variety of health problems.

You may not be aware of it, but every tense situation—or even memories of tense situations —causes a change in breathing. The more stressed you feel, the more shallow your breathing becomes. Consciously breathing deeply can relieve tension, quiet fear and relieve pain. So before you reach for aspirin or antacid tablets, do some breathing.

EMOTIONS AND HEALTH

There is a heavy price to be paid when feelings are denied or repressed. Lethargy, boredom and a lack of enthusiasm toward life may be the consequences. Those who are unaccustomed to dealing with feelings in healthy ways often seek out other means to cover up those feelings or distract themselves, such as alcohol, food, drugs, TV, unhealthy relationships or compulsive work.

Befriend your emotional self. Accept emotions as valuable signals that tell you something is in need of attention. *How to acknowledge emotions…*

- **Write an angry letter** and then tear it up.

- **Compose a poem** about your grief.

- **Draw, paint or even dance** to express your feelings.

- **Exercise vigorously.**

- **Talk about your feelings.**

- **Let fear be there.**

- **Let discouragement be there.**

Don't try to chase these emotions away. Look at them. Express them when it is appropriate to do so. Then move on.

SIMPLIFY YOUR LIFE

Becoming well in body, mind and spirit is not nearly as difficult as it may seem. Wellness is not a matter of accumulating something, like more research or experience.

Rather, wellness is realized by unburdening yourself of all those things that prevent the natural state of healthiness from being present. To become well is to appreciate simplicity. *Examples:*

- **One breath is precious**…one smile…one day of seeing the sun.

- **Simplify your life.**

- **Simplify your diet.**

- **Take time to rest your mind.**

- **See your loved ones as brand-new every day.**

HONOR YOUR BODY'S WISDOM

Inhabit your body. Learn to start listening to what it is saying to you and to trust what you hear.

Listening to others instead of yourself…or saying *yes* when you mean *no* are just two examples of the many ways you shortchange yourself. Wellness is about "coming home"— taking up residence inside your own body once again.

REPROGRAM YOURSELF

Current research in the field of psychoneuro-immunology verifies what folk healers have known for centuries—that thinking and emotions have a direct impact on the strength of the immune system.

The immune system is the first line of defense against disease. Strengthening your immune system consciously, through the use of imagery or nurturing self-talk, gives you a much better chance of maintaining whole-body health.

CONNECT TO THE EARTH FOR HEALING

When was the last time you sat on the ground or touched the earth in some way? This may seem silly, but physical contact with soil, natural waters, sunlight and fresh air is healing.

When stress has built up, a walk around the block is often all that is needed to restore perspective.

Beyond that, you connect with forces stronger than the individual self in nature, and this puts everything in perspective.

A PARTNERSHIP IN HEALING

There will be times in your life when you need the care and attention of a helping professional—a doctor, psychologist, social worker, etc.*

*Helping professionals interested in learning more about developing partnership relationships with their patients or clients can contact Wellness Associates, 828-251-5594. A book, *Wellness for Helping Professionals: Creating Compassionate Cultures*, is available from Wellness Associates.

When you're looking for such professionals, it's important to find people willing to take the time to answer questions and listen to your concerns. If you find someone who is unwilling to do this, switch to someone who will.

BOTTOM LINE

Getting started on these small changes will help you make a difference in your life. We hope that you will experience increased self-awareness and self-appreciation...have a sense of greater inner strength...and, above all, live a healthier life.

The Truth... And Your Health

Brad Blanton, PhD, a psychologist in private practice in Washington, DC, and the author of Radical Honesty. *Dell Trade Paperbacks.*

Revealing your true feelings lowers your risk for cancer and heart disease. Dishonesty seems to weaken the immune system, raising the risk of infectious disease.

Helpful: Before responding to any question, ask yourself, *Is what I am about to say truthful? ...Is it necessary?...and Is it kind?* By reflecting on these three questions, you'll be honest, while not hurting others.

All About Moods

Martin Groder, MD, a Chapel Hill, NC, psychiatrist and business consultant. He is author of Business Games: How to Recognize the Players and Deal with Them. *Boardroom Classics.*

We are living in a time of great expectations and big disappointments. When things don't go our way or stress at work or at home gets us feeling down, we become uncooperative, grouchy and even angry.

Though feeling blue or cranky is perfectly normal and healthy, there are times when we would like a bad mood to lift more quickly than nature will allow it to do.

WHAT ARE MOODS?

Moods result from a complex interaction between the internal brain chemistry and the external events you experience.

In the brain, three major neurotransmitters affect the way we feel...

●**Serotonin,** which acts as a mood stabilizer.

●**Dopamine and norepinephrine,** which act as stimulants.

While the full extent of how these three neurotransmitters work is not very well understood, we do know that they are being generated all the time and they naturally move in their own cycles.

The chemicals are also affected by external stimuli—such as foods, drugs and smells—which can cause rapid changes in the production and balance of the neurotransmitters.

This helps explain why people can plunge into bad moods after hearing bad news. Likewise, a person in a bad mood can snap out of it instantly after getting a phone call from a beloved or humorous friend.

SHAKING A BAD MOOD

While feeling sullen is important to the development of a sense of critical self-analysis, there are steps you can take to trick your mind into letting go.

Important: If none of the strategies I'm about to recommend brings relief and your bad mood persists for more than two weeks, see your doctor. The problem may be depression, which must be addressed and treated more aggressively.

Strategies for pulling yourself out of a bad mood...

●**Trace the source of your bad mood.** Common sources of bad moods include recent illness...loneliness...boredom...unrealistic expectations...failure to accomplish a goal...catastrophizing by making mountains out of molehills...and unacknowledged disappointment, guilt or anger.

In these cases, taking the time to analyze what was happening in your life before the bad mood occurred is useful. Knowing where the negative feelings come from gives you some sense of control, and uncovering the cause of your bad mood may actually give you clues on how to remedy it.

Example: One of my patients felt anxious and irritable but didn't know why. We talked about what had been happening during the past few days and discovered the patient's spouse was the target of unexpressed anger. The spouse had been spending money with little regard to the fact that the couple was trying to get out of debt. Once the source of the bad mood was identified, the patient was able to talk directly about it and felt better immediately.

Another often overlooked source of bad moods is having been in a good mood for too long. People who are involved in highly intense projects at work find themselves disappointed when the projects end. In these cases, what feels like a bad mood is simply lack of rest or a neutral mood, neither good nor bad.

●**Make a list of all the positives in your life.** When you're in a bad mood, you view everything in a negative light. Setbacks and letdowns become magnified while positive things aren't recognized at all.

Helpful: If you make a quick list of all the positive factors in your life, your negative perception will likely shift.

●**Exercise.** Physical exertion produces endorphins—natural chemicals in the brain that are responsible for creating good moods. Depending on the individual, the physical activity doesn't have to be strenuous—even a brisk 20-minute walk is sufficient to combat a bad mood. Just being outdoors will expose you to sunlight—another natural antidepressant.

Over time, exercise will make you look better and improve your overall health. And by providing a steady stream of endorphins, regular exercise will actually help protect you from future bad moods.

●**Socialize.** One of the biggest mistakes we make when feeling blue is to isolate ourselves, which can make a bad mood even worse.

Helpful: Force yourself to call someone… or even throw a simple party—take-out pizza will do—and invite some people you haven't seen in a while.

●**Seek humor.** Nothing dissolves a bad mood faster than laughter. Go to a comedy club…rent a funny video…or call a friend who has a great sense of humor.

Helpful: Make a recording of your complaining, and listen to it. Even the most seemingly tragic *woe-is-me* complaint eventually sounds ridiculous.

●**Do something nice for someone else.** Forget yourself by concentrating on someone else. Buy a present for a friend. Call someone you haven't talked to in years. Volunteer at a hospital or nursing home, where you'll likely see others who have much more serious problems than yours.

●**Change your immediate environment.** The simple act of moving furniture around will help freshen your attitude. Hanging new curtains, switching lamp shades, changing your bedspread or rearranging pictures will also give you an immediate lift.

●**Enjoy the arts.** For centuries, the arts have been civilization's tonic. It's hard to stay in a bad mood when gazing at a magnificent painting or listening to music you love.

Even fooling around with paints or a piano will divert you from your woes and give you another way to express yourself.

●**Spend time in a natural setting.** Being close to nature makes us realize that no matter how we feel, the sun still rises and sets each day.

Sitting on a bench in a garden, strolling on a beach or lying on a hillside and gazing at the sky will remind you there is a larger world out there than your own.

Secrets of Inner Strength

Joan Borysenko, PhD, the noted lecturer on health and spirituality and president of a Boulder, CO, educational firm, Mind/Body Health Sciences. A former cancer cell biologist at Harvard Medical School, she is author of *Minding the Body, Mending the Mind* (Bantam) and *A Woman's Book of Life* (Riverhead Books).

Ever notice how some people manage to stay on track despite suffering a serious illness, financial setbacks or other problems that would derail other people?

We spoke with Joan Borysenko, PhD, to learn more about such "emotionally resilient" individuals.

A cancer biologist turned mind/body researcher, Dr. Borysenko has spent decades studying emotional resilience. But her expertise on the subject also stems from personal experience.

She has flourished despite having had her share of misfortune—including a divorce, a near-fatal car accident and the suicide of her father, who was dying of leukemia.

How do emotionally resilient people differ from the rest of us? *Researchers have identified three key attitudes they all share...*

CHALLENGE

Emotionally resilient people view crises as opportunities for problem-solving—as challenges, not as threats to survival. I witnessed this phenomenon in my own life 14 years ago, when my three children and I ran aground while boating in Scituate, Massachusetts.

I immediately began to imagine the worst, thinking "We'll be stuck here all night."

But my 14-year-old son, Justin, was thrilled. "I'll rescue us," he said.

He had us step onto a sandbar, then began casting the anchor farther out in the river, pulling the boat along until we were afloat.

Justin's attitude was a wonderful example of emotional resilience. Mine was not.

CONTROL

Emotionally resilient people recognize that while they cannot control everything that happens to them, they can control their response to events.

They also know when to stop struggling... and when to just let things be. They personify Reinhold Niebuhr's famous serenity prayer: *God grant me the serenity to accept the things I cannot change, the courage to change the things I can and the wisdom to know the difference.*

COMMITMENT

Emotionally resilient people believe there is a higher purpose for even the most painful event.

That doesn't mean they view problems as intrinsically good. But they recognize that some good often does come from even the most traumatic events.

When my dad killed himself in 1975, I felt not only grief but also terrible guilt. As a cancer biologist, I felt I should have done a better job of helping him endure the difficult treatment process he was undergoing.

But I refused to give in to despair. I told myself that if I could help even one other family avert such a tragedy, my father's death would have meaning.

I quit my job at the lab and retrained as a behavioral medicine specialist. Then I founded a mind/body clinic at one of Harvard Medical School's teaching hospitals, beginning a new career helping patients and their families cope physically and spiritually with life-threatening illnesses.

A friend went through something similar when her son died in a car accident. To survive the wrenching pain, she forced herself to think about how her experience might help others.

She now volunteers as a support group facilitator, helping other parents who have suffered the loss of a child.

The late psychiatrist and Holocaust survivor Viktor E. Frankl maintained that it is the meaning that we ascribe to *negative* events that allows us to endure suffering without giving in to despair.

RESILIENCE CAN BE CULTIVATED

Emotional resilience doesn't always come naturally. It certainly didn't come naturally to me. *But it can be developed...*

●**Observe your usual response to emotional stress.** Do you "catastrophize?" Believe nothing you do will make a difference? Blame yourself?

Simply noticing these responses is often a starting point for change.

●**Learn more productive ways to respond to problems.** Whenever you feel worried or annoyed, ask yourself, "How does this situation challenge me? What can I learn from it?"

●**Take care of yourself.** When we're under severe emotional stress, we tend to abandon our healthful habits. But that is precisely when we need them the most.

No matter what else is going on in your life, always eat a balanced diet...exercise regularly ...and get plenty of sleep.

●**Feed your soul.** Each day, do something you find deeply pleasurable—whether it's walking in the park, listening to music or curling up with a book.

●**Find social support.** Sharing your problems with friends and/or family members is the best buffer against stress.

If you lack close relationships to call upon, join a support group. There's one for practically every crisis you may face.

To find a group in your area, consult a hospital social worker...or contact the National Self-Help Clearinghouse at 212-817-1822 or *www.selfhelpweb.org.*

●**Practice gratitude.** In her best-selling book *Simple Abundance* (Warner), Sarah Ban Breathnach recommends spending a few minutes each morning and evening listing five things for which you are grateful.

This will help you focus more on life's gifts instead of its burdens. I think it's a great idea.

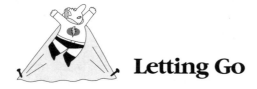 **Letting Go**

Jim Spira, PhD, director of the Institute for Health Psychology, San Diego.

People who freely express negative emotions may live longer after heart attacks. A Belgian study of 300 heart attack survivors found that those who held in their negative emotions—particularly anger and fear—were four times as likely to die within six to 10 years after their heart attacks than a group of survivors who spoke more freely.

Researchers speculate that the emotionally unexpressive types experience greater stress, which causes spasms in the arteries and increases the tendency of blood to clot—both of which contribute to heart problems.

A Survivor's Journey

Greg Anderson, founder and president of the American Wellness Project, Box 238, Hershey, PA 17033. He is author of *The 22 (Non-Negotiable) Laws of Wellness.* Harper San Francisco.

In 1984, at the age of 38, I was diagnosed with lung cancer. After having one lung removed, I learned that the cancer had spread to the lymph system. My doctor gave me a month to live.

But I've been cancer-free since 1989.

What accounts for my survival? Good medical care, including radiation therapy, of course. But I'm convinced that much of the credit goes to my strict adherence to what I call the "laws of wellness."

I've identified 22 laws. *Here are the six most important ones...*

THE LAW OF THE BODY

The body component of wellness hinges on oft-heard advice—avoid tobacco and alcohol ...eat a variety of foods...minimize consumption of fat, salt and sugar...exercise daily... and avoid being overweight.

The latest research shows that eating a low-calorie diet that limits meats of all types adds to both the quantity and quality of your life.

Ideal: 1,500 to 2,000 calories a day for most people, depending on how much you exercise.

THE LAW OF EMOTIONAL CHOICE

Whether or not you realize it, you're capable of choosing which emotions you allow to affect your life. You also have the power to let go of negative feelings.

Problem: We tend to let our emotions dictate our behavior and experiences. We react to situations and to people around us instead of taking responsibility for our own feelings.

Example: If your boss criticizes you at a meeting, you can feel angry for hours...or you can follow the law of emotional choice. It says to let go of the emotion, forgive the transgressor and dismiss the behavior.

Casting off negative emotions does *not* mean that you condone bad behavior. It means you are aware of the stress you encounter on a daily basis—and refuse to let it ruin your life.

THE LAW OF WIN-WIN

Numerous studies illuminate the harm that comes from social isolation and the benefit that comes from belonging…

●**Heart attack victims face a greater risk of death if they go home to an empty house** than if they go home to a spouse or pet.

●**Breast cancer patients who join a support group live longer** than those who don't.

●**People with lots of close friends have stronger immune systems** than people with few friends.

Social wellness means more than simply belonging. It means getting along with others… and cultivating caring, supportive relationships.

Problem: Most people operate with a "win-lose" mentality. They unconsciously believe that in any given encounter, one person wins…and the other loses.

Better: Heed the law of win-win. This law says that it's better to find not *your* way, or *my way*, but a way that's *mutually* beneficial. You'll create allies, not adversaries.

THE LAW OF LIFETIME GROWTH

Most people view aging in terms of biology. In fact, 80% or more of the aging process can be attributed to our attitudes and expectations.

If you think you're too old to do something or to try something new, you are. If you think you're young, you are.

Our self-image is immensely powerful. Consider an acquaintance of mine. He started a new business—at age 96. He even took a 30-year mortgage on an office building. *That's* wellness.

Pursuing your interests prevents boredom and depression…keeps you healthy…and distracts you from physical discomfort. And preliminary data suggest that intellectual activity helps prevent Alzheimer's disease. Strive to grow each day.

THE LAW OF LIFE MISSION

In a survey, 75-year-olds were asked, "What makes life worth living?" The most frequent answer was, "Having a sense of purpose."

Serving others—the law of life mission—is essential for personal fulfillment. Unfortunately, many of us are so busy that we never sit down to consider our purpose in life.

Your purpose is more than your job. Before I fell ill, I lived the life of a fast-paced corporate executive—the classic workaholic. Cancer helped show me my mission—to create wellness for myself and others.

I can't say I'm happy that I got sick. But my illness was clearly filled with many surprise benefits.

How can you discover your life mission? Think. Reflect on your personal creed—your philosophy about why you were put on this earth. And write out a mission statement.

Most people have three distinct missions…

●**Inner mission**—What you want to achieve in personal growth. Look to become a more positive, loving influence in the world.

●**Shared mission**—What you want to achieve in partnership with someone else. Perhaps it's to help raise a child in a loving environment or to redeem an errant social condition.

●**Unique mission**—The mission only you with your unique talents and abilities can accomplish. This mission should involve helping others—doing volunteer work, for example.

THE LAW OF PERSONAL PEACE

Spiritual wellness involves focusing on a higher level of understanding of yourself and others.

I'm talking about learning to love and be loved unconditionally…to express gratitude for your life…to forgive yourself and others for past transgressions or perceived failures…and to let go of resentment and anger.

Achieve personal peace by quieting your mind and spirit. For a few minutes each day, meditate, perform deep breathing, take a bath, pet an animal or pursue another quiet, contemplative activity.

FOLLOWING THE LAWS

Incorporate these laws into your life one at a time. Today, focus on one law. Tomorrow, another. The next day, another—until you have fully incorporated the spirit of wellness into your life. You'll enhance your health, enrich your life…and change the world.

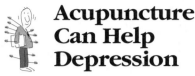

Acupuncture Can Help Depression

John J. B. Allen, PhD, assistant professor of psychology, University of Arizona, Tucson. To find an acupuncturist near you, contact the American Association of Oriental Medicine, 433 Front St., Catasauqua, PA 18032.

In a six-week study, patients given acupuncture experienced a 43% reduction in depressive symptoms. After treatment, more than half no longer met the criteria for clinical depression. That makes acupuncture just as effective as antidepressants and psychotherapy.

How to Put Much More Happiness in Our Lives

Bernie Siegel, MD, founder of Exceptional Cancer Patients in Middletown, CT, which provides information and therapeutic support to people with life-threatening and chronic illnesses. He is author of several books, including *Love, Medicine and Miracles* and *Peace, Love and Healing*. HarperCollins.

Each new year brings ambitious attempts to kick bad habits...live a healthier life ...and accomplish more at work.

But this year, instead of trying to reach many different and difficult goals, resolve to achieve just one—putting more happiness in your life.

Keep this resolution, and your life and immune system will improve, resulting in a healthier—and more prosperous—year. *Simple ways to put more happiness in your life...*

●**Change your attitude about your job and colleagues.** If you are stuck in a job you hate, explore your options for change and make an effort to switch to a career you will find more personally satisfying.

But if you can't change jobs—for financial or career reasons—change your attitude toward your job and the people with whom you work.

If you need motivation, listen to tapes...read uplifting books...and talk to inspiring people.

By behaving like the person you want to be, you can vastly improve your life.

The more you practice your new attitude, the better you'll become at reversing your bad moods and unhealthy feelings.

●**Make time for activities you enjoy.** Studies have shown that when people work on projects or hobbies that they enjoy, their blood chemistry is altered almost immediately in a positive way. When your blood chemistry is altered in this way, it increases your body's resistance to infections and life-threatening diseases.

Key: Engage in activities that make you lose track of time. Such activities depend on the individual—and can range from washing a car or painting a house to reading or exploring the Internet.

●**Change the way you think about failure.** Failure is a state of mind. When you fail to live up to your expectations or those of others, you can dwell on it until you feel terrible about yourself. Or you can choose never to feel this way again by thinking of failure as a redirection that leads to good things. Remember that "F" does not have to stand for *failure*. It can stand for *feedback*.

People who learn from upsetting events and then move on are happier and healthier than those who don't.

My wife has a wonderful saying—*Never consider yourself a failure. You can always serve as a bad example.* She knows that there is a use for everything—even failure—and that we can derive something good or beneficial from every unhappy life event.

●**Get fully in touch with your feelings.** Most of us are extremely adept at repressing issues with which we would rather not deal. We distract ourselves by cramming so many activities into our schedules that we never have time to get at the root of what is making us feel unhappy or anxious.

If you take the time to get in touch with your feelings, you can discover and heal the source of your psychological pain.

●**Keep a journal.** One of the best ways to get in touch with your feelings is to record them in a journal every day. Carry a pad and pen with you, and jot down anything that moves you as each day progresses—whether the events are happy or upsetting.

At the end of each day, read over your notes so you can remember how you felt at specific times and what may have caused those feelings. You may also want to add to your notes.

Studies have shown that people who write regularly in journals feel less stressed and are less susceptible to various diseases.

●**Treat yourself as you would treat a beloved pet.** Many people have problems treating themselves well. They don't forgive themselves easily for making mistakes and do not give themselves permission to enjoy life.

I tell people to take care of themselves as they would a pet.

Examples: Would you allow your pet to smoke? Drink too much alcohol? Become obese? Of course not. You make sure it gets exercise, good food, occasional treats and enjoyable toys. And most important, you give it lots of hugs and express your love.

Do not resolve to eat a healthy diet and get plenty of exercise to avoid dying. Eat a healthy diet and exercise because you care enough about yourself to do it.

Love yourself enough to enjoy the beautiful things in life without feeling guilty. Buy a new outfit. Take a day off from work and go to the movies. Lighten up, and spend some time playing.

●**Make a difference.** Individuals who help others several times a week often live longer, healthier lives. When you volunteer to help other people, you feel better emotionally and physically. You achieve a natural high.

●**Develop a childlike sense of humor.** Just as children are able to see the silly side of almost everything in life, you can use humor to get through the ordinary hassles and crises you face. Watching humorous movies and TV shows can boost your physical immunity.

If you despise your job and hate going back to work on Monday…or you are scheduled for a medical treatment you dread, your body will start releasing stress-provoking chemicals before you get to the office or hospital. You can neutralize this reaction by reading an amusing book, listening to a funny tape or just looking for the humor in life.

Take charge of your life, and decide which labor pains you are willing to experience in order to give birth to yourself.

Gambling a Problem?

Eric Hollander, MD, professor of psychiatry, Mount Sinai School of Medicine, New York City. His study of 19 compulsive gamblers 22 to 57 years of age was presented at a meeting of the American Psychiatric Association.

Compulsive gambling can often be controlled with the antidepressant *fluvoxamine* (Luvox). Among 10 gambling addicts who took the drug for two months, seven said they no longer had the desire to gamble. Fluvoxamine is also effective against compulsive shopping.

The Smart Way to Handle Negative Emotions

David K. Reynolds, PhD, a leading expert on Eastern psychotherapies in Coos Bay, OR. He has trained numerous instructors in Constructive Living worldwide and is the author of more than 30 books, including A Handbook for Constructive Living. William Morrow.

Most people try to fix negative emotions like anxiety, anger or sadness. Instead of solving our problems, however, this approach inevitably leaves us frustrated and confused. It doesn't work because *feelings are uncontrollable.*

But we can control what we do. This simple fact is the basis of a way of life called *Constructive Living.* By helping us focus on what we can control (our behavior) rather than what we can't (our feelings, other people, the past), Constructive Living makes life more satisfying and meaningful.

ROOTS OF CONSTRUCTIVE LIVING

Constructive Living is based on two schools of Japanese psychotherapy…

• **Morita therapy** represents the action side of Constructive Living. Developed in the early 1900s by psychiatrist Morita Shoma, it has its roots in Zen Buddhism.

• **Naikan therapy** is the reflective side. It was developed in the 1930s by Yoshimoto Ishin, a businessman-turned-priest.

Despite its origins, Constructive Living is *not* a therapy. It's a way of living learned through daily practice and observation.

THE IMPORTANCE OF ACTION

Like the weather, feelings are unpredictable. Sadness and anger come and go. So do joy and excitement. The most sensible approach to handling such feelings is to accept them... and *continue doing what you need to do.*

Example: If you're nervous about starting a new job, do not fixate on your anxiety or try to eliminate it. Let it encourage you to learn as much as possible about your duties beforehand. Your performance will be enhanced...and you will probably find yourself feeling less anxious.

Bottom line: Trying to change the way you feel makes no more sense than trying to will a storm to stop. Just wait.

While you wait, take action toward your goals. Doing so prevents you from dwelling on things you cannot control and brings a sense of accomplishment—which should lead to greater happiness and satisfaction. Even if it doesn't, focusing on your *purpose* and *behavior* rather than your feelings will give you a sense of calm and contentment.

THE PROBLEM WITH WESTERN PSYCHOTHERAPY

Conventional psychotherapists have things backward. They try to help their clients feel better so that they can take steps to improve their lives.

You don't have to feel good about yourself to make changes in your life. In fact, things usually work the other way—we feel better as a *result* of having made constructive changes.

Feelings that are labeled "negative" in psychotherapy often have very useful roles.

Example: Fear helps us avoid physical danger...anxiety prompts us to organize our thoughts before making a speech.

Acknowledging these feelings doesn't mean you must submit to them. You can feel shy and still invite someone out to lunch. You can fear flying and do it anyway. You can feel sad about the end of a relationship and still go to work.

MORITA EXERCISES

Exercise I: Next time you find yourself brooding about someone who treated you badly, do something useful and vigorous. Wash your car, for instance, or vacuum the house.

By the time you're done, the troubling thoughts will probably have passed...*and* you'll have accomplished something.

Exercise II: List all the chores you have to do, then tackle them in alphabetical order. The point is to *do*—not agonize about what to do.

Exercise III: Over the next 24 hours, try several activities that you haven't tried before —knitting, cooking a new recipe, painting, etc. This teaches you not to let fear or other feelings keep you from trying something new.

THE ROLE OF REFLECTION

Balancing the *Morita* side of Constructive Living is *Naikan*, the reflective side.

Naikan teaches us to revere all the gifts we have been given. It shifts our focus from ourselves to other people.

When we fail to get what we want, it's easy to feel unhappy. We feel that we haven't gotten our fair share. But nothing we have is exclusively ours.

Our bodies are a gift from our parents, who got their bodies from *their* parents. We are sustained by food grown and processed by people we've never met. Even our ideas are based upon the wisdom of others.

Conventional therapy encourages people to review the bad things that happened to them in the past—all the ways others hurt or disappointed them.

How much time do you spend thinking about the ways *you* hurt other people?

Even if your parents were neglectful, you owe them a debt for giving you life. The fact that you reached adulthood means that *someone* in your past took care of you.

The proper response to recognizing all that we have been given is *gratitude.* Rather than focusing on how much the world owes us, focus on how much we have received from so many sources.

NAIKAN EXERCISES

Exercise I: At the end of the day, spend 20 minutes recalling what people did for you that day…what you did for others…and any trouble you caused others. *Don't* devote time to reviewing troubles others caused you. Most of us are already skilled at that.

Exercise II: Once a week, find something broken and fix it. *Examples:* A leaky faucet, a jammed copier, etc. This is a way of expressing gratitude to the things that support you every day.

Exercise III: Think of someone you haven't been getting along with—a coworker, for example. Say "thank you" to that person 10 times a day.

Exercise IV: Every day, secretly perform a favor for a family member. If anyone detects your "secret service," find another secret service to do.

Example: Shine your spouse's shoes and return them to the closet.

We tend to do things for others with the idea that we'll get something in return. This exercise reminds us that the world doesn't owe us anything.

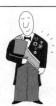

Overcoming Fear of Failure

Arnold Fox, MD, a specialist in cardiology and internal medicine for more than 30 years and a commissioner on the California State Board of Quality Assurance. He and his son, Barry Fox, PhD, are coauthors of several books, including *Beyond Positive Thinking: Putting Your Thoughts Into Action.* Hay House.

We generally understand that a chronic fear of failure can be detrimental to our careers or personal relationships. But recently, scientists have discovered that such negative feelings take a serious toll on our *physical* health, as well.

ADRENALINE AND CATECHOLAMINES

For better or worse, every thought in our head—positive or negative—affects our internal biochemistry. Fear, worry, self-doubt and other emotional "downers" do much of their behind-the-scenes damage by stepping up secretion of adrenaline and other hormones called *catecholamines.*

Even in individuals with perfectly normal hearts, catecholamines can trigger a condition called *paroxysmal tachycardia*—skipped or rapid heartbeat. This has been linked to sudden death.

Elevated catecholamines also boost cholesterol levels and blood pressure.

Result: Increased risk of heart attack and stroke.

Over time, chronically elevated levels of catecholamines raise the heart's metabolism, forcing it to work harder. The same chemicals reduce the body's output of insulin. Reduced insulin production raises the risk of both diabetes and atherosclerosis.

A steady flow of catecholamines also erodes the inner lining of small blood vessels. The vascular "potholes" resulting from this erosion fill up easily with platelets and cholesterol—even if cholesterol levels in the body are normal.

Our fear of failure can keep cholesterol at peak levels for long periods of time. *Illustration:* Cholesterol levels of medical students remain high even weeks after major exams.

Chronic worry also wreaks havoc on the immune system, reducing the effectiveness of our protective *T-cells.*

Anxiety can also stimulate the adrenal glands to secrete more cortisone, setting the stage for peptic ulcers.

CHANGING OUR PERCEPTIONS

To counteract the potentially deadly fear of failure, we must change our perceptions. *Key:* Realizing that failure itself is an unavoidable fact of life.

Each and every one of us has stumbled at some time or other. But that doesn't make us failures.

Even a long string of setbacks or mistakes doesn't qualify us for this sweeping, negative label. The scripts of our lives are filled with failures and unhappy scenes as well as successful and joyful ones.

Helpful: Replay and savor the positive scenes. Don't dwell on the negative scenes.

Review negative scenes only long enough to learn from them—and then move on.

People who view themselves as failures or chronic worriers are simply stuck in their negative scenes. They can't put the script down and move on to another page, so to speak.

A vicious cycle ensues, as the belief that they are failures and the constant fear of failing again discourage them from trying new experiences or persevering at tasks that can lead to more positive results. That holds true for their health, their careers and their relationships.

FINDING THE SILVER LINING

Mini-case study: Imagine two clerks in the same office, doing pretty much the same work.

One clerk thinks the work is beneath his talents and abilities. He resents having to take orders from a female boss and fears being viewed as a failure for having such a low-level job.

The other clerk, a child of recent immigrants, is glad to have a job that pays enough for her to attend evening classes and complete her college degree.

Although both clerks are performing the same tasks for the same pay, the first views the work as dreadful, the other as a great opportunity to get ahead.

To put it another way, the second clerk views her work as a *new, interesting* and *challenging experience* (NICE).

Clearly, the same stimulus can trigger NICE or negative feelings, depending on our perceptions. Positive perceptions allow us to control our world by altering our interpretations of situations and events. This helps us focus on our successes while gearing up for any difficult tasks that might lie ahead.

FOUR REASONS NOT TO GIVE IN TO FEAR

●**Internal messages—***You can't do it...You're not good enough...You'll never make it...*and *You're going to fail*—whether intentional or not, verbal or otherwise, sap our confidence, energy and creative juices.

When we give in to fear and worry, our mental eye is fixed only on images of failure, weakness and embarrassment, blocking out positive, encouraging images.

●**We are often less worried about failure itself than about how we will look to others** if we do fail.

But excessive concern with appearances robs us of our initiative and of the freedom to take control of our lives. It programs us to behave according to others' expectations—setting us up for chronic anxiety.

●**Fear of failure, self-doubt and other "can't do" emotions** are what I call "master" addictions. They can lead to smoking, overeating, alcohol and drug abuse and other potentially deadly habits.

●**The word "worry" comes from the Old English *wyrgan,* meaning "to strangle."** That's what we do when we worry—we strangle our ability to think and perform effectively, along with our strength, flexibility, enthusiasm and belief in ourselves.

Concern—an awareness of problems and a desire to overcome them—spurs us on and helps us find solutions to our problems. By contrast, worry keeps us from taking any action at all.

TAKING POSITIVE ACTION

To free yourself from the stranglehold of fear, uncertainty and doubt...

●**Remind yourself that everyone makes errors.** More important is what we do with those errors. Don't allow your mistakes or failures to color your self-image.

Instead, say, *This led to results I really didn't want. Next time I'll avoid that...and look for another way of behaving.*

Helpful: Set clear goals. Know where you want to go, then divide your journey into small, manageable trips.

Follow these three easy rules...

●**Don't sweat the little things.**

●**Everything is little.**

●**If you can't flee, go with the flow.**

●**Almost every problem has a lighter side** —look for it! Humor is a great healer. It helps you avoid "sweating" the minor irritants and hurdles in your life and serves to put matters in perspective.

Try smiling especially when you don't feel like it. You may have to act at first, but the happy feelings will soon follow. Act confident and upbeat—and soon you will be.

● **Take the focus of fear and worry off yourself.** Use your talents and strengths to help someone else—a child struggling with homework, an elderly neighbor, a troubled friend. Often the best way to feel better about yourself and your life is to do something for others—even if that means simply offering your companionship and support.

● **Don't wring your hands over the things you can't control.** Focus only on those things you *can* control.

● **Don't go it alone.** If a task seems overwhelming, ask for help. Doing so is not a sign of weakness, but of resourcefulness and strength.

Make yourself part of a community. Whether it's a family, neighborhood, house of worship or any other caring group, feeling that you belong is an effective antidote to fear.

How to Overcome Emotions that Hold You Back

Marilyn Mason, PhD, associate professor at the University of Minnesota and a corporate consultant and lecturer in Minneapolis. She is author of several books, including *Seven Mountains: The Inner Climb to Commitment and Caring*. NAL–Dutton.

Over the past 20 or more years, I have hiked up some of the world's highest peaks. When I started climbing many years ago, I wasn't much of an athlete. But over time, it was a thrill to see my stamina escalate...and my body strengthen.

More startling is how mountain climbing helped me gain greater control over my mind. I even learned to master my emotions—and anyone can do the same.

FACING YOUR FEARS

Fear is one of our deepest emotions. It can either motivate us or inhibit us from taking action. When fear overcomes us, it can cloud everything else we are experiencing or thinking. That can happen no matter how intelligent or well-balanced you are.

Fear helped our ancient ancestors recognize the danger of predators, inspiring them to flee and survive. Since we're rarely chased by lions today, fear has become a more complex emotion. Many times we are reacting to perceived dangers rather than real ones.

Fear can affect your thinking in many ways today—keeping you from pursuing an opportunity as well as telling you to flee danger.

Helpful: Whenever you sense that fear is preventing you from trying something new, ask yourself why you're afraid. Think about it. Write down your fear. Identifying your fears and recognizing when they are working against your best interests is a liberating experience.

Example: I was terrified before my first climb many years ago. Logic told me there was nothing to worry about—I knew the rope was more than strong enough to support my weight, and I had tremendous confidence in my climbing partner's ability to swing me back to the cliff if I slipped.

Getting ready, the more I thought about it, the more I realized that I wasn't scared of injury. I was scared that I wouldn't succeed—that I wouldn't be up to the climb. That surprised me—I never realized that I was so scared of failure. But as soon as I identified the fear, I was able to overcome it.

EMBRACING COMMITMENT

We live in a rapidly changing age, when technology permeates much of our daily existence. Technology has made us more productive and has increased the amount of information we experience and absorb.

But technology has also made us less patient. More and more happens in an instant today, so we become frustrated when phones are busy, ATM machines run too slowly or the checkout lines are long.

Our general impatience also prevents us from enduring temporary obstacles when pursuing larger goals. The easiest response to trouble at work or with a relationship seems to be giving up.

Helpful: Think about what really matters to you and remind yourself of its importance. Whenever you become frustrated with yourself or with forces you can't control, ask yourself if your goals are still desirable.

If the answer is *yes*, remind yourself that the greatest rewards are possible only if you're willing to stick it out through tough times. Life's greatest achievements are never reached without some struggle.

Example: Climbing Mt. Kilimanjaro taught me this. The mountain doesn't require a tremendous amount of technical climbing skills, just the desire to reach the top.

At first the climb is wonderful. The mountain is beautiful at low elevations. But before long, it's just volcanic rock with nothing to distract you from the next step in front of you except the increasing cold and thinning air. Succeeding requires stamina and focus on the result.

SEEKING SUPPORT

Despite the organizational shift at work from the individual to teams, the person who makes his/her own way is still greatly admired in our society. That's why many people feel like failures when they must ask for help.

But few people succeed on their own—even when it *seems* they did it alone.

Isolating yourself from others and being embarrassed to let others see the real you fosters dishonesty and limits your exposure to opportunity. You're more likely to cover up personal flaws than address them.

Helpful: Force yourself to open up by creating a personal board of directors. Speak with them individually twice a year—or when you need help or have a tough choice to make.

No one person has all the answers on his own. Good judgment depends on asking great questions of smart people.

Example: I've found that on difficult climbs, the encouragement of the group plays a big part in each individual's determination and success. I've come to realize that needing help now and then isn't a sign of failure. Climbing is a personal experience, but you can't do it alone.

DEALING WITH SETBACKS

We all suffer reversals now and then. That's part of life, and without them, we would never fully appreciate our triumphs.

But not everyone reacts the same way to setbacks. Some people see every failed expectation as a major failure, which causes them to belittle or berate themselves. This negative view can prevent you from taking actions or help you sabotage your efforts.

Helpful: Recognize that living life means taking chances. Taking chances, on occasion, means conceding defeat. When we have to make a decision, we do so based on the information available to us. Sometimes, we later find additional information which leads us to conclude our initial decision was incorrect.

When you suffer a setback, take a look at why you made the decision in the first place before labeling yourself a failure. Was it failure —or feedback?

Example: My first failure came on Devil's Tower, an almost mile-high rock monolith in Wyoming. I barely had been able to complete the first leg of the climb, and I knew more difficult sections lay ahead—so I turned back. I felt humiliated and defeated.

BOOSTING PERSONAL EXCELLENCE

Few things in life are as psychologically difficult as putting ourselves through an experience at which we failed in the past.

Revisiting a failed experience carries painful memories of personal failure. We automatically tell ourselves that we're bound to fail again, in many cases robbing ourselves of our best chance to succeed. Or we don't even bother trying at all.

Helpful: Prepare in advance for these apprehensions. Focus on what you learned on your first attempt, not how you were hurt.

Then consider how you've changed since your first try. Have you done additional research? Have you spent extra time practicing in preparation? Chances are, you're not the same person who failed the first time around.

Example: I returned to Devil's Tower a year later. There were still lingering doubts in my mind, but I had done a lot of climbing over the year, and I knew I was much more skilled than I was on my first attempt. I made it to the summit.

Extreme Shyness Is A Health Problem: How to Overcome It

Franklin Schneier, MD, associate director of the anxiety disorders clinic at the New York State Psychiatric Institute in New York City. He is coauthor of *The Hidden Face of Shyness: Understanding and Overcoming Social Anxiety.* Avon.

Everyone feels shy or anxious *sometimes* —whether it's butterflies in your stomach when you walk into a party or a cold sweat when it's your turn to give a toast.

Half of all people fear public speaking. Believe it or not, many say they would rather die than give a speech.

Social anxiety runs the gamut from occasional jitters to a disabling disorder that makes work and relationships impossible.

Wherever you fit in, taming those butterflies can vastly improve your quality of life.

WHERE BUTTERFLIES COME FROM

Anxiety is the body's automatic response to perceived danger. The brain signals the *hypothalamus*, a gland at the base of the brain that stimulates production of the adrenal hormones *cortisol* and *adrenaline*.

Once these "stress hormones" enter your bloodstream, your heart begins to race, your muscles contract and you break into a sweat.

Some people blush, as blood rushes into the capillaries in their cheeks. Others develop trembling hands or a queasy sensation in the stomach.

Many people escape these distressing sensations only by avoiding social situations. You may not even think of yourself as shy, just that you "don't like parties" or "don't enjoy making presentations."

Problem: Avoidance means missing out on opportunities for pleasure, satisfaction and career advancement.

It's *not* a matter of timidity or weakness. One of my patients had no trouble going into perilous situations in his work as a narcotics detective. But the need to testify in court left him paralyzed with fear.

WHAT ARE *YOU* AFRAID OF?

Two basic fears underlie most cases of social anxiety—the fear of embarrassment and the fear of being judged harshly. We're afraid we'll arouse anger, contempt or ridicule…say something that others will consider stupid…or just look foolish.

It's thoughts like these that give meetings and other social situations that have no physical risk a feeling of danger.

Making matters worse, we tend to become fearful of the bodily manifestations of anxiety. "I'll blush, and everyone will see it," we think …or, "My sweaty palms will reveal to everyone just how nervous I am."

Example: One of my patients, John G., was anxious about his upcoming wedding. Why? Because he would have to hold a glass of wine during the ceremony. He was afraid his hand would shake. The wedding guests would see he was a nervous wreck, he believed, and deem him a jerk.

TAMING YOUR BUTTERFLIES

The more you avoid situations that trigger anxiety, the more ingrained your fears become.

Avoidance is just the *opposite* of what you should be doing. To uproot your fears, you must confront them—by doing the very things that you find so frightening.

Helpful: Set reasonable goals, and take small steps toward those goals. If you're usually shy at gatherings, it's unrealistic—and counterproductive—to try to be the life of the party. Instead, aim simply to start a conversation or two.

OTHER HELPFUL STRATEGIES

● **Focus on your actions, not other people's reactions.** The person you try to engage in a conversation at a party may be receptive …or he/she may walk away. Either way, give yourself the credit you deserve for what *you* did—initiating the contact.

● **Become aware of the unrealistic thoughts that make you anxious.** Before making a toast or a business presentation, do you automatically shift into "low-confidence" gear? Do you think, "I'll mess up, and they'll laugh at me"?

In social situations, do you find yourself thinking, "I'll be tongue-tied and run out of things to say?"

In such cases, the best antidote is to think *realistically*. In your presentation, how likely are you *really* to mess up? Will people really laugh if you flub a line? Or will they appreciate your humanness and listen more closely?

Replace negative, anxiety-provoking thoughts with positive ones—"I've given presentations before, and they've been fine. If anything, I've gotten better since last time."

When my patient John G. contemplated his prenuptial jitters, he saw how unrealistic they were. If his hand did shake, he realized, his friends and family would not think he was a jerk. They would think he was moved by the occasion—and respect him all the more.

• **Rehearse situations that make you nervous.** If you're scheduled to give a speech, hone your talk beforehand using a tape recorder or a video camera. Stand in front of a mirror, or have a friend observe you.

In the case of John G., rehearsing his wedding with a family member helped him boost his confidence.

People who fear public speaking can gain priceless experience by participating (along with other fearful speakers) in programs offered by Toastmasters International. To find a chapter in your area, call 800-993-7732 or go online at *www.toastmasters.org*.

• **Develop skills that will give you confidence.** Read up on how to give an effective business presentation or speech. Observe people whose social graces you admire, making mental notes of what works for them.

Many adult-education centers offer courses in social skills. These classes teach you what to do at parties and on dates.

WHEN SELF-HELP FAILS

Many people who cannot control anxiety on their own benefit tremendously from cognitive-behavioral therapy. Via this form of therapy, you learn to identify and change negative, anxiety-producing thoughts...and to become more confident and outgoing.

In just a few months of individual or group therapy, you can learn skills that will help you for the rest of your life.

When cognitive-behavioral therapy isn't enough, I prescribe anxiety-reducing medication.

For *occasional* anxiety—if you have to give a talk once a month, for instance—the beta-blocker *propranolol* (Inderal) is often best. It blunts the body's reactions to adrenaline, helping to curb symptoms such as a pounding heart or queasy stomach.

Many musicians and other performers who suffer from stage fright get relief from propranolol.

When anxiety occurs on an everyday basis, I often prescribe *fluoxetine* (Prozac) or another *selective serotonin reuptake inhibitor* (SSRI). Anxious people who take SSRIs say they have fewer fearful thoughts and feel more comfortable in social situations.

If SSRIs fail—or if sexual problems or other side effects make them intolerable—I prescribe a tranquilizer like *clonazepam* (Klonopin)...or a monoamine-oxidase inhibitor antidepressant like *phenelzine* (Nardil).

Some people find that a few months of drug therapy is all that's needed. For others, long-term therapy is needed to maintain their improvement.

For a referral to a social anxiety specialist in your area, contact the Anxiety Disorders Association of America, 11900 Parklawn Dr., Suite 100, Rockville, MD 20852, 301-231-9350. *www.adaa.org*.

25

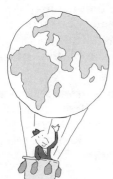

New Ways for the 21st Century

Alternative Medicine Moves Mainstream

James Gordon, MD
Georgetown Medical School,
Center for Mind-Body Medicine

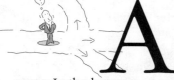

Americans' interest in alternative medicine and therapies has grown dramatically during the past few years. In the last year, more than one out of three people have used an alternative therapy to reduce stress and pain...and/or help cure an ailment.

The public's interest is so strong that the National Institutes of Health created the National Center for Complementary and Alternative Medicine, and many medical schools —including Harvard, Columbia and Stanford, as well as Georgetown, where I teach—now offer courses in alternative medicine.

As a physician, my concern is with finding the most effective synthesis of conventional and alternative medicines. Whenever I have

any doubt about my patient's condition, I always make sure a complete conventional diagnostic assessment is made before I begin a program of alternative therapies.

Among the alternative therapies that I have found particularly helpful...

RELAXATION THERAPIES

Many of these therapies can be self-administered and are extremely effective in reducing stress.

By reducing stress, you can lower blood pressure and improve your immune functioning. You may also be able to diminish the frequency and intensity of asthma attacks and migraine headaches and reduce chronic pain.

James Gordon, MD, clinical professor of psychiatry and of family medicine at Georgetown Medical School, Washington, DC. He is chairman of the Program Advisory Council, National Institutes of Health's Office of Alternative Medicine. Dr. Gordon is founder and director of the Center for Mind-Body Medicine, 5225 Connecticut Ave. NW, Washington, DC 20015, and author of *Manifesto for a New Medicine: Your Guide to Healing Partnerships and the Wise Use of Alternative Therapies.* Addison-Wesley.

467

All relaxation therapies begin with the induction of a relaxed state. You can achieve this in many ways—through deep-breathing exercises, meditation and even physical exercise. Once you are able to achieve a feeling of relaxation, you can move on to more complex therapies such as imaging or hypnosis, which are directed at specific conditions or symptoms. *How they work:*

•**Deep breathing.** Sit in a comfortable chair with your feet on the floor. Breathe deeply into your abdomen. Put a hand on your belly, feeling it rise and fall. Let the belly be soft. (Remind yourself by saying *soft belly* as you breathe in and out.) Begin with five or 10 minutes of this, and do it once or twice a day. Increase the amount of time as it suits you. After a while, you'll find that a few deep breaths will be enough to create a feeling of relaxation.

•**Meditation.** One simple form is called concentrated meditation. As you breathe in, repeat a sound like *one* or a word or prayer that is meaningful to you. Focus your attention on the sound or word.

•**Imaging.** You can use your mind's eye to visualize a relaxing scene, such as a placid lake or a beautiful mountain. You can also use images to affect specific physical functions. For example, visualize your immune system's white blood cells fighting an infection or imagine more blood flowing to a stiff joint.

•**Hypnosis.** This state of deep relaxation can have an impact on both physical and psychological conditions. It is generally administered by a practitioner, who helps you enter a state in which you are detached from the world around you and have an increased capacity to focus. He/she can also teach you strategies for "self-hypnosis."

Hypnosis requires that you be "suggestible" —open to someone else's instructions or your own and willing to allow your imagination to take over so that you disassociate yourself from the outside world and focus intently on whatever thought, scene, feeling or smell you are asked to conjure up.

Either the practitioner can give instructions that you will come out of the hypnotic state after a period of time, or you can give them to yourself. Contrary to popular fears, a person who is hypnotized cannot be forced to do something he would not ordinarily do.

How to find practitioners: Deep-breathing and meditation classes are commonly offered at holistic education centers, stress management clinics, community centers, community colleges and some hospitals and medical centers.

NUTRITIONAL/HERBAL MEDICINE

•**Vitamins and minerals.** Specific nutrients, especially the antioxidants in vitamins A, C and E, beta-carotene and selenium, may be helpful in preventing some kinds of cancer or the recurrence of some forms of the disease. Vitamin E has also been linked to a reduction in the risk of heart disease.

What I recommend to my patients: Vitamin E/400 international units (IUs), twice a day…vitamin C/1,000 milligrams (mg), once or twice a day…beta-carotene/a maximum of 25,000 IUs once a day…selenium/50 micrograms, twice a day.

I also urge my patients to consume 400 micrograms (0.4 mg) of folic acid a day. Folic acid is believed to prevent several birth defects and may reduce the risk of heart disease in men and women.

•**Herbs** contain ingredients that have specific pharmacological effects.

In both Western natural medicine and non-Western traditions, such as the Indian, Chinese and Native American, combinations of herbs are used to improve the functioning of various organs.

Keep in mind that herbs often take longer to work than traditional Western medicines. I advise my patients to look for improvements over a period of weeks or months.

It is important to work from an authoritative guide or herbal—a book about plants—especially with reference to their medicinal properties…and to take only the prescribed amounts. Herbs—like drugs—can have harmful side effects.

Good resources: *The New Holistic Herbal* by David Hoffman (Element Books) and *The Healing Herbs: The Ultimate Guide to the Curative Power of Nature's Medicines* by Michael Castleman (Bantam Books).

Herbal therapies may treat everything from allergies to migraines and improve physical and mental functions.

How to find a practitioner: Since herbalists aren't licensed, your safest bet may be to find a physician, nurse or licensed nutritionist who uses herbs in his practice. You can also check with friends who have found someone who is competent.

ACUPUNCTURE

Acupuncture is a part of Chinese medicine. It dates back thousands of years and is often used in conjunction with herbal medicine, dietary changes and relaxation techniques.

How it works: The practitioner inserts fine needles at key points along the body that are believed to connect to organs and affect virtually all body functions.

During acupuncture, our bodies' natural painkillers, called *endorphins*, are released, along with other chemicals. Acupuncture has an antidepressant effect, improves lung capacity, boosts the immune system and may enhance circulation. It is often used to alleviate pain and may be used as anesthesia for surgery. In hundreds of sites around the country, acupuncture is used to treat alcoholism and drug addiction.

How to find a practitioner: There are four times as many qualified nonphysician acupuncturists as physicians who practice acupuncture. Licensing requirements vary by state. To locate a qualified medical acupuncturist in your area, contact your state licensing board or the American Academy of Medical Acupuncture (800-521-2262 or *www.medical acupuncture.org*).

HOMEOPATHY

Homeopathy originated in Germany and was brought to the US in the early 19th century. Homeopathic practitioners treat illnesses by prescribing small, highly diluted doses of natural substances, which, in larger, more concentrated doses, would actually cause the patient's symptoms.

Example: A tiny amount of an allergen, a substance that triggers an allergic response, would be used to treat an allergy.

I've found homeopathic remedies particularly useful in boosting immune systems and in treating nausea and vomiting, colds and flu and emotional or physical shock.

Studies suggest that homeopathic remedies may also be effective in the treatment of hay fever, arthritis and diarrhea.

How to find a practitioner: Homeopaths are not licensed, except in Arizona. Some physicians, nurses and physician assistants currently use homeopathy in their practices.

Ask the practitioner where he has studied, whether he has passed some type of certification exam and how long he has been practicing homeopathy. As with any practitioner, you might want to ask if you can speak with patients whom he has already treated.

MANIPULATIVE THERAPIES

●**Chiropractic and osteopathy.** In both of these therapies, practitioners use their hands to manipulate bones in the spinal column, the neck, the head and the joints. By manipulating bones, practitioners feel they alter the functioning of the nervous and circulatory systems. They believe that manipulation affects all the internal organs, not just the musculoskeletal system.

●**Doctors of Chiropractic** (DCs) are licensed by each state and must complete two years of undergraduate study and a four-year course at a chiropractic college.

●**Doctors of Osteopathy** (DOs) receive a four-year education similar to that of a doctor. They also must complete a year-long residency and take the same licensing exams. DOs can prescribe drugs.

●**Massage therapy** can reduce muscle tension and stress, improve joint mobility and promote healing of some injuries.

Some states require that massage therapists be licensed or certified while other states do not. Look for a therapist who has a certificate indicating that he has passed the national exam of the American Massage Therapy Association.

Some licensed physical therapists and registered nurses now practice massage therapy.

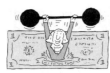

How to Get Your HMO to Cover Alternative Medical Treatment

Alan Raymond, vice president of public affairs for Harvard Pilgrim Health Care, an HMO, Brookline, MA, and author of *The HMO Health Care Companion: A Consumer's Guide to Managed-Care Networks.* HarperPerennial.

All HMOs rely on primary care doctors to provide or approve most care for their members. They also tend to cover only "medically necessary" and "nonexperimental" treatments.

Therefore, HMOs may not be willing to reimburse members for alternative medical treatments, such as acupuncture, biofeedback, massage therapy and chiropractic care.

But such treatments are growing in popularity. More than one-third of all Americans have already tried at least one of them.

Here's how to get your HMO to pay for alternative approaches...

●**Find out if the HMO must pay for the treatment in your state**, and under what circumstances. Some states now require that health insurers pay for certain treatments—especially chiropractic care. Your state's insurance department can fill you in.

●**Convince your primary care physician to recommend an alternative treatment.** Explain how it will likely succeed in treating your medical problem. Some HMOs will pay for alternative treatments—if you get a referral from your HMO doctor. Call the HMO to find out its policy.

●**Ask alternative treatment providers if they know of HMOs that cover their care.** Ask if they will allow referrals for alternative treatments. There may be limits—for example, chiropractic treatment for lower back pain may be covered, while the use of alternative therapies for chronic illness may not be.

●**Ask your employer to add alternative therapies to your benefits.** Some HMOs offer riders that expand coverage to include nontraditional therapies. It will cost your employer more, so you will probably see somewhat higher premiums as a result. The larger the number of your fellow employees who want such a benefit, the more likely it is your request will be granted.

●**If treatment is denied coverage, use tax-sheltered money.** Many employers offer flexible spending accounts, which permit you to set aside pretax dollars to pay for uncovered medical expenses.

Acupuncture and chiropractic care qualify, since the IRS has ruled that both are tax-deductible medical expenses. The IRS hasn't ruled on other treatments, so check with your employer. Also find out if you need a medical doctor's referral before getting your treatment.

Be careful when you set aside money in a flexible spending account. If you don't use all the money that is set aside by the end of the year, you forfeit the remaining amount.

Magnets Stop Pain... Ease Arthritis...Help Heal Broken Bones and More

Ron Lawrence, MD, a neurologist in private practice in Agoura Hills, CA. He is president of the North American Academy of Magnetic Therapy, 17445 Oak Creek Ct., Encino, CA 91316.

In China, France, Japan and especially in India, magnetic therapy has long been used to speed the healing of broken bones and soft-tissue injuries.

In the US, magnetic therapy is sometimes considered a form of quackery. But following the publication of several "pro-magnet" studies in the *Journal of Electro- and Magnetobiology* and elsewhere, a few pioneering doctors in this country are starting to use magnets in their practices.

Already, magnetic therapy has proven effective at treating slow-healing fractures and arthritic knees and necks. Studies also suggest that regular use of magnets may reverse osteoporosis...prevent heart disease...slow tumor growth...and boost mental function in some Alzheimer's patients.

I know from personal experience that people sleep better and wake up feeling more refreshed after a night on a magnetic mattress. I sleep on one myself!

Is magnetic therapy safe? *Absolutely.* Magnetic resonance imaging (MRI) machines routinely expose patients to magnetic fields as high as 15,000 gauss—with no negative effects. It stands to reason that a medical magnet rated at 200 to 800 gauss poses little threat.

HOW MAGNETS WORK

Studies have demonstrated quite clearly that when placed directly on the skin, a simple, handheld magnet works by…

•**Increasing blood flow.** It does so by stimulating cellular activity through the so-called "Hall effect." This is general heating of the magnetized area.

Some scientists think magnets improve the functioning of the autonomic nervous system, which could also stimulate blood flow to the affected area.

•**Diminishing pain.** This occurs via a combination of the Hall effect and possibly some stabilizing influence on the autonomic nervous system.

•**Speeding up the healing process.** It does so by boosting the body's synthesis of *adenosine triphosphate* (ATP), the "fuel" that fires all cellular processes…and by enhancing the blood's ability to carry oxygen.

MAGNETS VERSUS ARTHRITIS

Magnetic therapy helps relieve arthritis pain *and* slows the deterioration of cartilage inside arthritic joints.

For my patients with arthritis, I recommend sleeping on a magnetic mattress pad…or wrapping a flexible, magnetic bandage around the affected joint. If you do sleep on a magnetic pad, remove it for a day or two, every two to four weeks. This seems to prolong the beneficial effects.

HEADACHES AND BACK PAIN

Magnetic pillow liners appear to be an effective treatment for chronic headaches and jaw pain.

People with chronic back pain have obtained significant relief from sleeping on magnetic mattresses, and/or using magnetic seat cushions.

SOFT TISSUE INFLAMMATION

Tennis elbow, carpal tunnel syndrome and other tendon or ligament problems heal faster when wrapped in magnetic bandages.

In most cases, the magnet is wrapped into place over the affected area—and left in place until the pain disappears.

BROKEN BONES

In some hospitals, powerful electromagnets are being used to speed healing of stubborn bone fractures. Magnetic therapy also seems to promote regeneration of spinal disk tissue.

ASTHMA

Regular use of magnets helps prevent the violent allergic reaction in the lungs that is characteristic of bronchial asthma.

Helpful: Sleeping on a magnetic mattress …or wearing a magnetic bandage on your chest.

PUTTING MAGNETS TO WORK

The benefits of magnetic therapy are often apparent within the first hour of treatment. In others, three or four days of steady treatment are required.

For maximum benefit: Place magnets as close to your body as possible. The strength of the magnetic field drops off sharply with distance.

A variety of magnetic devices is now available—including mattress pads, seat cushions, pillow liners, magnet-studded bandages and simple handheld magnets.

Good source of medical magnets: Synergy for Life, Box 5962, Winston-Salem, NC 27113. 888-311-2963.

Chinese Medicine Works Well on Americans, Too

James S. Gordon, MD, author of *Manifesto for a New Medicine: Your Guide to Healing Partnerships and the Wise Use of Alternative Therapies.* Addison-Wesley. He is clinical professor of psychiatry and family practice at Georgetown University School of Medicine and director of the Center for Mind–Body Medicine, both in Washington, DC.

There's little doubt that Americans enjoy the most technologically advanced medical care in the world. Still, there's much we can learn from the Chinese system of medicine.

Scientific studies of China's ancient healing system are just beginning, and more are needed. But a growing body of research suggests that acupuncture, herbal remedies and other components of Chinese medicine do provide relief for many common ailments—even when Western medicine has failed.

Chinese medicine is helpful for everything from asthma and arthritis to migraines and menstrual cramps. It can help cure alcoholism and other addictions…and helps alleviate nausea and other side effects of cancer chemotherapy.

WHAT IS CHINESE MEDICINE?

The Chinese system of medicine is hard for Westerners to accept—or even grasp. More than a collection of exotic treatments, it's a unique way of looking at the world and the body.

The language Chinese physicians use to describe symptoms, diagnoses and physical processes is the language of the natural world. It uses terms like *earth, metal* and *fire* instead of the technical jargon familiar to most Western physicians and their patients.

Whereas Western medicine focuses on the specific disease entities and diagnostic categories, the Chinese system views the body as both expressing and fueled by a basic animating force called *qi* (pronounced *chee*).

This vital energy circulates constantly through *meridians*—lines along the body on which the acupuncture points lie. Chinese medical therapies are concerned with restoring the balance of qi.

Everything taking place in the organs and elsewhere in the body is considered to be interconnected to the individual's psychology, the time of day, season of the year—indeed, to *all* phenomena in the natural world.

The diagnostic techniques Chinese doctors use are alien to Western physicians. *They include…*

● **Touching and listening to the belly.**

● **Identifying imbalances in the body** by observing the patient's face and voice. For example, dark circles under the eyes might indicate a kidney ailment long before lab tests reveal it.

● **Observing not just one pulse**, but 12 different pulse points along the wrist.

● **Noticing the appearance, texture and moistness of the tongue.** A trembling tongue might suggest that qi is depleted.

ACUPUNCTURE

Acupuncture has proved helpful for a variety of ailments—irritable bowel syndrome… migraines…hot flashes…addictions. It can even serve as anesthetic during surgery.

The Chinese maintain that acupuncture redistributes the flow of qi, thereby affecting the activity of organs.

In Western terms, acupuncture induces the body to release natural anti-inflammatory substances and painkilling opiates.

To find a qualified acupuncturist in your area, ask your doctor or your friends for a referral. If your state requires licensing to practice acupuncture (about half of all states do), call the state medical board to make sure the person you're considering is licensed.

HERBAL REMEDIES

The Chinese use herbs…gold and other minerals…and animal products (such as dried fish, bile and bones) to restore balance to the body.

Example I: Ginseng eases stress, boosts immune function and enhances mood.

Example II: Certain mushrooms, including shiitake, strengthen the immune system.

Don't start taking massive doses of an herbal remedy just because you've read about it. That can cause dangerous—and perhaps fatal—side effects.

Chinese herbalists use *tiny* doses of many herbs. This strategy ensures maximum benefit while minimizing side effects.

If your doctor, acupuncturist or chiropractor is unable to recommend an herbalist, visit the nearest Asian-American neighborhood. The neighborhood pharmacist may be able to suggest someone. Many states require licensing of herbal therapists.

TAI CHI AND QI GONG

Tai chi (pronounced *tie chee*) consists of a series of smoothly connected postures. There are many different "forms," or sequences, of these movements.

Performed with rapidity, tai chi is a martial art. Done slowly and contemplatively, however, it increases energy, flexibility and mental clarity.

Tai chi instruction is offered at recreation centers, YMCAs, YWCAs and health clubs.

Qi gong (pronounced *chee gong*) is an integrated system of movement, breathing and visualization. It involves fewer movements than tai chi...and greater use of imagery.

In addition to its calming effects, qi gong seems to lower blood pressure...enhance immune function...and ease breathing in asthmatics.

Many Chinese medicine practitioners are trained in qi gong, as are a growing number of Westerners.

Placebo Power: How To Harness It

Howard M. Spiro, MD, professor of medicine and director of the Program for Humanities and Medicine at Yale University School of Medicine in New Haven, CT.

P hysicians have long observed that even very sick patients sometimes get better after taking a "sugar pill," or *placebo*.

For years, doctors viewed this placebo effect as an irrational element in an otherwise logical and systematic world of clinical medicine and medical research—a nuisance that needed to be explained away.

Now: Evidence is mounting that mental activity has a powerful effect on the body. Doctors are seeking ways to *exploit* the placebo effect for their patients' benefit.

We asked Dr. Howard M. Spiro, a nationally renowned gastroenterologist with a special interest in placebos, to tell us more about placebos and their expanding role in medical care...

●**What is a placebo?** Where treating patients is concerned, it's a pill that contains only inactive ingredients.

Prior to the 1960s, it was routine for doctors to give sugar pills to patients who complained of ailments that defied diagnosis. Patients were told, "Take this. It should help."

Anyone who got better after taking a placebo was assumed to be complaining of an ailment that didn't really exist.

Another important use of the placebo is in clinical trials of new drugs. Here the placebo gives researchers a way to "control" for non-medical factors that could affect the outcome of treatment—a patient's greater attention to health care during a study, for example, or simply the passage of time.

●**Why do placebos work?** One theory is that placebos help boost the body's production of the natural painkilling compounds called *endorphins*.

Another is that placebos simply distract the mind, keeping patients from noticing pain.

A placebo might foster the body's innate self-healing power simply by bringing to mind the emotional comfort associated with childhood memories of going to the doctor.

It's also possible that placebos do *nothing*—that the patient would have gotten better anyway, regardless of treatment. Given a few weeks or months, for example, up to half of all peptic ulcers heal *by themselves*—no matter what treatment is given.

●**Do doctors still give out sugar pills?** No. Today it's considered unethical to give a patient a drug without telling him/her exactly what it is.

However, placebo-like treatments are still being given to patients. Vitamin B-12 injections, for instance, are supposed to help fight fatigue and weakness.

I myself offer the injections to some patients. It would be unethical for me to tell a patient, "This treatment will cure you."

What I say is, "I suggest you get this shot. I can't promise it will help, and I can't tell you how it works. But other patients say the shot made them feel better."

●**How can doctors exploit the power of placebos without deceiving patients?** Doctors who speak optimistically to patients help them *feel* better...and this optimism may be associated with *physical* improvement as well.

Sadly, many doctors have forgotten the healing power of comforting words.

Doctors have also forgotten how to listen. At one time, listening was central to medical practice. But to many doctors, listening to patients now seems old-fashioned. They tend to rush to offer pills and procedures that are often unnecessary.

●**Does the doctor's style tie in with the placebo effect?** Absolutely. A good doctor-patient relationship is integral to the placebo effect and to healing. It fosters *catharsis*—the emotional release a patient feels after telling a doctor his troubles.

Interview doctors until you find one who listens well…and who has the time to talk to you.

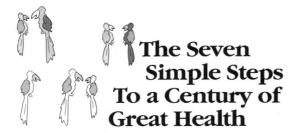

The Seven Simple Steps To a Century of Great Health

Robert D. Willix, Jr., MD, a traditionally trained physician and surgeon in a private alternative medicine practice in Boca Raton, FL. He is author of *Healthy at 100: 7 Steps to a Century of Great Health*. Shot Tower Books.

When Americans get sick, they go to the doctor and say, *"Fix me."* But—*only you* can fix *you*…and *you can!*

There is no biological reason we can't live to be a ripe old age, free of pain, illness and decay—still vital—and sexually active.

Working to balance modern scientific research and the ancient healing arts of India and China, I have developed a seven-step program to achieve that goal. Actively enhancing the link between mind and body will change the way you look, feel and live.

Follow my seven-step plan in any order you choose.

You start with the step that's least difficult for you and work on it as long as necessary—three months, six months, a year—until you're ready to try the next step.

As you move forward, reaping the benefits, observe the power you have gained in changing your life.

As with car repair and maintenance, the earlier you start my program, the more mileage you'll get. But it will definitely improve your health and outlook at any age.

Step 1: **Perform your own health risk appraisal.** To learn whether you're at greater risk of developing certain diseases than the general population, know your risk factors. With your health provider's help, choose actions to take or avoid to reduce your risk.

●**Physical status.** Do you have high blood pressure or high cholesterol? Both increase the risk of heart attack, stroke and premature death.

●**Family history.** Ask your close blood relatives how long other family members have lived. Find out if any of them had major chronic illnesses or conditions such as cancer, heart disease, osteoporosis, diabetes and degenerative arthritis.

Mistake: People with short-lived families resign themselves to an early death. That's totally unrealistic. Heredity accounts for no more than 10% of the chance of death.

●**Lifestyle.** Do you exercise and stretch regularly? How healthfully do you eat? Do you get enough rest and make an effort to avoid stress? Do you drink too much alcohol or use tobacco products?

Step 2: **Use antioxidants.** The most important medical discovery of the past 50 years is that antioxidants minimize the damage done by free radicals, agents in the blood that attack and weaken body tissues.

I am not impressed by a few imperfect studies debunking the remarkable effects of antioxidants. These studies do not refute 40 years of impressive research concluding that antioxidants help prevent heart disease, stroke, cataracts, skin wrinkling, senility and breast, lung and colon cancer—while slowing aging itself. For further proof, I could cite the remarkable positive effects that taking supplemental antioxidants has had on hundreds of my own patients.

The best source of antioxidants is organically grown fruits (three to five servings a day) and vegetables (three to four servings a day).

But if you're among the 90% of people who eat the typical American diet, which includes lots of meat and fat but few fresh foods, you need supplements.

Every day, take 500 to 2,000 milligrams of vitamin C, up to 10,000 international units (IU) of vitamin A, 400 to 800 IU of vitamin E and 12,000 to 25,000 IU of beta-carotene, which the body converts to vitamin A.

Step 3: Practice some form of aerobic exercise to keep your heart healthy. Exercise is a more powerful medicine than any drug. The evidence is overwhelming that people who exercise live longer and have less risk of death from heart disease. Exercise pumps oxygen through the body tissues. That's good for everyone and especially good for people with kidney disease.

Any exercise that is somewhat strenuous will do. Just be sure to raise your heart rate (you don't have to feel it pounding). You can ride a bike or walk. Do this for 30 minutes three times a week. After three months, you will feel better. Continue this regimen, working up to at least five days a week.

Step 4: Meditate for stress management and mind–body health. Stress, which many experts consider the most common cause of disease in this day and age, can rob you of life. By relieving stress, regularly practiced meditation becomes rejuvenating.

None of my accomplishments has had a stronger impact on my life than using meditation to neutralize the effects of stress on my nervous system.

At least once, preferably twice, a day meditate for 10 to 20 minutes.

Consider *tai chi chuan*…centering prayer… transcendental meditation…intoning a mantra. The aim is to create a quiet space between your thoughts. It requires conscious effort and is not the same as relaxing.

No time? Think again. Meditation will *increase* your productivity for the rest of the day. Its impact on the ability to absorb knowledge is tremendous.

Step 5: Practice weight training for stronger bones. Brittle bones (osteoporosis)

lead to falls, broken hips and a susceptibility to pneumonia while bedridden. And older people tend to have weak legs in general.

I call one simple exercise "chair-ups." Sit in an armchair. Can you raise yourself repeatedly, without touching the arms? Keep practicing until you can. That will strengthen your legs a great deal.

Step 6: Stretch and strengthen your back. Being supple will allow you to turn your head around while driving and not have a dangerous "blind spot." You can bend down to pick things up and stand up again without creaking and cracking.

Flexibility helps prevent the natural degeneration into stiffness that comes with aging… and helps prevent injury from accidents, the major cause of disability in older people, and back problems, suffered by 85% of American adults.

Stretch each and every day. Find a stretching routine you like and do it for two to five minutes shortly after getting up in the morning.

Keep trying to place your palms on the floor without bending your knees. The closer you can get, the more effective the stretch.

Step 7: Eat right. In my view, all extremes in nutrition are to be avoided. Low-fat diets alone don't make a difference. Eliminating any single factor won't keep you healthy. What's crucial is to maintain a balance of proteins, carbohydrates (pasta, whole grains) and plenty of organically grown fruits and vegetables. Eat more vegetable than animal protein. Read labels carefully and choose natural foods.

Look at where the food came from. Oatmeal and cream of wheat are closer to nature than sugar-coated bran flakes. When you see a box of cereal growing from a tree, you'll know it's a good food.

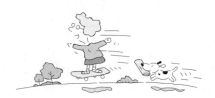

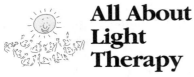

All About Light Therapy

George Brainard, PhD, professor of neurology and director of the Light Research Program at Thomas Jefferson Medical College in Philadelphia. He is a consultant for NASA and the National Institutes of Health on the behavioral aspects and therapeutic effects of light.

Touted as a quick fix for everything from insomnia to low sex drive, melatonin has fast become one of the biggest-selling nutritional supplements in US history.

For some individuals, however, the problem is not having too *little* melatonin—but too *much*. As a result, many people may be "overdosing" on this hormone.

MELATONIN AND DAYLIGHT

Melatonin is a natural hormone produced by the pineal gland, a pea-sized gland located at the center of the brain.

Melatonin synthesis is governed by *circadian rhythms*—the daily cycles of light and darkness to which each of us is exposed.

During exposure to sunshine or another bright light, the pineal gland stops making melatonin. That makes you alert.

In dim light or darkness in the evening, melatonin production soars. That's why we tend to get sleepy at night.

Problem: For many individuals, this melatonin production cycle has been disrupted. That's because so much of our time is spent indoors, under *artificial* light.

DISTURBED RHYTHMS

If you're not exposed to enough bright light each day, circadian rhythms may fall out of whack. This phenomenon is called *circadian rhythm desynchronization*.

Circadian desynchronization can also be caused by taking melatonin supplements...by jet lag...or by working odd hours.

Heart disease is twice as prevalent among night-shift workers as among those who work a normal nine-to-five shift.

In addition to heart disease, circadian disruption has been linked to...

- **Insomnia and other sleep disturbances**
- **Gastrointestinal problems**
- **Persistent drowsiness or fatigue**
- **Poor job performance**
- **Menstrual irregularities**

Light deprivation is also associated with a serious form of depression called *seasonal affective disorder* (SAD).

Psychiatrists now believe that SAD affects 10 million Americans (particularly during fall and winter, when time spent outdoors is at a minimum). Another 25 million are thought to have a milder, "subsyndromal" version of SAD called SSAD.

There have been hints that light deprivation may also be a factor in other disorders. Breast cancer, for instance, is far less prevalent near the equator—where the sun is brightest—than it is farther north or south. And breast cancer rates in the northern US are up to twice as high as rates in the South.

THE MODERN LIFESTYLE

Humans evolved to spend a great deal of time outdoors—and that meant lots of exposure to sunlight.

The electric light changed all that. Now our bodies are exposed mostly to artificial light... and most artificial light is far too dim to induce the pineal gland to stop making melatonin.

To stop making melatonin, the body needs about 2,500 lux (10 lux roughly equals the light shed by one candle).

Outside on a sunny day, light can reach 100,000 lux. By contrast, indoor lighting ranges from only 100 to 800 lux.

Implication: You may be working all day in light that's bright enough to see by—yet still be in "biological darkness" as far as your pineal gland is concerned.

THE NATURAL SOLUTION

Should you be worried about light deprivation? If you feel healthy, probably not. But if you are experiencing mood changes, fatigue, insomnia or daytime drowsiness, light deprivation might be an issue.

Simple solution: Get more natural sunlight. I urge my patients to take a 30-minute stroll outdoors each morning before work. Walking at lunch is good, too.

While indoors during the day, try to sit near a window in a well-lighted room.

BRIGHT LIGHT TREATMENT

Light deprivation can also be remedied with daily exposure to special artificial light (brighter than typical indoor lighting).

Typically, the minimum of 30 minutes up to two hours a day of "light therapy" will counteract light deprivation.

Especially beneficial: Exposure to bright light early in the morning, during the transition from sleeping to waking.

Various artificial light sources are now available. At present, most use white light—although other colors are under study.

•**Light boxes** consist of an array of fluorescent bulbs that collectively give off about 2,500 lux. The individual sits in front of the panel, about three feet away.

•**Work stations** are units angled overhead and placed closer to the eyes than a light box. They produce about 10,000 lux. They are comparable to light boxes in terms of effectiveness.

•**Light visors** are worn like a hat, with light shining onto the face. These devices permit mobility during light therapy.

•**Dawn simulators** slowly increase the light in your bedroom as you wake up. Several studies have shown this approach to be effective in relieving SAD.

For a list of light box manufacturers and treatment centers, contact the Society for Light Treatment and Biological Rhythms, Box 591687, 174 Cook St., San Francisco 94159. *www.sltbr.org.*

All About Prolotherapy

Robert G. Klein, MD, an internist and prolotherapist in private practice in Santa Barbara, CA...and Janice Guthrie, founder and director of the medical information and research firm, The Health Resource, 564 Locust St., Conway, AR 72032.

Chronic back pain, whiplash injuries to the neck and many other types of musculoskeletal pain that are not helped by physical therapy, painkilling medication or chiropractic manipulation can often be controlled via *prolotherapy.*

In this highly effective but little-known treatment, small amounts of an irritant solution—usually concentrated glucose—are injected into the painful area.

The resulting inflammation promotes growth of collagen, the protein that's a major component of ligaments, the cable-like structures that hold our joints together.

New collagen growth helps reduce pain and increases joint stability by strengthening the fibrous capsule around joints. It also brings significant improvement in joint mobility.

Many forms of chronic musculoskeletal pain are caused by ligament damage. Car accidents, falls or repetitive movements cause ligaments to loosen and/or tear. Prolotherapy is effective for most ligament-related pain.

SIDE EFFECTS

Prolotherapy patients generally feel fine for four to eight hours after the injections because a local anesthetic is given along with the irritant. The discomfort that usually follows slowly subsides over the next several days.

Many individuals who undergo prolotherapy experience pain, swelling, soreness, temporary stiffness and bruising at the injection site. Fortunately, discomfort can usually be minimized by medication, ice and massage.

Caution: Smoking makes the therapy less effective, as does use of aspirin and other anti-inflammatory drugs.

PRECISION COUNTS

Most patients need a series of injections over a period of several weeks or months. In some cases, prolotherapy is teamed with other forms of soft tissue treatment—such as physical therapy, joint manipulation or acupuncture.

Prolotherapy injections must be given *precisely* at the junction of a bone and a ligament. Misplaced injections are ineffective and possibly dangerous. If the irritant is inadvertently injected into the spinal canal, for instance, paralysis or even death could occur.

Consequently, prolotherapy injections must be administered only by a clinician thoroughly trained in the technique. Some say that orthopedic surgeons are ideal for administering prolotherapy injections. That's because they have a thorough knowledge of the location of ligaments and muscles.

FINDING A PROLOTHERAPIST

Only about 300 orthopedic physicians and osteopaths in the US and Canada currently use prolotherapy in their practices.

Among these practitioners is former Surgeon General C. Everett Koop, MD. He began using prolotherapy himself in the early 1960s, after another doctor used it on him to cure the once-intractable pain in his neck and arm.

For more information about prolotherapy, contact the American Association of Orthopaedic Medicine (800-992-2063). For a fee, you'll receive an informational packet including a list of qualified prolotherapists in your area.

INSURANCE COVERAGE

One prolotherapy session costs $75 to $300. The number of sessions needed depends upon both the severity of the pain and the patient's response to the treatment.

Some major health insurance companies now cover prolotherapy. Others decline coverage because they consider it to be an "unproven" or "experimental" treatment.

How to Harness the Amazing Power of Your Immune System

Henry Dreher, a medical and science writer who specializes in complementary medicine. He is author of several books, including *The Immune Power Personality: Seven Traits You Can Develop to Stay Healthy* (Plume) and coauthor with Alice Domar, PhD, of *Healing Mind, Healthy Woman* (Henry Holt).

The single best way to stay healthy is to strengthen your immune system. A strong immune system aggressively fights diseases ranging from common colds to arthritis and cancer. It can even prevent a wide range of ailments—particularly heart disease and cancer.

As the number of antibiotic-resistant bacteria increases, a strong immune system is your best defense against illness.

THE BODY'S POLICE FORCE

To help you understand your immune system, think of it as a police force of cells that conducts surveillance missions throughout the body. There are cells of different rank, and each has a different job to do. Like any good militia, all of the immune cells cooperate with each other to identify and arrest "invaders"— bacteria, viruses, cancer cells, etc. They also rush to each other's aid when necessary.

The cells' marching orders originate in the brain and certain organs, such as the thymus, a gland located behind the breast bone. The thymus acts as a "training school" for immature white blood cells.

Enemy viruses are captured by "field officers"—immune cells—including T-cells, B-cells and protein molecules called *antibodies*.

These immune "officers" communicate by spewing various "messenger" molecules that travel to other "troops" moving throughout your body.

When we don't have enough immune cells to conquer invading infections, we become ill. We can also become sick when our cells don't receive the proper messages because the different levels in the cell hierarchy fail to communicate with each other.

In the case of arthritis and other autoimmune diseases, our immune cells mistakenly attack our own cells, causing inflammation and crippling pain. Put differently, the police attack suspects who are really innocent.

SIZING UP YOUR IMMUNE SYSTEM

How can you tell if your immune system is dangerously weak?

Although there are numerous expensive tests that are used to diagnose immune deficiency, such specific conditions are rare. Most people have suboptimal immune function because they are run down.

An easier, more affordable way to assist your immune system's strength is to ask yourself a series of questions:

● **Am I constantly fighting bouts of colds,** the flu or bronchitis that last for two or more weeks at a time?

●**Am I fatigued throughout the day**…or on a regular basis?

●**Do I suffer from chronic conditions** such as allergies, asthma or arthritis?

If you answered yes to any of these questions, your immune system is probably flagging. Consult your doctor—but also consider taking several immune-boosting steps.

STRENGTHENING YOUR IMMUNITY

●**Improve the quality of your diet.** High-fat diets and a lack of vital nutrients compromise your immune system. That's because excessive intake of animal fats, such as red meats and whole-fat dairy products, trigger *free radicals*—unstable molecules that can harm immune cells.

Eating polyunsaturated vegetable oils, which are found in many snack foods, sauces, margarine and salad dressings, also produces free radicals.

●**To lower fat, cut back on red meats.** Instead, eat skinless chicken, fish and beans, which are excellent sources of protein.

●**Use moderate amounts of the safest oils**—olive and canola—instead of butter and other vegetable oils.

●**Eat more vegetables and fruits.** Nearly all are fat-free and contain nutrients that boost the immune system, such as vitamins A and C as well as phytochemicals. These compounds are found in plants and can fight disease.

Helpful: To get the proper amount of vitamins in your food each day, doctors advise that you eat a steamed vegetable side dish and a salad that includes dark leafy lettuce, peppers, bean sprouts, radishes and carrots at lunch and dinner. They also suggest you eat two to three pieces of fresh fruit each day.

●**Consider a vitamin/mineral supplement.** In a study of 96 people at the Memorial University of Newfoundland, some of the participants received a supplement with 18 nutrients while the other group received a pill with only calcium and magnesium in it. Those who received the larger supplement had fewer infections and half the number of sick days compared with others in the study. And… blood tests proved they had stronger immune responses to viruses.

Essential: Be sure that any multivitamin and mineral supplement contains the vitamins A, C, D and E…the B vitamins…beta-carotene…and the minerals zinc and selenium. Each nutrient plays a role in strengthening your immune system. Consult your doctor or nutritionist for doses.

Important: Avoid megadoses of specific vitamin supplements. Such doses can be dangerous —and won't boost your immune system any more than if you had taken the recommended amount.

●**Get into the habit of exercising daily.** Regular exercise has been shown to strengthen a particular group of immune cells that kills viruses and cancer cells. Researchers at the Harvard School of Public Health have shown that regular exercise can even prevent breast and gynecologic cancers among women.

Contrary to popular opinion, however, excessive exercise is not necessarily better for you. One study showed that excessive exercise— several hours a day of strenuous activity for five or more days a week—may actually dampen immunity, making you more susceptible to various ailments.

Better: Do about 30 minutes of aerobic exercise, such as walking, bicycling or swimming—three to five times per week. If that isn't possible, try a comfortable walking routine for 15 minutes a day.

●**Learn to reduce stress**—and control your emotional health. In a famous 1991 study published in *The New England Journal of Medicine*, scientists at Carnegie-Mellon University injected cold viruses into people and studied their stress levels. The researchers discovered that the chance of catching a cold was directly proportional to the amount of stress the volunteers had experienced.

Though most busy people can't avoid stress entirely, they can protect themselves from becoming consumed by it and learn to manage anxiety and pressure more efficiently. *Strategies…*

●**Write about your anxiety.** Holding in negative emotions has been shown to worsen stress levels and weaken immune cells.

James Pennebaker, PhD, of Southern Methodist University, has shown that one can bolster immunity and prevent illness by jotting down thoughts of fear, grief and anger about stressful events—both past and present.

Dr. Pennebaker suggests writing about such events for 20 minutes a day without stopping or censoring yourself.

By keeping a stress journal for three or four days, you will train yourself to identify toxic thoughts and unhealthy stress levels. You will develop a private way to release them and avoid letting them build up and aggravate and harm you.

•Teach yourself to be more assertive. Studies show that the patients who beat the odds against cancer and other serious illnesses are often assertive types who stand up for themselves and take charge of their own well-being. *Strategies for becoming more assertive...*

☐ **Use quiet contemplation or meditation** to develop an awareness of your needs and rights versus those of everyone else.

☐ **Engage in assertive communication** in which you clearly state your needs.

☐ **Learn to say *no*.** Conquer the habit of saying yes to every request or obligation when your energy is at stake. Remind yourself that your health comes first and taking on too much can risk your immune system.

•Practice relaxation. A study at Ohio State University showed that people who practiced relaxation techniques had stronger immune system cells. Two relaxation techniques that are easy to practice any time of day are *meditation* and *deep breathing*.

Useful exercise: Sit in a quiet room. Close your eyes and breathe deeply. Say the word *om* in your mind as you breathe in...and say the word *sah* as you exhale.

If your mind wanders, gently bring your attention back to your breathing. Allow each exhale to be an opportunity to let go of tensions in your body and mind. Practice this at least once a day for 20 minutes or whenever you feel that stress and tension have risen to an uncomfortable level.

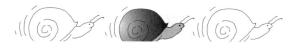

More About You... Your Immune System and Much Better Health

Henry Dreher, a health writer who specializes in mind–body and alternative medicine and author of *The Immune Power Personality: Seven Traits You Can Develop to Stay Healthy*. Dutton/Penguin.

Conventional take-a-pill, have-an-operation medicine has largely failed to combat chronic, painful conditions such as arthritis, asthma and allergies. And conventional medicine does not always have adequate treatment against cancer, AIDS and heart disease. But we can help fight illness...*with our minds*.

Relaxation techniques, exercise and good nutrition can help a lot, but they're not enough.

Short-sighted: Most corporate-sponsored stress reduction programs concentrate on relaxation techniques rather than facing up to sources of stress and working to solve them. The pivotal psychological factor in illness is not whether we'll encounter stress. That is a given. It's how we cope with stress.

As we grow older, our bodies find it harder and harder to fight disease as our immune systems begin their natural decline. Yet by developing certain aspects of our personality, which I call *Immune Power traits*, we can help fend off disease or reduce its symptoms.

All seven traits described below are directly or indirectly linked to a vigorous immune system. All are backed by scrupulous research showing that the mind can contribute to our risk of, and recovery from, almost any disease involving a dysfunctional immune system, from migraines to rheumatoid arthritis.

A person with an *Immune Power Personality* finds joy and meaning, even health, in the challenges of life. Stressful events are handled with acceptance, flexibility and a willingness to learn and grow.

We are all born with the potential to have Immune Power traits and can reawaken them at any age. It doesn't mean you have to change certain fixed parts of your personality.

The point is to draw on the strengths of your own character to assume challenges and cope with losses and other stressful events that you can't control.

SEVEN IMMUNE POWER TRAITS

Explore one new trait per week, continuing the previous ones. You're likely to find many of your headaches, stomach aches, back pain or other symptoms fading away.

●*ACE factor:* **Attend, Connect, Express.** Awareness of your mind-body signals—the opposite of repression and denial—strengthens the heart and the immune system.

●**Attend** to your feelings.

●**Connect** feelings to your consciousness.

●**Express** feelings appropriately. You may find out that you haven't been paying attention to the real cause of your ongoing distress.

●**Capacity to confide.** Sharing your concerns with others actually enhances your immune response. It's the opposite of being bottled up—verbally and emotionally. *Helpful:* Ask the person to listen in silence.

Exercise: For 20 minutes on three to four consecutive days, write down your deepest thoughts and feelings about the most traumatic event you can remember. If nothing comes to mind, choose an event that symbolizes a set of emotions that had a long-lasting effect on you.

●**Hardiness.** Hardy individuals can resist the slings and arrows of life. They seek support to bolster their self-worth...not to reinforce the *poor me* syndrome. *The hardy share the following three major characteristics:*

●**Commitment** and wholehearted involvement in their work, relationships and activities.

●**Control** over their life circumstances, facing problems with creativity and confidence. (Control freaks manipulate others...completely different.)

●**Challenge** (that may be in the occasion when stressful events strike). People with a sense of challenge adapt well to change.

To develop the three *C*s, focus your awareness on the sources of stress, then develop an action plan to restore balance. Sometimes no amount of focusing can lead to positive change.

Alternative: Compensatory self-improvement. Identify a related problem that you can resolve.

●**Assertiveness.** Standing up for yourself reduces your sense of victimization. Being a martyr can be a destructive way to treat your mind and body. Passivity is unhealthful in the long term.

Example: In many cases, AIDS and cancer patients who actively participated in their own care lived longer than those who did not.

●**Affiliative trust.** The desire and capacity for a positive, loving relationship based on mutual respect and trust actually boosts your defenses against a whole range of physical symptoms. Unconditionally giving love relaxes you...and changes your outlook.

Example: A 42-year-old man with severe heart disease, tired of surgery, forced himself to suppress his chronically hostile behavior by thinking through situations before reacting to them. He began to spend more time with his family. His chest pain and shortness of breath were quickly relieved and eventually disappeared.

●**Altruism.** Assisting others provides a *helper's high*, which promotes both health and spirit. *Adopt four characteristics of healthy helping:*

●**Personal contact.** Writing a check isn't the same as connecting with someone. Teach someone to read...serve food to the homeless...volunteer at a day-care center...offer advice to new business owners.

●**Frequency.** *The ideal frequency is about the same as for meditation or exercise:* Roughly two hours a week. Following a schedule will help you maintain your commitment.

●**Helping strangers.** We exercise more freedom of choice in helping strangers than family members or close friends. Bonding with strangers helps get rid of a sense of isolation.

●**Letting go of results.** Like any gift, your time should be given with no strings attached. Helping must be its own reward.

●**Self-complexity.** We boost our physical health by being able to draw support from many vital selves to sustain our energy, well-being and sense of purpose through painful times. For a sense of balance, foster diverse interests. People with more self-complexity have less depression and illness when self-esteem in one part of their lives is temporarily drained.

DRAW A BLUEPRINT

Find your own path to each of these health-promoting traits. If one is entirely out of character and unappealing to you, you may decide to reject it. Keep in mind, though, that the interconnections between traits provide the fullest benefits and a balanced life.

A positive aspect of one trait offsets the negative in another.

Example: A person who asserts his needs can give openly to others without becoming a victim.

Focus on the Immune Power traits where you need the most help.

Example: Someone who constantly yells at people would benefit from affiliative trust.

If you feel set in your ways, go about the process gently and patiently. Recognize that you can heal some wounds...even lifelong ones by confronting the aspects of your personality underlying them...gently and persistently.

Head Trauma Advance

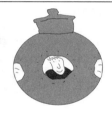

Guy L. Clifton, MD, chairman of neurosurgery, University of Texas Health Science Center, Houston.

Neurosurgeons have turned to hypothermia as an important treatment for potentially deadly head injuries.

How it works: The patient is wrapped in cool packs containing ice water. Over an eight-hour period, body temperature is lowered to 90°F, slowing metabolism and blocking trauma-induced chemical reactions that cause irreversible brain damage. Once the immediate danger passes—usually after 48 hours—the patient's body temperature is returned to normal. In a pilot study, 52% of the patients given hypothermia recovered completely, versus only 36% who received "normo-thermia," in which the patient is maintained at normal body temperature.

Heart Failure and Biofeedback

Debra K. Moser, RN, DNSc, assistant professor of nursing, Ohio State University, Columbus.

Heart failure patients benefit from biofeedback training, in which they learn techniques to raise their finger temperature. (Increased finger temperature is a sign of relaxation.)

Study: After a single 30-minute session, patients' blood vessels opened wider and their breathing slowed.

For a list of biofeedback practioners in your area, send a self-addressed, stamped, business-sized envelope to the Association for Applied Psychophysiology and Biofeedback, 10200 W. 44 Ave., Suite 304, Wheat Ridge, CO 80033.

Electrostatic Massage

Milton Hammerly, MD, medical director of the American Holistic Center, a group practice located in Littleton, CO.

Did you know that *static electricity* is an effective remedy for headaches, arthritis and other common sources of pain?

Physicians have long recognized that the human body is pulsing with minute electrical currents. If this flow becomes disrupted, "normalizing" it may promote healing. In fact, doctors have been using low-voltage electrical current to mend broken bones.

A similar effect can be obtained using static electricity. Sweeping a charged object across a painful or injured region of the body attracts a flow of healing electric current to the area.

Doing so also speeds circulation of fluid away from the area, thereby reducing swelling.

To do "electrostatic massage" (EM), you'll need a one-foot section of polyvinyl chloride (PVC) pipe, 1.5 inches in diameter...plus an ordinary painter's mitt. These items are available at hardware stores.

What to do: Rub the pipe vigorously with the mitt for one minute, then slowly sweep the pipe over the painful area. Move in a head-to-toe direction—one-quarter to one-half inch away from the skin.

I've used electrostatic massage in my practice for more than two years now—with remarkable results.

Ninety-two percent of sinus headache sufferers benefited from EM, as did 81% of fibromyalgia sufferers…76% of tension headache sufferers…75% of muscular pain sufferers…and 72% of osteoarthritis sufferers.

I usually recommend two 15-minute electrostatic massage sessions each day for as long as pain persists.

Abdominal Aneurysm Treatment

Peter D. Fry, MD, clinical professor of surgery, University of British Columbia, Vancouver.

Abdominal aneurysms can be treated without surgery. Until fairly recently, these weakened blood vessels had to be removed through a large incision running from the breastbone to the pelvis. Now, doctors thread a woven polyester tube called a *stented graft* through a small incision in the groin. The tube becomes a lining for the blood vessel at the point where it threatens to burst. This less-invasive procedure typically involves only a two-day hospital stay. Traditional surgery usually involves a more lengthy hospitalization.

"Super Glue" vs. Sutures

James Quinn, MD, clinical assistant professor of emergency medicine, University of Michigan, Ann Arbor.

Super glue may be better than sutures for closing many skin lacerations. In a study, doctors were able to close lacerations faster and with less pain when they used a medical version of the adhesive *octylcyanoacrylate* instead of sutures. The glued cuts healed just as well as cuts closed with sutures.

Bonus: Unlike sutures, which must be removed several days later, glue requires no follow-up care. It sloughs off in a few weeks.

Limitation: The glue is inappropriate for use on the hands, feet or joints.

Multiple Sclerosis Breakthrough

Todd Richards, PhD, associate professor of radiology, University of Washington, Seattle. His two-month study of 30 MS patients was published in *The Journal of Alternative and Complementary Medicine,* 12425 St. James Rd., Rockville, MD 20850.

Multiple sclerosis (MS) symptoms can often be controlled with a wristwatch-sized device that emits brief magnetic pulses. MS patients who wore the *Enermed* device for 10 to 24 hours a day for two months reported better bladder control, clearer thinking and more energy than similar patients who wore a placebo device.

Also: Hand function, mobility, sensation, muscle control and vision all improved for the Enermed group.

More information: Contact the manufacturer, Energy Medicine Developments, 866-ENERMED.

Nausea Relief

Hillary Steinhart, MD, assistant professor of medicine, University of Toronto.

A battery-operated device worn on the wrist relieves seasickness, morning sickness, chemotherapy-related vomiting and post-surgical nausea. Called *ReliefBand*, the $35 to $100 prescription device stimulates nerves in the wrist, keeping signals that trigger nausea from reaching the brain.

Only side effect: Tingling of the hand when the band is at higher settings.

Index

Bad breath
  avoiding, 61
  tongue scraping and, 61
Balloon angioplasty, 310
Balloons, dangers from, 158
Bananas, freeze peeled, 220
Barbecue, summer, 227
Basal energy expenditure,
    Harris-Benedict equations to
    determine your, 344
Basil, 423
Baths, medicated, 50
Bay leaf, self-healing and, 414
Beans in diet, 210
Bedtime snack, 216
Bed-wetting
  prevention of, 161
  stopping child's, 161
Beer
  alcohol in, 231
  stomach size and drinking
    of, 329
Bee sting, first aid for, 58
Behavior, sleep and, 157
Benign paroxysmal positional
    vertigo, 24
Benign prostatic hyperplasia
    (BPH), 203-4
Benzene as cause of chronic
    fatigue, 39
Beta-blockers
  heart attacks and, 87
  for heart disease, 76
  for high blood pressure, 41
  sex and, 259
Beta-carotene, 219-20
  benefits of, 249, 286-87
  cancer and, 239-40
  need for, 243
  sources of, 243
Bifocals, 363
Bike helmet, 62
Biking, stationary, 382
Biofeedback
  heart failure and, 482
  for incontinence, 53
  for migraines, 32
Biomarkers, aging and, 269
Birth control
  cystitis risk from
    diaphragms, 141
  emergency, 140-41
Birth control pills
  ovarian cancer and, 138-39
  safety of, 141
Birth defects, vitamins versus, 248
Bladder cancer, vitamin C
  and, 247

Bladder pain, relief from, 135-36
Bladder training, 52-53
Blood clots
  controlling, 67
  preventing, 226
Blood pressure. *See also* High
  blood pressure; Hypertension
    borderline high, 74
    congestive heart failure
      and, 280
    lowering, 64
    meditation in, 430
    natural ways of, 429-30
    taking your, 74
Blood tests
  for CA125, 138
  in detecting ulcers, 444
Blood thinners, antibiotics
  versus, 113
Blood transfusions
  donating blood for your, 190
  getting information on, 311-13
  human immunodeficiency virus
    testing and, 311
  reducing risks from, 191
Blood vessels, improved
  function of, 84
Blues versus exercise, 388
Boating
  carbon monoxide poisoning
    and, 313
  dangers in, 313
Body. *See also* Mind/body
  connection
    arthritis and mechanics of, 28
    health risk and shape of, 336
    learning to regulate your, 407
    reading messages from, 7-9
Bone density, 136
Borage oil, 434
Borderline high blood pressure,
  74
Bowel continence, aging
  and, 266
Bowel movements, better, 122
Bowel trouble, 8-9
Brain drain, 11
Bran in baths, 50
Bras
  breast cancer and, 130-31
  sports, 131
Breakfasts, 215
  better, 222
Breast cancer
  abortions and, 128
  bras and, 130-31
  checklist for preventing, 447
  chemotherapy and, 133

  in men, 208
  milk and, 130
  support groups for, 45-46
  surviving, 128-30
Breastfeeding, benefits from, 134
Breast implants, 132
Breast lumps
  benign, 131-32
  evaluating, 128
Breasts
  enlarged, in men, 23
  strategies for avoiding
    troublesome cysts of, 127-28
Breast-sparing surgery, 129
Breath, sweeter, 372
Breathing
  asthma and, 148
  elevation and, 57
Breathing exercises for stress, 174
Brothers, Joyce, secrets of
  winning ever-changing game
  of life, 9-11
Bunions, prevention and
  treatment of, 54
Bupropion, 420
Bursitis
  prepatellar, 29
  shoulder, 29
Butter, substitute for, 213
B vitamins for healthy heart,
  67-68
Bypass surgery, 77-78
  better, 78
  dangers in, 81

C

CA125, blood test for, 138
Caffeine. *See also* Coffee
  children and, 157
  in fighting jet lag, 6
  indigestion and, 21
  information on, 222-23
  surgery and, 194
  withdrawal symptoms of, 315
Calcitonin-salmon as alternative
  to hormone replacement
  therapy, 124
Calcium
  costs of, 245
  getting enough, 137
  increasing, 64
  need for, 243
  osteoporosis and, 240-41, 287
  in preventing heart disease, 65
  in reducing colon cancer
    risk, 37
  sources of, 231, 243
  women and, 136-37

Diet doctors, weight-loss secrets
and, 337-38
Dieting, 332-33
exercises versus, 378
trick for, 228
Diet pills for incontinence, 53
Digestion, poor, 390
Digital rectal examination, 35
Dihydroergotamine (DHE) for
migraines, 32
Dinner, 216
Disaster training, 17
Disease. *See also* specific
avoiding worry about, 3-4
hostility, stress and, 352
reducing risk of, 84
Disinfectant, dangers from, 310
Distilled water, safety of, 223
Disturbed rhythms, 476
Diuretics
for high blood pressure, 41, 72
sex and, 259
Divorce, men and, 208
Dizziness, 23-25
Doctors. *See* Physicians
Dogs
owning, in extending life, 273
stress management and, 174
Dosages, measuring, 110
Drawstrings, dangers from, 163
Dressing, methods of, 148-49
Drinks, safe, while traveling, 7
Drowning, 320
Drugs. *See* Medications
Dust, controlling, 356

E

Earaches when flying, 367
Ear and brain disorders, 24
Ear infections, 24
childhood, 162
chronic, 366
Earlobes, 367
Ear thermometer, dangers
from, 314
Eating. *See also* Diet
Dean Ornish's secrets to
healthier, 209-10
power, 225-26
Echinacea, 421
for colds, 19
as immunity boosters, 238
Echocardiogram, 73
improving, 82
Eggs
in diet, 213
in recipes, 228

Eldercare services, 281
Elderly. *See also* Aging
crime safety and, 287-89
liquid nutritional supplements
for, 223
mental ability maintenance
in, 273-75
mistakes in treating, 270-71
sex and, 256-58
shoes for, 278
Electrostatic massage, 482-83
Elevation, breathing and, 57
Emotions
expression of negative, 456
handling negative, 459-61
impact on health, 451-53
overcoming negative, 463-64
Empowerment, 401
Encepone for Parkinson's
disease, 271
Endoscopy, doctor's competency
of performing, 191
Energy, Deepak Chopra's secrets
of having boundless, 389-91
Entrainment, 2
Environmental control of
allergies, 356
Environmental toxins as cause of
chronic fatigue, 39
Episiotomy, 139
Erectile dysfunction, treating,
200-201
Erotica, sources for, 263-64
Erotic videos, 256
Erythropoietin (EPO), 313
Escherichia coli, 47
Esophageal cancer or
esophagitis, 151
Estrogen, 274
Alzheimer's disease and, 276
for incontinence, 53
in reducing colon cancer
risk, 37
Estrogen replacement therapy
(ERT). *See also* Hormone
replacement therapy (HRT)
Alzheimer's disease and, 275
and asthma, 126
Evening primrose oil, 434
Exercises, 373-88. *See also*
Health clubs; Walking
abdominal, 13
aerobic, 76, 79, 475
aging and, 51
for arthritis pain, 28, 381
asthma and, 381
benefits of, 156
versus blues, 388

for chronic pain, 26-27
dangers of too much, 375-76
developing habit, 387-88
versus dieting, 378
for fibromyalgia, 323
getting regular, 419
hearing and, 276, 365
for heart, 64, 85-86
impotence and, 258
incontinence and, 133
inexpensive methods, 378
versus insomnia, 382-83
Kenneth Cooper's plan for,
379
longevity and, 379
magic fives, 374-75
menopause and, 123-24
mental, 399
for migraines, 32
overrated machines, 385
in reducing colon cancer
risk, 37
rehabilitation, 25
relaxation, 430
right time to, 379
shorter sessions, 380, 383
sleeping better and, 385
smarter, more effective, 379
sticking with regimen of,
381-82
in stress management, 168
during television
commercials, 373-74
tubing and, 383-84
vitamin E and, 248-49
weight loss and, 328, 335, 386
for your eyes, 363
Extracapsular cataract
extraction, 361
Eyedrops, dangers with, 363-64
Eyedrop test in diagnosing
Alzheimer's disease, 268
Eyes. *See also* Vision
asthma and, 362
cataracts, 357, 360-61
complications of LASIK surgery
and, 191
corneal infections in, 359
diabetes and, 310, 359
diet and, 361, 364-65
examination for, 362-63
exercise your, 363
glaucoma and, 357, 362
itchy, 363
macular degeneration in,
278-80, 358
red, 363
reducing injury of, 364

Contents

Figures and Tables

Figures[1]

---

1 The figures and illustrations presented in this volume were drawn from images understood by the authors as public domain. Soviet-era propaganda art or illustrations within training manuals and state textbooks commissioned by the government of Ukraine, while attributable in some cases to individual artists, are considered public property. Reference, where appropriate, has however been given to both artist and year of completion of the piece or to the author/publisher of the volume or public archive/collection within which certain pieces are found or have been reproduced.

Tables

Acknowledgments

We gratefully acknowledge the financial support received from the Mykhailo Onufriiovych Samytsia Endowment Fund (Canadian Institute of Ukrainian Studies at the University of Alberta), the Simon Fraser University Publications Fund, the Prometheus Foundation, Dopomoha Ukraini, and the Wrzesnewsky, Dzulynsky, Korbutiak, and Hankivsky families. We thank the World Federation of Ukrainian Women's Organizations for the administration of funds supporting this publication.

We would also like to thank Marguerite Pigeon for her editorial assistance, Mykhaylo Salnykov for technical and emotional support throughout the project, and our colleague Diego de Merich for his indefatigable commitment and invaluable assistance in the preparation and completion of this edited collection.

Contributors

Tetyana Bureychak holds a *kandydat nauk* degree in sociology and is an associate professor at the Department of History and Theory of Sociology, National University of Lviv. Her research interests include studies of men and masculinities in the Soviet and post-Soviet periods, hegemonic masculinity, gender and nationalism, gender identities in the context of consumer culture, and gender representations in advertising.

Olena Hankivsky (Ph.D., University of Western Ontario) is an associate professor in the School of Public Policy at Simon Fraser University, Vancouver, where she is also the director of the Institute for Intersectionality Research and Policy. Her research interests are focused on social and health policy. She is an internationally recognized expert in gender mainstreaming, health determinants, violence against women, and intersectionality-based analysis. She is the author of *Social Policy and the Ethic of Care*, co-editor of *Women's Health in Canada: Critical Perspectives on Theory and Policy*, and lead editor of *Health Inequities in Canada: Intersectional Frameworks and Practices*. Her work has appeared in journals such as *Social Science and Medicine, Journal of Health and Social Policy, International Journal of Health Services, Canadian Public Policy,* and *Critical Public Health.*

Alexandra Hrycak (Ph.D., Sociology, University of Chicago) is an associate professor of sociology and chair of the Department of Sociology at Reed College in Portland, Oregon, where she teaches courses on feminisms, social movements, the collapse of communism, and consumer culture. Her research focuses on the role of women's activism, and more broadly, gender in post-Soviet democratization. She has been a recipient of grants from IREX, the U.S. Institute of Peace, the National Science Foundation, and the Kennan Institute for Advanced Russian Studies of the Woodrow Wilson Center. Her publications have appeared in edited volumes and in journals including *East European Politics and Societies, Journal of Communist Studies and Transition Politics, Studies in East European Thought*, and *Women's Studies Quarterly*.

Oksana Kis holds a *kandydat nauk* degree in history (specialization: ethnology) from the Ivan Krypyakevych Institute of Ukrainian Studies, National Academy of Sciences of Ukraine, Lviv. She is a senior research fellow at the Institute of Ethnology, National Academy of Sciences of Ukraine (in Lviv), an associate professor at the Ukrainian Free University (Munich), president of the Ukrainian Association for Research in Women's History, and a head of the Lviv research centre Woman and Society (an NGO). Her academic interests focus on women's history and feminist anthropology of Ukrainians, and her book *Women in the Traditional Ukrainian Culture, Second Half of the 19th – Early 20th Centuries* was published in Lviv in 2008. She has authored over 50 articles published in scholarly journals in Ukraine and abroad. Currently, she is conducting an oral history project on women's historical experiences in Ukraine.

Iryna Koshulap is a Ph.D. candidate in gender studies at the Central European University in Budapest, where she is working on her dissertation 'Women, Nation, and the Generation Gap: Women in the Ukrainian Diaspora in the United States.' Her research interests include diasporas, women and migration, gender and nationalism, masculinity, and gender regimes in Eastern and Central Europe.

Tamara Martsenyuk holds a *kandydat nauk* degree in sociology. Her research focuses on the social structure of society and, particularly, on gender relations. She teaches at the Department of Sociology at the National University of the Kyiv-Mohyla Academy. Her courses include Sociological Analysis of the Forms of Deviant Behaviour, Masculinity and Men's Studies, Gender and Politics, Social Problems in Ukraine and the World, and Gender Relations in Ukraine: Sociological Analysis. She is the author of some 30 academic papers. In addition to the implementation of gender equality in Ukrainian society, her research and activism interests also surround the promotion of diversity, overcoming xenophobia, and racism.

Svitlana Oksamytna holds a *kandydat nauk* degree in sociology, is dean of the Faculty of Social Sciences and Social Technologies, National University of the Kyiv-Mohyla Academy, and senior researcher at the Institute of Sociology, National Academy of Sciences. Her research interests are social stratification and inequality, intergenerational social mobility, educational inequality, and gender differentiation and stratification.

Sarah D. Phillips (Ph.D., Anthropology, University of Illinois at Urbana-Champaign) is an associate professor of anthropology at Indiana University. Her major publications include two books, *Disability and Mobile Citizenship in Postsocialist Ukraine* and *Women's Social Activism in the New Ukraine: Development and the Politics of Differentiation*, and an ethnographic documentary film, *Shapes in the Wax: Tradition and Faith among Folk Medicine Practitioners in Rural Ukraine*. Her geographical areas of specialization are Central and Eastern Europe, the former Soviet Union (especially Ukraine and Russia), and the United States. Her topical interests include post-socialist transformations, civil society and non-governmental organizations, development, gender studies, medical anthropology, disability studies, post-Chernobyl health and healing, revitalization of the Chernobyl 'exclusion zone,' and the anthropology of pharmaceuticals.

Olga Plakhotnik holds a *kandydat nauk* degree in social philosophy and is an associate professor in the Department of Philosophy at National Aeronautic University in Kharkiv, Ukraine. She also teaches courses on gender and education and gender aspects of social policy at Karazin Kharkiv National University. Her research interests are in social critical theory and feminist methodology, with a focus on education, sexuality, and feminist teaching. She is a recipient of international scholarships for research in gender studies from IREX (University of Illinois at Urbana-Champaign), Open Society Institute (Central European University), and DAAD (Free University in Berlin). She has published widely on gender and education issues and feminism in Ukraine. Currently she is writing a book on Western feminist pedagogy and its applicability in Ukraine.

Anastasiya Riabchuk is a Ph.D. candidate at the Ecole des Hautes Etudes en Sciences Sociales (dissertation on the social construction of homelessness in contemporary Ukraine), and a senior lecturer at the Department of Sociology, National University of the Kyiv-Mohyla

Academy. She teaches courses on social problems and qualitative methodology, and her research interests are in the fields of poverty, homelessness, and urban marginality. She is editor of the Ukrainian journal of social critique *Commons/Spilne*.

Marian J. Rubchak is a senior Fulbright scholar and currently senior research professor of history at Valparaiso University. She has travelled extensively throughout Ukraine and has written on women's issues, gender, and identity construction in a variety of contexts. Her most recent publication is an edited collection titled *Mapping Difference: The Many Faces of Women in Contemporary Ukraine*. Among her numerous articles is 'Ukraine's Ancient Matriarch as a Topos in Constructing a Feminine Identity' (*Feminist Review*).

Anastasiya Salnykova is a Ph.D. candidate in political science at the University of British Columbia, where she works on her dissertation 'Deliberative Democracy in Transition: Electoral Systems, Crucial Events and Discourses in Ukraine and Georgia.' She is also a senior lecturer at Kyiv-Mohyla Academy where she teaches multiculturalism. Her research interests are in post-communist democratization and political theory, with a focus on ethnic relations, institutional design, deliberative democracy, gender, and health. She has co-authored such academic papers as 'Gender Mainstreaming in Post-Soviet Ukraine: Application and Applicability' (*Journal of Communist Studies and Transition Politics*) and 'National Identity of Ukrainians: Dilemmas Cultural and Socio-Political' (in Ukrainian) published in *Political Management*.

Elena Semikolenova holds a *kandydat nauk* degree in linguistics and is an associate professor of linguistics at the Department of Interlingual Communication and Journalism at Tavria National University, in Simferopol, Ukraine. She is also a director of the Tavria Centre of Gender Studies and a senior fellow at the Crimean Centre of Education Management. Her research interests are in Slavic languages grammar, linguistic gender studies, gender stereotypes in communications and mass media, and gender analysis of school textbooks. She has published widely on linguistic gender studies and gender education in Ukrainian and international scholarly journals and edited collections.

Alissa V. Tolstokorova holds a *kandydat nauk* degree and is an independent expert on gender issues, providing research expertise to the International School for Equal Opportunities (ISEO) in Kyiv. She is a recipient of international scholarships for research in gender/women's studies and social sciences from the ERSTE Foundation (Vienna), SAIA (Comenius University, Slovak Republic), Swedish Institute (Stockholm University), British Government Chevening Scholarship (University of Leeds), and U.S. Department of State, Fulbright Junior Faculty Development Scholarship (George Mason University). She has also received short-term training in gender/ women's studies and social sciences in Germany, Bulgaria, Italy, Czech Republic, United States, Kazakhstan, and Slovenia. She is a member of 15 international professional associations and networks, has presented papers at over 35 national and 40 international seminars, workshops, conferences, congresses, and symposia, and is an author of over 130 publications.

Tatiana Zhurzhenko holds a *kandydat nauk* degree in social philosophy and is Elise Richter Fellow at the Institute for Political Science, University of Vienna, where she is researching the politics of memory in post-Soviet borderlands. She has taught at the V. Karazin Kharkiv National University and worked at the Kharkiv Centre for Gender Studies. She has widely published on gender politics and feminism in Ukraine. Her recent books are *Gendered Markets of Ukraine: The Political Economy of Nation Building* and *Borderlands into Bordered Lands: Geopolitics of Identity in Post-Soviet Ukraine*.

GENDER, POLITICS, AND SOCIETY IN UKRAINE

Gender in Transition: Legacies, Opportunities, and Milestones in Post-Soviet Ukraine

OLENA HANKIVSKY AND ANASTASIYA SALNYKOVA

The idea for gathering an edited volume on gender in Ukraine originated from our joint research into evolving post-Soviet Ukrainian gender policies and our respective research in the areas of sex trafficking, HIV/AIDs, and sociopolitical transformations in independent Ukraine. Scanning the literature in support of these projects, we came to the realization that in most edited publications on post-Soviet countries, Ukraine remained on the margins or simply absent from the analysis. And in published works on transition to democracy, the impact of this dramatic process on gender relations was ignored. In studies that did attend to questions of gender, the focus of investigations was typically on women only. There was, in short, something missing that would bring these threads of research together. This volume is an attempt to remedy that. Here, we combine brand new research into the gendered impact of transition with a detailed focus on a single country, Ukraine, and we do so from a broad perception of gender that goes beyond women only to include men, women, and the relations between the genders as they shift over time.

In the past twenty years, similarly to other former Soviet states, post-communist Ukraine has been undergoing what Taras Kuzio (2001) has termed a 'quadruple transition.' This transition has included four large-scale changes: (1) from communism to democracy, (2) from planned economy to free market, (3) from being part of an imperial state to building an independent state, and (4) from a suppressed national identity to identity revival (pp. 168–77). Transitions from communist to capitalist economic systems, along with the associated processes of democratization and changing social environment, have garnered much academic attention (Bunce 1995; Carothers 2002;

Kornai 1995; Kuzio 2001; Linz and Stepan 1996; McFaul 2005; Offe and Adler 1991; Perelli-Harris 2008; Rose 1998). For Ukraine, like other countries in transition, 'the time of transformations was not only a period of fast economic changes that resulted in the loss of everyday routines, welfare benefits, and job security, but also a period of transformations of cultural representations and changes of personal, collective, and public memories' (Lukić et al. 2006, 301).

In general, however, researchers investigating these transitions 'have explored the establishment of democratic institutions and processes with no reference to gender' (Johnson and Robinson 2007, 13), even though all elements of change in post-Soviet states have had significant and distinct effects on gender relations in the region. As Kuenhast and Nechemias (2004) explain, 'Societal transformation . . . encompasses more than political systems and economies. Social relations between men and women, young and old, rich and poor are also in transition' (p. 18). Thus, gender – a fundamental dimension of personal life, social relations, and culture (Connell 2007, vii) – is a critical but often overlooked factor in examinations of political, economic, and social changes within transitional states. As such, it is not possible to adequately understand the economic and political transformations in post-Soviet societies without considering the complex processes through which restructuring takes place in the gender order (Zhurzhenko 2008, 9), that is, the socially constructed constellation of dynamics between and within genders.

Despite the overall lack of attention to gender in the literature on transition, exceptions do exist. Beginning with Nanette Funk's groundbreaking work in 1993, *Gender Politics and Post-Communism*, a number of scholars have examined the specific history and experiences of women in post-Soviet countries (Corrin 1999; Einhorn 1993; Jähnert et al. 2001; Kuenhast and Nechemias 2004; Marsh 1996; Mogdhadam 1993; Occhipinti 1996; Rubchak 2011; Štulhofer and Sandfort 2005), and they have investigated gender dynamics in Central and Eastern Europe more broadly (Duffy 2000; Funk and Mueller 1993; Galligan et al. 2007; Gal and Kligman 2000; Jähnert et al. 2001; Johnson and Robinson 2007; Lukić et al. 2006; Pascal and Kwak 2005; Matland and Montgomery 2003; Rueschemeyer and Wolchik 2009). The range of studies to date has enriched understandings of the role of gender in post-authoritarian societies and, in particular, 'the dynamic interaction among gender and cultural, ethnic, social and political identities' (Kuenhast and Nechemias 2004, x). The analysis put forward by many such scholars highlights the challenges of searching for 'new identities and values to fill the ideological vacuum created by the collapse of communism' (Marsh 1996, 14). In the process these researchers have challenged the basic assumptions and arguments about gender that still dominate in the consolidated democracies of the West. Eastern European feminists and other scholars working in the field have long voiced objections to the imposition of Western analytical, methodological, and political principles on the examination of non-Western experiences (Blagojević 2003; Busheikin 1997; Havelkova 1996; Lukić et al. 2006; Slavova 2006; Marsh 1996; Muharska 2005). The inclusion of alternative perspectives in major debates about the discourses and practices of gender have therefore provided invaluable 'insights and correctives to Western feminism' (Funk 1993, 14).

For the most part, however, work in the area of gender and transition – whether explicitly focused on women or utilizing a woman-specific lens to look at gender relations – has prioritized women's experiences and the gendered effects of transition *on women*. Research questions whether 'the transition to democracy and a market economy opens doors or erects new barriers for women in post-Soviet society' (Kuenhast and Nechemias 2004, 1). It also asks whether and how women's lives are better or worse in the aftermath of the breakup of the Soviet Union. Investigations to date, while paying some attention to broader issues of gender, predominantly focus on women. Accordingly, less attention has been paid to the gender order in which men *and* women figure and are 'learning both new and old ways of living gender' (Johnson and Robinson 2007, 18). With few exceptions (e.g., Johnson and Robinson 2007; Gal and Kligman 2000; Štulhofer and Sandfort 2005), examinations of the gendered transformations occurring during transition in the post-communist region have, therefore, been limited to analyses of women's lives.

The focus on women, while important, yields only a partial depiction of gender. In its definition of gender, the United Nations Office of the Special Adviser on Gender Issues and Advancement of Women (2000) points out that:

> Gender refers to the social attributes and opportunities associated with being male and female and the relationships between women and men and girls and boys, as well as the relations between women and those between men. These attributes, opportunities and relationships are socially constructed and are learned through socialization processes.

They are context and time specific and changeable. Gender determines what is expected, allowed and valued in a woman or a man in a given context. In most societies there are differences and inequalities between women and men in responsibilities assigned, activities undertaken, access to and control over resources, as well as decision-making opportunities.[1] (UNEGEEW 2011)

Only by taking into account this changeable, large-scale set of dynamics can we truly characterize a society's *gender order*. Accordingly, examinations of societal transitions in many post-Soviet states should include both men and women and their relationships in all their diversity.

Against this backdrop, the aim of this volume is twofold: to build upon the path-breaking work in the gender and transitional field – especially in terms of highlighting non-Western perspectives – and to extend this developing body of literature by specifically investigating the effects of transition on the gender order in Ukraine. As such, while a few of the chapters focus on the tradition of examining the situation of women, most pay attention to the continual development and concomitant challenges of more and more various forms of gender, a choice that highlights the multidimensional and variable nature of gender, including what Johnson and Robinson (2007) call 'gender multiplication,' in which 'the market, globalization, a larger civil society and the like enable a diverse array of strategies and tactics that women and men may use to construct the version of gender that they believe will help them survive if not thrive' (p. 2). In this way, the volume advances a relational approach to gender that also emphasizes the gendering of men's lives. This latter focus fills an especially important gap in the literature. As Štulhofer and Sandfort (2005) have noted, 'What is often lacking in the analyses of the gender relations in post-communism is the fact that social reality changed drastically for men too' (p. 4). Referring explicitly to Ukraine, Janey et al. (2009) have recently argued that 'efforts will be needed to understand men and how they are responding to the demands of the post-Soviet era in a country that is trying to separate itself from its Soviet past, and redefine its identity' (p. 138).

Thematically, this volume is closely aligned with that of Johnson and Robinson (2007) whose collection explores several related questions: how gender is presented and performed after communism; the role of the state and market in establishing preferential gender constructions as well as in enabling new opportunities for gender identities, performances, and behaviours; whether state and market roles have changed since the communist period and in what ways; and finally, how transition from authoritarian state power to a weaker central state has affected gender ideologies (p. 6). Here, we build on these themes, with a particular focus on how the gender contract continues to be transformed through transition. But this volume is also a single-country study, presenting biographical, historical, and critical analyses of Ukraine. This choice is justified in several ways.

In the environment of burgeoning academic literature on gender politics and policy in Central and Eastern Europe, the case of Ukraine remains largely unexplored. This is a significant gap. From the perspective of the world community, Ukraine represents a bridge between Europe and Eurasia. It is also the largest country in Europe, with a population of over forty-six million people.[2] It has been referred to as the most democratic state in the post-Soviet space (Pifer et al. 2009; World Audit 2009; Campbell and Pölzlbauer 2010; Freedom House 2010). Indeed, Ukraine was one of the first countries to entrench gender equality in its Constitution (Gander and Magdyuk 2006, 37). At the same time, in today's Ukraine numerous inequities and complex issues along gender lines persist that reveal the interplay between local history, communist-era politics and economics, and transition. Membership of women in the Verkhovna Rada (Ukrainian parliament) is consistently low, at no higher than 8 per cent. In general, women occupy few positions of power in either the public or private sector. Furthermore, a veritable laundry list of disturbing statistics continues to emerge from Ukraine showing that it has one of the lowest fertility rates in the world (Maksymenko 2009; Perelli-Harris 2008), one of the highest rates of maternal and infant mortality in Eastern Europe (Betliy et al. 2007; Gander and Magdyuk 2006), the highest per capita prevalence of HIV/AIDS in Eastern Europe and Central Asia (UNAIDS 2008, 52; Booth et al. 2004), the worst human trafficking problem in the world (Trafficking in Persons 2009), and significant rates of poverty, with 35 per cent of the Ukrainian population living below the poverty line as of 2009 (CIA The World Factbook 2010).

The pressure of economic restructuring has taken a serious toll on the population's self-reported health (Gilmore et al. 2002), life expectancy (WHO 2006), chronic pain conditions (Tsang et al. 2008), mental and alcohol disorders (Bromet et al. 2005), and levels of distress and anxiety (Cockerham et al. 2006; Kohn et al. 2002). While the number of people who have migrated abroad for work between 2003 and 2008 is officially pegged at about 233,000, information from related areas like statistics that track temporary migration indicates that closer to 1.8 million people did so in that same period (Hampton et al. 2009, 35).

Ukraine has been among the countries most severely impacted by the global financial crisis that began in 2008 (Round and Williams 2010), and it is currently the third largest recipient of funds from the International Monetary Fund (United Nations 2010).

All of these trends and developments make Ukraine a unique context for examining issues of gender vis-à-vis transition. In a short time, gender relations in this country have been affected in a myriad of ways, leading, in particular, to the feminization of poverty, a serious prevalence of violence against women, and growing unemployment and poor health among men of working age.

Meanwhile, the process of forging an independent national Ukrainian identity has been challenging. Ukraine remains strongly shaped by its past and related political and ideological legacies. As Lukić et al. (2006) explain, 'In Ukraine, its 337 year history of Russian domination and Soviet rule ensures a more difficult process of independent state building' (p. 124). There is no doubt that Ukraine is considered the single most important post-Soviet state from a Russian perspective, as the buffer state between Russia and NATO countries. Ukraine hosts the Russian Black Sea Fleet and houses important infrastructure linking Russia to Europe, most notably gas pipelines. But the Russian legacy is only part of the story, as Ukraine simultaneously experiences ongoing pressures from the West as well. From a U.S. and European viewpoint, a strong independent Ukraine is an important source of regional stability (Woehrel, 2009; Kolisnichenko and Rosenbaum 2009). Negotiating these conflicting forces has meant that less attention has been paid to what are often perceived as secondary social issues, such as gender equality. In addition, the East-West tug-of-war, instrumentalized by various political actors (including politicians looking to lure an electorate with its own divided East-West loyalties), has created multiple divisions in Ukrainian society, including along the lines of gender. For example, NATO funding for Ukrainian nongovernmental organizations, (among them women's NGOs in Ukraine) has been perceived equivocally by different sectors of society. Moreover, in an attempt to increase their public support, pro- and anti-NATO proponents have capitalized on women's family sentiments by arguing that either a pro- or anti-NATO stance in the country could see Ukrainian soldiers sent to Iraq or Chechnya (T. Zhurzhenko, personal communication) respectively.

Ukraine's current approach to addressing gender parity is shaped by vestiges of Soviet ideologies. While Soviet gender policy guaranteed important political and socioeconomic rights for women and a commitment to full equality, it also perpetuated the traditional treatment of women. On the one hand, the Soviet ideological and economic system was beneficial for women, as it demanded full employment of the entire population, which eliminated the notion of a 'housekeeping wife.' The literacy level among both Soviet women and men approached 100 per cent, and the rate of higher education among women increased immensely. The Soviet state also provided health care and parenting support systems, as well as a network of housekeeping services. Politically, parliamentary quotas of at least 30 per cent for women were in place. As a result, in the mid-1980s, 36 per cent of members in the Ukrainian Soviet Parliament were women (Hrycak 2001, 153). On the other hand, the shortcomings in Soviet gender policies outnumbered their positive effects. The Communist Party claimed gender equality and vilified feminism as bourgeois (Johnson 2007, 395), thus denying the necessity of further work in the area. Despite legal guarantees of gender equality, the Soviet regime perpetuated the oppressive view that childbearing and family caregiving should be women's primary concerns. The formal equality practised in the Soviet Union led to the perception that women's rights were fully protected and, consequently, that no reforms in terms of gender equality were needed. Arguably, such perceptions underlie current resistance in transition countries like Ukraine to dealing with issues of discrimination and inequality.

The movement for Ukrainian independence, which started in the late 1980s, and afterwards the project of nation building, has caused a resurgence of nationalism. Patriarchal traditional gender images, roles, and narratives were revived, leading to what has been referred to as 'neotraditional gender' – that is, the idea that men and women have distinct roles in society (Johnson and Robinson 2007). For example, Pavlychko (1996) explains that feminism played an ambivalent role within Ukraine's nationalist movement for independence, one that became even more diluted after independence when state building became focused on both reasserting and inventing an ideal female citizen: a pure, maternal, self-sacrificing Ukrainian woman. As in many other post-Soviet states, a particular national ideology has developed in Ukraine's process of state building that is creating a resurgence of traditional gender divisions (Lukić et al. 2006). Consequently, 'at the level of mass consciousness, women are primarily seen as mothers whose place is in the family. Such stereotypes hinder real equality between women and men, and obstruct harmonization of professional and family roles for Ukrainian women' (Von Struensee 2002, 10). Ironically, this is in considerable contrast to women's experiences under a communist state where they simultaneously performed the 'triple role of "mother," "working class hero," and "socialist citizen"' (Lukić et al. 2006, 249). At the same time, post-communism idealizes pre-communist gender roles and has driven men out into the business world (Janey et al. 2009).

Debates have ensued about how to respond to these essentialist trends, and in particular, how to forge ideas and approaches to gender inequality that do not necessarily draw only from the Western tradition as point of reference. Indeed, as Galligan et al. (2007) point out, 'gender equality is a context-bound concept, shaped by the specific social reality that it inhibits' (p. 14). And yet, Western influences, both in terms of ideas, such as discourses of equality rights, and in terms of concrete action in the form of powerful equality development organizations, have affected Ukraine's approach and response to gender equality. For example, the Fourth World Conference on Women, in Beijing in 1995, the ideological agenda of which was set in largely Western feminist terms, is now considered to have been 'a watershed moment for the women's movement in Ukraine, as activists began to realize that the state is obliged under international law to take effective steps to protect women from violence and that state resources could be designed to defend women's rights' (WWICS 2007, 1). At the same time, throughout the 1990s the Ukrainian state 'formally acceded to gender-equality conventions – such as CEDAW [Convention on the Elimination of all Forms of Discrimination against Women] – but persisted in a quasi-Soviet maternalist approach to women's rights that diverged from the norms and practices of international organizations' (Hrycak 2005, 78). Initiatives were for the most part ineffective and contradictory, and the responsibility for their execution was left to underfunded government bodies concerned with social services.

The contradictory stances towards gender issues among Ukrainian policy makers are captured by the very formulation of the gender equality provision in the Ukrainian constitution. Article 24 of Ukraine's 1996 Constitution states:

Equality of women's and men's rights is ensured by providing women with opportunities that are equal to those of men in the sociopolitical and cultural spheres, in education and in obtaining professional accreditation, at work and its remuneration, special actions targeted at women's work safety and health, establishment of pension privileges, creation of conditions for combining work with motherhood, legal protection, material and moral support of motherhood and childhood, including paid vacations and other privileges to pregnant women and mothers.

Tamara Melnyk (personal communication, Sept. 2009) has argued that this provision contains a number of problems. First, it is focused on the problems of one of the genders, namely, women; only women's health, work safety, and special pension privileges are addressed. Second, emphasis is placed on women having equal opportunities in the cultural sphere, even though they already make up two-thirds of workers in that area, and therefore need no further promotion in this realm. Third, Article 24 uses the words 'motherhood' and 'childhood' in tight connection, hinting that a woman's role is primarily as a mother.

In the 2000s positive developments in gender policy began to take hold when the Ukrainian government introduced a number of crucial documents, including legislation to promote gender equality, and ratified and adopted a number of key international conventions and agreements: In May 2001 a special presidential decree About Upgrading the Social Status of Women in Ukraine was issued on the matter of women's equal rights and opportunities in public and political life. In July 2003 a *gender adviser* position was created within all ministries and regional governments. In 2005 the Law on Ensuring Equal Rights and Opportunities for Women and Men (often referred to simply as the Law on Gender Equality) was passed, intended to secure parity for men and women in all sectors. Moreover, it can be argued that the 2006 Cabinet of Ministers' Decree on the Concept of the State Program 'On Mainstreaming Gender Equality in Ukrainian Society 2006–2010' contained the beginnings of what is called a *gender mainstreaming* (GM) policy approach because it follows the basic idea of considering the status of both men and women in combating gender imbalance (Gander and Magdyuk 2006, 40–1). Besides legislative work, there have been three national action plans that have focused on gender in a host of areas. These plans have addressed policy making, labour market and career growth discrimination, programs for women victims of economic reforms, education for women about gender equality legislation, encouragement for women to participate in decision making and media, a focus on gender in the health sector, the establishment of policies related to human trafficking, production of annual reports on governmental actions, and monitoring of the dynamics with respect to gender issues. Ukraine is also a signatory of the U.N. Millennium Declaration, which has as one of its central goals the achievement of equality between women and men. Ukraine proclaimed that its goal is to reach an improved gender balance by the year 2015.

Of course, a crucial event in the past decade was the Orange Revolution of 2004, which appeared to signal a decisive shift towards Europe (White et al. 2010, 346). President Yuschenko proclaimed European integration to be among his highest priorities and one of his first decisions in office was to create the Ministry for European Integration (Karatnycky 2005). In the aftermath of 2004, legislation and measures pertaining to gender equality came into being that were congruent with the standards and norms of practices in the European Union, for example, the aforementioned 2005 Law on Gender Equality and the state program on establishing gender equality proclaimed in 2006. Concurrently, however, frequent restructuring of state institutions has resulted in blurred responsibilities for the development, implementation, and evaluation of gender policy. The only state institutions working on these issues today are the Ministry for Social Policy, and the Sub-Committee on International Relations and Gender Policy, which reports to the Parliamentary Committee on Human Rights, National Minorities, and International Relations. Everything else exists on paper only (Kisselyova and Trokhym 2007, 8).

Currently, Ukraine's path towards a European framework for gender equality has been interrupted with the election of Victor Yanukovych as president, in 2010, a change that again brings to light Ukraine's position at a political crossroads between Western and Eastern power and pressures. Besides running on a generally anti-Western and pro-Russian platform, Yanukovych also sent a clear message about his stance on the issue of gender when he refused to participate in pre-election debates with Yuliya Tymoshenko, comparing such debates to 'women's whim' (RIA Novosti, 20 Jan. 2010) and announcing that Tymoshenko should return to her kitchen (OSCE 2010, 5). Moreover, newly appointed Prime Minister Azarov has justified the absence of women in his government by pronouncing that 'conducting reforms is not women's business' (Harding 2010).

In sum, like in many other post-Soviet states, the fall of communism in Ukraine opened up opportunities to embrace democracy with its principles of human rights, inclusion, and non-discrimination, and in particular, to promote and protect gender equality. These opportunities have not been overlooked. The sheer amount of gender-related documents adopted in Ukraine, especially since 2000, is impressive; there are laws, national action plans, and parliamentary hearings on gender issues. State policy evolved from its first use of the term *gender* to the establishment of a state program on gender mainstreaming in just ten years, a significant achievement given the slow-moving nature of most government machinery. At the same time, however, formal priorities have not led to effective gender politics and practices. National and international developments and mechanisms are primarily on paper only. They are not implemented, and widespread marginalization and discrimination continue (Lukić et al. 2006; Buchanan 2003; Von Struensee 2002).

Furthermore, the state rhetoric has not yet fully moved to a relational perspective on gender roles. Gender equality initiatives focus on protecting women rather than on creating equal opportunities for both men and women and changing the relations between men and women (Gander and Magdyuk 2006, 39). With the exception of fatherhood provisions in the Family Code, government documents tend not to address men's problems in Ukrainian society, even though they are equally numerous and significant. Not surprisingly, then, despite the range of formal commitments and related programs and policies, Ukraine ranks 57th out of 146 countries in the 2011 U.N. Human Development Report on the gender inequality index (p. 140). (The gender inequality index measures inequality in achievements between women and men in three dimensions: reproductive health, empowerment, and the labour market.) The Committee on the Elimination of Discrimination against Women (CEDAW) still faults Ukraine for the lack of state efforts in the areas of fighting discriminatory stereotypes, ensuring women's representation and equal economic opportunities, and addressing the burgeoning women's health issues (United Nations 2010). Despite this blatant contradiction between formal commitment and weak implementation, however, few researchers have taken a closer look to understand why such a gap persists. Janey et al. (2009) explain that 'contemporary gender roles in Ukraine are influenced by a number of factors including Soviet ideology, Ukrainian history, the fall of communism, and dramatic changes in the Ukrainian economy. These elements interact within a larger context of a society that is in the process of establishing a national identity and distancing itself from a totalitarian past' (p. 139). Yet, such factors, among other explanatory causes, are only starting to be identified, understood, and fully interrogated, making this collection a particularly timely and important contribution to the literature.

The Ukrainian experience presented here will be of interest to scholars who investigate similar phenomena in other post-Soviet countries. It is true that it is impossible to generalize about gender in all the countries of the former Soviet Union because of the influence of disparate cultures, histories, and religions. As Rai (2007) points out, 'Different contexts bring different strains and tensions' (p. 270). Nevertheless, in writing about social identity and women's experiences, Duffy (2000) asserts that 'there are similarities shared across the countries of ECE [East-Central Europe] that entice scholars to examine women's situations at a fairly high level of abstraction. All the countries in this region, after all, have undergone drastic economic and political changes since 1989, resulting in considerable instability and social turmoil. In all . . . nationalist inclinations have strengthened . . . In all, there has been a recent retrenchment in government-guaranteed benefits . . . and (re)surfacing of what appear to be very traditional and patriarchal policy proponents' (p. 215).

Not surprisingly, then, Galligan et al. (2007) have argued that 'more comparative research remains to be carried out on the subject of gender and politics' (pp. 147–8). Moreover, Funk (1993) has observed the need for 'more thorough investigation of the similarities and differences across the postsocialist states' to compare and contrast the development of 'Slavophil versions' of gender equality (p. 14) in the midst of political, economic, and social turmoil. By focusing on Ukraine, this volume will facilitate such comparative analyses. At the same time, an in-depth examination of the Ukrainian case enhances the knowledge of academics, the NGO community, and international political bodies like the United Nations and regional groupings such as the European Union of how 'universal' gender principles play out in specific cultural and historical settings. Indeed, there is much to learn from the Ukrainian context about how specifically Western notions of gender and gender equality are 'appropriated, rejected or transformed' (p. 1).

This volume is unique in bringing together, for the first time, an interdisciplinary group of leading scholars and practitioners from political science, public policy, sociology, history, anthropology, education, linguistics, economics, women's studies, and philosophy to examine gender issues in the context of Ukraine. Although this is the first Western publication on the issues of gender and politics in Ukraine, gender studies do continue to develop within this country. As Zhurzhenko (2008) puts it, 'Feminism and gender studies have stopped being exotic in Ukraine: university courses on gender issues are taught, conferences are organized, dissertations get defended, articles and books are published. There have also been created several independent centers of gender (women's) studies, among which the ones in Kyiv, Kharkiv, Lviv and Odessa are most known' (p. 38). Here we feature research by leaders in the development of gender scholarship in Ukraine and in the West, alongside writings by new and emerging scholars whose contributions will continue to advance the field well into the future. The collection is far from comprehensive: our attempt has been to cover central areas of concern and their implications for a Ukrainian-specific gender order, including political participation, education, health, demographics, violence against women, economic inequality, homelessness, masculinities, fatherhood, sexual orientation, and gender mainstreaming. Until now, many of these areas have been woefully underrepresented in international volumes on post-Soviet gender relations.

As readers will observe, there is no uniform point of view on offer here. Each contributing author draws on a range of theoretical and methodological approaches – statistics, ethnography, interviews, content analysis, to name a few – from both non-Western and Western perspectives. The contributors also bring to the volume a range of writing styles and insights. Moreover, because many of the sources (including government laws, regulations, and documents) drawn on throughout this collection are in Ukrainian, unless otherwise indicated, the translations into English are by the authors themselves and, as a result, the terminology used may vary slightly. The diversity and breadth of scholarship are the strengths of this volume, as is the variety of topics covered, ranging from longer-standing debates and discussions to emerging gender challenges and issues facing Ukraine.

All of the authors of this volume are in agreement that the implementation of the gender policies adopted and the international documents ratified by Ukraine requires sustained attention. However, while understanding that gender equality cannot be realized solely through governmental instruments and interventions, the authors point out that all sectors must participate in the promotion of structural changes in Ukrainian society and especially in the development of effective educational initiatives to break down harmful gender stereotypes, such as those that have re-emerged or been further entrenched as a result of nationalistic discourses in post-Soviet Ukraine.

A majority of the contributors discuss the importance of including men in gender equality work. Gender justice requires transformations of masculinities and gender relations in both the public and private spheres. Although in Ukrainian laws and concomitant policies, gender still tends to be associated with women, men's issues are no less problematic and much less investigated to date.

Finally, another key issue that arises across the chapters is the role and consequences of international forces. The contributors stress that international governments and organizations have been vital to the development and adoption of numerous pieces of gender policy legislation. At the same time, the issue of the applicability of Western models to Ukraine remains in question and is addressed by several contributors. As they note, the problem of 'travelling models' is that they are not automatically effective or appropriate to the distinct realities of the Ukrainian context. Moreover, international aid for the development of gender equality initiatives has often undermined rather than furthered such work by creating new inequalities and elitism among gender NGOs and even demobilizing existing civil society. Most importantly, these developments, as highlighted by the collection, raise serious questions and concerns regarding the extent to which Ukraine should be expected to follow and adapt Western 'best practices' and, to the extent that it does not, whether it should be evaluated as 'falling short' in developing an appropriate and effective country response to gender equality.

Thus, taken together, all of the scholars contributing to this volume tackle the gendered effects of the Soviet legacy while addressing new problems and challenges, including decay in the general welfare system, the patriarchal nature of nation building, new forms of capitalism, and the power of European and North American influences in Ukrainian society. This collection furthers the understanding of the complex obstacles to challenges of operationalizing gender equality in a transitional society and, in particular, of creating contextually grounded approaches to advancing gender equality that reflect Ukraine's needs.

The volume is organized into four parts, each addressing an area of crucial importance to gender relations in any society, yet which have been largely overlooked in gender research in the post-communist region and Ukraine in particular. The areas are political processes and structures, socioeconomic transformations, educational policy, and emerging issues.

Part I addresses the political and institutional dimensions of gender in Ukraine, reflecting on the transformation of gender relations in the context of a transitional society's changing political order. It opens with Tolstokorova, who identifies the main stages of gender policy development in post-Soviet Ukraine and analyses the country's overall approach to gender policy by comparing it with four major gender policy models in the European Union. In keeping with Ukraine's complex political-historical situation, Tolstokorova finds that the policy model in use represents a kind of mosaic of other models. Next, in Chapter 2, Rubchak tightens the focus to analyse Ukrainian parliamentary hearings on gender issues and discusses their impact on Ukrainian society at both the elite and grassroots levels. Moving yet further from general aspects of the political system to particular issues of institutional design with respect to gender, in Chapter 3, Salnykova looks at the relationship between electoral rules and women's representation in Ukraine and analyses the effects of two rounds of electoral reforms on the gender balance in the Ukrainian political system. Interestingly, she finds that an electoral system of proportional representation works differently in Ukraine, compared with Western countries, and that the potential for electoral mechanisms to assist in women's representation depends in part on the will of Ukraine's women's movement. Part I concludes with Hrycak's examination, in Chapter 4, of global influences on the rise of national campaigns in Ukraine to combat violence against women and the responses of state actors at the national and local levels to advocates who work on the prevention of violence. Like Salnykova, Hrycak points to the importance of effective strategies by activists for taking advantage of circumstances to further their cause. Hrycak shows that, in the case of violence against women, advocates in Ukraine have effectively inserted their issue into ongoing efforts by politicians to woo voters by demonstrating their allegiance to either Eastern or Western values.

Part II delves into the underlying social structures and economic processes that influence gendered social relations in Ukraine. It opens with Zhurzhenko's discussion of new demographic discourses in Ukraine (Chapter 5), particularly those surrounding the country's very low fertility and high mortality rates (the latter especially among men).

Through an exploration of developments in policies and practices designed to address these issues, she assesses their complex impacts on gender inequality and concludes that fundamental change in family gender roles and models of masculinity must take place in order to alter Ukraine's demographic tendencies. This is followed by Kis's critical survey (Chapter 6) of works on Ukrainian women's history published in Ukraine since the early 1990s. Kis identifies the dominant narratives in these works within the wider sociocultural and political contexts and shows how some of these narratives, including that surrounding the matriarchal figure of *Berehynia*, have had a disturbingly powerful impact on political and public discourses. In Chapter 7 Phillips addresses class and the experiences of women social activists who struggled throughout the late 1990s to preserve their social worth. By following these women's stories the chapter examines how calculations of class have shifted during the post-socialist transition. Phillips also assesses the effects of these shifts on organizing strategies by NGOs that work in the interests of marginalized Ukrainian women. Ironically, she finds that the women who run the NGOs, whose own social worth has been put in doubt by what she calls the new neo-liberal order, can find themselves playing conflicting roles as both advocates of greater government support and agents of further class differentiation. In Chapter 8, Riabchuk looks at the issue of homelessness and how it is intertwined with gender realities and their particular impact on men in post-socialist transitions. Riabchuk's analysis powerfully demonstrates the connection between economic and political transition and social processes related to gender in Ukraine.

Part III is dedicated to education, which is an understudied aspect of gender-related processes in post-communism. In Chapter 9, Plakhotnik explores the development of Ukrainian gender policy in the educational sector, demonstrating the superficiality of governmental gender equality initiatives. She provides a rich narrative about key problem areas in the educational system, including the lack of gender awareness among educators, and she engages in a critical debate with so-called gender pedagogy, which claims to support gender equality but which, in fact does the opposite. In Chapter 10, Semikolenova presents findings from her analysis of Ukrainian textbooks used in Grade 1 classrooms in Ukraine's Autonomous Republic of Crimea. Showing the immense preponderance of gender stereotypes that these books transmit to young children, her seminal research is an eye-opener for gender equality-minded educators. Part III concludes with Chapter 11, in which Oksamytna looks at the impact of gender and social background – especially the level of education achieved by mothers, and not only fathers – on educational attainments and the transition from school to work in Ukraine, and how these factors have an impact on graduates' opportunities for employment and achievement in professional, managerial, and non-skilled jobs.

In Part IV we explore several emerging issues pertaining to gender in Ukraine. Hankivsky, in Chapter 12, examines the effects of gender on health issues in the Ukrainian population. She looks at the extent to which this crucial connection is captured by state gender and health policies and concludes that the government needs to change its current approaches and draw on a perspective that uses the social determinants of health to shape and direct health reform efforts. In Chapter 13, Bureychak provides a comprehensive overview of Soviet and post-Soviet Ukrainian images of masculinities, drawing our attention to the key implications that such constructs of gender have for men's experience. The theme of men's issues continues with Koshulap, who in Chapter 14 contends with prevalent Ukrainian discourses on fatherhood and their impact on fathering practices. By presenting findings from a qualitative study of new fathers, she shows how recent state support for more involved fatherhood has influenced men's perceptions of their role in the family. In Chapter 15, Martsenyuk analyses the results of sociological research on homophobia and attitudes towards representatives of the lesbian, gay, bisexual, and transgender communities. Part IV concludes with Chapter 16, where the co-editors, Hankivsky and Salnykova, evaluate existing gender equality instruments in Ukraine and, in particular, the beginnings of a gender mainstreaming approach.

The chapters in this volume should be read as individual pieces, each with its own theoretical interpretations and methodological approaches to a diverse range of topics. At the same time, we understand them as contributions that cohere within a framework that provides preliminary insights into the current situation and future challenges to the advancement of gender equality in Ukraine. It seemed appropriate, then, to speak to what might come next in terms of new areas of research and policy. The Afterword is our attempt to do so. We hope that academics and decision makers alike – among them, some of the contributors featured here – will pick up on the overall discussion of gender and transition in Ukraine and move it forward in their various fields.

REFERENCES

Betliy, O., O. Kuziakiv, and K. Onishchenko. 2007. *The Evaluation of Health Care System in Ukraine in the Context of Structural and Quality-Enhancing Reforms.* Revised Final Report MIR04 – 009. Moscow: EERC. Full text available at http://pdc.ceu.hu/archive/00004087/01/18_eng_070815_final.pdf (accessed 1 Feb. 2010).

Blagojević, M. 2003. Creators, Transmitters and Users: Women's Scientific Excellence at the Periphery of Europe. In *Gender and Excellence in the Making,* 135–45. Brussels: European Commission Research Publications.

Booth, R.E., S.K. Mikulich-Gilbertson, J.T. Brewster, S. Salomonsen-Sautel, and O. Semerik. 2004. Predictors of Self-Reported HIV Infection among Drug Injectors in Ukraine. *Journal of Acquired Immune Deficiency Syndromes* 35(1): 82–8.

Bromet, E.J., S.F. Gluzman, V.I. Paniotto, C.P.M. Webb, N.L. Tintle, V. Zakhozha, J.M. Havenaar, Z. Gutkovich, S. Kostyuchenko, and J.E. Schwartz. 2005. Epidemiology of Psychiatric and Alcohol Disorders in Ukraine: Findings from the Ukraine World Mental Health Survey. *Social Psychiatry and Psychiatric Epidemiology* 40(9): 681–90.

Buchanan, J. 2003. Women's Work: Discrimination against Women in the Ukrainian Labor Force. *Human Rights Watch* 15(5): 1–52.

Bunce, V. 1995. Should Transitologists Be Grounded? *Slavic Review* 45(1): 11–27.

Busheikin, L. 1997. Is Sisterhood Really Global? Western Feminism in Eastern Europe. In T. Renne, ed., *Ana's Land: Sisterhood in Eastern Europe,* 12–22. Boulder: Westview.

Campbell, D.F.J., and G. Pölzlbauer. 2010. *The Democracy Ranking 2009 of the Quality of Democracy: Method and Ranking Outcome. Comprehensive Scores and Score for the Dimensions.* Vienna: Democracy Ranking. Available at http://www.democracyranking.org/downloads/method_ranking_outcome_2009_A4.pdf.

Carothers, T. 2002. The End of Transition Paradigm. *Journal of Democracy* 13(1): 5–21.

CIA. 2010. The World Factbook. Available at: *https://www.cia.gov/library/publica tions/the-world-factbook/geos/up.html* (accessed 15 June 2011).

Cockerham, W.C., B.P. Hinote, and P. Abbott. 2006. Psychological Distress, Gender, and Health Lifestyles in Belarus, Kazakhstan, Russia, and Ukraine. *Social Science and Medicine* 63(9): 2381–94.

Connell, R.W. 2007. *Gender.* Cambridge: Polity.

Corrin, C., ed. 1999. *Gender and Identity in Central and Eastern Europe.* London: Frank Cass.

Duffy, D.M. 2000. Social Identity and Its influence on Women's Roles in East-Central Europe. *International Feminist Journal of Politics* 2(2): 214–43.

Einhorn, B. 1993. *Cinderella Goes to Market: Citizenship, Gender and Women's Movements in East-Central Europe.* London: Verso.

Freedom House (FH). 2010. *Freedom in the World 2010: Erosion of Freedom Intensifies.* Available at http://www.freedomhouse.org/uploads/fiw10/FIW_2010_Tables_and_Graphs.pdf (accessed 22 July 2010).

Funk, N. 1993. Introduction: Women and Post-Communism. In N. Funk and M. Mueller, eds., *Gender Politics and Post-Communism: Reflections from Eastern Europe and the Former Soviet Union,* 1–14. New York: Routledge.

Funk, N., and M. Mueller. 1993. *Gender Politics and Post-Communism: Reflections from Eastern Europe and the Former Soviet Union.* New York: Routledge.

Gal, S., and G. Kligman. 2000. *The Politics of Gender after Socialism: A Comparative Historical Essay.* Princeton: Princeton University Press.

Galligan, Y., S. Clavero, and M. Calloni, eds. 2007. *Gender, Politics and Democracy in Post-Socialist Europe.* Leverkusen: Barbara Budrich Publishers.

Gander, C., and L. Magdyuk. 2006. *Ukraine Gender Equality Review.* Ottawa: CIDA.

Gilmore, A.B., M. McKee, and R. Rose. 2002. Determinants of and Inequalities in Self-Reported Health in Ukraine. *Social Science and Medicine* 55: 2177–88.

Hampton, R., D. Ball, J. Pennington, and A. Nguyen. 2009. *Estimating the Extent of Out-Migration Human Trafficking in Ukraine.* Available online at http://digitalcommons.unl.edu/cgi/viewcontent.cgi?article=1016andcontext=humtraffconf (accessed 1 June 2010).

Harding, L. 2010. Ukrainian Women Berate 'Neanderthal' PM for Sexist Remarks. Guardian.co.uk, 24 March 2010. Available online at http://www.guardian.co.uk/world/2010/mar/24/ukraine-mykola-azarov-women (accessed 12 July 2010).

Havelkova, H. 1996. Abstract Citizenship? Women and Power in the Czech Republic. *Social Politics: International Studies in Gender, State and Society* 3(2/3): 243–60.

Hrycak, A. 2001. The Dilemmas of Civic Revival: Ukrainian Women since Independence. *Journal of Ukrainian Studies* 26(12): 135–58.

– 2005. Coping with Chaos: Gender and Politics in a Fragmented State. *Problems of Post-Communism* 52(5): 69–81.

International Herald Tribune (IHT). 2007. *International Herald Tribune Online.* Available at http://web.archive.org/web/20080316021607/http://www.iht.com/articles/ap/2007/02/19/europe/EU-GEN-Ukraine-Human-Trafficking.php.

Jähnert, G., J. Gohrisch, D. Hahn, H.M. Nickel, I. Peinl, and K. Schäfgen, eds. 2001. *Gender in Transition in Eastern and Central Europe: Proceedings*. Berlin: Trafo-Verlag Weist.

Janey, B.A., S. Plitin, J.L. Muse-Burke, and V.M. Vovk. 2009. Masculinity in Post-Soviet Ukraine: An Exploratory Factor Analysis. *Culture, Society and Masculinities* 1(2): 137–54.

Johnson, J.E. 2007. Domestic Violence Politics in Post-Soviet States. *Social Politics: International Studies in Gender, State and Society* 14(3): 380–405.

Johnson, J.E., and J.C. Robinson. 2007. *Living Gender after Communism*. Bloomington: Indiana University Press.

Karatnycky, A. 2005. Ukraine's Orange Revolution. *Foreign Affairs* 84(2): 35–52.

Kisselyova, O., and I. Trokhym. 2007. *A Gender Analysis of EU Development Instruments and Policies in Ukraine*. Kyiv: Network of East-West Women, Gender Watch. Available at http://www.neww.org.pl/download/EU_Gender_Watch_Ukraine.pdf.

Kohn, M., W. Zaborowski, K. Janicka, V. Khmelko, B.W. Mach, V. Paniotto, K.M. Slomczynski, C. Heyman, and B. Podobnik. 2002. Structural Location and Personality during the Transformation of Poland and Ukraine. *Social Psychology Quarterly* 65(4): 364–85.

Kolisnichenko, N., and A. Rosenbaum. 2009. Building a New Democracy in Ukraine: The Unacknowledged Issue of Ethnic and Linguistic Diversity in Public Administration Education and Training. *Public Administration Review* 69(5): 932–40.

Kornai, J. 1995. *Highways and Byways: Studies on Reform and Post-Communist Transition*. Cambridge, MA: MIT Press.

Kuehnast, K., and C. Nechemias. 2004. *Post-Soviet Women Encountering Transition: Nation-Building, Economic Survival, and Civic Activism*. Washington, DC: Woodrow Wilson Center Press.

Kuzio, T. 2001. Transition in Post-Communist States: Triple or Quadruple? *Politics* 21(3): 168–77.

Linz, J., and A. Stepan. 1996. *Problems of Democratic Transition and Consolidation: Southern Europe, South America and Post-Communist Europe*. Baltimore: Johns Hopkins University Press.

Lukić, J., J. Regulska, and D. Zavrišek, eds. 2006. *Women and Citizenship in Central and Eastern Europe*. Aldershot: Ashgate.

Maksymenko, S. 2009. Fertility, Money Holdings, and Economic Growth: Evidence from Ukraine. *Comparative Economic Studies* 51: 75–9.

Marsh, R.J., ed. 1996. *Women in Russia and Ukraine*. Cambridge: Cambridge University Press.

Matland, R.E., and K.A. Montgomery, eds. 2003. *Women's Access to Political Power in Post-Communist Europe.* Oxford: Oxford University Press.

McFaul, M. 2005 Transitions from Post-Communism. *Journal of Democracy* 16(3): 5–19.

Moghadam, V., ed. 1993. *Democratic Reform and the Position of Women in Transitional Economies.* Oxford: Clarendon.

Muharska, R. 2005. Silences and Parodies in the East-West Feminist Dialogue. *L'Homme. Zeitschrift für feministische Geschichtswissenschaft* [L'Homme: European Review of Feminist History] 16(1): 36–47.

Occhipinti, L. 1996. Two Steps Back? Anti-Feminism in Eastern Europe. *Anthropology Today* 12(6): 13–18.

Offe, C., and P. Adler. 1991. Capitalism by Democratic Design? Democratic Theory Facing Triple Transition in East-Central Europe. *Social Research* 58(4): 865–92.

Organization for Security and Co-operation in Europe (OSCE). 2010. *Ukraine Presidential Election.* Office for Democratic Institutions and Human Rights: Election Observation Mission. Interim report No. 4 (18–26 Jan.). Available at http://www.osce.org/documents/odihr/2010/01/42521_en.pdf (accessed 12 July 2010).

Pascal, G., and A. Kwak. 2005. *Gender Regimes in Transition in Central and Eastern Europe.* Bristol: Policy.

Pavlychko, S. 1996. Feminism in Post-Communist Ukrainian Society. In R. Marsh, ed., *Women in Russia and Ukraine*, 305–14. Cambridge: Cambridge University Press.

Perelli-Harris, B. 2008. Family Formation in Post-Soviet Ukraine: Changing Effects of Education in a Period of Rapid Social Change. *Social Forces* 87(2): 767–94.

Pifer, S., A. Aslund, and J. Elkind. 2009. *Engaging Ukraine in 2009.* Brookings Foreign Policy Paper No. 13 (March). Available at http://petersoninstitute.org/publications/papers/aslund0309brookings.pdf (accessed 2 March 2010).

Rai, Shirin, ed. 2007. *Mainstreaming Gender, Democratizing the State? Institutional Mechanisms for the Advancement of Women.* New Brunswick, NJ: Transaction Publishers.

RIA Novosti. Yanukovych Rejects Debate, Says Tymoshenko Can Show Off in Kitchen. 20 Jan. 2010. Available online at http://en.rian.ru/exsoviet/20100120/157628829.html (accessed 12 July 2010).

Rose, R. 1998. *Democracy and Its Alternatives: Understanding Post-Communist Societies.* Baltimore: Johns Hopkins University Press.

Round, J., and C. Williams. 2010. Coping with the Social Costs of 'Transition': Everyday Life in Post-Soviet Russia and Ukraine. *European Urban and Regional Studies* 17(2): 183–96.

Rubchak, M. 1996. Christian Virgin or Pagan Goddess? In R. Marsh, ed., *Women in Russia and Ukraine*, 315–30. Cambridge: Cambridge University Press.

Rubchak, M., ed. 2011. *Mapping Difference: The Many Faces of Women in Contemporary Ukraine*. London: Berghahn.

Rueschemeyer, M., and S.L. Wolchik, eds. 2009. *Women in Power in Post-Communist Parliaments*. Washington, DC: Woodrow Wilson Center Press.

Slavova, K. 2006. Looking at Western Feminisms through the Double Lens of Eastern Europe and the Third World. In J. Lukić et al., eds., *Women and Citizenship in Central and Eastern Europe*, 245–64. Aldershot: Ashgate.

Štulhofer, A., and T. Sandfort, eds. 2005. *Sexuality and Gender in Postcommunist Eastern Europe and Russia*. Binghampton: Haworth.

Trafficking in Persons. 2009. Country Ratings. Tier Placements. [Adapted from U.S. State Dept Trafficking in Persons Report, 17 June 2009]. Available online at http://gvnet.com/humantrafficking/00-Ratings.htm (accessed 15 June 2011).

Tsang, A., M. Von Korff, S. Lee, J. Alonso, E. Karam, M.C. Angermeyer, G.L. Guimaraes Borges, E.J. Bromet, G. de Girolamo, R. de Graaf, O. Gureje, J.-P. Lepine, J.M. Haro, D. Levinson, M.A. Oakley Browne, J. Posada-Villa, S. Seedat, and M. Watanabe. 2008. Common Chronic Pain Conditions in Developed and Developing Countries: Gender and Age Differences and Co-morbidity with Depression-Anxiety Disorders. *Journal of Pain* 9(10): 883–91.

UNAIDS. 2007. *A Global View of HIV Infection*. Available at http://data.unaids.org/pub/GlobalReport/2008/GR08_2007_HIVPrevWallMap_GR08_en.jpg.

– 2008. *Report on the Global AIDS Epidemic*. Joint U.N. Program on HIV/AIDS – WHO. Geneva: WHO.

U.N. Human Development Report. 2011. Available at http://www.beta.undp.org/content/dam/undp/library/corporate/HDR/2011%20Global%OHDR/English/HDR_2011_EN_complete.pdf (accessed Jan. 2 2012).

United Nations. 2010. *Concluding Observations of the Committee on the Elimination of Discrimination Against Women: Ukraine*. (CEDAW/C/UKR/CO/7). Available at http://www2.ohchr.org/tbru/cedaw/CEDAW-C-UKR-CO-7.pdf (accessed 25 July 2010).

United Nations Entity for Gender Equality and the Empowerment of Women (UNEGEEW). 2011. Available online at: http://www.un.org/womenwatch/osagi/conceptsanddefinitions.htm (accessed 15 June 2011).

Von Struensee, V. 2002. *Gender Equality: Legal and Institutional Framework on Women's Rights – Ukraine*. Originally published through the Public Interest Law Institute for the Transitional Societies Access to Justice Forum, 15 Jan. Available at www.pili.org/cgi-bin/a2j?_nameserve_vonstruensee).

White, S., I. McAllister, and V. Feklyunina. 2010. Belarus, Ukraine and Russia: East or West? *British Journal of Politics and International Relations* 12(3): 344–67.

Woehrel, S. 2009. *Ukraine: Current Issues and U.S. Policy*. Report 7–5700 prepared for the Members and Committees of Congress, 13 Aug. Available at http://ftp.fas.org/sgp/crs/row/RL33460.pdf (accessed 1 July 2010).

Woodrow Wilson International Center for Scholars (WWICS). 2007. *Women's NGOs in Ukraine and the End of Western Aid*. Available at http://www.wilsoncenter.org/index.cfm?fuseaction=events.event_summaryandevent_id=237920 (accessed 21 Aug. 2009).

World Audit. 2009. *Democracy Audit*. Available at http://www.worldaudit.org/democracy.htm.

World Health Organization (WHO). 2006. *Mortality Country Fact Sheet*. Statistical overview prepared by WHO. Available at http://www.who.int/whosis/mort/profiles/mort_euro_ukr_ukraine.pdf (accessed 22 July 2010).

Zhurzhenko, T. 2008. *Gendernye Rynki Ukrainy* [Gender Markets in Ukraine]. Vilnius: European Humanities University.

PART I

Politics and Gender

1 A Mosaic Model of Gender Democracy in Ukraine

ALISSA V. TOLSTOKOROVA

With the results of the 2004 elections, when pro-European forces came to power, Ukraine for the first time openly declared its commitment to follow the European way of development and to seek membership in the European Union (EU). Governmental policy aimed at European integration was confirmed by the Ukraine – EU Action Plan signed in 2005. According to the plan, the state assumed obligations to respect and implement program documents of the United Nations and the European Commission and to promote equality between women and men in social and economic life (Plan dij Ukraina – Evropejsky Sojuz 2005, 10). In this context Ukraine's movement towards European norms of democracy becomes a central concern to policy makers in the country, and this includes heightened awareness of gender equality standards within the European Union. Indeed, the protection and promotion of gender equality are among the key components necessary to meet the Copenhagen criteria, used to evaluate candidate states seeking membership in the European Union. Therefore, the goal of this chapter is to examine how Ukrainian public policy pertaining to gender equality compares with various models practised in the European Union by tracing the development of gender governance in Ukraine. To reach this goal, I first outline existing EU approaches to the promotion of gender equality as summarized by the EQUAPOL Project, which studied eight EU countries and identified four main models of gender mainstreaming (Braithwaite 2005).[1] Next I look into the history of the formation of 'parity democracy' in Ukraine, understood here as 'a form of social relationship in political and legal areas, which guarantees women equal social status with men on the grounds of actual representation at all the levels of all power structures' (MFYU

1998, 7). I identify the main stages of the development of gender equality policy and spotlight a 'gender mainstreaming paradox' (Novikova, 2006) in Ukraine, which implies that some key stakeholders in the advancement of gender equality, while claiming to be its major advocates, in effect, turn into its principal obstacles. Finally, I draw conclusions about the correspondence between the existing models of gender governance in Ukraine and in the European Union. My analysis clearly shows that, in practice, Ukraine's model is at best a mosaic or mixture of EU models of gender democracy. Its key challenges stem from the fact that the state has not yet sorted out its own national identity vis-à-vis gender and gender equality.

Experience of Gender Equality Policy in the European Union

Between 2002 and 2004 the EQUAPOL Project was undertaken in eight European countries (Belgium, Spain, France, Greece, Ireland, Lithuania, Sweden, and the United Kingdom), with the aim of evaluating the success of mainstreaming gender into European public policy. The strategy of gender mainstreaming (GM; for a detailed discussion of GM, see Chapter 16, in this volume) was introduced by the European Commission in 1996 as one of the policy instruments prioritized by its agenda for social policy. Gender mainstreaming is understood as 'mobilizing all general policies and measures specifically for the purpose of achieving equality by actively and openly taking into account at the planning stage their possible effects on the respective situation of men and women' (European Commission 1996). In the EQUAPOL final report (Braithwaite 2005) the existing approaches to gender governance were grouped into four principal models: the Swedish or 'integrated' model, the 'transversal' model, the 'Union-impetus' model, and the 'generic model' or 'equality beyond gender.' These models were also briefly outlined by Rugemer (2007).

(1) *The 'Integrated' Model or 'Swedish Gender Mainstreaming.'* As follows from the EQUAPOL report, this model approaches gender equality from multiple directions, embracing socioeconomic, political, cultural, civic, public, and private aspects of society. It consists in applying a whole package of measures aimed at achieving gender equality as an 'all-encompassing' policy goal, together with a variety of gender mainstreaming instruments used at all levels of governance. Under this model, the responsibility for developing gender policy is spread across different departments and sub-departments and is

shared with private and public sectors of society. To my mind the Swedish model comes closest to the understanding of GM by the European Commission and will be understood in this meaning in this chapter.

(2) *The Transversal Model.* This model implies that gender equality policy cuts across a variety of governance sectors. It relies on the tradition of 'positive actions,' also known as affirmative action, positive discrimination, or reverse discrimination. Within EU law and policy practice, the term 'positive actions' is used preferentially to signify a wide range of measures taken to compensate for present and past disadvantages that exist because of discrimination, with the goal of achieving 'full equality in practice' (European Commission 2007, 5). Belgium fits this model most closely, with France and the region of Andalusia in Spain fitting to a lesser degree. As noted in the EQUA-POL report, although initially positive action measures were aimed at promoting women's employment and human capital development, currently they are being applied to many other areas, such as in the fight against domestic violence in Spain; in recruitment policies in Belgium; as measures targeted at men, like development programs for boys in Ireland; or as measures for both women and men, such as those used to counteract gender stereotyping in France, Greece, and Spain.

(3) *The EU-Driven or 'Union-Impetus' Model.* This model is new and it emerged in response to pressures for greater gender equality both 'from below' and 'from above.' On the one hand, it considers the demand of women's and feminist organizations to approach gender from their perspective; on the other hand, it responds to the requirement to integrate a gender perspective as a condition of EU funding or membership. This model is significant for gender policy making in Lithuania, Ireland, and Greece, and to a lesser extent in Spain. One of the challenges that EQUAPOL identified with this model is a bureaucratic understanding of public policy pertaining to gender equality, which is seen as an end in itself with no connection to other dimensions of equal opportunity policies. Another challenge is that the conditions in the countries where EU gender interventions are being implemented may not necessarily be mature for the introduction of gender mainstreaming policies, which may have a negative impact on the progress towards a more gender-inclusive society.

(4) *The Generic Equality Model or 'Equality beyond Gender' Model.* This model is aimed at advancing equality in a wider sense than gender equity alone. It assumes that social inequality extends across gender

asymmetries and cuts across other forms of oppression such as class, race, ethnicity, age, and disability. This model promotes equality by attempting to restore the balance in favour of disadvantaged groups and by drawing on all possible sources of support, including financial ones, to 'build alliances across intersections of identity.' However, as is highlighted in the EQUIPOL report, adhering to this model bears a danger of losing the specificity of gender among other dimensions of disadvantage and treating the gender component the same as minority issues. This multidimensional approach is implemented, for example, in the United Kingdom.

Main Stages of Public Policy for the Promotion of Gender Equality in Ukraine

Comparing Ukraine's approach to gender equality with these EU models first requires an examination of the development and implementation of gender policy in Ukraine. Elsewhere I have identified four main stages in the evolution of state gender policy in Ukraine (Tolstokorova 2007a, 2008a). Here, taking a more nuanced view that better reflects this history as well as recent developments, I suggest that these stages may be further subdivided into phases, making six in all (see Table 1.1). Historically, a link is observable between these phases and the periods when major documents on gender issues in Ukraine were prepared, including reports on the Convention on the Elimination of all Forms of Discrimination Against Women (CEDAW) and the Beijing Platform for Action, as well as two national action plans. The goal of identifying key achievements in the promotion of gender equality during the development of these documents has enabled a gradual reconceptualization of state gender policies. In turn, this has created the knowledge base at key stages for a dialectical transition to new stages in Ukraine's evolution of gender equality policies.

Stage I (1992 to 1997): Policy in the Interests of Family, Children, and Women

PHASE 1 (1992 TO 1994): MOTHERHOOD POLICY
Throughout this period women were perceived by the Ukrainian state less as subjects than as objects of public policy. In demographic terms they were lumped together with children, youth, the elderly, and disabled persons, and treated as marginalized, deprived, vulnerable, and

Table 1.1. Stages of Gender Equality Policy in Independent Ukraine

Stage and Phase	Years	Developments
Stage I	1992–1997	Foundational period for state equality policy: policy for family, children, and women
Phase 1	1992–1994	Protective and family-centred approach to women: motherhood policy
Phase 2	1995–1997	Policy aimed at women as a self-contained branch of public policy
Stage II	1998–2000	Conceptual bifurcation of social policy into family policy and policy aimed at women
Stage III	2001–2004	Transformation of policy aimed at women into policy for the promotion of gender equality
Stage IV	2005–present	Policy of equal opportunities for women and men
Phase 1	2005–2008	Beginning of gender mainstreaming policy
Phase 2	2008–present	First steps towards fatherhood policy and focus on men's issues

requiring state protection and support. In sociopolitical terms womanhood was conceptualized as motherhood. Women were addressed solely within the context of family, marriage, and domesticity, and their position was primarily identified in terms of their reproductive and nurturing roles. This approach reveals a common tendency in the Central and Eastern European sub-region to 'address women's issues only in relation to family issues' (UNDP 2003, 13), both theoretically and practically. As a result, in post-socialist states, 'the concept of women as dependent on men and as responsible for nurturing and rearing the children has been widely reproduced by social policies' (Fábián 2006, 55).

During this phase, issues concerning women, family, children, and youth were deeply interwoven and tackled by the same branch of public policy. The state looked at them as one social group, and took a paternalistic approach, aiming at the *improvement of their position*. This protective attitude to women is known in social sciences as 'domestication' (Baker 1984; Harsch 2006) or 'familization' (Holland 1970; Saxonberg and Sirovátka 2006). In my opinion, it may be better defined as a family-centred approach, given that it departs from the assumption that 'woman's place is at home' (Kleberg 2007). It implies that women's social position and public policies developed in their interest should be considered primarily in terms of family policy and the well-being of the family.

This approach tends to limit women almost exclusively to the family domain, defining their social roles mainly in terms of maternity, caretaking, nurturing, and homemaking. It ignores the aspiration of women to seek self-realization beyond social reproduction. Instead of addressing family issues, the state shifts the full burden of responsibility for them to women. Among these issues are unequal distribution of domestic chores between the sexes, domestic violence, dependency on the breadwinner, and so on. This approach draws upon the protectionist principle or a safeguarding conception in relation to women's issues that reinforces the rhetoric of protection of motherhood and childhood and promotion of the situation of women. Such a paternalistic attitude towards women set Ukraine back decades in history. Even the mother-centred Soviet family policy of the 1930s, based on a highly repressive ideology, never dared to claim that a woman's place is at the family hearth, and it encouraged women to actively join the labour force (Chernyaeva 2007, 134).

The protectionist principle was embedded even in the Constitution of Ukraine. In particular, it prohibits women's labour in the so-called hazardous occupations based on the expressed claim that this is to safeguard mothers. In fact, this puts two hundred professions officially off limits to women (Kupryashkina 2000). Even more than that, Article 24 of the Constitution (adopted 28 June 1996), which enunciated equality of the sexes, is based on paternalistic language. It proclaims that 'Equality of women's and men's rights is ensured by providing women with opportunities that are equal to those of men in the sociopolitical and cultural spheres.' A linguistic representation of the concept of gender equality thereby portrays women as a dependent social group without its own political will, as consumers of a legislative system crafted by men. Viewed through a gender lens, the wording of this Article 24 raises a number of questions (Tolstokorova 2005, 10–11). First, why should opportunities be 'provided to' (*nadayutsia*) Ukrainian women? Are women seen as socially disabled individuals incapable of obtaining them by themselves and, therefore, in need of masculine guidance? And who is in charge of providing rights to women? Men? The state? Society? If men, why are they so privileged? If the stateor the society, why are women not subsumed as its integral part, equal in rights with others? If they are a part of the society, then here they are presented as both givers and receivers of their own rights. Hence, this wording suggests that civil rights in Ukraine belong primarily to men, but that these can be generously shared with women. It implies that men control civil rights and that women have to receive them from this legislatively privileged group. Thus, women are viewed as passive receivers of social gains – which are owned by men (Tolstokorova 2006, 195). Were the sexes truly represented as equals in Article 24, replacing the word 'woman' for 'man' would not change its implications. Yet, is it possible to imagine that the Constitution would read: 'Equality of women's and men's rights is ensured by providing *men* with opportunities that are equal to those of women in the sociopolitical and cultural spheres'? As empirical research shows, wording of this kind is perceived by speakers to be 'linguistically unacceptable' (Tschudi 1979).[2] This means that men and women are not perceived to be citizens of equal worth. Hence, in its current formulation, Article 24 represents men as 'the measure of all things' (MacKinnon 1991, 82) and as the social norm, defining legislative standards for other groups of the population.

Paternalistic and family-centred ideology is also reflected in the language of many other state documents of this period. The very titles of documents like 'Long-Term State Program for the Advancement of the Situation of *Women* and the *Family*, the *Protection* of *Motherhood* and Childhood' (1992, emphasis added) testify to this. Similar embedding of protectionist ideology occurs in the names of state bodies created to address women's issues during the period, like 'The Commission for the *Protection* of Health, *Motherhood* and Childhood,' the 'Sector for the Analysis of the Development of Health *Protection*, Issues of *Women* and *Family*' (1993, emphasis added), and the 'Committee for the Affairs of Women, Motherhood and Children' (1995). The ideology of this phase, which sought to protect women and improve their position, had a narrow and ambiguous conceptual framework from the outset. Critics have noted that it emerged in response to the acknowledgment that the position of women had deteriorated in the immediate post-Soviet period (UCIPR 2006, 73). Born as a kind of reaction, the ideology lacked both strategic consistency and precise mechanisms for its implementation (Levchenko 2003, 63–4; UCIPR 2006, 73). As for the family-centred approach to policy making, it is argued (Levchenko 2003, 66) that the positioning of women's issues within the family domain is unacceptable as long as women have their own interestsoutside the family, and therefore public policy must address more than issues of family and children if it is to meet women's needs. The ideological conflation of 'womanhood' and 'motherhood' also neglects the situation of childless women. At the same time, this approach waters down the role of fathers and their rights. In its entwining of a protectionist principle and a family-centred approach, the policy approach of this phase also exacerbated conflicts between the private and the public spheres and strengthened the belief that only women are competent to care for the family.

PHASE 2 (1995 TO 1997): POLICY AIMED AT WOMEN AS A SELF-CONTAINED BRANCH OF PUBLIC POLICY

The participation of the Ukrainian delegation in the Fourth World Conference on Women, in Beijing in 1995, and the work on its final documents became a cornerstone in the development of public policy in the interests of women and men in Ukraine. Beijing provided the impetus for the reorganization of the national machinery for the promotion of gender equality and enabled the conceptualization of a self-contained branch of public policy to address women's policy needs, one that was independent from policies in the interests of the family and children. Beijing also created the conditions for the transition to a new stage in the evolution of national gender ideology. This period was benchmarked by the foundation in 1996 of the Ministry for Family and Youth, which replaced the former Committee for Issues of Women, Motherhood and Childhood at the Office of the President of Ukraine. This measure showed that women's issues had acquired for Ukrainian decision makers the significance of policy issues requiring institutionalization at the highest levels of executive power. Within the new ministry an Office for Women's Issues was established, itself consisting of two departments – one targeted at the promotion of the sociojuridical work with women, the other at encouraging the civic, cultural, and educational participation of women. The creation of these departments reflected an emerging awareness of the necessity of developingseparate public policies aimed at women. The ministry's name, however, was evidence that the family-centred approach was still dominant.

The parliamentary hearings of 1995 were another landmark moment of this phase. They were focused on the implementation of the CEDAW in Ukraine. What emerged was a list of state institutions responsible for the development of national equality policy, as well as practical recommendations for the realization of this goal. This created the conditions for the formation of a systemic control mechanism for the promotion of gender equality in Ukraine (see more in Tolstokorova 2007a). This phase can be said to have ended with the publication of a research report on the issue of the development of gender democracy in transitional Ukraine (MFYU 1998), which marked the first attempt by the state to apply a gender-sensitive approach to the analysis of Ukrainian society, incorporating the issue of gender democracy enhancement into the societal agenda and outlining its key challenges.

Stage II (1998 to 2000): Bifurcation of Social Policy
into Family Policy and Policy Aimed at Women

In conceptual terms, the second stage represents a period of bifurcation of social policy into policies in the interests of the family and children, on the one hand, and policies in the interests of women, on the other (UNDP 2006, 12). In practice, each of these emerging branches of public policy was conceptualized by separate strategic documents. The first was backed up by 'The Conception of State Family Policy' and the all-Ukrainian program 'The Ukrainian Family,' the second by 'Draft Conception of Public Policy for the Promotion of the Situation of Women' and 'Draft National Strategies for the Promotion of the Situation of Women.' The two latter documents have never been adopted, signalling a missed opportunity in Ukraine to secure a conceptual framework for state policies for the promotion of gender equality. At the same time, these two documents had already lost their social currency by the time they might have come into being, insofar as they were inherently contradictory, placing the language of equality and equal opportunities for women alongside the outdated language of paternalism and state protection (Levchenko 2003, 63–4).

Changes in public awareness regarding the status of women throughout this stage were thus inconsistent. Although increasingly acknowledged as targets of public policy and addressed beyond the family-centred ideology, women were still viewed in line with the protective principle and as objects of governance, requiring the protection of the state, but not yet as self-sufficient players. This duality was showcased in phrasing enshrined in strategic documents adopted during this stage. Thus, the 'Declaration of a Conceptual Framework for State Policy towards the Family and Women in Ukraine,' adopted in 1999, confirmed that the state assumed the responsibility to guarantee equal rights and possibilities to the sexes, to eliminate all forms of discrimination against women, and to promote their ample and equitable participation in the political, economic, social, and cultural life of the society. At the same time, it limited the magnitude of 'ample' equality for women by highlighting the area of domesticity as their main sphere of interest and their civil responsibilities as being focused on family and children (UCIPR 2006, 77).

Stage III (2001 to 2004): Policy for the Promotion of Gender Equality

In early 2001 came a new milestone in the evolution of public policy for gender equality: the Presidential Decree on the Promotion of Social Status of Women in Ukraine. This document created a conceptual basis for transition to a new stage of development of gender democracy in Ukraine by tying the traditional objective of promotion of the status of women to a new goal of promoting gender equality in Ukrainian society. More importantly, it conceptualized women's issues outside the rhetoric of children, family, and youth (UCIPR 2006, 81). The decree placed a great deal of emphasis on the promotion of equal opportunities for women to take part in the social and political life of society on a par with men as a priority for public policy. It was the first time that women were represented as autonomous subjects of public policy, albeit passive ones – still beneficiaries of public policy rather than active players, insofar as the state was still expected to promote the situation of women and create opportunities for them.

As in the earlier stages, the conceptual evolution of public policy in the interests of women and men was mirrored in the language of state documents. Thus, the National Action Plan for 2001–2005 explicitly included the goal of 'promoting gender equality in society.' Public discussions during this period brought the rhetoric of women's rights to the forefront.

Also, during this period a project co-sponsored by several Canadian government agencies resulted in the development of a framework for gender equality policy.[3] Called 'Gender Equality in Ukraine in the Period of Current Socio-Economic Transformations,' and realized throughout 2002–03,[4] the project had three goals: (1) to conduct a robust analysis of the advancement of gender democracy in Ukraine; (2) to inform society about the progress of gender equality policy both nationally and internationally; and (3) to develop viable strategies for the promotion of equal rights and opportunities of women and men. In the Ukrainian context this was a unique research experience, since it was the first gender-targeted nationwide project. It began with all-nation sociological survey and included in-depth interviews with twenty experts in gender policy as well as focus-groupdiscussions with civil servants in five regional centres: Kyiv (centre), Odessa (South), Kharkiv (North-East), Donetsk (East), and Lviv (West).

Two program documents emerged from this work: the Draft Strategic Directions of State Policy for the Promotion of Gender Equality in Ukraine, and, as a supplement, Recommendations for the Implementation of Strategic Directions of State Policy for the Promotion of Gender Equality in Ukraine. The former document, based on the analysis of the latest Ukrainian statistics, public surveys, and expert evaluations offered a coherent, well-balanced conceptual framework for the advancement of gender equality policy in Ukraine, taking into account transformations in gender consciousness in Ukrainian society over the previous decade. It was a strategic paper aimed at harmonizing national theory and practice of gender policy making with recent conceptualizations of gender ideology from the international sphere and reinforcing the gender dimension of Ukraine's integration into the EU framework. It outlined four major pillars for the development of gender democracy in Ukraine and set up a political goal for their implementation. The four pillars of this approach are (1) the promotion of gender parity in the quality and level of life; (2) the advancement of equal rights and opportunities of women and men in major domains of life, including human rights and law, labour and economic relations, political and civic life, decision making, private (family) life, health care, and education and science; (3) the enhancement of gender roles and the transformation of stereotypes; and (4) the eradication of violence and human trafficking.

The major breakthrough in the Draft Strategic Directions of State Policy for the Promotion of Gender Equality in Ukraine was the acknowledgment of the principle of gender mainstreaming as the appropriate conceptual framework for gender equality policy in Ukraine. The document also defined the promotion of gender equality as a complex, systemic, and targeted activity of the state, set out its basic principles and the criteria for evaluation of how well the state carried out this promotion, identified the major goals, and put forth its key priorities (Tolstokorova 2008a, 2009a). These evaluation criteria were framed as the '3Rs principle' – *rivnist'* (equality), *rozvytok* (development), and *reorghanizacia* (reorganization). *Equality* in this document was understood as 'ensurance for all people, irrespective of sex, race, and capabilities, of equal opportunities for positive effects of the equal opportunities policy.' *Development* stood for 'multiplication of possibilities for choice.' Hence, *gender in development* was conceptualized as the elimination of gender inequality in social, economic, and political domains to create a foundation of sustainable development for society. *Reorganization,* meanwhile, implied a complex institutional transformation of the national machinery for the promotion of gender equality based on a dual-track approach, reconciling the principles of gender equity and advancement of the status of women. These provisions were reflected in a research monograph on gender mainstreaming, produced by the State Institute for Family and Youth (SIFY 2003). Its Chapter 3 provided a rigorous analysis of the content and main pillars of gender mainstreaming as an efficient instrument for public policy, examined earlier in my larger work (Tolstokorova 2003).

Although the two documents have never reached any branch of the national machinery for the promotion of gender equality, those few experts who had an opportunity to familiarize themselves with them noted that passing them into law could help to overcome the precarious situation of the 'absence of gender policy' in Ukraine. They proposed that the definition of gender policy offered in the 'Draft Strategies' should be accepted as a starting point for the implementation of such a policy (Levchenko 2003, 78). Indeed, if the documents were to be adopted as a conceptual framework for the promotion of gender democracy in Ukraine, they could enable its transition to a new stage, hallmarked by the implementation of European standards in the development of gender policy. At the time they were drafted, however, they were obviously too forward-looking, because neither the state nor the society were ready to progress to a new stage of gender democracy.

Stage IV (2005 to Present): Policy of Equal Opportunities for Women and Men

PHASE 1 (2005 TO 2008): BEGINNING OF GENDER MAINSTREAMING POLICY
During Phase I of this most recent stage, some elements of gender mainstreaming began to be enshrined in several key documents in Ukraine as well as through a growing body of legislative and administrative measures, although these fell short of officially acknowledging gender mainstreaming as a policy principle.

As a side note, there is no direct equivalent to the concept of *gender mainstreaming* in the Ukrainian language, which is why the UNDP office in Kyiv introduced the translation of the term into Ukrainian in two ways: first as *kompleksny pidhid do problemy rivnosti zhinok i cholovikiv*, or complex approach to the issue of equality between women and men, and later on, as *henderne integhruvannya*, or gender integration. Thus, gender experts' preference for the term *gender integration* over *gender mainstreaming* in Ukrainian public policy (as discussed in chapter 16 in this volume) is based on a terminological ambiguity, rather than on the absence of mainstreaming practices.

In July 2005 the Presidential Decree on the Perfection of the Work of Central and Local Government Bodies in the Promotion of Equal Rights and Opportunities for Women and Men was issued. Developed by the Ministry of Justice, it aimed to mainstream gender into the activity of all branches of government from top to bottom and outlined the functions of top state officials with regard to the promotion of gender equality. In particular, decision makers at the national and local levels were obliged to assign one of their deputies to carry out gender equality policies, and their duties included the integration of a gender component into the activity of their respective branches of government.

Another hallmark of this period was the adoption by the Verkhovna Rada (parliament of Ukraine) in September 2005 of the Law on Ensuring Equal Rights and Opportunities for Women and Men (often simply referred to as the Gender Equality Law), which came into effect in January 2006 after seven years of lobbying by grassroots women's organizations. In compliance with GM principles, the key objective of the law was the advancement of equality between women and men in all domains of social life. Article 4 stipulates the necessity to conduct a gender analysis of existing national legislation, also in line with GM. Additionally, the law incorporated recommendations by experts from the Council of Europe regarding the realization of a GM strategy in the Ukrainian context.

Critics of this law have argued that it is incapable of tangibly counteracting gender discrimination in society because it is only of a framework character and has neither an efficient mechanism for its implementation nor sanctions for its breach. After the adoption of the law, various amendments were required to the Civil, Labour, and Criminal codes. This resulted in the adoption of a number of new laws throughout 2007–08 to bring the codes into compliance with the Gender Equality Law. In 2009, based on a decree of the minister of justice, a complex analysis of the 2002 Family Code of Ukraine was undertaken to ensure that it complied with the principle of equality between women and men. The analysis focused on the legal foundations of marriage and property rights of family members, including children, foster parents, and other family members.

A resolution of the Cabinet of Ministers of Ukraine, issued in April 2006, was also important for the successful implementation of GM principles in Ukrainian public policy. It required the gender analysis of national legislation mentioned earlier with the intention of bringing this legislation into compliance with the Gender Equality Law. Already, a range of national laws have been evaluated and revised. In 2007 alone, ten state laws underwent gender evaluation.[5]

Efficient realization of a GM strategy in Ukraine is impossible without its implementation at the local and regional levels of governance. There are departments of affairs of family and youth at the regional, municipal, and district levels, and these are responsible for the implementation of state policies for equal opportunities in their territories. In 2006, in the course of a pilot project aimed at the enhancement of gender equality policy in four cities in Ukraine, a set of methodological recommendations was developed. They were targeted at the realization of gender equality policy at the municipal level – a first attempt at mainstreaming gender in local governance (Tolstokorova 2007b, 16). The project provided a unique opportunity to implement such innovative gender-awareness practices as gender-sensitive regional budgets; gender awareness in the organization of local information campaigns and task-oriented programs; and gender literacy training for civil servants and representatives of the media and business at the municipal level. Out of this came regional *gender portraits* – napshots that identified the main challenges to policy implementation and priority directions for further progress in the geographical regions under study.

There are, therefore, grounds to claim that throughout the first phase of Stage IV Ukraine made some tangible progress in the promotion of gender parity in key areas of life. It began to incorporate European norms of gender equality into its legal apparatus and made its first attempts to implement GM in major sectors of national governance. However, one paradox in the implementation of gender mainstreaming in Ukraine, which has also emerged in the Baltic states (Novikova 2006, 158–9), is the prevalence of an 'expert bureaucratic model,' as opposed to a 'participatory-democratic model' (Beveridge et al. 2000, 386). The development of national strategies for the advancement of gender democracy has been the prerogative of a narrow, closed circle of experts and civil servants, the so-called *femocrats* and *non-governmental individuals* (NGIs) who keep a tight grip over the funding – state and especially international – allocated for the promotion of gender equality. Their activities proceed without transparency or accountability to civil society, the academic community, the women's movement, or the general public. The result is unequal, uncompetitive, and unfair distribution of scarce resources in favour of the 'fully funded different few.' This creates constraints to the advancement of the principles of democratic and gender-equitable governance in Ukraine. This opinion is confirmed by experts who question, for example, how truly the coordination councils, which function under the auspices of the Ministry for Family and Youth, represent the interests of grassroots women's organizations (Levchenko 2003, 234).

Arguably, the placing of the interests of individual elites over social responsibility stems from an overall ideological vacuum in transitional Ukraine where, nearly two decades after independence, a clear national identity has yet to emerge, let alone a clear gender identity. This helps to explain why none of the three proposed national doctrines for the promotion of gender equality has ever been seriously considered in Ukraine.[6] At the same time it evidences the immaturity and 'materialist value orientations' (Inglehart 1997) of emerging women elites in Ukraine, tendencies seen in other new democracies in Central and Eastern Europe as well (Siemieńska 1999).

PHASE 2 (2008 TO PRESENT): FIRST STEPS TOWARDS FATHERHOOD
POLICY AND FOCUS ON MEN'S ISSUES

In 2002, the World Bank pointed to an emerging crisis in men's health in Ukraine that made clear the critical need to pay closer attention to men's issues in the country. The reality of this crisis was confirmed in 2006 by the findings of a research project sponsored by the United Nations Population Fund. It explored Ukrainian men's reproductive and sexual health and found that in many areas, including reproductive health, life expectancy, addictions, and employment, men faced greater threats than women, which in turn, affected the well-being and health of women and children. This is consistent with the results of still another project, by the Canadian Urban Institute (CUI and CIDA 2006, 7), showing that in addition to grave health challenges Ukrainian men face more problems than women in overcoming crises and confronting discrimination with regard to paternal rights. However, this long list of challenges was only recently acknowledged publicly, during the current stage of equality policy formation, and only after they had attracted the attention of NGOs focusing on the promotion of fathers' rights and fatherhood policy.

In 2008, issues of fathers' rights and responsibilities finally appeared prominently on the agenda of seminars and conferences on issues of responsible parenthood organized across Ukraine. They also received special emphasis at the First All-Ukrainian Public Forum called 'The Importance of the Father in the Family and Society,' held in Kyiv in September 2008. Participants at the forum drafted an open letter to the president of Ukraine wherein they expressed concerns about the crisis facing the institution of fatherhood in Ukrainian society and emphasized the necessity to overcome conservative gender stereotypes regarding the role of men in the family. Furthermore, they supported an initiative to celebrate Father's Day as a national holiday. This initiative, however, was not confirmed by the president. In September 2009, another campaign, 'I am Proud – I am a Father!' was launched under the auspices of the Father's Day initiative, the goal of which was to make Father's Day a national holiday in order to draw attention to paternity, strengthen the role of men in the family, and promote responsible fatherhood. There has been some support for this initiative by the state. In response to the campaign, later in 2009 the Ministry for Family, Youth, and Sports developed a Presidential Decree on Father's Day and submitted it for consideration by the Cabinet of Ministers.

One factor enabling this renewed focus on fathers' rights and responsibilities is the changing nature of Ukraine's workforce, specifically through the increasing feminization of labour migration (Tolstokorova 2009b). This change is seen especially in rural areas of Western Ukraine (resultant from this gendered out-migration, a large number of families there lost their female members of working age, who found employment in the EU as caregivers or domestic workers (Tolstokorova and Gál 2008). Consequently, in the demographic structure of many small villages tangible gender imbalances emerged, because their remaining population consists mainly of males, children, and the elderly. This situation entailed grave social challenges. Above all, it is the children left behind at home. Most often they stay with their fathers, but in the case of single mothers or when both parents are working abroad, children stay in the care of their grandparents or are even left unattended (Tolstokorova 2008b). There is also evidence of social des-adaptation among husbands of migrant women and single men who cannot find wives as a result of women's out-migration. These men are often unemployed. Large numbers of them resort to alcohol, drug use, and unprotected sex, thereby negatively affecting their reproductive health. As a result of these behavioural patterns, these regions have experienced a dramatic increase of male mortality.

Questions related to men's responsibility for themselves and their children have thus gained currency. Evidence shows that the impact of female out-migration on the Ukrainian family is changing the nature of masculinity (Cherninska 2006). Many husbands of migrant women find their roles as caregivers and as housekeepers acceptable, although largely only during the period of their wife's absence (Yarova 2006).

However, as was shown elsewhere (Tolstokorova 2010), this reconstitution of gender role models in transnational families and the emergence of the category of 'new fathers' (Coltrane and Allan 1994) do not automatically result in the 'modernization of fatherhood' (LaRossa 1997) and have not tangibly altered 'the culture of fatherhood' in Ukraine. Society must still conceptualize these transformations in gender arrangements and offer viable solutions for their regulation.

More recently, in 2009, a movement for men's rights has taken shape in Ukraine through a series of events, including a seminar called 'The Situation of Ukrainian Men' held in the Rada. This represented one of the first attempts on the part of the government to address the role of men in the family and society in the context of the masculinity crisis, itself partly a result of the deterioration of fatherhood roles throughout decades of totalitarian rule. As a follow-up to this initiative, the youth movement MODOS appealed to the president to replace 23 February's Day of the Motherland Defender with International Men's Day. Despite the odd ideological underpinnings of this appeal, which would see the image of the Ukrainian man as defender substituted with an abstract idea of an *international man* with no specific social identity, this initiative was nonetheless a step forward, as it highlighted the masculinity crisis and drew closer attention to finding solutions to it. Yet another event cementing the framework of the emerging men's movement was a press conference held to launch the National Network of Men-Leaders against Violence, held as part of a campaign called 'Stop Violence!' in March of 2009. There, prominent male figures in Ukraine, including politicians, public leaders, athletes, and artists, reinforced the idea of the responsibility of men in building a peaceful and non-violent society.

These initiatives, however, were generated mainly by the civil society, while the role of the state in promoting men's issues remained obscure. An analysis of the implementation of the 2006 State Program to Implement Gender Equality in Ukraine (SIFYD 2007), for example, showed that key stakeholders in the realization of public policy on gender equality, especially on the regional level, still tend to limit the concept of gender equality to women's issues, neglecting the challenges faced by men. Furthermore, those issues that were addressed with regard to women were themselves limited mainly to the private sphere and were based on traditional roles and images of women as mothers, beauties, and keepers of the family hearth, while areas of professional, political, and cultural realization by Ukrainian women went unattended to. Nonetheless, the timid steps towards promoting men's issues and rights in Ukraine may yet serve as an important precursor to a more inclusive gender movement. Such a movement would implicitly acknowledge gender as a 'two-sided coin, being as much an issue for men as for women' (World Economic Forum 2005).

Correspondence of the Ukrainian Experience with European Models

Analysis shows that the Ukrainian state applies a somewhat eclectic approach to the enhancement of gender democracy. More specifically, the variety of government practices of promoting gender policy in Ukraine and their correspondence to the EU models of gender governance may be summarized as described below.

(1) *Integrated Gender Mainstreaming*. Some elements of GM have been introduced in Ukraine, mainly during the most recent stage of gender democracy development, triggered by the adoption of the Gender Equality Law in 2005. Practically, GM has been applied via the measures of the Ministry of Justice aimed at a gender-sensitive analysis of Ukrainian legislation. Further, if we interpret GM broadly as 'gender-based analysis' (Hankivsky 2005, 997), there are grounds to claim that some elements of this model were implemented during the third stage of Ukraine's gender democracy evolution (2001–04), that is, during the realization of the Gender Expertise in Ukrainian Legislation project. That project published and disseminated background research papers

and methodological recommendations for the implementation in Ukrainian legislation of gender-sensitive expertise that took into account the specific national context. If, however, we abide by the 'Swedish model' of GM, then we must say that attempts to apply GM principles in Ukraine do not go very far beyond legislation, and that socioeconomic, political, and private/family domains, and civil society are neglected altogether with regard to gender. From this point of view, the efficacy of such a policy approach for Ukraine has been rather low, as confirmed by a decrease in the country's gender development index, as measured by the United Nations, which dropped from 67th place in 2001 to 76th place in 2008 (United Nations 2008).

(2) *The Transversal Model.* The Ukrainian government has utilized the transversal model quite extensively, since the principle of 'positive discrimination,' on which it is based, is enshrined in Ukrainian legislation and practised in policy design and realization. In particular, quotas are in place to guarantee places for women in the workplace, and a system of incentives for mothers has been introduced, as well as special measures aimed to support women's entrepreneurship (Tolstokorova 2007b, 24–6).

(3) *The EU-Driven Model.* The implementation of the EU-driven model will only become possible if Ukraine obtains the status of an EU candidate country, enabling access to EU Structural Funds to financially support the realization of gender equality policy. At present this is continuously suspended because of the absence of political will and a lack of coordinated efforts aimed at the enhancement of Ukraine's integration into the European Union on both sides of the newly emerged 'wall around the West' (Andreas 2000) created by the European bureaucracies.

(4) *The Generic Equality Model.* Currently the objective of restoring the balance away from inequalities resulting from age, disability, race, and ethnicity is not really on the Ukrainian state's agenda, especially given the present conditions of a durable political crisis, itself exacerbated by the ongoing global financial downturn. Some steps are being made in this direction, however. As an example, in 2006, I managed a project that set out to explore the gendered dimensions of the rights of people with disabilities in Ukraine. The project, sponsored by the Ministry for Family, Youth, and Sport, was one of the first attempts on the part of the state to seek equality beyond gender in the Ukrainian context.

Given the comparison above, we can say that the promotion of gender democracy currently implemented in Ukraine is a *quilt pattern* or *mosaic model* of equality policy that primarily makes use of elements from two of the aforementioned models of gender management: integrated gender mainstreaming and the transversal model. The state's gender policy has begun to integrate elements of the generic equality model, while the EU-driven model remains a remote possibility. Should the former two models be reinforced and implemented more thoroughly in the future, they could provide a good framework for state gender policy grounded on a 'dual-track approach,' that is, a combination of gender mainstreaming principles with specific actions in favour of either disadvantaged sex. This dual strategy, enshrined in the European Pact for Gender Equality, is actually recommended by the European Commission for the promotion of gender equality in current conditions.

Ukraine's eclectic model, however, has not emerged as a result of a purposeful, coordinated, and conscious effort by decision makers, aimed at mobilization of all available resources to ensure gender justice in society. Rather, it has resulted from the lack of a coherent conceptual framework or strategy for the development of gender democracy. Research on gender mainstreaming in Ukraine (Extröm 2002, 4, 8) suggests that this is because within Ukrainian society gender equality 'is seen as a solved issue,' while the 'attitude to feminism is complicated' and 'resistance is large and awareness is low' with regard to gender mainstreaming.[7]

Ukraine still lacks a clear national strategy for the advancement of gender equality, and much will need to be done to change that. Partly, acknowledgment is required by Ukrainian thinkers that despite tangible progress in this area in recent decades, neither the state nor civil society has reached European levels of gender awareness. Nor have they met international standards of gender justice. Some gender experts argue that GM strategies are simply alien to both state and society, compared with a more traditional family-centred, or women-protective strategy. After all, up to now, state gender policy has remained limited to outreach conducted by the Ministry for Family, Youth, and Sport. Meanwhile, strategies for the promotion of parity democracy in Ukraine remain to be developed.

NOTES

1 The full name of the project is 'EQUAPOL: A 5th Framework Programme Research Project funded by the European Commission – Gender-sensitive and women friendly public policies (a comparative analysis of their progress and impact).'

2 A psychologist, Finn Tschudi, found that statements such as 'Men can care for children just as well as women' were judged by interviewees as linguistically unremarkable, whereas statements like 'Women can care for children just as well as men' were assessed as bizarre.

3 These were the Embassy of Canada in Ukraine, the Canadian International Development Agency (CIDA), and the Canadian – Ukrainian Gender Fund.

4 I put forward the idea for this project and acted as its coordinator, organizer, and moderator of focus-group discussions and in-depth interviews. Furthermore, I developed strategic policy papers to be submitted for approval by the parliament of Ukraine and administered the final international research conference on the project's output (Tolstokorova 2002).

5 State laws submitted to gender analysis in 2007 included: Law on Annual Vacations, Law on State Support to Families with Children, Law on Employment of the Population, Law on Immigration, Law on Elections of People's Deputies, Law on the Status of a People's Deputy, Law on Civil Service in Local Bodies of Power, Law on Social and Legal Protection of Military Servants and Their Families, Law on Military Duty and Military Service, and Law on the Status of Highland Settlements in Ukraine.

6 These were Draft Conception of Public Policy for the Promotion of the Situation of Women (1999), Draft of National Strategies for the Promotion of the Situation of Women (1999), and Draft of Strategic Directions of State Policy for the Promotion of Gender Equality Promotion in Ukraine (2003).

7 Hankivsky and Salnykova draw similar conclusions in Chapter 16, in this volume.

REFERENCES

Andreas, P. 2000. Introduction: The Wall after the Wall. In P. Andreas and T. Snyder, eds., *The Wall around the West: State Borders and Immigration Controls in North America and Europe,* 1–14. Oxford: Rowman and Littlefield.

Baker, P. 1984. The Domestication of Politics: Women and American Political Society, 1780–1920. *American Historical Review* 89(3): 620–47.

Beveridge, F., S. Nott, and K. Stephen. 2000. Mainstreaming and the Engendering of Policy Making. *Journal of European Public Policy* 7(3): 385–405.

Braithwaite, M. 2005. *Gender Sensitive and Women Friendly Public Policies: A Comparative Analysis of Their Progress and Impact.* Final Report Project HPSE CT-2002 00136. Luxembourg: Directorate General for Research, Citizen and Governance in a Knowledge-Based Society, European Publications Office. Available at http://cordis.europa.eu/documents/docu mentlibrary/2747EN.pdf (accessed 1 Aug. 2009).

Cherninska, T. 2006. *Zhinocha migracia: zmina gendernyh rolej;* [Female Migra-
tion: Change of Gender Roles]. Foundation for Safe Society (in Ukrainian).
Available at http://fsb.net.ua/articles.php?lng=uaandpg=11 (accessed 8
Oct. 2006).

Chernyaeva, N. 2007. Proizvodstvo materej v Sovetskoj Rossii: Uchebniki
po uhodu za det'mi epohi industializacii [Production of Mothers in Soviet
Russia: Child Care Manuals of the Epoch of Industrialization]. *Gendernye
issledovania* [Gender Studies] 12: 120–38.

Coltrane, S., and K. Allan. 1994. 'New' Fathers and Old Stereotypes: Representations of Masculinity in 1980s Television Advertising. *Masculinities*
2(4): 43–66.

Canadian Urban Institute (CUI) and the Canadian International Development
Agency (CIDA). 2006. *Zvit schodo ocinyuvannya gendernyh ta molodizhnyh
problem* [Report on the Evaluation of Gender and Youth Challenges] Kyiv.

European Commission. 1996. *Incorporating Equal Opportunities for Women and
Men into All Community Policies and Activities.* COM(96)67final. Brussels:
European Commission.

– 2007. *Putting Equality into Practice: What Role for Positive Action?* Brussels:
European Commission.

Extröm, M. 2002. *Networks and Driving Forces: Ways to Implement Gender
Mainstreaming through Development Cooperation within Public Administra-
tion in Ukraine.* Master's Thesis, School of Public Administration, Göteborg
University.

Fábián, K. 2006. Bridges across the Public-Private Divide: The Welfare-Related
Activism of Hungarian Women after 1989. In E. Saurer, M. Lanzinger, and
E. Frysak, eds., *Women's Movements: Networks and Debates in Post-communist
Countries in the 19th and 20th Centuries,* 47–64. Cologne: Böhlau-Verlag.

Hankivsky, O. 2005. Gender vs Diversity Mainstreaming: A Preliminary
Examination of the Role and Transformative Potential of Feminist Theory.
Canadian Journal of Political Science 38(4): 977–1001.

Harsch, D. 2006. *Revenge of the Domestic: Women, the Family, and Communism in
the German Democratic Republic.* Princeton: Princeton University Press.

Holland, D. 1970. Familization, Socialization, and the Universe of Meaning:
An Extension of the Interactional Approach to the Study of the Family. *Journal of Marriage and the Family* 32(3): 415–27.

Ingelhart, R. 1997. *Modernization and Postmodernization: Cultural, Economic and
Political Change in 43 Societies.* Princeton: Princeton University Press.

Kleberg, M. 2007. *Views on Women: Home and Family Programming in Swedish
Television 1956–1969.* Stockholm University. Available at http://www.jmk.

su.se/contents/sidor/publikationer/avhandlingar/kleberg/summary.php (accessed 3 Sept. 2007).

Kupryashkina, S. 2000. Public versus Feminist: Enabling and Limiting Sides of Democracy for Women in Ukraine. *Online Alumni Journal.* June. Available at http://ames.gilan.uar.net/irex/iatp/journal/a2.html (accessed 23 June 2000).

LaRossa, R. 1997. *The Modernization of Fatherhood: A Social and Political History.* Chicago: University of Chicago Press.

Levchenko, K. 2003. *Genderna polityka v Ukraini: Vyznachennya, formuvannya, upravlinnya* [Gender Policy in Ukraine: Definition, Formation, and Governance]. Kharkiv: National University for Domestic Affairs.

MacKinnon, C. 1991. Difference and Dominance: On Sex Discrimination. In K.T. Bartlett and R. Kennedy, eds., *Feminist Legal Theory,* 81–94. Boulder: Westview.

Ministry for Family and Youth of Ukraine (MFYU). 1998. *Issues Concerning the Development of Democracy and the Maintenance of Equal Rights for Women and Men in Ukraine during the Transition Period.* Kyiv: MFYU.

Novikova, I. 2006. History, National Belonging, and the Women's Movement in the Baltic Countries. In E. Saurer, M. Lanzinger, and E. Frysak, eds., *Women's Movements: Networks and Debates in Post-communist Countries in the 19th and 20th Centuries,* 141–62. Cologne: Böhlau-Verlag.

Rugemer, C. 2007. A Measured Approach to Gender. *Research EU: The Magazine of the European Research Area* 52(June): 36–8.

Saxonberg, S., and T. Sirovátka. 2006. Failing Family Policy in Post-communist Central Europe. *Journal of Comparative Policy Analysis* 8(2): 185–202.

Siemieńska, R. 1999. Elites and Women in Democratizing Post-communist Societies. *International Review of Sociology* 9(2): 197–219.

State Institute for Family and Youth (SIFY). 2003. *Integhruvannya gendernogho pidhodu v derzhavnu polityku Ukrajiny* [Gender Mainstreaming in Ukrainian Public Policy], 32–43. Kyiv: SIFY.

State Institute for Family and Youth Development (SIFYD). 2007. *Zvit pro vykonannya u pershij polovyni 2007 roku derzhavnoi programy z utverdzhennya gendernoi rivnosti v ukrajins'komu suspil'stvi na period do 2010 roku* [Report on the Implementation of the State Program for the Promotion of Gender Equality in Ukraine during the 1st Half of 2007]. Kyiv: SIFYD.

Tolstokorova, A. 2003. *Kompleksne vprovadzhennya gendernyh pryncypiv u derzhavnu politylu jak shlyah do evropejs'kogho spivtovarystva. Indyvidual'ne naukove doslidzhennya* [Gender Mainstreaming in Public Policy as a Way to European Community. Working Paper]. Kyiv: SIFY.

– 2005. More Human Rights for Women: A Linguistic Perspective. *Kadin/ Woman 2000* (A publication of the Eastern Mediterranean University, Gazi Magosa, North Cyprus), 6(1–2): 1–28.

– 2006. The Linguistic Dimension of Gender Equality: A Human Rights Perspective. *Polissema: Revista de Letras do ISCAP* (A publication of the Instituto Superior de Contabilidade e Administraja), 6: 193–216.

– 2007a. Gender Equality in Ukraine: Between Declarations and Reality. In C. Sarmento, ed., *Eastwards/Westwards: Which Direction for Gender Studies in the 21st Century?* 40–76. Newcastle upon Tyne: Cambridge Scholars.

– 2007b. Nacional'ny mekhanizm obespecheniya ravnyh prav i vozmozhnostej zhenschin i muzhchin [National Machinery for the Promotion of Equal Rights and Opportunities for Women and Men]. In L. Leontyeva and A. Tolstokorova, eds., *Draft Report on the Realization in Ukraine of the United Nations Convention on the Elimination of All Forms of Discrimination against Women* (6th and 7th Joint Regular Report), 9–18. Kharkiv: Folio.

– 2008a. Modeli derzhavnoi gendernoi politky v Ukraini z tochky zoru Evropejskyh tradycyj gendernoi demokratii' [Models of State Gender Policy in Ukraine in Terms of European Traditions of Gender Democracy]. In D. Yagunov, ed., *Aktual'ni problemy evropejskoi integracii* [Current Problems of European Integration], 138–59. Odessa: Phenix.

– 2008b. Locally Neglected, Globally Engaged: Ukrainian Women on the Move. In R. Anderl, B. Arich-Gerz, and R. Schmiede, eds., *Technologies of Globalization,* 44–61. Publication compiled from the proceedings of the 'Technologies of Globalization' International Conference, Technical University, Darmstadt, 30–1 Oct. 2008.

– 2009a. Osnovnvye etapy formirovania koncepcii gendernoy politiki i modeli paritetnoy demokratii v Ukraine [Main Stages in the Development of Gender Policy and Models of Parity Democracy in Ukraine]. *Newsletter of the Pacific State University* (Vladivostok, Russia) 2(50): 99–113.

– 2009b. Who Cares for Carers? Feminization of Labor Migration from Ukraine and Its Impact on Social Welfare. *International Issues and Slovak Foreign Policy Affairs* 18(1): 62–84.'

– 2009c. *Multiple Marginalities: Gender Dimension of Rural Poverty, Unemployment and Labour Migration in Ukraine.* Paper presented at the FAO-IFAD-ILO Workshop 'Gaps, Trends and Current Research in Gender Dimensions of Agricultural and Rural Employment: Differentiated Pathways out of Poverty,' Rome, 31 March – 2 April, 2009. Available at http://www.fao-ilo.org/fileadmin/user_upload/fao_ilo/pdf/Papers/17_March/Tolstokorova-final.pdf.

– 2010.Where Have All the Mothers Gone? The Gendered Effect of Labour Migration and Transnationalism on the Institution of Parenthood in Ukraine. *Anthropology of East Europe Review (AEER)*, Special Issue, 'Gender in Postsocialist Eastern Europe and the Former Soviet Union,' 28(1): 184–214.

Tolstokorova, A., ed. 2002. *Formuvannya gendernogo parytetu v konteksti suchasnyh social'no-ekonomichnyh peretvoren.' Materialy mizhnarodnoi naukovopraktychoi konferencii* [The Promotion of Gender Parity in the Context of Current Socioeconomic Transformations]. Edited publication compiled from the proceedings of the International Research and Practice Conference, Kyiv, 5–7 Dec. 2002.

Tolstokorova, A., and Z. Gál. 2008. Problemy mighracijoi polityky central'noji ta skhidnoji Evropy v konteksti starinnya evropejs'kogo naselennya [Challenges to CEE Migration Policies in the Context of Aging Europe]. *Aghora: Perspectyvy social'mogho rozvytku reghioniv [AGORA: Prospects for the Social Development of Regions]* 7: 85–93. Kyiv: Stylos/Kennan Institute.

Tschudi, F. 1979. *Gender Stereotypes Reflected in Asymmetric Similarities in Language*. Paper presented at the Annual meeting of the American Association of Psychology, 1–5 Sept. 1979.

Ukrainian Centre for Independent Political Research (UCIPR). 2006. *Rozvytok demokratii v Ukrajini: 2001–2002 roky* [Development of Democracy in Ukraine, 2001–2002]. Kyiv: UCIPR.

United Nations. 2008. *The 2007–2008 Human Development Report*. Geneva: United Nations.

United Nations Development Program (UNDP). 2003. *Drafting Gender-Aware Legislation: How to Promote and Protect Gender Equality in Central and Eastern Europe and in the Commonwealth of Independent States (CIS)*. Bratislava: UNDP.

– 2006. *Integhracia genderu v nacional'ni derzhavni proghramy* [Integration of Gender into National State Programs]. Kyiv: UNDP.

World Bank. 2002. *Ukraine: Gender Overview*. Edited by N. Dudwick, R. Srinivasan, and J. Braithwaite. Washington, DC: ECSSD.

World Economic Forum (WEF). 2005. *Women's Empowerment: Measuring the Global Gender Gap*. Geneva: WEF.

Yarova, O. 2006. The Migration of Ukrainian Women to Italy and the Impact on Their Family in Ukraine. In A. Szczepanikova, M. Canek, and J. Grill, eds., *The Migration Process in Central and Eastern Europe: Unpacking the Diversity*, 38–41. Prague: Multicultural Centre.

2 Discourse of Continuity and Change: The Legislative Path to Equality

MARIAN J. RUBCHAK

> Try not to hurt anyone, or step on any toes. Use caution in public; forget the word 'I.'
>
> – Deputy Olena Kondrakova[1]

Ukraine's transition from socialism to a market-driven society began in 1991. On 24 August of that year the country was on the cusp of an epiphany – its successful declaration of independence. Sitting in our dining room was Pavlo Movchan, a poet with a history of dissidence in the Soviet Union, and one of a series of our house guests from Ukraine. As we listened in disbelief to this stunning news item on public radio, he suddenly leapt to his feet and exclaimed excitedly: 'I am an author of that declaration!'

The actual transitional process had been set in motion a year earlier, with public demonstrations for liberation from the tyranny of the Soviet regime already gaining momentum. During the first days of September, 1990, my husband and I, with our four daughters, were in Kyiv, where we witnessed the fulfilment of what had always seemed to us to be an impossible dream. On 3 September a massive political demonstration moved along Khreshchatyk, Kyiv's main thoroughfare. As we watched this amazing spectacle in what was still Soviet Ukraine, we witnessed wave after wave of right hands being raised, diffidently at first, then more boldly – until they became a sea of three middle fingers held aloft, signifying Ukraine's national symbol – the trident. Soapbox orators dotted Kyiv's central plaza, soon to be known as Maidan Nezalezhnosti (Independence Square), and clusters of people could be heard agitating for secession at various locations throughout the city centre. This astonishing demonstration set the tone for more changes to come. By 1991, with the Soviet Union imploding, secession was no longer an issue. The USSR had fractured into fifteen pieces, and with republic after republic declaring its independence, Ukraine fell away as a sovereign state.

This chapter is concerned with the ways in which the language of gender and women's rights discourses have been incorporated into the passage and ratification of new statutes designed to promote gender parity in Ukraine in the aftermath of 1991. I will focus on one aspect of that objective – the interplay between women as victims of discrimination and violent actions, and the significant rise in policies, legislation, and initiatives employed to introduce women's rights. Despite such well-intentioned efforts, however, the move forward has been slow, hampered by an inept criminal justice system, corrupt law enforcement agencies, negative stereotyping, and the government's unwillingness to implement gender-parity legislation. As is the case in other parts of the world, 'gender inequality has proven to be much more intractable than anticipated . . . and [the] quality of life [has] worsened' (Cornwall et al. 2007, 1). Ukraine 'is laden here, as are societies elsewhere, with its own historical baggage' which is inhibiting meaningful change (Kandiyoti 2007, 191).

Although comparisons with judicial systems and law enforcement agencies in other transitional countries would be instructive, the aim of this chapter is confined to examining the failure of a system to secure women's rights in one country – Ukraine – its progressive legislation notwithstanding. I scrutinize this process from a perspective of participant observation. My findings are supplemented by media accounts, official government reports, primary evidence posted on the Internet, and scholarly readings related to empowering the powerless in the post-Soviet Ukrainian reality. Through the use of this methodology, this chapter brings to life the mix of traditional beliefs and traditions with Western views of equal rights.

International Statutes in Ukraine

The Convention on the Elimination of All Forms of Discrimination against Women (CEDAW), adopted in 1979 by the U.N. General Assembly, is often described as an international bill of rights for women. It is also judged to be 'the most important piece of international legislation encoding women's rights, which commits 171 signing governments to respect a range of principles that have . . . led to positive reforms in constitution and civil codes' (Molyneux 2007, 235). Soviet Ukraine became a signatory in 1980, and ratified the convention the following year. On the eve of independence a decade later, complying with its obligation as a party to the Convention, Ukraine's government issued a periodic progress report on the advancement of gender equity. Instead of recording improvement in the status of women, however, the report referred to the state of Ukrainian society as one of 'outmoded stereotypes that reflect the role and purpose of women . . . still prevalent in society . . . [where] women are not prepared to fight in the political arena, and are incapable of standing up for their rights' (United Nations 1991, sub-section on Ukraine).

Early in the 1990s, a handful of forward-looking feminists, together with supporters of women's rights who shunned the feminist label, began laying the foundation for equal rights initiatives. A series of projects dedicated to raising public awareness of gender inequities were launched. One of the first was the establishment of a women's rights centre, Zhinochi Perspektyvy (Women's Perspectives), in Lviv in 1993. In 1995, Olena Suslova founded one of Ukraine's earliest non-governmental organizations (NGOs), Zhinochyi informatsiino konsultatyvnyi tsenter (the Women's Information Consultative Centre). It gathers information on gender and feminism, and generates public discourse based upon the accumulated data; the centre has sponsored numerous countrywide seminars for that purpose (AWID 2005). A second initiative, the Gender Integration Program, a project of Open World Practices of the Open Society Institute, funded by George Soros, was launched in March 1995 with the aim of creating an environment reflective of European standards of gender equality. These initiatives, combined with increasing numbers of special consciousness-raising projects, set the stage for a series of unprecedented parliamentary hearings on women's issues. The first of these has been described as an historic landmark in the country's quest for women's rights, and so it is, but it might also, and more precisely, be viewed as 'political theatre' staged by male legislators to publicize governmental compliance with the terms of the U.N. Convention.

Two events – a meeting of the Organization for Security and Co-operation in Europe (OSCE), held in Ottawa, Canada between 4 and 8 July 1995, and a conference in Kyiv titled 'Woman and Democracy,' held on 2 July 1995 – deliberated gender issues. The Ukrainian delegate to the OSCE meeting, Deputy Oleksandr Moroz (chair of the initial parliamentary hearing), concluded from the Ottawa proceedings that women's rights had been secured throughout much of the world. This prompted his prediction that such success would soon inspire Ukraine to follow suit. Moroz described this experience as a defining moment in his determination to work for an end to gender discrimination. The purpose of the second meeting was to craft a platform for Ukraine's delegation to the upcoming Fourth World Conference on Women's Issues, held in Beijing at the beginning of September 1995. Delegates were instructed to scrutinize the proceedings for ideas on women's rights.

Making Parliamentary History

On 12 July 1995, the politically oriented Zhinocha Hromada (Women's Society), Ukraine's Cabinet of Ministers, and Ukrainian representatives to the United Nations, sponsored the initial parliamentary hearings on women's issues (Parliament of Ukraine 1995).[2] Participants included members of Ukraine's ministries, the United Nations, the European Commission, the European Parliament, the Russian Duma, and Kyiv's foreign diplomatic community. Most of the speakers were Ukrainian activists, members of various NGOs, and government officials.

In his opening remarks, Chair Moroz mentioned the OSCE meeting, and reaffirmed his commitment to gender equality. His female colleagues in the Verkhovna Rada (parliament of Ukraine), he continued glibly, 'are only 16 in number, but they are working zealously for the cause.'[3] The sincerity of his alleged conviction, however, would have inspired greater confidence were it not for the fact that earlier Moroz had spearheaded opposition to the hearings among male parliamentarians. His characterization of gender equality as 'equal rights for women as women' also did nothing to dispel my scepticism of his change of heart, yet his references to 'women as women' clearly resonated with the female constituency, as the language of the women's demands during the hearings revealed.

The first speaker, Vice-Chair of the Parliamentary Commission on Human Rights Nina Karpachova, described the hearings as a positive preliminary step, signifying the government's readiness to champion affirmative action on ending discrimination. 'A new generation of women,' she announced, 'is prepared to lead this fight.' Judging from the agitated buzz among the men that erupted immediately throughout the assembly hall, the prospect of such female leadership unsettled the male legislators. Its mounting crescendo compelled the chair to admonish the men for disrupting proceedings. Appeals for a suitable environment where 'women can be women' reverberated countless times during the session, as did demands for protective measures to eliminate 'poverty with a woman's face,' and the unchecked discrimination against women. The Janus-like nature of the proceedings, illuminating special concessions for women on the one hand, and equal rights on the other, highlighted the paradoxical nature of the women's crusade for justice.

When foreign speakers – Norwegian Ambassador to Ukraine Øyvind Nördsledtten and Suani Hunt, U.S. Ambassador to Ukraine – alluded to discrepancies in the status of women between Ukraine and their own countries, Moroz countered testily: 'You have your countries and we have ours. Ukraine will follow its own path towards eliminating discrimination.' I should point out that many people in Ukraine still believe that Ukraine needs to develop its own feminist paradigm, rooted in national (native Ukrainian) traditions. As I sat pondering this exchange, I became acutely aware of another troublesome tendency – the incessant linkage of women to motherhood, persistent calls for creating conditions amenable to the integration of women's maternal obligations and professional lives, and presenting women's rights as concessions to their special needs as women, rather than human rights.

Startled out of my musings by an unexpected hush in the chamber, amid highly charged murmurs of intense expectancy, I watched Deputy Serhii Kiyashko reach under his seat to retrieve a floral bouquet. Striding purposefully to the front of the assembly hall, he placed the offering, described as a token of respect and admiration for his female colleagues, at the base of the podium. Kiyashko's 'homage to women' brought to mind the annual Veteran's Day ritual of laying a wreath at the tomb of the 'unknown soldier,' the fallen hero who had made the supreme sacrifice for his country. The deputy's gesture relegated women to this symbolic realm, where sacrifice is rewarded with a ceremonial gesture of appreciation. Although Chair Moroz expressed his displeasure with Kiyashko's action, he tempered it with: 'Even though women appreciate such chivalry, you have breached parliamentary discipline.' The finale of this 'theatre of the absurd' was played out by a beaming female deputy, who interrupted the session in her turn by performing a familiar domestic task – searching for a vase.

At day's end, I discussed this episode with several women; each hastened to assure me that she found such chivalrous acts appealing. In no way did the women deem themselves diminished as women by such pleasant 'tokens of esteem.' Indeed, they insisted that disavowing the custom would merely testify to their lack of femininity, a quality that defined them as women. When I pressed for their view of femininity, the best they could offer was: 'Why, to be a woman, of course.' 'And what does it mean to be a woman?' I persisted. 'Why, to possess feminine qualities, naturally,' was the response. This circular regression underscored my earlier conviction that many Ukrainian women seem unaware of themselves as social units whose identity is constructed by the opposite sex, within the male matrices of power, and manipulated by men for their own purposes. The vagaries of history have produced a culture and a philosophy of life which lead Ukrainian women to view such 'chivalry' in a positive light.

The demands of most of the day's female speakers still reflected essentialist convictions; only occasionally was this unmarked paradigm disregarded. For example, the head of Soiuz Robochykh Zhinok Ukrainy (the Working Women's Alliance of Ukraine), Nina Pokotylo, used her allotted time to censure male powerbrokers for violating the U.N. convention. Accusing them of corruption and mismanagement, she charged: 'You men who sneer at any woman aspiring to political office, what have *you* accomplished? Our society is in crisis. We need to bring women into the political process.' Thus, she highlighted a dilemma which would occupy legislators and women's rights advocates in Ukraine for the next decade and beyond, without appreciably narrowing the gap between declaration and deed.

Legislating Women's Rights

In 1997, the United Nations Development Project – a global development network – began its implementation of projects designed to promote equal rights and opportunities. Its staff provided policy support for gender-sensitive legislation, and enhanced official capacity for integrating gender issues into strategic planning. In 1999, the U.N. Representative Office, which operated in Kyiv on the authority of the U.N. secretary general, received its own formal status in Ukraine and began to implement a series of U.N.-sponsored programs. Larysa Kobelianska, a tireless advocate of women's rights and firm supporter of educational programs designed to increase public awareness of gender injustice, heads the UNDP Equal Opportunities Program. Her office is responsible for pioneering a wide array of creative projects on feminist activism. The most recent endeavour is an ambitious two-year Gender Education and Training Project (2009–2011), with a total of six hundred training sessions scheduled. The program targets teachers, government employees, and police officers (under the jurisdiction of the Ministry of Internal Affairs).

In 2000, Ukraine subscribed to the U.N.-sponsored '16 Days of Activism against Gender Violence,' running from 25 November to 10 December each year to advance the eradication of violence against women. That same year, Ukraine signed the U.N. Millennium Declaration, and unveiled a year-long nationwide public information campaign on gender awareness, 'Ukraine 2015: Millennium Development Goals.' The eight Millennium Development Goals, to be achieved by 2015, are drawn from the U.N. Millennium Declaration, General Assembly Resolution 55/2, signed by 147 heads of state and government during the Millennium Summit in 8 September 2000; goal number 3 is promoting gender equality and empowering women.

On 15 November 2001, the Rada followed this with the Law of Ukraine on the Prevention of Violence in the Family. It was preceded by a number of normative acts, including a presidential decree on 25 April 2001, aimed at upgrading the social status of women. A second law, creating a platform for reviewing acts or threats of domestic violence, came into effect in 2002. On 26 April 2003, the Cabinet of Ministers issued Decree 616, containing a plan for strengthening certain provisions in the foregoing laws. A year later, in collaboration with the Ministry of Family, Children, and Youth, the Ministry of Internal Affairs issued a decree establishing cooperation in efforts to expand gender equality throughout the various governmental institutions (Fedkovych 2005).

During the early years immediately following the dissolution of the Soviet state, domestic violence was either ignored or victims were charged with provoking it (Johnson 2007).[4] In 2001, Ukrainian legislation enshrined this injustice in Article 11 of the Law of Ukraine on the Prevention of Violence in the Family. It embodied the concept of a victim's 'provocative' behaviour as the source of domestic violence. In the interest of providing victims of such abuse with some protection, on 22 April 2002, the Ministry of Internal Affairs established a procedure known as 'Preventive Warning' for putting assailants on preventive record (already embedded in Article 10 of the law on 'Prevention of Violence'). Soon, however, even this expedient was being used to deny women's complaints ('He has been warned') or to deflect responsibility. Once the warning was lodged in a legal document, officials considered it adequate protection for women. In one way or another, and 'despite . . . enactments of new statutes police have failed to change their conduct' (Buzawa and Buzawa 2003, 71).

This reinforced externalization of such violence committed by male assailants, who responded to the charges with: 'She provoked me' (Buzawa and Buzawa 2003, 35). Historically, victims of domestic violence have failed to report the crime to police because of the latter's failure to respond appropriately (Buzawa and Buzawa 2003, 35). Although the phenomenon is recognized worldwide, in Ukraine it takes on a more sinister aspect. The absence of a viable law enforcement mechanism encourages police to turn a blind eye to evidence of violence, which is bad enough. What is even worse is that the police themselves often behave like the criminals. Law enforcement personnel are known to demand sexual favours from victims in return for registering their complaints, even to sexually assault women in police or other forms of state custody. For its part, the social stigma attached to sexual violence, stemming from an internal culture with a bias against 'airing one's dirty laundry in public,' simply dissuades reporting. Such deterrents, coupled with societal norms prone to condoning the assailants' actions and impugning the victim instead, create conditions that overwhelmingly favour the perpetrator (Network Women's Program 2009; Amnesty International 2007).

Hearing for a Second Time

To address such abuses, on June 2004, the Rada held a second set of hearings, titled 'The Status of Women in Ukraine: Reality and Perspectives.' On this occasion, Adam Martyniuk, first deputy head of the Verkhovna Rada, acted as chair. He opened the session – which was attended by media personnel, members of civic organizations, government officials, and foreign dignitaries of both sexes – with the bizarre 'Greetings to our bewitching guests. Consider yourselves at liberty to say whatever comes to mind; you may even sing if you wish.' Throughout the day he indulged himself in anti-women comments. Oddly enough, no one reacted to his barbs until, in a dramatic accusation, one of the final speakers, Tamara Melnyk, reproached him decisively. She was rewarded with a rousing ovation, and vociferous demands from the participants for an extension of her allotted time to allow a conclusion of her presentation. Smarting from Melnyk's criticism, the chair refused to extend it, yet when the next speaker, Communist Party Deputy Petro Symonenko, exceeded his allotted five minutes, the microphone was left open for him to continue speaking (Martyniuk and Symonenko are close Communist comrades). Only the women's chants of *'han'ba'* (shame) and rhythmic clapping compelled his retreat. As I strolled with a group of participants along the streets of Kyiv at the end of the day, I witnessed as people, apparently moved by the drama in the assembly hall which they had watched on television, approached Tamara Melnyk to congratulate her on her presentation.

Except for the fact that references to violence against women, the evils of sex trafficking, and policies detrimental to men were somewhat more in evidence during this round of hearings, the general rhetoric differed little from that of 1995. Once again, speaker after speaker linked women's mission in life to motherhood, called for an environment in which 'women could be women,' and for conditions conducive to the integration of their domestic and professional duties. Women's rights were still viewed as concessions to their unique needs. Male deputies continued to address women with the customary 'beautiful, charming, and weaker half.'[5] Deputy Leonid Chernovets'ky (mayor of Kyiv at the time of this writing), brought this patronizing tendency into relief by suggesting that women elect qualified men to advocate on their behalf. The women countered with demands for increased female political representation. On 8 September 2005, legislation to this effect was passed. Ukraine's landmark Law on Ensuring Equal Rights and Opportunities for Women and Men (after this, often referred to simply as the Gender Equality Law) was ratified. For the first time in Ukrainian history, a law defined discrimination based on sex, and provided judicial protection from such discriminatory tactics (Fedkovych 2005).[6]

Third Time Around

A third hearing, titled 'Equal Rights and Opportunities in Ukraine, Realities and Perspectives,' was convened on 21 November 2006. The hearing, attended by roughly equal numbers of male and female participants, was divided into two discrete parts – the first on violence and the second on equal rights and possibilities. During the lunch break, many of the men vanished. Ostensibly oblivious to the presence of males, Martyniuk (presiding as chair again) opened the assembly with another of his legendary non sequiturs: 'Today we find ourselves in the presence of a true matriarchy. One is simply dazzled by your amiable, smiling faces.'[7]

The first speaker, Minister for Family, Youth, and Sport Yuriy Pavlenko began with a reference to the '16 Days of Activism against Gender Violence' campaign noted earlier.[8] Even though violence against women is declining, he contended, there is an urgent need for changes to Ukraine's Criminal Code as a corrective to administrative violations and the inadequacies of past laws (Buzawa and Buzawa 2003, 112–15). He presented a list of proposed remedies against domestic violence, which included more severe sanctions against batterers, and maximum penalties for their crimes. The minister also advocated assistance to victims in the form of psychological support, hotlines, and crisis centres.

Leonid Hrach, head of the Parliamentary Committee on Human Rights, National Minorities, and Interethnic Relations, continued in a similar vein, but warned that the criminal justice system itself harbours assailants. He also drew attention to the severe underfunding of support agencies for women, railed against the evils of poverty 'with a woman's face,' and censured the political underrepresentation of female advocates in their own cause. His response to the mounting offences against women centred on pragmatic solutions, such as essential social services, but he too stopped short of plans for funding them.

Olena Bondarenko, head of a Parliamentary Sub-Committee on Gender Policy within the Parliamentary Committee on Human Rights, National Minorities, and Interethnic Relations, echoed the call for improved legislation. Challenging Pavlenko's exaggerated claim of declining violence, she insisted that it had simply been driven underground for lack of effective law enforcement procedures and correctional facilities. Bondarenko laid the blame squarely on Pavlenko's ministry, but did concede some progress. If the process is to move forward, she cautioned, additional crisis shelters, more violence-prevention measures, and closer cooperation among legislators, state policymakers, NGOs, activists, and concerned citizens, is imperative.

In a dramatic departure from most presenters, Bondarenko offered two real-life illustrations of the consequences of domestic violence. The first was that of a 16-year-old youth: unable any longer to stand by and watch his father savagely beat his mother, the young man committed patricide. A second example revealed that incessant beatings of a young woman by her father and brother had caused her to succumb to mental illness; this triggered a new cycle of violence. She beat her 18-month-old daughter so brutally that the infant had to be rushed to a trauma centre with severe brain damage and other multiple injuries.

Condemnations of domestic violence continued to dominate the first half of the proceedings, along with a near consensus that Ukraine's criminal justice system is ill-equipped to cope with the complexity and pervasiveness of such crimes. Its failure was attributed to a lack of properly trained personnel, virtually non-existent social services, and a government that ignores preventive programs, provides no assistance to victims, and includes no provisions in its budget for funding violence intervention. Some participants cited alcohol as the leading factor in the commission of violent crimes, a charge frequently repeated in the public sphere. Inexplicably, this allegation seemed to exasperate the chair. He reacted with scarcely controlled irritation, turning to the women with another of his baffling comments: 'Esteemed women! Restrain yourselves, don't give in to anger. I understand that your emotions might be heightened by such remarks made from the podium, but I remind you, these hearings are all about women, not the criminal conduct of violent men.'

The most provocative censure of the systemic breakdown – ranging from lawgivers to the judiciary, from the criminal justice system to the government – came from Deputy Victor Taran. He attributed the Ukrainian male's current predisposition to violence to the historical Russian custom of men brutalizing their women. By way of example, Taran cited one perverse manifestation of Russian brutality – homosexual antics parodying women engaged in bizarre violent acts, performed for the amusement of Stalin and members of his Politburo. This Russian addiction to violence against women, he charged, has been naturalized in Ukraine. Taran also disparaged the Ukrainian political system for the immunity it afforded male deputies. Under no circumstances do women receive such concessions, Taran argued. He described this male immunity as *nedotorkannist* (untouchability). With his time about to expire, Taran requested a few seconds more to complete his presentation, but was cut off by yet another of the chair's perplexing statements: 'Don't align yourself with the women,' he cautioned, 'lest you convey the wrong impression. As for women's "untouchability," please abstain from such catchphrases. Think about it, if women are truly "untouchable," who will give birth to our children?'

Was this some failed comedian, a person fatally obsessed with gibberish, or a man so obtuse as to feel no connection to the hearings that he was chairing? One participant became so incensed by Martyniuk's demeaning comments about women that she passed a note to the chair, reproaching him for reducing the proceedings to a 'female dog and pony show' (to use an American cliché).[9] Without disclosing its contents, but with scarcely concealed irritation, Martyniuk managed a restrained response: 'Esteemed women, you authors of such angry notes! I too am a participant here, with the same rights as you. I must ask you not to politicize these proceedings. This is a parliament, not a marketplace, even though we do enjoy freedom of speech.' In the end, no longer able to conceal his displeasure, the chairman trained his indignation onto one unregistered speaker who insisted on taking a turn at the podium. He addressed her with the derogatory 'little woman' (*zhinochko*, a term that infantilizes women), and when she persisted, he threatened to suspend the hearings. 'Because I can do this, you know,' was his defiant warning.

As petitions for change followed one another in rapid succession, they turned increasingly strident. Presenters repeated their insistence on deletion of the offensive Article 11 from the Law on the Prevention of Violence in the Family and they also urged lifting the fines against perpetrators, insisting that such penalties only compound domestic misery by depleting the family budget. Tetiana Yezhova, minister of Youth, Family, and Gender Politics in the Autonomous Republic of Crimea (the Cabinet of Ministers of Ukraine does not have such a ministry), injected sex trafficking into the deliberations, citing Ukraine as one of the leading suppliers of human flesh to the international sex industry. Her proposed solution lay in the economy. If women are to avoid the temptation of seeking a livelihood abroad where they are apt to be coerced into sexual slavery, she charged, they must be empowered to earn a decent living here. And she referred to Ukraine's catastrophic demographic imbalance (males constitute a mere 38% of the adult population and 40% of these are incapable of procreating). Inasmuch as men between the ages of 29 and 45 are four times as likely as women in that age cadre to die, she noted that they too are victims of the system.[10] Faulty economic policies, causing men to resort to alcohol or drugs, or to fall prey to debilitating diseases, bring an early death.

Deputy Mykola Tomenko[11] carried the earlier discussion of violence against women into the second half of the proceedings, designated for a dialogue on equal rights and opportunities. Referring to the negative stereotyping that marks parliamentary plenary sessions, he inquired: 'If this is the way our deputies behave, what can we expect from ordinary citizens?' He also raised a new question: Why had no woman addressed the problem of alimony or child support? Men seldom receive custody of their children, and they are notoriously negligent in paying child support. They can easily negotiate minimum assessments by declaring a fraction of their income or true financial worth. These same men also know that, even if they avoid making the court-ordered payments, retaliatory action is unlikely, regardless of what the law stipulates. The road to female poverty is littered with such cases.

The hearings experienced an unexpected reversal when the next speaker, Ol'ha Matvienko, professor of pedagogy at Shevchenko National University, began her presentation with the explanation that equality and replication are not coterminous, that genuine equality means each sex fulfilling its own distinct role. Women have no business, Matvienko asserted, aspiring to such noble male qualities as a strong intellect, an impressive body of knowledge, and limitless possibilities. They would do better to capitalize on their own discrete female roles of 'beautiful, loving caretakers' (Johnson 2007, 10). Naturally, women's lesser intellectual capacities are not altogether attributable to their sex, she concluded, they are also stymied by the absence of male role models (in many Ukrainian households) during a girl's formative years. Without a male to introduce them to rational thought, females will never develop what potential they do possess.

Returning the deliberations to the main issue, Tamara Melnyk (adviser to Minister Pavlenko) began her presentation with a reference to recent advances in gender equality. Although the expansion of women's rights remains largely on paper, she noted, when nothing concrete has been accomplished for so long, even the smallest gain represents progress. Relatively speaking, however, women are losing ground; advances in gender parity legislation have not translated to sweeping social progress. In any civilized country, Melnyk explained, rational gender policy is indexed by a decent standard of living for all, not some pandering to a Soviet-style technocracy that shamelessly exploits females. Moreover, Ukraine's catastrophic demographic decline is indisputable evidence of the government's callous indifference to the welfare of the *entire* citizenry. Ukraine needs clearly delineated gender priorities, sustained by a functional criminal justice infrastructure and unbiased law enforcement agencies.

An unequivocal condemnation of officialdom brought the session to an end. The final speaker, A. Komarova, referred to the incessant talk of non-functioning law enforcement agencies, a corrupt police force, and biased criminal justice system. She referred to President Yushchenko's address before the International Forum of Ukrainians in May 2006, in which he, too, described those same agencies as the most corrupt in the nation. In Yushchenko's judgment it is not individual perpetrators who are the real criminals, but rather the entire corrupt system, which unleashes so much violence against the entire people. If these so-called guardians of human rights cannot, or will not, reform themselves, Komarova asked, what kind of gender justice can we speak of?

In 2007, a year-long nationwide public information campaign titled 'Ukraine 2015,' mentioned earlier, was launched. On 4 March 2008, representatives from the Rada and the government, U.N. experts, and prominent media personnel met in Kyiv to discuss the UNDP project on equal opportunities and women's rights. Among its achievements during the first phase (2003–06) was the passage of normative laws on gender justice. On 15 September 2008, the second phase of the UNDP-led initiative, 'Equal Opportunities and Women's Rights,' was launched to consolidate earlier gains. For the first time since Ukraine's declaration of independence, an egalitarian gender strategy was included in the government's program of action. The groundbreaking Gender Equality Law of 2005, together with the 'Law on the Adoption of a State Program for Ensuring Gender Equality in Ukrainian Society for 2006–2010,' established a sound formal foundation for the work ahead. In an interview for the daily newspaper *Den'* (The Day), Professor Svitlana Oksamytna, dean of sociology at Mohyla National University in Kyiv, characterized this legislation as 'still in its declarative stage; but its passage indicates at least a modicum of reflection on the part of lawmakers' (Mykytiuk 2008).

Changing a stereotype is a fluid and protracted struggle, with its inevitable setbacks along the way, as official greetings on International Women's Day demonstrated so well. A stunning example of backsliding came in the form of a news item on 3 March 2007, on the Mykolaiv District Government website (in Russian: *Nykolaivskaia oblasnaia gosudarstvennaia administratsiia*). It was titled 'Woman-Worker, Woman-Mother, Wife-Guardian of the Ancestral Fire.' The item equates women with a legendary empowered 'hearth mother' (*Berehynia*), who has long since been divested of her original meaning, yet her legacy survives as a topos to delude contemporary Ukrainian women into believing in their own empowerment. Conversely, in a Kyiv newspaper early signs of a rising feminist consciousness appeared. On 3 March 2009, the following news item ran in *Den'*:

> Last year's 8 March greeting from the president so struck women [in the eastern Ukrainian city of Kharkiv] that they determined not to react post factum . . . instead of 'tender sentiments' [they declared] women would prefer . . . some assurance that Ukraine's Law on Guarantees of Equal Rights and Possibilities for Women and Men would be implemented. The women also wrote an open letter to all government personnel requesting a change in their customary form of address from 'my dears, most beloved, bewitching, tender, caring,' to terms that more accurately reflect their professional status.

Déjà-vu versus Change

Some two years after the third hearing, on 15 October 2008, I arrived in Kyiv to participate in an array of events on women's rights. My first stop was a Forum: Stop Violence meeting, held in Kyiv on 16 and 17 October. Recalling Minister Pavlenko's 2006 claim of progress on gender issues, which included crisis centres, I was dismayed to learn that the only such centre in Kyiv was scheduled for closing because of insufficient funding, while two regional centres had already been shuttered. Even at best, such shelters offer only thirty days of refuge for women age 35 and younger, with the result that many victims return to their abusive situations for want of an alternative. Still, one can argue, even these centres are better than nothing. Notwithstanding amendments to the 2001 Law of Ukraine on the Prevention of Violence in the Family, wherein Articles 10 and 11 put the onus on the victims, the entire legal system continues to favour male perpetrators of crimes. Current police responses to calls reporting domestic violence hover around 85 per cent, but few men are prosecuted, and fewer still are punished.

The forum proceedings brought to mind the series of parliamentary hearings – inspirational rhetoric on the urgency of reform, including much talk of the necessity for more effective legislation, the pressing need to establish social services for victims of violence, and the advisability of intervention – but still had no reference to a concrete plan for implementing legislation or for funding desperately needed services. Three of the foreign speakers, Francis M. O'Donnell and Jeremy Hartley, representatives of the United Nations in Ukraine, and William Taylor, U.S. ambassador to Ukraine, contributed Western ideas of a kind that would help raise the general awareness of gender injustice. Foreign participants had also advanced such ideas during the parliamentary hearings.

Later, participants congregated in clusters during coffee breaks or sat together in small groups around luncheon tables, for informal dialogue. They discussed equal rights, and proposed practical solutions for eliminating gender injustice, yet I sensed that some still had failed to avoid the trap of essentialism, not unlike the women at the hearings who so ardently defended those chivalrous male acts that 'defined them as women.' I left with a vague feeling that as much as the desired changes might continue to inspire stirring rhetoric, real hope for sweeping social progress would persist in eluding even the most committed activists for some time to come.

Instead of remaining for the second day of the forum, four of us travelled to the city of Vinnytsia for a two-day conference titled 'Perspectives for Developing Gender Education as the Realization of Democratic Changes in Ukrainian Society.' It was sponsored by the U.N. Development Program for Ukraine, the Swedish Agency for International Development (SIDA), the Vinnytsia State Administration, the Vinnytsia Administration of Family and Youth Affairs, the Vinnytsia Gender Education Centre, and Vinnytsia's National Technical University. Some fifty or sixty gender scholars, educators, and members of gender centres from around the country came together on 17 and 18 October to share their personal experiences in gender education and to evaluate its current state in Ukraine. They pointed to the fact that Western critical theories and feminist methodologies have been incorporated into their programs, talked about publishing projects (completed and contemplated), and suggested strategies for mainstreaming women's scholarship and stimulating further research; native Ukrainian traditions found no place in their discourse. A questionnaire was distributed that sought answers to queries on gender such as: What sorts of problems does it present in education? Has this approach produced any practical results? What can be done to address popular concerns? And finally, my numerous informal chats with the participants during coffee breaks and a final reception, revealed a surprising mastery of Western feminist ideas and the fact that the women were analysing their own situation in terms of global feminism. I also learned more about the breadth of their impressive outreach efforts in gender education.

The succeeding event was an eight-hour seminar at Kyiv's Court of Appeals on 21 October. It was designed for young graduates with law degrees who work in the Appellate Court. These are future judges in training who describe their professional activities as conducting research on upcoming cases and preparing briefs for presiding judges. Approximately sixty of these recent law graduates, divided into two groups, assembled in matching morning and afternoon sessions to hear female judges from the Appellate Court, legal scholars, gender activists, and a psychologist speak on gender politics, equal rights, and gender sensitivity in interpreting the law. The presentations were followed by a gender awareness exercise, in which real-life scenarios were used to test sensitivity to the scale of discrimination against women. Unlike the older generation of participants in the parliamentary hearings, with their different life experiences, the seminar revealed a new kind of Ukrainian citizen in the making. I witnessed the phenomenon of young people, unencumbered by traditional beliefs and prejudices, at ease with Western views of a just society, seeking to integrate their ideas on equal rights into Ukraine's discursive landscape.

The next day, 22 October, I was privileged to meet with a small group of pioneering feminists – women belonging to the previous generation. They were journalists, directors of gender programs, and feminist scholars, many of whom had spent time abroad as recipients of study and research fellowships or grants of one kind or another. We gathered for an informal chat session at the home of my hostess Tamara Melnyk to assess the country's progress in implementing the equal rights and opportunities that animated the parliamentary and forum dialogues, and to exchange views on feminist scholarship. This conversation, along with the Vinnytsia conference and Appellate Court seminar, reinforced my impression that the country's urbanizing culture was beginning to thrust the rustic *Berehynia* myth into the shadows. I realized that she was still 'out there,' together with other remnants of Ukraine's folk culture, and was not likely to fade away soon; the current proliferation of neo-pagan religions in Ukraine, and rising numbers of believers in them, testify to the still-viable role of tradition in Ukraine's cultural evolution. Still, it was obvious that new values were beginning to replace some traditional thinking on female identity construction, and that the younger generation, such as these legal scholars, was introducing a more innovative, more forward-looking perception of their world to Ukrainian society.

Events such as the parliamentary hearings and the forum, with their lofty rhetoric, admirable goals, stated determination to lift the status of women, and justified complaints against the slow pace of change, have been instrumental in generating some modest gains, and their appreciation of the need for equal rights and opportunities continues to intensify, yet that necessary first step, legislation, still awaits its implementation. In the words of Hilary Standing (in her discussion of gender mainstreaming): 'There has been an almost mechanical belief in the power of intention to determine the outcome of policy implementation' (2007, 107). In Ukraine, the 'power of intention,' enshrined in its progressive legislation, has yet to deliver the promised social change. Effective legislation is indispensable, but it takes more than statutes to achieve a transformative result.

Conclusions: Reflecting on the Future

Since the implosion of the Soviet empire, positive policy changes and scholarship on Ukrainian gender relations have represented upward momentum, yet the larger environment is still pointing in the opposite direction. Uninterrupted upward momentum calls for radical shifts in social relations. It is imperative for traditional discursive practices to interchange with the modern world. If it is to have an impact, gender discourse must reach the general population; it cannot simply be confined to the intellectual elite and political players. Gender-friendly legislation needs meaningful outcomes. A responsive criminal justice system is imperative. Corrupt institutions need to be reformed. Negative stereotypes need to be dispelled. In sum – good government must display the political will to see gender-friendly legislation put into action.

A new social movement effects change with difficulty, as it works its way through the people's resistance to new cultural beliefs (Dobash and Dobash 1992). The decades ahead will present even greater challenges to building gender justice.[12] Overcoming them will call for cooperation from all sectors of society. As they take stock of the progress over the past decades, the pioneering advocates of women's rights will find that they must now take their efforts to a higher level. To answer this call, they have broadened their sphere of consciousness-raising activity by introducing new and even more effective programs, aimed at reaching ever-increasing numbers of men and women.

NOTES

1 This was Deputy Nina Kondrakova's advice to women aspiring to a political career.
2 In addition to my notes taken as an observer, I had access to a draft copy of the proceedings provided by a participant: *Tretia Sesiia Verkhovnoi Rady Ukrainy* (Third Session of the Ukrainian Parliament), Bulletin No. 97, 1995.
3 There were, in point of fact, 17 (4.2%), not 16, female deputies in the Ukrainian parliament.
4 An Amnesty International Report of 2007 informed that Ukraine's Law on the Prevention of Violence in the Family dictated that victims of domestic violence must be given a warning against 'victim behaviour,' perpetuating the myth that women are to blame for any violence inflicted upon them.'
5 Women are beginning to challenge this practice as a 2009 posting on the Internet indicates. An activist group in Kharkiv went on record on 8 March 2009 to demand that women be addressed in a professional manner, reflecting respect for them. See Viktoria Kobyliat's'ka, 'Zhinky vyrishyly pryvitaty sebe sami,' *Den'*. Available at http://www.day.kiev.ua/290619?id source=270898&mainlang=ukr.
6 Passage of the law required six years of lobbying and eight separate drafts before legislators, who, after persistent refusal to acknowledge the existence of a problem, finally passed it (see Mykytiuk 2008).
7 A reference to Ukraine as a matriarchal society, with a history of alleged female centrality since prehistoric times, was used to convince women that Western-style feminism is redundant. For a comprehensive treatment, see Rubchak (1996, 2009).
8 The '16 Days of Activism against Gender Violence' is an international campaign emanating from the first Women's Global Leadership Institute sponsored by the Center for Women's Global Leadership in 1991. Participants chose 25 November to begin its annual observance.
9 She was Oksana Kis, a prominent ethnologist and feminist scholar.
10 These statistical data were obtained from Tamara Melnyk.
11 Coincidentally, the three most outspoken critics of gender injustice, Mykola Tomenko, Victor Taran, and Olena Bondarenko, all belong to the Yulia Tymoshenko political bloc. Although Tymoshenko rejects the feminist label as a self-descriptor, in her way of life she conforms to its principles.
12 The current Ukrainian government offers an illuminating example of how difficult it will be to dispel the old stereotypes, to change entrenched regressive ideas about a woman's 'proper place.' During the election campaign, Victor Yanukovych remarked that his competitor, Yulia

Tymoshenko, ought to pursue her whims in her kitchen, where women belong. His newly installed Prime Minister Mykola Azarov echoed this sentiment. When asked why there were no women in his cabinet he replied: 'Conducting reforms is not women's business . . . the current situation in Ukraine is too tough for women to handle' 'Feministky rozdiahly "Azarova" pered kabminom,' *Ukraina*, 22 March 2010. Also available at http://.unian.net/ukr/news-368344.html. His comments set off a fire storm of opposition, and the media stoked the fires with extensive coverage.

REFERENCES

Amnesty International. 2007. *Report 2007: The State of The World's Human Rights*. Available at http://report 2007.amnesty.org/eng/Regions/Europe-and-Central-Asia/Ukraine on 1/13/2009 (accessed 26 April 2010).

Association for Women's Rights in Development (AWID). 2005. *An Interview with Olena Suslova, Founder and Chair of the Board of the Women's Information Consultative Center (WICC)*. Available at http://www.awid.org/eng/Issues-and-Analysis/Library/Ukraine-and-the-recent-call-for-democracy-s-impact-on-women-s-human-rights/(language)/eng-GB (accessed 3 March 2009).

Buzawa, E.S., and C.G. Buzawa. 2003. *Domestic Violence: The Criminal Justice Response*. Thousand Oaks: Sage.

Cornwall, A., E. Harrison, and A. Whitehead. 2007. Introduction. In A. Cornwall, E. Harrison, and A. Whitehead, eds., *Feminisms in Development: Contradictions, Contestations and Challenges, 1–20*. London: Zed Books.

Dobash, R.E., and R.P. Dobash. 1992. *Women, Violence and Social Change*. London: Routledge.

Fedkovych, H. 2005. *Legislative Trends and New Developments*. Stop Violence against Women Website. Available at http://www.stopvaw.org/Legislative_Trends_and_New_Developments24.html (accessed 31 Dec. 2008).

Johnson, J.E. 2007. 'Contesting Violence, Contesting Gender: Crisis Centers Encountering Local Government in Barnaul, Russia.' In J.E. Johnson and J.C. Robinson, eds., *Living Gender after Communism*, 40–59. Bloomington: Indiana University Press.

Kandiyoti, D. 2007. Political Fiction Meets Gender Myth: Post-conflict Reconstruction, 'Democratization' and Women's Rights. In A. Cornwall et al., eds., *Feminisms in Development*, 191–200. London: Zed Books.

Molyneux, M. 2007. The Chimera of Success: Gender Ennui and the Changed International Policy Environment. In In A. Cornwall et al., eds., *Feminisms in Development*, 227–40. London: Zed Books.

Mykytiuk, O. 2008. 'Navishcho nam gender'? *Den.'* Available at http://www. day.kiev.ua/2253910/ (accessed 22 Sept. 2008).

Network Women's Program (NWP). 2009. *Sexual Assault.* Stop Violence against Women Website. Available at http://www.stopvaw.org/Sexual_Assault.html (accessed 3 March 2009).

Parliament of Ukraine (Verkhovna Rada). 1995. *Tretia Sesiia Verkhovnoi Rady Ukrainy* [Third Session of the Ukrainian Parliament]. Bulletin No. 97. Kyiv: Verkhovna Rada.

Rubchak, Marian J. 1996. Christian Virgin or Pagan Goddess? Feminism versus the Eternally Feminine in Ukraine. In R. Marsh, ed., *Women in Russia and Ukraine,* 315–30. Cambridge: Cambridge University Press.

– 2009. Collective Memory as a Device for Constructing a New Gender Myth. In L. Onyshkevych and M. Rewakowicz, eds., *Contemporary Ukraine on the Cultural Map of Europe,* 139–53. Armonk: M.E. Sharpe.

Standing, H. 2007. Gender, Myth and Fable: The Perils of Mainstreaming in Sector Bureaucracies. In A. Cornwall et al., eds., *Feminisms in Development,* 101–11. London: Zed Books.

United Nations. 1991. *Report on the Convention for the Elimination of All Forms of Discrimination against Women.* Available at http://www.stopvaw. org/10August2004.18.html (accessed 3 March 2009).

3 Electoral Reforms and Women's Representation in Ukraine

ANASTASIYA SALNYKOVA

Despite its significant advances in democratic reforms compared with other former Soviet states (World Audit 2009; Campbell and Pölzlbauer 2010; Freedom House 2010), Ukraine falls short of meeting the criteria for gender equality. In terms of women's political representation, Ukraine demonstrates poor results compared with world averages, ranking 112th in 2009 based on the proportion of women in the Verkhovna Rada (parliament of Ukraine) – worse than, for example, Côte d'Ivoire (108th), and only slightly better than Kuwait (114th). After the 2007 elections, only 8.2 per cent of Ukraine's parliamentary deputies were women, while the world average was 18.6 per cent. This result was also lower than any of the world's regional averages, including that of the Arab states, at 9.7 per cent (Inter-Parliamentary Union 2009). Thus, the need to improve gender equality in Ukraine's parliamentary arena is pressing.

In part, this requires a reassessment of the existing voting system, since voting systems are crucial institutional factors able to influence the number of women elected. The established view is that a single-member district (SMD) plurality system tends to reduce representation of women;[1] in contrast, proportional representation (PR), on average, leads to 10 per cent more women being elected (Electoral Reform Society 2009). Since gaining independence, Ukraine has undergone several electoral reforms and therefore presents an interesting case of recent electoral engineering. The country shifted from a majority to a mixed system in the 1990s and then from a mixed to a purely proportional system in 2005.

This chapter evaluates the effects of both these reforms on gender balance in political representation in Ukraine. It first provides a summary of the available knowledge on the interaction between electoral systems and women's representation. Another institutional tool, gender quotas, is also briefly addressed here. Then the case study of Ukraine is presented, followed by a discussion of probable outcomes of the current electoral system in terms of women's representation. The chapter concludes that PR has not created an automatic change in terms of women's representation in Ukraine, because other factors, including voter prejudices, internal political manipulations by political parties, and lack of mobilization in the women's movement, have played a role. Future improvement in gender representation will thus depend on deeper changes to enable the potential positive effect of proportional representation.

Electoral System and Women's Representation

There exists a wide consensus about the positive connection between a proportional electoral system and women's representation, while many of the single-member district systems are thought to produce obstacles for women's access to parliament. This consensus is based on both correlational evidence from comparative cross-national studies and an understanding of the specific mechanisms through which PR affects the decisions of political actors. Finally, the recognition of PR's superiority is also shared by feminist political theorists (Williams 1998; Guinier 1994; Young 2000; Phillips 1998), although this recognition is based mainly on a critique restricted to the reality of the U.S. political system.

Correlation between Proportional Representation and Women Elected

A series of studies have confirmed the association between a 'party list' version of PR and higher entry of women into elected office in established democracies (see Norris 2004; Rule and Zimmerman 1992; Lijphart 1994; Matland 1998). Among the countries defined as 'free' or 'partly free' by the Freedom House, the ten leaders in terms of women's representation all use PR electoral systems (Matland 1998, 106). Data for the year 2000 from 182 countries show that women made up an average of 15 per cent of members of parliament in countries using PR systems, compared with 11 per cent in those with mixed systems, and just 9 per cent in those employing plurality or majority systems

(p. 117). Moreover, among countries with mixed member proportional (MMP) systems, where some of the candidates are elected by majority and another portion by proportional representation, women's representation is usually higher in the proportional part of the system. Furthermore, when countries switch from a plurality or majority system to PR, there is an increase in women's representation. These correlations have also been confirmed in a study of changes to electoral systems in Central and Eastern Europe (Matland 2003). Finally, statistical analysis demonstrates that the role of the electoral system is independent of levels of socioeconomic and political development (Norris 2000, 2).

Nevertheless, it is known that PR is not enough; the relationship between the electoral system and women's representation is influenced by other factors as well. While there are several striking cases of women gaining significant representation in developing countries with PR systems, there are many more cases where no gains have been made despite PR. The non-effect of the electoral system variable confirms an observation made by Matland (1998), which is that while institutions or rules may benefit a particular group, an effect will occur only if the group is sufficiently well organized to take advantage of the situation (p. 107). In Russia, for example, consistently more women are elected through the SMD part of the ballot than through PR (Moser 2003, 153). In addition, more women have been elected in 'first past the post' systems, such as those in Australia and Canada, than in some highly proportional party list systems, such as those in Israel and Belgium. By itself the electoral system is neither a necessary nor a sufficient condition to guarantee women's representation. Nevertheless the electoral system functions as a facilitating mechanism that expedites the implementation of measures within parties, such as affirmative action for female candidates (Norris 2000, 2).

Mechanism of the Proportional Representation Effect on the Number of Women Elected

The theorized mechanism by which PR results in a positive effect on women's representation is made up of several elements, including PR's focus on political parties over individual candidates; the higher district and party magnitudes that characterize it; fewer wasted votes which, in turn, lead to a contagion effect in terms of women's representation; and greater competition. An additional mechanism for the representation of women that is facilitated by PR is the possibility of the introduction of gender quotas under this electoral system.

The PR system encourages participants in the electoral process to *focus on parties* and their policies, rather than on individuals. This party focus is seen as working for women because it shields them from built-in prejudices against women candidates among the electorate (Kethusegile-Juru 2003, 6). Yet the assumption that voters discriminate against women is not always correct. There are three levels of approval that any potential electoral contestant must pass: (1) self-selection, (2) selection by the nominating agent, and (3) selection by voters (Matland and Montgomery 2003, 20). Thus, when attitudes of the electorate are not discriminatory against women, or when an electorate is more in favour of women than the parties are, candidate-centred systems can actually facilitate women's representation (Larserud and Taphorn 2007, 11). Moreover, only a 'closed list' version of PR can combat voter prejudice; otherwise, in an 'open list' PR, voters can still express their preference for a male candidate when they choose individual candidates that they want to see on a party list.

Another important consequence of the party focus is that parties may help women organizationally and materially, and thus enable a run for office that they might not be able to undertake on their own in a single-member district. Conversely, because women often have fewer material resources than men, are less linked to informal networks of power, and find it more difficult to mobilize peers in support of their political aspirations, they may be disadvantaged by non-partisan competition (Birch 2003, 132).

A second element of the PR mechanism is the use of multi-member districts, which implies higher district magnitudes (i.e., the number of seats per district), and, as a result, higher party magnitude (the number of seats a party can win in a district) (Larserud and Taphorn 2007, 15). *Party and district magnitudes* affect party strategy when choosing candidates. Under PR, a woman candidate can be seen as a benefit to a party by attracting voters without requiring the most powerful intra-party interests, normally represented by men, to step aside, as would be required in a plurality or majority system (Matland 1998, 101). If parties can nominate more than one person, then they are more likely to nominate a balanced slate – in particular, in terms of gender – to attract a wider spectrum of voters. In contrast, if only one candidate is to be nominated, then it will often be the male incumbent, as he is seen as a more broadly accepted candidate. Moreover, since the top slots on candidate lists or in party hierarchies are often occupied by men, the bigger the party magnitude, the better the chances for women, as parties will then fill their subsequent seats with candidates other than their leaders (Larserud and Taphorn 2007, 10). The importance of district magnitude is illustrated by the case of Ireland, which uses the single transferrable vote (STV)[2] form of PR, but, due to small district magnitudes (three to five members per district), Ireland has lower levels of female representation than countries using plurality or majority systems, such as Canada, Australia, and the United Kingdom (Matland 1998, 106–7).

PR also functions with *fewer wasted votes*, which works in favour of women. If a plurality of votes is needed to gain a seat, as it is under the SMD system, then parties will be likely to give priority to their core group of voters. In contrast, in PR, where almost all votes count towards gaining the next seat, parties are more eager to appeal to all kinds of voters in a district, including marginalized groups (Larserud and Taphorn 2007, 11). Because of the winner-takes-all nature of the plurality system, parties are reluctant to introduce more women candidates even if their competitors do so. In contrast, under the proportional rule, such contagion does happen, since the marginal increase in a party's attractiveness to the wider number of voters can be more easily translated into seats under PR. In other words, because PR systems tend to produce more political parties, and thus the political distance between them is smaller, the threat that women voters could shift allegiances to another party is greater. As a result, party leaders feel a greater need to respond in kind when competitors start promoting women candidates (Matland and Montgomery 2003, 28). For example, the Norwegian Labour Party increased the number of women in winnable positions in those districts where it faced a challenge by the Socialist Left, the first party to adopt quotas in Norway. In contrast, in the Canadian SMD system, the Liberal Party has not been more likely to nominate women in those districts where the New Democratic Party had nominated women (Matland 1998, 102).

PR is also viewed as *enhancing competition* by creating more parliamentary parties. In a highly competitive environment, parties are likely to try to appear fair and gender-balanced in order not to lose votes to any of the parties whose policies are close to their own. It should be noted, however, that a very high number of parties in the legislature can work against the representation of women, as party magnitude goes down in that case (Larserud and Taphorn 2007, 11).

These four elements of the mechanism by which PR tends to produce more winning female candidates are important. However, the electoral system is not enough to ensure equal representation. An additional institutional factor important for women's representation is the *electoral threshold*, that is, the minimum percentage of votes required for a party to enter parliament. A high threshold discourages the creation of 'mini-parties,' which often elect only one or two representatives, who are usually male. In Israel, for example, despite a PR system and maximal district magnitude, women's representation is only average (15%). This may be partially attributed to Israel's low electoral threshold of 1.5 per cent (Matland 1998, 103–4). Thus, even though a multitude of parties increases competition, which in itself has positive implications for women's nomination, having too many parties jeopardizes this positive effect.

Another feature, that is not inherent in PR per se, is whether this electoral system is applied using open (voters choose which of the party's candidates are elected) or closed (the party determines the rank-ordering of candidates) lists. The question, in terms of women's representation, is whether in a particular context it is easier to convince voters to vote for women candidates or to convince party gatekeepers to include more women in prominent positions on the party list (Matland 1998, 104). Thus, in deciding between the closed versus open list versions of PR, it is crucial to understand that both the *supply* of women through party nomination and the *demand* for women politicians count (Wilcox et al. 2003, 43). For example, in Norway, where the parties are highly supportive of women candidates, preferential voting presupposed by open-list PR hurts women. In Poland, on the other hand, women do better with voters than they do with party committees; that is, the preferential vote leads to greater women's representation (Matland 1998, 105).

Finally, one of the reasons for PR's popularity among proponents of women's rights is that it is more appropriate for the introduction of *gender quotas* in the sense of places for women on candidates' lists. Thus, part of the causal power of PR in terms of female representation comes from quotas, the introduction of which is considered easier under a proportional electoral system. Gender quotas work best in combination with a proportional representation electoral system with closed lists, the zipper or zebra principle of candidate placement (meaning that every second candidate on the list is a woman), a high electoral threshold, and a high district magnitude, as those structures stimulate parties to balance their electoral roll to be as inclusive and representative as possible.

To summarize, based on comparative research, a consensus has emerged among researchers that PR electoral systems favour women's representation. This is mostly explainable by the elements of PR's electoral mechanism that have been outlined above. At the same time, however, this list of mechanisms is not exhaustive, and the correlation between PR and women's representation is not absolute. As Norris put it, we know that PR is associated with more women, yet the precise reasons for this pattern remain a matter of speculation (2004, 23).

Effects of Electoral Reform in Ukraine

As mentioned at the outset, the Ukrainian electoral system has changed twice: from a majority to a mixed system in the 1990s and to proportional representation in 2005. Thus, the 1994 parliamentary election was by majority: one deputy was elected from each constituency, with a run-off held between the two candidates who received the highest number of votes if no candidate gained an absolute majority in the first round (Birch 1997, 48). By 1998, a semi-proportional system was in place, in which half of the deputies were elected by a plurality of votes (i.e., the first-past-the-post system) in single-member districts, and half from national party lists, with a 4 per cent electoral threshold. The same system was used in the 2002 national election, with 225 deputies elected through SMD and the other 225 elected under the proportional system (Harasymiw 2006, 2). The electoral law that was in effect 2005–11 was introduced as part of a pact between the incumbent political forces and the Orange Revolution opposition in 2004. According to this arrangement, the entire Rada is elected through party lists and the electoral threshold was lowered to 3 per cent (Fisun et al. 2006, 52).

The consequences of introducing PR in Ukraine were unusual. According to Duverger's (1965) law – which states that proportional voting tends to produce a multi-party system and that plurality/majority voting, in contrast, leads to a two-party system – the new Ukrainian electoral system should have aided in the creation of a greater number of parties in the Rada. Given the examples in other settings, it was also expected that PR would bring along an increase in women's representation. However, these expectations were not realized. Under pure PR, the number of parties actually decreased. Even though no fewer than forty-five parties or party blocs were listed on the ballot for the 2006 elections, only five cleared the 3 per cent threshold (Harasymiw 2006, 4). Results from the subsequent early elections of 2007 were no different. The switch to pure PR in Ukraine has, therefore, been associated with less fragmentation in the party system, not the other way around (p. 9). This observation – as well as evidence from comparative research on Polish, Russian, and Ukrainian plurality voting systems, all of which failed to produce the expected bipartism, that is, a two-party system (Moser 1999) – suggests that the reach of Duverger's law is limited.

Another noticeable outcome of the change to PR was that the parties that did pass the 3 per cent threshold in Ukraine were bigger than those doing so in previous elections. In other words, PR did not produce better representation of previously marginalized groups by letting their parties into the Rada, but instead saw the success of the already dominant parties reinforced, irrespective of whether they represented diverse social groups. Although voters had a choice of more than forty parties on their ballots, popular support for small parties was negligible. In addition, those small parties predominantly expressed the ideological visions or personal ambitions of their leaders, rather than the interests of marginalized groups (Harasymiw 2006, 8).

Finally, the parties that got into Rada were not ideological in nature (with the exception of the Communist Party), while classically centrist and rightist parties did not meet the electoral threshold (Fisun et al. 2006, 53–4). Thus, the usual expectation that PR favours parties with more clearly formulated ideologies (Lijphart and Grofman 1984) was not met in Ukraine either.

In view of these peculiarities of the actual results of proportional representation in Ukraine, its impact on women's representation there merits special attention. It is necessary to analyse whether the mechanism of interaction between electoral rules and women's representation in Ukraine is similar to that at work in other European states. In general, the association between different electoral rules and women's representation demonstrates that the number of women deputies did, indeed, increase with the change towards greater proportionality (from SMD to MMP and from MMP to PR) in the Ukrainian case. As Table 3.1 makes clear, however, discrete improvements were not very significant. Moreover, reductions in women's representation took place twice: in 2002 and again in 2007. Finally, the overarching positive tendency might be explained by factors other than changes in the

Table 3.1. Women's Representation in Independent Ukraine, 1990–2007 (total seats = 450)

National Election (year)	Electoral System	Women Elected n (%)
1990	SMD	13 (2.8)
1994	SMD	18 (4.0)
1998	MMP	35 (7.8)
2002	MMP	29 (8.2)
2006	PR	37 (8.2)
2007	PR	35 (7.7)

Source: www.vru.gov.ua.
MMP = mixed member proportional; PR = proportional representation; SMD = single-member district.

electoral rules. After all, the positive trend towards greater political representation of women began even before elements of PR or pure PR were introduced. The percentage of women elected was growing gradually since independence, including the years in which SMD and MMP systems were used. Therefore, this growth cannot be attributed entirely to PR.

In her analysis of Ukraine's first round of electoral reforms, from SMD to MMP, prior to the 1998 elections, Birch argues that the increase in women's representation from 4 per cent in 1994 to 7.8 per cent in 1998 was clearly affected by the reform (2003, 139). That twenty-one women were elected through PR and fourteen through SMD in the latter year supports this view. Yet, the causal effect of the change in rules on the increase in women's representation is not certain. If PR itself was able to produce such an increase in women's representation, then we would expect it to do so with the shift from MMP towards pure PR as well. But as we can see in Table 3.1, the increase in women's representation between 2002 and 2006 was less than 2 per cent (from 6.4% to 8.2%).

Interestingly, a change from plurality to proportional elections has also led to fewer women elected on the local level in Ukraine. An activist working with local women candidates reported in an interview:[3] 'Women themselves expressed their concerns saying that under the current system it is more difficult to run; they need to build contacts with national parties and become someone's protégé.'

Some researchers have similar doubts about the causal link between PR and female representation. In her study of mixed electoral rules and women's representation in Russia and Ukraine until 1998, Andreenkova (2002) did not observe any advantages offered by any of the electoral systems as such. Similarly, Saxonberg concludes that while all the Eastern European countries that switched from majoritarian to mixed elections saw an increased level of women's representation, it is not clear whether the change in electoral rules accounted for this increase, or whether it was part of a general trend after the original drop in female representation in the first post-communist elections (2000, 148).

Future Trends

According to classifications made by the International Institute for Democracy and Electoral Assistance (IDEA), Ukraine's electoral system as of 2011, which is a closed-list PR with a single electoral district and no quotas, is considered to be an adequate model in terms of women's representation (Larserud and Taphorn 2007, 14).[4] This system is generally expected to increase the chances of women being elected. However, a closer look at how PR is expected to affect women's representation in Ukraine provides further insights.

In general, the party focus of electoral campaigns under PR is expected to help combat voters' prejudices against women candidates. In the Ukrainian case, however, this outcome is doubtful for two reasons. First, with no gender quotas in place or other responsibilities in terms of balancing gender representation, parties are not obliged to put forward more women on party lists. Moreover, if the population is prejudiced against women candidates, party gatekeepers will be especially reluctant to introduce more women on their candidates' lists, and therefore, parties cannot be expected to become leaders in combating such gender stereotypes. Although 10 per cent of the candidates for most major parties were women in 1998, they were so far down the lists that they had little chance of being elected on the basis of PR (Pavlychko 2000, 250). In contrast, many strong women candidates were elected that year as independents through SMD. Both the leader of the Progressive Socialists, Natalia Vitrenko, and ex-Prime Minister Yulia Tymoshenko entered politics through SMD (p. 251). And although their parties have failed, the leaders of two right-wing extremist parties – Yaroslava Stetsko, of the Congress of Ukrainian Nationalists, and Liudmyla Vansovska, of Menshe Sliv (Less Talk) – both won personal victories by gaining seats through SMD (p. 257).

A director of the major alcohol distillery Artemida, Hanna Antonyeva, won through SMD as well (p. 258). These individuals cannot run as independents under the party-based electoral law, and unless they can sustain their own parties (as Tymoshenko or Vitrenko do), they are doomed to lose political independence, even if they get on some other party's list of candidates.

A second reason to doubt the assumption that PR will combat voter prejudice is that evidence regarding voter attitudes towards women candidates in Ukraine is contradictory, and it is unclear whether there is anything for PR to combat. On the one hand, about 30 per cent of men in Ukraine strongly agree and 70 per cent agree that men make better leaders; 60 per cent of women also agree with this statement (Wilcox et al. 2003, 45). On the other hand, another survey demonstrates that only eight out of 1,741 citizens interviewed before the 1998 elections listed the sex of the candidate as the principal factor for their choice (Birch 2003, 198). Even in Russia, where the electorate arguably holds even more traditionalist views, gender stereotypes have been shown not to be an obstacle for women to do better in candidate-based competitions than through party lists; there, political parties represent the main obstacle to women candidates, not the electorate (Moser 2003, 160). Therefore, the mechanism of combating prejudices through PR is not expected to change the picture of women's representation in Ukraine significantly.

A third aspect that is worth special attention is the expectation that PR's increased party focus will lead to greater female representation because stronger parties will be more favourable for women who lack their own resources to enter politics. In the context of the growing feminization of poverty (Hankivsky 2008; Predborska 2005), as well as income inequality and structural imbalances in employment between men and women in Ukraine (see Chapter 11, in this volume), this mechanism could have positive results. On the other hand, the process through which party lists are formed in Ukraine is not transparent and is normally intertwined with major financial contributions or reciprocal services to the party from individuals who want to get on the list (Protsyk 2003). Such procedures nullify the socioeconomic levelling potential of PR and make it unlikely that it will counterbalance existing capacity discrepancies between potential male and female candidates.

Moving on to another mechanism of PR, Ukraine has *maximal district magnitude*, with the whole country being a single electoral district.

This feature of the voting system decreases the cost of introducing women onto party lists. Women can be nominated together with men so that incumbent men are not specifically challenged, and we can therefore expect that the magnitude mechanism will cause some degree of positive outcome in women's representation in Ukraine.

As for PR's *competition-enhancing mechanism* resulting from an increase in the number of parties, its effect will not be present in the Ukrainian case because, as we have seen, the introduction of PR has been associated with a reduction in the number of parties. There are still about five major parties in Ukraine, as well as a number of smaller ones, which is enough to create a competitive environment. This competition cannot be attributed to the introduction of PR, however. Moreover, the competition mechanism assumes that parties trying to attract more voters will attempt to look fair and thus nominate more women on their lists. But for this to happen, a demand from the voters is needed first, and this is not yet present in Ukraine; gender is not an issue discussed in electoral campaigns in Ukraine. Other issues such as NATO and EU membership, Russian as a second language, and economic reform have much greater currency, making it unlikely that gender will become a major issue in political competition any time soon.

Nevertheless, gender can become a second- or third-tier campaign issue. As the nature of the PR system produces fewer wasted votes, and thus provides incentives to appeal to marginalized groups, it can become an opportunity for a women's party to enter the Rada. At the moment, however, there is no such party in Ukraine, and the women's movement does not provide ground to hope for such a party in the nearest future. However, since in PR even a marginal increase in received votes translates easily into more seats in the Rada, it can become an incentive for parties to start playing the gender card in order to win at least a little bit more of a feminist vote, even from outside their own group of defined voters. In turn, this approach also has the potential to create a contagion effect, with other parties following the first mover. At the moment, there are no signs of this mechanism at work, but there are also no obstacles to it. For the contagion effect to start happening, a major party needs to be a first mover, a party that already has significant core support. To illustrate this point, in the 2002 and 2006 national elections, the Green Party of Ukraine used the zipper principle in its party list, but it did not manage to meet the electoral threshold nonetheless. During the 2007 elections, the Greens abandoned the zipper principle, demonstrating that for them it was only an electoral technology that did not bear fruit in terms of extra votes. The broader conclusion is that when gender is being picked up by a minor party, not only may it be of no use to that party, but it will also have no effect in terms of creating a contagion of nominating women candidates among other parties.

Given the *closed-list version of PR* in Ukraine, the potential to guarantee electoral results in terms of women's representation would exist if quotas were introduced. Until then, the list does not provide any such guarantees. To the contrary, the closed-list system, as well as the quota system, actually poses a danger in terms of putting *token women* in office who are entirely dependent on their party, and therefore will be reluctant to make any independent decisions, including those related to advancing gender equality. Discussion about the need to introduce open lists is ongoing in Ukraine, and an open-list system was supported by the former president, Viktor Yuschenko, in particular. At the moment, however, it is too early to say whether this change is probable.

As has been shown, PR by itself is not enough to solve the problem of women's representation, and it is quite possible that it may not bring the much-expected positive results in Ukraine. In fact, there are currently no signs of such change happening. Matland and Montgomery (2003) emphasize that we can expect women in countries with high magnitude PR to do better than women in less women-friendly systems. Yet as long as women are inadequately organized and public attitudes remain anti-feminist, women will be unable to fully utilize even favourable rules (p. 40). In the West, for example, electoral systems had no significant effect on the level of women's representation until the 'second wave' feminist movement in the 1970s. Strong women's movements have to convince parties in countries with PR to nominate more women candidates. If existing parties do not respond, the movement can simply create its own party (Saxonberg 2000, 148).

In Ukraine, the situation does not look promising with respect to action by the women's movement. Despite seven hundred registered women's organizations,[5] half of the gender experts interviewed for a recent research project reported that the women's movement in Ukraine is highly ineffective in promoting gender equality.[6] As one state official put it, 'The women's movement is not very influential and in recent years it got weaker.' An NGO employee echoed this negative judgment, saying, 'The women's movement is very disorganized;

there is no unity as in some countries.'[7] As a result, women's organizations have little influence on the state's handling of women's issues (WWICS 2007, 1), and they are not expected to make PR work for
women in Ukraine any time soon.

Because women's political representation does not increase automatically with a certain electoral system, it is early to be overly optimistic about the introduction of PR. On the one hand, in the Ukrainian
context, PR does open up a number of opportunities, and it is expected
that women's representation will benefit from the maximal district magnitude and fewer wasted votes aspects of the PR electoral
process. These mechanisms are expected to result in a greater number
of women nominated as well as a more salient role for gender issues
in campaigns. On the other hand, such features as closed lists and a
3 per cent electoral threshold can affect women's representation in
both directions. In addition, the party focus of the PR electoral process
is not expected to bring much change in relation to the broader Ukrainian context either in terms of combating prejudices or with respect
to counterbalancing the economic gap between genders. Similarly, the
enhanced competition mechanism is not working in Ukraine. Finally,
although expected to bring results over time, PR is not very effective in the Ukrainian context today, primarily because of the lack of a
strong women's movement capable of using this instrument for its own
benefit.

Dangers Ahead

The core problem with PR in the context of women's representation
is the danger of falling into the trap of a numerical approach. Policy
recommendations suggesting closed-list PR plus a quota system as an
optimal strategy (e.g., Larserud and Taphorn 2007, 12–13) assume that
a higher number of women in parliament is the desired end goal. This
view is in line with contemporary political theory that asserts the superiority of the politics of presence over the politics of ideas (e.g., Phillips 1998). This belief in the strength of numbers is also evident in the
attitudes of Ukrainian women's rights activists. In the words of one
former state official, 'when we have 35 per cent of women in the Rada
this will change everything because a woman's mind works better than
a man's.'

Yet, a high number of women politicians does not necessarily translate into an adequate representation of either women's interests or the

promotion of gender equality. As one parliamentary committee member commented, even quotas would not necessarily lead to that because 'the women who are going to be on the [political party candidates'] lists will be the wives and daughters of the oligarchs, and they will only press voting buttons when told to do so.' Indeed, despite the existence of quotas in the Soviet Union, and the presence of 36 per cent of women in the parliament in the mid-1980s (Hrycak 2005), no real improvements to gender equality took place, and as soon as quotas were removed, in 1990, women's representation dropped to nearly nothing, down to 2.8 per cent in Ukraine (Hrycak 2001, 2005).

In the 1998 elections, the Progressive Socialists, led by a woman (Natalia Vitrenko) and with the largest proportion of women candidates of all the major parties, made no mention of women in their program at all. The same was true for the Agrarian Party, also headed by a woman (Kateryna Vaschuk). The Women's Initiative Party saw women as mothers. In contrast, the conservative Rukh (People's Movement of Ukraine) Party vowed to promote the activity of women in civil society and business. Finally, the Green Party, with the smallest number of women on their candidates' list that year, devoted the most attention among all the parties to women's issues in their program, calling for equal rights, for women to work in leadership positions, and to have childbearing work counted for pension benefits (Birch 2003, 144–5).

The failure of the numerical approach to women's representation manifests itself in two ways. First, such instruments as closed-list PR and gender quotas (i.e., reserved seats) that ensure an increase in the number of women in parliament provide incentives for nominating token or proxy women instead of strong women politicians. Chowdhury (2002) submits that 'in a way, the word "reservation" has a passive connotation in that it refers to numbers without much reflection upon the interface between numbers and outcome' (p. 1). Reserving seats for women can even play out in a negative way by accentuating women's dependence in politics and reinforcing their marginality (Lowe-Morna 2003, 7–8).

Research has revealed many cases of purely symbolic representation of women, especially if the women elected have no power base in a constituency of their own or in strong movements outside the political institutions (Dahlerup 2006, 149). Such symbolic women feature on the party lists in Ukrainian politics as well. For example, Nina Matvienko, a pop-folk star popular among the middle aged and elderly, became Rukh's token woman. Not only was she inactive in terms of political work, she was also the epitome of traditional Ukrainian womanhood (Pavlychko 2000, 254). Other examples include the well-known Soviet actress Valeria Zaklunna, with the Communist Party; Soviet pop-star Sofiya Rotaru, with the Soyuz (Union) Party; famous actress Ada Rohovtseva, affiliated with the Liberal Party and Party of Labour bloc; Olha Sumska, the actress who starred in the first Ukrainian soap opera, with the Party of National Economic Development of Ukraine (ibid.); and the Eurovision song contest winner Ruslana, as well as another pop-singer Oksana Bilozir – both deputies from Yuschenko's Our Ukraine; and there are others.

To be fair, there are also success stories of women who felt isolated and powerless at the beginning of their careers, but eventually gained confidence and influence (Dahlerup 2006, 149). Even in these cases, however, advancement of women's interests or gender issues is not guaranteed. This leads to the second reason the numerical approach fails: in contrast to token women, who do virtually nothing in terms of actual decision making, there are also women who become politically active but are of no use to the women's rights movement, as they do not have the interests of women as a group among their personal and political priorities. For example, Valentyna Datsenko, a leader of the All-Ukrainian Party of Women's Initiatives, often expressed essentialist views about women's nature: 'Politicians squabble among themselves because they are men; politics need women because they are naturally peace-loving.' These traditionalist attitudes extended to the party's political program, which spoke of giving birth and bringing up children as the highest achievements in a woman's life. Ukraine's ex-prime minister, Yulia Tymoshenko, meanwhile, despite often being accused of manliness, is also a carrier of traditionalist gender views: 'The problem is not that we have too few women in politics; rather we have too few real men' (Pavlychko 2000, 256).

Most Ukrainian women deputies were not even supportive of the 2005 Gender Equality Law, which is why it took six years and pressure from the European Union for the Rada to finally adopt a mild version of it. In reference to the first gender bill proposed in 1999, one woman deputy said that Ukraine could not afford this law before it solved the problem of needy children (Hrycak 2005, 75). Women deputies ridiculed the notion of equal rights legislation, claiming that women are already equal if not over-emancipated and need to devote themselves more to motherhood (Hrycak 2001, 141). A scholar who worked on a draft of the law remembers: 'I could not appeal to women either. Lilia Hryhorovych – our "great genderist" today – was one of the first against the law. I had to fight with the women's movement at the time for the idea of gender equality.' This illustrates a major paradox: that women's representation often does not lead to the advancement of gender issues, which include both women's and men's interests in relation to one another and which require attention and transformation to bring about meaningful equality.

The next danger that could emerge in the future relates to the closed-list form of PR, such as that used in Ukraine. Although it is considered more effective for women's representation, it also suffers from a democratic deficit in other respects, such as poor accountability of elected officials to their constituency. As Norris (2000) has put it, underlying arguments about electoral systems are 'contested visions about the fundamental principles of representative democracy, the central normative criteria that an electoral system should meet, and whether the virtues of strong and accountable government are more or less important than social representation, including women and ethnic minorities' (p. 1). Therefore, in assessing the overall desirability of the list PR system, we need to consider not only women's representation in isolation, but also broader societal needs, so that women's rights do not come at the expense of some other rights. In addition, if voters, both men and women, prefer male politicians to female, even though their preference is the result of gender prejudices, it is undemocratic to force society into having more women in the Rada, in particular through quotas. A more democratic – and more effective – solution is working with people's attitudes directly, through education or the media, thus creating a demand for women in politics.

Finally, the introduction of proportional representation, and even more so the introduction of a quota system in the future, could become an incentive to wait passively for the desired result of increased female representation instead of mobilizing the women's movement to actually use institutional advantages to create the change. According to an interviewed parliamentary committee worker, such passivity followed the passing of the Gender Equality Law in 2005: 'Women's NGOs fought for the law for so long that when it was finally adopted, they took it as a happy end and did not know what to do next. In fact, the law is only the beginning.'

The main implication of this discussion is that the numerical approach to women's representation is not at all satisfactory, and achieving results in terms of gender equality requires transcending it. The instruments aimed at a numerical increase in women representatives do not account for the problem of token women and unenlightened women who are of little use to the program of advancing gender interests. In addition, there is a danger of promoting a democratic deficit when raising the number of women politicians through administrative means rather than by nourishing a change in voters' attitudes and in women's capacities. Finally, an overly optimistic view of PR may also carry the risk of creating undue passivity within the women's movement.

In her study of gender in development, Tiessen (2005) defines three approaches to gender mainstreaming: (1) technical or operational, (2) subtle, and (3) networking. The technical approach involves strategies such as gender-sensitive policies, increasing the number of gender advisers and providing gender-training sessions. The subtle approach involves strategies such as resistance and subversion conducted by women within a given organization. Networking refers to the building of coalitions and committees (especially ones that include sympathetic men) that make gender concerns a matter of group responsibility as opposed to just a personal commitment by individuals. The first approach is unlikely to lead to any notable advances in gender equality, whereas the second and third approaches have the potential to challenge mainstream and patriarchal norms (ibid.). Based on the present review of the introduction of PR in Ukraine, the change to the electoral system is clearly a technical solution, and by itself, it will not lead to the attitudinal shifts that are required for gender mainstreaming to be effective.

Conclusions

Despite the introduction of proportional representation in Ukraine, it is still too early to celebrate.[8] Analysis of trends in women's representation in association with a change in electoral rules demonstrates that, overall, the Ukrainian case is in line with established expectations. As the proportionality of the electoral system has increased over the years, the number of women elected to the Rada has also increased. At the same time, it is also clear that improvements following the introduction of elements of PR or pure PR have not been very dramatic and have been followed by reductions of women's representation. Therefore, it is more plausible that other significant factors have been at play as well, with PR not being a crucial force for the advancement of women's representation in Ukraine.

A closer look at the mechanism by which PR in Ukraine might affect women's representation gives us reason to be only moderately hopeful that, despite the social reality of discrimination against women, their political representation will increase, at least numerically. This expectation is grounded in the fact that PR does indeed open up a number of opportunities for women's representation, including maximal district magnitude and fewer wasted votes.

Nevertheless, it is also important to face the potential dangers associated with a move towards proportionality. The first danger is trading quantity for quality, which allows token women or women who are unaware of women's interests to 'represent' women in parliament. The second danger is the democratic deficit related to the lower accountability of elected officials in PR, as well as the lack of democratic spirit in mechanisms that force society to have more women representatives despite the will of voters. Finally, enthusiasm for PR could decrease the much needed mobilization of the women's movement if activists expect the institutional incentives to work by themselves.

The introduction of PR is only a technical solution that by itself will not effectively lead to gender equality in political representation. The crucial factors that can enable the electoral system's functioning to support gender equality are: strengthening of the women's movement's ability to pressure political parties; economic empowerment of women that decreases their dependence on men in general and on male party members in particular; and transformation of societal attitudes to create demand for women politicians and for women's issues and – even more importantly, gender issues – to be represented in mainstream politics. In a nutshell, deeper transformation and much more work is needed for Ukrainian society to reap the gender dividends promised by the introduction of PR.

NOTES

1 A single-member district (SMD) system can exist in the form of majority system or plurality system (also known as 'first past the post').
2 The single transferable vote (STV) is a voting system based on proportional representation and preferential voting. Under STV, votes are initially

allocated to the voters' most preferred candidate and then, after candidates have been either elected or eliminated, any surplus or unused votes are transferred according to the voters' stated preferences.

3 Author's interview with Oleksandra Sorokopud, August 2010.

4 Ukraine's system of 2005–2011 falls into IDEA's medium-fit category of models, meaning that it is not yet the best-practice system, but it is at least not antagonistic towards women.

5 This number used to be even higher, at more than 1,200, according to O. Sydorenko, *Zhinochi Organizatsiyi Ukrayiny: Dovidnyk* (Kyiv: Tsentr Innovatsiyi ta Rozvytku, 2001).

6 Interviews with 32 gender experts in Ukraine (from civil society, government, and academia) were conducted in 2006–7 for a research project on gender mainstreaming led by Olena Hankivsky and myself. The results of this study are most fully presented in Olena Hankivsky and Anastasiya Salnykova's Chapter 16 in this volume and in their article in the *Journal of Communist Studies and Transition Politics* 26/3 (2010), 383–408.

7 For more on the women's movement in Ukraine, see sources in n6 above. Also see Alexandra Hrycak (2005).

8 When this book was in press in 2011 the electoral system was changed back to a mixed one.

REFERENCES

Andreenkova, A.V. 2002. Women's Representation in the Parliaments of Russia and Ukraine. *Sociological Research* 41(2): 5–25.

Birch, S. 1997. Ukraine: The Perils of Majoritarianism in a New Democracy. In International IDEA, ed., *The International IDEA Handbook of Electoral Systems*, 48–50. Stockholm: International IDEA. Also available at http://twistedmatrix.com/users/z3p/files/esd_english.pdf (accessed on 28 Sept. 2009).

– 2003. Women and Political Representation in Contemporary Ukraine. In R. Matland and K. Montgomery, eds., *Women's Access to Political Power in Post-Communist Europe*, 130–52. Oxford: Oxford University Press.

Campbell, D.F.J., and G. Pölzlbauer. 2010. *The Democracy Ranking 2009 of the Quality of Democracy: Method and Ranking Outcome. Comprehensive Scores and Score for the Dimensions*. Vienna: Democracy Ranking. Available at http://www.democracyranking.org/downloads/method_ranking_outcome_2009_A4.pdf.

Chowdhury, N. 2002. The Implementation of Quotas: Bangladesh Experience – Dependence and Marginality in Politics. Presented at the International

IDEA Regional Workshop on the Implementation of Quotas: Asian Experience. Available at http://www.quotaproject.org/CS/CS_Bangladesh.pdf.

Dahlerup, D. 2006. Increasing Women's Political Representation: New Trends in Gender Quotas. In International IDEA, ed., *Women in Parliament: Beyond Numbers*, 141–84. Stockholm: International IDEA.

Duverger, M. 1965. *Political Parties: Their Organization and Activity in the Modern State.* Translated by B. North and R. North, with a Foreword by D.W. Brogan. London: Methuen.

Electoral Reform Society (U.K.). 2009. *Campaigns: Women.* Available at http://www.electoral-reform.org.uk/article.php?id=35 (accessed 20 July 2009).

Fisun, O., T. Mosentseva, and O. Drobotenko. 2006. Transformation of the Political System of Ukraine. In O.S. Vlasiuk, ed., *Ukraine: Strategic Priorities: Analytical Assessment-2006*, 49–55. Kyiv: National Institute for Strategic Studies. Also available at http://www.niss.gov.ua/book/Vlasyuk_mon/01–5.pdf (accessed 28 Sept. 2009).

Freedom House (FH). 2010. *Freedom in the World 2010: Erosion of Freedom Intensifies.* Available at http://www.freedomhouse.org/uploads/fiw10/FIW_2010_Tables_and_Graphs.pdf (accessed 22 July 2010).

Guinier, L. 1994. *The Tyranny of the Majority: Fundamental Fairness of Representative Democracy.* New York: Free Press.

Hankivsky, O. 2008. Globalization, Trafficking, and Health: A Case Study of Ukraine. In C. Patton and H. Loshny, eds., *Global Science/Women's Health*, 175–99. Amherst: Cambria Press.

Harasymiw, B. 2006. Ukraine's 2006 Parliamentary Elections in Dynamic Perspective. Paper presented at conference of the Canadian Association of Slavists, York University, Toronto, 29 May.

Hrycak, A. 2001. The Dilemmas of Civil Revival: Ukrainian Women since Independence. *Journal of Ukrainian Studies* 26(1–2): 135–58.

– 2005. Coping with Chaos: Gender and Politics in a Fragmented State. *Problems of Post-Communism* 52(5): 69–81.

Inter-Parliamentary Union. 2009. *Women in Parliaments Database.* Available at http://www.ipu.org/wmn-e/classif.htm (accessed 20 July 2009).

Kethusegile-Juru, B.M. 2003. *Quota Systems in Africa: An Overview.* Paper presented at the IDEA Workshop on the Implementation of Quotas: African Perspective, Pretoria, 11–12 Nov. Available at http://www.quotaproject.org/CS/CS_SADC_Overview_Bookie_27_7_2004.pdf (accessed 28 Sept. 2009).

Larserud, S., and R. Taphorn. 2007. *Designing for Equality: Best-Fit, Medium-Fit and Non-favourable Combinations of Electoral Systems and Gender Quotas.* Stockholm: International IDEA.

Lijphart, A. 1994. *Electoral Systems and Party Systems: A Study of Twenty-Seven Democracies, 1945–1990*. Oxford: Oxford University Press.

Lijphart, A., and B. Grofman. 1984. *Choosing an Electoral System: Issues and Alternatives*. New York: Praeger.

Lowe-Morna, C. 2003. *Beyond Numbers: Quotas in Practice*. Paper presented at the IDEA Workshop on the Implementation of Quotas: African Perspective, Pretoria, 11–12 Nov. Available at http://www.quotaproject.org/CS/CS_Lowe%20Morna-1-6-2004.pdf (accessed 28 Sept. 2009).

Matland, R.E. 1998. Enhancing Women's Political Participation: Legislative Recruitment and Electoral Systems. In International IDEA, ed., *Women in Parliament: Beyond Numbers*, 93–111. Stockholm: International IDEA.

– 2003. Women's Representation in Post-Communist Europe. In R.E. Matland and K.A. Montgomery, eds., *Women's Access to Political Power in Post-Communist Europe*, 321–42. Oxford: Oxford University Press.

Matland, R.E., and K.A. Montgomery. 2003. Recruiting Women to National Legislatures: A General Framework with Application to Post-Communist Democracies. In R.E. Matland and K.A. Montgomery, eds., *Women's Access to Political Power in Post-Communist Europe*, 19–42. Oxford: Oxford University Press.

Moser, R.G. 1999. Electoral Systems and the Number of Parties in Post-Communist States. *World Politics* 51(3): 359–84.

– 2003. Electoral Systems and Women's Representation: The Strange Case of Russia. In R.E. Matland and K.A. Montgomery, eds., *Women's Access to Political Power in Post-Communist Europe*, 153–72. Oxford: Oxford University Press.

Norris, P. 2000. Women Representation and Electoral Systems. In R. Rose, ed., *The International Encyclopedia of Elections*, 348–51. Washington DC: CQ Press. Available at http://www.hks.harvard.edu/fs/pnorris/Acrobat/WOMENELE.PDF (accessed 7 Sept. 2010).

– 2004. *Electoral Engineering: Voting Rules and Political Behaviour*. Cambridge: Cambridge University Press.

Pavlychko, S. 2000. Women's Discordant Voices in the Context of the 1998 Parliamentary Elections in Ukraine. In A. Bull, H. Diamond, and R. Marsh, eds., *Feminisms and Women's Movements in a Contemporary Europe*, 244–60. Basingstoke: Macmillan.

Phillips, A. 1998. *The Politics of Presence*. Oxford: Clarendon.

Predborska, I. 2005. The Social Position of Yong Women in Present-day Ukraine. *Journal of Youth Studies* 8(3): 349–65.

Protsyk, O. 2003. Semi-Presidentialism and Stability in Ukraine. *Europe-Asia Studies* 55(7): 1077–95.

Rule, W., and J.F. Zimmerman. 1992. *Electoral Systems in Comparative Perspective: Their Impact on Women and Minorities.* Westport: Greenwood.

Saxonberg, S. 2000. Women in East European Parliaments. *Journal of Democracy* 11(2): 145–58.

Tiessen, R. 2005. What's New about Gender Mainstreaming? Three Decades of Policy Creation and Development Strategies. *Canadian Journal of Development Studies* 26: 705–19.

Wilcox, C., B. Stark, and S. Thomas. 2003. Popular Support for Electing Women in Eastern Europe. In R. Matland and K. Montgomery, eds., *Women's Access to Political Power in Post-Communist Europe,* 43–62. Oxford: Oxford University Press.

Williams, M. 1998. *Voice, Trust and Memory: Marginalized Groups and the Failings of Liberal Representation.* Princeton: Princeton University Press.

Woodrow Wilson International Center for Scholars (WWICS). 2007. Women's NGOs in Ukraine and End of Western Aid. *Kennan Institute U.S. Alumni Series* 14. June. Available at http://www.wilsoncenter.org/index.cfm?fuseaction=events.event_summaryandevent_id=237920 (accessed 28 Sept. 2009).

World Audit. 2009. *Democracy Audit.* Available at http://www.worldaudit.org/democracy.htm.

Young, I.M. 2000. *Inclusion and Democracy.* Oxford: Oxford University Press.

4 Global Campaigns to Combat Violence against Women: Theorizing Their Impact in Post-Communist Ukraine

ALEXANDRA HRYCAK

Since the 1980s – when international women's organizations first placed the issue of gender violence on the agenda of international institutions – states have come under considerable international pressure to adopt the policy recommendations made by transnational campaigns to combat violence against women (Keck and Sikkink 1998). In 1992, gender violence was added to the Convention on the Elimination of All Forms of Discrimination against Women (CEDAW; Joachim 1999, 2007). In 1993, the U.N. General Assembly adopted the Declaration on the Elimination of Violence against Women. In 1995, the need for all states to take action to prevent violence against women was made a top priority for the Beijing Call for Action and the Beijing Platform for Action. A broad range of global campaigns and projects have mobilized at regional and national levels to place further pressure on states to develop policies to prevent gender violence. In response to the diffusion of the 'global policy scripts' that these international treaties and global campaigns against violence promote, activists have struggled to persuade states to pass legislation and implement comprehensive programs bringing them into compliance with their treaty obligations to take action to prevent violence against women. Despite extensive international pressure, however, these efforts have met with uneven success. In some countries, global campaigns to combat violence against women have resulted in extensive legislative and policy responses, in others, there has been relatively little or no response (Coomaraswamy 2003; Webhofer 2009).

Ukraine holds the distinction among post-Soviet countries of responding first and most extensively to the policy recommendations of global campaigns to address gender violence. In 1998, Ukraine became the first post-Soviet country (and one of the first countries in Europe) to formally criminalize human trafficking (Pyshchulina 2003; Lutsenko et al. 2005). In 2001, Ukraine introduced further changes to bring its human trafficking legislation into closer conformity with international treaties against trafficking. That year, Ukraine also became the first post-Soviet country to pass a law to combat domestic violence (Hrycak 2010a). After the Orange Revolution brought Western-leaning leaders to power in 2004, state officials further increased support for the prevention of violence, opening new shelters for victims of domestic violence and new crisis and rehabilitation centres that provided a wide range of services to battered or trafficked women. They also created gender advisory bodies within government ministries to provide access for women's rights advocates to introduce gender mainstreaming measures that would help harmonize Ukrainian law with the stringent standards of the European Union (Hrycak 2010b). Lawmakers passed comprehensive gender equality legislation, and gave women's and human rights groups the opportunity to discuss the shortcomings of the implementation of laws and policies with lawmakers and state authorities (e.g., through parliamentary hearings on gender violence and equality of opportunity held in November 2006; see Chapter 2 in this volume) and to amend the 2001 Law on the Prevention of Violence in the Family to bring it in line with the recommendations made by women's rights advocates and such human rights groups as Amnesty International.

Ukraine's early response to global campaigns to prevent violence against women, and its extensive recent efforts to respond further to pressure from domestic women's and human rights activists, are improbable and puzzling when compared with the later and less positive responses to global activism that have occurred in most countries in the former Soviet region. In recent years, most post-Soviet countries have passed legislation to criminalize human trafficking, in large part to avoid economic sanctions that the United States threatens to use against non-compliant states (Johnson 2009). But, as of 2009, there was still no specific legislation to prevent domestic violence in Armenia, Azerbaijan, Belarus, Estonia, Latvia, Lithuania, Russia, Tajikistan, or Uzbekistan.[1] Aside from Ukraine, the only post-Soviet countries that have passed laws to prevent domestic violence are the Kyrgyz Republic (in 2003), Georgia (in 2006), and Moldova (in 2007) (Fábián 2010; Hrycak 2010a, 2010b).

I argue in this chapter that Ukraine's response cannot be explained by the leading theoretical approaches to the effects of global campaigns on policy making: world polity theory, world civilization theory, and global feminism theory. If we follow the expectations of the world polity approach, which stresses that global norms and global policy scripts (disseminated via international organizations) are the primary influence informing policy regime choices, we would expect that *all* post-Soviet states would have acted quickly to develop policies that are in line with the international treaties they sign, including those that call for states to take action to combat violence against women (Boli and Thomas 1997). This is not what happened. If we follow the expectations of the world civilization approach, which argues that states adopt global policy scripts in order to signal their Western geopolitical orientation (Beckfield 2008), we would expect that the early adopters of anti-violence policies would have been Estonia, Latvia, and Lithuania, where government elites embraced a Western geopolitical orientation when they restored their independence and seceded from the Soviet Union. This is also not what happened. Finally, if we follow the expectations of global feminism approaches, which consider transnational feminist networks to be the main actors that help local women's groups develop the capacity to pressure states to enact policies to protect women's rights (Moghadam 2005), we would expect that the earliest adopter of global policies among post-Soviet countries would arguably have been Russia. In the post-Soviet region, Russia became the first target of global feminist advocacy. It has received the most extensive funding to support the activities of local advocates who promote global feminist frames regarding the prevention of domestic violence, and its local activists were also the first in the post-Soviet region to draft legislation against domestic violence (Hemment 2007; Johnson 2009; Johnson and Brunell 2006). However, more than forty draft laws later, legislation on the prevention of domestic violence has not been passed in Russia. Instead, Ukraine overtook Russia to become the leader among post-Soviet countries in passing and implementing policies to address violence against women.

Why did the Ukrainian state react earlier than others to pressure to address violence against women? Following recent calls to 'bring the state back in' to studies of women's activism (Randall and Waylen 1998; Stetson and Mazur 1995), this chapter sheds light on the development in Ukraine of special units charged with promoting women's rights – such as offices, commissions, agencies, ministries, and committees devoted to raising the status of women and promoting equality of men and women. Through a reconstruction of the process by which such organizationally based women's rights initiatives in Ukraine aided the development, revision, and implementation of policies to prevent violence against women, it lays the groundwork for future research to address two related puzzles. The first concerns Ukraine's early adoption of laws against various forms of gender-based violence. The second concerns why, despite this state's early adoption of these 'global policy scripts,' policies to combat violence remain partially unimplemented today.

The explanation suggested in this chapter for why Ukraine is an early adopter is consistent with the conclusions made by Keck and Sikkink (1998) in their cross-national studies of transnational advocacy networks. Keck and Sikkink argue that the influence of human rights campaigns on the behaviour of target states depends upon activists' ability to 'mobilize shame,' that is, use compromising information strategically at moments of government vulnerability or state legitimacy crisis. As I show below, such moral leverage is created for women's rights activists in Ukraine because government power holders are deeply divided over the country's geopolitical orientation. Consequently, government actors belonging to rival factions use evidence of their own responsiveness to accusations of non-compliance with international treaties to enhance their own moral leverage over their political rivals, thus creating periodic legitimacy crises.

The chapter explores domestic bids for legitimacy in relationship to two main dimensions of global advocacy campaigns that previous research confirms shape local openness to global women's activism: (1) international exposure to new global campaigns through international conferences and (2) the priorities of international funders. The chapter starts with an assessment of the impact of the Beijing World Conference for Women, which exposed all post-Soviet countries to new global policy scripts that raised the visibility and salience of violence against women. It then considers the mediating impact of international donors who singled out Ukraine as a priority country and violence against women as a focus for aid, thereby initiating projects that focused on implementing global policy scripts. It then moves on to explore the importance of increased political access given to women reformers who worked on developing a new legislative and policy framework for addressing violence against women. It next examines the problems that continue to prevent the establishment of programs to aid victims of violence. The chapter ends with suggestions for a theoretical framework that draws upon sociological studies of social movements and could be used to further explore the conditions under which global advocacy campaigns influence policy agendas in post-Soviet countries.

Before going further with this analysis, my standpoint on the complexities of Western intervention into post-Soviet transition needs to be acknowledged. This chapter is part of a larger research project that examines the impact of Western-funded initiatives that were established in Ukraine to address women's issues. Women's organizations in Ukraine have received considerable support from Western donors, with the largest sums devoted to the prevention of trafficking in women and somewhat smaller sums dedicated to fighting domestic violence. As I argue elsewhere, these two types of anti-violence initiatives are frequently billed as promoting women's political empowerment and strengthening support for women's rights. But they nonetheless also serve to promote Western government interests by preventing women from migrating abroad illegally to Western countries and aiding in the return of undocumented migrants to their communities of origin (Hrycak 2011). Anti-violence initiatives have provided aid to some migrants. They have also given rise to a complex field of women's organizations and an elite stratum of expert organizers and professional activists in non-governmental organizations (NGOs), who act as gatekeepers of Western aid aimed at strengthening civil society. Ironically, these projects have provided financial support mainly to professional NGOs that operate job skills seminars or offer training in self-empowerment, rather than to the grassroots women's voluntary associations that, at least according to their mission statements, Western women's NGO projects were designed to assist (see Hrycak 2006). As Hemment (2004) notes, in her research on such NGO development initiatives in Russia she has found that Western 'support for NGOs . . . comes with strings attached; NGOs that accept donor support are required to take on the responsibilities of the retreating state, picking up the slack for the radical free market,' meanwhile, generally, such 'NGO-ization' acts to 'demobilize social movements' by minimizing local concerns about the transition and creating 'new hierarchies [that have] allowed former elites to flourish' (p. 821).

As I demonstrate below, Western anti-violence projects have led to positive changes in state policy and legislation that protect women from abuse and can be used to prosecute human traffickers. But so far, initiatives to fight human trafficking and domestic violence have been unable to reverse the broader socioeconomic decline that is provoked by the neo-liberal reforms promoted by Western donors. They leave largely unaddressed the economic conditions that unleashed the tide of illegal immigration and contribute to rising rates of domestic abuse, conditions that are likely to be exacerbated further by privatization. Nor do anti-violence projects aid in reintegrating most of the migrants who are deported from Western countries through anti-trafficking programs and who are compelled to return home to communities plagued by economic insecurity. Instead of working to protect the rights of women migrants (most of whom go abroad to work as nannies or nurses), anti-trafficking crusades continue to direct resources towards rehabilitating the 'victims of sex slavery.' By continuing to code women who cross borders as victims of sex trafficking ('fallen women,' if not prostitutes), these projects to 'promote women's empowerment' may unintentionally disempower women by reaffirming damaging stereotypes, in some cases leading migrants to be labelled negatively and rejected by their communities upon their return.

Bearing in mind that Western aid to post-Soviet countries has had a range of consequences that are contradictory, complex, and often negative, it is my contention that anti-violence initiatives have also had decidedly different *policy* outcomes in Ukraine than in neighbouring countries. There is much to be gained, therefore, by investigating the surprising effectiveness of legal and policy reform initiatives in Ukraine.

Conceptualizing Violence against Women

Violence against women was not recognized as a political issue during the Soviet era. The leaders of the Communist Party claimed that Soviet women had achieved equality and emancipation and denied that any systematic violations of women's rights took place in the Soviet Union (Johnson 2009). In practice, state policies on women's issues served to bolster the participation of women in the labour force and reverse declines in the birthrate – while failing to address gender-based income inequality and a host of other issues affecting the status of women. When restrictions on independent organizing were relaxed in the late 1980s, advocates of new women's issues became active in public life and began organizing women and raising new issues (Hrycak 2002). But violations of women's rights attracted the interest of small circles of intellectuals and human rights activists. Instead of addressing gender discrimination, most of the women's groups that emerged during the late 1980s voiced various other concerns (Buckley 1997). In particular, women activists challenged the Soviet state to recognize violations of human rights that occurred during military service. Many activists also sought enhanced state assistance to mothers of large families, single mothers, mothers of disabled children, and other categories of needy mothers.

Violence against women first began to be viewed as a social problem in need of state action after the Soviet Union collapsed and the post-Soviet states were established. At that time, a broad range of international actors placed pressure on post-Soviet states to develop policies based on global human rights treaties. The most visible were international agencies such as the United Nations and the World Bank; foundations such as George Soros's Open Society Institute, the Ford Foundation, and the MacArthur Foundation; and development agencies and related projects sponsored by the United States, Canada, and other Western countries.

Pressure to adopt comprehensive policies to defend women's rights intensified in response to an external event: the Fourth World Conference on Women held in 1995 in Beijing. The Beijing Conference exposed post-Soviet states to new policy norms, models, and practices. The NGO Forum introduced post-Soviet women activists to new understandings of violations of women's rights and new tactics utilized by transnational advocacy networks to pressure states into honouring their international treaty commitments. Bringing states into compliance with the Beijing Declaration and with the mandates of international treaties (e.g., CEDAW) became a central focus for subsequent women's activism.

Participation in preparations for the conference and the NGO Forum triggered new political processes that enhanced the salience and visibility of violations of women's rights, creating potential political opportunities to place violence against women (and other new issues, such as gender equality) on the agenda of local women's organizations as well as their allies. Among the most crucial results of participation in Beijing was the collection of credible information on the status of women and its dissemination to potentially sympathetic actors in the state, international NGOs, intergovernmental organizations, and foundations. The gathering of credible information on an issue, which Keck and Sikkink (1998) call 'information politics,' is central to human rights work but had been suppressed in the Soviet era. All states that participated in the Fourth World Conference on Women were expected to hold public discussions and parliamentary hearings to examine the information that explored the status of women in their country (Rudneva 2000). State officials in Ukraine and other post-Soviet states were faced for the first time with the opportunity to collect, analyse, and publish data assessing the country's progress towards complying with CEDAW. Ukraine had ratified CEDAW in 1980. In accordance with its provisions, officials submitted periodic country reports to the U.N. Commission on the Status of Women on measures the state had taken to remove barriers standing in the way of equality for women. However, they had never conducted an independent assessment of the effectiveness of these measures, as earlier reports were submitted during the Soviet era, when the Communist Party leadership dictated the conclusions of reports to the United Nations.[2]

The preparations for Beijing thus created new discursive opportunities for advocates of women's empowerment. Women legislators, state officials, scholars, and heads of women's organizations were tasked with organizing the hearings, gathering data, providing testimony, and participating in identifying concerns they had about the status of women.[3] It was in response to these activities that violence against women first began to gain recognition as a distinct policy issue. Government representatives issued a series of specific recommendations for government activities to protect women's rights. Among the measures they called for was the establishment of shelters, crisis centres, and rehabilitation centres for battered women, as well as comprehensive legal and institutional reforms that would protect women from violence (Laboratoriia zakonodavchykh initsiiatyv 2004).

Beijing marked a crucial turning point for how women's organizations and state officials in post-Soviet countries discussed, understood, and worked on women's issues. Notably, participation in this event initiated a paradigm shift in how violence against women was framed. Domestic violence came to be seen as a distinct social problem that required legislative and policy remedies.[4] Yet, only some of the post-Soviet countries that participated in Beijing responded to the conference's mandates by passing legislation to address gender violence. Therefore, exposure to global policy scripts and frames cannot explain why countries adopt new policy models, nor can it explain why Ukraine stands alone among post-Soviet countries as an early adopter of global policy recommendations regarding violence against women.

International Assistance

Resources are needed to mobilize credible information and promote support for new causes. Funding is a second crucial force that greatly influenced the local impact of global campaigns to address gender violence and other women's issues. The Soviet state had long promulgated institutional arrangements that disabled potential loci of criticism or opposition and constrained efforts to engage in political reform. Surveillance, repression, and control over public expression left a legacy of 'atomization' and 'alienation' from 'meaningful political or collective activity' (Verdery 1991). There is widespread agreement that Western funding set women's rights activism in motion in post-Soviet states by offering grants, opportunities for travel, and other inducements to organizers (Hrycak 2002, 2006; Johnson 2009; Sundstrom 2005).

After the breakup of the Soviet Union and the end of the Cold War, Western donors became the key supporters of initiatives to promote state reform. They set up numerous projects to promote economic restructuring and political reforms and provide humanitarian assistance. They also provided crucial financial support for local human rights groups. The donors that became the most active in efforts at what came to be called 'civil society building' and 'democracy promotion,' for example, the United States Agency for International Development (USAID) and George Soros's Open Society Institute, dedicated significant resources to support local initiatives to address women's issues. At first, within the former Soviet Union, donors directed their activities mainly towards projects located in Russia. But in the mid-1990s, Ukraine rose in prominence as a target of Western aid after the Clinton administration made the country a centrepiece of its post-Soviet transition programs (Pishchikova 2006).[5] Once the U.S. government singled out Ukraine as a priority country for democratization, other donors followed suit.[6]

In the late 1990s, new pools of resources became available to pursue the two issues that commanded most interest among international donors: human trafficking and domestic violence (Richter 2002). The U.S. government was the first Western donor to make the prevention of human trafficking a priority of its post-Soviet foreign aid program. Prevention of domestic violence also became a principal focus for international aid at this time, because the U.S. government considered domestic violence to be a root cause of trafficking (Pishchikova 2006).[7] And because the U.S. government, and other Western donors, came to consider it to be a 'priority country,' Ukraine began receiving more direct funding for women's issues than it had in the early 1990s, when aid providers tended to cover most of the post-Soviet region through offices based in Russia.

The increasing centrality of violence prevention activities in Ukraine among Western women's initiatives is illustrated by the shifting aims of the main projects USAID funded to address women's issues in post-Soviet countries. The first major project USAID supported to strengthen women's activism in the post-Soviet region was the New Independent States – United States (NIS – US) Women's Consortium, a network of post-Soviet and U.S. women's NGOs headquartered in Moscow and. Washington, DC (Hrycak 2002).[8] The original mission of the consortium was to foster partnerships and exchanges between women's NGOs in the United States and post-Soviet countries, thereby strengthening the capacity of post-Soviet women's groups to provide training that would help local women to become political leaders, entrepreneurs, and providers of services to women, as well as advocates of changes in policies affecting women. In 1997, the consortium moved its office from Moscow to Kyiv. Subsequently, USAID narrowed the focus of its women's rights program to the prevention of human trafficking.

In 1999, USAID began disbursing multimillion dollar grants for anti-trafficking projects in Russia and Ukraine.[9] USAID projects to fight trafficking established nationwide networks of crisis centres and business incubators throughout Russia and Ukraine. They also funded a broad range of other activities related to violence prevention in Russia and Ukraine, including the development, refinement, and implementation of new policies on the prevention of trafficking that were coordinated through the American Bar Association – Central and East European Law Initiative (ABA–CEELI). USAID also provided additional support for other projects to strengthen local organizations working to fight trafficking and domestic violence. One such key program was the Project Harmony Domestic Violence Community Partnership Program. In 1999 and 2000, under the auspices of this program, groups of representatives of civic organizations and state agencies travelled from several Ukrainian cities to sister cities in the United States, where they received training in the prevention of domestic violence and human trafficking and visited crisis centres and shelters for battered women. Upon their return, they were given further financial and technical support to transplant these organizations to the Ukrainian context.

Another important source of funding that channelled resources towards projects addressing violence against women was the Ukrainian branch of philanthropist George Soros's Open Society Institute – the International Renaissance Foundation. The International Renaissance Foundation set national women's rights advocacy in motion in Ukraine in the early 1990s by sponsoring seminars that introduced Western conceptions of women's rights, by funding local projects to raise women's issues, and by facilitating attendance by women's advocates at the NGO Forum at the Fourth World Conference on Women and other international women's rights conferences. After Beijing, from 1996 until 2004, the Renaissance Foundation operated a project in Ukraine called 'Woman in Society,' which drew attention to new issues and transformed understandings of women's rights. Women in Society helped initiate interest in domestic violence, which was one of its priority issues. The program provided grants that helped local advocates who were interested in violence prevention to participate in international conferences and exchanges, engage in the development of crisis centres to aid victims of abuse, and participate in projects to change the state's handling of violence.

Also of central importance to initiating and sustaining these new efforts to reform the state's handling of violence against women was the women's rights program of the U.N. Development Program (UNDP) (Mel'nyk 1999). In 1997, as part of a broader U.N. initiative to provide assistance to post-communist countries, the UNDP Gender in Development Program started a project called 'Equal Opportunities in Ukraine,' whose aim was to promote the 'mainstreaming' of gender and human rights concerns in the organization's programs and activities (Smolyar 1999, 2001; UNDP 2003). A unit referred to as the Gender Bureau was placed in charge of this project's activities. The bureau was delegated the role of working directly with Ukrainian state agencies and government officials on programs to protect women's rights, in particular, developing comprehensive legal measures to address violence against women.

Western donors were crucial intermediaries in stimulating new forms of women's activism that raised awareness of violence against women among women activists in the newly independent states of the former Soviet Union. Most aid providers initially focused their energies on Russia, which became the first gateway to international assistance. However, by the late 1990s, they began to differentiate among post-Soviet countries and singled out Ukraine as a country whose transition was of particular significance. Simultaneously, international assistance providers began to encourage projects to address violence against women in Ukraine. International assistance facilitated exposure of Russian and Ukrainian women's rights advocates to global policy scripts through international conferences. It provided further incentives to direct attention to violence against women.

U.S. funding priorities had a dramatic impact on local women's movements in post-Soviet countries, encouraging both a proliferation of new groups and a shift among women activists away from other issues towards the prevention of domestic violence and human trafficking (Hemment 2004, 2007).[10] In both Ukraine and Russia, Western funding became the main source of support for a rapidly growing field of professional women's organizations (Suslova and Karbowska 2003; Sundstrom 2005).[11]

Generally, studies have found that Western funding has not been able to achieve its broader mission of empowering women as political actors (Hemment 2004, 2007; Henderson 2003; Hrycak 2002). Many activists, who previously had worked on other issues, began to identify the prevention of domestic violence as one of their priorities in order to vie for grants and other forms of support and encouragement. The intervention of Western donors raised the salience of domestic violence as a policy issue. But it has had complicated effects on local efforts to pass and implement national laws against violence, to reform the criminal justice response to violence, and to mobilize a public following for women's activism (Johnson 2009; Hrycak 2010b). In Russia, international assistance to women's rights advocates was extensive, enabling many valuable projects to be undertaken: crisis centres were established, public awareness campaigns were undertaken, and research on violence conducted. However, policy initiatives experienced little success, as illustrated by the fate of projects to pass a new law against domestic violence. In 1994, a draft law was submitted to the state Duma, but it failed to pass. Since then, more than forty drafts of a law against domestic violence have been rejected by the Duma, which has become increasingly dominated by anti-Western political blocs. As the Russian case demonstrates, sustained and extensive international assistance will not result in the passage of policies to combat domestic violence when political structures and participatory channels are closed to Western-style policy models. The following section turns to examine a crucial mediating factor that explains Ukraine's early adoption of legislation to combat violence against women: the openness of state actors to Western policy recommendations.

State Openness to Campaigns against Domestic Violence

Political openness is often assumed to encourage political activism, while 'closed' political opportunity structures are often assumed to discourage it. Crucial differences characterized the political opportunity structure activists faced in Russia and Ukraine. The early 1990s was a time of great optimism regarding post-Soviet democratization. Government elites throughout the former Soviet region exhibited openness to mobilization by civic actors, relaxed prior restrictions on political life, and declared commitments to Western and international policy models. But by the end of the 1990s, only Estonia, Latvia, and Lithuania had successfully democratized and were actively pursuing integration with the West. Meanwhile, the governments of all other post-Soviet countries had become noticeably more repressive and more hostile to Western ideals, although to varying degrees. Government repression of political opponents and civic groups and hostility to Western states and their efforts to promote democracy ranged from more moderate and intermittent in such countries as Ukraine and Moldova, to extreme in Belarus and, later, Russia. By the late 1990s, Russia, Belarus, and most of the countries of the Caucasus and Central Asia, were ruled by authoritarian regimes that expressed antagonism towards Western donors and their efforts to promote the development of legal and institutional reforms. Authorities unleashed an increasing wave of repression against civic groups, the media, and opposition politicians. In most post-Soviet countries, this wave of repression succeeded in consolidating political power in the hands of authoritarian leaders. But it backfired in Georgia in 2003, Ukraine in 2004, and the Kyrgyz Republic in 2006, when growing blocs of Western-leaning political groups successfully ousted authoritarian regimes through 'coloured revolutions.'

All post-Soviet countries that experienced 'coloured revolutions' also passed legislation to prevent domestic violence and exhibited greater responsiveness to their women's rights treaty obligations than did either the consolidated democracies of the Baltics or the post-

Soviet states that became authoritarian by the late 1990s. Why did this happen? In Ukraine, the efforts of political blocs to compete for power involved numerous contests for legitimacy: these created opportunities for women's rights advocates to become seen as potentially valuable allies. It was President Kuchma himself who created the most important political opportunity for women's rights activism by agreeing, in the mid-1990s, to establish a new state agency devoted to gender issues. A chief priority of the Beijing Platform for Action was the establishment of 'national machinery' to advance women's rights. CEDAW requires national machinery within the state apparatus to monitor the problems of women, to enhance women's rights, and to ensure equality of opportunity. There was, however, no state agency in Ukraine for coordinating state activities to advance women's rights (Mel'nyk 1999). Before attending the Beijing World Conference, ex-Party functionaries approached President Kuchma. Arguing that 'administrative structures' focused on 'gender equality' and 'women's problems' existed throughout the world and that Ukraine also needed to adopt such an approach, they requested that he create a state unit to coordinate policies in this domain.[12] He gave his consent. In 1995, at the national level, a new unit was formed to raise the status of women, mothers, and children: the Committee on Women, Maternity, and Childhood under the Authority of the President.[13] The following year, this structure was expanded, becoming the basis for the Ministry for Family and Youth, whose mandate was expanded to include the development and implementation of policy on the family, women, youth, and children (Kulachek 2005). The ministry proposed a number of legislative bills, presidential decrees, and government decisions that adapted global policy scripts to define and defend women's rights in Ukraine.[14]

The ministry was successful in placing violence and the other issues identified by the Beijing Action Plan on the state policy agenda. The National Action Plan for 1997–2000 to Improve the Status of Women in Society, for instance, outlined violence as a key area of concern for the status of women and defined mechanisms for fighting it. The ministry also created new access points for women's rights activists by establishing two expert advisory boards: a Gender Council and a Coordinating Council on Women's Issues. These two bodies brought together representatives of new women's NGOs to develop joint projects with state agencies and the Verkhovna Rada (parliament of Ukraine). One of their most important tasks was working with parliamentary deputies to draft legislation that would advance women's rights. The councils also worked to bring together women's rights groups and legislators who were interested in developing laws on gender equality and domestic violence.

The ministry developed the first measures to reform the state's handling of domestic violence. Its official policy recommendations closely followed the global policy script suggested by CEDAW and the Beijing Platform for Action. Following the recommendation of international gender experts, the ministry's representatives vowed to direct state funds to create a 'set of networks to link international organizations, foreign foundations, state officials, and local women's NGOs that were involved in advocacy against domestic violence, the reform of laws, and the provision of social services to victims' (Kolos and Danyleiko 1999). Second, they also promised funding to help local civic organizations provide support to victims of violence and unveiled a plan to offer seminars on domestic violence to raise awareness among state officials of the need to create a nationwide network of local crisis centres and shelters providing support for victims of violence. Ministry officials stressed that they planned to work on violence through the establishment of cooperative networks that brought together state officials and local women's NGOs. The measures recommended, and the discourse adopted in framing violence prevention as a cause, were quite new to Ukraine and other post-Soviet countries. They were called for by the Beijing Platform for Action and by international assistance providers.

Ministry officials encouraged women's NGOs to single out domestic violence and human trafficking as hot button issues. The increasing salience of gender violence became evident in 1998, at the First Congress of Women in Ukraine, an event the ministry sponsored and organized (Dovzhenko 1998; Kolos and Danyleiko 1999). A distinct sub-unit of the congress was devoted to discussing policies to prevent various forms of violence against women, in particular, human (or sex) trafficking. The congress issued resolutions calling on the public and the government to develop concrete solutions to fight violence against women and human trafficking. Among the steps the congress recommended were, first, for the Rada to amend the Criminal Code of Ukraine and other legislation in order to define three new categories of violence against women: domestic violence, forced prostitution, and trafficking in women. Second, the congress recommended that the state create particular institutions to assist victims of violence, including 'service networks, centres of rehabilitation for women who have suffered from violence, including within the family,' and that it support all the crisis centres for women that had come into existence in Ukraine (Dovzhenko 1998). As in the case of the 1995 recommendations of the parliamentary hearings, these proposals were based on the global scripts provided by international treaties and global campaigns to combat violence against women.

The openness of the Ukrainian state to Western policy proposals is further illustrated by efforts to create and refine new legislative and policy measures to fight human trafficking and domestic violence. In 1998, Ukraine became the first post-Soviet country to pass a law criminalizing human trafficking, Article 124.1 of the amended Criminal Code of Ukraine. The following year, Ukraine became the first post-Soviet country to launch a comprehensive state program to prevent and combat human trafficking. In 2000, specialized criminal investigation units were established within the Interior Ministry and Security Service to prosecute trafficking cases. The Ukrainian state subsequently responded with speed to international efforts to refine state handling of human trafficking. After Ukraine signed the U.N. Palermo Convention against Transnational Organized Crime, hearings were held in the Verkhovna Rada that later led to the passage of a draft law to amend the Criminal Code of Ukraine.

Ukraine's legislators also displayed considerable openness and relatively little resistance to global policy models, passing the first piece of legislation in post-Soviet countries to address domestic violence using the comprehensive approach called for by the Beijing Platform for Action (Government of Ukraine 2004).[15] A working group set up by the UNDP Gender Bureau helped to draft this law in the late 1990s. In 2000, the law's sponsors introduced it to the Rada and it passed its first reading with little opposition. In 2001, after a second reading elicited little debate, the Law on the Prevention of Violence in the Family was passed and entered into force.

Exposure to global policy models and the resources provided by international assistance to address violence against women together encouraged women's rights advocates in Russia, Ukraine, and other post-Soviet states to focus on domestic violence and human trafficking. But openness to Western models among state actors (particularly pro-Western legislators) was the third crucial facilitating factor that helps to explain why Ukraine became an early adopter of global policy recommendations for women's rights. At the same time that international assistance providers focused on pressuring Russia, Ukraine, and other post-Soviet states to enact policies to fight gender violence (specifically, domestic violence and human trafficking), authoritarian regimes throughout the region were growing increasingly hostile to Western policy recommendations. In Ukraine, however, the president and legislators both continued to support the passage of Western-style reforms. Campaigns to enact policies to address violence succeeded in politically divided Ukraine and in the few countries where authoritarian consolidation did not take place (Georgia and the Kyrgyz Republic). In sum, international resources and pressure appear to achieve the greatest policy success where the polity is decentralized, but they tend to fail when it is centralized.

Implementation of New Women's Rights Projects

New women's rights projects were initiated in Ukraine during a politically turbulent era when deep political divisions emerged over Ukraine's geopolitical orientation, initiating frequent symbolic contests for legitimacy. One political bloc embraced a pro-Western orientation and sought membership for Ukraine in both the European Union and NATO. Another bloc opposed this geopolitical orientation and expressed support for retaining close political and economic relations with Russia. Increased political competition between these two blocs created political opportunities for women reformers, but also limited their ability to implement new policies and establish new programs to assist women. This section focuses on problems that have befallen projects to address gender violence as the political fortunes of institutional sponsors have waxed and wane.

Implementing policies to prevent gender violence requires sustaining the commitment of high-level sponsors of new projects. The fate of the state agency charged with developing and implementing legislation and policies to prevent violence illustrates several of the main challenges such projects have faced in response to fluctuations in the commitments of their high-level sponsors in the government. The Ministry for Family and Youth was created in order to serve as the 'national machinery' for coordinating state efforts to implement treaties and laws addressing women's rights. As such, it was also the main state agency responsible for developing and implementing policies to address violence. But in 1999, before the ministry's projects had been implemented, it was dismantled. Paradoxically, this was done in order to demonstrate Ukraine's compliance with Western donors' neo-liberal agendas, which called for evidence that recipients were reducing the size of their states. Women's issues were bundled together with child and youth welfare as well as sports and tourism, and placed under the jurisdiction of a series of state agencies that were repeatedly dissolved.

In 2005, following the Orange Revolution (which ended Leonid Kuchma's time as president and led many of his allies to lose their government posts, at least temporarily, thus perhaps lessening the need to show symbolic support for Western-style women's activism), the government initiated a further reorganization of these units that resulted in the merging of the Ministry for Family, Children, and Youth with the State Committee on Sport and the establishment of a new ministry, the Ministry for Family, Youth, and Sport. Within this new ministry, the unit charged with addressing women's issues is small, has low status, and is devoted mainly to the family. Furthermore, the budget of the ministry is devoted mainly to organized sports, in particular, participation in the Olympics and other international athletic competitions (Kulachek 2005, 204).[16] In sum, the national machinery that was so crucial for the success of earlier campaigns to prevent violence against women lost the capacity to carry out its own policies. This administrative move has undermined the machinery for promoting gender issues, leaving state officials concerned with women's rights struggling to sustain themselves and reliant mainly on funding from international donors. In the absence of coordinated pressure from central state authorities, municipalities have failed to respond to new legislation and national government programs obligating municipalities to fund local organizations that provide services to survivors of violence. Indeed, the Kyiv municipal authorities have recently attempted to close the country's oldest shelter for battered women.

As mentioned above, moments of political vulnerability have been crucial determinants of the local impact of international pressure and assistance; however, as these examples suggest, in Ukraine, openness to reform appears to be cyclical and seems to occur mainly during moments of intense competition between Western-leaning political reformers and their opponents. The impact of transnational advocacy campaigns, global frameworks, and international pressure on state policy is thus clearly mediated by the structure of domestic political opportunities. Whenever Western-leaning parties or leaders have emerged victorious and taken control of the government, new political access points have been created for introducing new approaches to women's rights based on global policy paradigms. But before these changes have been implemented successfully, parties and leaders who oppose a pro-Western geopolitical orientation have retaken control over the government and cut off support for policies and programs associated with Western integration. A return has been initiated to a state policy that adopts a more traditional Soviet definition of women's issues, which identifies women with motherhood and the family. The government has reduced its support for fighting domestic violence and human trafficking because these issues are associated with 'gender mainstreaming' efforts intended to bring Ukraine closer to membership in the European Union.

Reformers' efforts at building new state agencies to address women's issues have nonetheless resulted in several achievements. First and foremost, they led to official recognition of several new women's issues, in particular, domestic violence and human trafficking. State acknowledgment, in turn, has spurred the development and refinement of new state policy that places greater priority on preventing violations of women's rights. State policy created new access points for partnerships between the state and civic groups, and this has created a potential new local source of support for the activity of civic organizations that raised women's issues. Such partnerships between state officials and local women's NGOs led to the passage of the 2001 Law on the Prevention of Violence in the Family and several other laws and state programs that made international treaties and global models the basis for Ukrainian policy on issues of violence.

However, the creation of state administrative structures to address women's issues also has had negative effects; once high-level political commitments shift when the balance of power tips away from Western-leaning political forces (Hrycak 2007). Leaders of women's rights groups, who worked with state agencies on the development of the law on domestic violence and related projects based on international women's rights advocacy, noted with bitterness that during President Kuchma's second term, it seemed that the women's movement lost its earlier leverage over the state and, as a consequence, was unable to monitor or participate in the implementation of the state programs that resulted from earlier collaboration with women's NGOs (Skoryk 2006). As the state became increasingly authoritarian, officials lost interest in partnering with civic actors and this, in turn, led to a decline in the overall activity level of civic organizations concerned with women's issues. Furthermore, just as in many other countries, the state agencies that came into being to advance women's equality for the most part were treated as peripheral and were bundled with an amorphous set of assistance categories that typically included children and mothers.

New political opportunities were created after President Viktor Yushchenko assumed office in 2004, and pro-Western politicians came to power. As mentioned earlier, state authorities increased support for state-funded hotlines, shelters, and other forms of practical support for victims of domestic violence. They also opened six new shelters for victims of domestic violence, eighteen new crisis centres that provided a wide range of services to women going through crises such as divorce or domestic violence, and twenty-four new centres for psychological and medical assistance. Gender equality legislation was passed, and gender advisory bodies were created within government ministries to provide expertise from women's rights groups on how to further harmonize Ukrainian and European Union policies. Women's and human rights groups also were given the opportunity to discuss the shortcomings of the implementation of laws and policies with lawmakers and state authorities through a Parliamentary Hearing on Gender Violence held in November 2006.[17] In 2007, as mentioned earlier, the Rada held the first discussion of a new draft law to amend the law on domestic violence to bring it in line with the recommendations made by women's rights advocates and Amnesty International (Amnesty International 2008). The Rada passed this amended legislation in 2008. The amendment was an important step forward for protecting women from violence, as it deleted a clause that could lead women to be blamed for provoking violence, and thus permit perpetrators to avoid prosecution (see Chapter 2 on discussion of this issue). However, with the decline of President Yushchenko's power, broader implementation of anti-violence programs has slowed.

Conclusions

What conclusions can be drawn from the preceding analysis of activities to combat violence against women? Ukraine's early and positive response to global advocacy around issues of gender violence makes Ukraine what social scientists call an exceptional or 'deviant' case – that is, one that behaves differently from the other cases with which it is generally compared. Typically, such cases are used to *disprove* a theory (because proving a theory would require more cases). They may also be used to suggest avenues for future research on omitted conditions or variables of interest in explaining an outcome that diverges from theoretical predictions. Indeed, I argue above that the case analysed here helps disprove the three main theories typically used to explain response to global policy regimes and transnational advocacy to combat violence against women: world polity theory, world civilization theory, and global feminism theory. World polity theory stresses exposure to global scripts and world civilization theory stresses the resonance of national and global values, while global feminism theory typically places greatest emphasis on ties to transnational feminist advocacy groups. I argue above that exposure to global scripts cannot account for Ukraine's divergence from other post-Soviet countries. All post-Soviet countries participated in the Fourth World Conference on Women held in 1995 in Beijing, the principal international policy event that introduced countries to global policy scripts and created normative pressure for them to adopt women's rights models in line with the Beijing Platform for Action. Support provided by international aid helped domestic reformers forge ties to foreign feminists, thus spurring local advocacy campaigns, but it alone cannot account for Ukraine's divergent outcome, as aid to Russia began first, and arguably exceeded aid to Ukraine.

Analysing a deviant case requires a focus on differences from other similar cases, as looking for 'differences in initial conditions' helps 'to account for differences in outcome' (Emigh 1997, 680). Studying an early adopter of transnational feminist advocacy projects also helps to shed light on the mediating conditions that enabled women's rights advocates in Ukraine to be more successful in using global policy scripts to reshape their country's gender regime than has been the case in other post-Soviet countries. So, if the main conditions pointed to by other theories are necessary but not sufficient, what is the crucial mediating condition that helps us to explain when we should expect global scripts to be adopted? I argue above that the crucial difference between such early adopters as Ukraine and such non-adopters as Russia lies in the structure of domestic political opportunity. Three of the post-Soviet countries that have passed laws against domestic violence experienced 'coloured revolutions' (Georgia in 2003, Ukraine in 2004, and the Kyrgyz Republic in 2005). Somewhat similarly, Moldova, the one exception, witnessed similar protests against alleged electoral fraud in 2009 in what some have called the Twitter Revolution. Shortly thereafter, Moldova also passed an act for the prevention of domestic violence. By contrast, non-adopters of such policies fall into two categories: the Baltic States (which made their turn to Western-style democracy before the wave of global advocacy against violence); and Russia, Belarus, and the remaining post-Soviet countries (all of which were becoming consolidated authoritarian regimes when the wave of global advocacy peaked).

My analysis suggests that domestic political opportunities for local anti-violence advocacy result less from Western aid itself than from deep divisions within the polity that render power holders in Ukraine more open to the policy proposals advocated by global women's rights advocates. This hypothesis is broadly in line with general social scientific findings on social movements in other regions of the world. Theorists of activism have found that infusions of external resources (such as those provided to post-communist countries by Western donors) are unable to explain the success of social movements and may even weaken them. Shifting political opportunities are far more important, because they significantly reduce the costs of mobilization by increasing perceptions that mobilization is likely to achieve success. Typically, the most important dimensions of shifting political opportunity are: (1) the opening up of access to the political system for new actors, (2) shifting political alignments among elites, (3) the appearance of new allies within the polity, (4) the emergence of splits within the elite, and (5) a decline in the state's willingness or ability to repress challengers (Tarrow 1998, 76). The relative openness of the political system, the stability of elite alignments, the presence of elite allies, and the state's capacity for repression all shape the ability of challengers to mobilize (McAdam et al. 2001). The emergence of social movements in post-Soviet countries as well as in other non-democratic contexts often follows favourable changes in a political system – such as the rise or success of opposition parties that may see alliances with new challengers as beneficial. Also important as initiators of such mobilization are 'negative opportunities' – such as the crises that eroded public support for regime elites in the countries that experienced 'coloured revolutions.' Indeed, future research should explore how deep and growing divisions within post-Soviet political systems have affected policy on other issues that are not coded as 'women's issues.'

A further crucial conclusion can be offered regarding globalization. Some scholars of globalization argue that the rise of supranational institutions and an increasingly integrated global economy signals the decline of the nation state, but this study suggests that such a conclusion is premature at best. The state still matters in conditioning the possibilities for activists not only to engage in political campaigns that cross national boundaries but also to put into practice the policies they recommend. Its response to global campaigns suggests that state-level actors are central to understanding the factors that mediate between supranational institutions and nation states. It is particularly important to 'bring the state back in' to study women's activism in post-Soviet countries, most of which are governed by authoritarian and semi-authoritarian political dynamics.

Finally, future research should look comparatively across countries to determine what mechanisms and approaches facilitate the implementation of new state programs against violence. Because adopting global policy models involves an encounter between local activists and ideas from elsewhere, it is instructive to examine what helps in the reception of new types of language and discourses that have developed within the new policy domain concerned with violence against women. As has been noted in analyses of global women's rights advocacy, many American phrases (e.g., 'gender,' 'empowerment,' 'training of trainers') and, more broadly, an American discourse of self-empowerment, have migrated from Western projects into the vocabulary of the NGOs that work on women's rights campaigns in post-Soviet states (Hrycak 2006). Similarly, various American phrases and discourses have made their way into state programs against trafficking and domestic violence in Ukraine. The adoption of new vocabulary solves some problems: most importantly, it creates new visibility and legitimacy for concepts that have no easy equivalent in local parlance. But it creates new problems as well. Law enforcement personnel in Ukraine have levelled much criticism at the confusing terminology employed in anti-trafficking legislation. Global policy models introduced new terms such as 'debt bondage,' 'sexual exploitation,' and 'exploitation of work' without providing guidance as to their definition or application. Prosecutors have complained that the law's provisions cannot be applied as long as the main elements of the crime had not been defined in practical terms. Similarly, law enforcement officers are normally given specific procedures to follow in enforcing new laws, but the initial legislation was not accompanied by instructions for handling cases of human trafficking. As a consequence of such problems of translation and application, prosecutors were initially reluctant to initiate cases against traffickers (Fedkovych 2007).[18] Considerable efforts have been made to further refine new anti-violence campaigns so that new policies can be used as intended. Donors have funded various programs to retrain law enforcement personnel and fine-tune legislation. Their efforts have met with some success, as with every passing year, more trafficking cases are prosecuted. Nonetheless, the most recent anti-trafficking legislation – which was intended to be an improvement over the previous law – continues to employ terminology that law enforcement personnel find unclear and confusing. Future research should explore the puzzle of implementation: what works and what does not work for bridging the discursive gap between recipients and producers of new state policy to prevent violence.

ACKNOWLEDGMENTS

Fieldwork and interviews were conducted for this project with leaders of women's NGOs in Kiev, Lviv, and Kharkiv. I am grateful to the women scholars and activists whom I interviewed, and to the International Research and Exchanges Board and Reed College for financial support.

NOTES

1 I have compiled this information mainly from the Stop Violence Against Women website (STOPVAW), available at http://www.stopvaw.org/ Country_Pages.html (accessed 5 April 2009). Another useful source is the Council of Europe's webpage on violence against women in members states, available at http://www.coe.int/T/E/Human_Rights/ Equality/05._Violence_against_women/.
2 For instance, the introduction to the initial report of the Ukrainian Soviet Socialist Republic (CEDAW/C/5/Add.11) at its 16th and 21st meetings, held on 5 and 10 August 1983 (CEDAW/C/SR.16 and 21) stated: 'As a result of the Great October Socialist Revolution, the principle of equality of the sexes had come to be applied for the first time in history and had become an integral part of the policy of the State.' Experts on the committee noted the strong similarity between the reports submitted by the Ukrainian SSR and the USSR, and also indicated in their review that statistics and data were not provided to assess progress towards gender equality.

3 For the text of this hearing, see http://www.rada.gov.ua/zakon/skl2/
   BUL23/120795_97.htm.
4 In the case of Ukraine, many prominent women's rights advocates I
   interviewed noted that Beijing initiated a dramatic shift in how the status
   of women was conceived (interview, League of Women Voters 50/50, Kyiv,
   3 May 2001; interview, National Council of Women, Kyiv, 12 July 2001;
   interview, president and founder, Ukrainian Women's Union, Kyiv, 8 June
   2001; interview, Women's Information Consultative Centre, Kyiv, 22 March
   2001; interview, Ukrainian Women's Studies Centre, Kyiv, 27 June 2005;
   interview, Kharkiv City Women's Fund, Kharkiv Oblast Diia, Kharkiv, 29
   May 2001).
5 During the crucial first decade and a half of independence, the U.S.
   government outspent all other Western donors in Ukraine. Using U.S.
   government sources, I estimate that the U.S. government provided over
   three billion U.S. dollars for various assistance projects since independence
   in 1991; see U.S. Overseas Loans and Grants, available at http://qesdb.
   usaid.gov/cgi-bin/broker.exe (accessed 9 May 2007).
6 For instance, Canada also later came to view Ukraine as a 'priority
   country' for democratization; indeed, it was the only country in Eastern
   Europe given this classification.
7 Western projects to halt illegal immigration tied together the issues of
   domestic violence and trafficking in women because they assumed that
   victims of domestic abuse could not remain in the country and fell into the
   hands of cross-border human trafficking rings.
8 The consortium was created using funding the Clinton administration
   earmarked for women's leadership training in the former Soviet bloc. In
   1994, Winrock received two initial grants: a $95,000 grant from the Eurasia
   Foundation, and a $750,000 grant from USAID. The consortium's initial
   aim was to create partnerships between established NGOs in the United
   States and newly formed women's groups located in post-Soviet countries.
   Through partnerships with a sister NGO in the United States, local NGOs
   were to learn to advocate on behalf of women.
9 In addition to these two anti-trafficking projects, in 1999 Winrock
   International started two other projects that were also related to the
   prevention of trafficking: Women's Economic Empowerment and
   Supporting Micro, Small, and Medium-Size Enterprise Development. The
   former was awarded a total of $3,612,399 in funding from USAID; the
   latter received $1,544,294.
10 Interview, Women's Information Consultative Centre, Kyiv, 22 March
   2001.

11 In Ukraine, the number of women's organizations increased from five
in 1991 to well over 1,200 by 2001 (Sydorenko 2001). Similarly, in Russia,
women's organizations experienced rapid numerical growth. However, the
impact of activities funded by Western initiatives has been complex and
hard to assess. Sundstrom, for instance, notes that, 'growth in numbers of
NGOs themselves cannot be considered an accurate indicator of movement
success, because foreign donors sometimes encourage growth in numbers
of organizations through their grant programs, but those numbers
may not indicate high levels of movement activity. Many organizations
remain hollow with few members and even one person forming several
organizations, largely as a result of donors' preference to grant funds to
many different organizations over time' (2005, 424).

12 In response to Beijing and other events that introduced them to
international women's rights activism, several of these state-builders
embraced new Western models of women's rights advocacy that focused
on achieving gender equality (interview, former deputy director, Ministry
of Family and Youth, Kyiv, 27 July 2001).

13 Interview, League of Women Voters 50/50, Kyiv, 3 May 2001.

14 In 1999, the ministry was transformed into the State Committee for Family
and Youth, which took responsibility for the status of women and gender
equality. A further series of reorganizations has taken place, with a variety
of state units given responsibility for women's issues.

15 The Law on the Prevention of Violence in the Family calls for the state to
provide funding to crisis centres, shelters, hot lines, and other facilities that
provide medical and social rehabilitation to victims of domestic violence.
It specifies conditions under which temporary restraining orders are to be
issued. It also requires perpetrators of domestic violence to attend training
sessions on non-violent behaviour patterns.

16 For more detailed information on the Ministry of Family, Youth, and Sport,
see http://www.kmu.gov.ua/sport/.

17 Women's rights advocates were concerned by the lack of state support
ensuring adequate short-term and long-term alternative housing for
victims of domestic violence as well as elements of the original law that
they deemed harmful to women.

18 According to information provided by the Ministry of Internal Affairs in
2001, only 30 criminal trafficking cases were filed during the first two and
a half years after the adoption of Article 124.1 in 1998 until 2001 (Rudneva
et al. 2005). Subsequently, the number of cases filed increased steadily:
2 in 1998, 11 in 1999, 42 in 2000, 91 in 2001, 169 in 2002, and 289 in 2003
(Lutsenko et al. 2005).

REFERENCES

Amnesty International. 2008. *Ukraine.* Amnesty International Country Reports. Available at http://thereport.amnesty.org/eng/regions/europe-and-central-asia/ukraine (accessed 8 Nov. 2008).

Beckfield, J. 2008. The Dual World Polity: Fragmentation and Integration in the Network of Intergovernmental Organizations. *Social Problems* 55(3): 419–42.

Boli, J., and G.M. Thomas. 1997. World Culture in the World Polity: A Century of International Non-Governmental Organization. *American Sociological Review* 62(2): 171–90.

Buckley, M., ed. 1997. *Post-Soviet Women: From the Baltic to Central Asia.* New York: Cambridge University Press.

Coomaraswamy, R. 2003. *Integration of the Human Rights of Women and the Gender Perspective: Violence against Women.* Addendum 1: International, Regional and National Developments in the Area of Violence against Women, 1994–2003. Paris: UNESCO.

Dovzhenko, V., ed. 1998. *Zhinka na porozi XXI stolittia: Stanovyshche, problemy, shliakhy sotsial'noho rozvytku: Zbirnyk materialiv Vseukrains'koho Konhresu Zhinok, Kyiv, 21–23 travnia 1998 roku* [Women on the Threshold of the 21st Century: Status, Problems, and Methods of Social Development: The materials of the Ukrainian Women's Congress, Kyiv, 21–23 May, 1998]. Kyiv: Ukrains'kyi instytut sotsial'nykh doslidzhen'.

Emigh, R.J. 1997. The Power of Negative Thinking: The Use of Negative Case Methodology in Building Sociological Theory. *Theory and Society* 26(5): 649–84.

Fábián, K., ed. 2010. *Domestic Violence in Postcommunist States.* Bloomington: Indiana University Press.

Fedkovych, H. 2007. *Violence against Women: Does the Government Care in Ukraine?* Budapest: Open Society Institute.

Government of Ukraine. 2004. *Ukraine: Beijing +10 National Reports on the Implementation of the Beijing Platform for Action.* Progress Report Prepared by the Government of Ukraine for the United Nations Beijing +10 Review in March 2005. Available at http://www.cities-localgovernments.org (accessed 26 May 2007).

Hemment, J. 2004. Global Civil Society and the Local Costs of Belonging: Defining Violence against Women in Russia. *Signs: Journal of Women in Culture and Society* 29(3): 815–40.

– 2007. *Empowering Women in Russia: Activism, Aid, and NGOs.* Bloomington: Indiana University Press.

Hrycak, A. 2002. From Mothers' Rights to Equal Rights: Post-Soviet Grassroots Women's Associations. In N. Naples and M.K. Desai, eds., *Women's Community Activism and Globalization: Linking the Local and Global for Social Change*, 64–82. New York: Routledge.

– 2006. Foundation Feminism and the Articulation of Hybrid Feminisms in Post-Socialist Ukraine. *East European Politics and Societies* 20(1): 69–100.

– 2007. Gender and the Orange Revolution. *Journal of Communist Studies and Transition Politics* 23(1): 152–79.

– 2010a. Transnational Advocacy Campaigns and Domestic Violence Prevention in Ukraine. In K. Fábián, ed., *Domestic Violence in Postcommunist States*, 74–122. Bloomington: Indiana University Press.

– 2010b. Orange Harvest? Women's Activism and Civil Society in Ukraine, Belarus and Russia since 2004. *Canadian American Slavic Studies* 44(1–2): 135–58.

– 2011. Women as Migrants on the Margins of the European Union. In M. Rubchak, ed., *Mapping Difference: The Many Faces of Women in Ukraine*. New York: Berghahn.

Joachim, J.M. 1999. Shaping the Human Rights Agenda: The Case of Violence against Women. In M.K. Meyer and E. Pruegl, eds., *Gender Politics in Global Governance*, 142–60. Lanham: Rowman and Littlefield.

– 2007. *Agenda Setting, the UN, and NGOs: Gender Violence and Reproductive Rights*. Washington, DC: Georgetown University Press.

Johnson, J.E. 2009. *Gender Violence in Russia: The Politics of Feminist Intervention*. Bloomington: Indiana University Press.

Johnson, J.E., and L. Brunell. 2006. The Emergence of Contrasting Domestic Violence Regimes in Postcommunist Europe. *Policy and Politics* 34(4): 578–98.

Keck, M.E., and K. Sikkink. 1998. *Activists beyond Borders: Advocacy Networks in International Politics*. Ithaca: Cornell University Press.

Kolos, L., and O.M. Danyleiko. 1999. Uchast' derzhavnoho komitetu Ukrainy u spravakh sim'i ta molodi v realizatsii polozhen' kompleksnoi prohramy po zapobihanniu nasyl'stvu v sim'i [The Participation of the State Committee of Ukraine for Family and Youth in the Implementation of the Comprehensive Program to Prevent Violence in the Family]. In O. Rudneva, ed., *Problemy nasyl'stva v sim'i: Pravovi ta sotsial'ni aspekty* [The Problem of Violence in the Family: Legal and Social Aspects], 83–6. Kharkiv: Pravo.

Kulachek, O. 2005. *Rol' zhinky v derzhavnomu upravlinni: Stari obrazy, novi obrii* [The Role of Women in State Administration: Old Models, New Perspectives]. Kyiv: Vydavnytstvo Solomiii Pavlychko 'Osnovy.'

Laboratoriia zakonodavchykh initsiiatyv [Laboratory of Legislative Initiatives]. 2004. *Svitova praktyka to Ukrains'kyi dosvid vykorystannia mekhanizmu parlaments'kykh slukhan' ta slukhan' u komitetakh iak instrument kontrol'noi funktsii parlamentu. Chastyna 3. Laboratoriia zakonodavchykh initsiiatyv, Prohrama spryiannia parlamentu Ukrainy Universytetu Indiany SShA* [World Practices and the Ukrainian Experience of Using Parliamentary Hearings and Committee Hearings as an Instrument for Monitoring the Functions of Parliament: Part 3. The Laboratory of Legislative Initiatives, Indiana University Parliamentary Development Project for Ukraine]. Available at http://www.parlament.org.ua (accessed 28 May 2007).

Lutsenko, Y., L. Matiaszek, S. Scanlan, and I. Shvab. 2005. *Trafficking in Ukraine: An Assessment of Current Responses*. Kyiv: UNICEF.

McAdam, D., S.G. Tarrow, and C. Tilly. 2001. *Dynamics of Contention*. New York: Cambridge University Press.

Mel'nyk, T. 1999. *Henderna polityka v Ukraini* [Gender Policy in Ukraine]. Kyiv: Lohos.

Moghadam, V.M. 2005. *Globalizing Women: Transnational Feminist Networks, Themes in Global Social Change*. Baltimore: Johns Hopkins University Press.

Pishchikova, K. 2006. *Lost in Translation: USAID Assistance to Democracy Building in Post-Communist Ukraine*. Doctoral dissertation, University of Amsterdam.

Pyshchulina, O. 2003. An Evaluation of Ukrainian Legislation to Counter and Criminalize Human Trafficking. *Demokratizatsiya: The Journal of Post-Soviet Democratization* 11(3): 403–11.

Randall, V., and G. Waylen, eds. 1998. *Gender, Politics and the State*. London: Routledge.

Richter, J. 2002. Evaluating Western Assistance to Women's Organizations. In S.E. Mendelson and J.K. Glenn, eds., *The Power and Limits of NGOs: A Critical Look at Building Democracy in Eastern Europe and Eurasia*, 54–90. New York: Columbia University Press.

Rudneva, O. 2000. Ukraine. In M. McPhedran, ed., *The First CEDAW Impact Study: Final Report*, 215–32. Toronto: York University Centre for Feminist Research.

Rudneva, O., G. Khrystova, I. Kononenko, O. Pyshchulina, and O. Kochemyrovska. 2005. *Alternative Report on CEDAW Implementation in Ukraine*. Kharkiv: Kharkiv Centre for Women's Studies.

Skoryk, M. 2006. Na shliakhu do hendernoi polityky [Developments in Gender Policy]. In Z. Bezpiatchuk, I.L. Bilan, and S.A. Horobchyshyn, eds., *Rozvytok demokratii v Ukraini, 2001–2002* [The Development of Democracy in Ukraine, 2000–2001], 71–92. Kyiv: Ukrainskyi nezalezhnyi politychnyi tsentr.

Smolyar, L. 2001.The Women's Movement as a Factor of Gender Equality and Democracy in Ukrainian Society. In O. Sydorenko, ed., *Zhinochi orhanizatsii Ukrainy: Ukrainian Women's Non-Profit Organizations*, 27–44. Kyiv: Innovation and Development Centre.

Smolyar, L., ed. 1999. *Zhinochi studii v Ukraini: Zhinka v istorii ta s'ohodni* [Women's Studies in Ukraine: Women in History and Today]. Odessa: Astroprynt.

Stetson, D.M., and A. Mazur, eds. 1995. *Comparative State Feminism*. Thousand Oaks: Sage.

Sundstrom, L.M. 2005. Foreign Assistance, International Norms, and NGO Development: Lessons from the Russian Campaign. *International Organization* 59(2): 419–49.

Suslova, O., and N. Karbowska. 2003. *'Zhinoche krylo' hromads'kykh orhanizatsii. Zaluchennia koshtiv dlia pidtrymky zhinochykh initsiatyv* [The Women's Wing of Civic Organizations: Fund-Raising to Support Women's Initiatives]. Available at http://portal.uwf.kyiv.ua/index.php/article/libraryview/36/1/4/ (accessed 28 May 2005).

Sydorenko, O. 2001. Zhinochi orhanizatsii Ukrainy: Tendentsii stanovlennia. In O. Sydorenko, ed., *Zhinochi orhanizatsii Ukrainy: Dovidnyk* [Women's Organizations in Ukraine: Developmental Tendencies], 45–52. Kyiv: Tsentr innovatsii ta rozvytku.

Tarrow, S.G. 1998. *Power in Movement: Social Movements and Contentious Politics*. New York: Cambridge University Press.

United Nations Development Program (UNDP). 2003. *Gender Issues in Ukraine: Challenges and Opportunities*. Kyiv: UNDP.

Verdery, K. (1991). Theorizing Socialism: A Prologue to the 'Transition.' *American Ethnologist* 18(3): 419–39.

Webhofer, R. 2009. *Wave Country Report 2009: A Reality Check on European Services for Women and Children Victims of Violence*. Vienna: WAVE Network.

PART II

Gender and Social Structures

5 Gender, Nation, and Reproduction: Demographic Discourses and Politics in Ukraine after the Orange Revolution

TATIANA ZHURZHENKO

Alarmist discourses about a 'demographic crisis' are not new in contemporary Ukraine. They have existed since the mid-1960s, when it became obvious that the decline in fertility in the European part of the USSR was not just a temporary response to the difficulties of the postwar era, but a stable tendency. Some pro-natalist political interventions led to a short-term improvement in fertility rates in the second half of the 1980s (Rivkin-Fish 2003). However, in the next decade the economic recession and neo-liberal reforms of the socialist welfare system, which caused economic insecurity and mass impoverishment, led to a dramatic deterioration of social and demographic indicators. Indeed, with its total fertility rate (TFR) of 1.2, Ukraine belongs to the group of European countries with very low fertility. Since 1993 the Ukrainian population has been shrinking: it dropped from 52.5 million in 1993 to 46.6 million in 2007; that is, by more than 10 per cent. By 2050 it is likely to have fallen to 29 million. Another problem is high mortality rates, particularly among males. Life expectancy in Ukraine for men is only 62.5 years, for women 74.2, a particularly large gender gap (the second worst in Europe after Russia). And, despite some progress in recent years, maternal and infant mortality rates remain relatively high.

In Ukrainian public and political discourses the 'demographic crisis' is associated with the shortage of labour resources and the 'brain drain,' with problems of the pension system due to aging of the population, and even with the issue of territorial integrity and national security. Labour migration of Ukrainians abroad, which affects first of all young educated people and women in their reproductive years, is another subject of public concern. The importation of labour as a possible solution is usually viewed with scepticism, because it might raise problems with social integration and even lead to ethnic conflicts.

As in other post-socialist societies, 'demographic anxiety' has been used by various political forces. The Communists and the left popu-lists have been using the discourse of a 'dying nation' for criticizing market reforms, whereas market liberals tend to blame the low fertil-ity in Ukraine on the poor economic conditions inherited from the Soviet era. Nationalists, for their part, usually see depopulation to be a result of the abandonment of traditional values by the Ukrainian eth-nos and connect it with the genocide politics of the communist regime, that is, the Holodomor (Great Famine) of 1932–33. As in other coun-tries of Eastern Europe, demography is at the core of reconstructing the nation, because it concerns such issues as territorial sovereignty, regional development, relations with the neighbours and the fam-ily, national culture, and interethnic relations. The discourse about a 'demographic crisis' in Ukraine is also highly gendered. Women are usually made responsible for low fertility because they selfishly prefer a professional career, consumption, and self-fulfilment to duty to their family. On the other hand, high mortality is perceived first of all as a men's issue. Ukrainian men are represented as an 'endangered species' because they have to carry the burden of breadwinner and are exposed to the risks of market capitalism. Therefore, the state's attempts to reg-ulate demographic dynamics have important implications for gender equality.

This chapter addresses gendered demographic discourses and poli-tics in Ukraine after the Orange Revolution,[1] an event that made mani-fest a new political approach to nation building. Feminist debates on demographic politics, gender, and transition draw on the classical com-parative study of welfare regimes by Esping-Andersen (1990) and their development in the post-socialist countries (Standing 1996; Deacon 2000). In Eastern and Central Europe, 'the new global ideology, conser-vative and populist endeavours and path-dependency, all play a part, resulting in producing faceless or mixed systems, some of them close to what is called "ill-fare"' (Ferge 2001, 127). From this point of view, demographic and family politics should be understood in the contexts of the neo-liberal deconstruction of the paternalist socialist state, the backlash of patriarchal values, and the emergence of new gender in-equalities (Klenner and Leiber 2009), as well as the heritage of Soviet pro-natalism (Rivkin-Fish 2010). Another important factor in the region is nation building and the return of nationalism. Nira Yuval-Davis (1997) revealed profound links connecting gender, nation, and demographic discourse and demonstrated that women not only provide the biological reproduction of the nation, but also carry the burden of its symbolic representation; this approach is certainly applicable to the Ukrainian case. I was also inspired by the work of Susan Gal and Gail Kligman (2000a, 2000b), who underline the central importance of gender and reproductive issues to political and economic transformations in post-socialist societies and combine the analysis of politics and institutions with the analysis of discourses. Last but not least, the anthropological approach to demographic politics (Douglass 2005; Rivkin-Fish 2003, 2010) offers a bottom-up analysis of the 'cultures of reproduction' and focuses on the meaning of children and parenting under different social conditions.

I start my analysis with the role of familialist and traditionalist values in the 'Europeanization' project proclaimed by the leaders of the Orange Revolution. As a next step, a closer look at new state initiatives aimed at stimulating fertility explains why, despite public anxiety about the demographic situation and despite the popular familialist rhetoric, pro-natalism remains half-hearted. Under conditions of a market economy and consumer capitalism, the socially and politically prioritized model of a 'responsible' middle-class parenthood and the changing gender roles put limits on traditional pro-natalist politics. Finally, I discuss the gender dimensions of demographic discourses and politics in Ukraine, their impact on family gender roles, women's economic status, and women's reproductive rights. This chapter is based on media materials, political speeches, and demographic research, as well as on expert interviews and focus groups conducted in Kyiv and Kharkiv in March 2009.

Ukrainian Nation Reloaded: Familialism with a European Face

According to Gal and Kligman (2000a) reproduction is at the heart of redefining a nation and of legitimizing a new democratic order, while Rebecca Nash (2005) points that 'reproductive politics is about geopolitical belonging' (p. 95). The Orange Revolution corresponds with both statements as it can be seen to be a project aimed at a new democratic quality of the Ukrainian nation and a pro-European geopolitical choice. The 'ideology' of the Orange Revolution, and the political rhetoric of its

leader Viktor Yushchenko, exemplified the dilemmas of nationalism/
traditionalism versus Europeanism embedded in the project of democratic reconstruction of the Ukrainian nation.

The dominant discourse of the Orange Revolution was the discourse
of the 'birth of the Ukrainian nation,' an emotionally loaded phrase
with a new feeling of 'Us.' In opposition to Leonid Kuchma's Ukraine,
characterized by the alienation of citizens from the state and associated
with corruption and fraud, the 'new' Ukrainian nation was reimagined
as a community united by love, trust, and common values, while the
new democratic leader presented himself as a caring father possessing
high moral authority. The 'birth of a nation' as staged on Kyiv's Maidan
Nezalezhnosti (Independence Square) referred to the powerful myth of
a 'new beginning.' Not by accident, one of the popular stories particularly loved by the 'Orange' media told about young couples who first
met on the Maidan. This narrative related a public event to the sphere
of intimate human emotions and, at the same time, to the symbolism
of procreation and the nation's future. Paradoxically, the metaphor of
the 'family,' referring to an 'organic community' united by common
origins and destiny, was central in reinventing the Ukrainian nation as
modern, democratic, and European.

In his election program Viktor Yushchenko promised Ukrainian voters a strong social policy. Among the priorities listed in his program 'Ten
Steps towards the People' was the promise of 'five million new jobs,' increased pensions and social benefits, reduced taxes, increased support
of families, and the defence of children's rights. This social program,
quite similar to the one suggested by his political opponent, Prime Minister Viktor Yanukovych, was, however, presented as a moral alternative to the cheap populism of the 'old regime.' References to 'family
values' and iconic images of his own family were actively used in the
election campaign. Yushchenko's pro-familial attitudes and his fertility
(he has two adult and three young children) represented his potential
as a man and a politician. President Yushchenko's young children in
particular became a symbol of the nation's future, of a new 'innocent'
Ukraine in contrast to the corrupted and alienated society burdened
with the Soviet past. His family sets an example to follow: it demonstrates that modern Ukrainians with higher education and professional
ambitions can have at least three children. His family also represents a
'truly Ukrainian family': it takes part in most important cultural events,
uses the Ukrainian language both in public and private, and often appears in Ukrainian ethnic clothes.

The familialist values supported by President Yushchenko correspond with his rather traditionalist attitude to gender issues. For
example, in May 2006, in one of his regular radio speeches (this time
devoted to Mother's Day and the International Day of the Family),
Yushchenko directly addressed the demographic situation in the
country. Characteristically, he began his speech with references to
the traditionally high value of the family in Ukrainian culture and
the highly respected status of the mother. As interpreted in this speech,
demographic policy was practically reduced to state support of
women as mothers, of children, and of families. Yushchenko (2006a)
stressed that the mission of the Ukrainian authorities is 'to preserve
the nation, and to do everything [to ensure] that every year more and
more healthy babies are born in Ukraine, that all children have strong
and happy families.' Praising the first steps of the state in this direction, he suggested that every Ukrainian family should now dare to
have two or three children. Although Yushchenko mentioned the need
for a modern system of preschool education, he did not actually go
beyond the traditional understanding of the family and the role of the
mother. He did not address issues of gender inequality or family violence, and at the end of his speech he referred to the notorious motto
'We should become 52 million!'[2] In another radio speech on the occasion of the Day of Children's Rights in June 2006, Yushchenko (2006b)
stressed the need to increase the child care allowances for parents with
children under 3 years of age, arguing again in a rather traditional way:
'In the first years of children's lives mothers should always be around.
The state should create all necessary conditions for this.' Characteristically, Ukrainian men were not addressed in their social role as fathers,
and the only appeal of Yushchenko to the male audience was related
to alcoholism: hard drinking, according to him, has never been part of
Cossack tradition.

Two important projects directly related to demography that have
been personally supported and supervised by Viktor Yushchenko reflect his preoccupation with both 'Europeanization' and familialism.
These are a comprehensive reform of the orphanage system, encouraging the adoption of orphans by Ukrainian families, and the charitable
program 'Warm Up a Child with Your Love!' focusing on social support
of families with many children.

The first project, known as the 'national adoption' program, is ad-
ministrated by the Ministry for Family, Youth, and Sport. This is an ambitious attempt to radically improve the material and social situation of

orphan children and children without parental care, to provide them with a family environment, and to raise their chances for social integration, better education, and employment opportunities. The core of the project is the deinstitutionalization of the state orphanage system inherited from Soviet times and its profound reform according to the European model. This implies that adoption, foster care, and 'family type' children's homes become the preferable forms of raising orphans. The funding mechanism has been reformed to support a child, not an institution (the so-called money follows child principle). The decree of the president proclaimed 2008 the Year of National Adoption. New legislation enacted in October 2008 encourages the adoption of orphans by Ukrainian families, guaranteeing them a one-time social benefit equivalent to the benefit parents receive now at the birth of the first child (12,240 UAH in 2008). One of the adopting parents is now entitled to a paid leave of fifty-six days, which is supposed to help with the integration of the child into its new family. 'National adoption' is advertised in the media, referring to examples of famous Ukrainians (such as 1996 Olympic champion Lilia Podkopayeva). New regulations enacted in 2009 make adoption rules for Ukrainians more transparent and less bureaucratic, while introducing additional requirements and controls for foreign citizens who wish to adopt a child in Ukraine.

The reform of the orphanage system is seen by the Ministry for Family, Youth, and Sport as a contribution to improving the demographic situation and as a budget-saving measure, given the inefficient management of the state orphanage system (Katrychenko 2008). But the project also carries particular ideological values, assuming that the family is the only natural environment for a child and claiming that Ukraine as a 'civilized' nation is able to care for its own children. The hidden ideology of the project connects familialism with the Europeanization of Ukrainian society while opposing both the 'false Soviet values' of communist collectivism and the ideological indoctrination in children's education. At the same time, the life chances of the majority of children in the state orphanages, who cannot be adopted because of serious health defects or psychological problems and who need professional treatment and rehabilitation, are rarely discussed. The reform is also supposed to stop the notorious corruption in the field of adoption and improve the reputation of Ukraine, which has become known as one of the biggest adoption markets. Last but not least, by giving priority rights to Ukrainian adoptive parents over foreigners it attempts to close this 'population leak.'

The second project – the charitable program 'Warm Up a Child with Your Love!' – was initiated by the president in December 2007. It has been implemented together with big business and is chaired by Yushchenko's eldest daughter, Vitalina. In 2008, the program focused on social support for families with many children: on improving their living conditions, providing medical services, helping with formalities, and so on. The program includes close monitoring of such families and their needs, and is creating a database (the so-called *pasportyzatsiia*). However, only families with ten or more children are eligible for material and social support. Needless to say, such families constitute only a tiny minority. For example, in the Kharkiv oblast, where the program works in partnership with the Olexandr Feldman Foundation, there are only nine such families. This program provides substantial help (e.g., funding a new apartment, renovating an old one, or installing a gas supply), but reaches only a very limited target group. Its main dimension is symbolic, as it contributes to the construction of the Ukrainian nation as a 'family,' with the oligarchs as patriarchal benefactors of the poor. At the same time, the charitable program honours traditional motherhood and promotes the value of childbearing.

Demographic Anxiety and Half-Hearted Pro-Natalism

From the mid-1990s, the dramatic worsening of the demographic indicators in Ukraine became obvious, but the capacity of the new state to deal with this issue was rather limited. Because of the economic crisis, even minimal family support payments were often delayed for months. Since 2001, the economic boom and growing public concern with the 'demographic crisis' brought the political elite to reconsider the possibilities of state welfare for population engineering. In June 2003, special hearings on 'the demographic crisis in Ukraine, its causes, and consequences' took place in the Verkhovna Rada (Ukrainian parliament). Underlining the alarming developments of the previous decade, including the rapid fertility decline and mortality increase, which 'hamper the economic development and threaten national security' (Parliament of Ukraine 2003), the Rada recommended the preparation of a program document dealing with demographic issues. It was supposed to take into account 'the experience of the advanced European countries' and was to be aimed at 'decreasing mortality, raising fertility, the protection, rehabilitation, and recreation of the Ukrainian gene pool, and at preventing migration, which worsens the demographic situation in Ukraine' (ibid.).

The 'Concept of Demographic Development of Ukraine' for the period 2005–15 was developed by the Institute of Demography and Social Research of the Ukrainian Academy of Sciences and approved by the Cabinet of Ministers (at that time headed by Viktor Yanukovych) in October 2004, at the peak of the presidential election campaign. After the Orange Revolution, the new political leadership ostentatiously gave priority to social issues and the Concept was developed into the 'Strategy of Demographic Development of Ukraine.' In May 2006, the new document was presented to the Rada and, a month later, was approved by the government. The Strategy explains the demographic crisis in Ukraine first of all by 'the fertility decline to a critical level.' As one of the first tasks, it proposes to reinstall 'family values' in Ukrainian society and to promote the two-child family as a model. At the same time, pro-natalist goals seem rather declarative, as no pathbreaking measures to achieve them are suggested. The Strategy declares as its main aim, not fighting depopulation, but 'improving the quality characteristics of the population' and the 'harmonization of the population's reproduction' (Parliament of Ukraine 2006).

In professional publications and debates, Ukrainian demographers are even more sceptical about pro-natalism. According to Ella Libanova (2008a), deputy director of the Institute of Demography and one of the main authors of the Demographic Strategy, decline in fertility and population aging are tendencies all across Europe, and the tools of a state to influence reproductive behaviour are rather limited. These tendencies reflect women's rising educational level and their professional career orientations, but also the new opportunities of self-realization and consumption which emerge as alternatives to childbearing. A similar position is shared by another Ukrainian demographer, Iryna Pribytkova (2008), who is also sceptical about the capacity of state policy to raise fertility significantly and change women's attitudes to childbearing.

If politicians are often tempted to call on Ukrainian families to produce more children, Ukrainian demographers do not insist on an absolute population size and propose, instead, to focus on improving health indicators. In Ukrainian demographic discourse it is not so much low fertility (which Ukraine shares with some other European countries), but high mortality, low life expectancy, and poor indicators of health that exemplify the 'backwardness' of the country. In this respect Ukraine differs from Russia, where the absolute population size has a geopolitical and strategic value for the political elites. Consequently, 'Europe' as a symbol of modernization plays a different role in Ukrainian and Russian demographic discourses. In the Russian debates 'Europe' is often seen as a source of individualism and moral decay undermining the Russian family. At the contrary, Ukrainian demographers see Ukraine following the pattern of low fertility as 'natural' for a European country.

Has Ukrainian policy become more pro-natalist since 2004? Politicians, public officials, and experts have different answers to this question. Indeed, in 2005, many of the family benefits and child care allowances were raised. The biggest sensation was certainly the radical increase of the one-time benefit paid upon child birth. From April 2005, the one-time benefit upon the birth of the first child was raised up to 8,500 UAH, a sum that is 11.7 times higher than it was in 2004. From January 2008, this sum was raised again to 12,240 UAH, while upon the birth of the second child a mother gets 25,000 UAH and upon the birth of the third (and every next) child – 50,000 UAH. A relative increase in the total number of births since 2006 has been interpreted by the Ukrainian president and his supporters as evidence for the success of the new policy and of people's growing optimism. At the opening of the local maternal hospital in Kryvyi Rih in March 2009, Yushchenko celebrated the new tendency of increasing fertility, explaining it as a success of state pro-natalist measures by stating: 'Never before in Ukraine was fertility stimulated at such a high level.'

While politicians view the new system of benefits as stimulating fertility, experts consider them, rather, an instrument of social protection for the most vulnerable social groups and have doubts about their sustainable effect on fertility. In the research monograph *Marriage, Family, and Childbearing Attitudes in Ukraine,* published in 2008 by the Institute of Demography, the authors explain the growing number of births since 2006 by the social and economic stabilization in the country and the post-crisis 'compensation' of postponed births as well as by the more numerous cohort of young women who are now reaching reproductive age (Libanova 2008b). Comparing the reform of 2005 with the pro-natalist measures introduced by the Soviet government in 1982, Ukrainian demographers argue that such policy can have only a short-term effect, as the measures cannot compensate for the low family income and changed attitudes to childbearing (pp. 33–4). Admitting that the new benefits upon child birth are supposed to stimulate fertility, the authors are sceptical about the possibility of a significant fertility increase, at least as long as the average family income remains low and the housing problem is not solved.

To summarize, for the first time in post-Soviet Ukraine, substantial economic incentives were introduced to increase fertility, but this measure has not been supplemented by a corresponding tax and investment policy or programs of social housing and child care. Moreover, pro-natalist incentives clash with the new challenges of post-communist transition that influence reproductive choices of families and individuals: consumer capitalism, new models and standards of parenthood, and the changing gender roles in Ukrainian society.

'Middle-Class Parenthood' and the Limits of Pro-Natalist Politics

Alison MacIntosh (1983) has summarized several barriers to installing pro-natalist policies in Western countries: (1) lack of public demand, (2) limits to the governments' ability to finance them, (3) doubts about the efficiency of material incentives as a means to encourage childbirth, and (4) a weak nationalist rationale. Carrie Douglass adds, in this respect, that 'in liberalizing democracies any restriction or pressure on individual liberty and autonomy seems inappropriate' (2005, 8). Drawing on interviews of experts and on focus groups conducted in Ukraine, I suggest one more argument: in the liberalizing post-Soviet state, reproduction becomes a class issue. Children are supposed to be born into families that can take full responsibility for their material provision, education, health, and preparation for adult life. The norm of 'middle-class parenthood' assumes that a couple should wait until it can 'afford' a child and offer it proper material and living conditions. Normative arguments around middle-class parenthood work through the media, advertising, and other forms of cultural production, turning child rearing into a 'consumption project.' Requirements of modern parenthood may include, for example, a separate child's room or a private nanny, extra English lessons, or expensive toys. The 'culture of responsibility' associated with middle-class parenthood poses particular expectations on parents. In the case of Ukraine, this culture of responsibility can include, for example, private medical consultations (because parents have little trust in the public health care system) or extra cooking for a child because of imagined and real dangers of environmental pollution or unhealthy food. This makes parenthood extremely time-consuming and financially demanding, and partly explains the persistence of the one-child family model.

Middle-class parenthood is not just a cultural phenomenon; it is also explicitly or implicitly encouraged by state institutions and policies. The Strategy of Demographic Development openly declares that one of its main aims is the 'formation of a "middle class" family model, which is characterized by material well-being, by investments in family, and by childbearing as a stimulus and object of such investments.' This approach is reflected, for example, in the state housing credit program for young families, which aims to help them finance a separate living space. The program offers its clients partial refunds of bank interest payments and is funded through the state budget. In 2005, after allegations of corruption, a new, more transparent regulation (based on a score system) was introduced. Because of the small budget of the program, only a very limited number of families can profit from it. Since 2006, the program has suffered from debts and insufficient funding. But, more importantly, the program is available only to those young people who already have a permanent and well-paid job. The main criteria are income level and the ability to repay loans. In fact, the program is oriented to well-educated and career-oriented young people under the age of thirty-five. The new regulation gives priority to young academics and promising athletes, while more children hardly improve the score. Only a minority of young families fit these requirements, which assume professional success and material well-being.

The ideology of middle-class parenting is reflected in the ambiguous attitudes that state institutions and society have towards families with many children. Demographers argue that the culture of high fertility has practically disappeared in Ukraine. At the same time, families with many children should be rewarded by the state as they can slow depopulation to some extent (Libanova 2008b, 20–1). However, the main reason such families get special attention is not demographic but social and economic. Household surveys demonstrate that there is a direct correlation between the number of children in a family and its level of well-being. The majority of families with three or more children live in poverty, and many of these families could not survive without state support, however limited it is.

In the late Soviet era, as a part of the pro-natalist agenda, families with many children were entitled to numerous privileges and benefits, most significantly concerning housing. Although high fertility was already stigmatized in urban Soviet society as old-fashioned and irrational behaviour, the state encouraged childbearing by supporting families with many children. Mothers of five or more children were rewarded with special medals; mothers of ten or more were honoured as 'Mother Heroines' and entitled to higher pensions. At first glance, politicians in post-Soviet Ukraine continue this kind of policy. In 1999, by presidential decree, Kuchma introduced 'Measures for Improving the Situation of Families with Many Children,' who, as part of this program, pay only 50 per cent for school lunches and child care and should have privileged access to higher education. In addition, regional authorities can introduce other forms of social support (and they often have done so, especially before elections). In 2001, the honorary title of 'Mother Heroine' was re-established. Viktor Yushchenko initiated a special charitable program aimed at social and material support of families with many children and introduced a special one-time benefit for 'Mother Heroines.'

In contrast to Soviet policy, however, which was motivated by pronatalist goals, in the Ukrainian approach, social protection dominates over encouraging births. In practice, families with many children can enjoy material support only if they belong to the low-income strata. But, only a few families fit the 'low-income' criteria, as they have to be under the (very low) official minimum wage. In 2008, only 150,000 families (9%) were registered as 'low income,' which does not correspond with the official statistics of poverty (Poda 2009). The new amendments from the end of 2008 make it even more difficult for a family to meet these criteria: a family cannot claim social support if one of its members does not work (or does not study) longer than three months, if it has a plot of land bigger than 0.6 hectare, owns another apartment, or has other sources of support. Almost 40 per cent of low-income families which get social support in Ukraine are families with many children. Experts warn that such families can be particularly hit by the economic crisis which began in 2008, because regional authorities have also introduced cost-saving measures.

Public servants responsible for the social support of families with many children often share common stereotypes about them as marginal and even deviant. In their eyes, such families behave irresponsibly because they count on state support and are not able to control childbearing. Such non-rational, non-modern reproductive behaviour does not correspond with the model of middle-class responsible parenthood. Local authorities focus their attention on the control and monitoring of such families, checking their eligibility for social support and their use of child allowances for the intended purpose. The honorary title of the 'Mother Heroine' can be awarded today only if a woman has raised her children at least until the age of eight and if, for example, none of the children has ever been criminally punished. This means she has to be not just a biological mother, but also a socially responsible one. For their part, the associations of families with many children present them as being 'more responsible' than one-child families. They praise the values of mutual support and altruism that dominate in their families and stress their contribution to improving the demographic situation. Thus, families with many children find themselves at the centre of various political dilemmas: between liberal ideology and familialism, between the state's pro-natalist desires and public fears of 'poverty proliferation,' and between traditionalist values supporting the extended family model and the modern ethos of 'responsible parenthood.'

Demographic Policy and Gender Equality

Women as bearers of children are the first to be affected by state efforts to regulate the demographic dynamics. This particularly concerns measures to raise fertility. There is an ongoing debate in gender studies whether or not pro-natalist ideologies and policies inherently conflict with women's rights and gender equality (Heitlinger 1991; Yuval-Davis 1997). Although, in some cases, pro-natalism is inspired by nationalism and neo-traditionalist ideology, reducing women's role to the biological reproduction of the national 'body,' in other cases welfare policies encouraging fertility can be women-friendly and gender-aware. Leslie King (1998) argues that 'pro-natalist programs are specifically relevant to women in at least three ways. First, pro-natalist policies may include measures to limit access to contraceptives as part of an overall plan to increase births. Second, policies can affect women's economic status through birth allowances, single-parent benefits, or state-run child care facilities that make it easier for women to participate in the labour force. Finally, pro-natalist policies can influence gender roles by promoting particular family forms, such as families where the mother remains at home with the children' (p. 33). A glance into Ukraine's newest demographic policies through this angle helps in understanding its gender dimension.

In Eastern Europe, at least two examples of pro-natalist politics were heavily based on denying women's control over their bodies: in the Soviet Union under Stalin and in Ceausescu's Romania. However, banning abortion (and limiting access to contraception) with the aim of increasing births was also practised in liberal countries, historically. In Poland, where the restoration of moral and religious values in the post-communist society was the main impetus of the anti-abortion initiatives, demographic considerations also played a role (Zielinska 2000). In contemporary Russia, the issue of low fertility and the still-high number of abortions are often discussed in connection with one another, as abortions are seen to be a potential 'resource' of increasing births. Conservative politicians as well as the Russian Orthodox Church consider sex education at school and knowledge about contraception harmful to Russian family morals, and abortions are seen as worsening the demographic situation; in some regions such educational programs have been suspended.

In this context, Ukraine is one of the few European countries where abortion has not become a political issue. As in Russia, in Ukraine, the high number of abortions is discussed in moral terms, but unlike in Russia, abortion is rarely connected to the problem of depopulation. Abortion issues concern the demographic situation only in one respect: the popularity of abortion is seen by experts to be the main reason for women's reproductive health problems, which contribute to low fertility. Mass use of abortion is seen as a regrettable Soviet heritage,[3] a barbaric habit to be overcome through education and the use of modern contraception. Indeed, the number of abortions in Ukraine has dropped almost by half in recent years (from 34.1 per 1,000 females of fertile age in 2000 to 17.3 in 2007) and by 80 per cent compared with 1991 (DKSY 2008, 185). However, the number still remains high compared with European indicators. Family planning workers stress that in Ukraine there is no systematic opposition to publicly funded sex education programs and propaganda of modern contraception.

With the exception of Western Ukraine, where some local initiatives have recently appeared, there is no pro-life movement in Ukraine. Opinion polls show little public interest in this issue, and they demonstrate that only a tiny minority of Ukrainians (even among religious persons) would support the idea of strengthening abortion regulations.[4] What is probably more important is the fact that there is no consolidated conservative political force in the country interested in raising this issue. Ukraine's regulations on abortion from 2006 are rather liberal, as they allow abortions to be carried out up to twelve weeks' gestation without restrictions. Between the twelfth and twenty-second weeks, women are eligible to request an abortion for health reasons and specific social reasons (such as pregnancy resulting from rape). Earlier regulations on abortion (1993) allowed abortions for health and social reasons until the twenty-eighth week and listed among social reasons three or more children in the family, divorce, death or illness of the husband during pregnancy, imprisonment of the husband, and so on. In fact, unemployment or a severe financial situation sometimes was also considered a sufficient reason. In 2006, the Cabinet of Ministers significantly reduced the list of social reasons for abortion, a fact that went practically unnoticed by the Ukrainian public. Because abortion in the second trimester remains an exception anyway, these restrictions can hardly be related to pro-natalist intentions. To summarize, even the radical opponents of abortions in Ukraine believe that the problem can be solved neither by banning measures nor by measures that would help to raise fertility. Thus, concerns with the dramatic demographic situation in Ukraine have not been translated into restrictive policies on abortion and access to contraception. On the contrary, sex education programs supported by the state, non-governmental organizations (NGOs), and international donor organizations seek to improve women's reproductive health as one of the factors of higher fertility.[5]

The next question concerns the way demographic policies in Ukraine (either already practised or just planned) might affect women's economic status and their situation in the labour market. Women's relatively low economic status and persisting discrimination against them remain a serious problem, despite their high level of education and active participation in the labour force. The gender wage gap in Ukraine is more than 30 per cent, and women constitute 68 per cent of the registered unemployed. Despite the new 2005 Gender Equality Law, an effective mechanism preventing gender discrimination in the labour market has not yet been created. Women with small children, especially those with low qualifications and without a work record, have little chance to get a job, and young married women, that is, prospective mothers, are particularly discriminated against in the labour market. The Labour Code guarantees women with small children the right to a part-time job, but employers often are not interested in providing such an opportunity, especially in the private sector.

Although increased child care allowances (and particularly significant benefits upon child birth) might improve the economic situation of women as legally acknowledged beneficiaries of state support (which is particularly relevant for single mothers), they can hardly improve women's status in the labour market in the long term. Moreover, the Ukrainian system of family and maternal benefits hardly encourages women to return to the labour market after maternity leave. It also does not encourage a combination of maternal duties with professional obligations, as it does not offer special compensation for kindergarten fees or for private child care, as in other countries. A policy aimed at providing mass availability and high-quality of child care would be much more important from a gender equality point of view (and at the same time would stimulate fertility). Some Western countries such as Germany also concerned with low fertility recently made significant investments in the child care system. In Ukraine, the Ministry for Family, Youth, and Sport recognizes the current shortage of places in the daycare centres. Many kindergartens were closed during the 1990s, when the demand for places in them was low and funding was insufficient, and their premises were privatized and used for other purposes. Today, property developers often do not keep up with the regulations that oblige them to provide child care facilities in new residential areas. The lack of available and good child care, especially for children with special needs and health problems, impedes not only women's careers but also the rise of fertility.

And finally the last question: how do demographic policies in Ukraine, particularly measures aimed at increasing fertility, affect gender roles in the family and in society? Are demographic politics in Ukraine gender sensitive? Krause (2005) points out the 'moralizing effects of alarmist demographic discourses': without naming them explicitly, women are made responsible for low fertility. Ukraine is not an exception in this respect. Moreover, public discourse in Ukraine is highly gendered: if women are held 'responsible' for low fertility, high mortality appears first of all as a 'men's problem'; as a result of the high consumption of alcohol, unhealthy lifestyle, and hazardous labour conditions, mortality among men, particularly those between the ages of 20 and 45, is much higher than among women. Both demographers and journalists tend to focus on women's childbearing attitudes as if men did not participate in reproductive decisions. They see women's emancipation as a main factor of low fertility without taking into account the changes in post-Soviet masculinity and men's social roles. At the same time, the problem of men's high mortality is usually discussed without taking into account women's and family problems. In many ways, this approach continues the old Soviet discourse on the 'crisis of masculinity' (Zdravomyslova and Temkina 2002), which presented men as an endangered species and passive victims. The problem with Ukrainian men as presented in the media is twofold: on the one hand, men are 'spoiled' by women from childhood on and remain infantile boys, unable to take responsibility for a family, looking for pleasure (alcohol, smoking), and enjoying risk; on the other hand, men suffer from permanent stress related to the high competitiveness and insecurity of the modern market economy, and from the all-too-heavy burden of being the breadwinner.

Both demographic problems, however – low fertility and high male mortality – should be approached jointly, as they require both radical changes in the dominant model of masculinity and an improvement in the social position of women. Ukrainian demographers have already suggested consideration of new forms of demographic policy, based not only on family values, but also on principles of gender equality. In particular, Scandinavian countries achieved one of the highest levels of fertility in Europe by creating opportunities for women to combine their maternal role with professional life and by actively involving men in child care. For example, in Norway men have a statutory right to be granted a father's portion of parental leave and they actively use it. An enlightened and gender-aware pro-natalism based on the active promotion of new gender roles can also be more effective in the long run. At the same time, promoting 'new' models of masculinity oriented to such values as family, health, and a safe way of life will contribute to reduce mortality.

A shift to such an approach can be found in Ukraine, both in state policy and in civil society. Along with women's NGOs, new men's groups and initiatives are emerging that deal with the issues of parenthood, children's rights and education, and family violence. Also successful are the so-called schools of fatherhood ('daddy schools') or schools for responsible parenting which promote new gender roles (supported by the Equal Opportunities United Nations Development Program in Ukraine). Several NGOs have launched an initiative on establishing a Father's Day in Ukraine (similar to Mother's Day) in order to bring attention to the issue of fatherhood. Problems like avoiding paying alimony, a father's right to regular contact with his child after divorce, among others, which have been silenced until now, have become the subject of public discussion. The Ministry for Family, Youth, and Sport also supports new gender roles in the family. Ukrainian law now allows fathers to make use of child care leave until the age of three years, and makes fathers eligible for all family and child care benefits. Moreover, amendments on the statutory right for fathers to ten days of paid leave upon the birth of child and for paid care leave in case of a child's illness are under consideration. However, because of women's lower wages, the choice of who takes a child care leave in most cases is decided automatically. Ukrainian men and Ukrainian families in general can only profit from these new opportunities if women's status in the labour market is improved.

Conclusions

Disturbing demographic tendencies, first of all a dramatic decline in fertility and a high mortality, have forced the Ukrainian political elites to reconsider the role of social welfare for population engineering, while the economic recovery at the beginning of this century has allowed the introduction of substantial material incentives for bearing children. The Orange Revolution endowed these reforms with the ideological values of Europeanization and neo-traditionalism. However, the pro-natalist ambitions of the Ukrainian state are limited, not only by economic and social insecurity, but also because of the changing gender roles and the dominant values of 'middle-class parenthood.' The new demographic policies are liberal regarding the reproductive rights of women, but they neither encourage women to combine a family and a professional career nor do they improve their economic status. The problems of low fertility and high men's mortality can only be solved by a gender-aware demographic politics that encourages new models of masculinity and new gender roles in the family.

ACKNOWLEDGMENT

I am grateful to the ERSTE Foundation (Austria) for supporting my research.

NOTES

1   For a review of earlier family politics and its gender implications in Ukraine, see Zhurzhenko (2004).

2 In the summer of 2005, about 500 billboards in Kyiv displayed the slogan: 'Let's make love! We should become 52 million!' It remained unclear who commissioned this 'social advertising,' but the action had significant public resonance.

3 Abortions were liberalized in the USSR in 1955.

4 See also the complete findings of a sociological survey published in *Natsional'na bezpeka i oborona* (National Security and Defence) 3 (2001): 21–4. Available at http://www.razumkov.org.ua/ukr/journal. php?y=2011&cat=159.

5 For example, the educational project 'Together towards Health' (2006–10), supported by USAID, is aimed at improving women's and men's reproductive health and it promotes modern practices of family planning.

REFERENCES

Deacon, B. 2000. Eastern European Welfare States: The Impact of the Politics of Globalization. *Journal of European Social Policy* 10(2): 146–61.

Derzhavnyj komitet statystyky Ukrainy/State Statistics Committee of Ukraine (DKSU). 2008. *Dity, zhinky ta sim'ia v Ukraini* [Children, Women and the Family in Ukraine]. Kyiv: DKSU.

Douglass, C.B., ed. 2005. *Barren States: The Population 'Implosion' in Europe.* Oxford: Berg.

Esping-Andersen, G. 1990. *The Three Worlds of Welfare Capitalism.* Cambridge: Polity.

Ferge, Z. 2001. Welfare and 'Ill-Fare' Systems in Central-Eastern Europe. In B. Sykes, B. Palier, and M. Prior, eds., *Globalization and European Welfare States: Challenges and Change,* 127–52. Basingstoke: Palgrave.

Gal, S., and G. Kligman. 2000a. *The Politics of Gender after Socialism: A Comparative-Historical Essay.* Princeton: Princeton University Press.

Gal, S., and G. Kligman, eds. 2000b. *Reproducing Gender: Politics, Publics and Everyday Life after Socialism.* Princeton: Princeton University Press.

Heitlinger, A. 1991. Pro-natalism and Women's Equality Policies. *European Journal of Population* 7: 343–75.

Katrychenko, T. 2008. Ne chuzhi dity [They Are Our Children, Too]. *Glavred* 47(96): 28–31.

King, L. 1998. France Needs Children: Pro-natalism, Nationalism and Women's Equity. *Sociological Quarterly* 39(1): 33–52.

Klenner, C., and S. Leiber. 2009. *Wohlfahrtsstaaten und Geschlechterungleichheit in Mittel- und Osteuropa.* Wiesbaden: VS-Verlag.

Krause, E.L. 2005. Toys and Perfumes: Imploding Italy's Population Paradox and Motherly Myths. In C.B. Douglass, ed., *Barren States*, 159–82. Oxford: Berg.

Libanova, E., ed. 2008a. *Borot'ba za kozhnu dytynu* [Fighting for Every Child]. Interview with Ella Libanova. Available at http://dialogs.org.ua/dialog. php?id=23andop_id=611#611 (accessed Feb. 2009).

– 2008b. *Shliub, Sim'ia ta Ditorodni Oriientatsii v Ukraini* [Marriage, Family, and Childbearing Attitudes in Ukraine]. Kyiv: ADEF-Ukraina.

MacIntosh, A.C. 1983. *Population Policy in Western Europe*. Armonk: M.E. Sharpe.

Nash, R. 2005. The Economy of Birthrates in the Czech Republic. In C.B. Douglass, ed., *Barren States*, 93–114. Oxford: Berg.

Parliament of Ukraine. 2003. *Rekomendatsii parlamentskyh slukhan 'Demografichna kryza v Ukraini: iiii prychyny ta naslidky'* [Recommendations of the Parliamentary Hearings 'Democratic Crisis in Ukraine: Its Causes and Consequences']. Available at http://zakon.nau.ua/doc/?uid=1071.610.0 (accessed 4 Sept. 2004).

– 2006. *Strategiia demografichnoho rozvytku v period do 2015 roku* [Strategy of Demographic Development for the Period until 2015]. Available at http:// zakon1.rada.gov.ua/cgi-bin/laws/main.cgi?nreg=879–2006-%EF (accessed 7 June 2007).

Poda, V. 2009. Maloobespechennykh v Ukraine pochti net [There Are Almost No Low-Income Families in Ukraine]. *Kommentarii*, 13 Feb.

Pribytkova, I. 2008. *Expert: Demograficheskaia situatsiia v Ukraine stabilizirovalas'.* [Expert: The Demographic Situation in Ukraine Is Stabilized]. Available at http://newsukraine.com.ua/news/101642/ (accessed 17 Nov. 2008).

Rivkin-Fish, M. 2003. Anthropology, Demography, and the Search for a Critical Analysis of Fertility: Insights from Russia. *American Anthropologist* 105(2): 289–301.

– 2010. Pro-natalism, Gender Politics, and the Renewal of Family Support in Russia: Towards a Feminist Anthropology of 'Maternity Capital.' *Slavic Review* 69(3): 701–24.

Standing, G. 1996. Social Protection in Central and Eastern Europe: A Tale of Slipping Anchors and Torn Safety Nets. In G. Esping-Andersen, ed., *Welfare States in Transition: National Adaptations in Global Economies*, 225–55. London: Sage.

Yushchenko, V. 2006a. *Mother's Day Address.* Address to the Nation by President Yushchenko, 13 May. Available at www.president.gov.ua/news/3206. html (accessed 20 June 2006).

– 2006b. *Address on Children's Rights*. Address to the Nation by President Yush-chenko, 3 June. Available at www.president.gov.ua/news/3400.html (ac-cessed 20 June 2006).

– 2009. *Narodzhuvanist' v Ukraini stymuliuiet'sia iak nikoly'* [Fertility in Ukraine Is Stimulated as Never Before]. 3 March. Available at http://ua.for-ua.com/ukraine/2009/03/05/150712.html (accessed 20 June 2009).

Yuval-Davis, N. 1997. *Gender and Nation*. London: Sage.

Zdravomyslova, E., and A. Temkina. 2002. Krizis maskulinnosti v pozdne-sovetskom diskurse [Masculinity Crisis in the Late Soviet discourse]. In S.A. Oushakine, ed., *O Muzhe(n)stvennosti* [On Masculinity], 432–51. Moscow: Novoe Literaturnoe Obozrenie.

Zhurzhenko, T. 2004. Strong Women, Weak State: Family Politics and Nation Building in Post-Soviet Ukraine. In K. Kuehnast and C. Nechemias, eds., *Post-Soviet Women Encountering Transition*, 23–43. Baltimore: Johns Hopkins University Press.

Zielińska, E. 2000. Between Ideology, Politics, and Common Sense: The Dis-course of Reproductive Rights in Poland. In S. Gal and G. Kligman, eds., *Reproducing Gender*, 23–57. Princeton: Princeton University Press.

6 (Re)Constructing Ukrainian Women's History: Actors, Authors, and Narratives

OKSANA KIS

Initial historical and ethnographic research on Ukrainian women emerged in the second half of the nineteenth century. At that time, a number of eminent Ukrainian scholars researched women's issues and published a range of original works revealing various aspects of the lives of ordinary Ukrainian women, on topics ranging from pre-marital sexual relations to women's status under the law.[1] In fact, research on women was one of the most advanced and rapidly growing areas of Ukrainian studies at the turn of the twentieth century. Those writings, however, had their shortcomings. As early as 1929, Kateryna Hrushevska (1900–1943), then a young historian and ethnographer, was expressing serious concern about the male bias inherent in these works. Her article, 'Towards a Study of Sex Groups in Primitive Societies' (1929) became a kind of academic manifesto for new – feminist – principles of research into the history and anthropology of women. Hrushevska identified the main problem of historical research as follows: 'It tends to treat women outside the cultural context.' Her insight into the androcentric (male-dominated) character of scholarship anticipated Simone de Beauvoir's idea of the female as a second sex. 'Since for some reason,' Hrushevska wrote, 'the men's world – male-public aspects of culture – happened to be researched more thoroughly it makes an impression that it is in fact the norm, whereas the women's realm constitutes just a variation, episode, or fragment' (pp. 26–8). Hrushevska stressed the need to take into account women's perspectives in order to create an accurate and complete picture of the past.

That very promising direction, however, was brutally disrupted in Soviet times, when the majority of Ukrainian scholars (including

Hrushevska) were repressed.[2] In Ukraine, basic principles of feminism were distorted by Soviet ideology and discredited by state-imposed, socialist practices.[3] This ultimately resulted in profound misconceptions of, and prejudices against feminist scholarship among Ukrainian historians. Ukrainian women's history stagnated as a subject; no significant research emerged during this period.[4] What took its place were publications on Soviet women's lives and achievements. Written by order of the Communist Party leadership, however, these were strictly ideologically framed and thoroughly censored to serve the goals of Soviet propaganda. As such, they can hardly be used as informative sources for reconstructing women's history during that time.

When the USSR collapsed, Ukrainian scholars recognized women's history as an underdeveloped research area. Desperately searching for a new start, they identified two possible jumping-off points: (1) they could return to works on women's issues by pre-Soviet Ukrainian historians and ethnographers (published in the Russian and Austro-Hungarian empires in the late nineteenth and early twentieth centuries), or (2) they could turn to writings emerging from the Ukrainian diaspora (published mainly in the United States and Canada after the Second World War). At that time, in the early 1990s, post-Soviet Ukrainian social sciences and humanities were in crisis; there was a methodological vacuum, theoretical chaos, and very poor access to the principal Western works on women's history. That crisis helps explain the admiration and uncritical perception by fledging historians of women in Ukraine of their predecessors' works.

During that first decade after the collapse of the totalitarian order, Ukrainian scholars struggled to fill gaps in their theoretical knowledge of, and research into Ukrainian women's pasts. This was by no means easy; the academy did not consider women's history as a fully autonomous field and therefore provided minimal (if any) support for it.[5] Despite this hostility, feminist historians continued their work, which has resulted in numerous scholarly publications, students' essays, doctoral theses, and even elective university courses taught all over Ukraine. Thus, it is undeniable that women's history has, in fact, become a research field of its own in contemporary Ukraine, although it is still maturing.

History is never a politically neutral subject, of course, and Ukraine's past remains a battlefield in many areas, including women's history. Politically invested approaches to and interpretations of Ukrainian women's historical legacies continue to influence the development of further research into the field, while the field itself has become an object of political manipulations and is used as a point of reference for those involved in developing instruments and policies to implement gender mainstreaming in Ukraine. But a true understanding of today's gender order is impossible without a clear understanding of the genesis and historical transformations of that order in this specific cultural context, and this, in turn, requires a clear view of women's history and how it has been interpreted over time.

In this chapter, I map Ukrainian women's history by exploring the origins and peculiarities of four prevailing narratives in the field. Each of these narratives constructs its own version of the past and carries particular political messages (both implicit and explicit). Based on a careful overview of the body of work on Ukrainian women's history published in Ukraine and available to Ukrainian readers (including original research by Ukrainian scholars and Ukrainian translations of foreign authors), these narratives are as follows:(1) *Berehynia*, in which adherence to an eternal Ukrainian 'matriarchal' past is stressed, as well as the concept of a feminine Ukrainian mentality; (2) *the great woman* narrative, where outstanding Ukrainian women are praised and their personal achievements lauded; (3) *national feminism*, which argues for a unique movement beyond existing feminist paradigms and explores women's contributions to the Ukrainian national cause; and (4) *woman's devotion*, which highlights ordinary women's experiences.

After describing each of these narratives in detail, I discuss the role of official/political history in framing women's history as a research field as well as the impact on the field of dominant national narratives. I demonstrate the extent to which women's history has been entwined with politics over time. I conclude that, in Ukraine, the feminist paradigm was not embedded in research on women's history during the 1990s, and thus the national discourse (with its patriarchal implications) has framed the field and determined its developments in terms of themes, approaches, interpretations, and conclusions. Finally, I address some recent problems and challenges faced by Ukrainian women's history.

Berehynia

The narrative of *Berehynia* is based on the idea of matriarchy as inherent to Ukrainian society from ancient times up to the present day. This idea first originated in the works of Ukrainian ethnographers and folklorists publishing at the turn of the twentieth century. At that time, the evolutionist theory of matriarchy was very popular in the social sciences, and Ukrainian scholars attempted to find and to expose its traces in Ukrainian culture.[6] These scholars highlighted women's special roles in ancient rituals and the relative autonomy women enjoyed in Ukrainian society as an indicator of how progressive this nation was compared with neighbouring nations. The influence of these writings was powerful, carrying over time. Ivan Franko, a distinguished Ukrainian ethnographer and poet, expressed these views in 1883 (in Franko 1980, 210): 'Since ancient times all the educated people who have looked closely at Ukrainian life have admitted that Ukrainians treat their women in a much more gentle, more humane and liberal way than their neighbouring nations. Women occupy very respected and honourable positions in the family.'

The Berehynia narrative was also strengthened by Ukrainian literature, which reflected the culture of a stateless nation and therefore often praised folk culture. In popular novels, Ukrainian writers at the fin de siècle (some of whom shared a feminist world view) created vivid portrayals of strong, self-sufficient, and powerful women.[7] Written in a realistic manner, these works were (and sometimes still are) perceived as a mirror of everyday life. Together, the ethnographic works and Ukrainian literature impacted Ukrainian mass consciousness during the time of the national revival in the 1980s; people began to believe that Ukrainian women always enjoyed broad rights, privileges, and respect in the family and society. None of those writers or scholars working at the turn of the twentieth century, however, used the actual term *Berehynia*.

The modern concept of Berehynia – a symbolic matriarch and guardian of Ukrainian national culture and ethnic identity – was invented much later. It seems to have emerged at the time of the Ukrainian national upheaval during perestroika in the late 1980s through the writings of several authors. It is quite remarkable that patriotically spirited male Ukrainian writers conceived of an allegedly ancient Ukrainian pagan goddess, Berehynia, to further their cause.[8] Works by these writers were widely read and cited, allowing the concept to filter into the public discourse of post-Soviet Ukraine. Although heterogeneous, representing a combination of pagan beliefs, matriarchal myth, and Christian ideas as well as popular folk motifs, Berehynia pretended to represent an 'authentic' Ukrainian femininity.[9]

In the early 1990s, at a time of a desperate lack of substantial studies of Ukrainian women's history, the idea of Ukrainian matriarchy was easily revived in the academy, and scholars took for granted the conclusions of their predecessors, including the (never proven) idea of the Ukrainian matriarchal past. Modern adherents of this concept saw themselves to be the heirs and successors of fundamental (and unjustly interrupted) research on Ukrainian women's history conducted a century before.[10] The actual history of matriarchy among ancient Ukrainians, meanwhile, was never examined in depth, and to this day no comprehensive study either confirming or disproving it has been published. Instead, in the 1990s, Berehynia spread unchecked inside academia and beyond. Authors of numerous publications on women's issues, regardless of their field of inquiry, steadily referred to the 'native traditions of matriarchy.' For example, in the chapter 'The Status of a Woman in the Historical Past' from her book *A Woman: Self-Fulfilment in the Family and Society* (1999), sociologist Natalia Lavrinenko fills her pages with unsubstantiated statements such as 'since the period of matriarchy' and 'the protracted remains of matriarchy among Ukrainians.' Even the most solid and substantial works written by professional historians are sometimes affected by the Berehynia narrative, as demonstrated in the volume *Women's Studies in Ukraine: A Woman in History and Today* (Smolyar 1999). The first chapter, 'Matriarchal Beliefs in Ukrainian Culture: Feminine Principles in Ukrainian Mentality,'[11] by Olena Lutsenko, repeatedly strikes the reader with groundless statements such as 'Ukrainian woman as the peculiar and independent female type,' and 'the image of Berehynia is deeply rooted in the matriarchal family cult of spirit-protectors' (pp. 15–17). The chapter also presents quotations from other works without any clear theoretical or critical approach. The narrative ultimately leads the reader to conclude that Ukrainian women always experienced exceptionally high social status and gender equality (if not all-out dominance) and that these realities are inherent to Ukrainian culture.

Normally, texts framed by the Berehynia narrative contain no analysis of empirical data. Instead, certain favourable historical facts about Ukrainian women (from archaeology, ancient history, rituals, religion, folklore, literature, history of law, and social history) are taken out of context, uncritically exaggerated, and used to confirm the inherently egalitarian (if not matriarchal) character of the gender order in Ukraine. Since Ukrainian women have allegedly never experienced discrimination, the logical conclusion the reader is left to draw is that a feminist approach is totally irrelevant to research on Ukrainian women's history.

This problem is caused mainly by the fact that, while adherents to the Berehynia narrative may be experts in various academic areas, they are not professional historians. As dilettantes in women's history, they merely repeat the opinions of prominent figures, some 'commonplaces,' or both, without ever questioning or critically reconsidering them. In fact, their pseudo-scientific 'historical' revelations become vehicles for the popularization of a distorted vision of Ukrainian women's past and the legitimization of outdated theories. The impact of these publications on mass consciousness is detrimental: invested with the authority of science, they appear as reliable and trustworthy references for schoolteachers, activists, and journalists who then spread further the dubious idea of an 'eternal Ukrainian matriarchy.'

Thus, while scholarship surrounding the Berehynia narrative is feeble, its impact on public discourse in Ukraine has been paradoxically important. During the 1990s, parties to literally every public discussion on women's issues applied the notion of Berehynia and corresponding rhetoric to argue for a special Ukrainian path to women's emancipation that precluded feminism. At the peak of its popularity in the late 1990s, Ukrainian politicians, both men and women, used and promoted the concept of Berehynia for various political purposes. This happened at all levels of political authority, in different forms, on a wide variety of occasions, particularly in International Women's Day speeches.[12] Thus, the official greeting from the former speaker of the Verkhovna Rada (Ukrainian parliament), Oleksandr Tkachenko, on 8 March 2000, entitled 'Berehynias of Our Immortal Family,' addressed Ukrainian women in the traditional way: 'Woman-Mother, Woman-Wife, a Berehynia of our family . . . I sincerely wish you eternal beauty, strong health, happiness, and a sincere love' (Tkachenko 2000). Three years later, Volodymyr Lytvyn, who is the current speaker of the Rada, congratulated women with similar language: 'Woman in her various representations – as mother, wife, sister, lover – is the most blessed among all of us . . . She is a crown of nature, a sacred object, mother, housewife, girlfriend, worker, Berehynia of a family hearth, embodiment of the highest human virtues . . . I wish you strong health, a spring mood, kindness and family happiness' (Lytvyn 2003). Local authorities reiterated this kind of address, as we can see in the following examples: 'The words "family," "kin," "mother," "Berehynia" are a single whole, namely, Life. Our mothers, eternal Berehynias of a family hearth, have the most beautiful eyes, the tender hands, and the most faithful hearts' (*Nikolayev Vecherniy* 2003); and 'the 8th of March is the holiday of our Berehynias. Our present and our future achieve-ments, the fortune of each family and the prosperity of the region de-pend on them' (*Reporter* 2003).

One of the most revealing cases of Berehynia's hold on the public consciousness was the construction of the Monument of Independence, erected in 2002 at Majdan Nezalezhnosti (Independence Square, in Kyiv, Ukraine's central symbolic space). The monument consists of the figure of a woman in Ukrainian national dress standing on a column and holding a snowball tree branch over her head,[13] a symbol of the triumph and glory of the independent Ukrainian nation. At the unveil-ing, which took place on the eve of Independence Day, then-President Leonid Kuchma called the figure 'the embodiment of the Berehynia of our Ukrainian family.' Other officials joined him in attesting to her maternal qualities (Kuchma 2002). Such rhetoric was quite typical of political discourse at the time of Kuchma's presidency: politicians tended to concentrate on one aspect of the Berehynia myth – the idea of Universal Motherhood – while neglecting other possible implications of the image.[14] A woman's 'natural' role as mother was applied to the nation-state and merged with notions of nation and patriotism. Such visual representations of the Berehynia narrative (in monuments, book illustrations, traditionalist women's organizations' logos, and so on[15]) all tend towards this kind of essentialism: the concepts of womanhood, motherhood, nationhood, and Christianity merge and ultimately dis-place other possible matriarchal implication (such as authority, respon-sibility, assertiveness, and power).

Over time, the Berehynia narrative, which originated as a part of Ukrainian national mythology, has thus become a core element of a new national ideology and has been incorporated into the official na-tional narrative. As such, it resists criticism and deconstruction.

The Great Woman

The second significant narrative of Ukrainian women's history was conceived by Ukrainian diaspora scholars like Oles Kozulia (1993), Oleh Luhovy (1993), and Ivan Kuzych-Berezovsky (1994), whose writ-ings were republished in Ukraine in the early 1990s. These works for-ward an epic narrative about the special role that Ukrainian women have played in the history and cultural advancement of the nation. They focus on the biography of Ukraine's most outstanding women from different historical epochs. Given the aforementioned shortage of research and publications on women's history in Ukraine in the early 1990s, these widely publicized books became very popular and helped frame the entire field.

The distinctive feature of these studies is the glorification of prominent Ukrainian women whose contribution to the national cause can be clearly defined and measured. The list includes iconic personalities and, occasionally, names of distinguished but forgotten women – writers, scientists, artists, educators, and philanthropists. This is perhaps the most important contribution of the biographical perspective: that it makes some unsung women visible in national history.

In recent years, one can observe a noticeable increase in the number and variety of biographies of women – historical personages and contemporary figures alike. These include original archival documents, stout monographs, edited volumes, conference proceedings, reference books, educational brochures, and even wall calendars. Scholarly editions vary in genre and publishing quality. Take, for example, two works: *The Outstanding Women of Ukraine and Their Contribution to the Progress of National and World Scholarship (From the Second Half of the 19th to the Mid-20th Centuries)* (2003), a monograph by Lyudmyla Shumrykova-Karagodina; and *Ukrainian Women in History* (2004), a volume edited by Valentyna Borysenko and produced by a collective of authors, including scholars, writers, and journalists. At first glance, the books are alike; both offer life histories of a range of outstanding Ukrainian women. However, Shumrykova-Karagodina's monograph is poorly printed (paperback, no illustrations, cheap paper, 300 copies), whereas Borysenko's volume is done exquisitely (hard cover, artistically designed, luxurious paper, huge circulation).[16] This striking distinction is easily explained: the latter came out as a part of the national program supporting so-called socially significant publications under the personal patronage of then-first lady Kateryna Yushchenko, whereas the former was published by Dnipropetrovsk University Press at the author's expense.

Why such a glaring disparity in publishing quality between two otherwise similar books? The answer lies in the texts. Borysenko's volume is clearly shaped by national historical discourse: all the heroines are ethnic Ukrainians, and their personal achievements are assessed based on their contribution to the overall consolidation and progress of the Ukrainian nation. The nationalist tone is supported by the book's illustrations as well. Shumrykova-Karagodina's biographies, on the contrary, describe each woman's attainments in a particular academic domain with little reference to the national cause. One may conclude from this comparison that the Ukrainian state encourages and supports studies in women's history that conform to the national paradigm and serve to further legitimize the nation.

In fact, only those female historical figures who have directly contributed to the national cause ultimately achieve the highest levels of recognition by the state. Usually, three names come to mind when discussing prominent Ukrainian women of the past: Queen Olha, Roksolana, and Lesya Ukrainka. The Grand Duchess Olha is invariably presented as a model of women's statecraft.[17] But, despite her versatile activities as leader of the first proto-Ukrainian state, Kyivian Rus, she is known first and foremost as the symbol of Christian women's devotion to the country. Ironically, the attempt by the state to show appreciation for this outstanding figure turned into another latent mechanism for women's marginalization. In 1997, President Kuchma issued a decree establishing the new insignia 'The Order of the Grand Duchess Olha.' This decoration was to be awarded to women 'for important personal merits in governmental, industrial, public, academic, educational, cultural, charitable, and other spheres of social activity, and for child rearing in a family' (Kuchma 1997). This implies that women's achievements in any of these areas are very special and incompatible with those of men, as if women can compete only among themselves. It is by no mere chance that the iconography for the insignia resembles the famous ancient inlay of Our Lady Preaching, from the Cathedral of Saint Sophia in Kyiv, which implies that certain Christian ideas are in play as well. Meanwhile, the public monument to Saint Olha brings tangible national and Christian ideas inscribed into the image of a strong (matriarchal) femininity.[18] The monument's location between Ukraine's two most honoured Orthodox cathedrals (St Sophia and St Michael the Gold-domed) further strengthens this complex of ideas.

The second emblematic figure of the great woman narrative is Roksolana, an enslaved Ukrainian woman who succeeded in gaining great authority in the Ottoman Empire in the mid-sixteenth century.[19] Despite Roksolana's highly mythologized life story and the problematic reconstruction of her biography, her public representation is as a model of women's self-sacrifice for the sake of the fatherland.[20] This idea was central to the epic 1997 TV mini-series about her, *Roksolana*, produced by the state-owned channel UT-1.[21] That enormous financial resources from the state budget were allotted to the production of *Roksolana* during a time of economic hardships testifies to the story's exceptional political significance in mobilizing women to the national cause. In 1999, this popularity continued when a monument to Roksolana was erected in her hometown to commemorate the patriotism of thousands of Ukrainian women trafficked abroad.

Lesya Ukrainka, an outstanding Ukrainian writer, is a third iconic figure in this tradition and a symbol of women's fortitude and national dedication, although her feminist views remained unknown until recently.[22] Because she was considered to be a classic writer in Ukrainian literature long ago, Lesya Ukrainka's name and works were celebrated even under socialism. She is one of a very few prominent Ukrainian women whom ordinary citizens always recall. In independent Ukraine, state commemorative practices include using portraits of the nation's most prominent figures on the national currency.[23] When the new currency, the Hryvnya, was introduced in 1996, all of the new banknotes (from 1 to 100 Hryvnya) featured male personages. A few years later, inflation required the introduction of a new 200-Hryvnya note. Lesya Ukrainka's likeness was selected to appear on this note.[24] Thus, partially by chance, a woman was symbolically valued more highly than the most outstanding men. From this point on, Lesya Ukrainka was virtually canonized in the pantheon of great Ukrainian national heroes.

There are a huge number of outstanding Ukrainian women whose personal achievements in various spheres deserve to be thoroughly studied and appreciated, but many of them do not fit into the narrative of 'the great woman,' which includes only those who have contributed to the national cause. Official political history affects Ukrainian women's history as a field when politics promote research and publication on a specific selection of female personages whose life stories are closely intertwined with Ukraine's national history. As a result, the nation-state effectively appropriates women's history, foisting its own – politically determined – principles on it.

National Feminism

In 1988, Martha Bohachevsky-Chomiak published a groundbreaking study entitled *Feminists despite Themselves: Women in Ukrainian Community Life, 1884–1939*, which was translated into Ukrainian and published in Kyiv in 1995. The study energized the field of Ukrainian women's history and led to a new branch of research into the history of the Ukrainian women's movement. Bohachevsky-Chomiak introduced the concept of 'pragmatic feminism' to describe the distinctive feature of this movement. She argued that pre-Soviet Ukrainian women activists contributed to women's emancipation by their practical activities even though they did not identify themselves as feminists in the West European sense. Bohachevsky-Chomiak showed that, during the period when Ukraine was a stateless nation (especially before 1939), the Ukrainian women's movement consciously subordinated the feminist agenda to the national liberation struggle.[25] This insight became a point of reference for subsequent research on the Ukrainian women's movement and constitutes the cornerstone of the narrative of national feminism.

Since the late 1990s, a number of substantial works exploring the activities of women's organizations in various regions of Ukraine in pre-Soviet times have followed. Some use a feminist framework and are notable for their thorough and comprehensive historical research (see, e.g., Smolyar 1998). In most cases, however, the authors' knowledge of feminist epistemology and methodology is questionable. As a result, their writings are factual and descriptive at best. The monograph *Women in Public Life in Western Ukraine* (1998) by Borys Savchuk stands as a vivid example of this type of research. The chapter 'Origins and Nature of World Feminism' cites hardly any recent studies; instead, it is based on citations from Brockhaus-Efron's *Encyclopedia* (1890 edition) and other century-old publications. The author's attempt to explore Ukrainian women's emancipation is striking for its lack of a theoretical basis. Savchuk praises female activists' contribution to the promotion of national education and national awareness among western Ukrainians while diminishing the importance of women's achievements in advancing the feminist agenda itself.

Ignorance of feminist scholarship often renders authors who work in this area helpless when it comes to analysing empirical data. If this was excusable in the early 1990s (a time of scarce access to basic theoretical works), it cannot be so now, particularly among experts in women's history. Thus, a recent monograph by the high-profile historian Oksana Malanchuk-Rybak, *The Ideology and Social Practices of the Women's Movement in Western Ukraine* (2006),[26] while factually rich and accurate, fails in its theorization: a scant eight lines are devoted to summarizing Joan Scott's contributions to women's and gender history, but a full eight pages detail Mykhaylo Hrushevsky's reflections on family relations among medieval Ukrainians.[27] In so doing, Malanchuk-Rybak

makes clear her political loyalties: Hrushevsky's historical work, although important, is simply not as relevant here, and it is to his position as a founding father of the Ukrainian nation that the author's
attention pays homage. This situation echoes practices during Soviet
times, when every scholar was expected to cite the 'brilliant theoretical ideas' of communist leaders, no matter what the research subject.
Furthermore, while Malanchuk-Rybak points to the intersection of nationalism and feminism as the major challenge for the ideological consistency of the Ukrainian women's movement, she fails to scrutinize
the origins, unique interplay, and long-term consequences in particular
contexts of this issue using modern theories of gender and nation. Instead, she offers hasty explanations of compromises in the women's
movement due to Ukrainian women's paramount dedication to the national cause. Names of authors like Nira Yuval-Davis, Cynthia Enloe,
Jill Vickers, and other scholars whose theoretical insights into current
debates on women/gender and nation are extremely relevant to the
analysis are never even mentioned. In the end, the women's movement
is presented as an essential part of the overall Ukrainian national liberation movement, and as such, it is appreciated mainly for its contribution to national consciousness-raising. Almost two decades after
Bohachevsky-Chomiak's groundbreaking work was published, Malanchuk-Rybak's conclusions do not add much to her conclusions: 'Feminism in the Western Ukrainian women's movement was closely related
to nationalism and patriotism. Actually, nationalism as an awareness
of a group's distinction and/or originality based on ethnic, linguistic,
and religious homogeneity . . . along with the necessity to maintain
and protect such an originality constituted a foundation for the functioning of feminist ideology' (Malanchuk-Rybak 2006, 456). Despite the
unquestionable factual value of this kind of research, it is essentially
descriptive. In it, the positivist, androcentric paradigm for studying the
past remains unquestioned. These scholars tend to use non-academic
instruments to interpret empirical materials. Their conclusions are pre-
dictable and opportunistic, catering to the dominant political discourse
instead of resulting from an unbiased and comprehensive critical analysis. Ultimately, the main message of publications on the history of the
Ukrainian women's movement is approval and justification for the subordination of the feminist agenda to the goals of the Ukrainian national
liberation struggle and nation building.

This has had direct implications for women's activism: during the
first decade of Ukrainian independence, some Ukrainian women's

NGOs attempted to follow their foremothers' steps, declaring that the subordination of women's issues was needed to meet the goals of nation building.[28] Their constitutions stressed the principal mission: 'to contribute to the revival of the Ukrainian nation and firmly establish it among the other free peoples of the world' (Zhinocha Hromada 1993, 2); to 'establish the democratic ideal and national awareness in the society, to preserve the territorial integrity and political sovereignty of Ukraine . . . to promote patriotic education of future generations . . . of the Ukrainian language and spirituality revival' (Olena Teliha 1997, 2); to 'struggle for the nation's physical and spiritual revival, to build an independent Ukraine as a national state' (Ukrainian Christian Women's Party 1993, 4); and to 'join in women's activities for the consolidation and development of the Ukrainian nation-state' (Nova Doba 1995, 1).

In short, within the post-Soviet paradigm for the social sciences, which continues to value ideological compliance over critical analysis, Ukrainian women and their Her-story are still used for political purposes: the narrative of national feminism serves to (historically) substantiate the priority of national interests over any other group interests and thus legitimizes the subordination of any social movement to the goals of nation building.

Women's Devotion

Recently, there has been a real publication boom in Ukraine of books about individual women's experiences of the recent past. Memoirs, autobiographies, biographies, diaries, personal correspondence, biographical reference books, and more have appeared. Their format and style vary greatly – from amateurish and journalistic essays, to professionally edited and published personal documents and biographies. Meanwhile, the everyday experience of ordinary women under state socialism and in post-Soviet times in Ukraine has yet to be properly studied. The monograph *Women in the History of Ukrainian Culture in the Second Half of the 20th Century* (2002) by Olena Styazhkina is the only exception.[29] In it, Styazhkina explores the gendered aspects of professional work and creativity and reconstructs the peculiarities of the daily life of several women – writers, musicians, and actors – within a wider artistic and cultural context. Unlike many others, Styazhkina is knowledgeable in the theory and methodology of women's history, so she consistently examines the empirical data through a gendered lens. However, this important study is limited to a particular category of women – artists – whose way of life is hardly typical of the majority of ordinary Ukrainian women.

Reference books still constitute the majority of publications on Ukrainian women. These normally consist of short biographical sketches of women who have excelled in different spheres – from motherly heroines to top politicians. *Women of Ukraine* (2001), edited by Maria Orlyk, is a leading example of this kind of work.[30] In each of its 2,500 entries, a photograph accompanies a brief description of the woman's key achievements and awards. The significance of her contribution to the particular domain is also stressed.[31]

Women's participation in and contribution to the national guerrilla movement in the mid-twentieth century is perhaps the favourite subject of recent publications in women's history,[32] especially in Western Ukraine.[33] Mainly presented in the form of individual initiatives, however, such studies are usually targeted towards more or less clearly articulated political and/or ideological goals, such as patriotic education of the youth, national consciousness-raising, exemplification of individual heroism during the national liberation struggle, and so on. Besides these numerous memoirs (both written recollections and oral testimonies), two other types of publications on this subject include biographical reference books of female partisans and works summarizing women's experiences in the guerrilla movement.

The former type is exemplified by the book *Ukrainian Women in the Liberation Struggle in the 1940s and 1950s* (2006), edited by Nadia Mudra.[34] It contains more than 1,600 entries – all short biographical notes about ordinary Ukrainian women participants in the Ukrainian Insurgent Army who dedicated their lives to the national cause. Beyond the essential biographical facts, however, there are few details of women's clandestine activities. On the one hand, this publication makes women's agency in the national liberation movement visible and thus partially enacts historical justice; on the other hand, it tells us next to nothing about the gendered peculiarities of women's contributions and practices in the guerrilla movement, or about their motives for, or the long-term effects of, such participation.

When it comes to understanding women's overall participation in the national liberation struggle, the situation is worse: no comprehensive research on this subject has yet been published. Individual, local studies are the only (feeble) attempts so far to summarize women's roles in the national underground movement, and their approaches raise many questions. *Death Gave Them Immortality* (2003) by Bohdan Savka is typical in this regard. The book presents a chaotic collection of biographical data, photographs, and personal documents assembled and published by a schoolteacher who fails to analyse or even properly edit or comment on the empirical material. Instead, we get highly emotional and moralist nationalist rhetoric. Life stories of women partisans are used to exemplify the extreme patriotism, self-sacrifice, and unconditional devotion to the nation of female champions of the struggle. Needless to say, reconstruction of women's history per se is not the central objective of this work; their stories are used to articulate and substantiate the utter superiority of national interests. For this reason, and because of other failings, this book is truly the anti-model of what a women's history should be.

The narrative of women's devotion contrasts that of the great woman. If glorification of some outstanding Ukrainian women is the distinctive feature of the latter, victimization of ordinary women is typical of the former. For Ukrainians, as for people in other emerging nations, the very idea of Nation is personified by a woman. She may serve as a symbolic representation of spiritual firmness and victory (as in the case of the Monument of Independence), but national tragedies and losses are also often imagined and visualized as a suffering woman. This is apparent in the most recent developments around official recognition of the tragedy of the Holodomor of 1932–33 (the Great Famine) and corresponding commemorative practices.[35] Holodomor memorials often feature an exhausted or dead woman's body, symbolizing the tribulations suffered by the nation. Scholarly publications on the tragedy, meanwhile, tend to exemplify the horrors of starvation with creepy stories of desperate women (Kis 2010). Thus, a strong association between womanhood and victimhood is constructed, and women's historical experiences are conceptualized mainly in terms of eternal suffering and loss.

The same trend is noticeable in studies on women's experiences in the Ukrainian national guerilla movement in the 1930s to 1950s. Although it is undeniable that women endured enormous hardships and losses at the time, it is wrong to reduce all their experiences to suffering only. Constructing an image of a Ukrainian woman as an eternally helpless victim of historical developments ultimately displaces the possibility of exploring and recognizing women's versatile agencies in history, their survival strategies, and their numerous practices of active or passive resistance or accommodation to circumstances. Such a one-sided view of Ukrainian women as passive objects of history is both incorrect and unjust.

A more promising trend in research into Ukrainian women's history from an individual perspective is the development of women's oral histories. These are increasingly being used in Ukrainian social sciences today. As a methodology, oral history has proven to be an effective tool for studying formerly overlooked or totally silenced aspects of the Soviet and post-Soviet past. The variety of oral history research projects in Ukraine also proves that gender is an essential category for fieldwork and analysis; women constitute the majority of Ukrainian oral historians and subjects, regardless of research area.[36] Thus, all kinds of women's experiences and views are coming to the fore, disclosing formerly muted women's perspectives on the past. Furthermore, feminist oral history is a growing research sub-field. A few research projects focusing especially on women's personal memories have recently been carried out in Ukraine (Kis 2007).[37] Feminist methodologies of this kind challenge traditional historiography in many ways, introducing unusual research topics and innovative methods of analysis, and drawing less conventional conclusions. Women's oral history can be a kind of gender-sensitive, alternative methodology for historical research, allowing first-hand women's historical accounts to be heard, studied, and included in the general historical record.

Oral history has problems of its own, however. The project 'Women's Oral History: The Restitution,' under the leadership of Halyna Datsyuk, exemplifies the advantages and shortcomings of doing women's oral history beyond academia.[38] The study resulted in a published volume containing twenty-eight fragments of women's recollections of the most significant historical periods – as defined by the national historical narrative – that they had witnessed and survived (Datsyuk 2003).[39] Thus, although some historical experiences of women are voiced, thereby balancing the existing gender bias in our knowledge of the recent past, the presentation of these memories fails to question the androcentric framework of historiography. In fact, the editor has chosen to publish certain fragments of women's stories *because* they appear to be meaningful in the framework of already constructed national history. Women's lives as such count less than their attendance to certain 'historically significant' events. In this way, we can see how women's oral history may be used as another supplement to official history.

The spontaneous 'feminization' of oral history in Ukraine, however, along with advancements in feminist oral history, create a sense of optimism, as this approach could create a substantial counterpoint to the traditional way of writing history in Ukraine. The study of the past from the perspective of individual women's lives can reveal the variety of women's agencies in recent Ukrainian history.

Conclusions

Rapid socioeconomic and political transformations in Ukraine, accompanied by progress in the field of gender studies, have resulted in a considerable rise in gender awareness in Ukrainian society. This trend has ultimately led to an increased public interest in publications on women's and gender issues that could be extremely promising and beneficial for the advancement of women's history. However, this will only happen if the authors are professional historians knowledgeable in modern feminist scholarship, which will ensure both factual accuracy and innovative critical approaches.

Right now, however, the outstanding feature of current publications in this area is the prevalence of dilettantes among the authors pretending to write the history of Ukrainian women. The urgent public demand for more women's histories remains mostly unnoticed by academia, which, because of persistent prejudices against women's and gender studies, has failed to answer the call with more quality research on the subject. This gap is quickly being filled with pseudo-scientific publications that imitate women's history in form, while profaning its substance.[40] This problem is aggravated by poor marketing (including publishing, distribution, and promotion) of academic publications on women's history. Indeed, a book can become a bestseller or fall into oblivion depending on factors that have little to do with its scholarly value. Oftentimes, fundamental studies on women's history are unavailable to readers only because of their limited circulation and poor distribution, whereas low-quality publications conceived exclusively as commercial projects flood the book market. The failure to properly present and deliver substantial research in women's history to its potential target group is fatal for the establishment of women's history as a solid field of research. If fundamental research is invisible to readers, it gives the impression that Ukrainian women's history cannot be serious scholarship.

There is one more blemish peculiar to many publications on Ukrainian women's history: too often they are spoiled by poor prefaces or introductions written by some high-ranking official who is totally ignorant of women's history.[41] Such introductory texts are usually replete with stereotypical rhetoric based on women's 'special' mission in making and maintaining the nation. An extremely essentialist notion of women is usually presented through two main points: first, the infinite variety of women's social roles is reduced to their 'natural' or 'eternal' maternal and aesthetic functions only; second, authors steadily use the word 'woman' or 'womankind' in the singular form (*zhinka, zhinotstvo*) which implies that Ukrainian women are to be seen as a mass, as a solid kind of undifferentiated homogeneous category – all alike, possessing the same basic features, assigned the same mission, sharing the same destiny. Women are discursively denied any differences (social, ethnic, age, regional, etc.), and their individualities, personal interests, needs, and aspirations are neglected. The obvious discrepancy between the messages in these introductions and the content of the books themselves (which explore the variety of women's activities and achievements beyond traditional gender roles) can confuse and disorient readers, failing to equip them with a much-needed conceptual framework.

In this situation of uncertain institutional affiliations, methodological weakness, dispersed human resources, and political affections, the only way to establish Ukrainian women's history as a solid academic field is through joint efforts by Ukrainian feminist historians. The Ukrainian Association for Research in Women's History (UARWH), a non-governmental organization of professional historians (conceived in August 2010) declares institutionalization of women's history as a relatively autonomous research field in historical scholarship in Ukraine to be its main goal. The Association's versatile activities aim at the 'support, promotion and coordination of research and teaching in women's and gender history in Ukraine' (Ukrainian Association 2010, 1). This would raise the quality of research work and help the field withstand the flow of pseudo-scientific dilettantish publications. Other goals of this association include counteracting the instrumentalization and political manipulations of women's history, strengthening academic integrity, and consolidation of feminist historians around Ukraine. Through such a union, Ukrainian scholars could finally join the international community of feminist historians through membership in the International Federation of Research in Women's History (established in 1987).[42]

In her recent book, Tatyana Zhurzhenko (2008) argues that the national discourse plays a crucial role in forming feminist scholarship in Ukraine. Zhurzhenko discusses scholars' compliance with the national narrative and uncritical inscription of Ukrainian women's history onto that framework. She concludes that contemporary women's history is simply an additional tool to sustain and legitimize the history of the Ukrainian state (pp. 44–9, 57–63). The national paradigm is manifested even in the book's design. Strikingly enough, even publications dedicated to women's history in modern times often use very traditional images of women for their covers and illustrations: a peasant mother holding a baby, a peasant girl holding an archaic harvest tool, or a conventionalized Madonna – all invariably in Ukrainian national dress, all alike (see Borysenko 2004; Genyk 2008; Smolyar 1999; Zherebkina 1998). In this way, the national discourse (and to some extent, a religious one) is strengthened by imagery that frames readers' perceptions of Ukrainian women as essentially traditional, perhaps even conservative bearers and guardians of national culture.

The majority of publications in Ukrainian women's history today ultimately strive to answer the question 'What is so *Ukrainian*?' instead of 'What is so *women's*?' in research on literally any aspect of Ukrainian women's past. Indeed, when shifting the focus from *women's* to *Ukrainian* in the designation *Ukrainian women's history*, authors substantially change the framework of their studies. Exploring women's historical experience is no longer the primary goal. Instead, women appear as just another element in the history of Ukrainian nation building. Women's interests and agencies per se are subordinated to the nation once again, as *Her-story* is instrumentalized for the sake of *His-story*.

NOTES

1 See, e.g., the works of Mykola Kostomarov, Pavlo Chubynsky, Ivan Franko, Volodymyr Ivanov, Petro Yefymenko, Olexandra Yefymenko, Volodymyr Hnatyuk, Zenon Kuzelia, Volodymyr Okhrymovych, Orest Levytsky, and others.
2 Kateryna Hrushevska's father, Mykhaylo Hrushevsky (see n27 below), was persecuted by Soviet authorities for Ukrainian nationalism. Kateryna Hrushevska was arrested by the secret police, the NKVD, in July, 1938, accused of subversive, anti-Soviet activities, and was condemned to eight years in a concentration camp plus five years of deprivation of civil rights. She died in the Gulag in March 1943.
3 The socialist project of emancipation of women from above and the manipulative motives behind it have been discussed in several publications of feminist scholars. See, e.g., Moghadam (1993), Buckley (1997), Edmondson (1992), Marsh (1996), Corrin (1992), Einhorn (1993), and Funk

and Mueller (1993). While acknowledging some emancipatory effects of Soviet gender policies (especially free access to education and opportunities for professional self-fulfilment), scholars are unanimous in their judgment of 'gender equality' under socialism as hypocritical: compulsory full-time employment combined with undiminished household and maternal duties created a double burden for women; various forms of gender discrimination persisted for female employees; and women played no more than a token role in politics and governance.

4 The only exceptions to this were historical studies of the family, in which Ukrainian peasant women's family roles and household functions received some attention.

5 Women's history is absent from the Ukrainian state register of academic disciplines. Students cannot specialize in women's history. Nor can an academic degree be awarded in this field. Naturally, such official non-recognition has impeded studies in women's history. Still, it has not totally blocked their progress.

6 Volovymyr Okhrymovych, a famous Ukrainian ethnographer, persistently attempted to prove the existence of matriarchal traits in the Ukrainian culture through studying the most archaic elements of family rituals and popular customs. For more detailed discussions of the origins of the idea of Ukrainian matriarchy and the *Berehynia* narrative in Ukrainian academic, public, and political discourses, see Kis (2006; abridged version, 2005).

7 For example, the authors Marko Vovchok, Olha Kobelianska, Lesia Ukrainka, Natalia Kobrynska, and others.

8 Vasyl Ruban's novel *Berehynia* (1992) reintroduced the idea of an authentic Ukrainian matriarchy to the public discourse. He worked on the historical novel *Berehynia* since 1968 and published its fragments in several literary journals, but the complete version was published only in 1992. Vasyl Skurativsky has also published a book with the same title about Ukrainian native traditions in 1987. As editor-in-chief of the magazine *Berehynia,* devoted to the study of Ukrainian traditions and folklore, he also promoted matriarchal ideas through a range of publications.

9 Marian Rubchak (2001) has explored *Berehynia* as the fusion of two images – the Virgin Mary and a pagan (pseudo)goddess – that has been used to elaborate a new national model of femininity in Ukraine.

10 Meanwhile, the feminist trend in research on women's history, initiated by Hrushevska and others in the 1920s, remained largely unknown because of restrictions on access to their works in Soviet times.

11 In fairness, this chapter contrasts sharply with the rest of the book, which is one of the most successful attempts to reconstruct the history of Ukrainian women in a holistic way.

12 Public perception of the meaning of International Women's Day (8 March) in post-Soviet Ukraine is distorted. It is regarded either as a celebration of spring, women's beauty and love (this view having been cultivated during the late Soviet period), or as a part of Soviet heritage and originating from the (foreign) socialist women's movement (with reference to Klara Zetkin). The latter view is widely shared by nationalist women activists who deny any association with socialism. The internationally accepted meaning of this day (namely, celebration of solidarity among women struggling for their rights) has been promoted over the past few years by feminist women's groups.

13 The snowball tree, especially if pictured as a branch with ripe red berries, is an essential Ukrainian national symbol.

14 The rhetoric of matriarchal essence lost its popularity after the Orange Revolution and has seldom been mentioned by politicians since.

15 For a detailed analysis of these representations, see Kis (2005).

16 Borysenko's luxurious edition is not affordable for the average scholar or even for academic libraries, so in 2006 the international charitable foundation 'Ukraine 3000' donated 230 copies to university libraries throughout Ukraine on the occasion of Mother's Day.

17 Grand Duchess Olha headed the first proto-Ukrainian state, Kyivian Rus in 945–57; she was known for her tough, successful style of governance, versatile diplomatic activity, and effective administrative and taxation reforms, which strengthened state authority. She was also the first Ukrainian governor to adopt Christianity and was canonized a saint by the Orthodox Church.

18 The monument to St Olha (by Ivan Kavaleridze) was erected in 1911, destroyed by the Soviets in 1919, and totally demolished in 1926. In 1996, the Kyiv city council decided to restore it.

19 Roksolana (ca. 1500–1566, likely named Nastya Lisovska) was an ordinary Ukrainian woman from the western Ukrainian town of Rohatyn who was enslaved by Tatars for a time. Owing to the outstanding qualities of her character, she became a beloved wife of the Ottoman sultan Suleiman II the Great in 1520. Alleviation of Ottoman aggression against East Slavic nations at that time is usually ascribed to Roksolana's influence over her husband's political decisions.

20 A museum devoted to Roksolana is slated to open in Rohatyn in 2010.

21 The series was directed by Boris Neberidze. In 2004, UT-1 produced a second series, *Roksolana: Sovereign of the Empire*. Olha Sumska, who played Roksolana, became a national sex symbol.

22 Lesya Ukrainka was a pen name for the writer Larysa Kosach (1871–1913), one of the key figures in Ukrainian literature. Although weak from years of suffering from tuberculosis, she maintained an active public life and worked tirelessly to promote the Ukrainian national idea. Her biography and works are studied in Ukraine and abroad, and numerous monuments as well as museums have been dedicated to Lesya Ukrainka all over the globe.

23 Of 99 commemorative coins minted by the Ukrainian national bank, Ukrainian women (including Queen Olha and Lesya Ukrainka) are portrayed on 7.

24 The 200-Hryvnya note appeared in 2001. In 2006, however, it was out-valued by a 500-Hryvnya note portraying yet another famous male Ukrainian historical figure.

25 Ukraine had no statehood of its own until the Ukrainian Soviet Socialist Republic was formed in the framework of the USSR (1922). Until 1939, however, a big part of the Ukrainian territories (Western Ukraine – Galicia, Bukovyna, West Volynia, Transcarpathia) were under the governance of other countries (Poland, Romania, Hungary).

26 In this work, Malanchuk-Rybak, a doctor of history and professor at the Lviv Academy of Fine Arts and expert in women's history since the late 1980s, does provide excellent archival research to substantiate her reconstruction of the history of various women's groups.

27 Mykhaylo Hrushevsky (1866–1934) was a prominent Ukrainian historian, author of the 10-volume *History of Ukraine-Rus*, and president of the Ukrainian National Republic – the short-lived independent Ukrainian national state, in 1917–18.

28 Martha Kichorowska Kebalo (2007) and Marian Rubchak (2001a, 2001b) have both shown how this willingness to subordinate women's agenda was passed down within the movement. More recently, however, many women's NGOs have updated their programs and adjusted their agendas in order to foreground women's issues.

29 This book's scarce circulation (300 copies) makes it almost unavailable to readers.

30 It is worth noting that Maria Orlyk is not a scholar. During the 12 years preceding the collapse of the USSR she was deputy prime minister of Ukraine. Later, she served as a leader of the national women's organization

Spika zhinok Ukrainy (The Union of Women of Ukraine), which actually carried out this publishing project.

31 Unlike many other publications on women's history, this one has a short editorial foreword explaining the criteria and process for selecting the persons to be included, and the way their personal data were obtained. It is also remarkable that these persons are not necessarily of Ukrainian ethnic descent. In this way, the book does not cater to the Ukrainian national narrative. In general, there is little to criticize in this edition, except, perhaps, its relatively high cost.

32 The mass national liberation movement under the leadership of the Organization of Ukrainian Nationalists (OUN) took place in the western Ukrainian territories from the mid-1930s until 1953; after 1942, its guerilla army, known as the Ukrainian Insurgent Army (UPA), fought for an independent Ukrainian nation-state against the Nazis and the Soviets.

33 In other regions, research and publications on Ukrainian women's history are considerably less politicized and are concerned mostly with women's professional achievements.

34 Nadia Mudra is an activist and former member of the OUN who survived the Gulag. She managed to collect biographical materials, put them together, and ultimately publish the two-volume edition despite her advanced age and health concerns. Her work represents a unique source for further research, especially given the extreme circumstances of her information gathering on women partisans, whose activities and networking were clandestine.

35 The state-organized artificial famine in the Eastern, Central, and Southern regions of Ukraine, which caused some 4 million deaths in 1932–33, has been recognized by the Rada to have been an act of genocide against Ukrainians.

36 Perhaps the higher life expectancy of women (72.5 years compared with 60.5 years for men) and their relatively better health determine the predominance of female narrators in virtually all studies that uses oral historical sources.

37 For example, the research project 'Twentieth Century Ukraine in Women's Memories' was conducted between 2003 and 2007 under the leadership of Oksana Kis as a part of the international project 'Women's Memories: Searching for Lives and Identities of Women under Socialism.' For more details, see www.womensmemories.net.

38 Halyna Datsyuk is president of the Kyiv Women's Centre 'Spadshchyna' (Heritage) and a journalist who teaches at Kyiv National University. The project she led was part of a joint international undertaking called

'Women's Oral Histories,' which included the majority of post-Soviet countries and was supported by the Women's Network Program of the Open Society Institute. Andrea Peto, a professor at Central European University, served as research adviser for the international research group.

39 Despite the obvious merits of this pioneering project, its academic value should not be overestimated. Evident flaws in the project design and documentation and its general methodological vagueness suggest that the members of the research team were novices in oral history. For instance, published memories are neither accompanied by interviewees' personal data, nor by the date and place of the interview or the questions that were asked. It is impossible to assess the relevance of chosen theoretical principles and techniques to the project's goals because they are not described in the preface. As well, there is no evidence that a common interviewing strategy or questionnaire was used for collecting women's retrospections, and there is no discussion of the ethical and legal issues surrounding the use of personal life stories.

40 Here I am not taking into account the popular publications designed for a general audience, but those which conform to the formal characteristics of a scholarly book (including pre-publishing reviews, references, bibliography, appendix, index, etc.) and therefore could be identified as a research work.

41 For instance, Volodymyr Lytvyn, the speaker of the Rada and vice-president of the National Academy of Sciences of Ukraine, was the author of the 'Foreword' for the first volume of the Vadym Bolhov's book *Portraits of Our Women Contemporaries* (2003). His reflections unequivocally testify to his total incompetence in women's history: 'Women have always been an embellishment of our country, the nation's pride and treasure. Their beauty, intellect, kindness, and love inspire men to be the worthy knights and lovers. Professionalism and steadfastness, self-sacrifice for the sake of their families and children have always been the fundamental features of womanhood. Ukrainian woman is a *Berehynia* of the family hearth, a reliable backing and support for a man, a mother of a defender of Fatherland' (2003, 1). Thus, Lytvyn's political status and academic authority serve to legitimize the most stereotypical perception of women's social roles.

42 UARWH was accepted as a collective member to the International Federation for Research in Women's History in August 2010. For details of the IFRWH's history, structure, and activities, see its official website: www.ifrwh.com.

REFERENCES

Bohachevsky-Chomiak, M. 1988. *Feminists despite Themselves: Women in Ukrainian Community Life, 1884–1939*. Edmonton: Canadian Institute of Ukrainian Studies, University of Alberta.
– 1995. *Bilym po bilomu: Zhinky v hromadskomu zhytti Ukrainy, 1884–1939*. Kyiv: Lybid. (This is the translated edition, printed in Ukraine, of the original English language text, cited above.)
Bolhov, V. 2003. *Portrety suchasnyts* [Portraits of Our Women Contemporaries], vol.1. Kyiv: Ukrainska academia heraldyky.
Borysenko, V., ed. 2004. *Ukrainian Women in History*. Kyiv: Lybid.
Buckley, M., ed. 1997. *Post-Soviet Women: From the Baltic to Central Asia*. New York: Cambridge University Press.
Corrin, C., ed. 1992. *Superwomen and Double Burden: Women's Experience of Change in Central and Eastern Europe and the Former Soviet Union*. Toronto: Sumach.
Datsyuk, H., ed. 2003. *Usna zhinocha istoriya: Povernennia* [Women's Oral History: The Restitution]. Kyiv: Zhinochy Tsentr 'Spadschyna.'
– 2007. *Istoriya staroi fotografii: vizualizatsiya zhinochogo dosvidu* [A Story of an Old Photo: Visualization of Women's Experiences]. Kyiv: Zhinochy Tsentr 'Spadschyna.'
Edmondson, L., ed. 1992. *Women and Society in Russia and the Soviet Union*. Cambridge: Cambridge University Press.
Einhorn, B. 1993. *Cinderella Goes to Market: Citizenship, Gender and the Women's Movement in East Central Europe*. New York: Verso
Franko, I. 1980. Zhinocha nevolia v ruskykh pisniakh narodnykh. (1883). In *Works in 50 Volumes* (works by Ivan Franko), vol. 26, 209–53. Kyiv: Naukova Dumka.
Funk, N., and M. Mueller, eds. 1993. *Gender Politics and Post-Communism: Reflections from Eastern Europe and the Former Soviet Union*. New York: Routledge.
Genyk, S. 2008. *150 vydatnykh ukrayinok* [150 Outstanding Ukrainian Women]. Ivano-Frankivsk: Lileya.
Hrushevska, K. 1929. *Pro doslidzhennia statevyh hromad v pervisnim suspilstvi* [Towards a Study of Sex Groups in Primitive Societies]. *Pervisne hromadianstvo ta yoho perezhytky v Ukraini* 1: 24–33.
Kichorowska Kebalo, M. 2007. Exploring Continuities and Reconciling Rupture: Nationalism, Feminism, and the Ukrainian Women's Movement. *Aspasia* 1: 36–60.

Kis, O. 2005. Choosing without Choice: Predominant Models of Femininity in Contemporary Ukraine. In M. Hurd, H. Carlback, and S. Rastback, eds., *Gender Transitions in Russia and Eastern Europe,* 105–36. Stockholm: Gondolin.

– 2006. Koho oberihaye Berehynia, abo Matriarkhat yak cholovichyy vynakhid [Who Is Protected by *Berehynia,* or Matriarchy as a Men's Invention]. *YA: The Bulletin of the Kharkiv Women's Centre KRONA* 4(16): 11–16; *Dzerkalo Tyzhnia* (23 April 2005).

– 2007. Vidnovlyuyuchy vlasnu pamyat: proekt 'Ukraina XX stolittya u pamyati zhinok' [Resuming the Memory: The Research Project '20th-Century Ukraine in Women's Memories']. *Ukraina Moderna* 11: 266–70.

– 2010. Holodomor 1932–33 rokiv kriz' pryzmu zhinochoho dosvidu [The Great Famine 1932–33 as Seen through the Prism of Women's Experiences]. *Narodoznavchi Zoshyty* nos. 5–6: 633–51.

Kozulia, O. 1993. *Zhinky v istorii Ukrainy* [Women in the History of Ukraine]. Kyiv: Ukrainsky tsentr dukhovnoi kultury.

Kuchma, L. 1997. *On Establishing the Insignia of the President of Ukraine 'The Order of the Grand Duchess Olha.'* Decree of the President of Ukraine, no. 827/97, 15 Aug. 1997. Available at the official website of the Supreme Council of Ukraine http://zakon.rada.gov.ua/cgi-bin/laws/main. cgi?nreg=827%2F97.

– 2002. Nekhay mits, bahatstvo i slava vitchyzny pryrostayut nashoyu pratseyu: Vystup Prezydenta Ukrainy na vidkrytti Monumenta Nezalezhnosti Ukrainy [May the Fatherland's Strength, Wealth and Glory Increase Owing to Our Work: The President of Ukraine's Speech at the Inauguration of the Monument of Independence of Ukraine]. *President* nos. 7–8: 6–11.

Kuzych-Berezovsky, I. 1994. *Zhinka i derzhava* [Woman and the State]. Lviv: Svit.

Lavrinenko, N. 1999. *Zhenshchina: samorealizatsiya v semye I obshchestve (gendernyy aspect)* [A Woman: Self-Fulfilment in the Family and Society (Gender Aspects]. Kyiv: Vipol.

Luhovy, O. 1993.*Vyznachne zhinotstvo Ukrainy: istorychni zhyttiepysy* [Prominent Women of Ukraine: Historical Biographies]. Kyiv: Dnipro.

Lutsenko, O. 1999. Matriarkhatni uyavlennia v ukrainskiy kulturi: zhinoche nachalo v ukrainskiy mentalnosti [Matriarchal Beliefs in Ukrainian Culture: Feminine Principles in Ukrainian Mentality]. In L. Smolyar, ed., *Zhinochi studii v Ukraini: Zhinka v istorii i siogodni* [Women's Studies in Ukraine: A Woman in History and Today], 10–18. Odessa: Astroprynt.

Lytvyn, V. 2003. Zhinkam Ukrainy [To Women of Ukraine]. *Holos Ukrainy,* 7 March.

Malanchuk-Rybak, O. 2006. *Ideolohiya ta suspilna praktyka zhinochoho rukhu na zakhidnoukraïnskykh zemliakh XIX – pershoï tretyny XX st.: Typolohiia ta ievropeiskyi kulturno-istorychnyi kontekst* [The Ideology and Social Practice of the Women's Movement in Western Ukraine in the 19th and First Third of the 20th Centuries: Typology and European Cultural and Historical Context]. Chernivtsi: KNYHY – XXI.

Marsh, R., ed. 1996. *Women in Russia and Ukraine.* Cambridge: Cambridge University Press.

Moghadam, V.M., ed. 1993. *Democratic Reform and the Position of Women in Transitional Economies.* Oxford: Clarendon.

Mudra, N. 2006 [2004]. *Ukrainska zhinka u vyzvolniy borotbi, 1940–1950 roky* [Ukrainian Women in the Liberation Struggle in the 1940s and 1950s], 2 vols. Lviv: Svit.

Nikolayev Vecherniy. 2003. Iz dnem materi ta mizhnarodnym dnem simyi [Greetings on the Occasion of Mother's Day and the International Day of the Family]. 13 May.

Nova Doba [New Epoch, Women's Association]. 1995. *Statutes.* Lviv: Nova Doba.

Okhrymovych, V. 1891. Znacheniye malorusskikh svadebnykh obriadov v istorii evolutsii semyi. [Significance of the Ukrainian Wedding Rituals in the History of the Evolution of the Family]. *Etnograficheskoye Obozreniye* 4(11): 44–105.

Olena Teliha [All-Ukrainian Women's Association]. 1997. *Statutes.* Kyiv: Olena Teliha.

Orlyk, M., ed. 2001. *Zhinky Ukrainy: Biohrafichny entsyklopedychny slovnyk* [Women of Ukraine: Biographical Encyclopedic Reference Book]. Kyiv: Fenix.

Reporter. 2003. Zi sviatom vas, dorohi zhinky Zakarpattia! [Happy Holiday, Dear Women of Trans-Carpathia!] 7 March.

Ruban, V. 1992. *Berehynia: Istorychnyy roman* [*Berehynia:* A Historical Novel]. Kyiv: Dnipro.

Rubchak, M. 2001a. Christian Virgin or Pagan Goddess? Feminism versus the Eternally Feminine in Ukraine. In R. Marsh, ed., *Women in Russia and Ukraine,* 315–30. Cambridge: Cambridge University Press.

– 2001b. Evolution of a Feminist Consciousness in Ukraine and Russia. *European Journal of Women's Studies* 8(2): 149–60.

Savchuk, B. 1998. *Zhinotstvo v suspilnomu zhytti Zakhidnoyi Ukrainy (ostnnia tretyna XIX st. – 1939* [Women in Public Life in Western Ukraine (From the Last Third of the 19th Century to 1939]. Ivano-Frankivsk: Lileya.

Savka, B. 2003. '*A smert yikh bezsmertyam zustrila. . .*' *Narysy, spohady, dokumenty pro uchast zhinotstva v natsionalno-vyzvolniy borotbi OUN-UPA 40–50 rokiv XX stolittya* ['Death Gave Them Immortality. . .' Essays, Memories, Documents on Women's Participation in the National Liberation Struggle of OUN-UPA in the 1940 and 1950s]. Ternopil: Dzhura.

Shumrykova-Karagodina, L. 2003. *Vydatni zhinky Ukrainy i yikhniy vnesok u rozvytok natsionalnoyi i svitovoyi nauky (druha polovyna XIX – seredyna XX st.)* [The Outstanding Women of Ukraine and Their Contribution to the Progress of National and World Scholarship (From the Second Half of the 19th to the Mid-20th Centuries]. Dnipropetrovsk: Dnipropetrovsk University Press.

Smolyar, L. 1998. *Mynule zarady maybutnioho. Zhinochy rukh Naddniprianskoyi Ukrayiny druhoyi polovyny XIX – pochatku XX stolittia* [Past for the Sake of Future: The Women's Movement in the Dnipro Region of Ukraine in the Second Half of the 19th to the Early 20th Centuries]. Odessa: Astroprynt.

– ed. 1999. *Zhinochi studii v Ukraini: Zhinka v istorii i siogodni* [Women's Studies in Ukraine: A Woman in History and Today]. Odessa: Astroprynt.

Styazhkina, O. 2002. *Zhinky v istorii ukrayinskoyi kultury druhoyi polovyny XX stolittya* [Women in the History of Ukrainian Culture in the Second Half of the 20th Century]. Donetsk: Skhidnyy vydavnychyy dim.

Tkachenko, O. 2000. Berehyni rody nashoho bezsmertnoho [*Berehynias* of Our Immortal Family]. *Holos Ukrainy,* 8 March.

Ukrainian Association for Research in Women's History, 2010. *Statutes.* Lviv: UARWH.

Ukrainian Christian Women's Party. 1993. *Program and Statutes.* Lviv: Ukrainian Christian Women's Party.

Zherebkina, I., ed. 1998. *Femina Postsovietica: Ukrainskaya zhenschina v perekhodny period: ot sotsialnykh dvizheniy k politike* [*Femina Postsovietica:* Ukrainian Women in the Period of Transition: From Social Movements to Politics]. Kharkov: Kharkov Centre of Gender Studies.

Zhinocha Hromada [Women's Community, International Organization]. 1993. *Statutes.* Kyiv: Zhinocha Hromada.

Zhurzhenko, T. 2008. *Gendernyie rynki Ukrainy: politicheskaya ekonomiya natsionalnogo stroitelstva* [Gendered Markets of Ukraine: The Political Economy of Nation Building]. Vilnius: European Humanities University.

7 Gender and Social Worth in Post-Soviet Ukrainian Civil Society

SARAH D. PHILLIPS

Middle-Class Fantasies

2 February 1999, Kyiv, Ukraine

Vania is to pick up Svetlana, Vira, and me at the designated meeting place – the trolley-bus stop nearest to Svetlana's apartment.[1] It's 9:30 a.m. We stomp our feet on the frozen snow to ward off numbness and tug our coat collars tighter to stave off the icy wind and blowing snow. Vania finally pulls up in his car. The burgundy Opel, a fairly new sedan, looks promising, but it soon becomes clear that this trip will be a slow one. Every few miles the car dies and Vania gets out to tinker with something under the hood, willing the engine back to life so we can travel on. Vania, the father of five children, is a member of Our House, the non-governmental organization (NGO) run by Svetlana and Vira to support 'large families' (*bahotoditni*, those with five or more children in most cases, but families with three or more children may in some instances be designated as 'large'). Situated in Kyiv, Ukraine's capital city,[2] their organization serves about seventy families and 225 children in total. Since Vania recently lost his job, Svetlana and Vira call him up whenever they need a driver for their NGO affairs, and they pay him a small sum for his trouble and for gas. I'm tagging along with the women as they scour the city for discount food items to include in food baskets which they are putting together for distribution to the members of their organization. If we find a good price, we will purchase what we can fit in the car today and then return tomorrow for the rest.

As we drive around to different bazaars and warehouses searching for discounts on bulk quantities of cooking oil, sugar, and *hrechka* (buckwheat groats), with frequent stops for engine tinkering, Svetlana and Vira begin an elaborate verbal exchange about their 'dreams and wishes.' They seem to go to another place as they imagine themselves in different life circumstances – lives released from denial and liberated from worries about how to put the next meal on the table. These dream narratives are fascinating windows into the lives that these women live; they are testaments to their poverty, the desires it engenders, and the dreams it snuffs out.

We turn the corner from Shevchenko Boulevard onto Khreshchatyk (a giant statue of Lenin to our left), and my friends conjure an image of a 'women's club' they would like to start. If they had a women's club, the moms in their organization could gather every so often to enjoy female fellowship and relax away from their home life and domestic chores. 'Yes,' Svetlana offers, 'we'll have soft and luxurious couches to rest our weary bones.' 'Oh sure,' adds Vira, jokingly, 'the women can lounge on the couches and drink tea with lemon.' In a more serious tone, Svetlana explains that many of the women in their organization (including themselves) suffer from a lack of female companionship, since most 'mothers of many children' are homemakers and cannot leave the home and their children very often. She tells me:

> Sometimes I think I should have been a psychologist or gone into psychiatry. Because I sit there so often and listen to women – we give them a chance to get everything off their chests. They can talk to us because we are in the same situation as they.

The women's fixation with the lemon continues throughout our quest around the city for discount foodstuffs. While we wander through a warehouse hoping to find wholesale cereals, Vira leaves the rest of us as she goes on a search for 'one little lemon, so we can have tea with lemon later.' She runs up to all the makeshift fruit stands around the warehouse in pursuit of the elusive lemon. She finally finds the right lemon at the right price and buys it, triumphantly carrying it to show our small collective. She cradles the lemon until we reach the car, her little symbol of the indulgences of life that she and Svetlana are so rarely able to enjoy.

After our shopping trip, I invite Svetlana and Vira to my apartment to continue our chat and finally enjoy that tea with lemon. They are surprised to see the ancient Soviet refrigerator ('Siberia') that came with my rented apartment. 'That thing sounds like a car motor,' Svetlana observes, and adds: 'So I'm not the only one who still has one of those energy-sucking dinosaurs.' As I prepare a snack, I try to keep Vira from seeing that I already have four or five lemons languishing in the bottom drawer of the refrigerator. Svetlana reflects on her own poverty: 'If you ask me what my children and I live on, I can't tell you because I don't know myself. Our expenses greatly outweigh our income.' Her teenage son, she explains, recently has aged out of the system of social welfare, so her family no longer qualifies as a 'large' one. This means that all three of her children have lost their right to collect a monthly allowance of 70 UAH (about $20 at the time).[3] Svetlana's eldest daughter gets a small sum in child support from her father each month, and Svetlana's youngest daughter receives 6.40 UAH (about $1.85 at the time) as the child of a single mother. Svetlana sews house slippers from scrap material and sells them for 2.50 UAH (about $0.70 at the time) a pair to make extra money. This is the extent of her family budget, and Vira once told me, in secret, that 'Svetlana's children go around hungry.'

Svetlana again begins to articulate her middle-class fantasies:

My dream is to have a big kitchen with a huge refrigerator that is never empty. And a couch right beside the refrigerator. I would be able to relax there and open the refrigerator and take out anything I want at anytime and just eat it, without having to worry about dividing it into four parts [for me and my kids]. Because there will always be more . . . And I dream about walking up and down the aisles of the Besarabs'kyi Market and being able to buy anything and everything I want.

Svetlana takes a spoon and dunks a round slice of lemon to the bottom of her teacup, squashing the lemon to release the tangy juice: 'All I want is a normal life.'

Svetlana and Vira are just two of the thousands of women who have taken up leadership roles in various types of civic organizations in Ukraine since Gorbachev, in the mid- and late 1980s, loosened the reigns on the right of Soviet citizens to associate freely. Their experiences raise important questions about the nature of Ukraine's post-socialist 'third sector' (as the NGO sphere is called in transnational 'development-speak') and about the impacts on women of the collapse of the socialist system and the introduction of a market economy. As women such as these activists have flocked to the non-profit sector, they have found themselves in the crosshairs of processes of *differentiation*, as the criteria for productive citizenship are reworked, and the rights and needs of various categories of citizens redefined. These women's struggles for social justice and their uneven success highlights some of the social costs of economic reforms centred on marketization, privatization, and welfare reduction, policies that entail a re-evaluation of citizens' productivity and deservedness, and a dramatic rearrangement of the state's acknowledged responsibilities towards different groups of citizens. The claims of people such as Svetlana and Vira, who called upon the Ukrainian state to provide the same level of social protection as they had enjoyed as 'mothers of many children' in the Soviet Union, have become increasingly devalued as the state is pulled back and social problems become privatized.

Processes of differentiation have had an especially marked impact on women, which is reflected not only in macroeconomic indicators and unemployment statistics (which generally show women to be the losers of the transition) but also in the large numbers of women who have sought refuge in NGOs as a forum to advocate for marginalized populations and eke out a meagre living. In the context of economic reform and the shrinking social safety net, it is mostly women who have been left to pick up the pieces of the dishevelled social welfare system; women have been compelled to engage in the care and defence of marginalized groups whose concerns and demands are increasingly delegitimized in the neo-liberal moment. Barbara Einhorn (2000) describes this situation as a 'civil society trap,' since so many women have been ushered into the low-prestige, low-paying (or no pay) ghetto of NGO grunt work (Einhorn 2000; Handrahan 2002; Liborakina 1998).

Across the former Soviet Union, in general, the NGO sphere appears to be dominated by women.[4] Despite popular assumptions that this is the case in Ukraine as well, in 2006, a survey of 610 civil society organizations in Ukraine showed no significant gender differences in NGO leadership (51% were directed by women, and 49% by men; Palyvoda et al. 2006). There were some regional variations, with a greater proportion of NGOs in Western and Eastern Ukraine led by women, and men dominating in Central Ukraine. However, there are significant differences in the types of NGOs commonly associated with women and those associated with men. In Ukraine, women tend to head social organizations that serve the interests of women, children, and families, and those that focus on 'solving social issues'; women are believed to possess 'natural' roles as mothers, caregivers, and guardians of the home and nation.[5] Many women-led organizations are 'mutual aid' associations (*hrupy vzaiemodopomohy*) that are simultaneously a support group and a humanitarian (charity) organization. Like Svetlana and Vira, scores of NGO directors are themselves members of a marginalized category (large families, the elderly, the disabled), and they may engage in NGO work as a form of precarious employment as they wage social justice struggles to help themselves and others. Men, on the other hand, are more likely to direct NGOs associated with human rights, civic education, politics, the state, and the economy, which represent much more prestigious and lucrative spheres than children's issues and 'solving social problems' (Palyvoda et al. 2006, 92).

During a long-term ethnographic study of women social activists and their NGOs from 1998 to 2005, I tracked the activities and narratives of eleven NGO activists in Kyiv to examine multiple aspects of Ukrainian civil society building after socialism, and the intersections of gender and class in particular (Phillips 2008). In this chapter, I focus on just two of these activists – Svetlana and Vira, of the organization Our House – to explore the discourses about gender and about class in this post-socialist, neo-liberalizing state that intersect to discount the 'value narratives' of disadvantaged women such as these, and relegate them and their concerns to a marginalized underclass (Patico 2005, 491). Their experiences reveal a little-explored side of the supposed 'democratization' processes of the post-socialist transition in states such as Ukraine.

Calculations of Class

As I spent more and more time with activists such as Svetlana and Vira, talking to them about their lives and their NGO activities, and accompanying them around the city to meetings and events and on shopping trips, I thought a lot about issues of class. Some of my acquaintances in the city would look askance at me when I told them I had been spending time with *bahotoditni* (large families) and *pensionery* (pensioners or retirees): 'What could you possibly have in common with them?' The lifestyles of some of the activists I knew were so different from those of my friends who were moving into the Ukrainian middle class. These were younger people: some had studied abroad; most had knowledge of foreign languages. They were either working for foreign firms or had started their own small businesses. By 2002 and 2003, many of my friends were buying newly built or renovated apartments and modest foreign cars, and taking vacations to exotic places such as South Africa, Egypt, and the United States. They had bank accounts, credit cards, and leisure time. Meanwhile, social activists such as Svetlana, Vira, and others remained socially vulnerable, despite the long hours they devoted to raise public awareness, lobby government officials, and procure humanitarian assistance.

Until rather recently (Schröder and Vonderau 2008), the literature on post-socialism has had relatively little to say about class (but see Gapova 2004, 2005, 2007; Lampland 2000). Certainly, important work has been undertaken to explore the myriad affects of marketization and privatization on different aspects of personal and communal life (Caldwell 2004; Rivkin-Fish 2005). But these processes have most often been examined through the lens of consumption or labour, without an explicit focus on the intricacies of new forms of class differentiation in the post-Soviet world (Caldwell 2002; Dunn 2004; Ghodsee 2005; Humphrey 1995; Patico 2002, 2005). This is curious given the history of the region, the importance of class to the socialist project, and its continued relevance during the transition period. As Dunn (2008, 228–9) has noted, 'just at the moment that Eastern European societies began to experience widespread income differentiation and the dramatic cultural elaboration of new social classes, the most effective theoretical language in which to critique rising economic and political inequality was suddenly devalorised.'

I see the NGO sphere as illuminating both emerging processes of class differentiation in post-Soviet Ukraine, and the ways in which persons – and women in particular – variably resist these differentiation processes. In the face of new state policies that shifted the criteria for calculating needs, deservedness, and ultimately social and economic class, the activists in NGOs such as Our House were struggling to prevent the development of a permanent underclass. They sought to position and reposition themselves (and the categories with which they were identified; in this case large families and, for Svetlana, single mothers) for recognition and redistribution through both practical strategies (mutual aid activities, lobbying) and strategies of re-education of the public. Through all these efforts, representatives of devalued categories of citizens struggled to prove their social worth. The advocacy efforts in which women were engaged were especially likely to involve such struggles, a fact that has important implications for how both gender and class identities are being shaped in post-socialist Ukraine.

Among the social activists I knew in Kyiv, accounting for the social worth of devalued categories of citizens (large families, pensioners, the disabled) often hinged on the assertion of claims and centred around 'needs talk' (Haney 2002). In Ukraine's contemporary conditions of privatization, welfare reform, and state retreat, making claims for various forms of support (social, state, from international NGOs) is a slippery business. Neo-liberal economic reforms are accompanied by processes of privatization and individualization that privilege models of 'active citizenship' and 'productive citizenship' over socialist-era models of citizenship based more on entitlement and the state's responsibility towards citizens. Concomitantly, citizens who received special recognition under socialism (mothers of many children, veterans, retirees) risk being moved into the category of 'non-productive,' and therefore potentially 'undeserving' of state assistance. To counter this positioning, women such as Svetlana and Vira have had to scramble to assert themselves as deserving of recognition and worthy of state support. As they felt themselves sliding into a stigmatized 'low-class' identity, these women sought both to procure material benefits for themselves and their consociates, and to counter the new definitions of 'deserving' citizenship. They mobilized accounts of their own social worth to deflect others' negative assessments of them, such as 'they are giving birth to the poor' or 'they are bread beggars' (Rus. *nakhlebniki*).

In their claims making, Svetlana, Vira, and other women strove to resuscitate the Soviet-era formulation of class differentiation, one that was based not so much on citizens' productive potential or economic capital but on access to cultural and social capital, and claims to entitlement. These activists stressed the state's obligation to care for their 'needs,' as they defined them. These entitlement-based claims may ultimately have little resonance in the new Ukrainian political economy. To understand the shifting politics of claims in post-Soviet Ukraine, and why the advocacy efforts of Svetlana, Vira, and many others have proved largely unsuccessful, it is necessary first to understand the shifts between Soviet and post-Soviet formulations of class difference.

In the Soviet Union, real differences in income between more- and less-educated workers were small, yet a distinction between the intelligentsia and the 'working class' was central to perceptions of difference, often labelled as one's 'level of culture' (*kul'turnist'*; Patico 2005, 483).[6] Therefore, social differentiation was based not primarily on monetary capital but rather on cultural and social capital, which were assessed by calculating education and qualifications, manners, taste, 'knowledge,' social ties, and access to information and resources (Bourdieu 1986). In today's conditions of neo-liberal market reforms, and an increasingly stratified society in terms of socioeconomics, this system of social differentiation has changed. Income and material wealth are slowly becoming the common criteria for distinguishing between 'classes,' and the success of reforms in Ukraine is being gauged in part by donor governments according to the growth of the Ukrainian 'middle class.' However, a certain amount of cultural capital is still crucial to qualify as a member of the elite, or even as middle class.

Although the situation has changed as more Ukrainians move into the market sphere and engage in business activities, during the early years of post-socialism many were highly sceptical of the new cliques of very wealthy 'businessmen' (*biznesmeny*) and the trappings of their wealth (Grant 1999; Humphrey 2002; Ries 2002). Those years saw the rise of Ukrainian nouveaux riches ('New Ukrainians') who had access to a range of goods and services not available to the average Ukrainian, such as lavish meals in expensive restaurants, the ubiquitous black Mercedes-Benz or SUV, protection services, and medical care in Kyiv's numerous privatized clinics. More often than not, wealthy New Ukrainians were not afforded respect by their less privileged compatriots (except out of fear) – they were ridiculed for their poor taste and tacky lifestyles, and criticized for their conspicuous consumption.

Because the New Ukrainians were perceived to be lacking 'culture' and education, to have poor taste, and to exhibit bad manners, they were actually perceived as 'low class,' despite their material wealth (Patico 2000, 77).[7] By denigrating the New Ukrainians as wealthy yet 'uncultured' and dim-witted, people asserted their own 'culturedness,' intelligence, and good taste, thus indicating that cultural capital is still an essential part of calculating class in post-Soviet Ukraine, despite the growing importance of economic criteria. In their efforts to stem the tide of class differentiation, activists such as Svetlana and Vira capitalized on this fact in their descriptions of themselves as impoverished, yet cultured and intelligent women.

Despite the emergence of economic capital as an increasingly important criterion for calculating one's class, social capital also remains a key aspect of class identity. In the shortage economy of the Soviet Union, networks (called *blat*, meaning connections, or 'pull' in Russian) were important mechanisms for social stratification. One's *blat* networks consisted of relatives, acquaintances, and friends who were placed in positions affording them access to goods and services in shortage. Those unable to cope with the new market, and those who have been most marginalized by its introduction, continue to mobilize the ideology and practice of 'mutual help,' in which networks and shared assistance are crucial for everyday life; this was the main idea undergirding the activities of the 'mutual-aid associations' in my study. A certain shift in the focus of *blat* networks, however, does reveal the emergence of money as a new source of power; namely, *blat* networks have shifted away from access to goods towards possibilities for accumulating income. In other words, *blat* is mobilized as a form of social capital that has the potential to produce economic capital.

What I want to explore here is how the making of classes in postsocialism is both a structural and a subjective phenomenon. As Dunn (2008, 230) argues, 'One of the central theoretical dilemmas posed by the anthropology of postsocialism . . . is how to talk about the kinds of freedom that market democracy presents for self-making and agency without neglecting a rigorous, deep investigation into the constraints posed by emerging structures of inequality and new forms of oppression.' By examining the 'claims talk' and self-narratives of female social activists resisting socioeconomic and political marginalization, I hope to contribute new insights into theories of the formation and reproduction of social inequalities after socialism (see Dunn 2008, 232), particularly the intersections of class distinctions and gender inequality (Gapova 2004).

(Re)producing Claims

In the late 1990s, faced with the tide of post-socialist, neo-liberal social welfare reform that was slowly washing away universal benefits and leaving instead needs-based assistance, NGO activists such as Svetlana and Vira made it a priority to protect the interests of their constituents and themselves as mothers of many children (Haney 2002; Whitefield 2003). Although officially they were considered unemployed (their NGO work was not officially remunerated, and they did not hold other jobs), which seemed to indicate that they would easily qualify for assistance via new procedures of needs-based assessments, they were nevertheless in precarious positions. Svetlana's two eldest children were aging out of the system, and soon she would receive a pension for only her youngest daughter (and this as a single mother, as she would no longer qualify as a 'mother of many children'). Svetlana thought this was unfair – her son was a university student and she had borrowed large sums of money from relatives to put him through school. He did not contribute to the family budget; rather (in Svetlana's words), he helped drain it. The same was true for the elder of his sisters, who was taking secretarial courses and was not working. Vira's situation was slightly better: her husband was a small business owner. Still, he supported the family of five on the profits of his business, since Vira was unemployed and their daughters were still in school. Moreover, in the late 1990s, Vira's husband was clearing only 47 UAH (about $12 at the time) per month, not enough for him to pay into the pension fund (to draw an eventual old-age pension) and not enough for the family to receive a housing subsidy. It was unclear to Vira whether her family would qualify for needs-based assistance.

Neither Svetlana nor Vira was eligible for unemployment benefits, since they had turned down jobs they had been offered through the unemployment office, jobs where, in their estimation, the salary would have basically equalled their cost of transportation to and from work. Both women were extremely worried about how they would support themselves in their old age; with reforms tying old-age pensions to wage amounts and length of service, their pensions would be tiny or non-existent (V. Iatsenko 2005; N. Iatsenko 2006). So they were desperately trying to assert their claims as persons deserving of recognition and redistribution from the state and from society at large. This was essential for them personally as mothers, and also as NGO activists as they sought to garner support from the state, businesspeople, and foreign sponsors for their organization.

Amid the impending implementation of income tests and needs-based social assistance, Svetlana and Vira were caught in a bind. Differentiation processes entailed in welfare reform are characterized by shifts in focus between what people (now 'clients') contribute to society (making them 'deserving') and what they lack (making them 'needy'). In their claims making, then, the women were negotiating 'needs talk' from two sides. On the one hand, they sought to position themselves as needing assistance as members of a vulnerable category of citizens (mothers of many children, and, in Svetlana's case, single mothers). To do this, they focused on their poverty and emphasized that they were 'needy.' However, in the context of new processes of welfare stigmatization, where being 'needy' is seen as a personal shortcoming, Svetlana and Vira also had to calculate and demonstrate their social worth (Haney 1999). Therefore, the women had to emphasize the contributions they made to society. They needed to be both deserving and needy, because it was unclear how the scales of reform would tilt.

Svetlana and Vira based most of their claims on their status as mothers. These NGO activists had come to womanhood in a pro-natalist, socialist state, where their role as mother was prioritized. As mothers who were each raising three children, Svetlana and Vira felt strongly that they were owed entitlements. During our interviews, Svetlana frequently calculated the various types of government pensions she had received during her maternity leaves, the same allowances on which any mother in the Soviet Union would have depended. The sense of entitlement she felt was universal to all working Soviet women, who were promised a range of benefits to help them reconcile their roles as both workers and mothers. Haney's description of the maternalist claims that women were accustomed to espousing in the Hungarian socialist welfare system also applies to the Soviet Union: 'These policies trained women on how to stake a claim in the welfare apparatus and on how to emphasize their identities as mothers when couching their appeals. They taught women that as mothers and caretakers, they had "special" needs. What is more, their needs were transformed into social rights through an entitlement system that guaranteed specific resources for mothers' (p. 154).

Svetlana and Vira saw no reason why, in post-socialism, their roles as mothers should have diminished in the eyes of the state. However, in the late 1990s, their emphasis on their status as mothers had less and less resonance, and their stories often echoed those of Haney's informants in Hungary, who desperately asserted, 'But we are still mothers!' (Haney 1999). It is important to note that during those years their motherhood-focused claims were devalued both by representatives of the social welfare system and by international foundations that supported women's NGO initiatives in Ukraine. The maternalist nature of their claims and self-identity was seen as out-of-date and out-of-step with the feminist mandate promoted by these organizations. Representatives of feminist-oriented international NGO development organizations operated on the assumption that a 'rights' platform was incompatible with maternalist organizing. This assumption overlooked the fact that women such as Svetlana and Vira were using a motherist argument to fight discrimination against certain categories of women (mothers of many children, single mothers), but this was not interpreted as a 'rights' platform by representatives of donor organizations, who dismissed their maternalist stance as backward.

It seems curious that the voices of women who had several children would be dismissed by the state in the context of Ukraine's ongoing demographic crisis. At the level of official rhetoric, pro-natalist policies have been articulated ever since the Second World War in an effort to maintain and increase population levels. However, in our interviews, Svetlana and Vira told me a different story. They recognized that 'mothers of many children' were privileged in Soviet discourse, and they were nostalgic for the entitlements and subsidies they had been extended, but they were also quick to point out the discrimination they had faced under the socialist regime. In spite of the Soviet state's pro-natalist ideology, they told me, large families had always been treated ambivalently. The women attributed the contemporary poor treatment afforded them by state and business representatives to stereotypes of large families that had existed during Soviet times. Vira said:

'When the big crisis happened a few years ago, *mnogodetnye mamy* [Rus., mothers of many children] were despised. We could buy four kilograms of sugar instead of only one, because we had three children. People in line said, 'They have babies, but who will feed them?' I tried to explain to them that I pay for what I get, so what difference does it make to them? I'm not taking food out of their children's mouths; they get their 'norm,' too. But they still hated us.'

Svetlana added:

Whatever government office we go into, we always hear, '*Narozhdaiut nishchikh*' [Rus., 'They are giving birth to the destitute']. People can't stand *mnogodetnye*. They think we are parasites, that we can't do anything except have babies.

Given Svetlana's and Vira's descriptions of the stigmatization of large families, it is ironic that, among the elite classes in Ukraine, having many children has become quite fashionable. Former President Yushchenko has five children, for example, and the wealthy businessman and powerful parliamentarian Petro Poroshenko has four children.

There is certainly a perception in Ukraine that large families are either very rich or very poor, a dichotomy that positions only certain social strata (the wealthy, self-supporting elite) as possessing a real right to have many children. Although Svetlana and Vira indicated that they had been poorly treated both during and after socialism, the root of this stigmatization had shifted. If during the Soviet period large families were shunned primarily in times of shortage, in post-socialist Ukraine poor families with many children were seen as inherently non-productive and thus, as Svetlana put it, as a 'burden on society.' So when their claims to special recognition as mothers were devalued, these women sought to emphasize their productive potential as well.

They did so primarily by emphasizing their role as workers, both during and after the Soviet period. In our interviews, both women spoke at length about their work histories – they had received a technical education (commensurate with a two-year degree in the United States) and worked at various blue-collar and semi-skilled jobs. During the late 1990s, they were fighting hard to establish an identity as 'employees,' even though they were officially unemployed and did not receive a formal salary as NGO organizers. This was a pressing issue, since, as persons recognized as 'volunteers' by representatives of the state apparatus, no provisions were being made to ensure their retirement pensions. According to Svetlana and Vira, state bureaucrats regarded them not merely as 'unemployed' but rather as *tuneiadki* (Rus.), literally 'female spongers' or 'female parasites.'[8] The women thought this was ironic, since they had searched for work in earnest but had been unable to find jobs paying a living wage.

According to Svetlana and Vira, when they went to the Kyiv City Administration to plead their case and convince the authorities that as 'social workers' working fourteen-hour days, they were, in fact, 'employed' and should be given certain benefits (specifically, they wanted to be allowed to pay into the pension fund), the response of the woman in charge of their case was as follows:

Social [Rus. *obshchestvennaia*] work isn't considered to be 'work'; it is a hobby. We thought that you were prosperous ladies, that you didn't have anything to do, and in order to get out of the house and away from housework, you decided to dabble in social work.

The two women, both of them nearly destitute, laughed at this (most certainly sarcastic) characterization of themselves as 'prosperous ladies,' probably a reference to the wives of factory directors and other elites during the early Soviet period (the *obshchestvennitsi*) who were volunteer social workers. They realized that the caseworker was making fun of them, and their appeals to receive state benefits as bona fide 'employees' were brushed aside.

It is important to note that even when the women emphasized their productive potential as workers (rather than their reproductive potential as women), these narratives were nevertheless shot through with thoroughly gendered talk. Svetlana frequently described herself as a 'workhorse' and detailed her gruelling life as a blue-collar factory worker (which included lifting boxes that totalled two tons a day), but she took care to emphasize that she had undertaken this work 'as a good mother.'

Accounting for Social Worth

As they sought to secure support for themselves and other large families, women such as Svetlana and Vira were marginalized as 'low class' and their social worth was questioned, but not primarily because they were poor. Rather, they were stigmatized because they drew on Soviet-era discourses of state support, entitlement, and 'needs' that are an anathema to the perceived transition to a free market society. The neo-liberal ideology of the new free market economy labels these women (welfare mothers, retirees, and others) as non-productive and non-deserving. They were thus excluded from elite NGO circles, whose members shared narratives of self-empowerment, entrepreneurship, productive citizenship, and self-sufficiency. Recognizing their marginal position, these women used talk to shore up their sense of self-worth and to initiate public re-education. In navigating the shifting meanings of 'needs' and deservedness, they focused on their intense suffering as they spun out stories of hard work, shaming, and discrimination. Therefore, they emphasized their impoverishment and neediness even as they stressed their past and potential productive contributions to state and society. While relating their experiences of sudden and extreme poverty, the women were eager to convey that the mere fact of their poverty did not make them deserving of the cruel treatment they often faced from state officials and business representatives.

Many of my conversations with Svetlana revolved around her attempts both to account for her poverty and to resist the way she was categorized as 'low class' in post-Soviet Ukrainian society. Her narratives were strikingly different from those of activists in my study who had become part of Westward-looking NGO networks, like the Soros Foundation, the New Independent States – United States (NIS – U.S.) Women's Consortium, and others, since Svetlana's hinged not on ideas of democracy and self-empowerment but on suffering and entitlement. Svetlana continually emphasized how she had suffered through the years, sometimes slipping into the speech genre of 'saints' lives' described by Ries (1997) in the Russian context. Articulating her stories of suffering, I think, was one way she sought to generate moral capital in a political economy that had left her by the wayside.

Svetlana had been the victim of two broken marriages; her first husband, whom she called 'a weak man,' beat her and even had his friends stab her when she threatened to leave and take their two small children with her. After their divorce, he stalked her and the children, and once attempted to kidnap their son from a playground. Her second marriage was short-lived; her husband decided to remarry his former wife, leaving Svetlana, then several months' pregnant. When her daughter (and third child) was born, she simply wrote 'single mother' on the birth certificate. She did not want to see the baby's father again, so she decided not to take him to court to prove paternity. This freed the father from any child support payments or responsibility for the child, something Svetlana later regretted (she had made the decision before perestroika, when she had 3,000 rubles in savings and, in any case, received 75 rubles a month from the state for the new baby).[9]

Svetlana also described in detail how hard she had worked to independently support her three children, and how she had accumulated personal savings before perestroika and the economic collapse. As she listed the various blue-collar jobs she had held, Svetlana countered popular stereotypes of 'mothers of many children' and 'welfare mothers' who supposedly do not work, only have babies, do not think about the future, and only live in the moment. Svetlana emphasized, however, that the economic crash of the late 1980s meant that all her hard work and planning were for naught. Almost everyone in Ukraine experienced the same near-overnight destitution and panic. Svetlana portrayed herself as no different from others and yet stressed that, as an overstretched single mother, she had few material possessions at the time, which made her situation especially precarious. In her words:

Within two months I became destitute. Inflation totally ate up my savings. After that my savings would have bought nothing more than a box of matches. After I had worked so hard and economized – I could have bought a box of matches or ridden on the trolleybus once. My savings turned into soap bubbles.

If, as others did, Svetlana had foreseen the economic crash and used her savings to buy durable goods (such as furniture, appliances, or building materials), her situation would have been better. But with the crash her savings quickly melted away, and Svetlana, still a single mother, remained destitute despite attempts to find work. She stayed on the rolls of the local unemployment office but gave up hope of finding a viable job. She saw no alternative but to depend on state allowances as a single mother, her first husband's alimony payments (which he rarely paid), and her daughter's small monthly allowance from the state as a 'fatherless' child. Her role as the director of Our House was also a survival strategy, since any humanitarian aid the group acquired would go to her family as well.

Svetlana wanted to prevent her children from slipping into the underclass that she felt she was becoming part of, and she saw education as key. Her son, a teenager in the late 1990s, was a student at an institute in Kyiv. Svetlana had borrowed large sums of money from relatives, friends, and acquaintances to pay for his tuition, and was pinning all her hopes on his receiving a good job upon graduation. The debts she had incurred caused her great stress that often escalated into health problems. Svetlana and Vira were incensed when legislative changes threatened to bar families of three or more children that included university students from receiving state benefits as 'large families.' When they protested, the response of caseworkers was demeaning:

svetlana: Do you know what they told us? The 'ladies' [Rus. *damy*] who take care of that? They said, 'It is a luxury to get an education. Let them go and work.' Where? Not having a specialty and not having an education? What will they work as? Racketeers, or at the [stock] exchange [Rus. *birzha*]? What can they work as?

vira: So it's like before, [people think] 'They are creating superfluous [Rus. *lishnie*] people.' Superfluous for society. That was the woman who was supposed to be defending the interests of our families. If she has such an opinion of us, what can we expect from everyone else?

Svetlana and Vira interpreted the caseworker's position that teenagers from poor families should 'go and work' instead of receiving an education as evidence of the differentiation of large families as 'low class.' They responded in the interviews with attempts to counter negative stereotypes about large families that were prevalent in the popular imagination. They spoke of members in their organization who were accomplished musicians, and they showed me the artistic work of children from large families who had won art competitions.

They described their members as 'cultured people' who came from 'old Kyivan families' that represented the 'impoverished intelligentsia.' The women often noted that the privatization of education and the offering of 'extracurricular classes' in music, dance, and art on a fee-paying basis (subjects that were a standard part of the curriculum in Soviet times) meant that children from large families and impoverished families in general missed out on opportunities to develop their creative and performance skills and learn about high culture.

Despite the women's continued attempts to 'shake things up,' as they put it, and insist on the rights of large families as a deserving category of citizens, they were fighting an uphill battle. The organization Our House had been unable to pay 4,000 UAH (about $1,100 at the time) to the state in rent arrears, and the office was requisitioned in 2001. When I met them again in 2002, Svetlana and Vira assured me that their organizing activities had been interrupted only temporarily, but meanwhile they had sought official employment. Svetlana had gone to work for a crisis hotline, a job she found emotionally rewarding but physically demanding – she had to work twenty-four-hour shifts and said she was practically not allowed to lie down. Her salary was very low, just $100 a month (less than half the national average). Vira remained unemployed. With the advocacy efforts of Our House all but suspended, the seventy large families the organization represented were left to fend for themselves.

Conclusions: Assessing Needs

In describing how these NGO activists have articulated claims and espoused value narratives to argue for their social worth and resist being positioned in devalued class identities, I do not mean to imply that they had somehow become stuck in a Soviet past or a 'socialist mindset,' unaware of the transforming political economy and changing ideologies of worth swirling around them. On the contrary, these women were keenly cognizant of post-socialist processes of differentiation that positioned them on the losing end of the transition, and they were astute observers of others' opinions of them as needy mothers of many children. They were not some 'old Soviet guard' who longed for a return to the Soviet Union or to state socialism. Perfectly aware that others might perceive them this way, activists such as Svetlana and Vira were careful to emphasize the ways in which they were precisely 'not Soviet.' Svetlana and Vira, ironically, actually launched a project of differentiation when they undertook a 'needs assessment' of their organization's members that mirrored, eerily, case workers' 'reviews,' which they themselves would likely face as mothers of many children.

In a 1999 interview, Svetlana described her motivation for differentiating her needy members from the non-needy:

Once I visited one of our member families (they had five children) and I was shocked to see how well they were living. They had *Evroremont* [European-style renovations], a computer, and beautiful furniture. When I saw this family that I was working to help, it made me ill [Rus. *mne plokho stalo*]. They could have helped [others] themselves, and here we were running around to find help for them . . . I went about in a trance for about a month. I thought, 'Svetlana, why in the world do you need this? What are you doing this for?' Here I was – and I fall into the poorest category of the families of our organization – here I was running my legs off to find help for such families, and then I find out that they are living the high life and could have helped others themselves! I took it really hard . . . [After the experience we had with that well-off family] we immediately called a meeting of the organization's officers and decided to do an evaluation of all the families. We went around to each family and assessed their needs. About four or five of them we felt do not need help from the organization. But we didn't take any of them off our membership roster. They are still members, and their children can participate in our holidays and trips, but we excluded [Rus. *iskliuchili*] them from our help.

In conducting her own needs assessment of member families, Svetlana was both a subject and an agent of state institutions mandated to undertake 'differentiation' of social assistance as part of social insurance reform. Her participation in this project – one that she and other 'mothers of many children' resisted on other levels – reveals the complex nature of the politics of recognition and redistribution in post-socialist Ukraine. It also shows how NGO activists have become both subjects and agents of the reform process, which has led to the formation of somewhat contradictory personal and social identities. As Svetlana and Vira worked in their office and interacted with other impoverished heads of families, there was a sense of the common struggles of the underclass of the newly poor. They delighted in each other's stories of scraping by and making do. These sessions escalated into veritable storytelling matches: Who was the ultimate mama-heroine-trickster? Whose creative means of surviving destitution would prevail? But when Svetlana and Vira scoured the capital city for sponsors, knocking on doors asking for support, suddenly they were 'low class,' 'insolent' women 'giving birth to the poor.' In other contexts, they were administrators of a particular kind of social justice, bureaucrats in their own right who were empowered to assess the relative needs of their clients in Our House.

To assert their claims, these NGO activists at times emphasized their needs and right to entitlements as special categories of citizens. However, they also leveraged the language of self-sufficiency, differentiation, and active citizenship that increasingly informs the social contract in conditions of market reform. Although they did tend to draw on ideas of entitlement in their value narratives, it should be noted that entitlement is not necessarily a passive stance. In asserting their own social worth and that of others like them, and in engaging in lobbying efforts and claims making, women such as Svetlana, Vira, and other activists I knew saw themselves as taking a stance of active citizenship. Ultimately, however, their efforts met with little success.

The narrative accounts of these activists, understood in their 'etymologically rich sense' as both narration and bookkeeping, allow us to track the post-socialist creation of difference, and the material effects of exclusion, including the marginalization and disempowerment of certain categories of citizens, namely, those viewed as 'unproductive' (Stark 1994, 21). Although these women worked hard to carve out their own place in the new political economy, they failed in establishing a higher status for themselves in the society and securing the material benefits that go with it.

One activist I knew said that 'user' organizations such as the mutual-aid associations for large families, pensioners, and veterans would 'fade from view' once the economic situation in Ukraine improved and people 'outgrew' these NGOs. This vision of the happy post-socialist march to capitalism obscures the forms of differentiation that are occurring in the country at large, and in the NGO sphere as well. It is comforting to tell ourselves that privatization and democratization benefit all of society, but the stories of Svetlana and Vira tell a different tale. Their stories complicate rosy assessments of 'reform' and 'civil society building' because they present the stark reality in which entire categories of people, many of them women, seem to have fallen through the cracks.

NOTES

1 All names are pseudonyms, to protect the identity of my research informants. I use the Russian variant Svetlana (rather than the Ukrainian Svitlana) to indicate this informant's self-identification as an ethnic Russian. Vira, in contrast, self-identified as an ethnic Ukrainian. Both women preferred to speak Russian, and accordingly, all our conversations took place in Russian.

2 When transliterating from the Russian, I use the designation 'Rus.' When no designation is given, the transliteration is from the Ukrainian.

3 This was the benefit for children in large families in 1999, when the exchange rate went from $1 = 3.43 UAH (the Ukrainian hryvnia, the official currency of Ukraine) in January, to $1 = 4.27 UAH in August, and $1 = 5.02 UAH in December. To give a sense of how much buying power 70 UAH carried, consider that in 1999 one kilogram of meat cost 7.06 UAH, one litre of milk cost 1.26 UAH, and a loaf of bread cost .70 UAH.

4 The 'feminization' of the 'third sector' of NGOs is common across post-socialist states. Tohidi (2004) outlines the reasons women in Azerbaijan are especially likely to undertake NGO organizing: women are excluded from opportunities to advance in politics and business, women have traditionally been responsible for mediating social problems, the civic arena is seen as less corrupt than official politics (and thus more appropriate for women), and women tend to possess vital networking and linguistic skills. These factors hold for the Ukrainian case as well. Handrahan (2002, 80) notes that 76% of the 28 NGOs she surveyed in Kyrgyzstan were led by women, and 96% of her respondents believed that women were leading NGOs nationwide.

5 In May 2000, e.g., an event called 'Kyiv Civic Organization Day' was held by Kyiv's Innovation and Development Centre to showcase the work of the various social organizations in the city. Of the 150 civic and charitable organizations represented at the exhibition, 40% were formed to protect the

interests of children, families, and women. Of the organizations with such an orientation, 68% were directed by women (Innovation and Development Centre 2000).

6 Patico (2005, 483) further notes that '*kul'turnost*' (culturedness) came to refer in the early twentieth century to a code of public conduct and a template for the proper relationship of individuals to material possessions, denoting a combination of polite manners, hygiene, and basic knowledge of high culture.'

7 Stereotypes of 'New Ukrainians' (as with those of New Russians) almost never refer to women. Patico has proposed that 'this may be related to the fact that being a New Russian implies not only wealth, but also particular activities (including crime) and displays (raspberry jackets, shaved heads, heavy gold jewelry) that are associated more with men than with women and very strikingly differentiate New Russian men from other Russian men' (2000, 77). In St Petersburg, Patico found that New Russian women were usually understood to be successful businesswomen or the wives and girlfriends of New Russian men.

8 *Tuneiadets,* or 'parasite,' is a Soviet-era concept. In Soviet discourse, practically every citizen was required to work and thus 'make a contribution to society.' Those who did not were labelled 'parasites,' and could be arrested and jailed. The idea of the *tuneiadets* arose from the false assertion that unemployment as such did not exist in the Soviet Union, in contrast to the United States and other Western countries. Homelessness was also officially non-existent, although there were homeless persons in the Soviet Union.

9 During the early 1990s, 3,000 rubles was a large nest egg in the Soviet Union, and 75 rubles a month was enough to take care of all the needs of Svetlana and her children.

REFERENCES

Bourdieu, P. 1986. Forms of Capital. In J.G. Richardson, ed., *Handbook of Theory and Research for the Sociology of Education,* 241–58. Westport: Greenwood.

Caldwell, M. 2002. The Taste of Nationalism: Food Politics in Post-socialist Moscow. *Ethnos* 67(3): 295–319.

– 2004. *Not by Bread Alone: Social Support in the New Russia.* Berkeley: University of California Press.

Dunn, E. 2004. *Privatizing Poland: Baby Food, Big Business, and the Remaking of Labor.* Ithaca: Cornell University Press.

– 2008. Subjectivity after Socialism: An Invitation to Theory Building in Anthropology. In I. Schröder and A. Vonderau, eds., *Changing Economies and Changing Identities in Postsocialist Eastern Europe*, 225–33. Berlin: Lit-Verlag.

Einhorn, B. 2000. Discussant's Comments. In M. Lazreg, ed., *Making the Transition Work for Women in Europe and Central Asia*, 107–13. Washington, DC: World Bank.

Gapova, E. 2004. O gendere, natsii i klasse v postkommunizme [On Gender, Nation, and Class in Post-communism]. *Gendernye issldeovaniia* [Gender Research] 13:101–18.

– 2005. Conceptualizing Gender, Nation, and Class in Post-Soviet Belarus. In K. Kuehnast and C. Nechemias, eds., *Post-Soviet Women Encountering Transition: Nation Building, Economic Survival, and Civic Activism*, 85–102. Washington, DC: Woodrow Wilson Center Press.

– 2007. On the Political Significance of the Sexual Division of Labour. *Aspasia: International Yearbook of Central, Eastern, and Southeastern European Women's and Gender History* 1: 231–5.

Ghodsee, K. 2005. *The Red Riviera: Gender, Tourism, and Postsocialism on the Black Sea*. Durham: Duke University Press.

Grant, B. 1999. The Return of the Repressed: Conversations with Three Russian Entrepreneurs. In G. Marcus, ed., *Paranoia within Reason: A Casebook on Conspiracy as Explanation*, 241–67. Chicago: University of Chicago Press.

Handrahan, L.M. 2002. *Gendering Ethnicity: Implications for Democracy Assistance*. New York: Routledge.

Haney, L. 1999. 'But We Are Still Mothers': Gender, the State, and the Construction of Need in Post-socialist Hungary. In M. Burawoy and K. Verdery, eds., *Uncertain Transition: Ethnographies of Change in the Post-socialist World*, 151–87. Oxford: Rowman and Littlefield.

– 2002. *Inventing the Needy: Gender and the Politics of Welfare in Hungary*. Berkeley: University of California Press.

Humphrey, C. 1995. Creating a Culture of Disillusionment: Consumption in Moscow, a Chronicle of Changing Times. In D. Miller, ed., *Worlds Apart: Modernity through the Prism of the Local*, 43–68. New York: Routledge.

– 2002. The Villas of the 'New Russians': A Sketch of Consumption and Cultural Identity in Post-Soviet Landscapes. In C. Humphrey, ed., *The Unmaking of Soviet Life: Everyday Economies after Socialism*, 175–201. Ithaca: Cornell University Press.

Iatsenko, N. 2006. Ella Libanova: 'U zhinky menshe trudovykh prav cherez nyz'kyi pensiinyi vik i nyzhchu, nizh u cholovikiv, zarplatu [Women Have Fewer Labour Rights because of an Earlier Retirement Age and Lower

Salaries than Men's]. *Dzerkalo Tyzhnia* [Weekly Mirror] 22(601). Available at http://www.dt.ua/2000/2650/53616/ (accessed 27 Sept. 2007).

Iatsenko, V. 2005. Pensiina reforma: U poshuku zdorovoho hluzdu ta spravedlyvosti [Pension Reform: In Search of Common Sense and Fairness]. *Dzerkalo Tyzhnia* [Weekly Mirror] 11(539). Available at http://www.dt.ua/2000/49592/ (accessed 27 Sept. 2007).

Innovation and Development Centre (IDC). 2000. *Den' Hromads'kykh Orhanizatsii Kyieva: Kataloh Uchasnykiv* [Kyiv Civic Organization Day: Catalogue of Participants]. Kyiv: IDC.

Lampland, M. 2000. Afterword. In D. Berdahl, M. Bunzl, and M. Lampland, eds., *Altering States: Ethnographies of Transition in Eastern Europe and the Former Soviet Union*, 209–18. Ann Arbor: University of Michigan Press.

Liborakina, M. 1998. The Unappreciated Mothers of Civil Society. *Transitions* 5(1): 52–7.

Palyvoda, L., O. Kikot, and O. Vlasova. 2006. *Civil Society Organizations in Ukraine: The State and Dynamics (2002–2005).* Kyiv: Macros.

Patico, J. 2000. 'New Russian' Sightings and the Question of Social Difference in St Petersburg. *Anthropology of East Europe Review* 18(2): 73–7.

– 2002. Chocolate and Cognac: Gifts and the Recognition of Social Worlds in Post-Soviet Russia. *Ethnos* 67(3): 345–68.

– 2005. To Be Happy in a Mercedes: Tropes of Value and Ambivalent Visions of Marketization. *American Ethnologist* 32(3): 479–96.

Phillips, S.D. 2008. *Women's Social Activism in the New Ukraine: Development and the Politics of Differentiation.* Bloomington: Indiana University Press.

Ries, N. 1997. *Russian Talk: Culture and Conversation during Perestroika.* Ithaca: Cornell University Press.

– 2002. 'Honest Bandits' and 'Warped People': Russian Narratives about Money, Corruption, and Moral Decay. In C.J. Greenhouse, E. Mertz, and K.B. Warren, eds., *Ethnography in Unstable Places: Everyday Lives in Contexts of Dramatic Political Change*, 276–315. Durham: Duke University Press.

Rivkin-Fish, M. 2005. *Women's Health in Post-Soviet Russia: The Politics of Intervention.* Bloomington: Indiana University Press.

Schröder, I., and A. Vonderau, eds. 2008. *Changing Economies and Changing Identities in Postsocialist Eastern Europe.* Berlin: Lit-Verlag.

Stark, D.1994. Recombinant Property in East European Capitalism. *Program on Central and Eastern Europe Working Paper Series no. 33.* Available at http://www.ces.fas.harvard.edu/publications/docs/pdfs/CEE_WP33.pdf (accessed 12 May 2011).

Tohidi, N. 2004. Women, Building Civil Society, and Democratization in Post-Soviet Azerbaijan. In K. Kuehnast and C. Nechemias, eds., *Post-Soviet*

Women Encountering Transition: Nation Building, Economic Survival, and Civic Activism, 149–71. Washington, DC: Woodrow Wilson Center Press.

Whitefield, S. 2003. The Political Economy of Welfare Reform and Poverty Alleviation in Ukraine. In W.W. Isajiw, ed., *Society in Transition: Social Change in Ukraine in Western Perspectives,* 401–25. Toronto: Canadian Scholars' Press.

8 Homeless Men and the Crisis of Masculinity in Contemporary Ukraine

ANASTASIYA RIABCHUK

Homeless persons are among the most economically marginalized and culturally stigmatized social groups in post-Soviet societies. The Russian abbreviation, *bomzh* (*bez opredelennogo mesta zhytelstva*, literally meaning 'without a permanent place of residence'), is a widely used label for the so-called underclass of unemployed, middle-aged or elderly single men with a lack of social ties, health problems, and alcohol or drug addictions. In post-communist societies the homeless are often portrayed as deviants who spread infectious disease, are involved in criminal or asocial behaviour (digging through garbage, sleeping in the hallways of apartment blocks), and who refuse to work or to receive treatment.

In 2004 in Ukraine, more than 80 per cent of all officially registered homeless people were male, according to the research project 'The Way Home.'[1] But this gendered dimension of homelessness has not been analysed in detail. Although many problems that affect homeless people (such as bad health, vulnerability related to life on the streets, and lack of services and affordable housing) are true for nearly everyone who is homeless, other problems are gender-specific. Glaser (1994) notes that, because life on the streets is especially dangerous for homeless women, many in this group have 'learned to stay in the shadow in order to survive [and their] plight has also tended to remain hidden from view.' On the other hand, because it is not socially acceptable for a woman to be on the streets, there are often better and more diverse services available for homeless women than for homeless men. According to Cramer (2005), housing officers, in their informal categorization of homeless clients, tend to see homeless women as the more 'deserving' group and distinguish between 'troublesome' male offenders and 'troubled' women in need. She concludes that 'homelessness is a site where gender is both experienced and constructed' (p. 738).

Men, meanwhile, are more likely to suffer from chronic homelessness and remain on the streets for longer periods of time:[2] 'Homeless men [. . .] receive only the most meagre responses to their problems. Their independence and the public perception of them as threatening, as alcoholics, and as mentally ill put this group last on the list for help,' notes Glaser (1994, 37). Writing about the stigmatization of homeless women in post-Soviet societies, Höjdestrand (2009) admits that 'homelessness is not a fertile soil for cultivation of socially accepted men either.' To her, the homeless man, stereotyped as a *bomzh*, is a powerless, emasculated figure analogous to the refuse spaces he inhabits, and far from what Connell (2005), in referring to 'the pattern of practice that allows men's dominance over women,' would call 'hegemonic masculinity' (p. 832). Although this pattern is not common in the statistical sense – only a minority of men can enact it – it is considered normative as the 'most honored way of being a man, [requiring] all other men to position themselves in relation to it' (p. 832). The practice of hegemonic masculinity includes both 'negative' and 'positive' aspects: violence and domination over women (and men with subjugated or marginalized masculinities) as well as the more revered work of 'bringing home a wage, sustaining a sexual relationship and being a father' (p. 840). From this perspective, homeless men can be considered to be extreme cases of 'failed hegemonic masculinity': lacking stable employment, suffering from poor health, and unable to provide for their families (or having cut ties with them), they fail to live up to the standard of the successful, strong, and economically stable man. Analysing the situation of homeless men in the context of recent debates about the so-called masculinity crisis in post-Soviet societies, therefore, contributes to both gender studies and homelessness research.

In this chapter, I examine the situation of homeless men in the capital of Ukraine, Kyiv, in the context of gender studies theories on the masculinity crisis, destructive masculinities, and failed masculinities. Drawing on qualitative data I compiled in 2003 and 2004 through semi-structured, in-depth interviews with sixty homeless people in Kyiv, I utilize the typology of men's responses to the crisis of masculinity that was developed by Tartakovskaya (2003), who distinguishes six male self-perceptions related to how men have dealt with this crisis. In doing so, I diverge from her analysis, however, in insisting that more emphasis should be placed on the economic component of homeless men's stories, as this component provides greater explanatory possibilities for capturing the context of a post-Soviet crisis of masculinity. Taking a neo-Marxist position, I conclude that post-Soviet homelessness must be understood as an extreme case of 'failed hegemonic masculinity' in the context of wider structural changes taking place during a transition to capitalism. From this theoretical position, de-proletarization, unemployment, and lack of social security during a transition to capitalism are the main causes of poverty, alcohol abuse, crime, and deviance. These structural factors, combined with the masculinity crisis in post-Soviet societies, contribute to disproportionately high numbers of men among homeless people. An analysis of these structural factors is essential for understanding the phenomenon of homelessness in the Ukrainian context, for challenging stereotypes, and for informing policy action.

Theoretical Debates on the Crisis of Masculinity in Post-Soviet Societies

For a long time, debates on gender inequality have focused on the negative effects of hegemonic masculinity for women who, as a consequence of it, find themselves subordinated. However, recent research has shown that strictly regulated norms and expectations are harmful to men, too. To name just a few of these harms, men often retire later than women, rarely get custody of their children in cases of divorce, suffer from greater stress and pressure related to the need to be economically successful, and are more frequently labelled as losers if they are unable to provide for themselves and their families. Moreover, in all industrialized societies, modernization, technological development, and the greater involvement of men compared with women in the public sphere has led to a higher death rate and lower life expectancy for men (Zdravomyslova and Temkina 2002, 432–51). Many have labelled the sum of these increasingly negative consequences of hegemonic masculinity on men a 'crisis' (Kon 2009; Edwards 2007).

In post-Soviet societies, evidence shows that men are, indeed, in an unfavourable position compared with women: they continue to have a shorter life expectancy; they take up destructive practices such as smoking, alcohol abuse, and unhealthy eating habits more often; and they are more likely to die from preventable causes (stress, accidents, or cardiovascular disease). In Ukraine, as of 2007, men's life expectancy is about 11 years below that of women (62.3 years versus 73.6

years), and the death rate for working-age men (20 to 45 years of age) is more than three times higher than for women in the same age group (Amdzhadin 2007). Bureychak (2008) explains these demographic data as being the result of a number of social factors, such as greater involvement of men in risky behaviour, dangerous work, and criminal activity; men are three times more likely than women to suffer from tuberculosis, five to six times more likely to have alcohol addiction, and seven times more likely to commit violent crimes.

These trends in contemporary Ukrainian society are deeply rooted and can be traced back at least fifty years. Debates about the masculinity crisis in Soviet society actually began in 1968 after a demographic report by Urlanis (1970) showed higher rates of illnesses and mortality among men, compared with women. A public campaign to 'take care of men' was launched, highlighting the following economic and social consequences of what was deemed to be a crisis of masculinity: inefficient use of male labour power, high costs for medical treatment of preventable illnesses caused by male destructive practices, problems related to divorce and child rearing by single mothers, and the social costs of alcoholism. In late Soviet discourse, 'crisis of masculinity' actually became a metaphor for deeper structural ills in society: 'The thesis about the crisis of masculinity suggests that there is a certain normative model of true manhood and a possibility to attain this model of a true man . . . The impossibility to fulfil traditional male roles, related to limitations on liberal rights (property, political freedoms, freedom of expression) were implicitly recognized to be the causes of the destruction of true masculinity, although this thesis was not openly stated until the late 1980s' (Zdravomyslova and Temkina 2002, 343–5).

This reference to liberal rights suggests that a more liberal capitalist model that respected men's rights and freedoms would at least partially resolve the masculinity crisis. However, from today's perspective, such claims can be interpreted as wishful thinking of the perestroika years; the transition to capitalism did not resolve the problems associated with the masculinity crisis, and in fact, aggravated them.

Tartakovskaya (2003) has made a comprehensive analysis of this aggravated masculinity crisis in post-Soviet societies. She conducted research on gender strategies in the labour market in Russia to show that although both men and women often find themselves in crisis situations as a consequence of the transition to capitalism, for men the crisis also implies the impossibility of living up to hegemonic masculinity, a failure that causes a very emotional reaction and even leads to self-doubt in men about their own gender status. Focusing on respondents' own attitudes towards their gender roles, Tartakovskaya introduces the concept of 'failed masculinity' to capture this self-doubt. As she notes, 'Masculinity is not only a theoretical concept from the field of gender studies but has a very personal cultural meaning for each man. It is a project, the realization of which requires great efforts and often even turns out to be impossible.' She classifies six types of self-perceptions that characterize men's responses to situations of failed hegemonic masculinity: 'losers who give up,' 'men who feel unjustly offended,' 'alcoholics,' 'escapists,' 'housewives,' and 'single fathers.'

All of these self-perceptions are shaped by difficulties encountered in the labour market except 'single fathers' and, to some extent, 'housewives.' I will therefore leave aside these last two categories for another discussion, as they exceed the scope of this chapter. For Tartakovskaya (2003), changes that have taken place in the 1990s and 2000s have worsened the crisis of masculinity that began during the Soviet era. Many traditionally male-dominated sectors of the economy, such as the military or machine building, have shrunk, and as a consequence, the professional and economic situation of previously successful men has deteriorated. Men have faced unprecedented economic, professional, and personal difficulties. As Tartakovskaya describes it, 'An unemployed or a working, but poor man is deprived of the main characteristics of his own gender competence and becomes "de-masculinized" and faced with a problem of self-identification in his family circle (provided he has a family), among other close relatives, employees and work colleagues.' This insight is supported by Ashwin (2001), who argues that men have had to meet certain prerequisites in both the Soviet and post-Soviet era before truly becoming 'successful,' namely, professionalization and attaining economic stability as a breadwinner – not only to feed his family, but as a sign of prestige and self-esteem. Therefore, post-Soviet men have a very limited set of legitimate social roles and are dependent on the overall situation in the labour market.

Tartakovskaya (2003) stops short of making a thoroughgoing link between unemployment, poverty, and the masculinity crisis, however. In fact, she denies that economic restructuring during the transition could be solely responsible for failed masculinity. Instead, she lays the blame on the inevitable discrepancy between masculine ideals and reality: 'Even if we look at our respondents who were somehow affected by the contemporary socioeconomic crisis in Russia, the phenomenon of "failed masculinity" is in no way its direct result. On the contrary, a possibility of "failure" is already present in the very concept of masculinity that suggests an internal hierarchy between "real," successful men and those who could not live up to this standard.'

But, as I will argue, Tartakovskaya's focus on the failure of masculine ideals does not sufficiently take into account the social suffering of many post-Soviet men that is the result of economic restructuring. Although I do not claim that the transition to capitalism *caused* the crisis of masculinity, in the tyology that follows I demonstrate that it has had negative effects on the economic and psychological well-being of many men, including on their self-perceptions, and has caused social problems such as rising rates of alcoholism and homelessness.

Homelessness as an Extreme Example of 'Failed Masculinity'

One of the signs of the masculinity crisis is the spread of destructive masculinities, as witnessed in alcoholism, aggressive behaviour towards work colleagues and family members, and criminal activities or vagrancy. In post-industrial societies, these masculinities are especially pervasive among working-class men, as traditional masculine identities related to industrial production become obsolete (Schwarz 1990). Beynon (2002) shows that work is a fundamental component of hegemonic masculinity, but given the current labour market, in which work has become less stable and more oriented towards the service sector where women are more welcome as employees, men who have lost 'real masculine work' in the field of industrial production are stigmatized (p. 87). If a woman, having lost her work, can find other sources of positive identification (as a good housewife, as a beauty, or as a mother), men's identity is almost solely defined by work. Consequently, long-term unemployment is more likely to cause depression, suicide attempts, and/or criminal and destructive behaviour, such as alcoholism and drug abuse among men.

In the Ukrainian context (as well as in other post-Soviet societies), the masculinity crisis and the decline of the industrial economy have occurred alongside two other trends. First, a period of transformation after the breakup of the USSR meant higher levels of stress and social suffering for the majority of the population (related to the need to adapt to changing social conditions). Second, the demise of the social state with guaranteed full employment was felt in an especially acute manner by middle-aged and older working-class men who lost their jobs through economic restructuring. Therefore, when speaking of the negative consequences of the transition, it is important to distinguish those that have resulted from transition itself (felt by men of various social groups), and those that are due to capitalism (felt primarily by working-class men). Homelessness emerges from a combination of these mutually reinforcing 'crises,' with the risk of ending up on the streets being much higher among long-term unemployed working-class men.

To capture these subtle differences, I will now employ Tartakovskaya's typology to organize the findings from my own study. As we will see, the men in my study tend to slide across categories of self-perception rather than belonging to just one.

Losers Who Give Up

In Tartakovskaya's typology of men's self-perceptions in response to the crisis of masculinity, 'losers who give up' appear to be most prominent. Men in this category are mostly victims of economic restructuring – they have either lost their previous jobs or experienced a significant decline in living standards. They perceive their current or past jobs as being of little value, have accepted their low socioeconomic status, and sometimes suffer from additional marginalization because of alcohol abuse. At the same time, as Tartakovskaya notes, such personal devaluation is often preceded by a period of resistance during which a man, unhappy with his situation, tries to keep up at least temporary employment, look after himself, and take care of his family.

Several respondents in my research appear to be living through this initial stage of resistance. In their self-description, they are far from 'losers.' Instead, they define themselves as 'hard workers.' Many of these men are insecurely employed in the Kyiv construction industry, making do with day labour. They cannot rely on a regular income and often have to live for several weeks without work. Forced temporary unemployment may also be caused by injuries, illness, or food poisoning (because of the low quality of food and alcohol consumed). In such periods, these men often find themselves isolated and alone in a large city, and they turn to homeless shelters and soup kitchens for help in survival. Although their living arrangements in Kyiv are never stable, in difficult periods the men may be literally homeless, sleeping in parks, train stations, or shelters for the homeless. Experiences of temporary homelessness in the context of overall insecurity are part of a downward spiral, with negative effects on personal appearance and well-being. For example, Daly (1996) notes, 'There is a continual deterioration in their situation – physical and mental health, stability of friends or family, legal problems, financial and emotional independence, job prospects' (p. 158). The majority of homeless people are chronic alcoholics and 80 per cent suffer from tuberculosis.[3] 'One can only be on the streets for seven – eight years maximum,' says a doctor who helps street homeless in Moscow, 'after that comes death' (Yeroshok 2008).

Despite their experiences of homelessness, insecure housing arrangements, breaks in social ties, and stress that often leads to substance abuse, day labourers in the construction industry refuse to identify themselves as *bomzhi* (those who 'gave up') and fear the prospects of such degradation of their status. One of my study participants said:

> Don't think that I'm some kind of a *bomzhi* here! Yes, I go to these soup kitchens for bomzhi – I have to survive somehow! If they feed for free, why not come? But no, I'm not a bomzhi, I'm a hard worker! I work hard day and night, building apartments for you, Kyivites . . . Yes, building for you and not having anything myself . . . I live right there, at the construction site . . . it's cold there, chalk and sand everywhere. But anyway, I still look after myself. I wash myself every day, and shave. Look at me – do I stink? Do I have scruffy clothes? Am I drunk? Well, I tell you – if I drank and didn't look after myself, nobody would hire me to do the work![4]

If being a *bomzhi* means drinking, not looking after oneself, and refusing to work – something a person can be blamed for – a 'hard worker,' on the contrary, is poor through no fault of his own, not *because of* a failure to adapt, but *despite* all adaptation efforts. This perception is very important among respondents when positioning their own responses to negative change. Viewed structurally, however, we can see that these casual workers in the construction industry form an 'excess reserve army of labour' for whom 'economic advancement translates into a regression of material conditions and a curtailment of life chances,' while 'survival based on a mix of casual labour, welfare support and illegal activities trumps regular wage labour participation' (Wacquant 2007).

Another way in which day labourers distinguish themselves from *bomzhi* is by emphasizing the temporal nature of their status as opposed to those who are chronically homeless. Even when the casual male workers in this sample go through a difficult period, they still believe that things will improve shortly. As one of them said:

> Well, with the *bomzhi* it's hopeless . . . There's no way they will ever change their lives. As for us, hard workers, yes, there are difficult periods, when we sleep in shelters and go to these soup kitchens for bomzhi, but as the saying goes 'after the rain comes the rainbow' – we know that a good period will follow shortly. There will never be any good periods for the *bomzhi*, they can't work, they just gave up.

However, among those who do currently identify as *bomzhi*, many also perceived themselves as having been 'hard workers' at some point in the past. Their stories show that the distinguishing line between categories of self-perception (between hard workers and bomzhi, losers who give up and those who haven't given up yet) is unstable, and that any small injury, illness, or family conflict in a wider context of instability may lead a 'hard worker' to 'give up.' A 32-year-old homeless man from a small town in the Vinnytsia region recalls how he came to work at a construction site in Kyiv because there was no work in his hometown. In the summer he slept by the river, but in the winter he had difficulties finding a place to sleep, because apartment rent was too high even for a group of workers, and he had promised to regularly send money back home to his family. One night he slept at the train station and was robbed and beaten up by a group of street children, so he couldn't return to work the following day and lost his job, which made him feel 'miserable' and contributed to his alcohol abuse. He explained:

> I couldn't go back home either, you know, without the money . . . it's not right . . . what kind of a man am I? I felt miserable . . . Well, I started drinking, and, well, here I am . . . So I guess I'm a *bomzhi* now.

He concludes that he is very unhappy with his situation and drinks even more 'because it's all so depressing.'

Men Who Feel Offended at Being Unjustly Treated

In my sample, as well as in Tartakovskaya's study, men who did not receive positive evaluations of their work (either informally or through formal material and symbolic rewards) often came to lack self-esteem. Some left their jobs and remained unemployed for prolonged periods. Perceived betrayals by a wife represent another reason for which some of the men feel 'unjustly offended' (as such betrayal also challenges sexual potency). One of the men described his situation like this:

> Can you believe it, what a bastard! Son of a b. . . tch! He wanted to rape my wife – of course I didn't let him! I took a hammer and hit him on his head, this jerk. Who knew that he would die? So they put me in jail. Usually you get a life sentence for murder, but with me, because it was 'unintended murder,' I got 12 years. And my wife? She, b. . . tch, while I was in jail, evicted me from my flat; back then it was possible. So I come back and she, b. . . tch, won't let me in! Saying, 'Go away, Zhenia [pseudonym], I don't need you.'[5]

This case presents a violent scenario of family breakup and eventual homelessness beginning with the respondent's taking offence at his wife's behaviour (although the wife's point of view is lacking here, not allowing for an idea of the whole picture). A more 'peaceful' resolution to a similar conflict is related by Vitaliy, who said:

> Am I homeless? That's an interesting question. Actually, I am local, from Kyiv, but now I unwillingly became a vagabond. I left my home, could not live with my wife after she betrayed me . . . Of course, I could fight over my part of the flat in court, but I would have to hire a lawyer – and where would I find the money for that? And I don't want to quarrel with my wife – let her do whatever she wants with her beloved one, I can some-how manage to survive on the streets. Actually, it's not a matter of food or other 'material' things. I have no friends; I am alone. A knife in my pocket and no one will touch me. I collect bottles. No, it's not a matter of food or money. I go to the Victory Church – they have such preaching! Yes, people help me but it's not about help. Most of all I lack communication and rest – I have everything else.

In this passage, Vitaliy is resentful about his wife 'betraying him' with another man – he feels offended, but wants to preserve a sense of pride. He therefore presents himself as independent, not needing any-one's assistance and lacking nothing but human relationships and an opportunity to rest. Later in the interview, Vitaliy mentions that his children sometimes come to see him and wish to help him, but he refuses or even tries to give his children some pocket money. He ex-plained:

> On the contrary, I myself try to help them – my daughter is studying in a technical college, so I give her some money for her studies.

We do not know to what extent he can financially help his children, but it is important for Vitaliy to present an image of himself as a strong, proud, and independent man who is not in need of assistance. Both Zhenia and Vitaliy highlight their masculinity. At one point, Vitaliy ex-claimed:

> Am I a man or what? What man can stand his wife in bed with another?

Such defensive postures appear to permit some homeless men to better cope with changes that have been, in reality, beyond their power, but which have threatened their sense of manhood.

Alcoholics and Escapists

One psychological strategy for dealing with a situation of crisis is es-capism or infantilization – the failure to take responsibility for one's actions. Among the homeless men I interviewed, there were occasions when laying blame on external circumstances out of their own control masks another side of the story that would show their own degree of responsibility for events. Thus, in describing a wife's betrayal or deci-sion to kick them out of their house, few men mention possible reasons for such a response by their wives, whether because of alcohol abuse or failure to contribute to the household budget. Other men described having their documents stolen or being fired from work, but did not admit to any lack of initiative in renewing documents or securing a new job. For example, one man said:

> I'm not a *bomzh*, am I? I just fell down low. I started drinking, had noth-ing to do . . . And now something happened to my kidneys, they hurt real bad, I can't walk or sit – they hurt all the time. If I could lie in bed for

a while and get some treatment, then I could work. I am only 56 years old, and I am not a bomzhi. I arrived in Kyiv only 28 days ago. Police caught me. They say: 'Go to work or go home!' But how can I work? I can't – that's what I tell them. And I can't go home either – my wife would kill me if she saw me in such condition. So what am I to do?

Such descriptions of wives unwilling to see a drunk husband or forcing a man to leave his home are common among respondents. Meanwhile, criminal behaviour by the men sometimes leads to imprisonment, after which reintegration into society is extremely difficult. According to official statistics, about one-third of all homeless Ukrainians are ex-convicts (Cabinet of Ministers of Ukraine). In my own study, about a quarter of the respondents reported having served prison sentences.

Redistribution versus Recognition

Based on my study of homeless men in Kyiv, men's self-perceptions – and perceptions they have of other homeless individuals – tend to blend more than one of the types of responses to 'failed masculinity' that Tartakovskaya (2003) identifies in her typology. Men who end up on the streets may quickly give up in practical ways, but self-describe as working hard for something better; they may abuse alcohol and have an escapist attitude while also harbouring resentment towards their former wives, employers, or real estate agents, whom they claim are responsible for their condition of homelessness. However, as we have seen, the men also continue to adhere to a strong sense of masculinity, and they often justify their actions with reference to preserving it.

Thus, these men reflect on their experience, articulate their 'failed masculinity' to themselves and to others, and actively respond to the situation, although their choices can be limited. Speak (2004) notes that for many homeless individuals in developing countries, there is a degree of choice available: this is especially true among those who are homeless for short periods, who may choose homelessness 'as a means of improving their more permanent living conditions' and there is 'little indication of personal inadequacy or family dysfunction' (p. 469). The question of choice arose with the respondents in this study as well. Some chose to sleep in parks or shelters to save money. Many preferred to stay in the city instead of going back home, even in difficult periods when they were out of work. They kept looking for employment in order to justify the sacrifices they made by leaving home, or to avoid the embarrassment and criticism of their masculinity that might have occurred there. Some turned to panhandling or crime in order to keep the 'promise' they had made to their families and to send them money regularly. One man described his situation like this:

> Yes, there were times when I was out of work. It was wintertime, cold, and grim . . . I thought – maybe I should return home? But then I said NO, I came here, I told my family I'll provide for them, and I have to keep the promise. So I was begging in the underground, like those *bomzhi,* and I . . . well, don't tell that to anyone, but I . . . well, I got into a few shops with friends, and I was stealing wallets from foreigners. But you have to understand – I told my family, I'd be sending them money. They didn't even know that I was out of work and I didn't want to tell them, so they thought it was the money I made on the construction site.

This shows how important it is for marginally employed workers to be able to provide for their families – this man would rather steal or panhandle than have his family find out that he does not have work and cannot fulfil his 'promise' as a breadwinner.

We also see from the interviews that homeless men who have at least some temporary employment and have preserved family ties resist being labelled *bomzhi*. This label itself can symbolize failed masculinity and personal weakness of homeless men who 'give up.' In post-Soviet societies there is a tendency to draw a clear dividing line between the *bomzhi* and normal or ordinary citizens. Homelessness is seen to be a complete absence, not only of a permanent residence, but also of social ties, of a work ethic, of respect for social norms, and of individual responsibility. Such an attitude is in line with conservative explanations of homeless people as 'different' from the normal majority, and parallels Bahr's classical study on disaffiliation among men (1970; see also Bahr and Caplow 1973). Homeless men are also seen to be 'different' as men – as not living up to the standard of hegemonic masculinity.

My research shows that homelessness does not happen 'overnight' but often results from a series of occurrences. The first is often unemployment, lack of opportunities in their place of residence, the need to support a family, or all three at once. Wacquant (2007) describes this trend as 'de-proletarianization' – denial of access to wage-earning activities that is an inevitable by-product of the decline of industrial production and uneven economic development. The second occurrence is immersion in an unstable environment marked by a high risk of injury, victimization, unofficial casual labour, and lack of affordable housing. Further occurrences may include the use of survival strategies such as alcohol abuse, participation in crime, saving money on housing by sleeping in public places or in crammed conditions, and frequenting homeless shelters and soup kitchens. When we retrace these steps, however, it becomes clear that the primary causes of homelessness are economic and that people who are already in marginal positions – unskilled workers and the unemployed – are at a much higher risk of becoming *bomzhi*.

Tartakovskaya's typology of responses to situations of 'failed masculinity,' her own research on men who are in marginal positions in the Russian labour market, and our research on homeless men in Ukraine together reveal a much greater link between the structural and the symbolic aspects of gender inequalities than Tartakovskaya herself is willing to admit. Economic redistribution to decrease inequalities is no less important than recognition of gender differences if we wish to at least partially neutralize the negative effects of the current masculinity crisis. As Fraser and Honneth (2003) rightly observe:

> The demise of communism, the surge of free-market ideology, the rise of 'identity politics' in both its fundamentalist and progressive forms – all these developments have conspired to decenter, if not to extinguish, claims for egalitarian redistribution. In this new constellation, these two kinds of justice claims are often dissociated from one another – both practically and intellectually. Within social movements such as feminism, for example, activist tendencies that look to redistribution as the remedy for male domination are increasingly dissociated from remedies that look instead to recognition of gender difference. And the same is largely true in the intellectual sphere . . . scholars who understand gender as a social relation maintain an uneasy arm's-length coexistence with those who construe it as an identity or a cultural code. This situation exemplifies a broader phenomenon: the widespread decoupling of cultural politics from social politics, of the politics of difference from the politics of equality.

Fraser and Honneth conclude that this is a false decoupling, and that both redistribution and recognition are required to achieve greater social justice.

In this chapter, I have also stressed the importance of both a cultural and structural analysis when looking at homelessness among men using the concept of failed masculinity. By neglecting the economic problems that cause men to lose employment, break family ties, and end up on the streets, we fail to notice all the men who are at risk of homelessness, many of whom will 'give up' and become *bomzhi*. We also overlook the fact that the masculinity crisis would be less acute and all would benefit from more equal development, greater job security, and affordable housing. Fewer men would have to come to Kyiv and other large cities in search of work, fewer of those who do come would have to 'choose' homelessness as a survival strategy, and fewer of them would end up chronically homeless. Indeed, as of this writing, taking into account economic factors of existing gender-related problems is part of the state's Program to Implement Gender Equality until 2010 (Cabinet of Ministers of Ukraine 2006).

Therefore, it is important to look at the masculinity crisis among post-Soviet homeless men in the context of economic restructuring. Unequal economic development among regions and along the urban-rural axis, high unemployment rates, exploitation and lack of social security in the shadow economy, and lack of affordable housing for workers are among the underlying causes of homelessness. Homeless and other marginalized men also challenge expectations of hegemonic masculinity and reveal contradictions between ideology, real life experience, and self-perceptions, pointing to structural rather than individual causes of homelessness and failed masculinities in post-Soviet Ukraine.

NOTES

1 This research is on homelessness in 20 Ukrainian cities. Information about the project is available at http://homeless.net.ua/ua/index.php. A similar proportion of homeless men and women has been found in police statistics: among the 17,221 homeless people registered by the Ukrainian police in 2005, 14,560 were men and 2,661 were women. This information was retrieved from http://www.helsinki.org.ua/index.php?id=1138900432.

2 Although men are the focus of this chapter, it is important to touch on the devastating dimensions of homelessness for women as well. Glaser (1994) notes that although women constitute a minority of the homeless, they

suffer disproportionately from physical and psychological abuse and are less resistant to harsh living conditions [0] and to alcohol. Although women, in general, have a higher life expectancy than men, the situation is reversed for the homeless: women who do end up on the streets have a much higher death rate than men in similar conditions. In his research on homelessness, Ropers (1988) found that women, on average, were homeless for shorter periods but reported more health problems, and their health deteriorated rapidly on the streets. In her research on homelessness in Russia, Höjdestrand (2009) also found that homelessness is much more stigmatizing to women because of the taken-for-granted 'incompatibility of homelessness and femininity' that 'reveals itself in the general silence in official discourse and among non-homeless Russians about the existence of homeless women. Since they can hardly be imagined, there is nothing to say about them, and those who, against all odds, are spotted are in a figurative sense considered to have forfeited their womanhood.'

3 In 2006, the death rates of working-age men in Ukraine were three times higher than in the European Union, and half of all deaths were preventable, including those caused by suicide, poisoning by drinking low-quality alcohol, cardiovascular disease, and tuberculosis – diseases related to stress and poverty. See Smertnost' Naseleniya Ukrainy v Trudoaktivnom Vozraste (Mortality of the Working-Age Population in Ukraine), available at http://www.demoscope.ru/weekly/2008/0327/tema01.php.

4 These interviews were carried out as part of the research towards my B.A. The results are discussed in more detail in Riabchuk (2005).

5 All names have been changed to protect the participants' privacy.

REFERENCES

Amdzhadin, L. 2007. Genderni Vidminnosti Zdorovya Ukrayintsiv [Gender Differences in Ukrainians' Health]. In M. Skoryk, ed., *Genderni Peretvorennia v Ukrayini* [Gender Transformations in Ukraine], 131–8. Kyiv: UNDP.

Ashwin, S. 2001. Utvyer zhdyeniye muzhskoy idyentichnosti na rynkye truda sovryemyennoy Rossiyi [Affirmitation of Masculine Identity in the Labour Market of Contemporary Russia]. *Rubyezh* no. 16–17: 5–24.

Bahr, H. 1970. *Disaffiliated Man*. Toronto: University of Toronto Press.

Bahr, H., and T. Caplow. 1973. *Old Men Drunk and Sober*. New York: New York University Press.

Beynon, J. 2002. *Masculinities and Culture*. Buckingham: Open University Press.

Bureychak, T. 2008. Crisis of Masculinity in Theoretical and Empiric Perspectives. In *Gender Theories, Gender Practices: Building Bridges,* 20–7. Kharkiv: Raider.

Cabinet of Ministers of Ukraine. 2006. *State Program to Implement Gender Equality until 2010,* points 16, 17, and 18. Decree of 7 Dec. Available at http://zakon.rada.gov.ua/cgi-bin/laws/main.cgi?nreg=1834-2006-%EF.

Connell, R. 2005. Hegemonic Masculinity: Rethinking the Concept. *Gender and Society* 19(6): 829–59.

Cramer, H. 2005. Informal and Gendered Practices in a Homeless Persons Unit. *Housing Studies* 20(5): 737–51.

Daly, G. 1996. *Homeless Policies, Strategies and Lives on the Street.* London: Routledge.

Edwards, T. 2007. 'Crisis, What Crisis?' Sex Roles Revisited. In *Cultures of Masculinity,* 7–24. London: Routledge.

Fraser, N., and A. Honneth. 2003. *Redistribution or Recognition?* London: Verso.

Glaser, I. 1994. *Homelessness in a Global Perspective.* New York: Hall.

Höjdestrand, T. 2009. *Needed by Nobody: Homelessness and Humanness in Postsocialist Russia.* Ithaca: Cornell University Press.

Kon, M. 2009. Krizis maskulinnosti i vozniknovenije 'muzhskogo voprossa' [Crisis of Masculinity and the Appearance of the 'Men's Question']. In *Muzhchina v meniajushchemsia mirie* [Man in a Changing World]. Moscow: Vremia, 13–26.

Riabchuk, A. 2005. *Zayvi lyudy: bezdomni na vulycyakh Kyeva* [Homeless in the Streets of Kyiv]. Kyiv: Chetverta Khvylya.

Ropers, R. 1998. *The Invisible Homeless: A New Urban Ecology.* New York: Human Sciences Press.

Schwarz, O. 1990. *Le monde prive d'ouvriers.* Paris: PUF.

Speak, S. 2004. Degrees of Destitution: A Typology of Homelessness in Developing Countries. *Housing Studies* 19(3): 465–82.

Tartakovskaya, I. 2003. Nyesostoyavshayasya maskulinnost' kak tip povyedyeniya na rynkye truda [Unrealized Masculinity as a Behaviour Type on the Labour Market]. In L.N. Popkova and I.N. Tartakovskaya, eds., *Gendernye Otnosheniya v Sovremennoi Rossii: issledovanita 1990 godov* [Gender Relations in Contemporary Russia: Studies of the 1990s]. Samara: Samara University Press. Available at http://library.gender-ehu.org/hms/attach.php/t__articles.files/id__271/Tartakovskaya.pdf.

Urlanis, B. 1970. Beregite Muzhchin! [Take Care of Men!], *Literaturnaya Gazeta,* 29 June.

Wacquant, L. 2007. *Urban Outcasts: A Comparative Sociology of Marginality.* Cambridge: Polity.

Yeroshok, Z. 2008. *Brodyagi* [Vagabonds]. Available at http://www.novayaga
zeta.ru/data/2008/15/18.html.
Zdravomyslova, E., and A. Temkina. 2002. Krizis maskulinnosti v pozdne-
sovetskom diskurse [Crisis of Masculinity in Late Soviet Discourse]. In
S. Oushakine, ed., *O muzhe(n)stvennosti* [On Masculinity], 432–51. Moscow:
Novoe literaturnoe obozrenie.

PART III

Gender and Education

9 Gender Policy and Education in Contemporary Ukraine: Discourses and Controversies

OLGA PLAKHOTNIK

Gender studies aim to deconstruct traditional notions of the normative feminine and the normative masculine in diverse realms – in philosophy, science, art, and everyday practices. Education is an especially salient area for critique since schooling can fix sociocultural clichés in place and reproduce social inequalities. In Ukraine, the role of formal education in gender equality has not been adequately examined. Researchers in the field of post-Soviet studies have looked at the problem of gender and education from diverse methodological perspectives using, for example, essentialist, postmodernist, and broad sociological and pedagogical approaches. In contrast, this chapter is based on a socio-constructionist approach,[1] and it uses two perspectives to ground its analysis of education: open (or institutional) and hidden gender discourses.[2]

I understand 'gender' within a social constructionist paradigm (Berger and Luckmann 1966) as the social organization of sex differences, or as 'knowledge, which is used to signify body difference' (Scott 1986). I also take as a starting point the discursive nature of education and, in particular, of curriculum, which allows the possibility to divide discourses in educational space between open and hidden. I follow the methodological insight of Foucault, who equated schools to prisons based on the level of repression seen in both (1975, 138). Finally, I employ the critique put forward by a postmodern educational project – that is, the critical pedagogy movement represented, in particular, by Illich (1971), Giroux (1981), and McLaren (1995) – that emphasizes the connection between education and policy and addresses issues of race, gender, and other social inequalities in education.

My first analysis, of open gender discourses, shows that although Ukraine has a state gender policy in education it is very superficial and inconsistent, especially in the area of primary and secondary education. The analysis of hidden gender discourses, meanwhile, shows how important supports for gender inequality are necessarily included into educational spaces in Ukraine. They are discernible in the content of curricula and textbooks, in the features of gender stratification in the teaching profession, and in the structure of educational institutions. The chapter concludes by examining the field of 'gender pedagogy' in modern Ukraine, as one possible solution to current gender problems in education, and offering a critique of this approach.

Open Discourses of Sex and Gender in Ukrainian Education

During the years of post-communist transition, the Ukrainian educational system has been transformed significantly, and this includes changes to the gender regime of Ukrainian schools and universities (Zhurzhenko 2004; Hrycak 2005; Hrycak and Rewakowicz 2009). According to the World Economic Forum's *Global Gender Gap Report* for 2008, the sub-indices of educational attainment in Ukraine are high, and Ukraine ranks 34th among 130 countries in this area (Hausman et al. 2008). This means that women and men have mostly equal access to multiple levels of education.[3] At the same time, this recognition of equal access reinforces the false public opinion that Ukrainian education is gender-equal. In reality, the situation is far more complex and problematic, beginning with the legislative framework regarding education.

The main legislative act regulating gender policy in Ukraine, the Gender Equality Law of 2005,[4] provides descriptions of key concepts such as equal opportunities for men and women, gender discrimination, sexual harassment, and gender equality, which correspond with the tenets of equal opportunities discourse. A special chapter on education in the law (Chapter V, Art. 21) emphasized that:

- The state guarantees equal conditions for women and men in entering educational institutions, evaluating knowledge acquisition, and getting grants and student loans.
- It is necessary to publish textbooks and handouts that are free of gender bias.

- It is necessary to enhance the culture of gender parity and equal distribution of professional and family duties and work.
- It is necessary to conduct gender expert evaluation of existing syllabi, textbooks, and handouts.
- Courses and modules devoted to gender equality issues should be included in university curricula.

While these are important statements about gender parity, they remain no more than declarative, as does the law in its entirety. Arguably, additional legal documents issued by specific ministries must still follow for gender parity to take effect. In fact, as of this writing, the Ministry of Education has not issued a single document related to implementing the Gender Equality Law in the educational sector. The only exception is a set of guidelines devoted to the Annual Lesson on Gender Equality initiated by the United Nations Development Program (UNDP) Equal Opportunities Program in cooperation with the Ukrainian Ministry of Education and Ministry of Family, Youth, and Sports in 2007 to teach schoolchildren about the fundamentals of gender equality. Moreover, the Ministry of Justice, which works on gender expertise in legislation,[5] has not addressed any of Ukraine's education-related statutes, even though it had a gender expert evaluate fourteen documents in the 2007–08 academic year.[6] The Ukrainian Law on Education (no. 1060-XII), for example, urgently needs such expertise, as it demonstrates a high degree of gender insensitivity.[7] Article 3 declares equal rights for education as follows: 'All Ukrainian citizens have a right free of charge to education in state educational institutions independently of their sex, race, nationality, social, and property state.' This is the only place where the word 'sex' is used in the law. The document also lacks any notion of gender or gender equality principles and, therefore, fails to take into account new trends in understanding that distinguish between 'sex' and 'gender,' proof that the law needs to be updated according to Ukrainian state gender policy.

In another example from this same outdated education law, Article 56 declares that teachers and other school staff are obliged 'to bring up students with respect for parents, *women*, older people, *folk traditions*, the national, historical, and cultural values of Ukraine, the state and *social order* of Ukraine, and to inculcate careful attitudes to historical, cultural, and natural environment' (emphasis added). This passage raises a number of questions. Why are women treated as a special group in need of obligatory respect? What folk traditions and from what time and place in Ukrainian history should be respected, given that some of those traditions are discriminatory? Why should students respect the social order if it is not satisfactory in many aspects, including the status of gender?

Thus, the Ministry of Education's official gender policy remains superficial. As for the implementation of gender policy in educational institutions in Ukraine, I will now analyse primary and secondary schools, followed by universities. As I will show, the 'gender situation' at each of these levels of education is markedly different.

Open Gender Discourses in Schools

As mentioned earlier, equal access to primary and secondary education in Ukraine leads to the public perception that there are no gender problems within the school system. However, on closer analysis, the issue of gender policy implementation at the level of primary and secondary schools is actually very problematic and even more so than at the university level. One reason for this is the lack of transparency surrounding Ukrainian schools in comparison with universities. Civil society has little influence on public school education because, in accordance with Article 6 of the Law on Education, political and religious organizations are not allowed much access to children in schools. In practice, however, most civil organizations are typically not welcomed into school space. Moreover, parents have little influence on the content and forms of teaching; many simply trust professionals in educational issues. As well, Ukrainian school administrations are fully dependent on the ministry's regulations; their activities are delineated by ministerial orders or decrees. Until the ministry makes clear that it has the intention to implement gender awareness in the school curriculum, which is far from the case now, no major changes can be expected in this regard.

Partly as a result of this unwillingness, gender instruction for schoolteachers is virtually non-existent. All Ukrainian teachers undergo obligatory professional development at least once every five years at what are called the Institutes for Teachers' Professional Development. There is an opportunity in this process to increase teachers' knowledge about gender issues and develop their professional and personal gender sensitivity by including courses on gender. Teaching gender to teachers is the most comprehensive and effective way to make schools more gender-friendly. But until now, this opportunity has been missed. For example, the curriculum of the Kharkiv Institute for Teachers'

Professional Development includes only *two hours* of lectures on gender issues, and then only for history teachers. Moreover, these two
hours were only included in the curriculum as the result of a private
initiative by one of the institute's instructors, who had studied gender
within a non-formal gender-training program at a pro-feminist wom-
en's non-governmental organization (NGO). Thus, gender issues are
represented in the institute's curriculum without ministry guidance
and in the context of total dependence on the part of the institute's administration on ministry orders. Even if the Ministry of Education were
to agree to advance teacher training in gender issues, there remains the
question of who would 'teach the teachers,' as there are a limited number of gender experts at that level in Ukraine.

As a result of the lack of training, Ukrainian schoolteachers and staff
have poor knowledge of gender equality principles, and they hardly
recognize gender inequalities in educational contexts. As I have argued
elsewhere (Plakhotnik 2007), there are two main tendencies in the perception of gender issues on the part of teachers: (1) to believe that there
are no gender inequalities or related problems in schools, and (2) to
believe that men are discriminated against in the teaching profession
based on the larger number of women teachers. Ukrainian schoolteachers also lack understanding of the concept of hidden curriculum and
generally see no gender issues in schools.

A recent survey by Govorun and Kikinezhdi (2008) of teachers' gender competence in Ukraine showed that 75 per cent of teachers agreed
that girls must be prepared for the roles of mother and housekeeper,
and boys for the role of breadwinner. Also, 63 per cent of teachers
agreed that men are usually better leaders than women, while 60 per
cent said that they believe that all professions should be categorized as
either 'male' or 'female.' Another survey, conducted by Plakhotnik and
Gubina (2009, 68), confirms these results, showing that almost 50 per
cent of Ukrainian teachers in social sciences and the humanities agree
that it is necessary to prepare girls for the roles of mother and housekeeper, and boys for the role of breadwinner. These researchers also
found that nearly 50 per cent of respondents agreed that the sex of a
child predetermines his or her gifts and the way he or she learns and
should be taught. More than one-third of teachers surveyed held the
opinion that a woman's main destiny is to be a good wife and mother.
Such attitudes dramatically undermine gender equality and contribute
to sexist speech and practices, as further demonstrated by the following
examples.

As mentioned earlier, in September 2007 the UNDP Equal Opportunities Program, in cooperation with the Ukrainian Ministry of Education and Ministry of Family, Youth, and Sports, introduced a Gender Equality Lesson into the curriculum for students at all primary and secondary schools. The stated aim of the lesson was to inform children and youth about gender issues using such key concepts as gender, gender equity, and gender equality. The UNDP proposed the idea and published a special illustrated textbook for pupils along with methodological guidelines for teachers; the Ministry of Education supported this idea and placed an e-version of the teacher guidelines on its website.[8] The ministry also agreed to conduct a lesson in gender equality at the beginning of every school year. To date, the ministry reports that this has been done three times, in 2007, 2008, and 2009.

However, the quality of the supplied teaching materials is questionable as evidenced by the quality of materials cited on the Ministry of Education website (Plakhotnik 2010). The teachers, who, as has been shown, understand gender issues poorly, are expected to teach gender equality to the children using these flawed materials which are written in a far too theoretical manner and are void of concrete examples. As a result, teachers often prepare their own lessons reproducing their own, often incorrect, understanding of gender, gender issues, and gender equality. As Kisselyova and Mussienko (2008) show, many teachers understand gender policy in a very limited manner to mean taking sex difference into account in the teaching process (SPD Losynska 2008, 108), and Ukrainian schools rarely have gender experts among teachers and staff. This reality is further illustrated by a survey reported by Plakhotnik and Gubina (2009, 73–4) that asked teachers to evaluate the gender equality lesson mentioned above. Thirty-six per cent of teachers said this was the first they had heard about such a lesson; 27 per cent knew about the lesson but were not sure whether it had ever been conducted in their school; and just 15 per cent had actually conducted the lesson themselves, while 17 per cent had not, but said the lesson was being taught in their school. These data demonstrate that when the gender equality lesson is conducted – as the Ministry of Education reports that it is – it is not widely discussed among teachers. A 2009 report of another survey, of first-year students of Ukrainian universities (Guslyakova et al., 2009, 47) showed that only 5 per cent of recent high school graduates had received the ministry-sponsored gender equality lesson, which raises further questions about whether the lesson was, in fact, taught after 2007, as has been officially reported. These data demonstrate that, in practice, the gender equality lesson has been mostly ineffective and, if badly taught, could actually confuse students' ideas of gender equality.

Unfortunately, even innovative projects aimed at reconstructing Ukrainian education also ignore gender. For example, one current large-scale project entitled Equal Access to Quality Education (started in 2006 and planned as a 10-year project) conducted by the Ministry of Education and sponsored by a loan from the World Bank focuses on the deconstruction of social inequalities (based on ethnicity, place of residence, wealth, and other differences) in secondary education – that is, every social inequality except gender inequality. This type of framework ignores the fact that people's lives are the outcome of intersections of different social locations, power relations, and experiences in which gender figures prominently.

Despite the ample evidence showing how little is being done to increase gender awareness in schools, it is important to acknowledge that some innovative and successful non-formal gender educational practices are taking place outside of public schools in Ukraine. Among them is the School of Equal Opportunities (Kovalko et al. 2002), an international NGO established by youth in 2000 that uses different forms of work, such as festivals or rallies, to communicate ideas about gender equality.[9] Their Interactive Gender Theatre is a well-known program. Another interesting set of gender educational practices that work under the rubric of 'empowering education' have been undertaken at several schools and colleges.[10] The idea here is to apply an empowering pedagogy to give girls an awareness of their potential and the possibility that they could develop their talents, and to give boys a greater awareness of their attitudes and values and encouragement towards social responsibility (Semikolenova et al. 1999, 2001). These practices, however, are concentrated in several big cities (mainly Kyiv) and have limited influences on gender relations in education in Ukraine at large. The methodology and experience of these practices have not yet been analysed or widely discussed within the Ukrainian community of gender experts.

Hidden Curriculum in Education: Theoretical Background

The concept of 'hidden curriculum' is the most significant contribution of critical pedagogy (Jackson 1968). A hidden curriculum refers to implicit (unrecognized) knowledge content, as opposed to the open, explicit content that is transmitted from teacher to students in an educational setting. Hidden curriculum is translated non-verbally or is concealed in the deep structures of discourse (Apple 1971; Bourdieu and Passeron 1990; Althusser 1998). Hidden curriculum can include messages communicated by the organization and operation of schooling, quite apart from official statements of school missions and subject area curriculum guidelines. Messages usually convey attitudes, values, beliefs, and behaviours. According to Illich (1971), schools actively use hidden curriculum to suggest to students an ideology of passive consumption, that is, a non-critical perception of the existing social order. Hidden curriculum thus teaches children that their role in life is 'to know their place and to sit still in it' (Giddens and Griffiths 2006, 704).

Hidden curriculum is discursive but not necessarily communicated in language. Rather, we can think about it using the terms of Foucault (1972), who said: '[Discourse] is made up of a limited number of statements for which a group of conditions of existence can be defined. Discourse in this sense is not an ideal, timeless form . . . it is, from beginning to end, historical – a fragment of history . . . posing its own limits, its divisions, its transformations, the specific modes of its temporality' (p. 117). This interpretation gives us grounds for considering discourse to be not only a 'complicated unity of linguistic form, knowledge and reality' (van Deik 1989, 121), but also a fixed ordering of reality, the kind of world view that is realized in extremely varied practices that extend beyond the verbal. As Foucault understood, discourse not only reflects or describes the world, it creates it.

To fully comprehend hidden discourses, however, we still have to take account of the official ones. Karasyk (2000) distinguishes between different kinds of 'institutional' discourses in contemporary society, of which educational institutional discourse is one example. Such institutional discourses break down into binary oppositions of 'central versus marginal,' where 'central' denotes the legitimized content of discourse. In the case of education, 'institutional' means all that is connected with the goals of education and structural communication between a 'teacher' and a 'student.' Any sociocultural space contains hidden discourses in addition to the institutional ones. In education, these hidden discourses may communicate certain messages about violence, corporeality, sexuality, and others that are taboo for official pedagogical policy, like discourses of power, inequality, and discrimination, including on the basis of gender. Hidden curriculum discourse transmits social inequalities that cannot be spoken of in official institutional discourse.

Another way to think of hidden curriculum is as a metacommunication which is a means of social control (Stubbs 1976). Hidden curriculum includes the following elements: (1) the organizational culture of an institution, (2) the content of subjects, and (3) the teaching style (Wood 1994). These three dimensions of hidden curriculum not only reflect stereotypes of gender and disability, but also reinforce social inequality by constructing identities according to symbolic classifications of feminine and masculine, disabled and able-bodied.

When Hall and Sandler (1982) investigated verbal and non-verbal communicative practices in education, they found that dominant forms of teaching were based on masculine communicative patterns, which overlook women's ways of learning and talking. The numerous examples of unequal attitudes of teachers towards students of different sexes in class were also insignificant, since they resulted, according to Hall and Sandler, in a 'chilly climate' for girls in the educational process.

It is important to underline that gender analysis of hidden curriculum is not limited to quantitative measures like counting male versus female names in textbooks, or how long teachers will wait for an answer from a male versus from a female student. This is only a starting point. More important is the complex evaluation of the consequences of teaching and its effect on social growth among girls and boys. Teachers can undertake this evaluation of their own conduct and act accordingly. This is called 'gender sensitivity,' the ability to recognize and, to some extent, model the verbal, non-verbal, and objective influences of a socio-cultural environment and to reflect on the ways in which teaching forms and methods affect the formation of students and their gender identity.[11] Gender sensitivity also includes the ability of a teacher to recognize and react to cases of gender discrimination. According to Reardon (2003), gender sensitivity or 'gender justice' contains: (1) gender competence and (2) an ability to react constructively to cases of gender discrimination.

Hidden Curriculum in Schools

Despite its covert nature, it is possible to investigate three aspects of hidden curriculum: (1) the organization of the educational establishment, including (gender) relations between teachers and (gender) stratification of the teaching profession; (2) the content of syllabi and textbooks; and (3) the style of communication in teaching (Wood 1994; Yarskaya-Smirnova 2000; Plakhotnik 2005).

In terms of *gender stratification of the teaching profession*, I refer to the aforementioned *Global Gender Gap Report* for 2008, which shows that 99 per cent of primary school teachers and 79 per cent of secondary school teachers in Ukraine are female (Hausman et al. 2008). Likewise, according to the 2007 statistical report called *Women and Men in Ukraine*, the education sector was made up of 69 per cent women compared with just 31 per cent men (DKSU 2007, 72). Such feminization of the teaching profession is not unique to Ukraine and is common throughout the contemporary world. Unfortunately, statistics on the sex of school heads/ principals in Ukraine and data on teaching subjects are not public. My requests to the Ministry of Education and Science for this information have been unsuccessful. An informal count made on all the Kharkiv public secondary school websites, however, shows that 15 per cent of school directors in that city are men (24 of 156). Department heads in all nine districts of the city are women. These data can be interpreted as an additional illustration of the near-total feminization of secondary school teaching. Yet, given the lack of information at the moment, it is difficult to evaluate the vertical (across administrative levels) and horizontal (across subjects) gender stratification in Ukraine's educational system.

The question of which teachers teach what subjects is also an important one in terms of hidden discourses. We can say that women more frequently teach humanities, and men are mostly teachers of sciences and physical education. It is also interesting that as of 2006 the average salary of women in education is equal to just 83.8 per cent of the average salary for men in this field (KDSU 2007, 71), which means that although men are a minority, they nevertheless hold higher positions than women in education and receive higher levels of remuneration. This situation directly and indirectly reinforces to students a set of ideas about 'normative masculinity' as dominating and 'normative femininity' as subordinating.

With regard to gender bias found in *the content of curriculum, textbooks, and handouts* for pupils and students, analysis shows disturbing trends. For example, according to state-determined standards, Ukrainian secondary schools should divide pupils by sex for delivery of different curricula about physical training and career orientation. The different syllabi for career orientation (see Figures 9.1 and 9.2) even have different, sex-differentiated titles: 'technical work' for boys and 'serving work' for girls.

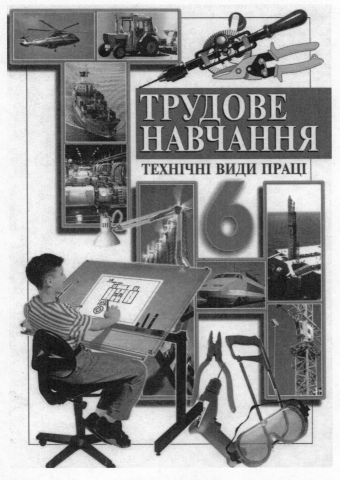

Figure 9.1. Cover image of *Work Training Grade 6: Technical Kinds of Work* (boys). Source: Madhizon et al. (2006).

A number of researchers have undertaken evaluations of the contents of textbooks from a gender perspective.[12] The well-known gender analysis of school textbooks was ordered by the United Nations Educational, Scientific, and Cultural Organization (UNESCO) and conducted in 1986 (Mishel 1991, 72). Ukraine was one of the target regions

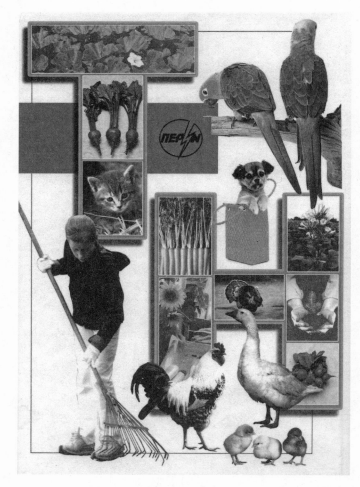

Figure 9.2. Cover image of *Work Training Grade 6: Service Kinds of Work* (girls). Source: Denysenko et al. (2006).

of the mentioned analysis, but there were no significant outcomes of this project due to significant political transformation related to the collapse of the Soviet Union. Similar work was later done in independent Ukraine (Chuhym 2001; Males 2004), Russia (Barchunova

1995; Voronina 2005; Smirnova 2005), and other post-Soviet countries. All this research has come to similar conclusions: that school textbooks in post-Soviet educational systems are mostly non-sensitive to gender. The majority of them actually contained traditional gender stereotypes, therefore aiding in the construction of gender biases among students.

Govorun and Kikinezhdi (2008), who conducted a content analysis of textbooks and handouts approved by the Ukrainian Ministry of Education for primary and secondary schools, found totally divergent representations of boys and girls and men and women in the text and images of these materials. This was apparent in traditional representations of suitable occupations. Astronauts, drivers, scientists, and engineers were represented by men, while homemakers, nurses, teachers, and doctors were represented by women. In stories and even in descriptions of math problems, women and girls were mostly passive victims of circumstances, or they assisted men in their activities. If girls were doing anything, it was usually sewing, housekeeping, or caregiving. Men and boys, meanwhile, were constructed as active, full of energy, and doing sports and outdoor activities (usually socially important ones), and they were portrayed overall as independent.

As another salient example, illustrations in the *Bookvar*,[13] a Ukrainian alphabet book in wide use in schools, are differentiated by sex 80 per cent of the time. Men appear in more illustrations in this book (65%) than women and are depicted as state leaders, politicians, scuba divers, doctors, and so on. Similar gender representations are common in popular children's magazines in Ukraine as well as history textbooks for teenagers, which portray males in dominant positions of power and policy- and decision-making processes, while reducing the role of women in history. This tendency is changing in the newest textbooks and other publications, but the process is very slow and inconsistent.

The third area where hidden curriculum can be analysed is in the *style of communication in teaching.* However, this is the most difficult to measure. Unlike in the West, such an analysis is only beginning in Ukraine. But I suggest that the existence of firmly entrenched gender biases in the minds of teachers, the evidence of which I outlined above, necessarily results in a significant difference in teacher attitudes towards girls and boys. The exploration of these issues is the focus of my forthcoming research project.[14]

Gender in Universities: Open and Hidden

Gender policy and the overall gender situation at the university level in Ukraine is markedly different from that in primary and secondary schools. At the beginning of the 1990s, gender issues were 'discovered' within post-Soviet academic circles, and since then, there have been big changes in the implementation and institutionalization of gender studies in Ukrainian universities. The majority of articles and books analysing the development of gender studies in Ukrainian universities draw positive conclusions, and they identify significant progress in this area during the past decade (Prykhodkina and Golubeva 2007; Sukovata 2007); at the same time, some authors, including myself, still have a rather sceptical opinion (Zherebkina 2003; Plakhotnik 2009). Since the 1990s, the number of gender studies centres at universities (mainly in large cities such as Kharkiv, Kyiv, Lviv, Odessa, and Lutsk) has grown significantly. At the same time, these centres exist as NGOs or professional associations rather than as part of the university structure. As a result, there are no gender studies (or women's studies) university departments in Ukraine. Meanwhile, Ministry of Education reports show a growing number of compulsory and elective gender courses for students at different levels and in different areas of study. The content and impact of such courses, however, have yet to be studied, and there are still no Master's programs in gender studies in any of the Ukrainian universities. Nor is there a gender research track on the official list of specializations of the Highest Qualification Attestation Commission of Ukraine. Nonetheless, there is an increasing number of defended candidate and doctoral dissertations on gender-related topics.[15]

Meanwhile, implementation of gender policy at universities remains controversial. Although it is possible to observe significant progress in this area, the lack of official recognition and institutionalization of gender issues is also evident. For instance, while technically, gender issues in the area of education are the mandate of the Ministry of Education, gender polices are actually implemented by the Ministry of Family, Youth, and Sports. Every year, the administration of each Ukrainian university reports to the latter ministry on its progress in implementation. These reports track the number of gender courses (or modules of courses), published articles and books, and seminars and conferences. This requirement could result in a positive change in gender policy and gender consciousness if it encourages greater implementation. However, it can also lead to performative reporting that does not correspond to the reality of university life (Zherebkina 2003). Indeed, this is evidenced by the fact that the standard university curriculum does not contain mandatory gender courses. Implementation of such courses depends largely on the enthusiasm of particular scholars and the support of faculty administration. Teaching gender courses, however, is only a part of the problem. The other issue is the real (unconscious) influence of the university's 'hidden curriculum.' As Prykhodkina and Golubeva argue, 'The university itself is the source of gender asymmetry, patriarchal behavioural models for youth. The structure of universities and the distribution of career hierarchies there are the example of male governance and male domination . . . Ukrainian universities really are like mirrors, which reflect male domination as a basis of social gender order' (2007, 29). In this sense, gender courses in university curricula can be seen as problematic: although students conduct critical analyses of the social (gender) order in such courses, they do so within the unchanging university (gender) structure that bespeaks the impossibility of progress in gender equality issues.

Vertical gender stratification is also an important part of the 'hidden curriculum' in Ukrainian universities. As the data on this issue are scarce and not readily available from the Ministry of Education, it is only possible to judge its status based on data collected in 2009 by the Kharkiv Regional Gender Resource Centre.[16] According to their study of Kharkiv universities (25 in total), the proportion of women among faculty deans was 23.6 per cent (46 of 195). The proportion of female department chairs was slightly higher, at 26.5 per cent (251 of 952). Thus, male domination of decision-making positions in Kharkiv universities is clear. Similar situations are probable all over Ukraine.

More data on the gender distribution of university positions have emerged from Franko Lviv National University (collected by V. Sereda in 2006), as shown in Figures 9.3 and 9.4.[17] In Figure 9.3, we can see that women are best represented at the lowest levels of university positions, where they actually outnumber men, but that they hold virtually none of the highest posts, as professors and chairs. In Figure 9.4, we note a similar trend: for both degrees and titles, the more prestigious the level, the fewer women there are.

One hope for overcoming patriarchal attitudes in Ukrainian universities could be within the European Union – Ukraine framework. In particular, the Bologna Process for university education includes,

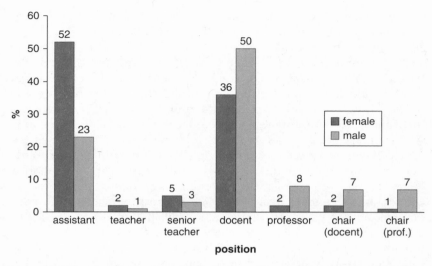

Figure 9.3. Gender distribution of university positions at Franko Lviv National University 2006. Source for data: Sereda (2006).

among other things, widespread distribution of European values of human rights and liberty.[18] However, despite their familiarity with European norms and standards of education, almost no Ukrainian philosophers of education, theorists, or administrators connect these with the question of gender policy in this area.[19] As an example, a recent book by established Ukrainian philosopher Klepko called *Philosophy of Education in the European Context* provides an analysis of the development and main features of recent educational policy in Europe and the conditions and opportunities for their application in Ukraine. But despite this work's significant impact on the development of Ukrainian education, it both ignores gender inequality and perpetuates negative gender stereotypes. This is evidenced in the following passage: 'The situation, when some particular person is unable to use his or her university education at the labour market, can be considered to be an indicator of poor quality of the entire educational system. But sometimes it should be distinguished as a positive phenomenon, some potential of personal capital. For example, women's university education does not have to be necessarily realized on the labour market: instead of this it can be realized in child care' (Klepko 2006, 253–4).

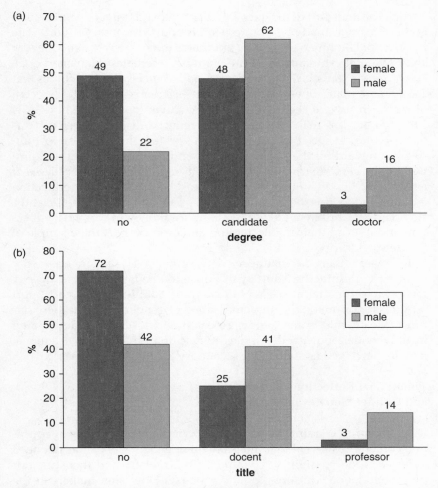

Figure 9.4. Gender distribution of degrees and titles at Franko Lviv National University 2006. Source for data: Sereda (2006).

From such a perspective, women's education is only an enhancement to traditional roles within the private sphere and not an opportunity to realize women's full potential as citizens who actively and meaningfully engage in public life as equals.

An important part of the question of gender and university education is the transition made by young people from education to work. The majority of Ukrainian university graduates today are women: for every sixty-five male students there are eighty-one females (Hausman et al. 2008). Yet the statistical report *Women and Men in Ukraine* concludes that the average salary of women is between 59.4 per cent and 91.3 per cent of men's in several segments of the Ukrainian labour market (KDSU 2007, 71), far less than par. These data reflect a disturbing reality: this better-educated social group of women sees few improved opportunities as a reward for their achievements, and their high potential is limited by the gender structure of the labour market and gender biases of employers.[20] Taking into account that most Ukrainian higher education is state-funded, this means public moneys are being spent inefficiently. As noted by Chukhym (2003, 28), 'to invest money in women's education and not use their intellectual potential properly is the example of a state spendthrift.'

To review, there is an uneven landscape in Ukrainian university education. Despite the Ministry of Education being the official agency responsible for this area, the Ministry for Family, Youth, and Sport requires reporting on the implementation of gender policy in these settings. Meanwhile, some gender research and teaching is developing in universities. But gender issues remain marginalized in academia, usually perceived as something secondary or simply fashionable.

Theoretical Reflections on Education and Gender Debates in Ukraine

Discussions on Ukrainian educational policy and philosophy at education conferences reveal that the problem of gender policy has not been reflected upon enough by Ukrainian philosophers and theorists, nor by practitioners, educators, policy makers, or decision makers in the educational sphere. There is a pressing need to systematically address a number of theoretical and methodological problems in this area, as these problems are having a significant impact on the implementation of gender policy. One issue is that the majority of studies on gender and education in post-Soviet Ukraine follow the tenets of equal opportunities discourse,[21] which is connected to an Anglo-American egalitarian version of feminism, as opposed to a European (mainly French) essentialist feminism represented in the works of de Beauvoir (1973), Irigaray (1985), or Cixous (1976). Yet, a number of contemporary gender theorists stress that, in some cultural contexts, other gender discourses besides Western ones can be more appropriate. For example, Sunderland and Kitetu (2000, 37) attest that 'it makes sense for gender activists working in education to look for and draw on *other, pro-female* discourses when an equal opportunities discourse is inappropriate. Here [in Kenya], the avowedly problematic discourse of "privileged femininity" may bring with it a range of emancipatory possibilities for girls.'

Another gender theorist, Zherebkina, explains that the Ukrainian situation is somewhat opposite to the Western one: 'In Western feminist theory the accentuation of the "primary basic" (the "woman's essence," for example) took place first, and then it has been deconstructed (for instance, by Butler's theory of performativity [or] Braidotti's concept of nomadic subjectivity . . .); [in Ukraine] we have got the opposite situation: this primary basic simply doesn't exist here' (2003, 251). Zherebkina concludes that clichés of Western gender discourse are problematic for Ukraine and argues that gender discourses in the West and in post-Soviet space are fundamentally different because of the different historical circumstances in which feminism and gender studies have developed and are applied, including in Ukraine (and in Russia, for that matter; pp. 249–51). In her opinion, the official Soviet ideology of equality repressed the question of sexual difference and did not address women's individual experiences (in contrast to feminist movements in the West). After the fall of the Soviet Union, asexuality of public discourse was replaced by an overemphasis on sexual difference and what Zherebkina calls the 'naturalization' of sex (pp. 19–22), in the sense of treating it as essential or natural.

Another issue worthy of a special attention is the understanding of gender issues among Ukrainian theorists of pedagogy. Much theoretical and applied research today is related to what is deemed 'gender pedagogy,' which conceptualizes what its authors consider to be key gender principles in education (Govorun and Kikinezhdi 2003; Severyna 2005). It is interesting that in this pedagogical discourse there is almost no discussion of gender theory in the educational context. Instead, a number of texts are devoted to 'implementation of a gender approach in pedagogy' (Kutova 2008; Cokur and Ivanova 2006; Olijnyk and Danylenko 2004; Petryshyna 2002). Such authors conclude that 'gender studies have now become an organic part of pedagogical science, and gender issues are implemented in different branches of pedagogy,' meaning that the researchers perceive implementation of gender policy in the educational sphere to be steadily progressing (Cokur and Ivanova 2006, 22).

Such assumptions about implementation can be challenged, however. First, the formulation of principles of gender pedagogy on offer here is not comprehensive. The majority of such texts are based on a methodological mixture emerging from essentialism, social constructivism, humanism, and other traditions, resulting in a lack of methodological consistency (see, e.g., Krave 2003). But the most dangerous tendency is the renaming of essentialist sex-role divisions as fashionable gender ones by authors who espouse gender pedagogy (see, e.g., Nechay et al. 2004). Krave's well-known textbook, aptly named *Gender Pedagogy*, defines the tasks of gender education as 'teaching the norms of sex-to-sex communication for youth, forming of corporeal identity, and the features of male and female psychology' (2003, 174). At the same time, Ukrainian gender pedagogy exists mostly in isolation from Ukrainian gender studies. No articles emerging from the gender pedagogy field have been published in the past ten years in Ukraine's only post-Soviet journal in gender studies, *Gendernye issledovaniya*. Nor is research on 'gender pedagogical' issues represented in the most significant volumes in post-Soviet gender studies. The fields of 'gender studies' and 'gender pedagogy' seem not to be intersecting at all, and thus gender pedagogy does not represent any critical approach to social reality, but is rather an essentialist educational technique. Moreover, Ukrainian gender pedagogy operates from a positivist paradigm. The critical pathos of gender theory has been eliminated by its proponents and replaced with bureaucratized formulas that offer something like 'recipes for practical use' teaching girls 'normative femininity' and boys 'normative masculinity' (Plakhotnik 2007). There is also a tendency in gender pedagogy texts to avoid feminist rhetoric, or to distinguish feminist and gender pedagogy as something totally different from what they are doing (Prykhodkina 2008). At the same time, proponents of gender pedagogy attempt to link their ideas with Ukrainian history, as if the former flows naturally from the latter. For example, they attempt to justify parts of the Soviet pedagogical experience in terms of 'gender approach' principles (Petrenko 2007). Govorun and Kikinezhdi (2003) go so far as to suggest that the educational philosophy of Makarenko and Sukhomlynsky (pedagogical practitioners from the early Soviet era) demonstrated clear gender-sensitive attitudes in understanding sex differences. These attempts are part of a larger nationalistic discourse in contemporary Ukraine, which can be called a 'revival of gender equality' (Kis 2005, 27). In contrast, the content analysis of five volumes of Sukhomlynsky's main works demonstrates the opposite tendency: there is a clear sex-role approach, as opposed to a gender-sensitive approach, in conjunction with traditional Soviet rhetoric of 'respect for women.'

As these examples demonstrate, although problems with gender equality in schools (and in education as a whole) are evidently connected with the gender competence and sensitivity of educators, the deeper causes of these problems lie with knowledge production in society, in part led by divergent intellectual movements. Drawing on ideas of social constructionism (Berger and Luckmann 1966) and the genealogical and archaeological studies of Foucault (1972, 1975), many scholars in feminist epistemology (Fricker 1998; Harding 1986, 1991, 1998; Haraway 1988) argue that the system of knowledge production has a masculine character. The strong patriarchal tradition in education keeps 'old' academics and administrators in power, as in the case in Ukraine, and thus this problem cannot be solved 'from above.' Overall, then, my analysis of the attempts of Ukrainian proponents of gender pedagogy to consider gender in education illustrates numerous theoretical and methodological weaknesses that greatly undermine the ability of existing pedagogy to advance transformations to gender equality in education.

Conclusions

Ukraine has, through its own actions and by absorbing ideas from elsewhere, made steps forward in gender equality policy in education. In spite of articulated intentions and some real steps towards the implementation of gender policy in Ukraine, as this chapter has demonstrated, this movement is insufficiently strong for overcoming both open and hidden discourses of gender inequality in Ukrainian education. At the same time, however, there are also grounds to hope for future improvements in gender equality, given the country's openness to Western influences and experiences, including those related to gender.

NOTES

1 This term entered the sociological vocabulary through Peter Berger and Thomas Luckmann's *The Social Construction of Reality* (1966). For Berger and Luckmann, the basic features of social order are captured in the principle

that 'society is a human product. Society is an objective reality. Man is a social product.'

2 The implications of gender theory for education have been investigated in post-Soviet spaces by, e.g., Chukhym (2001), Kon (2008), Voronina (2005), Yarskaya-Smirnova (2000), and Zherebkina (2003). The problem of the theory and practice of gender policy in education has been researched by Kutova (2008), Lutsenko (2004), Males (2004), Oksamytna and Khmelko (2007), Popova (2001), Prykhodkina (2008), and Shtyleva (2008), among others.

3 For more analysis of this point, see Chapter 10, in this volume.

4 Zakon Ukrayiny, *Pro zabezpechennia rivnykh prav ta mozhlyvostei zhinok i cholovikiv* (Law of Ukraine on Ensuring Equal Rights and Opportunities for Women and Men). Available at http://zakon.rada.gov.ua.

5 *Gender expertise* is, for the purposes of this chapter, understood as *gender analysis*. The term is widespread in Ukrainian discourse on gender legislation, and it is used in the Gender Equality Law.

6 For more details about this process, refer to the Ukrainian-language Ministry of Justice website at http://www.minjust.gov.ua/0/law_gendpravexp.

7 Zakon Ukrayiny, Pro osvitu, Ukrainian Law on Education (no. 1060-XII), available at http://zakon.rada.gov.ua.

8 For a copy of this pamphlet, refer to the Ukrainian Ministry of Education website at http://www.mon.gov.ua/education/average/new_pr/metod_rek_1.rtf.

9 More information is available from their website at http://www.gender-ua.org/index-uk.html.

10 The Empowering Education Program (led by Olena Suslova and Olena Kurganoskaya) was supported by the Open Society Institute as part of the Gender Education Project within the International Women's Program. The project was finished in 2006, but more information is still available from its website at http://empedu.civicua.org/.

11 The terms *gender sensitivity* and *gender-sensitive teaching* are commonly used in post-Soviet and European contexts. North Americans tend to call this *non-sexist teaching*.

12 For a more in-depth discussion of this issue, see Chapter 10, in this volume.

13 *Bookvar* is usually the first textbook in primary school, which is aimed to develop children's reading skills. See Chapter 10 in this volume for an analysis of *Bookvar*.

14 'Discourses of sex and gender in post-Soviet schools' is supported by the Centre for Advanced Studies and Education (CASE).

15 For a recent list of these, see http://www.gender.univer.kharkov.ua/diss/.
16 I am grateful to Tetyana Isaeva, the director of the Kharkiv Regional
    Gender Resource Centre, for sharing this information.
17 I am grateful to Victoria Sereda from Franko Lviv National University for
    sharing these data, which were presented by her at the Winter School in
    Sociology, Kharkiv, 2006.
18 The Bologna Process is an all-European reform initiative aimed at estab-
    lishing a European Higher Education Area by 2010. Forty-six countries
    are taking part in this process in cooperation with a number of inter-
    national organizations, including the Council of Europe. More informa-
    tion is available at http://www.coe.int/t/dg4/highereducation/ehea
    2010/bolognapedestrians_en.asp.
19 For example, during the 2008 international conference 'Implementation of
    Western Educational Standards in Post-Soviet Countries' (Kyiv, 21–2 April)
    my presentation on gender-sensitive teaching was the only one devoted
    to gender issues (and was accepted by other conference participants as a
    strange and exotic topic).
20 Similar conclusions are discussed in Chapter 11, in this volume.
21 For more information on equal opportunities discourse, refer to the
    EUROPA Glossary at http://europa.eu/scadplus/glossary/equal_treat
    ment_en.htm.

REFERENCES

Althusser, L. 1998. Ideology and Ideological State Apparatuses. In J. Rivkin
    and M. Ryan, eds., *Literary Theory: An Anthology,* 294–304. Malden:
    Blackwell.
Apple, M. 1971. The Hidden Curriculum and the Nature of Conflict. *Inter-
    change* 2(4): 27–40.
Barchunova, T. 1995. Sexism v Bukvare [Sexism in School Primers]. *EKO* 3:
    12–21.
Beauvoir, S. de. 1973. *The Second Sex.* New York: Vintage.
Berger, P., and T. Luckmann. 1966. *The Social Construction of Reality: A Treatise
    in the Sociology of Knowledge.* New York: Doubleday.
Bourdieu, P., and J.-C. Passeron. 1990. *Reproduction in Education, Society and
    Culture.* New York: Sage.
Chukhym, N.D., ed. 2001. *Genderna ekspertyza normatyvnyh kursiv i navchal'nyh
    program social'no-gumanitarnogo cyklu* [Gender Expertise of Normative
    Courses and Syllabi for the Social-Humanities Cycle]. Kyiv: Vydavnychyj
    centr Kyi'vs'kyj universytet.

Cixous, H. 1976. The Laugh of the Medusa. Translated by Keith Cohen and Paula Cohen. *Signs* 1(4): 875–93.

Cokur, O., and I. Ivanova. 2006. *Genderna pedagogika – nova osvitnja tehnologija* [Gender Pedagogy as a New Educational Technology]. Available at http://osvita-ua.net/school/upbring/1657 (accessed 2 Nov. 2007).

Denysenko L., O. Hnedenko, N. Kalinichenko, A. Romanchuk, M. Turov. 2006. Trudove Navchannia: Obslugovuyuchi Vvydy Pratsi. Pidruchnyk dlia 6 Klasu Zahalnoosvitnih Navchalnyh Zakladiv [Work Training: Service Kinds of Work. Textbook for Grade 6 for Public Schools]. Kyiv: Pedahohichna dumka, Cover Image.

Derzhavnyj komitet statystyky Ukrainy/State Statistics Committee of Ukraine (DKSU). 2007. *Zhinky i choloviky v Ukraini. Statystychnyi zbirnyk* [Women and Men in Ukraine. Statistics]. Kyiv: DKSU.

Foucault, M. 1972. *The Archaeology of Knowledge*. London: Routledge.

– 1975. *Discipline and Punish: The Birth of the Prison*. New York: Random House.

Fricker, M. 1998. Rational Authority and Social Power: Towards a Truly Social Epistemology. *Aristotelian Society Proceedings* 98: 159–77.

Giddens, A., and S. Griffiths. 2006. *Sociology*. Cambridge: Polity.

Giroux, H. 1981. *Ideology, Culture and the Process of Schooling*. Philadelphia: Temple University Press.

Govorun, T., and O. Kikinezhdi. 2003. Genderna ideologija u navchal'no-vyhovnomu procesi [Gender Ideology in Educational Processes]. *Osvita i upravlinnja* [Education and Government] 4: 56–68.

– 2008. *Gender u social'no-psykhologichnomu vymiri: Chastyna 1*[Social-Psychological Aspects of Gender: Part 1]. Available at http://helsinki.org.ua/index.php?id=1200305760 (accessed 4 March 2009).

Guslyakova, L., I. Danylenko, O. Plakhotnik, and M. Sukhomlyn. 2009. *Genderni problemy ochyma studentstva: Analytichna dopovid'* [Gender Problems in Students' Eyes: Analytical Report]. Kharkiv: Raider.

Hall, R.M., and B.R. Sandler. 1982. *The Classroom Climate: A Chilly One for Women?* Washington, DC: Association of American Colleges.

Haraway, D. 1988. Situated Knowledges: The Science Question in Feminism and the Privilege of Partial Perspective. *Feminist Studies* 14: 575–99.

Harding, S. 1986. *The Science Question in Feminism*. Ithaca: Cornell University Press.

–1991. *Whose Science? Whose Knowledge?* Ithaca: Cornell University Press.

– 1998. *Is Science Multicultural? Postcolonialisms, Feminisms, and Epistemologies*. Bloomington: Indiana University Press.

Hausman, R., L. Tyson, and S. Zahidi. 2008. *The Global Gender Gap Report*. World Economic Forum. Available at http://www.weforum.org/pdf/gend ergap/report2008.pdf (accessed 23 Jan. 2009).

Hrycak, A. 2005. Coping with Chaos: Gender and Politics in a Fragmented State. *Problems of Post-Communism* 52(5): 69–81.

Hrycak, A., and M. Rewakowicz. 2009. Feminism, Intellectuals and the Forma-tion of Micro-Publics in Postcommunist Ukraine. *Studies in East European Thought* 61(4): 309–33.

Illich, I. 1971. *Deschooling Society*. London: Marion Boyars. Available at www. preservenet.com/theory/Illich/Deschooling/intro.html.

Irigaray, L. 1985. *This Sex Which Is Not One*. Translated by Catherine Porter. Ithaca: Cornell University Press.

Jackson, P.W. 1968. *Life in a Classroom*. New York: Holt, Rinehart and Winston.

Karasyk, V.I. 2000. O tipah diskursa [About Types of Discourse]. In *Yazykovaya lichnost': Institucional'nyi i personal'nyi diskurs* [Language Person: Institu-tional and Personal Discourse], 5–20. Volgograd: Peremena.

Kis, O. 2005. Kogo oberigaje Berehynja, abo Matriarhat jak cholovichyj vy-nahid [Who Is Protected by *Berehynja*, or Matriarchy as Male Invention]. *Dzerkalo tyzhnja* 23: 27.

Kisselyova, O., and N. Mussienko. 2008. Genderna osvita v Ukraini: Dosy-agnennya, prgalyny i vyklyly. Analitychna dopovid' [Gender Education in Ukraine: Achievements, Deficiencies, and Challenges. Analytical Report]. Kyiv: SPD Lozynksa.

Klepko, S. 2006. *Filosofia osvity v evropeis'komu konteksti* [Philosophy of Educa-tion in the Europen Context]. Poltava: POIPPO.

Kon, I. 2008. *Razdel'noe obuchenie – plyusy i minusy* [Sex-single education – education – pluses and minuses]. Available at http://www.polit.ru/ lectures/2008/11/18/kon.html.

Kraveć, V. 2003. *Genderna pedagogika: Navchal'nyj posibnyk* [Gender Pedagogy: Handout]. Ternopil': Dzhura.

Kutova, N. 2008. *Rozvytok vyshhoi' osvity zhinok u SShA v 1970-h rokah XX – na pochatku XXI st.:gendernyj pidhid* [Development of Higher Educa-tion for Women in the USA from the 1970s in the Twentieth Century to the Beginning of the Twenty-First Century: A Gender Approach]. Kyiv: Universytets'ke vydavnyctvo Pul'sary.

Lutsenko, O. 2004. *Genderna osvita i pedagogika* [Gender Education and Pedagogy]: Osnovy teorii genderu [Basics of Gender Theory], 476–503. Kyiv: KIS.

Madhizon, V., H. Kondratiuk, H. Levchenko, O. Romanchuk, M. Turov, and D. Zakatnov. 2006. Trudove Navchannia: Tehnichni Vydy Pratsi. 6 Klas:

Pidruchnyk dlia Zagalnoosvitnih Navchalnyh Zakladiv [Work Training: Technical Kinds of Work. Grade 6: Textbook for Public Schools]. Kyiv, Irpin; VTF Perun, Cover image.

Males, L.V. 2004. *Osnovy g'endernogo analizu v dyscyplinah sociogumanitarnogo cyklu: Metodychni rekomendacii'* [Fundamentals of Gender Analysis in the Disciplines of the Socio-humanities Cycle: Handout]. Kyiv: Zlatograf.

McLaren, P. 1995. *Critical Pedagogy and Predatory Culture.* New York: Routledge.

Mishel, A. 1991. *Doloi stereotipy! Preodolet' seksizm v shkol'nyh uchebnikah* [Off with Stereotypes! To Overcome Sexism in School Textbooks]. Paris: UNESCO.

Nechay, S., N. Shevtsova, and L. Trygub. 2004. *Khrestomatiya navchal'nyh program z gendernogo rozvytku* [Reader of Syllabi in Gender Development]. Kyiv: Foliant.

Oksamytna, S., and V. Khmelko. 2007. Social'ne pohodzhennia ta osvitnia nerivist'v Ukraini [Social Origins and Educational Inequality in Ukraine]. *Naukovi zapysky NAUKMA: Sociologichni nauky* [Social Sciences] 70: 39–46.

Olijnyk, V.V., and L.I. Danylenko, eds. 2004. *Genderni pidhody do upravlinnia zakladamy serednyoi osvity: Navchal'nyi posibnyk* [Gender Approach in the Management of Secondary Educational Institutions: Handout]. Kyiv: Logos.

Petrenko, O.B. 2007. Klasyky ukrai'ns'koi' pedagogiky pro gendernu osvitu j vyhovannja shkoljariv [Authorities of Ukrainian Pedagogy on Gender Education and the Upbringing of Pupils]. *Visnyk* 10: 211–22.

Petryshyna, L.V. 2002.*Gendernyj pidhid – vazhlyvyj chynnyk demokratyzacii' osvity'* [Gender Approach as an Important Factor in Democratizing Education]. Available at http://www.edportal.org.ua/books/Conference_2002/Petryshyna.pdf (accessed 4 Sept. 2005).

Plakhotnik, O. 2005. Gendernyj vymir suchasnoi' osvity: Zdobutky amerykans'kyh feministychno-pedagogichnyh studij [A Gender View of Contemporary Education: The Experience of American Feministic-Pedagogical Studies]. In S. Klepko (ed.), *Amerykans'ka filosofija osvity ochyma ukrai'ns'kyh doslidnykiv* [American Philosophy of Education from the Ukrainian Researchers' Point of View], 128–33. Kyiv: Poltava.

– 2007. *Marginal'nye diskursy v obrazovatel'nom prostranstve post-sovetkoi shkoly* [Marginal Discourses in the Educational Space of a Post-Soviet School]. M.A. Thesis, European Humanities University, Vilnius.

– 2009. K voprosu ob institutsializatsii gendernykh issledovaniy kak uchebnoy discipliny v sovremennoi Ukraine [About the Institutionalization of Gender Studies in University Curricula of Contemporary Ukraine]. *Gendernye Issledovaniya* [Gender Issues] 19: 156–65.

– 2010. Shkil'ni genderni uroky yak dzerkalo ukrains'koi gendernoi polityky [School Gender Lessons as a Mirror of Ukrainian Gender Policy]. In *Genderna osvita v Ukraini: dosvid, problemy, perspectyvy* [Gender Education in Ukraine: Experience, Problems, Perspectives], 167–72. Kyiv: Tsentr Ukrainoznavstva KNU imeni Tarasa Shevchenka.

Plakhotnik, O., and S. Gubina. 2009. K voprosu o gendernykh ustanovkah i gendernoi kompetentnosti uchitelei [On the Question of Gender Attitudes and Gender Competence of Teachers]. In *Sbornik materialov konferencii 'Genderni peretvorennja v Ukraini: osmysljujuchy strategiju i taktyku* [Gender Transformations in Ukraine: Rethinking Strategies and Practice], 66–75.

Popova, L. 2001. Chto nuzhno znat' vospitatelyam o tom, kak mal'chiki i devichki nauchayutsya byt' muzhchinami i zhenshchinami [What It Is Necessary for Teachers to Know Regarding How Boys and Girls Are Learning to Be Men and Women]. In: *Gendernyi podhod v doshkol'noi pedagogike: Teoriya i practica. Chast' 1.* [Gender Approach in Preschool Pedagogics. Part 1]. Murmansk: Obrazovatel'nyi tsentr.

Prykhodkina, N.O. 2008. *Pedagogichni umovy realizatsii gendernogo pidhodu u fahoviy pidgotovtsi studentiv humanitarnykh special'nostey. Avtoref.dys. na zdobuttya n.st. kand.pedagogichnyh nauk* [Pedagogical Conditions for Implementing a Gender Approach in the Professional Training of Students Specializing in the Humanities. Doctoral dissertation in Pedagogy]. Kyiv: Universytet Menedgmentu Osvity.

Pryhodkina, N.O., and M.O. Golubjeva. 2007. Strategii' vprovadzhennja idej gendernogo pidhodu v osvitnju praktyku VNZ Ukrai'ny [Strategies for Implementing the Idea of a Gender Approach in Educational Practice in Ukrainian Higher Education]. *Pedagogichni, psyhologichni nauky ta social'na robota* [Pegagogical, Psychological Sciences, and Social Work] 71: 29–34.

Reardon, B.A. 2003. *Education for a Culture of Peace in a Gender Perspective.* Paris: UNESCO.

Scott, J. 1986. Gender: A Useful Category of Historical Analysis. *American Historical Review* 91(5): 1053–75.

Semikolenova, E.I., O.I. Suslova, and G. Daugon. 1999. *Upolnomochennoe obrazovanie. Posobie dlya trenerov* [Empowering Education: Handout for Instructors]. Kyiv: Dovira.

Semikolenova, E.I., O.I. Suslova, and G. Docjuk. 2001. *Shkola rivnyh mozhlyvostej: Navchal'nyj metodychnyj posibnyk* [School of Equal Opportunities: Handout]. Kyiv: Ukrai'ns'ki encyklopedichni znannja.

Sereda, V. 2006. Genderno-chutlyve vykladanya: sproby, problemy, znakhidky [Gender-Sensitive Teaching: Attempts, Problems, Findings]. Presentation for

Winter School for Junior University Teachers in Kharkiv National University, 8–9 February.

Severyna, S.O. 2005. Rozvytok gendernoi osvity v shkoli [Development of Gender Education in Schools]. *Teoretychni i prykladni problemy psyhologii* [Theoretical and Practical Problems of Psychology] (9): 135–41.

Shtyleva, L. 2008. *Factor pola v obrazovanii: gendernyi podhod i analiz* [in Russian]. Moscow: Per-Se.

Smirnova, A. 2005. Uchimsya zhit' v obschestve. Gendernyi analiz shkol'nyh uchebnikov [Let's Learn How to Live in Society: Gender Analysis of School Textbooks]. Moscow: Olita.

Stubbs, M. 1976. *Language, Schools and Classrooms.* London: Wiley.

Sukovata, V. 2007. Feminists'ka metodologija jak polityka osvity: konstru-juvannja novyh gendernyh identychnostej v ukrai'ns'kij vyshchij shkoli [Feminist Methodology as Educational Policy: Constructing New Gender Identities in Ukrainian Higher Education]. *Sociologija: Teorija, metody, marketyng* 3: 202–22.

Sunderland, J., and C. Kitetu. 2000. Gendered Discourses in the Classroom: The Importance of Cultural Diversity. In A. Yamashiro, ed., *Temple University of Japan Working Papers,* 26–40. Tokyo: Temple University of Japan.

van Deik, T. 1989. *Yazyk. Poznanie. Kommunikaciya* [Language. Perception. Communication]. Moscow: Progress.

Voronina, O., ed. 2005. Gendernaya ekspertiza uchebnikov dlya vysshei shkoly [Gender Expertise of Textbooks for Higher School]. Moscow: Soltex.

Wood, J.T. 1994. *Gendered Lives: Communication, Gender and Culture.* Belmont: Wadsworth.

Yarskaya-Smirnova, E. 2000. Gendernoe neravenstvo v obrazovanii: ponyatie skrytogo uchebnogo plana [Gender Inequality in Education: The Notion of a Hidden Curriculum]. *Gendernye issledovaniya* [Gender Studies] 5: 295–301.

Zherebkina, I. 2003. On the Performativity of Gender: Gender Studies in Post-Soviet Higher Education. *Studies in East European Thought* 55(1): 63–79.

Zhurzhenko T. 2004. Families in the Ukraine: Between Postponed Modernization, Neo-Familialism and Economic Survival. *Contemporary Perspectives in Family Research* 5: 187–209.

10 Gender Analysis of School Textbooks in Ukraine

ELENA SEMIKOLENOVA

Formal education should provide opportunities for young people to develop abilities and skills. It should also help to level the social playing field, providing the same possibilities for advancement to children from diverse economic and ethnic backgrounds, as well as to all genders.[1] However, in practice, education often emphasizes and affirms existing social inequalities by reproducing them among students (Giddens 1999, 489). This is true with regard to gender equality. Various aspects of the educational process, both explicit and subtle, from the choice of examples and illustrations in school textbooks, to the formulation of assignments and even the grammar and syntax of teachers' speech can foster a gender-biased perspective on the world that starts in kindergarten and runs through all levels of learning. For this reason, analysing the gender balance in education is an important area of study, as it is the prerequisite for rectifying that balance. This, in turn, is a key opportunity to advance gender equality in the larger society.

In this chapter, I examine the gender balance in the Ukrainian school system by analysing school textbooks. First, I provide some context for this work, looking at what is being done to address gender equality in education in today's Ukraine. I then explain the theory and methodologies that informed my analysis. I present the results of my analysis of textbooks used in Grade 1 classrooms in Ukraine's Autonomous Republic of Crimea. Finally, I discuss these findings and look at one possibility for remedying the gender imbalance in textbooks.

Overall, the chapter demonstrates how abundant and deeply rooted gender-biased information is in the new school textbooks of independent Ukraine. As I argue, addressing this problem through gender and educational policies is of primary importance if gender equality is to be advanced and not hindered for the next generation of Ukrainians.

Background

In Ukraine, equal rights to education are protected by the 2005 Gender Equality Law.[2] However, the existing educational system does not comply with the law's provisions. Educational institutions are supposed to provide 'inculcation of gender equality culture, and equal distribution of professional and family responsibilities' (Gender Equality Law, Art. 21). And yet, the actual policies and practices of educational institutions do not currently contribute to these goals. In great part, this is because the majority of textbook authors, teachers, and school staff lack an understanding of gender issues.[3] As a result, gender stereotypes are being transmitted and consolidated in the classroom (Semikolenova and Shilina 2006a).

The Gender Equality Law states that 'the central executive body for science and education shall organize expert analysis of curricula and textbooks for educational institutions as to their compliance with the principle of equal rights and opportunities for women and men' (Art. 21). Such an analysis would provide an opportunity to investigate discourses of educational literature and uncover concrete examples of gender asymmetry, gender neutrality, and gender sensitivity reflected in textbooks and manuals, as well as the specific character of their translation at different stages of education and in the framework of different subjects of study. As Riabova (2005) puts it, 'The discourse of school textbooks is one of the main resources of "creating gender," an intellectual space where notions of male and female are formed' (p. 123). Thus, findings from textbook analysis would reflect the expressed goals of the Ukrainian state and would reveal aspects of the society's broader gender consciousness as well as changes in gender relations in post-Soviet Ukraine.

However, up to now, very little of this 'gender critique of education' (Plakhotnik 2007) has been carried out. In 2004, the Ministry of Education and Science of Ukraine (MESU), with the support of the Canada – Ukraine Gender Fund, did conduct a curriculum competition for teaching gender issues. The goal was to implement gender education in high schools and to train gender-issue specialists. The winning curricula are now published as the *Anthology of Curricula on the Issues of Gender Development* (MESU 2004). But, although the anthology contains some examples of gender-sensitivity in the social science and humanities curricula, most entries are of poor quality or adhere blatantly to anti-gender equality principles.[4] Thus, in the texts of some programs such terms as *gender-role education*, *sex education*, and *gender education* were not differentiated and were given as synonyms. Many of the tasks proposed by the curricula for students actually reproduce patriarchal stereotypes instead of combating them. In one example, the curriculum proposes the following to teachers: 'Select differentiated tasks in mathematics for boys and girls. For example: "Put the same number of blocks as that of dolls" (for girls), "Put the same number of blocks as that of cars" (for boys), "Are there enough vases for the flowers?" (for girls), "Are there enough wheels to make cars?" (for boys)' (MESU 2004, 140). Other examples from the anthology include:

- 'To extend the children's idea about norms of masculinity and femininity one can conduct the lesson on creating stories "Country of Masculinity" and "Country of Femininity."' (p. 138)
- '. . . conducting discussions separately with boys and girls "Our Women's Secrets," "Our Men's Secrets," as well as [in] solving problem situations in the form of a game teach the child to find such variants of behaviour that meet society's requirements to be representative of a certain sex.' (p. 138)
- 'It is useful to conduct physical education events, where boys demonstrate their strength, agility, and speed, while girls compete in flexibility, grace, and musicality.' (p. 139)
- 'Besides joint games and toys it is necessary to think about equipment for games considering the child's sex.' (p. 140)

Importantly, several of these study programs, including the one from which the above quotes are taken, are recommended by the Ministry of Education and Science of Ukraine for use in all schools. This will bring more harm than benefit, however, as they only reinforce gender asymmetry and hierarchy among the children (Riabova 2005, 9). This governmental initiative, therefore, cannot be considered successful in terms of advancing gender equality. Its failure points again to the fact that many educators in Ukraine, including authors, editors, and illustrators of school textbooks, are steeped in gender stereotypes, and this is reflected in the content and design of their educational materials.

Meanwhile, non-governmental organizations (NGOs) in Ukraine are also tackling the problem. In 2009, the Program of Equal Opportunities and Women's Rights in Ukraine began a wide-ranging gender analysis of school textbooks, manuals, and curricula. The project brings together advocates and professionals, such as teachers, school administrators, specialists of regional institutes of postgraduate pedagogical education, and teachers from higher educational institutions, all of whom aim to develop the principles, criteria, and standards of gender analysis of school textbooks and curricula.

But more work remains to be done. Preliminary steps have been taken internationally to study gender imbalance in school materials more closely. Researchers like Kimmel (2006) have looked at gendered classrooms that produce gendered individuals in the U.S. context, while Smirnova (2005) has studied Russian textbooks to demonstrate the level of gender stereotypes use in them. For both these researchers, it is clear that school textbooks portray severe gender imbalance. The present analysis and that of Govorun and Kikinezhdi (2008) mark the beginnings of this crucial work in the Ukrainian context.

Theoretical Approach and Methodology

Gender expertise of school textbooks generally focuses on the following aspects: the choice of topics, content of texts, peculiarities of how the teaching materials are presented, analysis and interpretation of events, choice of subjects and how they are interpreted, how assignments and questions are formulated, illustrations, and language.[5] Although each of these components is important, the order in which they are to be examined depends on the school grade that a particular textbook is designed for: elementary, secondary, or high school.[6] For example, in elementary school, the content of illustrations is paramount due to the peculiarities of children's perception. The content of texts and examples, as well as assignments and the formulation of questions are next in importance for this age group. For secondary and high school textbooks, however, the choice of topics and the presentation of materials, as well as the suggested interpretation of certain events are more significant, given the more sophisticated learning skills of students in this age group. Meanwhile, language usage, such as grammar and syntax, are equally consequential in textbooks of all levels of study because these structural elements convey a specific set of ideas about the world (Taranenko 2005).

When conducting a gender analysis it is also important to consider textbooks for all study subjects, not just social sciences, which might, on the surface, seem most relevant for gender expertise. For example, the Ukrainian mathematics textbook for Grade 1 (Bogdanovych 2007) contains problems based on situations pertaining to mothers and grandmothers, but not a single problem where a father is the main character. The Grade 6 Ukrainian literature textbook (Bandura 1997) includes works of fifteen writers and poets, only one of whom is a female writer: Mariya Vilinska, known under the male pseudonym Marko Vovchok.[7] And, when writing of human beings, a textbook called *The Fundamentals of Health* refers primarily to males (Voronina 2003). Thus, it is clear that the potential for transmitting either gender-balanced or gender-stereotypical messages is available in any subject area.

Overall, it is possible to differentiate four broad types of textbooks with regard to gender. There are 'gender-blind' textbooks in which gender is entirely omitted. 'Gender-marked (stereotypical)' textbooks address gender, but in a stereotypical manner, where men and women are not represented equally. A third type is 'gender-marked (mixed),' in which some gender stereotypes are represented, but which also contain some gender-balanced information. And finally, there are 'gender-sensitive' texts, where content is based on the perspective of gender equality, the gender component is addressed consistently, and information on men and women is presented in an objective and balanced way.

I used these categories to consider a subset of school textbooks for Grade 1 currently used in Grade 1 classrooms in Ukraine's Autonomous Republic of Crimea. Almost all of these are in Russian, since the language of instruction in over 90 per cent of the schools in the Russian-speaking region of Crimea is Russian. In this sense, this subset of textbooks can be considered regional. At the same time, in terms of their content, only two of these textbooks are truly regional – meaning that their content and design differ from analogous textbooks used elsewhere in Ukraine. The first is an alphabet textbook containing Russian texts for Russian-speakers; the second is a Ukrainian language manual for Russian-speakers. The rest of the books are translations of textbooks written originally in Ukrainian and approved by the Ministry of Education for use in all Ukrainian schools, regardless of region. Thus, although the subset analysed here is regional, it is also representative of the general situation in the country. The main features of the books in the subset are summarized in the Appendix.

My primary method for analysing these textbooks was content analysis. Specifically, I divided the basic units of analysis (illustrations, text, assignments, etc.) according to the spheres of social life that their content represented, for example, family, school, outdoors, or public transportation. Second, I grouped the units of analysis according to the gender of those they depicted, that is, girls or boys, women or men, or several of these together. Third, I cross-tabulated the collected data to demonstrate the correlation between specific spheres of social life (indoors versus outdoors) and the participants' gender markers (female versus male). I also introduced the parameter of age to demonstrate that depiction of gender differences is similar for both children and adults.

The 'indoors' sphere was further broken down into two sections: 'household and family duties' and 'leisure activities' (games, pastimes, hobbies, toys). Each section was looked at while taking gender and age markers into account. The 'outdoors' sphere was also broken down into 'leisure activities' and 'work outside the home,' which referred to adults.

I also compared the content of illustrations and texts with common stereotypes divided into the following categories:

- Stereotypes concerning *family and professional roles,* in which the family sphere is marked as female, the professional sphere as male
- Stereotypes connected with differences in the *content of labour,* according to which women are destined to perform supporting, service/care work, while men's activities are creative, formative, and leading
- Stereotypes of masculine and feminine *qualities and personal features,* in which a girl's image emphasizes emotionality, politeness, and neatness, while a boy's image emphasizes activity, independence, and leadership skills (Smirnova 2005, 8)
- Stereotypes reflecting *particularities of pastimes,* where girls play with dolls, knit, and embroider, while boys play with cars and planes, go fishing, and play football and hockey.

Finally, I also analysed the school textbooks from the linguistic point of view to assess whether syntax and grammar used in children's manuals is gender-marked.

Results

In the following sections, I describe the findings from my analysis. As will be shown, one of the most dramatic results is how frequently women are confined to the home space in school texts and illustrations. The cost of this confinement is seen in the depiction of professional life in the textbooks, where boys grow up to choose from a large range of careers, while girls can expect far fewer options.

Representations of Home- and Family-Related Duties by Gender and Age

Table 10.1 outlines the kinds of typical household activities engaged in at home by adult women and men as seen in the Grade 1 textbooks that I analysed. As the left-hand column of the table makes clear, judging from the content and illustrations in these textbooks, all housework is done by mothers and grandmothers. Most often, they cook and shop for groceries. There are a lot of pictures in the books in which family members sit at the table while mother serves food. Grandmother's destiny, besides all the housekeeping, is to take care of small grandchildren. These duties are reflected in the following math problems: 'Grandmother baked several layers for a cake . . .,' 'Grandmother and Nikita went to the store . . .,' 'Grandmother is buying a dozen eggs . . .,' 'Mother bought 2 kg of cucumbers, 3 kg of tomatoes, and 4 kg of apples. What did mother buy more of – vegetables or fruit?'

There are virtually no household duties assigned to fathers and grandfathers in the textbooks. Illustrations that depict them in a home environment are few. Their everyday responsibilities are woodworking and gardening (see Figure 10.1).[8] The alphabet textbook contains the following description: 'There is a garden near the house. There are plums, apple trees, and pears there. Father and Tolia [the boy's name] work in the garden. Father has a saw. He cut off branches and Tolia watered the raspberry bushes.' Only one textbook, *The Fundamentals of Health*, has an illustration in which the whole family, adults and children, clean the apartment.

All of women's household work is carried out inside the house, in a closed space. In contrast, men's activities take place near the house, in an open space. If mothers and grandmothers appear outside the house, it is usually because they are required to leave for grocery shopping purposes. This rigid allocation of space reflects findings from textbook analyses conducted in other contexts. In Kimmel's analysis, for example, men and women are shown to have their own sphere of responsibility: 'his' area is in open air, such as the yard or garden; 'her' area is always in enclosed premises such as the kitchen, laundry room, bedroom, or bathroom (2006, 208).

Table 10.1. Household and Family Duties of Adult Family Members as Seen in Grade 1 Textbooks

Women (Mothers and Grandmothers)	Men (Fathers and Grandfathers)
• Cooking • Serving food • Washing dishes • Buying foodstuffs • Cleaning the house • Taking care of plants • Baking cookies and pies • Beating cream • Decorating cakes • Laying a festive table • Taking care of small children • Taking care of ill children • Meeting husband after work • Grandmothers feed grandchildren, walk with small grandchildren, read books to grandchildren	• Woodworking (sawing and planing boards) • Working in the garden (planting trees, tying branches, etc.)

Household duties for girls mainly repeat those of adult women (see Table 10.2). Girls either help mothers and grandmothers in the kitchen or perform these chores themselves. Girls very frequently water house flowers and take care of them. Meanwhile, like their fathers, boys' household duties include woodworking and garden duties. The textbook *Me and Ukraine* presents two pictures on one page that capture these distinct roles: a girl waters flowers, a boy planes a board (see Figure 10.2). The Ukrainian language manual, however, contains two pictures in which a girl and a boy serve a table and do the dishes together (see Figure 10.3). However, these are rather exceptions from the general trend. In pictures from the alphabet textbook, only girls do housework; boys help mothers and grandmothers with grocery shopping instead.

Indoor Leisure Activities by Gender and Age

Mothers' and grandmothers' pastimes are limited to knitting socks and reading books (but not newspapers). Fathers and grandfathers sit in armchairs or on sofas reading newspapers and books, but more often newspapers (see Table 10.3). Men are thus represented as more

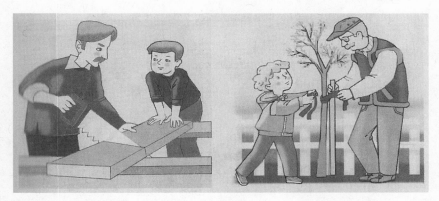

Figure 10.1. An illustration from *Fundamentals of Health*. Source: Boichenko and Savchenko (2007, 45).

interested in world events than women. In all the textbooks, only men and boys play chess.

The illustration used to depict 'family leisure time' in the textbook *Me and Ukraine* shows a father and grandfather playing chess and a son watching their game. Grandmother sits on the sofa with her small granddaughter and reads her a book (which is considered to be rest for the grandmother). In the background, a mother stands in the kitchen at the stove (see Figure 10.4). The picture is followed by a discussion question: 'How does the family rest?' Thus, it prompts students to invest in this gendered arrangement. More gender-balanced illustrations are presented in other textbooks. For example, in *The Fundamentals of Health*, the entire family is involved in a morning workout.

Inside games and activities differ for girls and boys (see Table 10.4). Girls play with dolls or, like mothers and grandmothers, knit and embroider. For example, consider the following math problems: 'The doll had 4 dresses. Marina sewed 3 more dresses. How many dresses does the doll have now?' 'Zoya washed 4 doll dresses and 2 more blouses. How many items did Zoya wash?' 'Masha had 5 toys. She was given several more toys, and now she has 11 toys. How many toys was Masha given?'

Boys' activities are more creative. They sit at computers, work with Meccano toys (Lego-like toys), create models for cars and ships, and play chess. Math problems that use boys in their description reflect this perception of their creativity: 'A boy had 10 stamps. He gave

Table 10.2. Children's Household Duties as Seen in Grade 1 Textbooks

Girls	Boys	Girls and Boys Together
• Helping mother or grandmother in the kitchen • Cutting vegetables • Washing dishes • Setting the table • Watering flowers • Walking the dog	• Planing boards • Woodworking • Working in the garden • Helping mother or grandmother with grocery shopping • Walking the dog	• Planting trees in the garden • Planting sprouts in kitchen garden

7 stamps to his friend . . .' 'Misha has 15 stamps, and Grisha has 7 stamps less . . .' 'Vova cut 5 triangles and 2 squares. Misha cut 3 squares and an equal number of triangles . . .'

Children often spend free time at home together. At first glance, all their joint indoor pastimes seem gender-neutral. However, if they watch TV, the boy holds the remote control. Boys also hold books in their hands more often than girls. If they read together, more often the boy is reading and explaining, while the girl listens. In one example, we learn that 'Oleg and Natasha are frequent visitors to the reading hall. It is quiet in the hall, there are bookshelves everywhere. Choose and read . . . What are you reading now, Oleg? sister asks. *Magic Tree*, the book by Kornei Chukovsky. *And Natasha can't read yet*. She looks at the pictures . . .' (emphasis added). This distinction is made even though the illustration shows children of about the same age. In such depictions, even reading ceases to be neutral and becomes gender-marked. The only gender-neutral activities that seem to exist in the world of these books are drawing and work with paper and scissors. As Kimmel puts it, daily activities are the means by which children recognize what it means 'to be a boy' or 'to be a girl' (2006, 205). Thus, depictions of children's games and sports in textbooks 'express and contain gender inequality expectations transmitted further in the process of gender relations in adult life' (ibid.).

Outdoor Leisure Activities by Gender and Age

Family rest outside the house is more diverse than what is depicted as their indoor activities. Outdoor leisure involves attending movies and visiting the zoo, hiking in the forest, and having a picnic at the

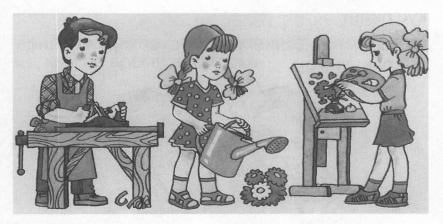

Figure 10.2. An illustration from *Me and Ukraine*. Source: Bibik and Koval (2002, 14).

riverside. During these activities, fathers and grandfathers become more visible. For example, the alphabet textbook describes the following situations: 'Zina with her father attended the Zoo.' 'Vasylko with his grandfather go to the pond.' 'Lena and her father were walking in the forest.' 'Marichka is happy. Today she goes to the mountains with her father.' Even here, women are haunted by the ghost of cooking: in illustrations under the sections 'Your Family' and 'Family Pastime' in the textbook *Me and Ukraine*, a family relaxes at the riverside, but the girl and the mother are positioned near a pot, while father is at an easel, and grandson and grandfather are returning from successful fishing.

In all textbooks, a great number of illustrations are devoted to children's outdoor pastimes and games (see Table 10.5), and pictures of girls are as frequent as those of boys. However, girls' activities are monotonous. As at home, these are often games with dolls and the care of flowers. In some textbooks, like *Me and Ukraine*, interactions between girls and flowers are repeated on virtually every page; they plant flowers, water flowers, make bouquets and garlands, hold flowers in their hands, and smell flowers. The majority of girls' outdoor occupations are static; they do not have an arc or developing plot. Girls' pastimes become more dynamic if they play with boys, who are regularly engaged in outdoor team games, walks, or rides.

As Table 10.5 clearly shows, boys' pastimes are very diverse – and frequently depicted. In the 'Family Leisure' section of *Me and Ukraine*,

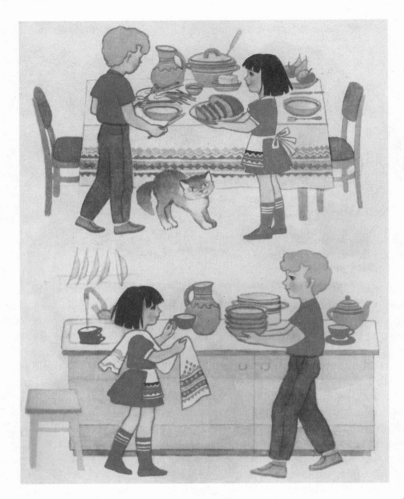

Figure 10.3. An illustration from *Ukrainian Language*. Source: Khoroshkovska and Okhota (2002, 71).

for example, there are only illustrations of boys. They go hiking, gather mushrooms, and build a sailing ship. Fishing is one of the most preferred hobbies: boys go fishing, come from fishing, hold fishing rods, haul in fish, etc. In one example from the alphabet textbook, we hear that 'At dawn Kostia and his grandfather Matvei go to the pond. They stop under the old willow . . . Here is the first one caught. How

Table 10.3. Adult Pastimes (Inside and Outside the Home) as Seen in Grade 1 Textbooks

Women (Mothers and Grandmothers)	Men (Fathers and Grandfathers)	All the Family Together
• Knitting socks • Reading books	• Reading newspapers or books • Sitting at the dinner table • Sitting in an armchair or on the sofa • Playing chess	• Watching TV • Going to the movies • Walking in the forest • Going to a riverside or beach

big! – Kostia is happy.' Similarly, in a math textbook young readers are presented with the following problem: 'A boy caught 5 perches, and the girl caught 2 perches *less*. How many perches did the girl catch?' This girl has other shortcomings: she also picks fewer plums: 'Vitia gathered 11 plums and Olia – 2 plums *less*' (emphasis added).

Images of boats are quite frequent: boys build boats, play with boats, make paper ships, and let them sail. This theme is further elaborated in romanticized texts: 'Morning is close. Fog. A sail boat is adrift. There are two sailors [*in masculine form*] in the boat. One steers, another sets sail . . .' 'Yakov Petrovich is the captain of *Mriya*, a motorized ship. He leads his ship far into the sea. Today the motorized ship *Mriya* arrives at Yalta. Mother, Andreika, and little Yasochka will come to meet him.'

Almost all boys' occupations are connected to movement and riding. Boys use cars, bicycles, skates, scooters, boats, etc. They also actively engage in different types of sports. In the textbook *The Fundamentals of Health*, the 'Sports' section depicts only boys in its illustrations. Boys play football, hockey, and water polo. In the alphabet textbook, we get another example of boys' active play: 'Iliusha and Andriusha [*2 boys*] like to play hockey very much. They are captains of their yard teams . . . And now is the game. Players quickly run across the field . . . – Goal! – their friends Niura and Liuba [*2 girls*] are happy.' The textbook also provides commentary to this text: 'Chess develops the brain and wit and hockey – strength, courage, and endurance. The song justly says: "Real men play hockey, cowards don't play hockey." '

All boys' games and pastimes are dynamic. They are also directed; many of these activities assist in the choice of future professions. Thus, prompting questions accompanying illustrations of young people's activities include: 'Which of these boys dreams to serve in the navy?' 'Who

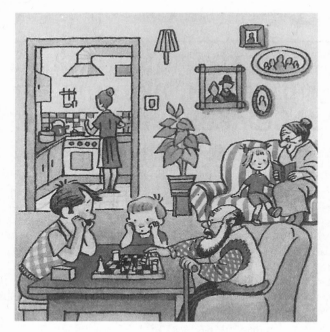

Figure 10.4. An illustration from *Me and Ukraine*. Source: Bibik and Koval (2002, 29).

is driving fruit to the shop?' 'Who learns to take photos?' and 'Who wants to become a pilot?' The general answer is mostly 'Boys.'

Kimmel observes, in the depiction of children's games, that boys play to get power, while girls play to make sure everyone is having a good time (2006, 203). This is also evident in the pictures in the textbooks that I analysed, where roles in games are divided in a way so that a boy would be a leader (a war general or a bus driver), with a girl playing a supportive role (a field nurse, or a ticket seller). As researchers have pointed out, in their games and play, boys and girls study and emulate the models of behaviour that they are expected to follow as future men and women (ibid.).

Work Outside the Home by Gender and Age

The most stark examples of discriminatory gender depictions in the textbooks relate to professions and types of jobs (see Table 10.6).

Table 10.4. Children's Pastimes (Games and Activities) as Seen in Grade 1 Textbooks

Girls	Boys	Girls and Boys Together
• Playing with blocks • Playing with dolls (dressing, feeding, nursing, putting to bed, walking, etc.) • Embroidering • Knitting • Drawing	• Sitting at the computer • Constructing models of cars, ships, rockets, etc. • Playing with Meccano toys • Reading • Drawing	• Reading • Watching TV • Drawing • Working with scissors and paper

Judging from illustrations alone, the most popular female profession is that of schoolteacher, depicted dozens of times in all textbooks. A total of three illustrations depict males in this profession, and these were teachers of mathematics and computer science. This dramatically skewed view reproduces the more general social perception that the 'hierarchy of sciences' has a masculine character: the 'hard' sciences, like mathematics or physics, are respected and prestigious, while 'feminine' areas, like literary studies, are much less so (Voronina 2003, 73). Among the other most frequent 'female' professions are baker and doctor, as well as jobs in the service sector.

In contrast, as can be seen in the right-hand column of the Table 10.6, the range of 'male' professions is much greater, from tractor operator to agronomist, and firefighter to astronaut. Male professions are depicted as more prestigious, romantic, heroic, and creative. Acquiring them presupposes a high level of qualification and professionalism, as well as the ability to work with advanced equipment. Interestingly, although cooking and sewing in the home are considered to be women's duties, the public-sphere professions of cook and tailor are represented by men, thereby further reinforcing the value of men's activities outside the home and diminishing women's work within the family.

Perhaps unsurprisingly, then, given these depictions, the textbook that deals explicitly with work futures, called *Career Education*, presents the most rigid gender stereotypes (Yarskaya-Smirnova 2000). The book consists of five sections, each of which is devoted to a particular professional sphere. Table 10.7 lists the kinds of work described in these spheres and whether they are represented by illustrations of men or women.

Table 10.5. Children's Leisure Activities Outside the Home as Seen in Grade 1 Textbooks

Girls	Boys	Girls and Boys Together
• Playing with dolls • Skipping rope • Caring for flowers • Watering flowers • Gathering flowers into bouquets • Twining garlands • Looking after trees • Embroidering	• Fishing • Hiking • Gathering mushrooms • Playing with a ball • Riding bicycles • Riding scooters • Skating • Diving • Flying kites • Playing with paper toy ships • Breeding pigeons • Conducting chemical experiments • Taking photos • Joining sports • Playing football • Playing water polo • Play hockey	• Reading • Walking in the park or forest • Gathering mushrooms • Taking part in team games • Playing with a ball • Bathing in a river • Skating • Sledding • Throwing snowballs • Making snowmen • Feeding birds in winter • Take part in concerts: singing and dancing

This breakdown reflects the traditional attribution of action, strength, intellect, rationality, and organizational skills to men. In another example, the book describes three broad categories of work, each of which is also accompanied by an illustration: to show intellectual labour, we see a boy reading a book; for physical labour, a boy holds a spade and a girl holds a rake in a kitchen garden; for artistic labour, a girl is shown drawing. Meanwhile, near the section of text that describes the value of labour, only male professionals are depicted: a blacksmith, carpenter, miller, potter, and tailor. The text speaks to these in the following way: 'Their work is valuable for a city and a village, valuable for the whole country.' This is in accordance with the widely held opinion in society that 'boys should grow independent and self-sufficient to explore the environment and cope with it' (Kimmel 2006, 200). Female images, meanwhile, are characterized by shows of care for others, support, sympathy, and diligence. In the world of these textbooks, professional life is far from paramount for women; the most important thing for them is family.

Table 10.6. Professions and Types of Labour as Seen in Grade 1
Textbooks

Women	Men
• Teacher	Agriculture-Related
• Doctor	• Agronomist
Agriculture-Related	• Forester
• Farm worker	• Harvest collector
• Calf-tender	• Beekeeper
• Milkmaid	• Tractor operator
• Poultry maid	• Combine operator
Other (Mainly Service Sector)	• Shepherd
• Sales assistant	• Miller
• Hairdresser	Other
• Seamstress	• Builder
• Baker	• Carpenter
• Painter	• Locksmith
• Assistant stationmaster	• Turner
• Craftsperson	• Steeplejack
	• Blacksmith
	• Potter
	• Driver
	• Gardener
	Service Sector
	• Cook
	• Tailor
	• Postman
	Creative
	• Artist
	• Designer
	Romantic and Heroic
	• Sailor
	• Skipper
	• Cosmonaut
	• Policeman
	• Firefighter
	Computer-Related
	• Computer operator
	• Programmer
	• Accountant

Gendered Representations of Toys

Almost all toys represented in the textbooks that I analysed are clearly
gender-marked (see Table 10.8). As Kimmel points out, many toys 'are

Table 10.7. Professions by Gender in Illustrations in the Textbook Career Education (Yarskaya-Smirnova 2000)

Sphere	Professions	Represented by
Human – nature	• Gardener • Agronomist • Forester	Only men
Human – human	• Doctor • Hairdresser • Teacher	Only women
Human – sign systems	• Operator • Accountant	Only men
Human – technology	• Tractor operator • Astronaut • Driver	Only men
Human – art/creativity	• Artist • Gardener • Craftsperson	Two men, one woman (craftsperson)

designed to be sold as girls' toys or boys' toys. Girls are given dolls and dollhouses; boys get trucks and building blocks, and are told that they are "sissies" if they want to play with girls' toys' (2006, 202).

Illustrations showing girls with dolls are repeated dozens of times. All games with dolls are static and limited to caring for them. In such games girls reproduce all types of household work performed by their mothers and grandmothers in the home: dolls are bathed, dressed, fed, nursed, taken for walks, put to bed, etc. Examples from the alphabet textbook demonstrate similar biases: 'Polia has a doll Lida. Polia picked up the doll to wash it. She sat the doll at the table and set the table . . ."Sit here, Lida" . . .' 'Ivan has new flippers. Inna has a new doll.'

Boys' toys are different in content, purpose, and quantity. Among them are a lot of different Meccano toys, and means of transportation, such as cars, planes, and ships. Games with these toys presuppose movement. Boys' toys also include 'bad toys' such as slingshots, thus communicating to the children that violence is more acceptable for boys than it is for girls. Even if children are shown playing together, the rigid

Table 10.8. Toys Held and Played with Inside and Outside by Boys and Girls as Seen in Grade 1 Textbooks

Girls	Boys	Girls and Boys Together
• Dolls	• Ball	• Ball
• Dishes	• Blocks	• Blocks
• Furniture	• Cars	
• Teddy bears	• Rackets	
• Stuffed rabbit	• Planes	
• Ball	• Ships	
• Toy blocks	• Wooden horse	
	• Kite	
	• Paper ships	
	• Slingshot	

division of their toys remains intact. This is true for textual references as well. The alphabet book contains the following scenario: 'Denis made a house. Sasha built a rocket, and Timur made a sailing boat.'

It would make sense that any toy could be available for play by any child, but in reality toys are divided by invisible borders of sexual difference between children (Kimmel 2006, 246). Textbook authors themselves 'push' children to the stereotypical choice of toys. Thus, pictures in the textbook *The Fundamentals of Health* show a doll, a teddy bear, a mirror, a comb, a handbag, a toy bed, toy dishes, a plane, a train, a robot, a truck, a ball, and a skipping rope (see Figure 10.5). Children are asked which of these a girl would choose, and which a boy would choose.

As children seek approval from teachers, they will obviously try to choose 'correctly.' Meanwhile, of all the toys represented on the pages of the textbooks under analysis, only two were gender-neutral: balls and blocks.

Gendered Language

The final content analysis conducted for this study was to look at linguistic structures used in the textbooks. The major finding here is that in all the books there is a high frequency of words used in the masculine gender. In the Ukrainian language, as in others, many words

2. Розглянь малюнок. Які іграшки, на твою думку, вибере хлопчик, а які — дівчинка?

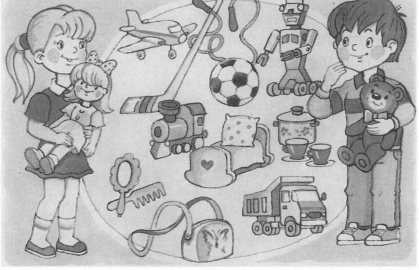

Figure 10.5. 'Look at the picture, which toys do you think a girl will choose? What about a boy?' An illustration from *Fundamentals of Health*.
Source: Boichenko and Savchenko (2007, 39).

can be used both in feminine or masculine form. The textbook authors do not choose the feminine forms as often. Thus, for example, the books address student readers using only the masculine gender form, despite the fact that half of these readers are girls. The very opening of the majority of the textbooks reads: 'Dear friend!' 'Young friend!' or 'Dear first-grader!' – all in the masculine form in Ukrainian or Russian. But examples aren't limited to these initial addresses. There are many others: 'As a young engineer [*masculine*] think what construction a racing car can have'; 'Compete with your classmates [*masculine*] in speed and length of movement of a toy car'; and 'Student's [*masculine*] work place should be convenient.' Thus, gender imbalance is built into the very structure of the language of these books.

Discussion

The results described above are alarming. They show that an abundance of gender-stereotypical content is being presented to children. Among the materials analysed here, there are no gender-sensitive textbooks, and none are even gender-blind. All of the textbooks are gender-marked and nearly all are stereotypical. Importantly, this stands in contrast with the Soviet period in Ukraine, during which time school literature was more gender-blind because of the predominance of communist ideas, which overrode other ideological discourses, including traditional gender ones. The findings presented here thus demonstrate the need for deep reform in the area of education in Ukraine.

At the outset, I discussed steps being taken in this regard in Ukraine to date, particularly with regard to analysing textbooks. I showed that more work needs to be done in this area, noting that this study is but one contribution. Here, I want to briefly review efforts being made to go the next step: that is, to replace textbooks found to be gender-stereotypical. I will then discuss one possible direction for policy reform in relation to the problem of gendered language in school textbooks.

Certain successful attempts do exist in the non-governmental sector with regard to the production of new, gender-balanced textbooks. For example, in 1996, the Women's Information Consultative Centre started the Empowering Education Program for secondary schools. This program was based on the idea of gender justice and non-violence and was directed at creating the conditions for students to acquire group self-organization skills by education through immediate experience (Suslova 2002). The program's authors, without rejecting the existing forms and methods of transmitting knowledge, suggested expanding the possibilities of modern pedagogy by taking into consideration the principle of gender justice. The textbook does not teach any absolute truths, but rather teaches children to find out those truths for themselves. It also teaches how to build relations and cooperate with other people following the principles of trust, partnership, equality, and non-violence.

In 2003, the study program Fundamentals of Dialogue built on this work. Designed for secondary schools, the program was approved by the Ministry of Education and Science of the Autonomous Republic of Crimea. The related textbook (Semikolenova et al. 2008) was published with the support of the Ministry for Family, Youth, and Gender Policy of the Autonomous Republic of Crimea, and educators started to implement the ideas of empowerment, equality, and non-violence in Crimean schools.

A third program, called Equal Opportunities and Women's Rights in Ukraine,[9] has the promotion of gender standards in education as one of its most important objectives. The project coordinator, Larysa Kobelyanska, initiated the publication of the educational manual *We Are Different – We Are Equal: Basics of Gender Equality Culture* for students in Grades 9 to 12 (Semikolenova 2007). The manual is intended 'to overcome stereotypical views on the roles of women and men in family and society, and form students' outlooks free from gender bias and prejudice' (ibid., 2). The textbook has since received official approval by the Ukrainian Ministry of Education and Science.

All of these efforts are important steps forward in creating gender-sensitive programs and textbooks available for use in schools. Although they represent only the tip of the iceberg, and much more work is needed to balance Ukraine's educational sector in terms of gender, these initiatives represent an important example that can be emulated.

Textbook Language: Future Directions

While the work of analysing textbooks for gender balance and then replacing them is ongoing, one important consideration is language. As mentioned in the results section, currently, children are nearly always addressed by their textbooks in the masculine form. This hints at the potential in the Ukrainian language itself for inclusion or exclusion. According to Ukrainian grammatical rules, masculine gender forms of words are preferred when persons of both sexes or a group of people are being described or addressed. Like many modern languages that differentiate genders, Ukrainian uses nouns of masculine gender to denote men and women both in the plural and the singular. Thus, speakers usually say: *'Teachers of our school . . .'* using the masculine gender, even though there may only be female teachers in that particular school. Similarly, city, regional, and national contests for excellence in teaching annually award the prize for Teacher of the Year using the masculine gender, even if a woman wins. And TV contests for children that are broadcast every Saturday by the 'Inter' Ukrainian channel deem one viewer 'The Smartest,' also using the masculine gender, even though both girls and boys take part in these competitions.

Until recently, this situation was justified in several ways. First, it was argued that gendered language reflected existing social divisions of labour between men and women, with a prevalence of men's labour in certain positions and professions, like lecturer, engineer, general, or priest (Vinogradov 1972, 65). Second, it was argued that the Ukrainian language lacks the resources to invent words to name professions in either the feminine gender form or neutrally (Schmelev 1997, 367).

But some sociologists, psychologists, and linguists now argue that such a 'mechanism of exclusion' is not innocently grammatical. Usage of masculine forms of nouns when women are also being designated contributes to ignoring women not only in the language but in the 'picture of the world' as well (Desinova 2002, 232–3). When women inhabit professions or positions with only masculine titles, this results in instilling into native speakers, children among them, the idea that these women are taking someone else's job. Some researchers argue that this has a greater influence than even crude forms of discrimination, as language penetrates deeper layers of consciousness (Gabrielian 1993). In a similar vein, Edward Taylor argued that attention to grammatical gender is crucial because words hold great power over the human mind and might be the greatest drivers of mythological development (1989, 141).

On this basis, certain linguists insist that existing language norms must be rethought and changed, arguing that consciously shaping language to take gender into account should be basic to contemporary language policy (Pomonariv 2001a, 2001b; Semikolenova and Shilina 2006b). To some extent, this is happening in the Ukrainian language. For example, such words as *khudozhnytsia, likarka, vchytelka, dyrektorka, redaktorka, aktorka, agronomka, vyhovatelka, budivelnytsia* (the feminine gender forms for artist, doctor, teacher, director, editor, actress, agronomist, educator, and construction worker) and the like are now used in common speech and mass media. The list of such words is constantly lengthening by 'forming new units or borrowing them from the language of Western Ukrainian diaspora: for example, *liderka, rezhyserka, spikerka, premyerka, derzhsekretarka, . . . chlenkynia, mystkynia* [feminine gender of leader, producer, speaker, prime minister, state secretary, member, artist]' (Taranenko 2005, 23).

In fact, the Ukrainian language is rather flexible and resourceful in producing feminine gender forms (Vykhovanets and Gorodenska 2004, 91). These new feminine gender words eventually take on normative status and are recommended for use by many Ukrainian linguists.[10] Thus, linguistically it is possible to reduce the level of gender bias in the language of textbooks. Work now needs to be done to communicate this idea to the authors of school textbooks.

To conclude this discussion, it is worth mentioning that Ukraine's educational policy is still under development. Even among the textbooks analysed for this study, the number of copies published in 2007 varied greatly across subjects, from 25,000 to 75,900 copies. This is illustrative of the fact that, until now, the area of textbook production and dissemination has lacked planning and control, even at the local level. Standardization only began very recently. It was only in 2004 that the Cabinet of Ministers of Ukraine adopted the State Standard of Elementary and Complete Secondary Education.[11] Yet, there are still no state standards regarding school textbooks or their content. In this context, the findings of this and similar studies of the gender balance of existing textbooks, as well as the recommendations discussed in this section with regard to increasing gender-neutral language and developing new textbooks, together have the potential to contribute to the development of state educational standards based on the principles of gender equality.

Conclusions

The material analysed in this chapter demonstrates how abundant and deeply rooted is gender-biased information in the new school textbooks of independent Ukraine. Addressing this aspect through both gender and educational policies is of primary importance if gender equality is to be advanced and not hindered among the growing generation of Ukrainians.

Some attempts at advancing gender equality through school textbooks have already been made. However, the governmental project in this area has reinforced gender biases rather than combated them. In contrast, non-governmental initiatives in textbook expertise and gender-sensitive programs and manuals have been more successful, yet of limited scope so far.

The chapter argues that future reform in this area has to follow a dual-track approach: textbook expertise and the creation of new texts and study programs. In doing so, both content and form have to be taken into consideration. Thus, both texts and illustrations need to be gender-balanced, together with the language in terms of grammar and syntax.

Appendix

Table 10A. Analysed Grade 1 Textbooks Used in Ukrainian Russian-Language Public Schools

Authors and Titles	Language	City and Publisher	Year	No. Printed
Vakulenko and Gudzhyk, *Bookvar* (Alphabet)	Russian; original text for Russian schools	Kyiv: Osvita	2004	57,200
Khoroshkovska and Okhota, *Ukrayinska Mova* (Ukrainian Language), 2nd ed.	Ukrainian; original text for Russian schools	Kyiv: Osvita	2007	75,900
Bibik and Koval, *Ya i Ukrayina. Vikonechko* (Me and Ukraine: A Little Window), 2nd ed.	Russian; translation from Ukrainian	Kyiv: Geneza	2007	60,350
Bogdanovych, Matematyka (Mathematics)	Russian; translation from Ukrainian	Kyiv: Osvita	2007	65,880
Boichenko and Savchenko, *Osnovy Zdorovya* (Fundamentals of Health), 2nd ed.	Russian; translation from Ukrainian	Kyiv: Geneza	2007	75,050
Veremiychuk, *Trudove Navchannia* (Career Education)	Russian; translation from Ukrainian	Kyiv: Pedahohichna Dumka	2007	25,000

NOTES

1 Article 26 of the 1948 United Nations Universal Declaration of Human Rights cites the provision of education as a priority of the international community in the twenty-first century, while Article 29 of the 1989 Convention of the Rights of the Child emphasizes that 'education of a child should be directed to the development of the child's personality, talents and mental and physical abilities to their fullest potential; . . . as well as to the preparation of the child for responsible life in a free society, in the spirit of understanding, peace, tolerance, *equality of sexes*, and friendship among all peoples, ethnic, national and religious groups' (emphasis added).

2 Zakon Ukrayiny, *Pro zabezpechennia rivnykh prav ta mozhlyvostei zhinok i cholovikiv* (Law of Ukraine on Ensuring Equal Rights and Opportunities for Women and Men), available at http://zakon.rada.gov.ua.

3 See Chapter 9 in this volume for further discussion of teachers' understandings of gender.

4 E.g., O. Kis's 'Gender Studies,' and T. Doronina's 'Gender Trends in Literary Studies: Theoretical and Methodological Basics and Interpretation Practices.'

5 Outside of the Ukrainian context this is known as *gender analysis*.

6 In Ukraine, school education is comprised of three stages: elementary school (grades 1 through 4), secondary school (grades 5 through 9), and high school (grades 10 and 11).

7 This is despite the fact that Ukrainian culture is unimaginable without its remarkable women writers, yet they are not included in the school program.

8 Woodwork is a stereotypically masculine activity, and no matter how outdated it is at the moment in both urban and rural settings, with very few men actually owning woodworking instruments or ever engaging in this activity, in the textbooks it still remains among the jobs most associated with men's roles.

9 The project was co-funded by the European Union, the Swedish International Development Cooperation Agency, and the United Nations Development Program. The project's national implementing partner is the Ministry of Ukraine for Family, Youth, and Sports. For more information, visit http://gender.undp.org.ua.

10 For example, by linguists such as Kateryna Gorodenska, Nina Ozerova, Yury Pradid, Elena Selivanova, Aleksandr Taranenko, Ivan Vykhovanets, Svetlana Yermolenko, and Anatoly Zagnytko.

11 'Derzhavnyi standart bazovoyi i povnoyi zagalnoyi serednioyi osvity' (State Standard of Elementary and Complete Secondary Education), available at http://www.mon.gov.ua/education/average/drzh_stand.doc.

REFERENCES

Bandura, O., and Y. Kucherenko. 1997. *Ukrayinska Literatura: Pidruchnyk dlia Shostogo Klasu* [Ukrainian Literature: Textbook for Grade 6]. Kyiv: Osvita.

Bogdanovych, M. 2007. *Matematyka: Pidruchnyk dlia Pershogo Klasu* [Mathematics: Textbook for the Grade 1]. Kyiv: Osvita.

Boichenko, T., and O. Savchenko. 2007. Osnovy Zdorovya: Pidruchnyk dlia 1 Klasu Zagalnoosvitnih Navchalnyh Zakladiv [Fundamentals of Health: Textbook for Grade 1 of Public Schools]. Kyiv: Heneza.

Bibik N., and N. Koval. 2002. Ya I Ukrayina: Vikonechko. Pidruchnyk dlia 1 Klasu [Me and Ukraine: the Window. Textbook for Grade 1]. Kyiv: ACK.

Denisova, A., ed. 2002. *Slovar Gendernyh Terminov* [Gender Terms Dictionary]. Moscow: Informatsiya – XXI Vek.

Doronina, T. 2004. *Gender Trends in Literary Studies: Theoretical and Methodological Basics and Interpretation Practices*, in *Khrestomatiya Navchalnyh Program z Problem Hendernoho Rozvytku* [Anthology of Curricula on the Issues of Gender Development] by Ministry of Education and Science of Ukraine. Kyiv: Foliant.

Gabrielian, N. 1993. *Meditatsii Na Temu Feminizma: Vsplyvayuschaya Atlantida* [Meditations on Feminism: Emerging Atlantis]. *Obschestvennye Nauki I Sovremennost'* [Social Sciences and Modernity] 6: 171–8.

Giddens, A. 1999. *Sotsiolohiya* [Sociology]. Translation from English by V. Shovkun and A. Oliinyk. Kyiv: Osnovy.

Govorun, T., and O. Kikinezhdi. 2008. *Gender u social'no-psykhologichnomu vymiri: Chastyna 1*[Social-Psychological Aspects of Gender: Part 1]. Available at http://helsinki.org.ua/index.php?id=1200305760 (accessed 4 March 2009).

Khoroshkovska, O., and H. Okhota. 2002. Ukrayinska Mova: Pidruchnyk, 1 Klas [Ukrainian Language: Textbook, Grade 1]. Kyiv: Heneza.

Kimmel, M. 2006. *Gendernoye Obschestvo* [The Gendered Society]. Moscow: ROSSPEN.

Kis, O. 2004. *Gender Studies*, in *Khrestomatiya Navchalnyh Program z Problem Hendernoho Rozvytku* [Anthology of Curricula on the Issues of Gender Development] by Ministry of Education and Science of Ukraine. Kyiv: Foliant.

Lebedinskaya, I., ed. 2003. *Problema Hendernoyi Rivnosti v Pedahohichnii Osviti* [The Problem of Gender Inequality in Pedagogical Education]. Kyiv: Foliant.

Ministry of Education and Science of Ukraine (MESU). 2004. *Khrestomatiya Navchalnyh Program z Problem Hendernoho Rozvytku* [Anthology of Curricula on the Issues of Gender Development]. Kyiv: Foliant. Niemanis, A. 2003. *Vprovadzhennia Hendernyh Pidhodiv* [Implementation of Gender Approaches]. Kyiv: KIC. Available at http.//www.undp.sk/genderlibrary.

Plakhotnik, O. 2007. Gender and Education: Survey of Literature. *Gendernye Issledovaniya* [Gender Studies] 15: 331–5.

Ponomariv, O. 2001a. Imennyky Zhinochogo Rodu u Nazvah za Profesiyamy [Feminine Nouns in Job Titles]. *Filosofsko-Antologichni Stufiyi: Spetsvypusk* [Philosophical Anthropological Studies: Special Edition], 183–6. Kyiv: Stylos.

– 2001b. *Kultura Movlennia* [Speech Culture]. Kyiv: Lybid.

Riabova, T. 2005. Gendernaya Ekspertiza Uchebnikov s Uchebnyh Posobii po Istorii i Literature [Gender Expertise of Textbooks and Manuals on History and Literature]. In O. Voronina, ed., *Gendernaya Ekspertiza Uchebnikov dlia Vysshei Shkoly* [Gender Expertise of University Textbooks], 123–40. Moscow: Solteks.

Semikolenov, V., E. Semikolenova, and O. Suslova. 2008. *Osnovy Dialoga* [Fundamentals of Dialogue]. Simferopol: DiAiPetri.

Semikolenova, O., ed. 2007. *My Rizni – My Rivni: Osnovy Kultury Hendernoyi Revnosti* [We Are Equal – We Are Different: Fundamentals of Gender Equality]. Kyiv: KIC.

Semikolenova, O., and A. Shilina. 2006a. Henderna Osvita v Serednii Shkoli: Deklaruvannia chy Vprovadzhennia? [Gender Education in Secondary School: Declaration or Implementation?] In O. Suslova and E. Rakhimkulov, eds., *Zakonotvorchist': Zabezpechennia Rivnyh Prav ta Mozhlyvostei Zhinok I Cholovikiv* [Lawmaking: Ensuring Equal Rights and Opportunities for Women and Men], 145–55. Kyiv: Zapovit.

– 2006b. Hendernyi Aspekt Suchasnoyi Movnoyi Polityky: Mizhnarodnyi Dosvid ta Ukrayinski Perspektyvy [Gender Aspect of Contemporary Language Policy: International Experience and Ukrainian Prospects]. *Movoznavstvo* [Linguistics] 4: 32–40.

Shmelev, A. 1997. Dve Strategii pri Vybore Roda Anaforicheskogo Referenta [Two Strategies in Choosing Anaphoric Reference]. In T. Bulygina and A. Shmelev, eds., *Yazykovaya Kontseptualizatsiya Mira: Na Materiale Russkoi Grammatiki* [Language Conceptualization of the World: On Material of Russian Grammar], 363–8. Moscow: Shkola 'Yazyki Russkoi Kultury.'

Smirnova, A. 2005. *Uchimsia Zhyt' v Obschestve: Hendernyi Analiz Shkolnyh Uchebnikov* [Learning to Live in Society: Gender Analysis of School Textbooks]. Moscow: Olita.

Suslova, O., ed. 2002. Upovnovazhuvalna osvita: Posibnyk dlia treneriv [Empowering Education: Trainers Manual]. Kyiv: Dovira. Available at http://empedu.org.ua.

Taranenko, O. 2005. Pryntsyp Androtsentryzmu v Systemi Movnyh Koordynat I Suchasnyi Hendernyi Rukh [Androcentrism Principle in the System of Language Coordinates and Contemporary Gender Movement]. *Movoznavstvo* [Linguistics] 1: 3–25.

Taylor, E. 1989. *Pervobytnaya Kultura* [Primitive Culture]. Moscow: Politizdat.

United Nations (UN). 1948. *Universal Declaration of Human Rights*. Available at http://www.un.org/en/documents/udhr/index.shtml

– 1989. *Convention of the Rights of the Child*. Available at http://www2.ohchr.org/english/law/crc.htm

Vinogradov, V. 1972. *Russkii Yazyk: Grammaticheskoye Ucheniye o Slove* [Russian Language: Grammar Study of Word]. Moscow: Vysshaya Shkola.

Voronina, O. 2003. Osnovy Gendernoi Teorii i Metodologii [Fundamentals of Gender Theory and Methodology]. In E. Faizulaeva and N. Kurganovskaya, eds., *Gendernoye Obrazovaniye* [Gender Education]. Post-conference publication, 4–5 Nov., Bukhara, Uzbekistan.

Vykhovanets, I., and K. Gorodenska. 2004. *Teoretychna Morfologiya Ukrayinskoyi Movy* [Theoretical Morphology of the Ukrainian Language]. Kyiv: 'Pulsary' University Press.

Yarskaya-Smirnova, E. 2000. Gendernoye Neravenstvo v Obrazovanii: Poniatiye Skrytogo Uchebnogo Plana [Gender Inequality in Education: The Notion of a Hidden Curriculum]. *Gendernyye Issledovaniya* [Gender Studies] 5: 295–301.

11 Educational Achievement, Social Background, and Occupational Allocations of Young Men and Women in Ukraine

SVITLANA OKSAMYTNA

The relationship between gender and inequality in educational and occupational attainment was the focus of much research interest in both Western European and some post-socialist countries throughout the second half of the twentieth century and has remained an important area of study since (see, e.g., Breen and Jonsson 2005; Erikson and Jonsson 1996; Domanski 2006; Ishida et al. 1995; Shavit and Blossfeld 1993; Shavit and Muller 2003). Yet, these issues have not been adequately addressed in Ukraine, where gender-based educational inequalities were not typically the focus of academic investigations during Soviet rule and where, today, significant gaps exist in the research with regard to how educational qualifications differently affect occupational and socioeconomic class status among men and women, and the influence of social background on educational opportunities.

This chapter begins to address these knowledge gaps by presenting findings from the Youth in Transition Survey (YIT) in Ukraine, carried out in 2007 by the Kyiv International Institute of Sociology (KIIS).[1] The survey sampled four thousand Ukrainians between the ages of 15 and 34 who had left school within the previous six years (2001 to 2006). The results highlight a number of important phenomena that can be summarized, in brief, as follows: (1) men and women in Ukraine have equal access to higher education; (2) Ukrainian women tend to achieve higher levels of education; (3) equal access to higher education has, nonetheless, failed to disrupt traditional segregation of young people by gender into particular areas of education; and (4) post-education, regardless of their chosen fields, men achieve more advanced positions and receive greater remuneration. Also, as will be shown, the YIT results strongly correlate social background with educational achievement in Ukraine – where social background is defined by the educational level of one's parents, one's place of residence, and one's social class. The latter finding holds for both men and women. Thus, based on this survey, we can conclude that social origin (and not gender) is the determining factor in access to education in Ukraine. But as the YIT data also show, gender does influence what people study and how well they do in the labour market once formal education is complete.

To fully explore these findings first requires a brief overview of the rapidly changing context in which Ukrainians undertake higher education, followed by a description of the design of the Youth in Transition Survey.

Ukrainian Education: Recent Trends

Recent decades have been characterized by intense educational expansion in many developed countries, creating greater educational opportunities for both women and men. In some European countries, female educational attainment has caught up with and even surpassed that of men. In Ukraine, female students became more numerous than male students well before independence, during the final decades of Soviet rule. However, educational expansion, in terms of an increase in the quantity of educational institutions, occurred mostly in the post-Soviet period in Ukraine. According to the State Statistics Committee of Ukraine (DKSU), since 1991, the number of higher educational institutions has been continuously increasing, as has the number of students. Colleges and universities – which in Ukraine are referred to as the 'third and fourth levels of accreditation' – increased in number from 149 in the 1990–91 academic year to 351 by the beginning of 2007–08, with an accompanying growth in the number of students, a number that increased by 2.7 times in the same period, from 881,300 to 2,372,500 (DKSU 2009). In fact, over the past two decades, the number of students at the college and university levels has tripled per 10,000 inhabitants in Ukraine: from 170 in 1990–91 to 178 in 1995–96; up again to 284 in 2000–01, then 466 in 2005–06, and finally to 512 in 2007–08 (Council for Cooperation in Education 2005). According to this measure, with regard to increasing access to higher education, Ukraine has exceeded the progress made in the majority of states formerly under Soviet rule (and now members of the Commonwealth of Independent States, or CIS), as well as that of several countries that are far more economically and politically developed.[2]

Given such massive educational expansion, it is important to evaluate to what extent this process has been characterized by gender equality or gender discrimination at different stages by examining the following factors: access to education, the structures and processes involved in the educational system, and the level of labour market outcomes of education.

Measuring Educational Attainment and Social Background

The Youth in Transition Survey measured educational attainment using an abridged version of the CASMIN educational schema (Shavit and Muller 2003) to assist with comparative mobility analysis.[3] Respondents could identify their highest level of educational attainment, as well as that of their parents, using the following four categories:

1bc *Incomplete secondary or lower* – completed elementary education; completed elementary education plus basic vocational qualification; completed secondary plus intermediate general qualification; completed secondary plus intermediate vocational qualification
 2b *Full secondary* – compulsory in Ukraine; completed full general secondary education or general secondary education plus vocational qualification[4]
 3a *Lower-level higher education* – e.g., technical college diplomas, non-university teaching certificates
 3b Full higher education

Areas of study were divided into the following nine categories from which respondents could choose: general programs; education; humanities and arts; social sciences, business, and law; sciences; engineering, manufacturing, and construction; agriculture; health and welfare; and services.

With regard to work, the YIT survey determined occupations by presenting respondents with nine options based on the International Standard Classification of Occupations (ISCO-88), a well-known tool for organizing jobs into clearly defined fields according to tasks and duties. These nine fields were: legislators, senior officials, and managers; professionals; technicians and associate professionals; clerks;

service workers and shop and market salespeople; skilled agricultural and fisheries workers; craftspeople and related workers; plant and machine operators and assemblers; and non-skilled workers.

Meanwhile, respondents could self-identify as being part of one of six social classes, a list that parallels the occupations listed above and which is based on the Erikson, Goldthorpe, and Portocarero (EGP) approach to class analysis (Shavit and Muller 2003, 17). These six classes are:

I *Upper service* – higher-grade professionals, administrators, and officials in the public sector

II *Lower service* – lower-grade professionals, higher-grade technicians, lower-grade administrators and officials, managers in small firms and services, and supervisors of white-collar workers

IIIab *Routine non-manual* employees in administration and commerce, and routine non-manual workers in services

IVabc *Small proprietors and artisans* with or without employees, and self-employed farmers

V + VI *Skilled workers*, lower-grade technicians, and supervisors of manual workers

VIIab *Semi-skilled and unskilled manual workers*, including agricultural labourers.

Results

As mentioned at the outset, the survey targeted young people aged 15 to 34 who had left school and entered the labour market within the previous six years, meaning that at the time they were surveyed their job status was 'employed.' Results for the youngest respondents (under age 20) must be considered in light of the higher likelihood that these respondents might return to their studies in the future, thereby possibly altering their level of educational attainment and social position. However, this possibility aside, the survey still shows distinct differences in levels of educational attainment between young women and young men, as seen in Table 11.1. In particular, among the women surveyed, a larger proportion (28.0%) had obtained at least a lower-level higher education compared with men (21.7%). This was also true of the highest category of educational attainment, full higher education (29.7% of women vs. 23.8% of men). More men

Table 11.1. Educational Attainment of Men and Women Aged 15–34 and Their Parents

Educational Attainment	Women and Men Aged 15–34		Their Parents	
	Women (%)	Men (%)	Mother (%)	Father (%)
Incomplete secondary or less	8.1*	10.8*	11.8	12.5
Full secondary	34.2**	43.8**	34.0**	41.5**
Lower-level higher education	28.0**	21.7**	34.2**	27.5**
Full higher education	29.7**	23.8**	19.9	18.5
N	2,091	1,734	3,935	3,478

Source: KIIS, *Youth in Transition Survey in Ukraine* (2007).
*P = .01.
**P = .001.

(43.8%) than women (34.2%) gave full secondary as their highest level of education attained. At the other end of the spectrum, we can note that quite a large number of the young people surveyed (8.1% of women and 10.8% of men) had entered the labour force without completing their secondary school education, even though completion is mandatory in Ukraine.[5] However, as mentioned earlier, we can also assume that some of these individuals will return to finish their secondary education in evening or vocational schools at a later date.

YIT participants were asked about their parents' level of educational attainment. Results, shown in the right-most columns of Table 11.1, demonstrate a relatively higher level of attainment among mothers compared with fathers. The largest proportion of respondents' mothers (34.2%) had incomplete or basic (lower-level) higher education, and almost exactly the same proportion (34.0%) had a full secondary education. Nearly 20 per cent of mothers had achieved full higher education (completed college or university), while the lowest proportion of the mothers, just 11.8 per cent, had an incomplete secondary education. With regard to the young adults' fathers, results from respondents who answered the survey questions about their parents' education showed that a similarly small proportion of fathers

Table 11.2. Mothers' and Fathers' Educational Attainment: Same or Different (Cell Values as % of the Total Sample)

Mother's Educational Attainment	Father's Educational Attainment			
	Incomplete secondary or less	Full secondary	Lower-level higher education	Full higher education
Incomplete secondary or less	**8.1**	1.8	1.0	0.5
Full secondary	1.6	**26.1**	4.0	2.1
Lower-level higher education	1.8	10.4	**17.5**	4.3
Full higher education	0.6	3.3	4.99	**12.0**

Source: KIIS, *Youth in Transition Survey* (2007).

(just 12.5%) as sons (10.8%) had failed to complete their secondary education. And, like mothers, about 20 per cent of fathers (though slightly less, at 18.5% vs. 19.9%) had gone on to complete their college or university education. But the educational attainment of the fathers contrasted distinctly from that of mothers in two ways. First, most respondents' fathers by far (41.5% vs. 34.0% of mothers) were found to have completed just their secondary education. And second, a lower number of respondents said their fathers had incomplete (lower-level) higher education (27.5% vs. 34.2% of mothers). Thus, among the parents of the young adults surveyed, mothers are more educated than fathers. As mentioned earlier, greater inclusion of women in education occurred in Ukraine during the final decades of Soviet rule. These results demonstrate the breadth and lasting impact of that change.

The majority of young respondents came from a homogeneous family educational background: 63.7 per cent (a sum of diagonal cell values) of parents had attained the same level of education (see Table 11.2). However, nearly a quarter of these young people (22.6%, the sum of cell values below the diagonal) had mothers who had attained a higher educational level than the father. It was only in the minority of cases (13.7%, a sum of cell values above the diagonal) that the father's level of education was higher than the mother's. This finding contrasts starkly with research results emerging from other settings. For example, according to Pfeffer's (2008) data from twenty developed countries, for families in which one parent has a higher level of education than the other parent, the situation is generally reversed: in 26 per cent of cases, the father's education level surpasses that of the mother, while the mother's exceeded the fathers' in just 15 per cent of cases. Ukraine thus presents a peculiar case where the mother's educational level is the same or higher than that of the father's in the majority of cases (86.3%). This is especially significant given that in many sociological studies the influence of parents' educational qualifications on children's education has only been measured based on the fathers' education, and not on that of mothers. The presented data, however, show that many mothers exceed fathers in their level of education attained and thus the impact of mothers' education on their children's educations should necessarily be considered.

Gender Differences in Areas of Study and Occupations

Findings from the Youth in Transition Survey show significant gender differences in the subject areas that young men and women choose to focus on in their studies. The survey approached this question using an index of dissimilarity, that is, an index showing what proportion of men or women would need to change their area of study in order to achieve equal gender distribution in the range of study areas.[6] As noted earlier, for the purposes of the survey, this range was divided into nine generalized categories (listed in the left-most column of Table 11.3). According to the YIT data, the index of dissimilarity for the nine categories equals 32 per cent: this means that one-third of young men or women aged 15 to 34 would have to change their area of education in order to achieve gender parity in those areas. We can also note that gender segregation would be even higher if the fields and branches of education were classified in more detail, with each of the sub-branches having a different gender profile. This has been shown to be the case in Smyth's (2002) study of a number of European countries.

Based on these results, we can divide the areas of education in Table 11.3 by the intensity of their gendering as being areas of 'female intensity' (more than 60% female), 'mixed intensity' (40% to 60% female), or 'male intensity' (below 40% female). Thus, health and welfare is far and away the most female-intensive area of study in Ukraine

Table 11.3. Distribution of Young Men and Women across Areas of Education

Area of Education	Men (%)	Women (%)	N
General programs	49	51	498
Education	28	72	306
Humanities and arts	21	79	121
Social sciences, business, and law	24	76	834
Sciences	40	60	94
Engineering, manufacturing, and construction	73	27	1,009
Agriculture	60	40	153
Health and welfare	11	89	186
Services	41	59	353

Source: KIIS, *Youth in Transition Survey in Ukraine* (2007).

(89% female), followed by three areas where women dominate in the classroom with more than 70% representation: humanities and arts (79%); social sciences, business, and law (76%); and education (72). According to these results, the most male-intensive area of study in Ukraine is engineering, manufacturing, and construction, with just 27 per cent female participation, followed by agriculture, which is at the threshold between male-intensive and mixed, at 40 per cent female participation. The same breakdown (60%–40%), though reversed, can be seen in the sciences, where the survey found that 60% of those choosing science were women.

Thus, the YIT findings support other evidence that institutions of higher education remain internally gender-segregated in Ukraine. For example, according to the State Statistics Committee of Ukraine (DKSU 2009), among young Ukrainian men it is typical to choose military sciences (99% of all university students acquiring this profession are male), transportation (80% men), national security (80%), computer sciences (74%), and engineering (74%). Young women, meanwhile, show a preference for professions in the social sciences (79% of all university students choosing this major are women), humanities (78% women), arts (77%), medicine (73%), and pedagogy (72%). Also in parallel with the Youth in Transition Survey results, according to the same Statistics Committee study, specialties such as natural sciences

Table 11.4. Distribution of Young Men and Women by Occupation

Occupational Fields	Men (%)	Women (%)	N
Legislators, senior officials, and managers	52	48	146
Professionals	29	71	667
Technicians and associate professionals	43	57	312
Clerks	18	82	188
Service workers and shop and market salespeople	29	71	687
Skilled agricultural and fisheries workers	76	24	50
Craftspeople and related workers	79	21	536
Plant and machine operators and assemblers	84	16	251
Non-skilled workers	67	33	335

Source: KIIS, *Youth in Transition Survey in Ukraine* (2007).

and agriculture are the most gender-neutral. One difference between the YIT results and those found by the Statistics Committee is that the latter study found legal studies to also be relatively gender-neutral, while Table 11.3 shows that the present survey found law to be among the more female-intensive areas of study. However, this is likely explicable by the fact that the YIT analysed only a sample of the population, not the whole population, as the Statistics Committee did. Table 11.3 reveals a gender typology by area of education, which is similar to that of other European nations, especially in Eastern Europe (Smyth 2002). More similarities with Europe emerge with regard to occupation by gender. Categorized according to the International Standard Classification of Occupations, or ISCO-88 scale (listed in the left-most column in Table 11.4), the YIT survey found that, as in other European settings, agricultural, handicraft, machine operating, and non-skilled (manual) jobs tend to be dominated by men in Ukraine, while women tend to predominate in professional, clerical, and service jobs.

Two occupational fields, senior officials and managers, and technicians and associate professionals, are gender-mixed, which reflects patterns of gender distribution in other European countries. Ukraine diverges from other settings, however, with regard to senior officials and managers, a category of occupations that is mixed in Ukraine, while more male-intensive in other European countries (Smyth 2002, 15).

Despite these numbers, we know that men's average income in Ukraine, as measured by the industry average for the country, dramatically exceeded the corresponding level for women (by 21.7%) as of 2007. Although some variation exists across sectors, men receive higher remuneration than their female counterparts, even in so-called female-intensive sectors. For instance, in the educational sphere (where 77% of those employed are women) and health care and social welfare (83% women) average earnings by men are nonetheless 15 per cent higher than women's earnings (DKSU 2008). Thus, there is a disconnect between the YIT survey findings, which show women working across occupational fields in high numbers – sometimes higher than the European average – and the financial gains they receive based on this integration.

Social Background and Class Status of Higher Education Graduates: Gender Aspects

Higher-level education is normally attained by persons between 24 and 34 years of age. By this age, the majority of young people who wish to (and can) achieve higher education will have done so. Table 11.5 narrows the survey results to this demographic of respondents in order to assess these Ukrainians' levels of educational attainment and that of their parents. What emerges most strongly here is the very large proportion of women (51.9%) and men (52.9%) in this age group who have completed the highest levels of education. If we compare this to what the respondents said about their parents' level of education, we can see that only about half as many mothers (25.2%) and fathers (23.9%) had attained such a high level. Table 11.5 also shows that respondents found themselves in the lower categories of educational attainment two to three times less often than their parents; this points to a significant increase in opportunities for higher education in Ukraine. If we look at the values for the two highest levels of education, almost 80 per cent of young people in this age range thus have either lower-level or full higher education.

To break this intergenerational change down in terms of gender, we need to assess what educational opportunities, or what level of educational mobility, is flowing down to young women versus young men from fathers and mothers depending on the parents' social status (as measured by mothers' and fathers' own educational attainment). Tables 11.6 and 11.7 present the proportions of intergenerational relationships between each of the parents and their children's educational

Table 11.5. Educational Attainment of Men and Women Aged 24–34 and Their Parents

Educational Attainment	Women and Men Aged 24–34		Their Parents	
	Women (%)	Men (%)	Mother (%)	Father (%)
Incomplete secondary or less	1.7*	3.3*	7.8	8.7
Full secondary	17.5	19.1	28.5**	35.5**
Lower-level higher education	28.9*	24.8*	38.5**	31.8**
Full higher education	51.9	52.9	25.2	23.9
N	989	645	1,776	1,616

Source: KIIS, *Youth in Transition Survey in Ukraine* (2007).
*P = .05.
**P = .001.

status. In other words, they show the level of educational mobility (or immobility) of the sons and daughters relative to their fathers and mothers.

Table 11.6 shows that the majority of children whose father had at most either an incomplete or complete secondary education display upward educational mobility (cells above the diagonal). These respondents were more or less evenly distributed among the three higher levels of educational attainment. Sons, however, ended their education at the full secondary level more often than daughters, who more often continued on to obtain a higher education. Nearly one-third of respondents whose fathers had a lower-level higher education maintained their father's achievement by completing this same level of education themselves, while many more, 52 per cent of men and 58 per cent of women, were upwardly mobile in this regard, rising to the level of full higher education. A smaller number expressed downward mobility, entering the labour market with less education than their father (cells below the diagonal). This was true twice as often for sons as it was for daughters. Finally, among the children of the top educated fathers, 70 per cent managed to reproduce this same full higher educational level. A minority finished at the level of an incomplete or lower-level higher education (more often daughters) or full secondary.

Table 11.6. Educational Mobility of Men (Upper Part of Table) and Women (Lower Part of Table) Compared with Their Fathers (% by Row)

Father's Educational Attainment	Men and Women Aged 24–34				
	Incomplete secondary or less	Full secondary	Lower-level higher education	Full higher education	N
Incomplete secondary or less	**13.5**	37.8	21.6	27.0	42
	11.6	29.8	27.3	32.2	85
Full secondary	4.3	**34.8**	29.7	31.2	202
	2.7	**30.4**	31.2	35.6	310
Lower-level higher education	2.4	18.2	**27.3**	52.2	169
	0.6	10.7	**30.5**	58.2	281
Full higher education	2.6	10.5	15.7	**71.2**	160
	1.0	8.3	20.6	**70.1**	187

Source: KIIS, *Youth in Transition Survey in Ukraine* (2007).

Table 11.7 shows a parallel comparison between survey respondents' educational achievements and that of their mothers. Immediately, we can see similar results emerge, indicating that a mother's education is as important as a father's for her children's educational mobility.

From these two tables it is evident that educational mobility processes are rather gender-blind for young people in Ukrainian society. What is more, mobility rates for women and men are approximately the same as in other developed countries (Pfeffer 2007). Overall, social background and parental education are much more influential for children's educational opportunities than is their gender. In order to determine the probability that children will obtain higher education depending on the educational levels of their mothers and fathers, I have applied an ordinal regression. What I found was that young men's and women's social background essentially determines their chances to obtain a full higher education. So, for example, the probability of children whose father and/or mother have a higher education obtaining the same educational level is approximately 80 per cent (see Table 11.8). At the same time, only about one-third of children who have a low-educated father have similar educational prospects.

Table 11.7. Educational Mobility of Men (Upper Part of Table) and Women (Lower Part of Table) Compared with Their Mothers (% by Row)

	Men and Women Aged 24–34				
Mother's Educational Attainment	Incomplete secondary or less	Full secondary	Lower-level higher education	Full higher education	N
Incomplete secondary or less	**15.4**	37.2	17.9	29.5	42
	11.2	39.7	21.6	27.6	89
Full secondary	3.9	**41.8**	24.6	29.7	171
	2.7	**34.9**	31.9	30.5	281
Lower-level higher education	3.7	23.1	**29.9**	43.2	225
	0.9	12.9	**34.9**	51.2	371
Full higher education	2.3	10.8	16.7	**70.3**	181
	1.2	5.9	16.5	**76.5**	214

Source: KIIS, *Youth in Transition Survey in Ukraine* (2007)

If we factor in place of residence, we see that geographical origins moderate the influence of social background as measured by parental educational levels, but not crucially. Thus, children from rural areas (31% of respondents in the YIT survey) have much better chances of obtaining a higher education, as long as their parents have already reached that level, compared with children from bigger towns and cities (69% of YIT survey respondents) whose parents have only a secondary education. Apparently, living in a big town or city, with their almost unlimited opportunities to access information sources, libraries, and additional education, does not on its own equalize educational opportunities. Social background remains the determining factor.

Along with education, social background can be measured by an individual's class status. The YIT survey results show that although men and women have similar distributions of educational qualifications, there are some gender differences with respect to social class. These are outlined in Table 11.9, which uses the Erikson, Goldthorpe, and Portocarero (EGP) approach to measure class using six categories of occupational fields (outlined at the beginning of this chapter). As we can see, even at the same level of education, men and women survey respondents identified themselves as belonging to different classes. Young female respondents with a full secondary education

Table 11.8. Probability of Completing a Full Higher Education Depending on a Parent's Level of Education

		Women and Men Aged 24–34	
Educational Attainment		Men	Women
Incomplete secondary or less	Mother	.31	.33
	Father	.38	.40
Full secondary	Mother	.35	.36
	Father	.39	.43
Lower-level higher education	Mother	.58	.57
	Father	.64	.62
Full higher education	Mother	.80	.80
	Father	.77	.75

Source: KIIS, *Youth in Transition Survey in Ukraine* (2007).

said they belonged to class III (routine non-manual labour) five times more often than men with the same educational level. At the same time, men more often appear to belong to classes V + VI and VIIab (qualified and non-qualified manual labour). The main trend with regard to the class of women with lower-level higher education is their concentration within class III, routine non-manual labour (at 43%) and class II, lower service, including lower-grade professionals (at 28%). Over half of men with an incomplete secondary education said they belong to classes V + VI and VIIab (manual labour). Evidently, a considerable number of young males are overeducated for the manual occupations they perform, especially semi- and non-skilled labour. Similarly, many young women are overeducated for the routine non-manual jobs they perform. Regretfully, until now there has been no rigorous investigation at the national level into this issue of correspondence between education and type of employment in Ukraine. The conclusions that I suggest here are indirect, since they are based not on the type of employment data per se, but rather on data about class belonging, which in turn, are based on the type of employment attained.

Full higher education, meanwhile, opens doors to occupations and employment statuses that belong to the highest classes in the EGP scheme, I and II, or upper and lower service classes. In general,

Table 11.9. Social Class Status by Educational Attainment and Gender (% by row)

Educational Attainment	Social Class Status of Women and Men Aged 24–34						
	I	II	III	IVabc	V + VI	VIIab	n
Men (N = 585)							
Full secondary	0.0	0.9	7.9	10.5	36.8	43.9	114
Lower-level higher education	9.3	15.9	11.9	5.3	29.8	27.8	151
Full higher education	37.2	32.2	7.8	5.9	11.6	5.3	320
Women (N = 881)							
Full secondary	1.3	5.5	41.7	2.0	29.1	20.5	151
Lower-level higher education	11.5	28.0	42.9	0.4	9.6	7.7	261
Full higher education	28.4	48.2	17.5	1.9	2.8	1.3	469

Source: KIIS, Youth in Transition Survey in Ukraine (2007).

occupations of almost 77 per cent of young women and 70 per cent of men who had attained a full higher education were within these service classes. However, there exists a noticeable gender disparity. Young men said they belong to the upper service class (I) more often relative to young women with the same level of education, who tended to say they occupy positions belonging to the lower service class (II). These positions have lower pay and worse career prospects. Women are thus receiving less remuneration and face weaker prospects in the labour market based on the same level of education. It also means that equally educated woman reach 'the glass ceiling' more quickly and more often than men.

We can therefore conclude that despite gender equality in access to education, in modern Ukraine, marked gender differences can be observed between women and men who have received the same level of education. One of the possible explanations of such an outcome may be that men and women tend to choose different areas of study, which predetermines their participation in particular occupations and labour market segments to a larger extent than does their level of education. Thus, the more conventional a woman's educational specialty is, the lower her income will be, and the poorer her career opportunities and social status. Yet this explanation, although valid, does not account for all the evidence, since men who hold accreditation in the same educational field as women tend to achieve greater career advancement as well. Therefore, the stable differences in socioeconomic achievement between men and women in Ukraine cannot be fully explained either by their levels of education or their educational field of choice. Culturally embedded gender stereotypes associated with different positions within the labour market also play a role. Reproduction of occupational gender segregation is also determined by the lack of efficient state gender policies, including educational policies, equal opportunities policies, anti-discrimination policies, and policy to enable a balance between family and work life, including provisions for part-time work and publicly funded child care.

Conclusions

Equal educational opportunities, regardless of an individual's social background or gender, are tightly connected with the ideas of social justice and social equality in developed democratic countries. They are generally regarded to be an inherent part of social integration, stability, and ongoing societal development. This chapter utilized recent data from a large survey, Youth in Transition, to assess gender equality at multiple levels of the Ukrainian educational system, with particular attention paid to access to higher education, structural characteristics of the educational process itself, and the relationship between educational attainment, class, and occupational advancement. As we have seen, the data highlight significant gender differences in these areas, as well as a number of negative tendencies in educational opportunities and accessibility in contemporary Ukrainian society.

As noted in brief at the outset, four trends were clear. First, gender is not a significant determinant of access to educational opportunities for Ukrainians. All levels of education are equally accessible for both men and women. What is more, in the cohort under investigation, women actually surpassed men in terms of attaining higher education. Second, social origin, as defined by one's parents' education and place of residence, does directly impact educational opportunities. This inequality holds across genders. With regard to the impact of parents' education, in particular, a mother's educational qualifications influence her child's opportunities for educational advancement as much as a father's do. Third, despite equal access to education by gender, the educational system remains unequal. Gender differences are easily observable in the choice of area of study, a reality reflected in other European countries, and especially Eastern Europe. In Ukraine, engineering, manufacturing, and construction courses are male-dominated, while education, humanities and the arts, social sciences, business, and law, and health and welfare courses are female-dominated. Finally, compared with women, men in this cohort held higher professional and managerial positions across all sectors and areas of employment regardless of their chosen field of education or their level of education. Thus, gender inequalities in socioeconomic class remain and will continue unless the state intervenes to redress them.

Returning to the observation made at the beginning of this chapter that higher education in Ukraine has expanded at a rapid rate, we can conclude that this expansion has not been accompanied by equalization of opportunities, including the chance to obtain higher education regardless of social background, or the possibility of enjoying the results of such education regardless of gender. One's chances of attaining higher education are much better for young women and men whose fathers and mothers have already reached those levels. The data show this to be true even for secondary education, which has been compulsory for the late Soviet and post-Soviet cohorts. Gender, meanwhile, remains an important factor in what young Ukrainians choose to study, what kinds of jobs they get afterwards, what they can expect to earn from those jobs, and how far up the ladder they can expect to climb before hitting a glass ceiling.

NOTES

1 Kyiv International Institute of Sociology is a private, for-profit research institution. Further information is available at http://www.kiis.com.ua/.
2 According to the CIS data, between 2000 and 2002, the corresponding number for Germany was 262; Japan, 313; Italy, 314; Austria, 327; Canada, 394; Sweden, 404; Norway, 423; Poland, 466; United States, 494; and Finland, 540 (Council for Cooperation in Education 2005).
3 To keep the results statistically significant I have combined the original 1a, 1b, and 1c categories of the schema into a single 1abc category. Similarly, I have united the 2a and 2b categories into a single 2ab.
4 Unlike in many other countries, both developed and developing, where only nine years of education are compulsory.

5 This can be explained by the fact that not all village schools provide full secondary education, and those students who do not want to or have no possibility to go to school in a different location often quit their education altogether. This situation is also perpetuated by the fact that there is no monitoring of this issue by the state, and there are no official sanctions for persons who decide not to get full secondary education.
6 The index of dissimilarity is calculated by summing up the absolute differences in the proportion of females and males in each educational area and dividing the total by two.

REFERENCES

Breen, R., and J. Jonsson. 2005. Inequality of Opportunity in Comparative Perspective: Recent Research on Educational Attainment and Social Mobility. *Annual Review of Sociology* 31: 233–43.

Council for Cooperation in Education. 2005. *Vysshieie proffesionalnoie obrazovanije (2004/2005 uchebnyi god)* [Higher Professional Education (2004/2005 School Year)]. Soviet po sotrudnichestvu v oblasti obrazovanija gosudarstv-uchastnikov SNG [Council on Educational Cooperation of CIS Countries]. Available at http://www.cis.unibel.by/index.php?module=subjectsandfun c=viewpageandpageid=157 (accessed 1 March 2009).

Derzhavnyj komitet statystyky Ukrainy/State Statistics Committee of Ukraine (DKSU). 2008. Dity, Zhinky ta Simya v Ukraini [Children, Women and Family in Ukraine]. *Statystychnyj zbirnyk* [Statistical Bulletin]. Kyiv: DKSU.

– 2009. *Osnovni pokaznyky dijalnosti vyshchykh navchalnykh zakladiv Ukrainy na pochatok 2008/09 navchalnogo rokuy: Statystychnyj biuleten* [Basic Indicators of Institutions of Higher Education in Ukraine by the Beginning of the 2008/09 School Year: Statistical Bulletin]. Kyiv: DKSU.

Domanski, H. 2006. Barriers of the Selection to Secondary and University-Level Education. *Polish Sociological Review* 4: 471–87.

Erikson, R, and J. Jonsson, eds. 1996. *Can Education Be Equalized? The Swedish Case in Comparative Perspective.* Boulder: Westview.

Ishida, H., W. Muller, and J. Rider. 1995. Class Origin, Class Destination, and Education: A Cross-National Study of Ten Industrial Nations. *American Journal of Sociology* 101(1): 145–93.

Konstantinivskij, D., V. Vakhshtain, D. Kurakin, and J. Roshchnina. 2006. Dostupnost kachestvennogo obshchego obrazovanija v Rossij:

Vozmozhnosti i ogranichenija [Availability of Qualitative General Education in Russia: Opportunities and Restrictions]. *Voprosy obrazovanija* [Educational Issues] 2: 186–201.

Pfeffer, F. 2007. *Intergenerational Educational Mobility in Comparative Perspective.* CDE Working Paper No. 2007–09. Madison: Center for Demography and Ecology.

– 2008. Persistent Inequality in Educational Attainment and Its Institutional Context. *European Sociological Review* 24(5): 543–65.

Shavit, Y., and H.P. Blossfeld, eds. 1993. *Persistent Inequality: Changing Educational Attainment in Thirteen Countries.* Boulder: Westview.

Shavit, Y., and W. Muller, eds. 2003. *From School to Work: A Comparative Study of Educational Qualifications and Occupational Destinations.* Oxford: Oxford University Press.

Smyth, E. 2002. *Gender Differentiation and Early Labour Market Integration across Europe.* Mannheim Centre for European Social Research (MZES) Working Paper no. 46. Available at http://www.mzes.uni.mannheim.de/publications/wp/wp-46.pdf (accessed 10 March 2009).

PART IV

Emerging Issues

12 Gender and Health in Ukraine

OLENA HANKIVSKY

The collapse of the Soviet Union has had enormous implications for health in Ukraine (Cockerham et al. 2006; Gilmore et al. 2002; McKee 2005). As with all former Soviet states, slow socioeconomic progress coupled with deteriorating social security and health care systems have contributed to high morbidity, lower life expectancy, and growing health inequities within the population. According to the World Bank (2009a), 'Ukrainians are not only dying younger but also have fewer years lived in full health relative to their European counterparts' (p. 11), resulting in what has been referred to as a national health crisis. All citizens, but especially those who are most vulnerable (e.g., people with disabilities, rural residents, refugees, and ethnic minorities), who had grown to depend on the state for their health care, now often lack the knowledge, experience, and capacity to promote their own good health (Gander and Magdyuk 2006). Moreover, the current state of the health care system and ineffective policies and programs have contributed to specific gendered health implications, especially among Ukrainian men, whose life expectancy is among the worst in the world. As has been highlighted elsewhere, 'There is a need for raising public awareness of important health issues, one of the most serious being the health situation for men' (SIDA 2003, 71).

In this chapter, I provide a brief overview of the current situation in Ukraine, outline selected leading health issues and challenges, and critically examine the responses of the Ukrainian government, international organizations, and health researchers to understand how to best address the health crisis. I will argue that proposed reforms to date are inadequate as they focus primarily on the health care system and modification of high-risk and health-compromising behaviours, without linking these to the social context of people's lives, and in particular, the social determinants of health (SDH) – an internationally recognized framework for working towards better health and health equity. I argue that for transformative change to occur in Ukraine, policy solutions need to be framed within a comprehensive SDH framework that allows for a better understanding of how gender and other important factors affect the way people live, their consequent chance of illness, and their risk of premature death (WHO 2008). At the same time, the presentation of such an overview is also intended to point to specific areas, which are pressing population health issues that require not only changes at the level of policy but also the development of strategic programs of research to produce the necessary knowledge base and evidence to fully inform policy reform in the Ukrainian health sector.

Background

Ukraine is considered to be in a demographic crisis because of its high death rate relative to its low birth rate. In 2007, the country's population was declining at the fourth fastest rate in the world (CIA 2008), *a rate that is currently the highest in Europe* (World Bank 2009a; emphasis added). While the overall health status of the general population was fairly good before the breakdown of the Soviet Union in 1991, Ukrainians now spend almost 13 per cent of their lives in poor health, compared with Poles (8%) or Slovenians and Czechs (9%) (pp. 7–8). The average life expectancy is now 62.3 years for men and 73.6 years for women, a decline in life expectancy of approximately 4.5 years for men and 2.2 years for women (Skoryk 2007).

The statistics show that the burden of transformation has been gendered, with men being disproportionately affected (Skoryk 2007; World Bank 2009a; SIDA 2003). The life expectancy gap of almost 12 years is a significant gender issue and, when compared with males and females in the European Union (EU), the life expectancy in Ukraine is 14 and 8.2 years lower respectively (World Bank 2009a). Within the territory of the former Soviet Union, the situation is worse only in Russia and Kazakhstan. The highest at-risk cohort is workers who are between 40 and 60 years of age. To illustrate: Ukrainian men age 40 years and older have a 31 per cent risk of dying before their 60th birthday (Word Press 2008). Men's mortality in Ukraine is comparable to countries with a five times lower gross domestic product

(GDP) per capita than in Ukraine (World Bank 2009a). In turn, this results in significant human and economic costs for individuals, their families, and the nation as a whole.

The outlook for Eastern Europe including Ukraine remains bleak, especially for men. For example, data from the *Global Burden of Disease Report* indicate that either no change or indeed a further decrease in life expectancy at birth among men of the 'former socialistic economies' of Europe is expected for 2020 (cited in Weidner and Cain 2003, 768). At the same time, according to the 2009 World Bank report *An Avoidable Tragedy: Combating Ukraine's Health Crisis* (2009a), if diseases were cured in their early stages, then 80 per cent of deaths could have been prevented among working-age men and 30 per cent among working-age women. In fact, the World Bank estimates that about 50 per cent of deaths under the age of 75 in Ukraine could be prevented with adequate prevention and treatment (p. 9).

Major Health Issues: Selected Examples

Health challenges in Ukraine include a number of health-compromising behaviours, as well as a number of non-communicable and chronic diseases. It has been determined that 94 per cent of deaths are caused by three risk factors: (1) smoking, (2) alcohol, and (3) violation of safety requirements (World Bank 2009a). The prevalence of smoking is very high among the Ukrainian population; more than 62 per cent of the population above the age of 15 are regular smokers (p. 9), and smoking is a growing problem among disadvantaged socioeconomic groups, among youth and younger women, and among those who live in Eastern Ukraine (World Bank 2009a; Ukrainian Ministry of Health [MoH] 2009). In terms of smoking, Ukraine, and in particular its Southeastern region, has the highest rates of tobacco use in all the former Soviet republics (Poznyak et al. 2002). Interestingly, medical workers smoke only slightly less than the general public does (MoH 2009). Government interventions have included a state program (2008–12) on decreasing tobacco use, educational courses in Grades 1 to 9, and awareness campaigns, all of which have had little impact on the overall rates of smoking (MoH 2009).

Moreover, the Ukraine – World Mental Health Survey found that one out of every three men and one out of every twelve women consume alcohol heavily (Webb et al. 2005). Similarly, Bromet et al. (2005) noted that 26.5 per cent of the male population of Ukraine reported an alcohol disorder in their lifetime. Alcohol has been found to cause 12.3 per cent of all disability adjusted life years (DALYs), which represent the sum of years of potential life lost due to premature mortality and the years of productive life lost due to disability, in Ukraine (World Bank 2009a, 9) and 13.6 per cent of deaths (p. 30). Even though national action plans for tobacco control and reduction of alcohol consumption exist, there has been little in the way of effective implementation (p. 30).

Furthermore, as the World Bank (2009a) has reported, non-communicable diseases and chronic conditions, often linked to high-risk behaviours, including excessive drinking and tobacco use, are responsible for the bulk of mortality in Ukraine. For example, it has also been reported that the majority of poisoning and trauma cases, including workplace and car accidents, result from alcohol abuse (SIDA 2003). Additionally, there has been a sharp rise in cardiovascular disease (CVD) and other diseases directly related to alcohol and tobacco consumption (Gander and Magdyuk 2006).

At present, the primary cause of health decline in Eastern Europe appears to be a dramatic increase in heart disease (primarily coronary heart disease), which has assumed epidemic proportions (Weidner and Cain 2003, 768). In Ukraine, ischemic heart disease was responsible for nearly 40 per cent of all deaths in 2005 (World Bank 2009a, 21).

It should also be noted, however, that communicable diseases, most notably HIV/AIDS and tuberculosis (TB) have reached epidemic proportions and are a growing threat to the health of the Ukrainian nation. Ukraine is presently at the epicentre of HIV infection in Europe, with an estimated prevalence of nearly 500,000, or 1.5 per cent, of the adult population (MoH et al. 2006). Although the government has implemented national program on the prevention and cure of HIV infection (for 2009–13), the virus continues to spread within the general population, and this has resulted in a substantial increase in HIV infection among women and children born to infected women. More than one-third (36%) of people who live with HIV infection are women of reproductive age (Skoryk 2007). In response, the government of Ukraine has developed what can be considered as generally sound legislation and policies; however, these are not always effectively implemented or adequately resourced. Moreover, the lack of awareness and correct information about the disease, as well as continuing stigma and discrimination against those who are diagnosed with HIV/AIDS, have impeded prevention and intervention efforts (Hankivsky 2009). The scale of epidemics continued to grow between 2004 and 2007, increasing by 10 per cent to 15 per cent annually (Skoryk 2007).

In terms of tuberculosis, despite the fact that this problem is a state priority under the control of the president of Ukraine, the spread of tuberculosis and mortality caused by it are at the epidemic level. The levels of the spread of TB and mortality due to it are eight to ten times higher than in most EU countries.[1] Several factors influence the difficulty in containing tuberculosis. According to Vassall et al. (2009), reduction in service funding, reduced economic status of the population, and the concurrent spread of HIV/AIDS have all led to increases in cases of TB (see also Drobniewski et al. 2005). Tuberculosis epidemics are much influenced by the epidemiology of HIV/AIDS in Ukraine. More than 30 per cent of those with HIV/AIDS have tuberculosis, and about 50 per cent of them die from it. Reported prevalence rates have more than doubled since the collapse of the Soviet Union, from 32 per 100,000 in 1990 to 80.9 per 100,000 in 2004 (Vassall et al. 2009). Similar to the situation with HIV/AIDS, tuberculosis has not been curtailed, largely because of the lack of effective and preventive health care measures (Betliy et al. 2007).

Responses and Current Challenges

Much of the demographic decline in Ukraine is fuelled by an ineffective health care system and the rise of unhealthy lifestyles (World Bank 2009a). In evaluating the current situation in Ukraine, Rekha Menon, senior economist at the World Bank, has recently concluded that 'compared with cities in other European countries, Ukrainians lead less healthy lives and receive poorer support from health services' and that 'premature mortality among adult Ukrainian males could be avoided through behaviour changes but public awareness of health risks is low. The solution to this challenge is complex, and involves a combination of focus on primary health care and prevention and broader system wide changes in how health services are delivered and financed' (p. 1).

To date, there have been numerous initiatives aimed at improving the health of the Ukrainian population, including reform of the health care system. In the past twenty years, the health care system has shifted from a reasonably effective curative system aimed at serving the entire population to a system that is broken, where little investment is made into primary health care services, and where even less investment in terms of health policies and promotion prevents the system from responding to contemporary health demands. In essence, it has changed very little in recent years (Betliy et al. 2007; Semigina and Kishkina 2006; De Bell and Carter 2005; Lekhan et al. 2004), and it is unable to respond to the current and changing health needs of the population.

In 2006, government spending on health care as a proportion of GDP was 7 per cent (WHO 2009). However, most spending (86%) is allocated to hospitals and specialized facilities. Nevertheless, those who work in the system complain of inadequate funding, especially in terms of buying new equipment and medical supplies, poor sanitary conditions, difficulties in recruiting and retaining health professions, and the low salaries offered to health care workers (Gatehouse 2009; Abbott and Wallace 2007; Betliy et al. 2007). A major obstacle to health care reform in Ukraine is the lack of a skilled workforce in health care management and public health. This is not surprising given that there is currently only one school of public health in the National University of Kyiv-Mohyla Academy and twenty-two medical schools in the country.

For citizens, the health care system – intended to be state funded under the Constitution of Ukraine – now imposes private payment for all treatment and services. The cost of services is prohibitive for most Ukrainian citizens, especially those in lower income groups (Gatehouse 2009; World Bank 2009a; Abbott and Wallace 2007; Betliy et al. 2007). In 2005, around 13 per cent of households reported that they were unable to access necessary health care services; 77 per cent claimed this was due to the costs of consulting a doctor, and 95 percent reported being unable to purchase the necessary medical devices (Betliy et al. 2007). According to the World Bank, 'Ukraine's health system is complex, inefficient, highly inequitable and of low quality' (2009a, 9). The situation is only worsening in the current global financial crisis and political turmoil because of the drop in value of the Ukrainian currency and significantly reduced budgets for health care spending, especially in terms of buying power for medicines by the state.

Beyond the formal system itself, and in addition to the plans and programs targeting tobacco and alcohol use, HIV/AIDS, and tuberculosis mentioned above, Ukraine has attempted a number of other initiatives at the national level. As early as 1992, Ukraine established Principles of Legislation on Health Care, which were aimed at regulating all aspects of the development and implementation of health policy in Ukraine, as a way of meeting international standards and human rights obligations. According to this legislation, the Ministry of Health is responsible for the following: (1) setting standards for health care provisions; (2) defining rules for accreditation of public and private health care establishments; (3) licensing health care professionals and pharmaceutical producers and distributors; and (4) determining the list of pharmaceuticals that can be purchased by public health care establishments. Commenting on the implementation of the Principles of Legislation on Health Care, Betliy et al. (2007) have observed that 'not all its provisions are fulfilled in real life' (p. 10).

In 2000, the president of Ukraine approved the Concept of Health Care Development in Ukraine, which recognizes the need to take into account population health care needs and setting standards in the health care sector. In 2002, the first national health strategy, 'Health of the Nation 2002–2011,' was adopted, in accordance with European World Health Organization (WHO) standards and policy; however, no financial resources were allocated for this program, leaving its implementation to local governments (SIDA 2003). In December 2005, a Presidential Decree on Urgent Measures Regarding Health Care System Reform was introduced. As part of the current President's Economic Reform Plan (2010) Ukraine has embarked on the most ambitions health reform plan since independence (Tarantino el al. 2011). Its goals are to optimize the network of health care institutions, reform health financing, and strengthen the system of standards and quality control at the central level. Significantly in its current conception – Health of the Nation: Ukraninian Dimension Program 2012–2020 – the government is beginning to acknowledge the significance of social determinants of health. While this recent initiative is promising, its development will have to be carefully monitored and evaluated. As the World Bank director for Ukraine has recently cautioned, 'Ukraine has made repeated attempts to launch health sector reforms, but their implementation has been slow and fragmented' (World Bank 2009b, 1).

Importance of a Wider Perspective: The Social Determinants of Health

Although having an effective health care system is important, the health outcomes of a population are not completely dependent on the state of such a system alone. As in all other jurisdictions, they are influenced by the 'circumstances in which people grow, live, work, and age, and the systems put in place to deal with illness,' and 'the conditions in which people live and die are, in turn, shaped by political, social, and economic forces' (WHO 2008, iii). Thus, a population health approach takes into account the complex interactions among factors that contribute to health. While lists of social determinants of health vary by jurisdiction, they typically include factors such as income and social status, social supports, education, economic and social environments, personal health practices and coping skills, early life experiences, genetics, health services, gender, and culture. And in post-Soviet countries, including Ukraine, the social determinants of health are of particular importance given the rapid and fundamental changes to the fabric of Ukrainian society and of its economy.

The changes brought about as a result of the collapse of communism are evidenced in growing poverty, social and economic inequities, and rising unemployment, crime, and violence. In their study on health and well-being in post-Soviet Ukraine, Abbott and Wallace (2007) identified cultural trauma to be a consequence of transition, leading to a breakdown of social trust and agency and contributing to insecurity and uncertainty in daily life. To illustrate, they report:

> They [Ukrainians] talk repeatedly about the daily struggle for survival – poverty; poor health; unemployment; a decline in trust; a decline in close relationships with neighbours; an increase in selfishness; politicians who do not care about them; not being able to afford a good diet, clothes, or education for their children or to pay the charges for medical treatment; an increase in consumption of alcohol and in cigarette smoking, including drinking and smoking by women and young people; and an increase in the use of hard drugs by the young. The present is compared unfavourably with the past. Young people are especially concerned about the lack of employment opportunities and often report poor health. They also complain about the environment, the poor water supply, the lack of street cleaning in the towns, pollution from cars and the impact of nuclear accidents. (p. 186)

A major outcome of such changes, especially in terms of the new political order, is that citizens feel unable to improve their lives and, in turn, their health (p. 183). As one male respondent explained: 'The transition to democracy brings about the problem of the loss of paternalism.

That is, we used to know that the state would provide a flat, work and so on and now the state's guardianship has vanished. Now we are on our own. We must rely on ourselves – but we can't and we become depressed' (p. 188). Abbott and Wallace conclude that residents of Ukraine perceive their living conditions and health as very poor and that 'there is a strong interaction between the poor quality of life after the economic and political collapse and the views of individual citizens about their ability to take responsibility for their health' (p. 181). These findings are supported by an earlier study, which noted that 43 per cent of women and 25 per cent of men reported their health as poor or very poor (Gilmore et al. 2002). The low material situation and control over life as a result of the changing political and economic circumstances were found to be key contributing factors (ibid.).

Although these developments signal the need for a broader conceptualization of health in the Ukrainian context, one that is consistent with a population health perspective that prioritizes the social determinants of health, Semigina and Kishkina (2006) have observed that 'this is a challenging matter for Ukrainian health policy since it was and still is predominantly medically (treatment) oriented and devoted to the advancement of medical care services' (p. 28). Moreover, these tendencies are replicated in a number of evaluations of the health care crisis, which focus on how to correct deficiencies and improve the efficacy of the health care sector (Betliy et al. 2007; Semigina and Kishkina 2006; Haidayev 2007). As argued in a recent study by the World Health Organization (2008), 'Traditionally, society has looked to the health care sector to deal with its concerns about health and disease. Certainly, maldistribution of health care – not delivering care to those who most need it – is one of the social determinants of health. But the high burden of illness responsible for appalling premature loss of life arises in large part because of the conditions in which people are born, grow, live, work, and age. In their turn, poor and unequal living conditions are the consequence of poor social policies and programmes, unfair economic arrangements, and bad politics' (p. 1).

A number of scholars have called for more attention to 'healthy lifestyles' among the population (Kryszyna et al. 2009; Haidayev 2007), as well as for more research on preventive care (Semigina and Kishkina 2006). The World Bank (2009a) has similarly asserted that 'many of the causes of premature-death and disease in Ukraine are linked to risk-factors which are largely modifiable and preventable' (p. 9). In turn, it has recommended the implementation of 'a comprehensive disease management model' (p. 10), although acknowledging that transformative changes cannot be achieved through the health care system alone but require intersectoral initiatives to modify the environment, behaviour, and health services (p. 38).

This acknowledgment does point to the fact that, while many Ukrainians want to accept personal responsibility for their health, including leading healthier lives, 'they do not see how to exercise this responsibility in their present economic circumstances' (Abbott and Wallace 2007, 201). A medical expert interviewed in Abbott and Wallace's 2007 study observed that 'the main thing [to improve health] must be to improve the standard of living – it must be sufficient to satisfy the main needs of people. Then we could start talking about improving the state of health' (p. 201). And in 2003, in the Swedish International Development Cooperation Agency (SIDA) report on gender issues in Ukraine, the authors observed the interconnected nature of health and the economy by arguing that 'if health does not improve, the risk is that the economy will continue to be an obstacle. If the economy does not recover, neither will the health of the population' (SIDA 2003, 76). Not surprisingly, then, economic reform is often prioritized as a precursor for improving the health of Ukrainians (Haidayev 2007).

Although a strong relationship exists between the state of the economy and health, it is not the only factor that influences and shapes population health outcomes. Arguably, 'economic growth is without question important, particularly for poor countries, as it gives the opportunity to provide resources to invest in the improvement of the lives of their population. But growth itself, without appropriate social policies . . . brings little benefit to health equity' (WHO 2008, 1). In addition, health strategies, which prioritize health care system reforms, lifestyle risk factors, and disease management, are important, especially given the state of the health care system in Ukraine and the epidemic in communicable diseases such as HIV/AIDS. However, they may tend to marginalize the processes by which structural factors at both micro and macro levels shape health outcomes. Any prescriptive change is, however, inextricably part of complex social relations of gender, socioeconomic status, ability, ethnicity, and sexuality. Thus, a myriad of factors outside the health care system, and *in addition to* the state of the economy must be recognized as impacting on health, including morbidity and mortality.

Not surprisingly, Weidner and Cain (2003) have argued that 'the experience of Eastern Europe should serve as an important example of how societal-level change can influence the health of a population' (p. 770). And of particular importance are the differential impacts that these changes have had. Weidner and Cain further elaborate by pointing out that 'the speed with which mortality rates changed, especially for middle-aged men, clearly point away from a biological or genetic explanation for the changes that occurred. Rather an explanation may be found by looking at the social context of people's lives during a period of great social unrest and examining their responses to it' (p. 770).

As such, there is a pressing need for Ukraine to approach its health crisis using a comprehensive social determinants of health framework. Others have made similar observations. According to McKee (2005), 'The collapse of the Soviet Union was a massive natural experiment that has provided many insights that help our understanding of the determinants of population health' (p. 374). Moreover, Gilmore et al. (2002) have argued that 'knowledge of the determinants of health is needed to underpin our understanding of the potential causes of the decline of life expectancy and to develop appropriate health and social policy responses within Ukraine' (p. 2179). And Betliy et al. (2007) have asserted that 'policies should also aim at promoting the health of the population' (p. 42). In these calls, less attention, however, is paid to gender as a key explanatory determinant or to how the order and power relations it creates in conjunction with other factors such as those associated with socioeconomic status, geography, ethnicity, age, and sexual orientation, translate into damaging health consequences.

Gender, Men's Health, and Women's Health

In other jurisdictions, such as Canada, which is internationally recognized for its pioneering work in the area of social determinants of health, the inclusion of gender as a key health determinant was considered a crucial development in questioning previously unquestioned norms and structures that influence gendered experiences of health and which affect vulnerabilities to illness, health status, access to preventive and curative measures, burdens of ill health, and quality of care (Hankivsky and Christofferson 2008). Gender can be understood to be 'the array of socially constructed roles and relationships, personality traits, attitudes, behaviours, values, relative power, and influence that society ascribes to two sexes based on a differential basis. Gender is relational, that is, gender roles and characteristics do not exist in isolation, but are defined in relation to one another'

(Health Canada 2000, 14). Moreover, gender is also understood to be a primary signifier of power (Scott 1986).

Accordingly, then, in the realm of health, gender should not be equated with women's health as is often the case in health research and policy literatures (Bates et al. 2009; Hankivsky 2007). In the context of men's lives, for example, gender, and the resultant social norms and cultural expectations of masculinity, affect men's emotional and psychological health, and often cause risky and unhealthy behaviours that, in turn, lead to reduced longevity (Sen and Östlin 2007, 1). Societal ideals of masculinity, specifically, 'hegemonic masculinity,' have detrimental health effects. As Courtenay (2000) states, 'In exhibiting or enacting hegemonic ideals with health behaviours, men reinforce strongly held cultural beliefs that men are more powerful and less vulnerable than women; that men's bodies are structurally more efficient than and superior to women's bodies; that asking for help and caring for one's health are those for whom health and safety are irrelevant' (p. 1398).

In most countries, men have a lower life expectancy and higher morbidity in relation to some diseases (Lohan 2007; Tsuchiya and Williams 2005). However, the situation is more pronounced in Ukraine, with the gap between female and male life expectancies growing (World Bank 2009a), and yet the ways in which gender affects men's health are still in nascent stages of investigation, recognition, and systematic policy response.

In terms of the Ukrainian context, evidence on gender differences in health is still emerging. What is now widely acknowledged is the significant gap in life expectancy. However, there are varied other effects in relation to health, including the experiences of illnesses and diseases. For example, there are a number of diseases that prevail among the male population. These include myocardial (cardiac) infarction and strokes, blood circulation system illnesses, and infectious diseases (Skoryk 2007, 135). The risk of getting AIDS correlates with gender and age: youth, especially young men, are the primary risk group (p. 135).

Gender extends to also influence the way in which the population responds to its environment. Perhaps the most significant impact of the transition period in Ukraine has been the changing labour participation among males. Rising unemployment rates have undermined men's traditional role as breadwinner (Gander and Magdyuk 2006), resulting in a loss of identity, and leading to stress and other high-risk and health-compromising behaviours consistent with the stereotypical conceptions of masculinity (Weidner and Cain 2004), including tobacco use and increased alcohol consumption. For example, Ukraine belongs to the countries with the highest level of smokers among men (Skoryk 2007), and alcohol use has also been shown to contribute to higher rates of mental and behavioural disorders, among others, in men (SIDA 2003).

A number of studies include qualitative data. Abbott and Wallace (2007) cite the following from a male respondent who links the use of alcohol and tobacco to the management of stress: 'You have a drink and the headache is gone. So it is a kind of medicine and not harmful for a middle aged person. I can drink alcohol – if something is wrong I go drinking' (p. 197) and, 'Of course everyone is going to say that people smoke, drink and take drugs, but again you have to mention the problem of stress. It is tough for us. People get very depressed' (p. 198). Significantly, more socially disadvantaged males are at particular risk for smoking, especially those with lower education, poorer economic situations, and less social support (Pomerleau et al. 2004, 1583).

According to Abbott and Wallace (2007), 'Men's actions – their heavy and binge drinking and excessive smoking – can be seen as a way of reasserting some measure of control and choice over their lives and life-styles: a way of coping with stress, and one that is culturally available and "scripted" for men but not for women' (p. 184). Cockerham et al. (2006) have similarly noted that 'in post Soviet societies it is appropriate masculine – but not feminine – behaviour to drink alcohol' (p. 2392). Not surprisingly, heavy drinking as a response to stress is also linked to cultural male norms and male socializing (p. 2392).

Moreover, in Ukraine, as in other jurisdictions, strong stereotypes among the population prevent men from disclosing or seeking help for their physical and mental health issues (Springer and Mouzon 2011; O'Brien et al. 2005; Weidner and Cain 2003). Consequently, when faced with the onset of disease, such as cardiovascular disease, this has dire consequences by delaying diagnosis and treatment. It also means that, as Weidner and Cain (2003) explain, 'interventions solely aimed at reducing traditional coronary risk factors are unlikely to have a dramatic impact on the cardiovascular disease epidemic in Eastern Europe. Rather, behavioral interventions designed to increase social support, decrease depression, and improve lifestyle behaviors and coping skills appear to be more promising venues for prevention. Considering that these psychosocial factors are differentially linked to notions of masculinity and femininity, the design of gender-specific interventions may be required to yield effective outcomes' (p. 770).

Finally, it is also worth noting the gendered nature of suicidality in Ukraine; for example, the rate of increase in the number of suicides is greater in the male population than in the female. Geography also seems to play a role. At a 2006 parliamentary hearing, it was reported that in Crimea more men died from suicide than from heart attacks (Skoryk 2007, 132).

While there is a need to pay special attention to men's health in the context of Ukraine, women's health also needs to be addressed. This is because women's higher average length of life compared with men's is not necessarily an indicator of their better health. According to data in annual reports about the Ukrainian population's health and activities of medical and preventive institutions of the national health care system, women's morbidity in a large number of disease classes is significantly higher than men's (UNFPA 2009). Abbott and Wallace (2007) note that women report higher levels of psycho-social stress, poorer physical health, and higher incidence of long-term illness, and they submit that 'while men die, women survive, to struggle on with a poor quality of life and poor health' (p. 184). Women who do survive to old age typically experience poverty and other hardships because the support systems that existed during the Soviet era simply do not exist now (SIDA 2003). Many elderly women in Ukraine have little food or economic and health security. One of the female respondents in the study by Cockerham et al. (2006) explain, 'If you experience economic hardship, no matter how hard you try to be healthy, there is nothing you can do about your diet' (p. 2392).

In terms of women's health more generally, there are a number of key issues. Rates of maternal and infant mortality are among the highest in Eastern Europe (Betliy et al. 2007; Gander and Magdyuk 2006). According to the Institute of Pediatrics, Obstetrics, and Gynecology, 40 per cent of Ukrainian women cannot carry through a normal pregnancy, and every sixth woman is infertile.[2] In recent years, women also have been suffering from a greater variety of illnesses than men and experiencing certain illnesses at different rates than men; for example, women suffer from urogenital system illnesses at a rate that is 4.2 times higher than for men. Women get tumours 1.7 times more often, and they have endocrine pathology 1.8 times more often than men. The female population seeks medical attention for blood diseases and hemogenic organ diseases 32 per cent more often; among working-aged women, the incidence of anemia is noticeably greater compared with men. Twenty per cent more women than men come for medical help with blood circulation problems. And, women are also very vulnerable to varicosity disease, migraine headaches, vegetovascular dystonia (autonomic neuropathy), pneumonia, bronchial asthma, and diabetes (Skoryk 2007). In recent years, the incidence of breast cancer has doubled in the population (Maistruk and Bannikov 2009). This is coupled with the fact that many women, especially those living in rural areas, do not receive early diagnosis which is key to effective treatment and survival.

The prevalence of smoking among women is continuing to increase, especially among women living in urbanized areas who are exposed to tobacco advertising campaigns (Pomerleau et al. 2004, 1583). HIV/ AIDS is rapidly spreading to the female population (Hankivsky 2009; SIDA 2003). And, of particular importance in the Ukrainian context, is violence against women in its many forms. According to SIDA (2003), 'how bad the real picture of gender violence is in Ukraine is still unknown' (p. 7). However, the increase in poverty and unemployment since independence and the breakdown of family structures and relationships has increased women's vulnerability to violence and trafficking (Hankivsky 2008; Gander and Magdyuk 2006).

In sum, however, the main gender health differences in Ukraine which are reported are higher mortality among working-aged men, and as a result there is a disproportionate number of surviving elderly women than men in the country; men tend to suffer from fewer illnesses, but they are vulnerable to diseases leading to more deaths. This is just the tip of the iceberg, and government responses to date demonstrate the limited extent to which issues of gender in relation to other social factors and processes are recognized and addressed.

In 2003, in its publication *Gender Issues in Ukraine*, SIDA reported that, in terms of government actions: 'Attention is dedicated to the health problems of women and children, such as implementation of screening programmes for early detection of various gynaecological conditions, pregnancy complications and an upgrading of obstetrical services. Men's health problems are addressed indirectly in the elements dealing with improving mental health, preventing suicides, organizing anti-alcohol campaigns and introducing healthy lifestyle (spiritual, physical and mental) education in schools' (p. 76).

In terms of the first government foci on reproductive health issues – reproductive health is an important health issue in Ukraine and, in particular, starting in the 1990s, a key aspect of the nation-building process (Kuenhast and Nechemias 2004, 5). The issue has taken on specific significance, as Zhurzenko describes in detail in Chapter 5 of this volume, because Ukraine is now among the countries with the lowest fertility rates in the world (Maksymenko 2009). Additionally, Ukrainian women use abortion as a form of fertility regulation at higher rates than women in the rest of Europe (Criswell 2009). In 2010, the CEDAW Committee in its review of Ukraine identified the large number of unwanted pregnancies and the high rate of abortions as areas of concern requiring sustained policy intervention (CEDAW 2010). Reproductive health has also become a specific issue of concern for Ukrainian men as well. According to the U.N. Population Fund (2009), Ukrainian men avoid dealing with issues of sexual and reproductive health which places them and their partners at risk for unwanted pregnancies and sexually transmitted diseases. Although important, women's health and men's health needs, however, extend beyond their reproductive functions. Moreover, reproductive health – for both women and men cannot be reduced to analyses of biological or health care systems. For example, in Ukraine, reduced reproduction is largely influenced by the lack of social and economic resources and other financial supports required to cover the costs of bearing and rearing children. And yet, in general, there is little attention paid to population health needs, including social determinants of health. In particular, there is no structure or related policies within the health care system that systematically responds to or monitors the gender aspects of population health (Skoryk 2007). Significantly, despite the mortality statistics and concomitant health issues, 'the crisis in men's health in Ukraine and other post-Soviet countries has not been adequately addressed by government or NGOs' (Gander and Magdyuk 2006).

A comprehensive social determinants of health approach, which takes into account the importance of gender and its interactions with other social factors and processes, needs to be implemented in health research, policy, and system-wide reforms. Specifically, in terms of men's health, 'there is a need to train doctors about men's health issues, provide more preventive care through specialized services, and lobby government to allocate resources to the problem. Special strategies and tools are also needed to educate the public about men's health needs and issues' (Gander and Magdyuk 2006, 30). There is also a need to 'work with boys and men through innovative programmes for the transformation of harmful masculinist norms, high risk behaviours, and violent practices' (Sen and Östlin 2007, ix). In all such undertakings, it is essential that researchers and policy makers recognize that men are 'not a monolithic category and the ways in which gender shapes men's health depend as well on its intersections with other social and structural locations' (Bates et al. 2009, 2).

Arguably, issues related to either men's health or women's health must be addressed through 'actions both outside and within the health sector, because gender power relations operate across such a wide spectrum of human life and in such inter-related ways' (Sen and Östlin 2007, xii). And while gender should be taken into account, the diversity in and among females and males needs to be taken into account when developing policies, prevention, and intervention measures and conducting health research. Importantly, analyses that cre-ate evidence to inform policy directions ought to address the associations between gender and other factors, namely, age, employment status, region, ethnicity, and sexuality. At the same time, successful interventions will require policies that are feasible within the Ukrainian context, taking into account the history, culture, and contemporary understandings and responses to issues of gender (World Bank 2009a).[3]

Conclusions

Given the current health crisis in Ukraine, the onus is on the government to rethink its approaches to the specific health challenges of this region. And time is of the essence. As the World Bank (2009a) has aptly put it, 'To safeguard the health of the population and prepare itself for the health challenges of the next half century, the Ukrainian government needs to undertake drastic measures' (p. 57). In its report, *Closing the Gap in a Generation: Health Equity through Action on the Social Determinants of Health*, the World Health Organization (2008) has suggested that in order to address health inequities, responsibility for action on health and health equity must be placed at the highest level of government to ensure its coherent consideration across all ministerial and departmental policy making. This ought to result not only in efforts to reform a health care system, services, and health-related behaviours. Such efforts should be framed within a comprehensive social determinants of health perspective, one that identifies interactions of gender with other characteristics of vulnerable populations, not only at the individual level but also at structural levels, thereby capturing fully the multiple contexts that shape lives and health outcomes. To ensure that such efforts are effective, Ukraine also requires sustained research to provide the necessary evidence base to inform the development of policies and effective strategic plans that will improve the health and well-being of Ukrainian women and men.

NOTES

1 For more detailed information and comparative statistics, visit the website of the Committee on Combating HIV/AIDS and other socially dangerous diseases at *http://stop-aids.org.ua* (accessed 18 Aug. 2009).
2 See also the short video *Movchannia Nemovliat* [Silence of Babies]. Available at http://noabort.org.ua/2006/11/28/mov4a/ (accessed 29 Aug. 2009).
3 For a further analysis of this point, see Hankivsky and Salnykova's analysis of gender mainstreaming in Ukraine (Chapter 16 in this volume).

REFERENCES

Abbott, P., and C. Wallace. 2007. Talking about Health and Well-Being in Post-Soviet Ukraine and Russia. *Journal of Communist Studies and Post-Transition Politics* 23(2): 181–202.

Amdzhadin, L. 2007. Genderni Vidminnosti Zdorovya Ukrayintsiv [Gender Differences in Ukrainians' Health]. In M. Skoryk, ed., *Genderni Peretvorennia v Ukrayini* [Gender Transformations in Ukraine], 131–8. Kyiv: UNDP.

Bates, L.M., O. Hankivsky, and K.W. Springer. 2009. Gender and Health Inequities: A Comment on the Final Report of the WHO Commission on the Social Determinants of Health. *Social Science and Medicine* 69(7): 1002–4.

Betliy, O., O. Kuziakiv, and K. Onishchenko. 2007. *The Evaluation of Health Care System in Ukraine in the Context of Structural and Quality-Enhancing Reforms.* Revised Final Report MIR04 – 009. Full text of report available at http://pdc.ceu.hu/archive/00004087/01/18_eng_070815_final.pdf (accessed 1 Feb. 2010).

Bromet, E.J., S.F. Gluzman, V.I. Paniotto, C.P.M. Webb, N.L. Tintle, V. Zakhozha, J.M. Havenaar, Z. Gutkovich, S. Kostyuchenko, and J.E. Schwartz. 2005. Epidemiology of Psychiatric and Alcohol Disorders in Ukraine. *Social Psychiatry and Psychiatric Epidemiology* 40(9): 681–90.

CIA. 2008. Field Listing – Population Growth Rate. *CIA World Factbook.* Available at *https://www.cia.gov/library/publications/the-world-factbook/fields/2002. html* (accessed 5 July 2008).

Cockerham, W.C., B.P. Hinote, and P. Abbott. 2006. Psychological Distress, Gender, and Health Lifestyles in Belarus, Kazakhstan, Russia and Ukraine. *Social Science and Medicine* 63: 2381–94.

Convention on the Elimination of All Forms of Discrimination against Women (CEDAW). 2010. *Concluding Observations of the Committee on the Elimination of Discrimination against Women.* Concluding remarks from the 45th Session (18 Jan. – 5 Feb. 2010). Full text available at http://daccess-dds-ny.un.org/doc/UNDOC/GEN/N10/292/82/PDF/N1029282.pdf?OpenElement (accessed 5 July 2010).

Courtenay, W. 2000. Constructions of Masculinity and Their Influence on Men's Well-Being: A Theory of Gender and Health. *Social Science and Medicine* 50(10): 1385–1401.

Criswell, R. 2009. *Motivations and Obstacles to Use of Contraceptive and Abortion Services in Ukraine.* Presentation to the International Conference on Family Planning – Research and Best Practices, Kampala, Uganda, 17 Nov. 2009. Available at http://www.fpconference2009.org/media//DIR_169701/15f1a e857ca97193ffff82f5ffffd524.pdf (accessed 1 July 2010).

De Bell, D., and R. Carter. 2005. Impact of Transition on Public Health in Ukraine: Case Study of the HIV/AIDS Epidemic. *British Medical Journal* 331: 216–19.

Drobniewski, F., V. Nikolayevsky, A. Asmolov, Y. Bazhora, and S. Servetsky. 2005. Increasing Trends in HIV and TB Rates in Odessa and the Ukraine. *International Journal of STD and AIDS* 16: 374–8.

Dye, C., M.A. Espinal, C.J. Watt, C. Mbiaga, and B.G. Williams. 2002. World-wide Incidence of Multidrug-Resistant Tuberculosis. *Journal of Infectious Diseases* 185: 1197–1202.

Gander, C., and L. Magdyuk. 2006. *Ukraine Gender Equality Review.* Prepared for the Ukraine Program. Ottawa: CIDA.

Gatehouse, G. 2009. *Ukraine's Healthcare System Falters.* Report for the BBC News Online. Available at http://news.bbc.co.uk/2/hi/europe/8182795. stm (accessed 5 Aug. 2009).

Gilmore, A., M. McKee, and R. Rose. 2002. Determinants of and Inequalities in Self-Perceived Health in Ukraine. *Social Science and Medicine* 55(12): 2177–88.

Haidayev, Y.O. 2007. Derzhavna Polityka u Galuzi Ohorony Zdorovya [Public Policy in the Area of Health]. *Ukrayins'kyi Meduchnyi Chasopys [Ukrainian Medical Journal]* 4(60), Issue 7–8: 4–8.

Hankivsky, O. 2007. Gender-Based Analysis and Health Policy: The Need to Rethink Outdated Strategies. In M. Morrow, O. Hankivsky, and C. Varcoe, eds., *Women's Health in Canada: Critical Perspectives on Theory and Policy,* 143–68. Toronto: University of Toronto Press.

– 2008. Globalization, Trafficking and Health: A Case Study of Ukraine. In C. Patton and H. Loshny, eds., *Global Science/Women's Health*, 175–99. Amherst: Cambria.

– 2009. The Challenge of HIV/AIDS in Ukraine. In C. Pope, R. White, and R. Malow, eds., *HIV/AIDS: Global Frontiers in Prevention/Intervention – An Interdisciplinary Reader*, 96–112. New York: Routledge.

Hankivsky, O., and A. Christoffersen. 2008. Intersectionality and the Determinants of Health: A Canadian Perspective. *Critical Public Health* 18(3): 271–83.

Health Canada. 2000. *Gender-Based Analysis Policy*. Ottawa: Minister of Public Works and Government Services.

Iyer, A., G. Sen, and P. Östlin. 2008. The Intersections of Gender and Class in Health Status and Health Care. *Global Public Health* 3(S1): 13–24.

Kryszyna, N.P., V.L. Veselskiy, N.Y. Kondratyuk, and O.V. Kryzyna. 2009. Family Medicine of Ukraine at the Present Stage of Reforming Health Care. *Health of the Nation* [Ukraine] no. 1–2.

Kuehnast, K., and C. Nechemias, eds. 2004. *Post-Soviet Women Encountering Transition: Nation Building, Economic Survival, and Civic Activism*. Baltimore: Johns Hopkins University Press in conjunction with the Woodrow Wilson International Center for Scholars.

Lekhan V., V. Rudiy, and E. Nolte. 2004. *Health Care Systems in Transition: Ukraine*. Copenhagen: WHO Regional Office for Europe on behalf of the European Observatory on Health Systems and Policies.

Lohan, M. 2007. How Might We Understand Men's Health Better? Integrating Explanations from Critical Studies on Men and Inequalities in Health. *Social Science and Medicine* 65: 493–504.

Maistruk, G., and V. Bannikov. 2009. *Breast Cancer Problem in Ukraine*. Available at http://www.whfp.kiev.ua/prbl_eng.shtml (accessed 3 Aug. 2009).

Maksymenko, S. 2009. Fertility, Money Holdings, and Economic Growth: Evidence from Ukraine. *Comparative Economic Studies* 51: 75–99. McKee, M. 2005. Understanding Population Health: Lessons from the Former Soviet Union. *Clinical Medicine* 5(4): 375–8.

Medical News Today. 2009. *Condom Price Increases in Ukraine Cause Concern about Spread of HIV, Other STIs*. (10 Feb. 2009). Available at *http://www.medicalnewstoday.com/articles/138455.php* (accessed 1 Aug. 2009).

Ministry of Health (MoH) Ukraine (with Ukrainian AIDS Centre, WHO, International HIV/AIDS Alliance in Ukraine, U.N. Program for HIV/AIDS, Geneva, Switzerland). 2006. *Report on the National Consensus Estimates on HIV and AIDS in Ukraine as of End of 2005*. Kyiv: MoH.

Ministry of Health (MoH) Ukraine. 2009. *Kontrol nad Tutunom v Ukrayini* [Tobacco Control in Ukraine]. National report. Kyiv: MoH.

O'Brien, R., K. Hunt, and G. Hart. 2005. Men's Accounts of Masculinity and Help-Seeking: 'It's Caveman Stuff.' *Journal of Epidemiology and Community Health* 59: 873–6.

Pomerleau, J., A. Gilmore, M. McKee, R. Rose, and C.W. Haerpfer. 2004. Determinants of Smoking in Eight Countries of the Former Soviet Union: Results from the Living Conditions, Lifestyles and Health Study. *Addiction* 99: 1577–85.

Poznyak, V.B., V.E. Pelipas, A.N. Vievski, and L. Miroshnichenko. 2002. Illicit Drug Use and Its Health Consequences in Belarus, Russian Federation and Ukraine: Impact of Transition. *European Addiction Research* 8:184–9.

Scott, J. 1986. Gender: A Useful Category of Historical Analysis. *American Historical Review* 91 (Dec.): 1053–75.

Semigina, T., and O. Kishkina. 2006. Public Health Policy and Public Health Research in Ukraine: Linked, Interlinked or Unlinked. *UDK* 614(477): 28–33.

Sen, G., and P. Östlin. 2007. *Unequal, Unfair, Ineffective and Inefficient Gender Inequity in Health: Why It Exists and How We Can Change It*. Final Report to the WHO Commission on Social Determinants of Health. (Sept.). Available at http://www.who.int/social_determinants/resources/csdh_media/ wgekn_final_report_07.pdf (accessed 4 Aug. 2009).

Skoryk, M., ed. 2007. *Genderni Peretvorennia v Ukrayini* [Gender Transformations in Ukraine]. Kyiv: UNDP.

Springer, K.W., and D. Mouzon. 2011. 'Macho Men' and Preventive Health Care: Implications for Older Men in Different Social Classes. *Journal of Health and Social Behavior*. Published online 13 April, 1–16.

Swedish International Development Co-operation Agency (SIDA). 2003. *Gender Issues in Ukraine: Challenges and Opportunities*. Kyiv: SIDA.

Tarantino, L., S. Chankova, J. Rosenfeld, S. Routh, and E. Preble. 2011. Ukraine Health Assessment. Available at: http://www.healthsystems2020org/ content/resource/detail/82461/(accessed 15 Dec. 2001).

Tsuchiya, A., and A. Williams. 2005. A 'Fair Innings' between the Sexes: Are Men Being Treated Inequitably? *Social Science and Medicine* 60(2): 277–86.

UNFPA. 2009. *Ukraine's Report*. United Nations Population Fund. Available at *http://www.unfpa.org.ua/en/icpd10/* (accessed 4 Aug. 2009).

Vassall, A., Y. Chechulin, I. Raykhert, N. Osalenko, S. Svetlichnaya, A. Kovalyova, M.J. van der Werf, L.V. Turchenko, E. Hasker, K. Miskinis, J. Veen, and R. Zaleskis. 2009. Reforming Tuberculosis Control in Ukraine: Results of Pilot Projects and Implications for the National Scale-Up of DOTS. *Health Policy and Planning* 24: 55–62.

Webb, P.M., E.J. Bromet, S. Gluzman, N.L. Tintle, J.E. Schwartz, S. Kostyuchenko, and J.M. Havenaar. 2005. Epidemiology of Heavy Alcohol Use in Ukraine. *Alcohol and Alcoholism* 40(4): 327–35.

Weidner, G., and V.S. Cain. 2003. The Gender Gap in Heart Disease: Lessons from Eastern Europe. *Men's Health Forum* 93(5): 768–9.

Word Press. 2008. *Russian Women Speaking English*. Available at *http://russian-womenspeak.wordpress.com/2008/03/10/ukrainian-demographic-statistics-comparable-to-russian* (accessed 1 Aug. 2009).

World Bank. 2009a. *An Avoidable Tragedy: Combating Ukraine's Health Crisis – Lessons from Europe*. Kyiv: World Bank.

– 2009b. Ukraine Is in the Midst of an Unprecedented Demographic Decline Compounded by a Health Crisis, Says a New World Bank Study. World Bank Press Release, Kyiv, 25 June. Available at http://web.worldbank.org/WBSITE/EXTERNAL/COUNTRIES/ECAEXT/0,,contentMDK:22225837˜menuPK:2246556˜pagePK:2865106˜piPK:2865128˜theSitePK:258599,00.html?cid=ISG_E_WBWeeklyUpdate_NL (accessed 4 June 2010).

World Health Organization (WHO). 2008. *Closing the Gap in a Generation: Health Equity through Action on the Social Determinants of Health*. Commission on Social Determinants of Health Final Report – Executive Summary. Available at http://whqlibdoc.who.int/hq/2008/WHO_IER_CSDH_08.1_eng.pdf (accessed 12 Nov. 2009).

– 2009. *Ukraine – World Health Statistics*. Available at http://www.who.int/countries/ukr/en/ (accessed 4 Aug. 2009).

13 Masculinity in Soviet and Post-Soviet Ukraine: Models and Their Implications

TETYANA BUREYCHAK

Over the past two decades, gender relations have become an issue of growing public and academic interest in many post-Soviet states, including Ukraine. This can be clearly traced in the simultaneous increase in gender studies publications and research and dissertations on gender issues, as well as in the introduction of gender studies courses into university curricula and the establishment of academic and research gender studies centres. At the same time, most of these projects have focused on women and femininities, primarily discussed in relation to patriarchy and gender inequalities. Masculinity, meanwhile, remains on the fringe of academic discussion in Ukraine to date. Yet the social, cultural, economic, and political changes experienced by Ukrainian society during its Soviet and post-Soviet history have had a powerful influence on the experiences of both women and men. Gender analysis focused primarily on female experiences does not capture the complexity of gender relations. This chapter contributes to the study of masculinities by looking at Soviet and post-Soviet gender regimes through their framing, normalizing, and prioritizing of particular notions and models of masculinities. Models of masculinities are understood here as exemplars or ideals of masculinity that contribute to the construction of the normative and discursively central notion of masculinity – what is called 'hegemonic masculinity.' The chapter offers an overview of gender politics in the Soviet Union; a discussion of dominant models of masculinity popularized in that period follows, as well as a look at their influence on men's experiences; finally, the chapter analyses masculine ideals in Ukraine in the post-Soviet period and considers to what extent they exist in reaction to the past or open up possibilities for men in the future.

Soviet Gender Policy and Ideals of Masculinity

With regard to gender politics, most scholars divide the long, seventy-year era of Soviet rule into three distinct periods: 1918–30, which was a time of Bolshevik experimentation in the sphere of sexuality, marriage, and political involvement by women; 1930–50, characterized by intensive economic involvement of women and, at the same time, a rollback towards traditional family relations and pro-natalist (i.e., targeted at the increase of birth rates) state policy; and 1950–80, which saw the liberalization of gender politics and the emergence of criticism of gender relations, much of which, however, was censored (Lapidus 1977; Rotkirch 2000; Kon 2005; Zdravomyslova and Temkina 2007a).

Despite the stark differences between these periods, scholars have also defined some of the overall features of the Soviet gender regime. Probably the most important of these was the dominant role of the state in defining and controlling gender relations. For this reason, Zdravomyslova and Temkina (2007a, 96) define the USSR's gender regime as 'etacratic,' that is, fundamentally shaped by state power. This shaping occurred via two major mechanisms: defining gender norms in legislation and enabling guarantees of state control over gender relations. One means by which the Soviet state guaranteed the latter control was to make private matters public. This, in turn, required the destruction of the patriarchal family and traditional gender relations within it. As a consequence of this policy, the traditionally dominant position of men in the private sphere was undermined. According to Zdravomyslova and Temkina (pp. 104–5), alienated fatherhood was especially promoted by the Soviet policy of 'defamilialization' in the period of the 1920s and 1930s. The policy reimagined the Soviet family as a union of two comrades—members of the big Soviet family and labour collective. Liberation of sexual relations during this period was aimed at ruining the family as the basis of bourgeois society and at rejecting individualism in the name of communist society. Although Stalin's regime reversed the policy and proclaimed the family as a basic unit of socialist society, the position of men in the family remained marginal.[1] According to Tartakovskaya (2005, 128–9), this was aided by a range of state-led shifts, among which were the following:

(1) Mass involvement of women in the labour force. This allowed women to be more socially and economically independent from

men, which led to the lowering of men's authority in the family,
since a man could no longer be the sole breadwinner and unconditional head of the household.

(2) Politicization of motherhood. This placed most responsibility for
raising children with mothers, and neglected the father's role,
which resulted in the legitimization of women's control over
children. It also contributed to the weakening of fathers' authority by reducing their role to an economic function: providing financial resources to the family (alongside universally employed
mothers), or paying alimony in cases of divorce.

(3) Various approaches to control men's behaviour. Women and
even children were occasionally recruited to assist in the state's
attempts to eradicate socially inadequate types of men's behaviour (alcoholism, marital infidelity, violence, and so on).

In the Soviet period, gender equality policies thus adhered more closely
to communist ideology than to principles of justice and gender egalitar-
ianism. The Soviets focused a lot of their effort on dealing with the so-
called women's issue (*zhenskiy vopros*), promoting women's education
and protecting their right to paid labour, as well as creating a network
of social services (public catering networks, kindergartens, and day-
cares, etc.). But little was done to overcome the vertical and horizontal
gender segregation of labour, women's limited access to power, their
insignificant participation in politics, or to relieve them of the burden of
most of the domestic work (Tartakovskaya 2005). While the policy of the
'new household' was initiated with the aim of liberating women from
'kitchen slavery' and mobilizing them into the workforce (Zhurzhenko
2008, 85)–men's participation in the household was never a part of this
policy–state support proved to be extremely inefficient (Gerasimova
and Chuikina 2004), and household duties continued to be distributed
in a traditional way, with most tasks carried out by women. Men's participation in the household was occasional and related to traditional
men's duties, such as changing electric bulbs, taking out the rubbish
bin, mending household equipment, and doing renovations. According to Slesarv and Yankova, gender inequality in the Soviet household
was therefore preserved because of an inefficient state service sector
and adherence to old patriarchal norms that saw girls raised to serve
the family (cited in Zdravomyslova and Temkina 2007a, 134). Men's
passivity contrasted with women's activity in the household, and this

imbalance caused a diminishment of men's investment in, and their alienation from the family (Chernova 2007, 166). The high level of divorces and alcohol addiction among men were some of the negative phenomena in the private sphere.

Spreading the Word about the New Soviet Man

Propaganda in the form of official rhetoric as well as printed, visual, and music media that suggested specific frames for Soviet masculinity and femininity played a crucial role in promoting the state's gender ideology (Haynes 2003). The visual mode of propaganda was especially powerful in the first decades of the USSR because of the necessity of establishing new ideological narratives for a broad and largely illiterate audience. This was equally true with regard to messages aimed at men (Bonnell 1999). The Soviet Union promoted specific idealized modes of masculinity deemed most appropriate to its aim of building a society of social equality and prosperity. This ideal was based on strength of mind and body and unconditional devotion and heroism in the name of state principles. The ideal, via various personifications, was widely conveyed, and every single Soviet man was socialized into one or more idealized masculine roles, including Defender of the Motherland, selfless worker, athletic man, and builder of communism, each of which merits further description. Another ideal, leader of the country, although masculine, was promoted rather as an abstract object of worship that represented the highest virtues of communist society and ideology.[2]

Defender of the Motherland

Soviet men received a steady stream of messages from their militaristic state, which insisted that men's self-fulfilment was possible only through service to the motherland (Tartakovskaya 2005, 128, 130). The first appeals to this defender ideal occurred during the creation of the Red Army in 1918, which was to become a stronghold of the new Soviet state and its ideals. According to Lenin, this was an army of liberation for a proletariat that would adhere to principles of internationalism. To be a defender of the motherland required the highest level of devotion to state ideals and readiness for self-sacrifice, including willingness to die for the motherland (Yuval-Davis 1997).

The idea of 'real' men as defenders intensified considerably in the post – Second World War period, when this image became particularly appealing because of the halo of victory and pride surrounding it. A strong and unconquerable Soviet state contributed to a symbolic increase in the status of masculinity among individual Soviet men. In times of peace, service to the motherland was extended beyond its original military function. A 'real' Soviet man thus had to be ready for unconditional and selfless participation in any state project (Tartakovskaya 2005, 128). Military discourse was altered to promote struggles for bountiful harvests, record-breaking industrial production, and labour heroism. At the same time, cowardice, weakness, and laziness were deemed the most negative characteristics that a man could possess. Soviet posters played a significant role in the visualization and promotion of the defender of the motherland ideal; Figures 13.1 to 13.3 illustrate examples.

Selfless Worker

Discouraged to play a significant role in the family under Soviet rule, men were banished to the public sphere. To a large extent, this was the area where they could find fulfilment. Although men's success in the professional sphere is traditionally measured by the achievement of high social and financial status, in the USSR, men's professional self-fulfilment was not necessarily associated with these indicators. Soviet ideology prioritized social needs over personal ones, as well as spiritual over material motivations (Magun 1998). As a result, the outcomes of personal efforts and achievements of men were measured by their input into the abstract of 'building a better future.' Ideas of selflessness and heroism were therefore intricately woven in with labour for Soviet men (see Figures 13.4 to 13.6). The selfless worker ideal was supported by numerous stories about Stakhanovite miners, daredevil aviators, and record-breaking collective farm workers. These were widely circulated through Soviet media and art. Based on events in the lives of real people, the success stories were nonetheless distorted and embellished to fit the socialist discourse (Haynes 2003, 3).

Selfless labour required men to be flexible and mobile. A man was considered a 'military unit' in Soviet ideology; he was expected to be ready to leave his home at a moment's notice and set up elsewhere to carry out the work of the Communist Party (Chernova 2007, 142–4). This emphasis on a man's mobility secured the possibility of his participation in socialist construction projects, the conquering of virgin lands, and the patrolling of state borders. As well, while their labour was mandatory, men were expected to go beyond just fulfilling this requirement to achieve extraordinary results and beat existing records in their fields of endeavour.[3] Record-breaking productivity was encouraged by the state in every possible way, including awards for labour achievements – comparable to military awards for achievements in battle.

Athletic Man

The cult of the healthy, strong, trained male body was a feature of Soviet education. Images of athletic men were also part of heroic and patriotic Soviet propaganda (Kon 2001). A strong body was the condition for dedicated work and effective labour. A strong male body also symbolized physical and moral advantage. In contrast, enemies of the USSR (capitalists and bourgeois) were always depicted as physically unattractive, with badly proportioned bodies – too short and fat, or too long and thin. Physical strength was supposed to be reached through strict discipline, regular sports activities, and hardening of the body (Gilmour and Clements 2002; see Figures 13.7 to 13.9).

Builder of Communism

This model for masculinity informs all of those discussed so far, since it provides the impetus for labour and service to the motherland. The moral code of the builder of communism was officially introduced as a part of the Third Program of the Communist Party of the Soviet Union in 1961.[4] This code stressed devotion to communism, love towards the socialist motherland, conscientious labour, respect for public duty, humane relationships, collectivism, and brotherhood, as well as intolerance of injustice, dishonesty, and careerism (see Figures 13.10 to 13.12).

Leader of the Country

The ideal of leader of the country, incarnated in the figures of Lenin and Stalin, had different functions from the other Soviet masculine ideals. It was not intended as attainable by ordinary men, but rather as an object of worship. Leaders of the country were not ordinary men. They were symbolic figures who played the role of wise leader, teacher of communism, strategy genius of the socialist revolution, and inspiration for the fight of Soviet people for socialist society and the building of communism (see Figures 13.13 and 13.14). According to Kon (2006), this mythological image of a great leader, father, and teacher symbolically compensated for the model of traditional fatherhood, which was difficult to achieve during times of totalitarianism (pp. 506–7).

Soviet ideology sought to redefine traditional masculine ideals, preserving and emphasizing some of the elements and abolishing others in ways that would best serve the regime. This picking and choosing led to an odd configuration: the Soviet man should be strong, brave, and devoted to his principles when it came to loyalty to the state, patriotism, and devotion to communist values, but he should refrain from applying traditional masculine qualities like energy, initiative, and independence with regard to critical assessments of these communist principles. Thus, the Soviet regime promoted a composite of traditional masculinity and communist ideology, while requiring that men remain under the total control of the state. The most conspicuous results of this were a decrease of men's traditional authority within the family (which had both positive and negative effects in terms of gender equality) and their alienation from the private sphere. It also led to men's mobilization for full-value participation in labour and and in the building of communism. This participation was encouraged through a range of symbolic rewards and promotions within power hierarchies.

Models for Ukrainian Men in the Soviet Era

Since one of the aims of Soviet ideology was the creation of a new community called the 'Soviet people,' ethnic and cultural differences were in most cases omitted from Soviet propaganda. However, aspects of the Soviet vision of Ukrainian masculinity can be discerned through analysis of Soviet cinema. Based on her review of images of Ukrainian men in Soviet films between 1940 and 1980, Semikhat (2009) assembled a list of traits that were typically inherent in these characters. A Ukrainian man is often depicted as a solidly built, middle-aged man of rural origin who did not complete school. He holds an ordinary, often marginal position within the professional hierarchy. His origin and education do not provide him with enough cultural capital to be an independent and self-sufficient character. In terms of personal qualities, the Ukrainian

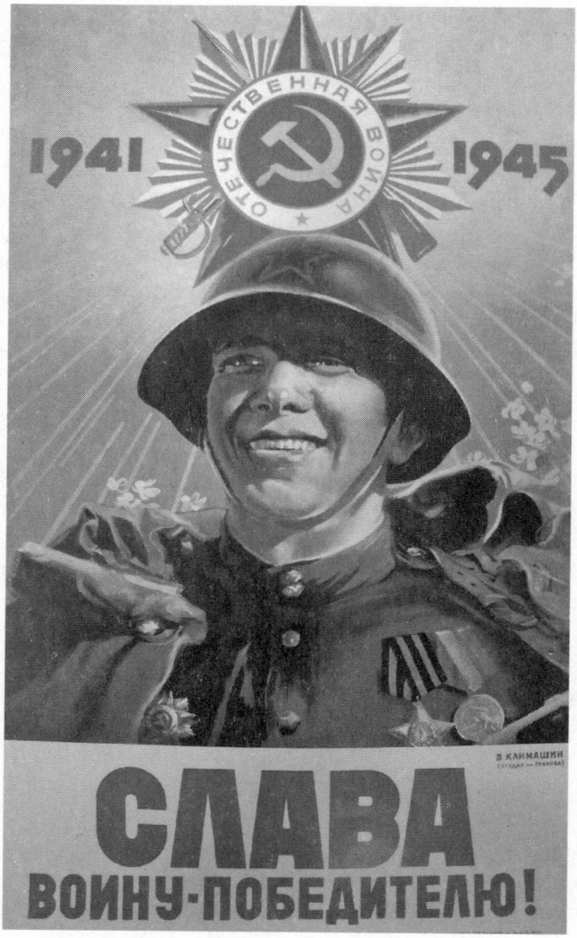

Figure 13.1. Glory to the Warrior-Victor! (1945). Artist: V. Klimahin; source: a reproduction from the author's personal collection.

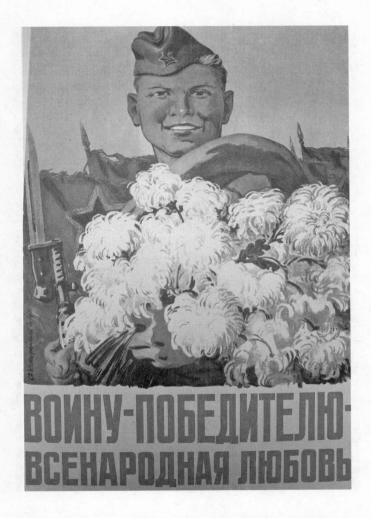

Figure 13.2. The Love of the Whole Nation to the Warrior-Victor (1944).
Artist: A. Kokorekin; source: the Soviet Posters Archive of the Davis Center
for Russian and Eurasian Studies, Harvard University.

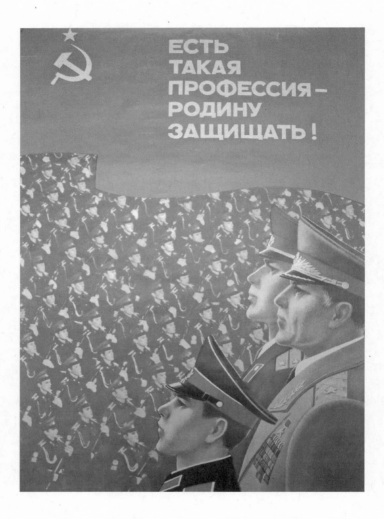

Figure 13.3. This Is a Profession – Protect the Motherland (1984). Artist: D. Denisov; source: the Soviet Posters Archive of the Davis Center for Russian and Eurasian Studies, Harvard University.

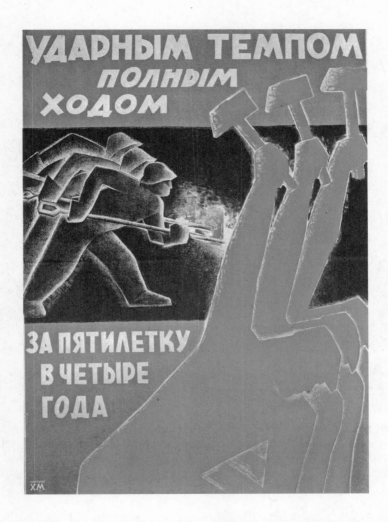

Figure 13.4. With Intensified Speed Let's Do Our Five-Year Plan in Four Years (1930s). Artist: unknown; source: a reproduction from the author's personal collection.

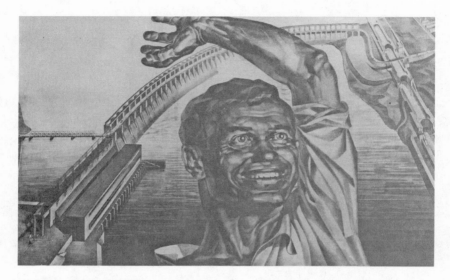

Figure 13.5. There Are No Fortresses that Cannot Be Conquered by the Bolsheviks and Stalin. Building of the Dneprostroy Dam Is Finished (1932). Artist: A. Strakhov-Braslavsky; source: Bonnell (1999, 69).

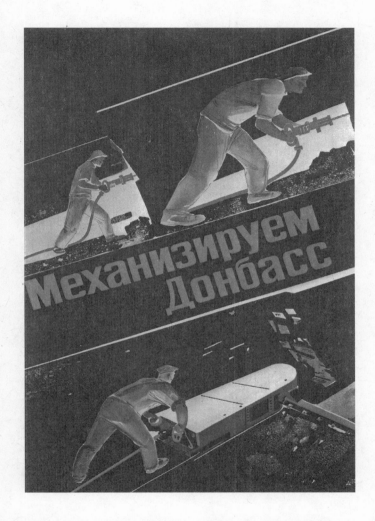

Figure 13.6. We Will Mechanize Donbass (1930). Artist: A. Deineka; source: Bonnell (1999, 53).

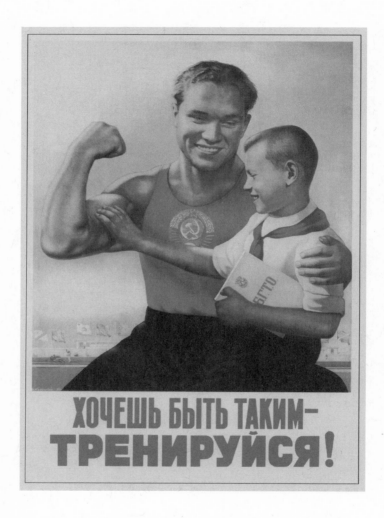

Figure 13.7. Train Yourself If You Want to Be Like This! (1951). Artist: V. Koretsky; source: a reproduction from the author's personal collection.

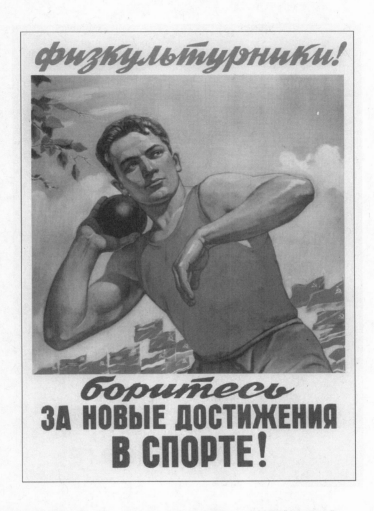

Figure 13.8. Fight for New Achievements in Sport! (1955). Artist: L. Golovanov; source: a reproduction from the author's personal collection.

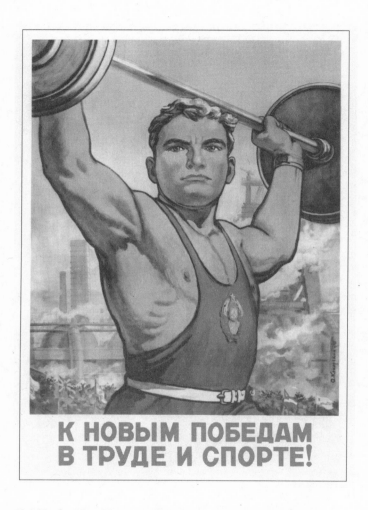

Figure 13.9. To the New Victories in Labour and Sport (1955). Artist: A. Kokorekin; source: a reproduction from the author's personal collection.

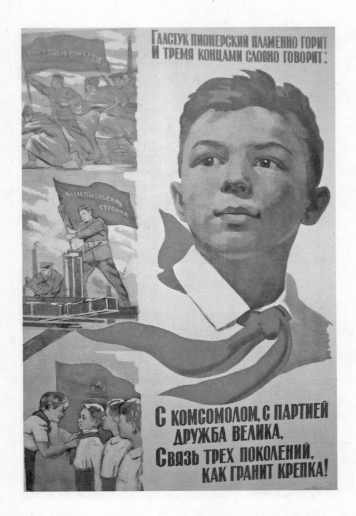

Figure 13.10. Pioneer's Tie (1961). Artist: A. Dobrov; source: Lafont (2007, 27).

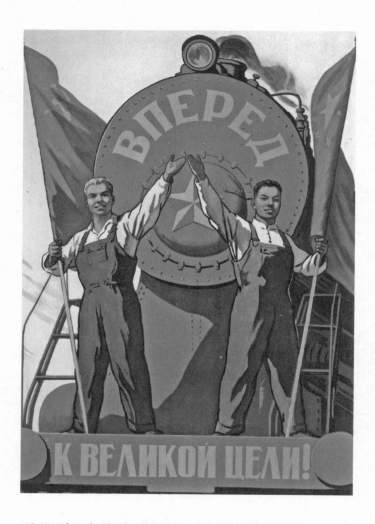

Figure 13.11. Ahead – To the Great Goal! (1959). Artist: M. Soloviev; source: Lafont (2007, 184).

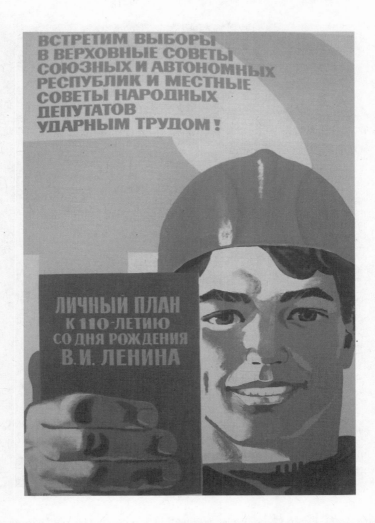

Figure 13.12. Personal Plan for the 110th Anniversary of Lenin's Birth (1979).
Artist: A. Dobrov; source: Lafont (2007).

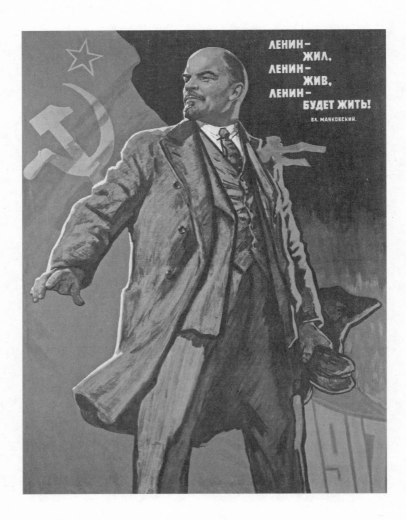

Figure 13.13. Lenin Lived, Lives, and Will Live! (1967). Artist: V. Ivanov; source: a reproduction from the author's personal collection.

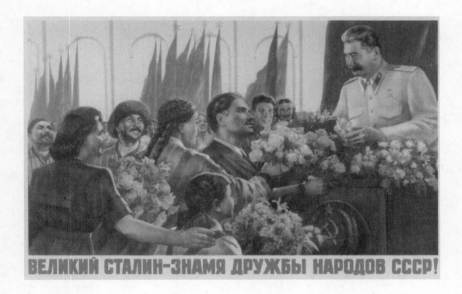

ВЕЛИКИЙ СТАЛИН-ЗНАМЯ ДРУЖБЫ НАРОДОВ СССР!

Figure 13.14. Stalin. 'Dear Stalin – Happiness of People!' (1949). Artist: V. Koretsky; source: a reproduction from the author's personal collection.

man is a positive character – kind and friendly, but sometimes an infantile simpleton. These traits are usually supplemented by others stereotypically ascribed to Ukrainians, such as wearing an embroidered shirt, eating *salo* (lard), and speaking Russian with a bad Ukrainian accent. This often makes him an object of jokes by his colleagues. He tries to be like a Russian, but he is not Russian yet (pp. 249–50). Thus, in Soviet films Ukrainian masculinity is presented as less prestigious compared with a successful Soviet model of a man. Applying the terminology of Connell (1995), Ukrainian masculinity was subordinated to hegemonic Soviet/Russian masculinity.

Soviet Man over Time

Although the dominant models of masculinity did not change considerably in the Soviet era, their reception and the levels of critical interpretation towards them did. Zdravomyslova and Temkina (2002) argue that the evolution of the gender order in the late Soviet period (1970s and 1980s) led to a discursive crisis of masculinity, that is, a discrepancy between the ideals of Soviet masculinity and the ability to fulfil them. As Soviet ideology weakened, models for men such as Defender of the Motherland or builder of communism were seen as irrelevant and were thus devalued. At the same time, other traditional masculine ideals from the pre-Soviet moment and modern Western masculinity were equally unachievable because of the lack of appropriate ideological and economic conditions. Social anxiety about inappropriate roles of men and women became particularly pronounced in discussions in the press, films, and academic publications in this late period.

Particular criticism was directed towards the so-called masculinization of women and the feminization of men (Kon 2006, 507). Men's low life expectancy, high death rates, poor health, alcoholism, and increased display of harmful habits were used as examples of a deteriorating masculinity. There were proposals to enforce strict state control and compulsory medical check-ups to combat men's poor health (Zdravomyslova and Temkina 2002, 436–9). However, these were never enacted. Discourse surrounding the 'weaker' man was also based on the inability of Soviet men to fulfil their traditional family roles – to serve as sole breadwinner, head of household, and good father. Thus, the Soviet redefinition of traditional masculinity according to the socialist agenda, while having some positive effects on gender equality, also created gender identity problems among Soviet men. Moreover, women, tired from carrying a double or triple burden of work and home life, began to reconsider the traditional ideal of the strong man as possibly desirable. Their longing for a return to traditional ideals was arguably primarily driven by the hope of lightening their duties, since with a traditional man they would no longer be entirely responsible for household and family as well as labour. This reasoning has the potential to shed additional light on the causes of gender neo-traditionalism in post-Soviet Ukrainian society and on women's acceptance of the return to patriarchal values.

Ideas about the need for change in the Soviet gender regime became especially popular during the wave of political liberalization in the 1980s to early 1990s. The collapse of the Soviet Union in 1991 led to the loss of the dominant role of the state in regulating social relations (Zdravomyslova and Temkina 2007b, 176) and opened up the possibility – and expectation – of change. Soviet gender norms were criticized as having been coercive and inadequate, and the attempts to create a 'new man' and a 'new woman' were seen as brutal experiments that had set out to ruin natural relations between genders. As a result, the search for new models of gender relations and ideals in the post-Soviet moment in many cases totally negated the Soviet gender experience.

Masculinity in Post-Soviet Ukraine

The Ukrainian state created after the collapse of the Soviet Union officially embraced democratic values. At the same time, in contrast to most Western European democratic countries, post-Soviet Ukraine has seen an increase in the popularity of traditional views about men's and women's roles. Accordingly, men's success is measured by achievements in professional life, while the primary realm of women's self-fulfilment is the family and keeping home and hearth. The post-Soviet period has thus been characterized by the growing legitimization of men's dominant position in the public sphere and more encouragement for women to move into the private sphere. These views have received particular support from the national media, as well as from political, religious, and non-governmental organizations (NGOs).

Traditional gender models have often been presented as a way to revitalize the Ukrainian nation, to preserve the family, and to renew moral traditions that the Soviet system destroyed. Some theorists have called this post-Soviet return to tradition in the gender regime (Zdravomyslova and Temkina 2007b, 177) a 'patriarchal renaissance' (Attwood 1996;

Watson 1993). This renaissance emphasizes the negative consequences of the artificial obliteration of gender differences during Soviet times as a means of promoting a traditional gender order, which proponents consider to be the 'authentic' gender norms and ideals that the Soviet system ruined. Thus, the search for 'true' Ukrainian femininity and masculinity in post-Soviet times can also be deemed neo-traditionalism – that is, harkening back to gender models from Ukraine's past and offering them as gender ideals for today.

Ukrainian Female and Male Ideals: Berehynia and the Cossack

These ideals include *Berehynia* (family guardian, the woman's ideal) and Cossack (warrior, the man's ideal). Their common function is to help construct a national identity and a version of history in which Ukrainian people struggle for an independent culture, language, and traditions. Although placed side by side, these female and male ideals actually have significantly different origins. The image of *Berehynia* refers to ancient history and archaic beliefs, yet Kis (2004) contends that it is an ideological invention of Ukrainian writers at the beginning of 1990s. In contrast, the Cossack ideal refers to a real, although generalized character from the Ukrainian past: Cossacks were a military community, which played an important role in European geopolitics and Ukrainian history between the fifteenth and eighteenth centuries.

The Cossack model has been significantly idealized in its contemporary interpretation. Current Cossack values give them the shape of noble heroes – bravery, courage, independence, and a devotion to principles and national values. Cossacks have been compared to knights in Western European history (Kosenko 2006, 576), glorifying traditional male qualities like dominance, leadership, courage, physical endurance, and sexual potency. For those promoting this ideal, these values are desirable for 'real' Ukrainian men (Bureychak 2006).

The Cossack idea has been introduced into discourses and practices of education. Beginning from early childhood, little boys are taught to restrain their feelings, because, as the popular saying goes, 'Cossacks do not cry.' As well, various sports groups for boys and young men, like *Spas* (meaning 'Saviour') or *Sokil* (meaning 'Falcon'), have opened in recent years and emphasize becoming physically strong like the Cossacks. 'Combat *hopak*,' a Ukrainian Cossack dance combining elements of martial arts, is one means through which this strength can be achieved. An invention of the late 1980s, this mixture of dance and

fighting is designed to be an integral part of raising healthy and patriotic male youth. 'Healthy youth are the future of Ukraine,' writes
Volodymyr Pylat, the founder of combat *hopak*, in his manual on the
sport (1994, 336).

The popularity of the image of the Cossack has also made it attractive for local Ukrainian manufacturers, who have transformed it into a
Ukrainian brand. Today the Cossack is used to mark public spaces related to consumption, such as restaurants that offer Ukrainian cuisine,
as well as to advertise locally produced Ukrainian goods and services.
Some of the examples of this kind of application of the Cossack image
are presented in Figures 13.15 and 13.16.

The popularity of the Cossack image rests on its ability to oppose
Soviet ideals while fighting for Ukrainian national values and an independent state. Yet, closer consideration of the qualities ascribed to
the Cossack reveals similarities to those of the Soviet models of men

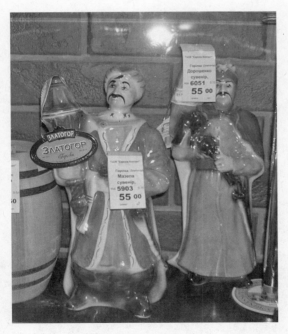

Figure 13.15. 'Mazepa' and 'Doroshenko' Vodka. A photograph taken by the
author, Lviv, Ukraine, 2007.

(defender of the motherland, physically strong man, and builder of communism). The Cossack presents a militaristic ideal, devotion to state principles, and heroic masculinity. There are two major differences between the new Ukrainian masculine ideal and the Soviet models of masculinity, however. First, they are based on different ideologies (nationalist versus communist). Second, they suggest different roles for the state in regulating the ideological portent of the image. The Cossack suggests a less coercive state position. Nonetheless, he is a retro-ideal based on a symbolic reconstruction of the imagined past.

Western Ideals of Masculinity in Today's Ukraine

The collapse of the Soviet Union not only made it possible to articulate a national ideal of masculinity in Ukraine, but it also opened up space for and promoted the popularity of masculine images emerging from Western culture. Media and advertising play an important role in the

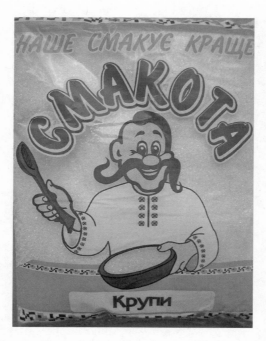

Figure 13.16. Sugar – 'Cossack' Brand. A photograph taken by the author, Lviv, Ukraine, 2008.

introduction and spread of these images in Ukraine. Powerful superheroes, successful businessmen, and 'New Lads' are all ideals of Western masculinity that appeal to independence, control, and individual freedom respectively.[5] Unlike with the Cossack, which opposes Soviet ideals only superficially, the attractiveness of these images in post-Soviet Ukraine, especially in the first years of independence, has been connected with their fundamental difference from Soviet ones. They refer to Western lifestyle values, which symbolically represent ideals of success and prosperity. The common feature between these Western masculine images and the Cossack ideal is that they offer a new version of traditional masculinity as a model of masculinity for today.

Another Western ideal that has recently been promoted by advertising in Ukraine, as it has been throughout Europe, is the erotized, metrosexual man,[6] or man as an object of women's gaze.[7] The primary audience for this advertising consists of young, well-to-do, urban, consumption-oriented men. These images stress the importance of grooming and aspiring to an attractive appearance – practices traditionally associated with femininity. It would be premature to say that metrosexuality has been accepted as normal by the majority of Ukrainian males; however, its growing public visibility is transforming existing ideals about men, who are not traditionally supposed to demonstrate interest in their appearance. It also gradually promotes tolerance for practices that build men's physical attractiveness. At the same time, metrosexuality does not necessarily challenge or undermine hegemonic masculinity, since grooming practices and focus on appearance can simply be employed as additional resources for the enhancement of social status among professionally and financially successful men.

Revived Religious Ideals and Traditional Gender Roles

On the other end of the spectrum, very traditional gender roles and ideals promoted by the Orthodox Church have also experienced a surge in popularity and a kind of revival in post-Soviet times. Annual all-Ukrainian sociological surveys reveal that at least 87 per cent of the population considered themselves religious in the past five years (Golovakha and Panina 2008, 75). Most of these people affiliate with the Orthodox Church, which has not undergone the same modernization processes as Western Christianity. As a result, Orthodox gender ideals support traditional stereotypes of man as a breadwinner and woman as family guardian. As seen in Table 13.1, these stereotypes are reflected

Table 13.1. Opinions of Men and Women on Who Should Be the Head of the Family (%)

Answers	Men	Women	Average
Man	66	57	61
Woman	8	10	9
Both	16	20	18
Neither	3	4	4
Difficult to answer	7	9	8

Source: All-Ukrainian opinion poll conducted by the Institute of Sociology, National Academy of Science of Ukraine, 2007 (UNDP 2007, 71).

in the attitudes of many Ukrainians who took part in a recent survey about family roles. This result, showing that Ukrainians see men as the natural heads of the family, is supported by another survey finding, as seen in Table 13.2, related to who should be responsible for contributing most to family income.

Traditional ideals also impact attitudes towards parenthood. In most cases, a woman is considered to be the primary caregiver for children. Although contemporary Ukrainian legislation provides equal rights to parental leave for men and women, most often it is the mother who takes it. Men are discouraged from taking parental leave and involving themselves in child care because of stereotypes surrounding men's incompetence in this area, and because of the absence of positive examples of involved fatherhood in Ukraine. Economically, it is an advantage for men to continue working, since they generally have higher incomes and better opportunities for promotion and career advancement. In fact, traditionally, good fatherhood has been equated with (and, to an extent, limited to) financial support. These stereotypes are supported and promoted at the highest official levels in Ukraine.[8] Nonetheless, in recent years a growing number of fathers have taken parental leave; but this number remains very small (around 3%).[9]

Recent survey results also point to the dominance of traditional ideas about gender roles in the public sphere. Table 13.3 breaks down survey results that show Ukrainians' opinions about who should lead in which public sphere – men or women?

These results demonstrate that responsibilities related to child care and cultural work are considered more suitable for women, while responsibilities related to power, status, and prestige, such as in business

Table 13.2. Opinions of Men and Women on Who Should Earn the Most Money in the Family (%)

Answers	Men	Women	Average
Man	66	65	65
Woman	7	8	7
Both	21	18	19
Neither	1	1	1
Difficult to answer	6	8	7

Source: All-Ukrainian opinion poll conducted by the Institute of Sociology, National Academy of Science of Ukraine, 2007 (UNDP 2007, 71).

and politics, are considered the domain of men. These views map onto dominant views about qualities inherent to men and women. Thus, kindness, friendliness, discipline, diligence, and communication are considered to be more typical of women, whereas career orientation, high professionalism, and aggressiveness are more often seen to be men's characteristics (UNDP 2007, 54). In practice, these ideas convey many advantages to men in the sphere of employment and career, increasing their chances for jobs and advancement. Perhaps unsurprisingly, then, the transition to a market economy in Ukraine has brought with it an increased salary gap between men and women. According to data from the State Committee of Statistics, as of 2007, this gap was still in place, with men's average salary in all spheres being around 30 per cent more than that of women (DKSU 2007, 71).

Men in Crisis?

While benefiting from these advantages, men also experience higher expectations of success in the public sphere. In fact, the collapse of the USSR only intensified the pressure to emulate a work-focused masculine ideal. But that ideal was harder to attain because of the adverse economic conditions in Ukraine, which were most dramatic in the early and mid-1990s. This was a time of massive unemployment, descending mobility, and deterioration of living standards for most of the population. The resulting loss of social status for men was painful (Shevchenko 2002). Many men sought escape. As a result, this period was marked by an increase in alcohol and drug addiction. Many began to express

Table 13.3. Opinions on Whether Society (Selected Spheres) Would Function Better if Headed by a Woman or by a Man (%)

Spheres	If Headed by a Woman	If Headed by a Man	No Difference
Education	44	9	47
Culture	44	7	49
Social policy	45	14	41
Institutions that provide services to families and children	67	4	29
Politics	9	53	38
Big business	6	55	39
Law	9	37	54

Source: All-Ukrainian opinion poll conducted by the Institute of Sociology, National Academy of Science of Ukraine, 2007 (UNDP 2007, 37).

concern with the state of men's health, as they were living much shorter lives, experiencing much higher rates of illnesses such as tuberculosis (MFYSU 2006, 16), and committing suicide in greater numbers (KDSU 2007, 24). As of 2007, the average life expectancy of Ukrainian men was 62.3 years, almost twelve years less than that of women and among the lowest in Europe (Amdzhadin 2007). This number reflects early mortality among able-bodied men. In particular, Ukrainian men aged twenty to forty-five years die at a three times higher rate than women of the same age due to a range of genetic and social factors, including greater involvement by men in high-risk activities such as crime and employment in health-hazardous industries (MFYSU 2006, 16) like many construction and heavy metallurgy. Violent deaths are also many times more common for men than for women.

With regard to addiction, alcoholism is six to seven times more prevalent among Ukrainian men than women (MFYSU 2006, 18). Rural areas of Ukraine, where permanent employment is difficult to secure, and where vodka is commonly used as payment for men's assistance in household or farming tasks, are particularly affected by widespread alcoholism. Furthermore, public consumption of strong alcoholic drinks (at gatherings of friends or family or at work parties) is considered to be a way of displaying and proving masculinity. Thus, the refusal to drink is an obstacle to being a 'real' man. Drug addiction is also a bigger problem for men than women (p. 19).

One of the social reasons for men's poor health relates to traditional expectations of men's physical toughness (Thompson and Pleck 1986), which presumes physical strength, endurance, and firmness. Men often try to live up to this through activities intended to intensify masculine characteristics, like increasing muscle mass by pumping iron, doing martial arts, and participating in endurance sports. A more passive way to contend with this expectation and a more common one is for men to become attached to national sports teams and celebrity athletes (such as Ukrainian football teams, world boxing champions like the Klitschko brothers, and the world's strongest man in 2004, Vasyl Virastiuk). But expectations of toughness promote an exaggerated idea of men's physical endurance, which makes them inclined to disregard their health problems and not ask for medical help in time. Asking for help and public manifestation of weakness are often considered to be confessions of one's own 'weak' masculinity. Thus, current gender standards support men's unrealistically positive self-assessments of their health, their fear of looking weak, and their inclination towards risk in order to prove 'real' masculinity. Men pay the price for these behaviours with poor health, and sometimes with their lives.

The norm of physical toughness also requires that men express aggression in certain situations where choosing not to demonstrate violence could be considered to be a 'non-masculine' action. Reinforcing oneself via aggression is often used as a way to compensate for a man's inability to fulfil oneself otherwise. Much research indicates that men who are inclined to aggression often have low self-esteem and low social status (Burn 1996, 173–5). Criminal activity is generally gender-marked, and contemporary Ukraine is no exception in this regard. The number of men convicted for premeditated murder is more than seven times higher than the number of women (KDSU 2007, 86). A similar gender gap can be observed for other types of crimes (p. 86). Numerous studies show that most crimes are committed by young, often unemployed, working-class men (Edwards 2006, 11). Sometimes, lack of access to power, money, and resources also encourages men to compensate through family violence. According UNDP data, every third woman in Ukraine is a victim of violence from her male partner (Yabchenko 2009). Despite this high incidence, domestic violence is rarely discussed with regard to preventing men's aggression in Ukraine. The focus is on outcomes and support of victims, mostly accomplished by women's

NGOs. Until recently, the only men's NGO working on the prevention of domestic violence was Men against Violence, established in 2004 in the city of Kherson and consisting of thirty members. In March 2009 another similar NGO, the National Network of Men-Leaders against Violence, was founded in support of the United Nations multiyear international campaign 'Unite to End Violence against Women.'

Men's destructive behaviour and the crisis of Ukrainian men are the subjects of much popular literature and mass media in Ukraine; see, for example, the articles 'Devaluation of Men or Who Should Ukrainian Women Marry?' (Godovanets 2008) and 'Men Should Enter the Red Book!' (Pokotylo 2006), which create an image of men as extinct species. However, the nature of the crisis remains highly contested (Bureychak 2008). There is a difference between a 'crisis of masculinity' connected with changes to, and attempts to undermine hegemonic masculinity, and a 'crisis of men' (i.e., of men's experiences), which relates to destructive behaviour, stress, depression, aggression, violence, poor health, suicides, and so on. Although a crisis of masculinity may influence a crisis of men, there is no causal link. The destructive experiences of modern Ukrainian men are connected not with the crisis of masculinity (as a crucial reconsideration of the notion of masculinity), but with too-narrow, strict, and rigid norms of traditional masculinity that are promoted in modern Ukrainian society as a part of revitalizing and constructing a modern national identity, but which are difficult to attain for a number of reasons, including their being unrealistic and the lack of resources given an adverse economic situation.

Conclusions

The construction of masculinity in Soviet and post-Soviet Ukraine inevitably reflects state ideology, cultural norms, and social ideas dominant at the particular period. Even though both Soviet and post-Soviet ideals of masculinity appeal to traditional masculine ideals, their meanings and the conditions under which they are emulated vary considerably. The construction of modern Ukrainian masculinity often occurs as a rejection of the Soviet system and involves the invention of masculine ideals that correspond to a new Ukrainian national identity. In recent years, one can observe the intensification of traditional or patriarchal expectations of men's conduct. This is legitimized as a way to reconstruct an 'authentic' Ukrainian model of masculinity that was undermined by the Soviet regime. The common feature of both periods is that men hold more power and resources compared with women. At the same time, the pressure to succeed in the public and professional spheres makes men vulnerable in terms of health and socially destructive behaviour.

NOTES

1 Only in the 1980s did fatherhood issues somewhat reappear on the state agenda. For detailed discussion of this period see Chapter 14 in this volume.

2 More personifications existed, such as Soviet superheroes like Chekists or KGB-ists, but it is beyond the scope of this chapter to discuss them all.

3 Setting records and achievement in labour were built into the Soviet five-year economic plans. Labour competitions were also a part of state ideology aimed at proving the superiority of the USSR over capitalist countries.

4 *Moral'nyi Kodeks Stroitelya Communizma* (Moral Code of Builders of Communism), available at http://dic.academic.ru/dic.nsf/ruwiki/250607.

5 'New lad' is a concept of new masculinity that appeared and started to be promoted by men's magazines (such as *FHM*, *Maxim*, and *Loaded*) since the 1990s. Arguably, the emergence of an anti-feminist 'new lad' ideal can be a reaction to the 'new man' model – a narcissistic and pro-feminist man – that was popularized in men's magazines in the 1980s.

6 Mark Simpson (1994) refers by *metrosexuality* to a type of masculinity concerned with attractive appearance, shopping, and a wish to attract other people's attention and win their admiration.

7 Traditional conventions of looking define men as the subjects of gaze, thus conferring the symbolic power of gaze, while women are the object of looking. As John Berger puts it, in 'Ways of Seeing' (1972), men 'look at women. Women watch themselves being looked at' (p. 46). Thus, the advent of the attractive and eroticized man who is oriented towards being looked at by women undermines traditional ideas about whose gaze is powerful.

8 In his presentation to the roundtable discussion 'On the State of Men in Ukraine' before the Verkhovna Rada (Ukrainian parliament), on 19 February 2009, Olexandr Marchenko, president of the International Centre of Fatherhood and head of an all-Ukrainian Civic Committee on Family and Responsible Fatherhood, stressed that responsible fatherhood involves the participation of a man in the conception, games, school life, and sexual education of the child, the child's entrance into society, and being

a grandfather. Marchenko also emphasized that the crisis of fatherhood in Ukraine can be overcome by encouraging men who support their families and are good fathers, by which he meant fathers who provide financial support and spiritual education to their children. The participation of fathers in child care was never mentioned in the presentation. See www. civicua.org/main/data?t=2&c=1&q=1168230.

9 For more on this issue, see Chapter 14 in this volume.

REFERENCES

Amdzhadin, L. 2007. Genderni vidminnosti zdorovya ukrayintsiv [Gender Differences in Ukrainians' Health]. In M. Skoryk, ed., *Genderni Peretvorennia v Ukrayini* [*Gender Transformations in Ukraine*], 131–8. Kyiv: UNDP.

Attwood, L. 1996. The Post-Soviet Women in the Move to the Market: A Return to Domesticity and Dependence? In R. Marsh, ed., *Women in Russia and Ukraine*, 255–68. Cambridge: Cambridge University Press.

Berger, J. 1972 *Ways of Seeing*. London: BBC and Penguin Books.

Bonnell, V.E. 1999. *Iconography of Power: Soviet Political Posters under Lenin and Stalin*. Berkeley: University of California Press.

Bureychak, T. 2006. Kozak yak genderno-natsionalnyi marker Ukraininskoi consumerystskoi kultury [Cossack as Gender and National Marker of Ukrainian Consumer Culture]. *Methodologiya, teoriya ta praktyka sociologichnogo doslidzhenna ukrainskogo suspilstva* [Methodology, Theory and Practice of Sociological Research of Ukrainian Society] 2: 241–7.

– 2008. Kryza maskulinnosti v teoretychniy ta empirychniy perspectyvi [Crisis of Masculinity in Theoretical and Empiric Perspectives]. In *Genderni teorii ta genderni praktyky: nalagodzhuyuchy mosty* [Gender Theories and Gender Practices: Building Bridges], 20–7. Kharkiv: Raider.

Burn, S.M. 1996. *The Social Psychology of Gender*. New York: McGraw-Hill.

Chernova, Z. 2007. Model 'sovetskogo' otsovstva: diskursivnye predpisaniya [Model of 'Soviet' Fatherhood: Discursive Prescriptions]. In E. Zdravomyslov and A. Temkina, eds., *Rossiyskiy gendernyi poryadok: sociologicheskiy podhod.* [Russian Gender Order: Sociological Approach], 138–68. St Petersburg: Publishing House of the European University.

Connell, R.W. 1995. *Masculinities*. Cambridge: Polity.

Derzhavnyj komitet statystyky Ukrainy/State Committee of Statistics of Ukraine (DKSU). 2007. *Zhinky I choloviky v Ukraini: Statystychnyi zbirnyk* [Women and Men in Ukraine: Statistical Digest]. Kyiv: DKSU.

Edwards, T. 2006. *Cultures of Masculinity*. London: Routledge.

Gerasimova, E., and S. Chuikina. 2004. Obshchestvo remonta [Society of Renovation]. *Neprikosnovennyi zapas* [Reserve Stock] 34(2): 70–7. Also available at http://magazines.russ.ru/nz/2004/34/ger85.html.

Gilmour, J., and B.E. Clements. 2002. 'If You Want to Be Like Me, Train!' The Contradictions of Soviet Masculinity. In B.E. Clements, ed., *Russian Masculinities in History and Culture*, 210–22. New York: Palgrave.

Godovanets, O. 2008. Deval'vatsiya cholovikiv, abo za kogo vyhodyty zamizh ukrains'kym zhinkam? [Devaluation of Men or Who Should Ukrainian Women Marry?] *Glavred*, 24 July. Available at http://glavred.info/archive/2008/07/24/114129–7.html.

Golovakha, Y., and N. Panina. 2008. *Ukrainske suspilstvo 1992–2008: Sociologichnyi monitiryng* [Ukrainian Society 1992–2008: Sociological Monitoring]. Kyiv: Institute of Sociology NAS.

Haynes, J. 2003. *New Soviet Man: Gender and Masculinity in Stalinist Soviet Cinema*. Manchester: Manchester University Press.

Kis, O. 2003. Modeli konstruyuvannya gendernoi identychnosti zhinky v suchasniy Ukraini [Models of Construction of Gender Identity of Woman in Contemporary Ukraine]. *Ji* 27: 37–58. Available at http://www.ji.lviv.ua/n27texts/kis.htm.

Kon, I. 2001. Muskulistaya masculinnost: Atletizm ili militarism? [Muscular Masculinity: Athleticism or Militarism?] *Gendernye issledovaniya* [Gender Research] 6: 114–27.

– 2005. *Seksualnaya kul'tura v Rossii* [Sexual Culture in Russia]. Moscow: Airis-Press.

– 2006. Rossiyskiy muzhchina I ego problemy [Russian Man and His Problems]. *Mezhdiscyplinarnye issledovaniya: Sociologiya, psyhologiya, sexologiya, antropologiya* [Interdisciplinary Research: Sociology, Psychology, Sexology, Anthropology], 506–17.

Kosenko, L. 2006. *Kozaky: Lytsarkiy orden Ukrainy* [Cossacks: Knight Order of Ukraine]. Kyiv: Shkola.

Lafont, M. 2007. *Soviet Posters: The Sergo Grigorian Collection*. Munich: Prestel.

Lapidus, G.W. 1977. Sexual Equality in Soviet Policy: A Developmental Perspective. In D. Atkinson, A. Dallin, and G.W. Lapidus, eds., *Women in Russia*, 115–38. Stanford: Stanford University Press.

Lenin, V. 1918. *Decree of Soviet People's Commissars about Organization of Workers and Farmers Red Army*. 15 Jan. Available at http://www.aha.ru/~mausoleu/documents/army80.htm.

Magun, V.S. 1998. Rossiyskie trudovye tsennosti: Ideologiya i massovoe soznanie [Russian Labour Values: Ideology and Mass Consciousness]. *Mir Rossii* [*World of Russia*] 4: 113–44.

Ministry of Family, Youth, and Sports of Ukraine (MFYSU). 2006. *Zaluchennya cholovikiv do zberezhennya zdorovya v Ukraini. Analitychnyi zvit* [Involvement of Men in Health Care in Ukraine: Analytical Report]. Kyiv: MFYSU.

Pokotylo, O. 2006. Cholovikiv–v Chervonu knygu! [Men Should Enter the Red Book!] *Den'* [Day] no. 174, 12 Oct.

Pylat, V. 1994. *Boyovyi hopack* [Martial Hopack]. Lviv: Galytska Sich.

Rotkirch, A. 2000. *The Man Question: Loves and Lives in Late 20th Century Russia*. Helsinki: Department of Social Policy, University of Helsinki.

Semikhat, E. 2009. Media-obraz ukraintsa: Opyt sociologicheskogo issledovaniya sovetskogo kino [Media Image of a Ukrainian: Experience of Sociological Research of Soviet Films]. In *Naukovi studii L'vivskogo Sociologichnoho Forumu 'Tradicii ta innovatsii v sociologii'* [Academic Studies of Lviv Sociological Forum 'Traditions and Innovations in Sociology'], 246–52. Drogobych: Provit.

Shevchenko, O. 2002. Esli ty takoi umnyi, to pochemu takoi bednyi? Utverzhdaya muzhestvennost' technicheskoi intelligentsyi [If You Are So Smart, Why Are You So Poor? Affirmation of Masculinity by Technical Intelligentsia]. In S. Oushakine, ed., *O Muzhe(n)stvennosti* [On Masculinity]], 288–302. Moscow: Novoe literaturnoe obozrenie. Available at http://www.gender-studies.info/sbornik/muzhest/14.htm.

Simpson, M. 1994. Here Come the Mirror Men. *Independent*. 15 Nov. Available at http://www.marksimpson.com/pages/journalism/mirror_men.html (accessed 18 Aug. 2010).

Tartakovskaya, I. 2005. *Gendernaya sociologiya* [Sociology of Gender]. Moscow: Variant.

Thompson, E.H., and J.H. Pleck. 1986. The Structure of Male Role Norms. *American Behavioral Scientist* 9: 531–43.

United Nations Development Program (UNDP). 2007. *Genderni stereotypy ta stavlennya gromadskosti do gendernyh problem v ukrainskomu suspilstvi* [Gender Stereotypes and Social Attitudes to Gender Problems in Ukrainian Society]. Kyiv: UNDP.

Watson, P. 1993. Eastern Europe Silent Revolution: Gender. *Sociology* 27(3): 471–87.

Yabchenko, M. 2009. Choloviky lidery obyednuyut'sya, shchob zupynyty nasyl'stvo proty ukrainskyh zhinok [Men-Leaders Unite in Order to Stop Violence against Ukrainian Women]. Available at http://www.undp.org.ua/ua/media/1-undp-news/769-ukrainian-celebrities-join-un-led-stop-violence-against-women-campaig (accessed 17 Aug. 2010).

Yuval-Davis, N. 1997. *Gender and Nation*. London: Sage.

Zdravomyslova, E., and A. Temkina. 2002. Krizis masculinnosti v pozdne-
sovetskom diskurse. [Crisis of Masculinity in Late Soviet Discourse]. In
S. Oushakine, ed., *O Muzhe(n)stvennosti* [On Masculinity], 432–51. Moscow:
Novoe literaturnoe obozrenie.

– 2007a. Sovetskiy etakraticheskiy gendernyi poryadok [Soviet Etacratic
Gender Order]. In E. Zdravomyslova and A. Temkina, eds., *Rossiyskiy gendernyi poryadok: Sociologicheskiy podhod* [Russian Gender Order: Sociological Approach], 96–137. St Petersburg: Publishing House of the European
University.

– 2007b. Sovetkie gendernye kontrakty i ikh transformatsyia v sovremennoi
Rossii [Soviet Gender Orders and Their Transformation in Modern Russia].
In E. Zdravomyslova and A. Temkina, eds., *Rossiyskiy gendernyi poryadok:
Sociologicheskiy podhod* [Russian Gender Order: Sociological Approach], 169–
200. St Petersburg: Publishing House of the European University.

Zhurzhenko, T. 2008. *Gendernye rynki Ukrainy: politicheskaya ekonomia
natsyonal'nogo stroitelstva* [Gendered Markets of Ukraine: Political Economy
of National Building]. Vinus: EGU.

14 Cash and/or Care: Current Discourses and Practices of Fatherhood in Ukraine

IRYNA KOSHULAP

> The family, childhood, motherhood, and *fatherhood* are under the State's protection.
>
> – Constitution of Ukraine, 1996, Article 51 (emphasis added)

It is hard to assess how many men in Soviet times and in the early years of Ukrainian independence had to tramp the grass behind maternity hospitals as part of their rite of passage to fatherhood, but the experience of waiting for the news about the newborn under the hospital windows is believed to have been almost uniform. It was a part of Soviet folklore and continues to feed numerous jokes, caricatures, and comic episodes in various movies and television shows. Indeed, the personnel-and-expecting-mothers-only entry to the maternity hospitals and wards (for the sake of sterility and hygiene), the prevailing medical ethics of having more important things to do than providing updates to the relatives of the woman who has just become a mother (or has she yet?), and the limited visitation times for family to see the newborn and mother (and then only through a prison-like glass wall) made young fathers' pilgrimage to the windows of maternity hospitals all the more poignant.

Not only poignant, however, but also overwhelmingly acceptable, raising no reaction apart from some innocent humour around the topic of the tipsy young men. The blatant exclusion of fathers from any access to their children in the first days of their lives was merely a reflection of the existing expectations the society had about a father's share in his child's upbringing. Nurturing, child care, and emotional attachment to a baby were never legitimate parts of Soviet hegemonic masculinity. The overall marginal meaning given to fatherhood was communicated in state legislation and welfare policy – both directed at protecting and supporting the mother and child without recognizing father's rights or encouraging his responsibility towards his children. Consequently, the prominence given to fathers as equal parents in the new Family Code,[1] and the promotion of 'conscious fatherhood' (*svidome bat'kivstvo*) by the government of Ukraine in the mid-2000s, marked what can be evaluated as revolutionary changes. At the same time, little attention has been paid to determining whether, with these newly recognized rights and duties, Ukrainian men were ready to shoulder the burden of fatherhood.

In this chapter, I offer a closer look at the ideals behind the 'new father' in contemporary Ukraine and show that 'conscious fatherhood' has come to integrate two competing images – a traditional view of the primary role of a father as breadwinner, and ideas of involved fatherhood, which stress the importance of the father–child connection – to address needed changes to children's development, men's emotional fulfilment, and more egalitarian and harmonious family life. While maintaining the requirement that men be breadwinners, in conscious fatherhood, involved parenting has been proclaimed to be 'in the best interests' of men themselves, and, for the first time, nurturing and primary caregiving are conceived as legitimate aspects of fathering. Most importantly, for the first time, the whole discussion on fathers' involvement has outgrown the pages of expert literature on parenting and entered government policy making and popular discourse.

The father-nurturer, however, has turned out to be a challenging role for young men in Ukraine to embrace; despite being seen as highly desirable, fathers' involvement in child care is the exception rather than the norm. To complement existing statistics – which seem to prove that traditional gender stereotypes related to the 'proper' distribution of family roles take a lifetime to change towards more egalitarian views – this chapter presents a discussion of the experience of young fathers in ten Ukrainian families who welcomed their first child during the period when fatherhood began to receive enhanced attention from the state and the public. As different as their stories are, they all bring to light the main contradictions between the ideal and lived practices of fathering, compelling us to reflect upon the influence that public discourses have on individual men's lives.

Images of Fatherhood in Ukraine: Past and Present

Fatherhood and Gender Equality in the USSR

As a sociocultural coding of men as parents, 'fatherhood' involves certain discourses and practices that define the rights and obligations as well as the status of fathers (Hobson and Morgan 2002, 10). It is generally agreed that during the Soviet era, notwithstanding fluctuations in state ideology, men were perceived to be workers, soldiers, and citizens, and there was no place for fatherhood in their profile (Ashwin 2000). Recent changes in the state and public discourses on fatherhood in Ukraine have been influenced by a number of factors, including the Soviet legacy in the area of social provision, the country's economic development, and the ideals of modernity and Europeanness.

To say that in the Soviet Union fatherhood did not become an object of explicit state politics does not mean to claim that the state was a bystander in the processes that shaped it. As some researchers have argued, the whole project of women's emancipation and the state's efforts to engage women in paid labour were triggered not so much by a true commitment to gender equality or urgent economic necessity as by the need to challenge the rule of the father-patriarch, who stood in the way of the state's new ideology regarding other family members (Kukhterin 2000). By proclaiming marriage to be a union of equal partners and by recognizing the rights of children born out of wedlock as early as 1917, the state made its first confident steps towards deeming individual fathers redundant (Ashwin 2000, 14–15).[2] These policies were further supported by declaring the protection of mothers and children to be mainly the duty of the state and by adhering to an economic model that engaged dual-earner families.

Having stripped fathers of their traditional authority as patriarchs and having weakened their role as breadwinners, the state did not, however, propose new responsibilities for men within the family. Instead, achievement at work and success in the public sphere laid the basis for the masculinity of the new Soviet man. The domestic sphere became associated with women, who very soon were expected to both take up full-time paid employment and maintain the burden of housework and child care by themselves, with some assistance from public services. This gender division of care-work was maintained with remarkable consistency through all the changes in state family policies over the decades of Soviet rule.

Some favourable circumstances for a slow rehabilitation of men's inclusion into the private sphere started to emerge in the 1980s, when lower birth rates in the European part of the USSR made the country's leaders pay attention to the family once again. Provisions were introduced in 1981–82 aimed at encouraging families to have more children, but they were designed with the same traditional gender expectations in mind – a longer maternity leave for women, as primary caregivers, to combine their work and family life, as well as additional child care allowances to compensate for the loss of the wife's salary, and thus to buffer the additional financial burden put on the family. By that time, however, the state's failure to provide sufficient public facilities that could help women juggle their paid employment and motherhood had become evident. A survey conducted in 1978 showed that over the previous decade available public facilities had reduced women's engagement with household work by only 5 per cent (Zhurzhenko 2002). Never backing away from its commitment to develop a more efficient system of public support in the near or distant future, the state looked for alternative resources, leading to renewed attention towards men and their contribution to the life of a family (p. 56).

The family policies that came out of this renewed attention never went so far as to make specific mention of fathers or fatherhood. The expert literature on family and child care, however, in the form of manuals for young parents, which acted as 'soft' propaganda for the state,[3] did begin to address men's parenting responsibilities by introducing and testing some new ideas in the safer context of a limited but very targeted readership. Literature on family and parenting published during the 1980s began to remind men that they had equal rights and responsibilities for their children's upbringing and that a proper fulfilment of their parental role was their 'moral duty and legal obligation' (Soloviev 1988, 5). Husbands were encouraged to take up an equal share of domestic work as part of this obligation, as opposed to 'helping out' their wives on occasion. Still, even the most outspoken advocates of fathers' involvement with children saw the father's role as complementary to that of the mother. This distribution was explained by natural differences between the sexes: 'It has always been important to organize family's leisure time, especially at weekends and holidays. This is where the father with his male's managerial experience comes into the picture. There is one simple reason for this – mother is preoccupied with other activities which are not of a lesser importance . . . In other words, while the mother is cooking dinner, father is engaged with children' (p. 13).

Describing the new generation of men who were ready to embrace some child care duties as 'proud,' 'thoughtful,' 'self-respecting,' 'most prudent,' 'energetic,' and 'creative,' the authors of these manuals took particular care to underline that involved fatherhood did not mean feminization of men and was quite compatible with traditional masculine features. To substantiate this, examples were provided to show that men could use their 'craftsman' skills in this process: 'The creativity with which some [fathers] invent different gadgets is amazing. One of them made an alarm lamp that indicates that the diapers need to be changed. Another set up a mike on the balcony so that the baby's cry could be heard in the room. And such examples are numerous' (Grebeshova et al. 1990, 26).

Involved fatherhood was presented as a challenge and an achievement for a modern man whose experience with child care was limited at the beginning, but who could easily master this 'unsophisticated science' (Kaliuzhyn and Deriugina 1990, 65). It proved hard to make nurturing sound compatible with masculinity, however, especially since most of the expert literature was heavily imbued with traditional ideas about the father's role as educator and mentor rather than caregiver. Analysing the shifts in gender roles in the public and private spheres during perestroika, Meshcherkina (2000) concludes that men were reluctant to take up housework or child care because they saw these as a 'women's job.' The total feminization of caregiving and teaching professions, together with the continuing glorification of motherhood, supported this view, which was shared by the majority of women, too; women expressed highly traditionalist views on family gender roles despite advocating for gender equality in the public sphere (ibid.).

The unwillingness of men to accept a greater share of housework and child care in response to women's increasing involvement in the paid labour market has been continuous across post-Soviet and Western countries. Similarly, a surprisingly high number of women have remained unwilling to relinquish their role as the primary parent and housekeeper (Kukhterin 2000, 72; Kay 2006; Hobson and Morgan 2002). Current research no longer tries to explain this through the idea of false consciousness, but rather shows that motherhood can be more fulfilling and empowering for women than many advocates for change have wanted to admit (Dienhart 1998). This does not mean that men should be limited in their parenting involvement; in the end, they are the ones who can gain from it despite the sacrifice that is required to raise a child.

Changing Images of Fatherhood in Post-Soviet Ukraine:
Coding a New Father in the Family Code

Changes in family and gender politics in independent Ukraine have had multiple effects on the institution of fatherhood. 'Protection of women' – the main, underlying principle of Soviet gender politics – was replaced by ideas of gender equality and human rights, and the family was proclaimed to be at the core of nation building. The state was to create 'favourable conditions' for the revival of 'family values,' which were said to have been ruined by the Soviet ideology (Zhurzhenko 2004). Starting from the mid-1990s, state family policies explicitly guaranteed not only the sovereignty and autonomy of a family's decision making, but also equality and partnership between women and men in all spheres of life; that is, the policies were designed to provide women and men with equal opportunities in the labour market and in the private sphere, including parenting and a fair division of family duties. For Ukrainian men, this meant official recognition of their right to fatherhood, which was now protected by the law and, unlike through Soviet equal-rights policies, included the right to be a primary caregiver.

The need to provide fathers with the same rights to shorter work-days in full-time employment, parental leave, and various subsidies was first voiced during perestroika. However, these and other rights were not granted to fathers until the 1990s. By 1992, 'support for mothers with many children,' for instance, was transformed into an 'allowance for mothers/fathers who look after three or more children under sixteen' (Alekseenko et al. 2004, 183). Maternal leave was replaced with parental leave, which includes a job guarantee and pen-sion entitlement, and can be used by either parent or shared. Most family benefits are now payable to a 'parent who is looking after the child' rather than to a mother (p. 183). Furthermore, the equality of rights of both parents is stated in the 1996 Constitution, and the underlying principle of the new 2002 Family Code is to eliminate any preferential rights in custody or claims for alimony for either parent.

It was this recognition of men's parenting rights that was seen to be among the most progressive provisions of the Family Code and was considered a big step forward to gender equality in Ukraine. As it serves national interests, the commitment to extend gender equality has also been used as a marker and proof of Ukraine's 'European choice.' On its official website, the Ministry of Justice of Ukraine opens the discussion of the changes in family regulations with, 'Being on the crossroads between the East and West, Ukraine slowly but steadily walks towards Europe' (Pavlova 2007). The authors of the Family Code stressed that they used 'the best European experience' when drafting regulations related to family issues, and that the new law was compatible with European legislation (Parliament of Ukraine 2000; Konovalov 2004).

'European,' however, has come to be applied to nearly any context. Perceived as a synonym for 'new' and 'modern,' it has been used not only to qualify provisions that have been adopted in accordance with international norms, but also to deny any connection with Soviet practices, even in cases where a new law closely resembled an old one. For example, with regard to the Family Code, this rhetoric of 'European approaches' helped to justify some more conservative rather than modern attitudes to family and presented an overwhelmingly generalized view of the 'European' experience, neglecting the diversity of family law across Europe. Defining marriage as a union between a man and a woman and claiming this to be in line with the European standard, Ukrainian lawmakers obviously missed the fact that six European Union countries legally recognize same-sex marriages and many more give same-sex civil unions identical or very similar rights to marriage.[4]

'Conscious Fatherhood'

Ukrainian legislators, however, rightly noticed that without more active promotion of a positive image of involved fatherhood, and without the introduction of some direct incentives, men would not rush to embrace their new rights and responsibilities in the family. This has been a shared experience of all European countries, which are still trying to put official 'parental equality' into practice.[5] Even in Sweden, where men have been reminded of the benefits of active parenting since the early 1970s, the introduction of 'father month' or 'daddy month' as a part of parental leave in 1994 did not go as smoothly as expected and required further campaigning and additional incentives for families to use it eagerly (Bergman and Hobson 2002; Hearn 2006, 132).

In Ukraine, with its decades-long history of marginalized fatherhood, there could be no expectation of quick and easy change. Shortly after the adoption of the new Family Code, the Ukrainian Parliamentary Committee on Gender Equality (2006) recommended more active promotion of 'conscious fatherhood' that would raise the social status of fathers and eliminate gender discrimination in the family. Suggestions ranged from amendments that would encourage men to take parental leave, to the establishment of an official Father's Day, and the introduction of 'schools for daddies' that would prepare men for fathering.

None of the above have been implemented so far, with the exception of the few 'schools for daddies' established in some local communities as a result of the efforts of non-governmental organizations (NGOs). At the same time, several projects have been introduced by different state bodies to popularize the idea of 'conscious fatherhood.' In 2006, the Ministry for Family, Youth, and Sport, which has as one of its priorities the promotion of a father's role in the family, ran a social advertising campaign called 'Holding the Father Tighter by the Hand' (Z bat'kom za ruku mitsnishe). Big posters depicting two silhouettes easily identifiable as a father and little son going fishing could be found in every big city and small town in Ukraine. In 2005, the mayor of Kyiv introduced an award for single fathers who were raising their children by themselves: Each year, during the official celebration of the International Day of Families in Kyiv, ten young fathers received a certificate of merit and 1,000 UAH. Winners of this Single Daddy of the Year award were selected based on 'the father's success in the child's upbringing, his achievements in the social sphere, the child's achievements at studies and extracurricular activities, and the family's welfare and living conditions' (Office of the Mayor of Kiev 2006). In 2008, the financial part of the award was doubled, and its terms were revised to include single mothers along with fathers. This move could arguably allow placing the single fathers, who often stand out as something exotic and extraordinary, into the broader context of one-parent families. At the same time, by choosing to use 'single fathers and single mothers' throughout the new mayor's decree, instead of the generic 'parent,' as well as by establishing ten separate awards in each category, it was ensured that the fathers who raise their children without spousal support continue receiving recognition and assistance.

For a while, it even became popular among male state officials to tell personal stories about their participation in their children's upbringing. Their message: that a tight work schedule cannot serve as an excuse – being a good father is one of the main responsibilities of a modern man. To quote the Minister of Family, Youth, and Sport of the time, 'It is very important that a father finds time for communication with his children. That's why, whenever I have a spare moment, I try to spend that time with my sons. And that's why I often take my wife and children to different events in which I have to participate' (Pavlenko 2006). President Viktor Yushchenko (2006) often took up the job of personally popularizing the idea of conscious fatherhood: 'Being a father of five and a grandfather of two, I try to spend all my free time, even if it's not more than a couple of hours per week, with my children. Often we spend this time doing sports and games, we go swimming together, ski, play some ball games, and hike. I know that these are the best and the happiest moments for my kids.'

When one of the most popular TV anchormen, Oles' Tereschenko, became a father, it was highlighted as 'the most welcome news of the day' on the evening news. In addition to information on the baby's weight and the usual congratulations to the parents, the broadcast noted that the father was beside his wife during the eight-hour delivery. Oles' confessed that it had not been an easy decision to take, but it was worth it – he really felt as if they both were giving birth to the child, the reporter detailed. This is one of a growing number of examples of favourable media representations of a father's responsible attitude to his parenting role. Be it a discussion of the importance of the introduction of Father's Day (Korrespondent 2007) or a personal story of a stay-at-home dad, fathers' involvement in nurturing and caring for their children is welcome, even if sometimes proponents have to admit, with regret, that this is much more of a trend in the West than in Ukraine (Husachenko 2006).

There is some evidence that a pinch of pessimism about the willingness of Ukrainian fathers to join the trend is not totally groundless. In terms of sheer numbers, only 1 per cent of one-parent families are male-headed, and only up to 3 per cent of children stay with their father after divorce, while custody is granted to fathers almost exclusively in cases when a mother abandons the child (Ukrainian Parliamentary Committee 2006). Another media product, a documentary *Who Will Sing a Lullaby* (*Khto zaspivaie kolyskovu*; Rudik 2006), filmed with the support of the International Ukrainian Women's Fund and the Open Society Institute, depicts the challenges and misunderstandings that men face if they decide to take parental leave and shows the resiliency of the belief that child care is a 'woman's job.'

As these examples demonstrate, understandings of fathers' involvement with children can range from the more traditional paradigm, where it complements a mother's caregiving (playing, going fishing), to the role of a father-caregiver who can be a substitute for the mother (Single Daddy Award, schools for daddies, encouragement of fathers to take parental leave). It is the latter perception that is the most challenging to establish after the decades of feminization of child care. However, history shows that even the most persistent gender stereotypes could take less than a generation to vanish (Dienhart 1998). After all, while at the beginning of 2007, a husband present at a delivery made the news, in 2008, some city hospitals reported that over 80 per cent of couples opted for partner labours.[6]

Breadwinners Despite Themselves?

In the new discourses around fatherhood, a man's role as bread-winner is rarely mentioned, except in relation to divorced and non-resident fathers. This has happened not because decades of women's employment have erased the expectation that a man should provide for the family – this expectation is simply taken for granted, and thus is not seen as requiring additional acknowledgment. Access to paid work undoubtedly enhanced women's financial independence. However, studies of the Soviet labour market as well as the most recent reports on gender equality in Ukraine confirm the persistence of a nearly 30 per cent pay gap and high job segregation throughout the history of women's employment in this country (Ashwin 2000, 13; Kukhterin 2000, 73). As a result, a man's 'natural' role as the family's main breadwinner has rarely been challenged, even though few men can actually boast of being the only family providers. In a way, their work and money has long been the only legitimate contribution to the family and household that husbands and fathers have been able to make. This becomes particularly obvious in cases of long-term unemployment, which causes feelings of shame and helplessness for men as they fall out of the labour market and, with few exceptions, fail to find a position in the household that would be acceptable for them and their family (Ashwin and Lytkina 2004).

In granting more independence to individual families, the Ukrainian government has also toyed with the idea of shifting most of the financial burden connected with child rearing to parents. A new approach to the distribution of responsibilities among the state, family, and society was spelled out in the government program 'Children of Ukraine' (1996),[7] which specified that the family 'should be the main source of financial and emotional support, and of psychological security.' The state took up the obligation to promote the legal and social protection of children, but assumed direct responsibility only for certain categories of children, primarily those being raised without parental support or in 'problem families.' In line with this, alimony payments were regulated to make it more difficult to evade them and to create stricter penalties for non-payment (Alekseenko et al. 2004, 165).

Liberal approaches have not gained enough support in Ukraine, however, and the ensuing yet temporary shift from universal family welfare to a means-based system was mainly dictated by the need to optimize the limited economic resources available at that time. While most of the family allowances provided under previous Soviet legislation were kept and some new provisions were added, state family support remained nominal for a long time and was more of a declaration of intention than an effective system that would reduce the cost of having children. The decreased value of allowances resulting from inflation and constant delays in payments made the situation even worse. One example of the government's helplessness in the context of economic deficit was the Presidential Decree on the Improvement of the Welfare of Families with Many Children (1999),[8] which did not increase family support payments for these families, as might have been expected, but only required a timely payment of the family benefits (Zhurzhenko 2002, 154).

Under such circumstances, the role of the father as breadwinner became much more important, especially during the initial period when the mother had to withdraw from the labour market and rely on child care payments while looking after the baby. Beginning in 2005, riding a new wave of pro-natalist politics, which aimed to increase birth rates in a country that was experiencing a continuous population decline, child allowances were increased considerably compared with previous years. However, this has never been discussed as a new opportunity for men to relieve their worries about providing for the family and free more of their time for looking after their children. Maybe this is because state support has not yet reached a high enough level; but whatever the reason, as my interviews show, cash and care has not been conceptualized as an either-or option for fathers yet.

Fathering a Baby in Modern Ukraine: Insiders' Opinions

State politics represent only one of the discourses around fatherhood; these set certain conditions for, but do not determine the actual practices of fathering. In assessing men's performance as fathers, researchers point out the important role of personal experience and the models of parenting set forth by one's own family, conditions created by the market economy, religious beliefs, not to say attachment to the child's mother (Lupton and Barclay 1997, 140; Ostner 2002, 165; Dienhart 1998).

There is evidence to claim that, in Ukraine, the idea of 'conscious fatherhood' is currently countered by prevalent gender stereotypes that favour traditional views on the distribution of roles between the parents. According to a recent survey, when it comes to questions of parenting, the majority of men (93%) and women (96%) support the idea that both parents should take equal part in a child's upbringing. In addition, 87 per cent of men and 83 per cent of women believe that fathers can be as good and caring parents as mothers. However, the age of a child turns out to be important in this assessment, and when the question is placed with regard to the care of a small child (under 3 years of age), only 54 per cent of men and 58 per cent of women agree that a father can cope. Besides, 13 per cent of men and 11 per cent of women add that they cannot imagine such an arrangement for their family anyway.[9]

Drawing on interviews with ten couples who have young children,[10] I examine the actual versus desirable involvement of fathers in their children's upbringing, their understanding of parental responsibilities, their emotional attachment to the child, and their perception of the compatibility of child care with masculinity. I name three major types of fathering based on fathers' participation in child care. However, I also focus on discourses that can be traced across these groups and that appear to be formative for the men's perception of their role as fathers.

Before making any generalizations about the role of the state and other discourses in the construction of fatherhood in Ukraine, it should be noted that this study embraces only the experiences of married, first-time fathers who live in the Western region of Ukraine; the differences that may exist across groups with other educational, ethnic, or religious backgrounds remain unexplored here. The choice of the sample group is based on several factors, including the generally accepted idea that the politics of fatherhood are usually directed at middle-class men. Men belonging to different minority groups (ethnic, sexual, and so on) can be denied benefits offered by the system, and their practices of fatherhood can be described as deviant in contrast to the hegemonic ones. In addition, the conditions and practices of fathering change through a man's lifespan, being influenced by the child's growing independence (Curran and Abrams 2000; Hearn 2006, 253), as well as by changes in employment patterns for both parents and the entry of other children into the family (Lupton and Barclay 1997, 141). To exclude these variables from the study, I focused on early-stage, first-time parenting and existing discourses around that experience.

Given the homogeneity of the families interviewed and the limited number of interviews, the sample cannot be seen as representative. Instead, it offers insight into the perception of state policy by fathers, the direct and indirect effects that those policies and discourses have on the division of child care duties within the family, and the issues that still need to be addressed to make the state policies that are related to fatherhood more efficient.

Fathers, Dads, and Daddies

In all the families that participated in the study, it was the mother who took the parental leave and stayed with the child most of the time. When it came to discussing the father's role in raising children, the ideas expressed by both men and women resonated with the general public discourse on conscious fatherhood; fathers' actual partici-pation in child care varied noticeably, according to the same interviews. Borrowing some of the terminology from earlier research (Hovorun et al. 2004), one can single out three types of fathers among my interviewees: the 'father-nurturer,' the 'child's best friend,' and the 'helping hand.'

As the promising code-name 'father-nurturer' suggests, this type of father could be a substitute for a mother in any activity. It was a matter of very little surprise that in my sample there was only one father who, although not a primary caregiver, took up the equal parenting role and found it rewarding. Despite working two jobs, he tries to use every available opportunity to spend time with his daughter. He manages the baby with confidence without seeking advice or assistance from his wife and is proud of being such a skilful parent. Since his wife was very weak after the delivery and could hardly get up from bed, he took a two-week leave from work to help with the baby: 'That's when I learned how to hold her, change diapers, put her to bed – how to be a real father.' He refers to this learning process as having been a challenge at the beginning, but unlike other fathers, who often felt embarrassed when they could not cope with the baby or had to ask for help, our 'father-nurturer' perceived it to be a natural process and did not feel any discomfort:

> When the baby arrives no one knows how to do certain things [. . .] mothers have to learn it as well. Then the better you come to know your baby, the easier it becomes. You can tell the hunger cry from the hey-you-I-need-my-diaper-changed cry from the I'm-bored-from-lying-in-my-bed-all-alone one.

Fathers for whom the role of the 'child's best friend' was most compelling engage with their child's upbringing at a later stage, when it becomes 'interesting' to play with the baby. They compare their experiences of fatherhood with 'returning to their own childhood,' when even reading a fairy tale is turned into a performance with every animal having its own voice. Neither housework nor child care belongs to a father's profile for them, which is why they find it difficult to 'bond' with the baby during the first year. A child is like a family guest who causes trouble and is the wife's responsibility. Another apt comparison is to say that the baby is like a caterpillar that will eventually turn into a playful butterfly, and the fathers in this group seem to be waiting patiently for that moment to arrive (Hovorun et al. 2004, 78). Or, as one of the fathers put it:

> A child is such a thing which you wouldn't like to break, you can hurt it. I wouldn't risk doing something wrong, so it's better to be on the safe side. As the child grows up, learns some basic things, it becomes more interesting. I can take it for a walk, for example. I also get more used to it, learn some things and professionalize as a father. So the interaction between us grows.

It is important to mention here that wives in this group do not demand much of their husbands, believing that a father has little to offer during the first year of a baby's life, or that mothers are 'naturally better' at child care.

Most men in my study fall into the third category of a 'helping hand' father, for whom patterns of behaviour and attitudes can range between those of a father-nurturer and those of a father-playmate. Despite being quite active fathers, they remain in secondary roles and are helping their wives rather than substituting for them. In general, men in this group say that they can do any domestic work, if their wives need help, and can look after the baby, if they have time for it.

Early physical contact with the baby right after birth seems to be among the important factors that help men develop emotional ties with their child and engage in their care in the early stages. Those men who were present during the delivery and/or had to take care of the child right afterwards, as well as those who attended prenatal classes were better at 'bonding' with the newborn and more willing to take up the nurturing role.[11]

Why Can't Men Nurture?

Although the above examples show that the actual practices of fathering vary considerably, most of the parents were quite unanimous in their definition of a good father. That he should 'spend time with the child' was by far the most frequent answer given by both men and women. And even though this could imply a number of different activities, from bathing and putting the baby to bed to going out for a walk together, more often than not the answers revealed that it did not matter how the time was spent as long as it was spent together with the baby. Just 'being there' to help raise the child or to set an example seemed to be the best thing a father could offer to confirm his love and responsible attitude. This was directly or indirectly contrasted with the father's responsibility to earn money, which was important, but could not justify the father's absence. Describing his childhood, one of the male interviewees complained:

> My brother and I saw our father only on Sundays. He worked, he had lots of money – his pockets were always packed full with it, but there was no father around.

A number of the interviewed fathers saw their responsibilities to make a living and participate in the upbringing of the child as competing, and they acknowledged that the latter was more important for them than the former. Mothers also named their husband's work as impeding their 'real' involvement. One mother said:

> He works Saturdays, so he spends only Sundays with the child. What kind of participation in the upbringing is that? The father should be there, should teach the child, educate him, be an example.

'To set his own example' was representative of these families' expectations concerning a father's involvement in the upbringing as well. 'Teaching' and 'educating,' either through 'explaining things' or 'setting his own example' were named as the most important roles for fathers. At the same time, child care, if mentioned at all, was discussed in terms of 'helping' the wife or 'being able to substitute for the mother in almost everything.' Thus, it is the mother who is considered to be a primary caregiver, while the father's duty is education of the child. This division of roles between parents is visible in sharper contrast if the responsibilities of a 'good mother' are added to the analysis. First of all, unlike a father, for whom the time he should spend with the child and the particular duties are not specified, for a mother, as some parents confirmed, the expectation is clear that she should 'give all her time to the child' and 'the child should be in the first place for her.' Most of her duties are reduced to nurturing, with only one mother mentioning that in addition to making sure that

> the baby should have the diapers changed on time, be fed and not to cry. . .
> a good mother has to play with the child, to develop him or her.

Both men and women clearly define a mother's primary responsibilities as nurturing and caregiving, but men tend to describe these duties in general terms. Instead of saying what a good mother must do, they usually specify personal characteristics that a good mother should exemplify, including been 'caring,' 'patient,' 'compassionate,' 'kind,' 'loving,' and 'hardworking.' In this way, they perceive mothering as requiring some traditionally feminine qualities. One of the fathers even used the term 'maternal instincts' when talking about a good mother:

> First, all her maternal instincts should be okay; that is, the child should be in the first place for her and then everything else. And it is difficult to add anything to it.

A number of the interviewed women observed that even though their husbands felt comfortable displaying emotions when they were with the baby at home, they avoided doing so in public, sometimes, as one mother described, to the extent of passing the pram to the mother whenever the baby started crying so that nobody would think the father was the one who was soothing the child. This last example can also be interpreted in terms of the fear many young fathers harbour that they may not be able to manage the baby in the right way, as they generally lack experience doing it. Such fear abets a vicious circle where limited contact with the baby prevents fathers from learning all the necessary skills, while not knowing how to manage the baby discourages them from taking up child care. Forwarded by both fathers and mothers, a standard justification for this reluctance was that a father could change the diapers or prepare some food, but, as one of the men in the study put it:

> The mother spends more time with him [the baby] and knows how to do it better.

Want to Be European?

Although 'a good father is a good father everywhere,' as one male interviewee said, 'there can be a difference between an average Ukrainian and Western fathers,' said another. He explained:

> Our parents want to interfere more, want to 'discipline.' In the West, I guess, though I've never been there, parents and kids are more autonomous, more equal in their rights. Our kids know their place and look up at/to their parents; over there it's the opposite.

Half of all references to 'the West' or Europe made in the interviews included this idea of higher equality of rights, not only between parents and children, but between the parents themselves; and although in general more women paid attention to these assumptions, men shared the view, too. One of them said:

> In the West, a woman cannot be considered a servant, men and women don't have such rigid roles there, while in Ukraine we see the traditional view on duties in the majority of families – husband earns money, wife

does shopping. Well, husband can also shop with her if they need to carry a lot of bags from the store [laughing].

Another area of discussion that was brought up in relation to 'Europe' was the connection between fathers, child care, and emotional attachment. Several interviewees mentioned that European fathers were 'kinder' and 'joking all the time,' while Ukrainian fathers were rather reserved. 'Maybe we were just raised like that,' said one mother. Five out of twenty interviewees noted that fathers were 'better respected' in other countries, not in terms of having greater authority, but in their ways of experiencing fatherhood. They could have fun and enjoy being fathers. As one of the male interviewees put it, he would like to participate in all those '"father and son ballroom dances" and other ridiculous things they do together on Father's Day,' but cannot, as there is no Father's Day in Ukraine yet.

No one mentioned any financial responsibilities for fathers when reflecting on the European practices of parenting: all the comments were about care, not cash. State support was also discussed in the context of encouraging men to become involved fathers, with little reference to social payments or any other type of family benefits, and such support was seen as positive and needed. One interviewee explained:

> From what we know, maybe the main difference is that the state encourages fathers' involvement. They organize prenatal courses for the couple where fathers also do some exercises, have to wear a belly to feel what it feels to be pregnant themselves. In our country, no one encourages fathers to attend those courses. They are called *Shkola materynstva* (motherhood schools) – what father would go there?

Conclusions

The popularization of the idea of 'conscious fatherhood,' which embraces a man's involvement in child care alongside his breadwinning obligations, is quite recent in Ukraine. It took form under the influence of a number of contradictory discourses and aims at promoting the status of fathers in a society where, as statistics show, egalitarian views on the distribution of rights and responsibilities in the public sphere are combined with traditionalist expectations about family gender roles. It is hard to argue that state-led discourses have a defining influence on day-to-day practices of fathering; but as incomplete and often contradictory as the state promotion of 'conscious father-hood' has been, the qualitative data in my study demonstrate that it has affected at least perceptions among individual fathers, and therefore, it should be seen as an important first step towards the legitimization of fathering and men's attachment to their children as a part of proper masculinity.

More willing to take up additional financial responsibilities than to look after a newborn, the young fathers in my study, however, see the real or imagined opportunities of spending time with children enjoyed by German or Swedish fathers as an example to look up to. The most common difficulties that men in Ukraine face on their way to involved fatherhood are the absence of male role models from their own child-hood that they can draw from, and gender stereotypes that depict nur-turing or emotional involvement as feminine and thus endangering their masculinity. Many fathers, even those who do not adhere to the traditional distribution of parental roles, find it 'safer' to wait until the child grows up enough to be worthy of their attention and to leave all the child care responsibilities to mothers until that time. One may want to conclude that men in Ukraine are far from being ready to enjoy the right of parental leave; but it may be more accurate to say that gender equality in both the public and private spheres should be promoted and enforced as a whole before men and women can embrace the idea of a truly shared parenthood. Indeed, when one of my male interview-ees heard the question, 'Would you consider taking the parental leave instead of your wife if she was earning more than you?' and snapped back, 'I cannot imagine where she could earn more than me,' he was probably being quite sincere and accurate in his assessment of women's career opportunities in today's Ukraine.

For gender-conscious legislation to become a success story, it must be seen as a beginning, not the end of the campaign for shared par-enting. The hospitals that proudly announce a considerable increase in the number of partner labours had to redesign the delivery rooms as well as train their personnel to make it possible for fathers to be present during the birth of their child. Prenatal schools for parents that manage to engage fathers-to-be in their courses made an effort to de-sign classes that would be relevant for both parents and to create a sup-portive atmosphere for them. There is still a considerable amount of work to be done to transform the public sector into a father-friendly environment, starting with kindergartens and schools that must no longer assume that mothers are the only involved parents in the child's education and upbringing, and progressing to family-friendly employment policies that would be equally aimed at women and men.

NOTES

1 *Simeinyi kodeks Ukrainy* (Family Code of Ukraine), 2002, available at http://zakon.rada.gov.ua/cgi-bin/laws/main.cgi?nreg=2947–14. Official English translation available at http://www.mfa.gov.ua/data/upload/publication/usa/en/7148/family_kideks_engl.pdf.
2 Aimed at women's emancipation, these provisions were made in two decrees passed in 1917 by the Bolsheviks.
3 For more on the use of the manuals on parenting in the Soviet Union to promote 'appropriate' gender norms see Chernyaeva (2000).
4 Zhurzhenko (2004, 25) argues that Western framing was also used to justify a 'return' to traditionalist ideas about gender roles at the beginning of the 1990s, when the image of a Soviet working woman was opposed to an American 'happy housewife' of the 1950s, which was presented as the Western model to follow.
5 For a discussion of the challenges that the United Kingdom and Sweden have faced in the implementation of equal rights for both parents, see, respectively, Collier (2008) and Bergman and Hobson (2002).
6 Kyiv City Hospital reported that, in 2008, fathers were present for their partner's delivery in 84% of cases; similarly, Uzhgorod City Hospital said their achievement was 85%. In both cases, the hospitals encouraged the couples to consider this option; they also invested in special personnel training and redesigned the wards and delivery rooms for that purpose. For more on this change, see http://clipnews.info/newstopic.htm?id=766.
7 Natsionalna prohrama 'Dity Ukrainy' (State program *Children of Ukraine*), from 18 Jan. 1996. Available at http://zakon.rada.gov.ua/cgi-bin/laws/main.cgi?nreg=63%2F96.
8 Ukaz Prezydenta Ukrainy *Pro zakhody shchodo polipshennia stanovyshcha bahatoditnyh simei* (Presidential Decree on the Improvement of the Welfare of Families with Many Children), 12 Nov. 1999. Available at http://zakon.rada.gov.ua/cgi-bin/laws/main.cgi?nreg=1460%2F99.
9 The survey was a part of a government-run project, 'Formation of Gender Parity in the Context of the Current Socio-Economic Change' (cited in Alekseenko et al. 2004, 156).
10 This part of the study is based on twenty semi-structured interviews with first-time parents (10 fathers and 10 mothers) who, at the time, had a child

under 12 months of age. The age of the interviewees ranged between 21 and 27 years for women, and 22 and 29 years for men; they were all urban middle-class professionals with a university-level education. The couples lived apart from their extended families, and the mother was taking the parental leave. Including mothers in the research allowed the possibility of a more accurate picture of gender roles in the family, the father's actual participation in child care, and the prevailing discourses on fatherhood and motherhood that circulated in the family.

11 This observation resonates with findings from other studies on fatherhood; see, e.g., Lupton and Barclay (1997).

REFERENCES

Alekseenko, T., O. Balakireva, Y. Halustian, and S. Holiuk, eds. 2004. *Simya v umovakh stanovlennia nezalezhnoyi Ukrayiny (1991–2003)* [Family in the Context of the Establishment of Independent Ukraine]. Kyiv: Derzhavnyi instytut problem sim'i ta molodi [State Institute for the Family and Youth Development].

Ashwin, S., 2000. Introduction: Gender, State and Society in Soviet and Post-Soviet Russia. In S. Ashwin, ed., *Gender, State and Society in Soviet and Post-Soviet Russia*, 1–29. London: Routledge.

Ashwin, S., and T. Lytkina. 2004. Men in Crisis in Russia: The Role of Domestic Marginalization. *Gender and Society* 18(2): 189–206.

Bergman, H., and B. Hobson. 2002. Compulsory Fatherhood: The Coding of Fatherhood in the Swedish Welfare State. In B. Hobson, ed., *Making Men into Fathers: Men, Masculinities and the Social Politics of Fatherhood*, 92–124. Cambridge: Cambridge University Press.

Chernyaeva, N. 2000. Proizvodstvo materei v sovetskoi Rossii: uchebniki po uhodu za detmi epokhi industrializatsii [Production of Mothers in Soviet Russia: Manuals on Child Care during the Industrialization Era]. *Gendernye Issledovaniya* [Gender Research] 4: 120–38.

Collier, R. 2008. *Fragmenting Fatherhood: A Socio-Legal Study*. Portland: Hart.

Curran, L., and L. Abrams. 2000. Making Men into Dads: Fatherhood, the State, and Welfare Reform. *Gender and Society* 14(5): 662–78.

Dienhart, A. 1998. *Reshaping Fatherhood: The Social Construction of Shared Parenting*. Thousand Oaks: Sage.

Grebeshova, I., N. Ananieva, and S. Gribakin. 1990. *Vash rebenok*. [Your Child]. Moscow: Meditsyna.

Hearn, J. 2006. *European Perspectives on Men and Masculinities: National and Transnational Approaches*. New York: Palgrave Macmillan.

Hobson, B., and D. Morgan. 2002. Introduction. In B. Hobson, ed., *Making Men into Fathers: Men, Masculinities and the Social Politics of Fatherhood*, 1–21. Cambridge: Cambridge University Press.

Hovorun, T., V. Kravets, O. Kikinezhdi, and O. Kiz', eds. 2004. *Henderni aspekty usvidomlenoho bat'kivstva* [Gender Perspectives of Conscious Fatherhood]. Ternopil: Navchal'na Knyha.

Husachenko, I. 2006. Tatusi stayut' mamamy [Daddies Become Moms]. *Dzerkalo Tyzhnya* [Mirror of the Week] no. 15, 22–8 April.

Kaliuzhyn, G., and M. Deriugina. 1990. Vazhnaya missiya – byt' ottsom [The Important Mission of Being a Father]. In V. Soloukhin, ed., *Nastol'naya kniga molodykh roditelei* [Reference Book for Young Parents], 64–6. Minsk: Vysshaia shkola.

Kay, R. 2006. *Men in Contemporary Russia: The Fallen Heroes of Post-Soviet Change?* Burlington: Ashgate.

Konovalov, D. 2004. Simeynyy kodeks Ukrayiny – shlyah do Evropy [Family Code of Ukraine – The Way to Europe]. *Yurydychnyi Zhurnal* [Law Journal] 10: 34–9.

Korrespondent. 2007. Ukrainskim muzhchinam sdelayut prazdnik [Ukrainian Men Will Have Their Special Holiday]. Daily Online Newspaper *Korrespondent*. 18 Jan.

Kukhterin, S. 2000. Fathers and Patriarchs in Communist and Post-Communist Russia. In S. Ashwin, ed., *Gender, State and Society in Soviet and Post-Soviet Russia*, 71–89. London: Routledge.

Lupton, D., and L. Barclay. 1997. *Constructing Fatherhood: Discourses and Experiences*. New York: Sage.

Meshcherkina, E. 2000. New Russian Man: Masculinity Regained? In S. Ashwin, ed., *Gender, State and Society in Soviet and Post-Soviet Russia*, 90–117. London: Routledge.

Office of the Mayor, Kyiv. 2006. Official Announcement. http://kmv.gov.ua/press.asp?Id=67301 (accessed 14 March 2009).

Ostner, I. 2002. A New Role for Fathers? The German Case. In B. Hobson, ed., *Making Men into Fathers: Men, Masculinities and the Social Politics of Fatherhood*, 150–167. Cambridge: Cambridge University Press.

Parliament of Ukraine. 2000. *Verkhovna Rada Ukrayiny, Transcript of the 47th session*. 12 May. Available at http://www.rada.gov.ua/zakon/skl3/BUL35/120500_47.htm (accessed 21 Jan. 2007).

Pavlenko, Y. 2006. V kariernykh pytannyah do rodychiv stavlyusya zhorstkishe, nizh do inshykh. [In the Issues Related to Career, I Am More Demanding towards My Kin than towards Others]. Interview. Available at http://ua.for-ua.com/interview/2006/10/06/100059.html (accessed 9 May 2011).

Pavlova, L.M. 2007. *Realizatsiya pryrodnoho prava na shlyub, simyu, materynstvo ta batkivstvo* [Realization of the Natural Right to Marriage, Family, Motherhood, and Fatherhood]. Available at http://www.minjust.gov.ua/0/3666 (accessed 17 March 2007).

Rudik, N., director. 2006. *Khto zaspivaie kolyskovu. . .* [Who Will Sing a Lullaby. . . . Documentary. 29 min. Ukraine.

Soloviev, N. 1988. Otets v sovremennoi semie kak predmet sotsiologicheskogo issledovania [Father in a Modern Family as a Subject of a Sociological Study]. In S. Rapoport, ed., *Otets v sovremennoi semie* [Father in a Modern Family], 4–14. Vilnius: Institut Filosofii, Sotsiologii i Prava AN Litovskoi SSR [Institute of Philosophy, Sociology, and Law of the Academy of Sciences of the LSSR].

Ukrainian Parliamentary Committee on Gender Equality. 2006. *Rivni prava ta rivni mozhlyvosti v Ukrayini, realii ta perspektyvy: Rekomendatsii parlaments'kykh slukhan'.* [Equal Rights and Equal Opportunities in Ukraine, Present and Future: Recommendations of the Parliamentary Committee]. Kyiv: Verkhovna Rada Ukrainy.

Yushchenko, V. 2006. *Proclamation on Family Day*. 15 May 2006. Available at http://www.president.gov.ua/news/data/25_8199.html (accessed 21 Jan. 2007).

Zhurzhenko, T. 2002. Staraya ideologiya novoy semyi. Demograficheskii natsionalizm Rossii I Ukrainy [Old Ideology of the New Family: Demographic Nationalism of Russia and Ukraine]. In S. Oushakine, ed., *Semeynye uzy: modeli dlya zborki* [Family Ties: Do-It-Yourself Models], 268–96. Moscow: Novoe Literaturnoe Obozrenie.

– 2004. Strong Women, Weak State: Family Politics and Nation Building in Post-Soviet Ukraine. In K. Kuehnast and C. Nechemias, eds., *Post-Soviet Women Encountering Transition*, 23–43. Baltimore: Johns Hopkins University Press.

15 Ukrainian Societal Attitudes towards the Lesbian, Gay, Bisexual, and Transgender Communities

TAMARA MARTSENYUK

In this chapter, I explore attitudes towards homosexuality in contemporary Ukrainian society. Taking a sociological approach, I analyse aspects of the lesbian, gay, bisexual, and transgender (LGBT) communities of Ukraine, Ukrainian attitudes towards them, and homophobic public discourses in the country today. This analysis usefully problematizes existing ideas about heteronormativity in understandings of gender issues in general and gender politics particularly.[1,2] Given that up to now there has been a lack of debate in Ukraine and a paucity of research on LGBT issues in Ukrainian universities and in the Academy of Sciences,[3] the chapter makes an important contribution in bringing together existing research and advancing the terms of debate on this issue.

Shortly after gaining its independence in 1991, Ukraine repealed criminal responsibility for non-violent male homosexual intercourse between adults. It was the first of the former Soviet republics to do so; Russia followed suit two years later, in 1993.[4] At that time, LGBT communities within these two and other post-Soviet countries were faced with the task of trying to convince the majority of the population and state authorities of the truth of statements such as the following: 'Along with race, national and religious affiliation, gender and other characteristics, sexual orientation and gender identity are inherent elements of everyone's dignity and personality and, thus, should not be a ground for discrimination or violation of rights' (Tagankina and Petrov 2009, Introduction).

Nearly twenty years later, this task is ongoing. Homosexuality is still largely considered a deviant behaviour in Ukrainian society, as analysis of public opinion survey data clearly demonstrates. Meanwhile, homophobia receives tacit and explicit support from state officials and the media, and it is 'normal' and acceptable that a politician responsible for the protection of human rights would utter 'hate speech' against homosexual people in public (Martsenyuk 2009).

In response to this situation, the LGBT communities have organized and are represented by a number of different non-governmental organizations (NGOs). In fact, taken as a whole, these communities are becoming institutionalized. LGBT NGOs are typically the only organizations commissioning and/or conducting research on issues related to homosexuality, as well as on issues of discrimination and violations of human rights. It is in this context that I present the results of initial research into LGBT issues, with particular attention to illustrating an alarming increase of homophobia in Ukrainian society in recent years. I tackle the difficult question of why, far from becoming more tolerant of homosexuality, public opinion in Ukrainian society has actually become less so.

First I should note that, like elsewhere in the world, LGBT communities in Ukraine are complex in diversity and organization. These communities represent many different people and their relationships, many of which are further marginalized even within community designations. For example, transgender and bisexual people (about whom we have the least information and sociological data) are, for the most part, invisible among so-called sexual minorities, both in the general public and inside LGBT communities. Notwithstanding this diversity, for the sake of clarity, when I refer to 'LGBT communities' in this chapter I refer primarily to gay- and lesbian-identified people, and I take as my starting point an understanding that membership within LGBT communities typically means to recognize one's own sexual and/or gender identity, and/or to share that information privately and/or publically.

LGBT Communities in Ukraine

As mentioned above, contemporary Ukrainian LGBT communities are now in the process of institutionalization. Since Ukrainian Independence, the number of LGBT NGOs has increased and become geographically diverse. According to the latest data provided by the Gay Forum of Ukraine, there are twenty-four officially registered LGBT organizations in Ukraine and twenty informal LGBT groups.[5] During 2009 and 2010 alone, six LGBT organizations appeared (both in Kyiv and in different regions of the country). While the first LGBT NGOs started their activities at the end of 1990s (the Nikolayev Association of Gays, Lesbians, and Bisexuals, or 'LIGA,' was established in 1996;[6] the Nash Mir Gay and Lesbian Centre,[7] in 1999), a quarter of all existing LGBT NGOs in Ukraine appeared in the past two years. Today in Ukraine there are many types of LGBT NGOs working at the national level (the Gay Forum of Ukraine,[8] the Gay Alliance of Ukraine,[9] and others), the inter-regional level (Nash Mir Gay and Lesbian Centre for Kyiv, Donetsk and Lugansk oblasts, etc.), and down to the local (either oblast or city levels).

Despite this wide regional coverage of LGBT NGOs, there remain regional disparities. The smallest number of NGOs are in Western Ukraine, where there are only two – half that found in other regions (there are five NGOs in the Northern region, five in Central Ukraine, four in the South, and four in the East).[10] The limited presence in Western Ukraine, which is the more religious and traditional part of the country, could be attributable to the difficulties of organizing public activities in this region (i.e., mobilization of members of the LGBT community and the peaceful functionality of this type of NGO). People there tend to support the values of the traditional patriarchal family. In addition, according to the latest data provided by the Gay Forum of Ukraine, while there are thirty-two service organizations in Ukraine directed towards men having sex with men (or MSM),[11] thirteen of which are also LGBT NGOs;[12] only one MSM-service NGO operates from the Western oblasts, which is perhaps indicative of the difficulty in reaching a so-called critical mass there of people in need of support.

LGBT activists unite their forces and ideas in LGBT organizations in order to have the legal opportunities to defend their human rights, particularly at the state level. There are approximately 150 activists within the LGBT community, and LGBT organizations members hail from approximately sixty Ukrainian cities (Women's Network 2009). According to an evaluation by Svyatoslav Sheremet (leader of the Gay Forum of Ukraine), in Ukraine there are between 800,000 and 1,200,000 LGBT community members. Some of these individuals belong to same-sex couples, which are estimated to number between 100,000 and 200,000 (Maymulahin et al. 2009, 25).

However, there are no official (state) statistical data to support such estimates. These numbers refer only to people who identify themselves as practising homosexual 'risk behaviour' for HIV/AIDS infection. The International HIV/AIDS Alliance in Ukraine conducts research and evaluates the size of most-at-risk populations vulnerable to HIV infection, among whom are men who are having sex with men (AIDS Alliance Ukraine 2008, 86). We should thus distinguish between identity and behaviour as two different characteristics of homosexual people. Not all people who practise homosexual behaviour identify themselves as homosexuals. In the case of MSM, not all men who practise homosexual behaviour (that could be 'risk behaviour' for HIV/AIDS infection) identify themselves as homosexual men.

According to the various results, and taking into consideration the high level of stigmatization of MSM that leads to underestimation of the size of the MSM group, the total number of MSM at the country level in Ukraine appears to range between 117,000 and 430,000 (Balakiryeva et al. 2006, 38). Although, as mentioned, most research on homosexual behaviour is conducted to evaluate risk behaviours in relation to HIV infection, other aspects of LGBT issues are researched predominantly by LGBT NGOs themselves (or through cooperation with other NGOs, mostly international ones). Attention paid by the international community to members of the LGBT community (particularly to homosexual men), especially through NGOs that finance strategies for the prevention of HIV/AIDS infection in Ukraine has been deemed by some to be a type of 'victimization' of this community, as problematic. On the other hand, some leaders of the LGBT movement of Ukraine believe that, without international HIV/AIDS support, LGBT communities would not have the same strength in terms of financial and human resources.[13] MSM-service NGOs provide not only medical support but also information (e.g., legal consultation) and opportunities for mobilizing activists (e.g., through encouraging participation in events). Thus, even while working only for homosexual men and mainly with regard to HIV/AIDS issues, MSM-service NGOs encourage a wider number of activities and support for LGBT communities as a whole.

On 13 June 2008, three organizations that had experience both in working with homosexual issues and developing a common strategy to advance Ukrainian LGBT communities co-founded the Union of Gay Organizations of Ukraine (UGOU).[14] The goals of the UGOU are the following: (1) to unite the efforts of its participants in advocating for the rights and freedoms of gay people; (2) to mobilize the LGBT communities towards building civil society in Ukraine; and (3) to improve the effectiveness of preventing HIV infection among homosexuals. The UGOU provides support to fledgling LGBT organizations and works to educate LGBT activists.

The LGBT NGOs that are most active in the public sphere aim to work both with their members and with other LGBT people in particular, as well as with the whole Ukrainian society and state in general. The Nash Mir Gay and Lesbian Centre mentioned above has two main goals: (1) the protection of human rights and freedoms of homosexuals and the improvement of their legal protection at the state level, and (2) the improvement of society's attitude towards homosexuality and homosexuals. The Centre also monitors homosexuality issues in Ukrainian society and organizes public events such as conferences. In 2005, Nash Mir organized the large international conference, 'Our World: Extending the Borders,' which included a roundtable discussion on 'New Homophobic Trends in Central and Eastern Europe,' at which LGBT activists and researchers from across Europe and the post-Soviet nations were present. The most recent international conference took place at the end of 2008 with the topic 'Gay and Lesbian Rights Are Human Rights,' and covered a wide variety of issues from human rights and homophobia to tolerance issues in education.

The Informational and Educational Centre Women's Network,[15] meanwhile, works on gender issues, feminist theory and practice, and human rights within the lesbian community of Ukraine. Its strategic goals are to participate in the formation of state policy related to lesbianism; to form tolerant attitudes within Ukrainian society towards lesbians; and to provide informational, educational, and consulting services to lesbians, their relatives, and friends, as well as to interested specialists. Being outside of MSM-service, lesbian NGOs are less 'visible' and therefore get less financial support from international NGOs.

The NGO called 'Insight' is an LGBT organization in Ukraine that includes representation for transgender people.[16] Insight was founded in June 2007 and became officially registered on 26 May 2008. Its mission is to represent and lobby for the rights of LGBT communities at the national and international levels. Its four strategic program areas are (1) information and education, (2) advocacy, (3) health, and (4) organizational capacity building. In 2010, Insight presented its first research results on transgender people in Ukraine.[17]

From this breadth of organizations, we can see that during the past few years LGBT communities have become more 'diverse,' that is, have included active work not only with homosexual men (MSM-service) but also with lesbians and transgendered people. Other features of the movement include the drive towards consolidation, including close cooperation among active LGBT NGOs, the creation of the Union of Gay Organizations of Ukraine, and so on; strategic planning (e.g., the Strategic Program of LGBT Community Development is now in place[18]); and compromise with state authorities by homosexual leaders (particularly Svyatoslav Sheremet, president of the Gay Forum of Ukraine). This latter feature has been the case specifically with regard to two main issues: (1) the organization of large public manifestations of gay pride, which leaders have agreed not to carry out because Ukrainian society is not 'ready' to tolerate this; and (2) legal marriage, which is currently not being advocated for – in its place the idea of legal registered partnerships has been put forward (Sheremet 2008).

Still more can be said of the Ukrainian LGBT movement as a whole. For example, it lacks cooperation with other parts of civil society, other NGOs that work with human rights issues, women's NGOs, and so on. In order to avoid marginality, therefore, LGBT communities should align themselves more closely with Ukrainian civil society. In my opinion, this could be accomplished through the organization of more common activities to help overcome xenophobia and to educate Ukrainian society (first of all, younger generations) to be more tolerant.

LGBT Issues in Public Opinion

In this section, I provide an overview of research on LGBT issues (predominately public opinion surveys) that has been conducted in the past five years. As discussed earlier, studies about homosexuality in Ukraine are done mostly by representatives of LGBT communities. During the one-year period between October 2004 and October 2005, the organization Nash Mir (2005) conducted a project to monitor, report on, and protect the rights of the LGBT communities in Ukraine by systematically examining human rights violations on the basis of sexual orientation in Ukraine. The results showed that 90.4% per cent of Ukrainian citizens noted that they had experienced one or more instances of discrimination on some basis (p. 13). Discrimination by health and age were most often cited (58.9% and 52.6% respectively), while sexual orientation was indicated as a basis of discrimination by 14.4 per cent of Ukrainians. Among young people (those under 35 years of age), 21 per cent of respondents indicated sexual orientation as a potential source of discrimination (p. 27).

Table 15.1. Opinions in Ukraine on the Human Rights of Homosexual People, 2002 and 2007

In your opinion, should homosexual citizens of Ukraine have the same rights as the rest of the population?	March 2002 %	March 2007 %
Yes, everyone should have equal rights.	42.5	34.1
No, some restrictions are needed.	33.8	46.7
I am not sure.	23.7	19.2

Source: Nash Mir, *Ukrainian Homosexuals and Society: A Reciprocation. Overview of the Situation: Society, State and Politicians, Mass-Media, Legal Position, Gay-Community* (Kyiv: Atopol, 2007), 67.

At the request of Nash Mir, another public opinion survey was conducted in March 2007 about Ukrainian attitudes towards equal rights for homosexual citizens.[19] This survey, the results of which were published in a report called *Ukrainian Homosexuals and Society* (2008), took up earlier polling work done in 2002 and thus provided insights into how the public's views had changed in the five-year interim. Results from the 2007 survey (see Table 15.1 below) show that the number of people who oppose the idea of granting homosexual people in Ukraine the same level of rights as heterosexual people *increased* by 13 per cent, from 34 per cent in 2002 to 47 per cent in 2007 (Nash Mir 2007, 67). Nonetheless, in general one-third of the Ukrainian population said it supports equal rights for homosexual citizens.

When asked about specific rights for LGBT people, such as registered same-sex partnerships (see Table 15.2) and raising children (see Table 15.3), more Ukrainians said they were against same-sex partnerships or child rearing by homosexuals than when asked a general question about human rights. In 2007, only 16 per cent of respondents supported the idea that homosexual people should have their relationships officially recognized by the state, while the proportion of those who were against this increased to 52 per cent from 40 per cent in 2002.

With regard to homosexual people raising children, which could be considered the most sensitive measure of intolerance towards LGBT communities, in 2007, less than one-fifth of respondents supported the idea that homosexual citizens have a right to raise children, which is 5 per cent less than five years earlier. The proportion of Ukrainians who were against this right increased in the five-year period, from 49 per cent in 2002 to 60 per cent in 2007 (see Table 15.3).

Table 15.2. Opinions in Ukraine on Registered Same-Sex Partnership for Homosexual People, 2002 and 2007

Do you think homosexual citizens should have the same right as heterosexual couples to have their relationship officially registered?	March 2002 %	March 2007 %
Yes, they should have such a right.	18.8	15.8
No, they should never, ever be given such a right.	40.2	52.3
There should be exceptions (individually considered).	13.6	11.4
I am not sure.	27.4	20.5

Source: Nash Mir, *Ukrainian Homosexuals and Society: A Reciprocation. Overview of the Situation: Society, State and Politicians, Mass-Media, Legal Position, Gay-Community* (Kyiv: Atopol, 2007), 67.

The report also described levels of homophobic attitudes by different socio-demographic groups within Ukrainian society (Nash Mir 2007, 68). For example, Ukrainian women were typically more in favour of equality for homosexual people than Ukrainian men. As well, people with higher education showed greater tolerance towards homosexual people, with double the number of affirmative answers from people with higher education compared with respondents with primary or incomplete secondary education. In 2007, 39.1 per cent of those with incomplete or complete higher education said they supported equality for homosexuals, compared with about half that number (21.5%) among people with primary or incomplete secondary education.

In general, these results show that respondents in all age groups have become more homophobic during the recent five-year period under study. Nevertheless, young people aged 16 to 29 years still remain the most tolerant of LGBT people. The final report warns: 'Here are seen the most clearly negative tendencies: if in 2002 respondents favouring equality for homosexuals comprised 63.2 per cent among [those] 16–19 [years of age] . . . (19.5 percent being against), then by 2007 we see that the proportion of positive answers for this age category has decreased to 40 percent (42 percent being against). This tendency is one of the most dangerous that the poll has uncovered' (Nash Mir 2007, 68). In just a five-year period, intolerance among teenagers had doubled, a tendency that can be perceived to be rather challenging for the future of Ukrainian democratic society.

Visible regional differences in people's attitudes to LGBT rights issues also emerge in the survey. The greatest tolerance towards homosexuals is seen among people in Kyiv and Crimea; less tolerant are people in the Eastern region of the country; and the most homophobic are the Western and Northern regions of Ukraine. For example, among the respondents who supported equality for LGBT people, the breakdown by city/region is stark: Kyiv (58.2%), Eastern region (25.4%), Northern region (15.6%), and Western region (27.2%) (Nash Mir 2007, 68). These differences can be largely explained by the level of urbanization of each region. The Western and Northern parts of Ukraine hold more conservative views on gender and sexuality issues and in general traditionally have higher levels of religiousness compared with other Ukrainian territories (ibid.). Given the earlier discussion regarding regional aspects of LGBT NGO activity in Ukraine, these survey results make clear why there are only a few LGBT and MSM-service NGOs in the Western part of the country (one of the most homophobic).

To conclude, Ukrainian citizens became less tolerant towards LGBT people during the period between 2002 and 2007. Attitudes towards homosexual people are not homogeneous across Ukraine and depend on the respondents' socio-demographic characteristics. It is also important to note that approximately 20 per cent to 30 per cent of respondents (depending on the question) were unsure of their answer when asked about the rights of homosexual people. This could mean that in Ukrainian society there is a lack of debate on the issue of homosexuality and the human rights of LGBT communities in general.

Another comparative public opinion survey on the topic of homosexuality, which showed differences in views between the years 1991 and 2006, was carried out by the Kyiv International Institute of Sociology (KIIS).[20] KIIS presented results of this large survey in a document entitled, *Opinions and Views of the Ukrainian Population on the Eve of the Referendum about Independence and after 15 Years*. Within this survey, one block of questions concerned homosexual people and AIDS. These results showed that homosexuals are still stigmatized as a group. According to the KIIS data, the level of tolerance towards homosexuals has not changed significantly over time (see Table 15.4). To the question 'Do you agree or disagree with the statement that "Society should treat homosexuals the same as other people?"' the proportion of those who disagreed decreased only slightly from 34.9 per cent in 1991 to 28.5 per cent in 2006, and the proportion of those who agreed remained stable, at 33.7 per cent in 1991 and 33.3 per cent in 2006.

Table 15.3. Opinions in Ukraine on the Right of Homosexual People to Raise Children, 2002 and 2007

Do you think that homosexual citizens have a right to raise children?	March 2002 %	March 2007 %
Yes	21.5	17.1
No	49.2	60.2
I am not sure.	29.3	22.7

Source: Nash Mir, *Ukrainian Homosexuals and Society: A Reciprocation. Overview of the Situation: Society, State and Politicians, Mass-Media, Legal Position, Gay-Community* (Kyiv: Atopol, 2007), 67.

What are the reasons for such a change in public opinion attitudes towards homosexuality in Ukraine? I would argue that the following three main factors have had an influence on the formation of intolerant attitudes of Ukrainians to LGBT communities:

(1) The decriminalization of homosexual behaviour in 1991 and the activism of LGBT communities during the post-Soviet period
(2) Negative public discourse, including hate speech (on the basis of sexual orientation) by Ukrainian politicians; media portrayals of LGBT issues as deviant and abnormal; and a lack of diverse information on homosexuality and homosexuals (i.e., beyond the discourse surrounding HIV/AIDS and Ukraine's demographic crisis)
(3) The negative position of the Ukrainian church (mainly Orthodox Christian) towards homosexuality and the impact of homophobic initiatives like the so-called movement, 'Love against Homosexuality.'

Decriminalization and Silence

On 18 December 2008, the U.N. General Assembly proclaimed for the first time the Statement on Human Rights, Sexual Orientation and Gender Identity. The statement was signed by sixty-six countries.[21] Ukraine was not among them and did not support the statement. In justification of the government's decision, Vasyl Kyrylych, the Ministry of Foreign Affairs spokesman, made the following comment in an interview given to STB Television on 19 December 2008: 'We don't have such a

Table 15.4. Opinions on the Statement: 'Society Should Treat Homosexuals the Same as Other People,' 1991 and 2006

	1991 %	2006 %	Change %
Disagree absolutely	27.6	19.5	−8.1
Rather disagree than agree	7.3	9.0	+1.7
Both disagree and agree	8.9	16.3	+7.4
Rather agree than disagree	7.1	13.5	+6.4
Agree absolutely	26.6	19.9	−6.7
Difficult to say	22.6	21.9	−0.7
Total	100.0	100.0	

Source: Kyiv International Institute of Sociology (KIIS), *Opinions and Views of the Ukrainian Population on the Eve of the Referendum about Independence and after 15 Years* (Kyiv: KIIS, 2007). See www.kiis.com.ua.

problem and we do not need to discuss it. Since this phenomenon was decriminalized in Ukraine, there has been neither punishment, nor persecution.'

The idea that one of the so-called solutions to the perceived problem of homosexuality is to keep silent and avoid the issue of LGBT people's rights because it is not as important as other social problems has been promoted in other post-Soviet countries too, including Russia, as can be seen from the following statement: 'The Russian government prefers to ignore and keep quiet about the problem of discrimination based on sexual orientation and gender identity' (Tagankina and Petrov 2009, section 3.4).

Information War: Ukrainian Media and Politicians Marginalize Homosexuality

Intolerance towards LGBT people is also influenced by official state discourse (as broadcast by the media). Several LGBT NGOs have understood the importance of keeping track of this discourse and analysing it. Thus, they monitor examples of 'hate speech' in Ukrainian society (society-wide homophobia, including the actions of several governmental bodies, as well as anti-gay statements by political leaders and homophobic groups). The International Lesbian and Gay Association (ILGA) is one of these groups, and in 2007, they put out a press release entitled 'Hate Speech by High-Ranking Politicians in Ukraine' (ILGA Europe 2007). In Ukraine, Nash Mir has also done this kind of monitoring. According to their work, since mid-2006, the mass media have carried a considerable number of statements by politicians about homosexuals and their rights (Nash Mir 2007, 75).

Homophobia is also typical of Ukrainian politicians of any ideology.[22] In February 2007, there was a clear example of hate speech based on intolerant attitudes towards homosexual people from an official whose responsibility it is to protect human rights in Ukraine. The Communist Party member Leonid Grach, Chair of the Parliamentary Committee on Human Rights, National Minorities, and Interethnic Relations, stated in an official capacity that 'the state must protect society against evil, violence and particularly against homosexuality and lesbianism.'[23] In reply to his statement towards homosexuality, Ukrainian LGBT organizations addressed a letter to Grach in which they called for him to respect and protect the rights of homosexual people; Grach not only did not change his attitude, he continued to express new hate speech towards homosexuals.

Likewise, in answering a question about same-sex marriages, Olexandr Turchynov, who, at the time was the second most important figure in the bloc of Yulia Tymoshenko declared: 'We are categorically against! It is a big sin.' After a journalist commented that this answer was more typical of the Conservative Party, Turchynov added: 'I do not agree. If a man has normal views, then you label him a conservative, but those who use drugs or promote sodomy – you label them progressive. All of these are perversions' (Nash Mir 2007, 69). Other examples of politicians' homophobic comments abound, such as the following: 'Personally, I won't support political ideas and demands of homosexuals . . . I believe that we need to protect the family and spiritual values of Ukrainian society' (MP Socialist Mykola Danilin in 2006), and 'Personally I think, that gays and lesbians violate all norms of morality. It is a physical failing that is necessary to hide, not to expose' (a member of the Parliamentary Committee on Social Policy and Labour, Vasyl' Khara, Party of Regions) (Nash Mir 2007, 69). On 14 December 2006, the President of Ukraine, Viktor Yushchenko, was asked during an Internet conference: 'What do you think about the legislation of same-sex marriages in Ukraine?' The president replied: 'Can I answer in one word? – Complicated.' He added, 'Though by this I would not like to give a differing opinion from that which is given by the society and law' (Nash Mir 2007, 69).

According to Russian sociologist Igor Kon, sexuality discourse used to be a controversial phenomenon for post-Soviet countries (particularly for Russia). In discussing sexual liberation and attitudes towards homosexuality, Kon identifies two polarities in these countries: 'conservative traditionalists, nationalists, and communists, with a common blending of sexophobia, homophobia, anti-Semitism, and anti-Americanism, on one side, and liberal "Westerners," on the other side' (Kon 1999, under the heading 'Unity of Opposites'). Kon concludes that, for the state, the main task is either to reconcile these two views or to choose 'the proper one' for its politics.

Religious Discourse and LGBT Rights

Meanwhile, the LGBT community in Ukraine has had to face ongoing challenges from powerful religious groups that shape public opinion about homosexuality. The same-sex marriage issue is one of the most controversial issues arising in Ukraine between LGBT supporters, state authority, and the Church. In response to what they felt was an unfair stance towards same-sex marriage, on 21 August 2006, LGBT NGOs sent a public letter to the president of Ukraine and to legislative and executive officials that reads, in part:

> We, the leaders of non-governmental and charitable organizations working for gays and lesbians in Ukraine, appeal to you with this letter in response to the recent initiative of His Excellency Lubomyr Huzar, Head of the Ukrainian Greek Catholic Church, which was put forward by him on June 2nd this year at the session of the All-Ukrainian Council of Churches and Religious Organizations. Cardinal Huzar proposed to elaborate and adopt amendments to current legislation, which would entrench the concept of a 'married couple' as a union exclusively between a man and a woman, and which would legislatively define the concept of 'sexual minorities.' This would allegedly serve to prevent the creation of same-sex families in Ukraine, legalization of same-sex marriage, and the upbringing of children in such families.

> We treat all religious organizations, registered in Ukraine, with respect and tolerance. Undoubtedly, both the Ukrainian Greek Catholic Church and other religious organizations have the right to formulate and

publicly express their opinion on homosexuality and homosexual behaviour. However, it is necessary to consider that any intolerant statements can provoke incitement of hate towards homosexual citizens and can lead to violence against them. (Nash Mir 2007, 71)[24]

Moreover, in this open letter, LGBT NGOs emphasized that homosexuality is neither a disease nor a personality disorder, nor is it a criminal offence. They demanded a 'civilized attitude' towards people of homosexual orientation, following the example of most countries in the free democratic world (Nash Mir 2007, 72). Among other things, LGBT activists asked for the following: that a legislative prohibition of discrimination on the basis of sexual orientation in all spheres of public life be introduced; that same-sex marriages between citizens of Ukraine or between citizens of Ukraine and foreigners, lawfully contracted in another country, as well as civil partnerships, lawfully registered abroad as valid be recognized; and that the rights and needs of gays and lesbians be taken into account while drafting and implementing normative and legislative acts.

LGBT NGOs received answers from several ministries that, on the one hand, mentioned the problem of 'preconceived attitudes towards gays and lesbians on the basis of their sexual orientation' (Ministry of Ukraine for Family, Youth, and Sport; Nash Mir 2007, 74). On the other hand, the issue of the protection of the human rights of LGBT people was considered to be not very urgent compared with other social problems in Ukraine: 'Today the question of the legalization of same-sex marriages is not timely. And personally I am against such legalisation,' said Minister for Family, Youth, and Sport Yuriy Pavlenko, in an interview with NTN News, on 16 November 2006.

Hate speech with reference to sexual orientation has become normal state discourse in Ukraine, especially in the media. Such discourse is supported by initiatives like 'Love against Homosexuality.' Since 2003, this organization has conducted public activities and issued press statements in Kyiv to further its homophobic agenda.[25] In 2007, it launched an initiative to establish criminal prosecution for the spread of information supportive of or leading to the popularization of homosexual behaviour on the ground that it threatens the national security of Ukraine (Nash Mir 2007, 75). This appeal was sent to the country's legislative institutions and prime political actors, including the president, the prime minister, and members of the Verkhovna Rada (Parliament of Ukraine). In October 2007, in Kyiv, a march was held under the slogan 'For the Moral Cleanliness of Ukrainian Society,' organized by the Embassy of the Blessed Kingdom Divine for All Nations[26]. Nearly five hundred persons marched from Kyiv's central square to the offices of the president of Ukraine.

Love against Homosexuality stated that they had in their possession a letter from the Parliamentary Committee on Freedom of Speech and Information that addressed propaganda of so-called sexual perversions in mass media: 'Such situation urges the government to take resolute and immediate measures to stop the popularization of homosexuality, lesbianism, and other sexual perversions that do not conform to societal moral principles' (Love Contra 2008a). Love against Homosexuality blames homosexual people for spreading HIV/AIDS in Ukraine and publishes articles with titles such as 'AIDS Kills Gays' on their official website (Love Contra 2008b).

In the Report on the Situation of LGBT People in Ukraine submitted to the Parliamentary Assembly of Council of Europe Monitoring Committee from ILGA Europe, the following summary of the current situation was provided:[27] homophobic attitudes in Ukrainian society are intensifying; mainstream politicians increasingly oppose the fundamental rights of LGBT people with intolerant language, and their statements go unchallenged by persons in authority; the Legal Department of the Supreme Court, instead of upholding fundamental rights, and defending a vulnerable minority, opposes proposals to protect LGBT people from discrimination in intolerant terms; and all leaders of mainstream faith organizations in Ukraine have now united in opposing the rights of LGBT people, expressing their opposition in disturbingly intolerant language.

Fighting Homophobia

On 25 April 2007, members of the European Parliament debated and adopted a new Resolution on Homophobia in Europe in which homophobia is compared with other forms of xenophobia: 'homophobia can be defined as an irrational fear of and aversion to homosexuality and to lesbian, gay, bisexual and transgender (LGBT) people based on prejudice and similar to racism, xenophobia, anti-Semitism and sexism' (European Parliament 2006, subsection A). Moreover, the language of the resolution acknowledges that homophobia manifests itself in the private and public spheres in different forms, such as hate speech and incitement to discrimination, ridicule, and verbal, psychological, and physical violence, persecution, and murder, as well as discrimination in violation of the principle of equality and un-justified and unreasonable limitations of rights, which are often hid-den behind justifications based on public order, religious freedom, and the right to conscientious objection (European Parliament 2006, subsection B).

According to the results of the first specialized study of the legal situ-ation of LGBT communities in Russia, made by the Moscow Helsinki Group in cooperation with the Russian LGBT Network in 2007–08, the situation with homophobia as a part of general xenophobia is even more subtle: 'the tolerant attitude of the government and the society towards discrimination of LGBT people contributes to the legitimacy of neo-Nazi and religious fundamentalist groups which are rather homo-phobic' (Tagankina and Petrov 2009, under the heading 'Conclusions and Recommendations').

To focus attention on homophobic attitudes that continue to be widespread in many countries, including post-Soviet countries, spe-cial dates and events are devoted to this issue. May 17 has thus been designated as the International Day against Homophobia. The Inter-national Lesbian and Gay Association chose this time of the year to launch a report on state homophobia around the world in order to raise awareness of the extent of institutionalized homophobia (ILGA 2007). On this day in Ukraine, LGBT NGOs (and others that work on human rights protection issues) organize special events, such as Queer Week, an annual festival of LGBT culture, to fight stereotypes about LGBT communities and draw attention to the problem of homophobia in Ukrainian society. But these initiatives have rather local impacts and are not organized on the state level. For official bodies (even those that are supposed to work with human rights protection in general), the rights of LGBT communities are a marginal problem that is not seen or discussed.

LGBT Community Rights: State Politics towards LGBT Issues in Ukraine

Founded in 1978, ILGA is now a federation of more than 670 groups in over 110 countries campaigning for lesbian, gay, bisexual, transgender, and intersex rights.[28] It is a worldwide network of national and local groups dedicated to achieving equal rights for LGBTI people every-where. Amnesty International believes that 'all people, regardless of their sexual orientation or gender identity, should be able to enjoy the full range of human rights' (Amnesty International USA 2009).

In 2006, a group of international human rights experts met in Yogyakarta, Indonesia, to outline a set of international principles relating to sexual orientation and gender identity. The result was the 'Yogyakarta Principles: a universal guide to human rights which affirm binding international legal standards with which all states must comply.' In the introduction to the Yogyakarta Principles (2007, 6), it is mentioned that 'all human beings are born free and equal in dignity and rights. All human rights are universal, interdependent, indivisible and interrelated. Sexual orientation and gender identity are integral to every person's dignity and humanity and must not be the basis for discrimination or abuse.' These Yogyakarta Principles were a focus of discussion in Kyiv in October 2008 at the International Conference on Human Rights Issues for LGBT people, where the theme was Gay and Lesbian Rights Are Human Rights.

The key points in the development of a LGBTI human rights legal doctrine can be categorized as follows: (1) non-discrimination, (2) protection of privacy, and (3) the ensuring of other general human rights protection to all, regardless of sexual orientation or gender identity (O'Flaherty and Fisher 2008). Amnesty International (2009) calls on states 'to take all necessary legislative, administrative, and other measures to prohibit and eliminate prejudicial treatment on the basis of sexual orientation or gender identity at every stage of the administration of justice'; it also seeks 'to end discrimination in civil marriage laws on the basis of sexual orientation or gender identity and to recognize families of choice, across borders where necessary.'

LGBT communities in Ukraine are also working to establish human rights legal doctrine to protect privacy rights on the basis of sexual orientation and gender identity issues. Yogyakarta Principle 24, 'The Right to Found a Family,' notes: 'Everyone has the right to found a family, regardless of sexual orientation or gender identity. Families exist in diverse forms. No family may be subjected to discrimination on the basis of the sexual orientation or gender identity of any of its members' (Yogyakarta Principles 2007, 27). LGBT NGOs (e.g., Nash Mir) stress the need for the discussion of human rights topics in state politics related to sexuality and family. First of all, they underline the absence of anti-discrimination articles in the 1996 Constitution (Art. 24), the Labour Code (Art. 2.1), and the Criminal Code (Art. 161) (see Nash Mir 2007, 81). In particular, these groups are concerned that the list prohibiting unequal treatment of citizens and discrimination does not contain the concept 'sexual orientation.'

Ukrainian LBGT communities have also tried to lobby for official recognition of same-sex unions in Ukraine, which are not recognized either in the form of official marriages or as civil marriages. According to ILGA Europe webpage data, legal recognition of same-sex relationships can be categorized into the following four main types: (1) *marriage,* as is the case in Belgium, the Netherlands, and Spain, where the rights, responsibilities, and legal recognition given to same-sex couples who marry is the same as for different-sex couples who marry; (2) *registered partnership,* as is the case in the Czech Republic, Denmark, Finland, France, Hungary, and Iceland, where a particular form of registration is often exclusively open to same-sex partners although some countries have also made it available to different-sex partners; (3) *registered cohabitation,* which is often available to both same-sex and different-sex couples and requires that the couples prove that they have lived together for a determined period of time before they can accede to their registration; and (4) *unregistered cohabitation,* such as in Croatia, France, and Portugal, where very limited rights and responsibilities are automatically accrued after a specified period of cohabitation – these rights are almost always available to unmarried different-sex couples as well (ILGA Europe 2007b). As discussed earlier, however, in Ukraine, none of these forms of recognition are in place, and the debates between the LGBT community, religious forces, and the state are ongoing.

The human rights of people in LGBT communities in Ukraine are being neglected in other areas as well. For example, rights are frequently abused in the labour market. Results of interviews with nine hundred homosexuals conducted in 2005 demonstrate that 'often homosexuals face problems in the workplace, and during contacts with representatives of law enforcement bodies' (Nash Mir 2007, 82). For example, 78.2 per cent of respondents who were employed or had tried to find a job noted that they faced one or another violation of their rights, unequal treatment, and a prejudiced attitude towards them in the labour sphere. Mostly, this took the form of refusal of employment or dismissal (p. 82). Moreover, 61.5 per cent of respondents who had to contact representatives of Ukrainian law enforcement bodies during the previous year noted one or more violations of their rights (p. 82).

In the sphere of education there is also a negative attitude towards LGBT people. According to the results of the same round of 2005 interviews conducted by Nash Mir, approximately three-quarters of 'open' homosexuals felt themselves subjected to a prejudiced attitude on the part of teachers or other pupils (p. 85).

Finally, privacy and information rights are subject to abuse. Of the gays and lesbians surveyed by Nash Mir, 23.4 per cent said that their right to privacy had been violated (p. 86). Particularly, information about their sexual orientation had been shared without their permission. In the main, this confidentiality had been violated by police officers, colleagues at work, or other persons to whom previously private information had become known. Homosexuals could be blackmailed in order to force them to provide information, to leave their job, and so on (p. 86). In the U.S. State Department's *Country Reports on Human Rights Practices* (2007), in the chapter entitled 'Other Societal Abuses and Discrimination,' the authors refer to Nash Mir's explicit concern with 'ongoing police abuse of gays, threats by police to inform gays' families and employers of their lifestyle, and the lack of access to medical treatment and information for gay men on prevention of HIV/AIDS' (U.S. Department of State 2008, under the heading 'Other Societal Abuses and Discrimination').

Much work remains to be done in these areas. At the end of 2007, the LGBT community submitted a draft review of the Labour Code to the Rada that was adopted at first reading on 20 May 2008. The anti-discrimination article of the draft did not include prohibition of discrimination on the grounds of sexual orientation. One of the authors of the draft review of the Labour Code, the Chair of the Parliamentary Committee on Labour and Social Policy, Deputy Vasyl Khara (Party of the Regions), said in one of his interviews: 'Personally, I think that gays and lesbians violate all norms of morality. It is a physical defect that should be concealed, not flaunted. On the other hand, what they [sexual minorities] are demanding is a European norm that is likely to be included in the draft of the Code. I am against it, though.' Despite numerous appeals by the Nash Mir Centre to the Rada concerning the urgent need to include prohibition of discrimination on the grounds of sexual orientation in employment, the issue was not included in the draft (Nash Mir 2008).

All these examples of human rights violations on the basis of sexual orientation and gender identity show that, in Ukraine, there are no legislative, administrative, or other measures to prevent this situation. In September 2008, Ukrainian LGBT organizations proposed a *Plan of Actions to Combat Discrimination on the Ground of Sexual Orientation and*

Gender Identity in Ukraine to a number of governmental agencies. This document contains a long list of actions that must be taken to ensure civil rights and freedoms for LGBT people; however, this proposition received no constructive response (Nash Mir 2008). Not only at the local (country) level, but also at the European level, the Ukrainian state is not ready to support human rights issues on the basis of gender identity.

Conclusions and Further Discussions

Compared with twenty years ago, in post-Soviet Ukraine, the activities of LGBT NGOs have become more visible in the 'public eye,' while the organizations themselves are more institutionalized and official, which has a reality that has played the most important role for the LGBT rights movement in Ukraine. While the stronger, more solid movement may account for a stronger voice for members of the LGBT communities, it may also definitely provoke public opinion (formed mainly by the media) towards homosexuality and challenge heteronormativity that is standard in Ukrainian society. Despite all the evidence outlined above of intolerance towards LGBT community members and the lack of protection for their rights, state officials in Ukraine responsible for human rights issues do not even keep statistics concerning the violation of rights among LGBT people in Ukraine. This represents an important gap in research. In order to combat discrimination against vulnerable groups of people, public opinion about attitudes towards these issues should also be studied more widely and the results made public. These results could be presented together with other statistics on discrimination as part of the European Commission Eurobarometer Special Surveys. In these reports, attitudes towards vulnerable groups are studied thoroughly according to different socio-demographic and cross-cultural perspectives.[29] Such sociological research on discrimination could be helpful for adopting measures that provide equal opportunities for everyone in fields such as employment and education where, as we have seen, LGBT community members are now suffering abuse.

On the other hand, LGBT organizations should try to cooperate actively with the research community and with universities. Information and knowledge sharing benefit from the promotion of human rights issues. As results of sociological research demonstrate, better educated people tend to be more tolerant.

Public opinion surveys and statistical information are the main tools used to demonstrate attitudes towards discrimination in Ukraine. Right now in Ukraine, such sociological research is carried out in great part by LGBT NGOs themselves and predominantly with funding from international grants. In general, the international community is more interested than are Ukrainian authorities in monitoring uman rights on the basis of sexual orientation and gender identity.

In closing, as this chapter has demonstrated, homophobic attitudes in Ukraine are intensifying. One of the primary reasons for increased homophobia in Ukraine is state discourse led by politicians who are themselves homophobic. Since 2006, there has been an increasing number of hostile statements (hate speech) uttered by Ukrainian politicians about LGBT rights. It is therefore incumbent upon Ukrainian politicians in particular and society in general to take Eurointegration as a direction for state development. In order to advance the rights of LGBT communities in Ukraine, increased social tolerance as evidenced through non-homophobic state discourse and human rights policies that specifically promote protections for LGBT people must be encouraged and implemented at the highest official levels.

NOTES

1 *Heteronormativity* is understood here as a norm-building system that discriminates against, neglects, and denies everything that is not heterosexual (Alsterhag 2007, 13).

2 Although I believe that debates over terminology are extremely important in gender studies – and queer studies especially, given the marginality of gender studies in Ukraine – it is beyond the scope of this chapter to unpack and discuss the complexities in terminology typically used to describe and differentiate meanings in gender and sexuality, such as 'gender identity,' 'sexual identity,' 'queer issues,' etc.

3 In Ukraine, only a small number of researchers have worked on queer and LGBT community issues; e.g., Mariya Mayerchyk and Viktoriya Sukovataya.

4 For a more complete discussion of discrimination based on sexual orientation and gender identity in Russia, see Tagankina and Petrov (2009).

5 This is according to the Gay Forum of Ukraine. Svyatoslav Sheremet, personal communication, 28 April 2010.

6 Nikolayev Association of Gays, Lesbians, and Bisexuals, or 'LIGA.' See http://www.gay.nikolaev.ua.

7 Nash Mir website at http://www.gay.org.ua/.

8 For more information, see the the Gay Forum of Ukraine website at www. lgbtUA.com.

9 For more on the Gay Alliance, visit http://ga.net.ua/.

10 Svyatoslav Sheremet, president of the Gay Forum of Ukraine, personal communication, 28 April 2010.

11 This category includes men of any sexual orientation who identify themselves as practising homosexual 'risk behaviour' for HIV/AIDS infection.

12 List of MSM-service organizations of Ukraine (updated database), Gay Forum of Ukraine, as of 28 April 2010.

13 This view emerges from recent field work I conducted, in April and May 2010, with members of the LGBT movement in Ukraine. I interviewed ten leaders of the movement from Kyiv, Kharkiv, Lviv, Donetsk, and Cherkasy.

14 Groups in the union include the Gay Alliance, Gay Alliance Cherkasy, and Nash Mir Gay and Lesbian Centre. For more information, please visit the Union of Gay Organizations of Ukraine website at http://gay.org.ua/activity/union-e.htm.

15 Informational and Educational Centre Women's Network website at http://www.feminist.org.ua/english/basic.php.

16 Insight website at http://www.insight-ukraine.org.ua.

17 Situatsiya Transgenderov v Ukrayine: Otchyot po Issledovaniyu (Situation of Transgender People in Ukraine: Research Report), Kiev, 2010. Available at http://insight-ukraine.org.ua/media/TRP_report.pdf.

18 The program was approved on 7 November 2009. It contains ten areas for implementation (social, political, legal, organizational, informational etc.).

19 The poll was representative in terms of age and sex of the Ukrainian population: 1,200 respondents between 16 and 75 years of age took part. The mathematical accuracy of the sample is ± 3%.

20 For full survey details, see http://www.kiis.com.ua.

21 For more information, see http://ilga.org/ilga/en/article/1211.

22 For the purposes of this chapter, I employ a rudimentary definition of homophobia as an irrational fear of, aversion to, or discrimination against homosexuality or homosexuals.

23 Author's translation from Ukrainian. Excerpt retrieved 11 April 2007 from the website ForUm at http://ua.for-ua.com/analytics/2007/02/14/112933.html.

24 The letter was signed by heads of the following organizations: Gay Forum of Ukraine, Women's Network, LIGA, Nash Mir, Gay Alliance, and Chas Zhyttya Plus.

25 For more detail on the activities of the Love against Homosexuality organization, see their website at http://love-contra.org/.

26 See http://www.godembassy.org/en/embassy.php.

27 Information on submitted findings was received directly by the author from administrators at the Nash Mir Gay and Lesbian Centre in Kyiv, Ukraine: Submission to the Parliamentary Committee Monitoring Rapporteurs on the situation of LGBT people in Ukraine, and the need to make strong recommendations on combating sexual orientation and gender identity discrimination. See ILGA Europe.

28 In biomedical terminology, intersex is commonly used to label a wide variety of chromosomal, gonadal, and genital characteristics that are deemed 'anomalous,' according to the narrowly defined scientific and medical norms of female and male sexes.

29 One of these reports, Discrimination in the European Union, examines the six legally prohibited forms of discrimination on the basis of sex, ethnic origin, religion or beliefs, age, disability, and sexual orientation. As a result, perception of the different forms of discrimination is measured among Europeans. In general, discrimination in the European Union is widespread (European Commission 2007, 4). Particularly, discrimination on the basis of sexual orientation is the third most widespread form of discrimination (after discrimination on the basis of ethnic origin and disability); 50% of respondents (EU citizens) perceived discrimination on the basis of sexual orientation to be widespread (p. 4).

REFERENCES

AIDS Alliance Ukraine. 2008. *Monitoring Povedenija Muzhchin, Kotoryje Prak-tikujut Sex s Muzhchinami Kak Komponent Epidnadzora Vtorogo Pokolenija* [Monitoring the Behaviour of Men Who Are Having Sex with Men as a Component of Epidemic Control of Second Generation]. Available at http://www.aidsalliance.org.ua/ru/library/our/monitoring_reports/pdf/report_MSM_rus.pdf (accessed 30 July 2009).

Alsterhag, S. 2007. *Open Up Your Workplace: Challenging Homophobia and Het-eronormativity*. A Publication of TRACE (The Transnational Cooperation for Equality). Available at http://www.homo.se/upload/homo/pdf_homo/HelaOpenupyourworkplace.pdf (accessed 10 Aug. 2009).

Amnesty International. 2009. *Sexual Orientation and Gender Identity.* Available at http://www.amnesty.org/en/sexual-orientation-and-gender-identity (accessed 5 Aug. 2010).

Amnesty International USA. 2009. *Lesbian, Gay, Bisexual and Transgender Human Rights.* Available at http://www.amnestyusa.org/lgbt-human-rights/about-lgbt-human-rights/page.do?id=1106573 (accessed 4 Aug. 2009).

Balakiryeva, O.M., L.M. Gusak, H.V. Dovbakh, O.O. Lavryenov, V.I. Paniotto, T.V. Petrenko, N.B. Pogorila, T.O. Saliuk, S.V. Sydiak, D.O. Khutkyi, and T.S. Shamota. 2006. *Evaluation of the Size of Most-at-Risk Populations Vulnerable to HIV Infection in Ukraine.* Kyiv: ICF International HIV/AIDS Alliance in Ukraine. Available at http://www.aidsalliance.org.ua/ru/library/our/monitoring_reports/pdf/size_en.pdf (accessed 2 Aug. 2009).

European Commission. 2007. Discrimination in the European Union – Summary. *Special Eurobarometer.* Available at http://ec.europa.eu/public_opinion/archives/ebs/ebs_263_sum_en.pdf (accessed 6 Aug. 2009).

European Parliament. 2006. *Homophobia in Europe: European Parliament Resolution on Homophobia in Europe.* P6_TA[2006]0018. Brussels: European Parliament. Available at http://www.ilga-europe.org/europe/news/ilga_europe_welcomes_europarliament_s_resolution_on_homophobia_in_europe/full_text_of_the_adopted_resolution (accessed 4 Aug. 2009).

ILGA. 2007. *State-Sponsored Homophobia.* Available at http://www.ilga.org/news_results.asp?FileCategory=9andZoneID=7andFileID=1058 (accessed 1 Aug. 2009).

ILGA Europe. 2007a. *Press Release: 'Hate Speech by High-Ranking Politicians in Ukraine.'* Available at http://www.ilga-europe.org/europe/guide/country_by_country/ukraine/hate_speech_by_high_ranking_politician_in_ukraine (accessed 1 Sept. 2009).

– 2007b. *Marriage and Partnership Rights for Same-Sex Partners: Country-by-Country.* Available at http://www.ilga-europe.org/europe/issues/lgbt_families/marriage_and_partnership_rights_for_same_sex_partners_country_by_country (accessed 10 Aug. 2009).

KIIS. 2006. *Dumky i Pogliady Naselennya Ukrayiny Naperedodni Referendumu shchodo Nezalezhnosti ta cherez 15 Rokiv* [Opinions and Views of the Ukrainian Population on the Eve of the Referendum about Independence and after 15 Years]. Available at www.kiis.com.ua/txt/doc/30112006/press30112006.doc (accessed 30 July 2009).

Kon, I. 1999. Sexuality and Politics in Russia, 1700–2000. In F.H. Eder, L. Hall, and G. Hekma, eds., *Sexual Cultures in Europe: National Histories.* Manchester:

Manchester University Press. Also available at http://sexology.narod.ru/publ012.html (accessed 6 Aug. 2009).

Love Contra. 2008a. *Palka v koliosa sodomii ot ukrainskih narodnyh deputatov* [Grit in Sodomy's Machine from Ukrainian People's Deputies]. Available at http://love-contra.org/index.php/news/issue/146/ (accessed 30 July 2009).

– 2008b. *Spid 'kosit' Geyev.* [AIDS Is 'Mowing Down' Gays]. Available at http://love-contra.org/index.php/expert/issue/195/ (accessed 30 July 2009).

Maymulahin, A.Y., M.G. Kasyanchuk, and Y.B. Leshchynskyy. 2009. *Odnopoloye Partnyorstvo v Ukrayine: Otchyot po Issledovanyiyu* [Same-Sex Partnership in Ukraine: Research Report]. Donetsk, Atopol.

Martsenyuk, T. 2009. *Strah Rozmayittya: Natsional'ni Vlastyvosti Tolerantnosti i Homophobiyi* [Fear of Diversity: National Peculiarities of Tolerance and Homophobia]. *Krytyka* 12(11–12): 145–6. Available at http://krytyka.com/cms/upload/Okremi_statti/2009/2009–11–12/10–13–2009_11–12.pdf.pdf (accessed 24 May 2010).

Nash Mir. 2005. *Gay Rights and Human Rights: Report about Discrimination on the Grounds of Sexual Orientation in Ukraine.* Kyiv: Nash Mir. Available at http://gay.org.ua/publications/report2005-e.pdf (accessed 4 Aug. 2010).

– 2007. *Ukrajinski Homosexualy i Suspilstvo: Vzajemne Pronyknennya. Oglyad Sytuatsiji: Suspilstvo, Derzhava i Polityky, ZMI, Pravove Stanovyshche, Gay-Spilnota* [Ukrainian Homosexuals and Society: A Reciprocation. Overview of the Situation: Society, State and Politicians, Mass Media, Legal Position and the Gay Community]. Kyiv: Atopol.

– 2008. *Human Rights Violations Based on Sexual Orientation in Ukraine.* Available at www.gay.org.ua/publications/gay_ukraine_2008-e.doc (accessed 5 Aug. 2009).

O'Flaherty, M., and J. Fisher. 2008. Sexual Orientation, Gender Identity and International Human Rights Law: Contextualizing the Yogyakarta Principles. *Human Rights Law Review* 8(2): 207–48. Also available at http://www.yogyakartaprinciples.org/yogyakarta-article-human-rights-law-review.pdf (accessed 5 Aug. 2009).

Sheremet, S. 2008. *Address by S. Sheremet, President of the Gay Forum of Ukraine.* Speech given at the International Conference 'Gay and Lesbian Rights are Human Rights!' Kyiv, 4–5 Oct.

Tagankina, N., and I. Petrov. 2009. *Discrimination Based on Sexual Orientation and Gender Identity in Russia: The Russian LGBT Network.* Available at http://www.lgbtnet.ru/news/detail.php?ID=4336 (accessed 1 Aug. 2009).

U.S. Department of State: 2008. Country Reports on Human Rights Practices: Ukraine. Available at http://www.state.gov/g/drl/rls/hrrpt/2008/eur/119110.htm (accessed 2 Aug. 2009).

Women's Network (Ukraine). 2009. *Informational and Educational Centre 'Women's Network.'* Available at http://www.feminist.org.ua/info/lgbtinfo.php#1 (accessed 2 Aug. 2009).

Yogyakarta Principles. 2007. *The Yogyakarta Principles: Principles on the Application of International Human Rights Law in Relation to Sexual Orientation and Gender Identity.* Principles adopted by the International Panel of Experts in International Jurisprudence in Yogyakarta, Indonesia, 6–9 Nov. 2006. Full text available at http://www.yogyakartaprinciples.org/principles_en.pdf (accessed 1 Aug. 2009).

16 Mainstreaming Gender Equality in Ukraine: Tensions, Challenges, and Possibilities

OLENA HANKIVSKY AND ANASTASIYA SALNYKOVA

In the context of Ukraine's movement towards integration with the European Union (EU), and its efforts to adhere to European norms, gender equality has gained significant political importance. Ukraine was one of the first countries in the world to adopt a constitutional guarantee of gender equality and since then it has signed numerous international documents to affirm the country's commitment to creating institutional mechanisms for promoting its realization (Kisselyova and Trokhym 2007). However, with the exception of a few reports from non-governmental organizations (NGOs) and sporadic governmental reports to the United Nations, virtually no attention has been paid to evaluating the implementation of gender equality instruments and, in particular, what could be considered the beginnings of a gender mainstreaming (GM) approach in Ukraine.[1]

Since 1995, gender mainstreaming, which requires the systematic evaluation of the differential impact of all policies and governmental actions on the situations and needs of women and men, has been recognized internationally as the desired approach for achieving gender equality in the public sphere. Despite its potential, however, evaluations of GM to date (Beveridge and Nott 2002; Daly 2005; Hafner-Burton and Pollack 2000; Pollack and Hafner-Burton 2002; Rees 2002; Shaw 2005; Squires 2005; Veitch 2005; Walby 2005; Woodward 2008) reveal a number of substantive shortcomings, particularly with regard to the conceptualization of GM and to the inadequate implementation of this strategy, leading some scholars to question its overall utility (Hankivsky 2005; Powell 2005). Although GM has been examined in developed countries, including the EU states (Booth and Bennett 2002; Mazey 2002; Woodward 2003; Carney 2003), assessment of GM in the development context, including within transitional, post-Soviet countries, is rudimentary or non-existent (Galligan et al. 2007). This chapter addresses this significant gap and contributes to the understanding of GM within the political interplay of gender and the dynamics of emerging democracies in post-communist countries such as Ukraine.

The discussion is based on thirty-two in-depth interviews that we conducted with experts from three sectors: officials employed by the state, representatives of NGOs (both international and local), and scholars in the field of gender studies. Analyses of key governmental and non-governmental documents and scholarly literature are also a basis for this discussion. The chapter begins with an overview of the concept of gender mainstreaming in the Ukrainian policy context. It then moves on to provide an assessment of Ukrainian society as well as the three areas that are considered crucial in the successful implementation of GM: (1) governmental and national machinery; (2) women's or equality organizations; and (3) academic research in gender and women's studies. The chapter ends with respondents' policy recommendations regarding the future of gender equality in Ukraine.

The chapter reveals some of the key reasons why, despite the impressive amount of formal equality policies and legislation in Ukraine, these have not translated into meaningful social or political change. Although education, improved implementation, monitoring, and research are identified (among other factors) as necessary prerequisites for improving Ukraine's response to gender equality, the research also demonstrates the challenges of implementing a transnational strategy such as gender mainstreaming within a national context in a way that is responsive to current socioeconomic circumstances, language, culture, and traditions, especially in relation to gender issues. The findings point to the limitations of adopting Western-style policy tools without adequate attention to the context and specific social realities of countries that are transforming from communism to democracy, and the chapter provides concrete suggestions as to how these challenges can be addressed.

Gender Mainstreaming in Ukraine: Overview of Perceptions

Even with calls to expand GM in Ukraine (Hankivsky 2008), and assertions that Ukraine is making attempts to mainstream gender into its policies and programs,[2] gender mainstreaming is not an official term in any of Ukraine's laws or policies. Although 'certain steps and efforts to mainstream gender have been . . . undertaken by the national

government with the support of international institutions and in partnership with civil society' (Kisselyova and Trokhym 2007, 3), it is also
the case, as one of the study participants from the government explained, that

> the GM concept is used but not that much in state structures . . . I know
> the GM concept, but not through state channels; I picked it up from NGOs
> and through self-education.

Even though gender mainstreaming may be used by certain gender experts working within government and the NGO community, and even
though it may be implicit in the government's strategies, it is not yet
part of the mainstream discourse.

In government documents, equal rights and opportunities and gender equality are emphasized. To illustrate: the Preamble of the Gender
Equality Law aims 'to achieve parity status for women and men in all
the areas of social functioning through legal provision for equal rights
and opportunities for women and men, liquidation of sex-based discrimination and use of special temporary arrangements targeted at ex-
termination of the disparity between opportunities for men and women
to realize their equal rights.'[3] Article 3 of the law states that 'the state
policy of ensuring equal rights and opportunities for women and men
is targeted at: establishment of gender equality.' The last gender strategy, 'Gender Equality in Ukrainian Society 2006–2010,' has as one of its
aims adapting the legislation of Ukraine to be in accordance with EU
legislation in the area of gender equality. In other sectors, 'gender integration' or simply referring to 'gender issues' is the preferred approach.
As an international NGO employee reported, 'We don't use gender
mainstreaming, instead we use "gender integration."' And a local NGO
activist explained, 'We would rather talk about gender issues.'

It is also important to point out that the term 'gender' itself is new
for Ukrainian language and society. As a researcher revealed during an
interview, it was only in 1995 that the term 'entered into the consciousness of society and started to be used.' Not surprisingly, the interview
participants highlighted that the term is poorly understood across sectors. According to one state official,

> Civil servants don't know the meaning of the word 'gender' . . . some-
> times even women's organizations don't understand these gender things
> clearly.

Moreover, a university professor stated, 'I doubt that even the Family and Youth Minister knows what gender is.' As was evident throughout the interviews, the lack of understanding also translates into a certain negativity and resistance towards gender-related issues. As one researcher put it, 'Gender for the state is like a red cloth for a bull.'

The majority of participants mentioned that gender is perceived to be synonymous with women's issues, which makes it open to ridicule. Reporting on her communications with state officials, a research centre director told us: 'They say that women thought [gender] up so that they have something to talk about.' Further, ignorance in terms of gender, according to one university instructor, 'is extremely widespread at the level of the public service workers and teachers.' This respondent further elaborated:

> A couple of years ago a dean in my university said that since we do not have an equivalent for the word 'gender' in the Ukrainian language we do not have such a problem in Ukraine.

One state official explained that people do not realize the existence of discrimination:

> When we ask people if there is gender discrimination, they say 'no'; but when we ask specifically about applying for jobs or getting bank credits they change the answer to 'yes.' This is because we are taught that there is no gender problem in our country.

These attitudes are evident at the highest levels of politics. When the first Gender Equality Law was proposed in 1999, it failed to get political support and was rejected in 2001. One state official recalled:

> As they discussed the law in the Rada (parliament of Ukraine) even [Deputy] Samoilyk, who was one of the submitters of the draft law, said that 'when we live better, there will be no need for gender,' and another deputy said that he was against the law since as believers we are to be against women influencing politics.

A former state official and activist recollected that the next time the Gender Equality Law was on the parliamentary agenda:

The session moderator from a communist party, Adam Martyniuk, said with cynicism: 'Colleagues, don't leave yet. We've just adopted the law on extinct species, now let's also quickly vote to protect women.'

And a local NGO activist reported to us:

> When we asked the newly appointed provincial head why gender equality was not among his priorities, he said, 'Because gender is not a Ukrainian word and our reality is different.'

Significantly, a common theme among the majority of respondents was that the concepts of gender, gender equality, and gender mainstreaming are seen to be a Western paradigm, imposed by Western organizations: 'gender is seen as something foreign [and] something only countries that have nothing else to do are worried about.' Therefore, there is the widespread perception that 'gender equality is thought of as not relevant for Ukrainian society' (university professor) and ' as something American' (NGO representative). One woman activist told us:

> Gender policy is not natural for Ukraine. We have a different history; we had Princesses Olha and Anna. Women could always take care of themselves. They don't go to politics today, because their dignity doesn't fall low enough to engage in it.

Assessing the Status Quo: The Application of Gender Mainstreaming

Comparing Ukraine's progress with other European countries, Serhiy Plotyan, Chief Consultant of the Parliamentary Committee in European Integration, has concluded that 'regardless of the prolonged cooperation in the framework of the European Council and the declared direction towards European integration, our country has not reached European standards in the sphere of gender equality' (Plotyan 2006, 109). As one of the study participants stated:

> As far as GM in Ukraine is concerned, apart from the efforts of NGOs, there are few results because few people understand what it is and what it is for.

To grasp the current state of affairs in Ukraine, it is necessary to evaluate both the achievements and obstacles to moving forward on issues of gender equality in Ukrainian society in general and, in particular, within three pillars of society that are considered key to successful gender mainstreaming: (1) academic gender and women's studies research and education, (2) women's or equality organizations, (3) and national machineries for gender equality (Einarsdóttir 2003).

Ukrainian Society

Economic insecurity is one key reason that gender is not a priority in Ukrainian society. This point was made by one-third of the respondents and is evidenced in the following statements by our interviewees:

> Economic instability is a problem. All thinking is about survival. (NGO employee)

> The general understanding in society is that all social programs are secondary to economic issues. (NGO employee)

Socioeconomic changes following the breakup of the Soviet Union have been challenging in general, but particularly difficult for women, who have become increasingly excluded from the social and political forefront (Pyshchulina 2004) and who experience increases in the feminization of poverty (Hankivsky 2008; Predborska 2005). In addition, women's work patterns have changed with both paid work and domestic responsibilities increasing (Cockerham et al. 2006). Such a transitional shift has been interpreted as 'a process of "aggressive remasculinization"' (Yakushko 2005, 590) in the development of Ukrainian society. Additionally, sexist images and ideologies are on the rise, and, according to former Deputy Minister for Family, Youth, and Sport Ludmyla Lukinova, 'stereotypes of public perception create a very powerful barrier in achieving gender equality in our society' (UNU 2010).

The presence and consequences of stereotypical perceptions of gender roles were reported by the overwhelming majority of the study participants, as illustrated by the following statements:

Not all men think that women have to be equal in all aspects . . . there's lots of stereotypes that remain. (Research centre director)

We live in a stereotypical patriarchal society. (State official)

Women here are talked about as physical bodies. (University professor)

In Ukraine, as in many other jurisdictions, there is a strong sense that anything to do with gender is necessarily linked to women or feminism, as evidenced by the following quotes from two of our interviewees:

Gender is perceived as something that only concerns women who try to squeeze men out.

The notion of gender has a female face whether we want it or not.

These assumptions permeate all levels of society. Recent studies indicate that college students and young professionals endorse highly stereotypical attitudes towards women and men (Yakushko 2005). One state official explained that 'the presence of discrimination is denied in Ukraine, everyone keeps talking of the image of woman-*Berehynia* on a pedestal.'[4] The perpetuation and celebration of this image and its inconsistency with gender equality is illustrated by former President Yushchenko's message on International Women's Day in 2007: 'This day is marked worldwide. The international community and free mass media draw our attention to the problem of gender inequality. March 8 is officially recognized by the United Nations Organization, and 2007 has been declared a year of equal opportunities in the European Union,' he said. 'On the other hand, I want us to never forget that the most precious and important things in our life are associated with women. They are our source of inspiration, tenderness, and love, and guardians of our homes and our country.'[5]

Significantly, gender stereotypes are also normalized among women. As a policy decision maker explained, 'Women themselves believe in the *Berehynia* myth and deny the fact of discrimination.' This is further sub-stantiated by the following statements from two of our interviewees:

There are many gender-insensitive women. (Gender researcher)

Women don't understand that inequality exists. (NGO activist)

Similarly, Predborska (2005) observed that gender inequality is firmly entrenched in the conservative views of many Ukrainian women. According to close to half of the participants in our study, the mass media play a key role in perpetuating harmful stereotypes, as can be seen from the following statements:

> The media keep spreading patriarchal stereotypes, especially in women's and men's magazines, but not only. (Activist)

> The media, especially TV series on (pro-)Russian patriarchal channels prevent youth from understanding gender issues. (University professor)

Overall, participants highlighted that there is little knowledge of gender in Ukrainian society, as well as of governmental initiatives that have been developed to work towards gender equality. Most telling is the lack of awareness about the existence of Ukraine's Gender Equality Law. According to one university professor,

> We had a national survey . . . about the equality law for men and women: 62 per cent had never heard of it and 31 per cent knew about it but did not know its contents.

Gender Education and Research

Gender is a novel problem in academic studies in the region (UNDP 2003, 84). Consequently, it is not surprising that interviewees offered statements such as the following:

> Gender studies are marginalized, not taken seriously. (Researcher)

> Education is not performing well in the function of advancing gender equality. (NGO employee)

Moreover, attempts to unify efforts across the country have failed. According to one university instructor and activist, 'There was a failed attempt in 2000 to create an association of gender studies.' Another university professor explained that 'there is an idea to create an interdisciplinary centre for gender studies, but there are not enough specialists.' These statements are consistent with previous conclusions drawn by Shymchyshyn (2005) that 'feminist theory cannot easily penetrate university curricula because it seriously questions the male-oriented ideology of Ukrainian society as well as the university, which serves as one institution for implementing this ideology' (p. 173).

Yet it is important to acknowledge the progress made in the past decade. In the words of one state official, 'In terms of gender integration into university education, there are big chang-es.' For example, the first university course 'Fundamentals of Gender Studies' was endorsed by the Ministry of Education and Science in 2003. It is not yet a mandatory subject, but for the departments willing to include it, a state-recommended program has been developed and is readily available. Similarly, the first textbook on gender studies published in Ukrainian is now available.[6] As one university professor explained,

> It is good to finally have something. I include some chapters from it in my course, even though I don't agree with some others.

Another university instructor and an activist described the many achievements at the micro-level:

> Six gender courses are being taught at the Culture Studies program in Lviv University, one of them on masculinity studies.

Moreover, a gender researcher reported that 'up to twenty gender courses are taught in the Karazin University.' Similarly, another researcher reflected on the recent changes, stating:

> Five years ago gender was not a topic considered appropriate for a philosopher. In contrast now, as our department chair heard of the EU grant on gender, he started considering a course on gender for our department.

The United Nations Development Program (UNDP) has also helped in organizing educational gender centres at universities. There is one at Kyiv Technical University, and there are more in four other regions. Up to thirty such centres work on university premises across the country as NGOs.

At the same time, there remain significant challenges in terms of academic education and research. In the words of one policy maker, 'I am convinced a lot of courses remain on paper. They're not taught at university.' This is echoed in the recollection of one university professor, who said:

> The President of the University doesn't want to include a gender course into the curriculum, saying that this is feminism.

It is difficult to teach courses and hard to fit them into the study plan of the Ministry of Education and Science. And even when courses are offered, as one NGO director made clear, it is also the case that

> gender is often taught either from an extreme feminist or traditionalist perspective [and] even students in the universities where gender studies are taught often treat gender as a discipline only, not something to be implemented in real life.

Resistance to gender equality penetrates all levels of education, which is alarming in the context of a need to bring up a more gender-sensitive generation. One university professor reported:

> In teachers' guides for elementary schools you can find different suggested exercises for boys and girls. The teachers' instructions for Crimean kindergartens encourage developing patience and friendliness in girls. And when it comes to maths it is suggested to ask girls to count flowers and boys – cars or so.[7]

Finally, gender research is underdeveloped and often of poor quality. In the words of a university instructor:

> Now everyone tries to include the word 'gender' into their titles and to justify it they simply count the number of men and women, but gender is not just about counting; quality research is lacking.

There is also 'a lack of good statistics on gender,' as one of the gender researchers pointed out. It is important to highlight that there is no national program to support gender research, and very little financing is available for such enterprises (UNDP 2003). The precarious nature of the situation was made clear by an NGO director, who informed us that

> Two key people [academics] who started gender work in Ukraine and did so at their own cost simply died.

Consequently, there is a lack of gender researchers and specialists in the country. As a result, 'even interested state officials don't have many specialists to get advice from because the educational system is not preparing such specialists' (gender researcher). The general lack of available research and gender specialists greatly impedes any effective knowledge transfer to the policy sector and undermines efforts for moving towards greater gender equality.

Women's Movement or Equality-Seeking Organizations

Although close to seven hundred women's organizations exist in Ukraine,[8] half of all respondents reported that there is no strong women's movement or effective organization that is able to lobby for issues of gender equality. This is made clear in the following statement made by an NGO activist and university professor:

> There is no strong women's organization to influence the situation.

The 1980s witnessed the emergence of the first independent women's organizations, many of which focused on the goal of Ukraine's independence and, for the most part, used maternalist discourses in their advocacy work. This proved an effective strategy in recruiting Ukrainian women who had never been politically active. Post-independence, this central force lost direction and momentum. As Hrycak (2005) explains, 'Ukraine's independence left women activists struggling to understand what role they could or should play in public life' (p. 72).

In the 1990s, after the Fourth World Conference on Women, where gender mainstreaming was first endorsed at an international level, Ukraine experienced an influx of international organizations supporting equality initiatives in the country. Ukrainian organizations started to be shaped by these foreign actors and took up Western gender terminology to secure funds, which were often tenuous and time-limited. These trends 'cut short the development of promising feminist groups, and created an elite of NGO experts who stopped speaking in local idioms' (Hrycak 2006, 97). For example, a gender research institute director reported:

> The only centre that was getting stable support over ten years is the one in Kharkiv. However, its impact is low because it does not cooperate with the Ukrainian authorities, and is pro-Russian.

Similarly, an NGO representative complained: 'A very narrow circle of organizations have access to big money, and their work is not very effective or noticeable.' In contrast, other organizations on the ground were left without significant financial support which was justified by the donors who referred to them as 'local traditions' (Hrycak 2006, 85).

In the responses of a number of participants, foreign funds have also been faulted for imposing a cookie-cutter approach to gender equality:

> They have a standard approach to all, without exploring the specifics of the Ukrainian situation. (Researcher)

> GM can't have a universal glossary, we need special terminology for every field . . . Every person has a gender-sensitivity door; but for everyone it is located in different places. (NGO representative)

Moreover, many respondents noted that access to funding often required accommodation to the specific agendas of foreign agencies. To illustrate, one researcher explained:

> At first we were a women's organization because we got an American grant, then we collaborated with the Canadian fund and they required a broader mandate, so we changed to a gender organization.

Another NGO worker complained about how difficult it is to have to adhere to changing funding paradigms and priorities of foreign donors and foundations:

> Four or five years ago the Canada – Ukraine Gender Fund stopped supporting women's organizations and focused on gender. But you can't shift like this here; we don't even have a history of the women's movement, we can't go in line with the global tendencies yet.

Despite the problematic aspects of foreign funding, its positive impact is also tangible. One university professor told us:

> All gender themes remain alive thanks to the support and pressure from international bodies. If not for this, even the formal documents might not have been adopted yet.

Indeed, a lack of funding from the Ukrainian government is generally recognized: 'women's organizations don't do enough lobbying because of small institutional capacity.' Many organizations have simply ceased to exist because they were not able to secure adequate funding. In the words of one state official:

> During independence struggles women's movements consolidated but later disintegrated because of economic problems.

Furthermore, according to an NGO representative, 'the state doesn't allow NGOs to make money or to become self-sufficient.' This seemed to be corroborated by another state official and activist, who observed that 'Canada and the United States support us, why not our own government?'

The lack of coordination and networking between existing organizations was also cited as a serious impediment by numerous interviewees, as the following statements show:

> There are some organizations that work on this, but they are not united. (University instructor)

> Women don't support each other. There is no consolidation of the women's movement. (State official)

Not surprisingly, there are serious divisions between organizations. Moreover, there is little sharing of information, and most organizations don't know about each other (Johnson 2007). Perhaps, most importantly, as one local activist put it, 'Women have lost hope that it is possible to achieve something through the women's movement.' Finally, the lack of coordination between women's organizations and the government was also mentioned. One NGO employee recalled that 'the Justice Minister signed the decree to create legal gender expertise but invited us – the experts – to the discussion only after.' As a result, women's organizations have little influence on the state's handling of women's issues (WWICS 2007).

Government and National Machinery

All thirty-two interviewees stated that the passing of the Ukrainian Law on Providing Equal Rights and Opportunities for Women and Men in 2005 was a watershed in gender equality. Yet each expressed serious doubts about the potential of the law to make transformative change. A number of respondents claimed that the passage of the law was only due to international pressures and expressed views such as the following, by two state officials:

> The passage of the law was influenced by the understanding that without gender regulations we're not going to get to Europe.

> The world is putting pressure on Ukraine, that is why some things are getting done but they aren't taken too seriously.

As a consequence, the law's potential efficacy in Ukraine is doubted, as can be seen from the following statements:

> The law was adopted, but internally the state power doesn't believe in it. (University instructor)

> We have a law but we don't have a change of consciousness. (State official)

In a similar vein, one researcher argued:

> The law will not affect anything, because the officials do not know what to do with this gender, for them gender means spying on the relations between men and women in bed.

And a university professor stated that 'the law is not enough, there is an urgent need for a strategy of gender development.' Moreover, while many respondents noted the existence of national plans for gender equality, more than one-third had serious reservations about their value. Many did not see these plans as translating into any type of meaningful state policies, as can be seen by statements like the following:

> We don't even have a well-developed state policy regarding gender. (Researcher)

> There is no government policy targeting GM. (University instructor)

> There is an action plan on who does what, but there is no common underlying platform on the goals and principles. (Researcher)

Not surprisingly, almost all of the respondents also bemoaned the lack of implementation of both the law and national gender plans. This was summarized by a research centre director, who said, 'There is the law and there is its implementation. These are two different things.' Similarly, one NGO director reported:

> Gender policy is not implemented across ministries. Our gender policy is formal. There is no good central body to deal with the issue. The ministry is only preoccupied with the social protection of women which is not enough.

As illustrated by the following, half of the respondents reported that the lack of implementation is linked to the absence of sanctions for non-compliance:

> There is no monitoring and no punishment for not implementing. (NGO representative)

> Severity of the law is compensated by the 'unnecessarity' of obeying it. (Researcher)

And for one-third of respondents, the key obstacle to implementation is a lack of funding and resources.

Besides insufficient financing, the coordinating structures have been subjected to frequent organizational changes (Kisselyova and Trokhym 2007, 6). About half of the respondents mentioned that frequent restructuring of power institutions creates organizational chaos and prevents effective work. Over the eighteen years of independence, the Ukrainian state machinery responsible for gender issues has been restructured ten times (Hrycak 2005). From 2004 to 2010, the institutions responsible for gender included the Department of Gender Policy in the Ministry for Family, Youth, and Sport, which was charged with 'participation in development and ensuring implementation of the state policy on issues of family, children, youth . . . equality of rights and opportunities of women and men, prevention of violence in the family,' as well as the Sub-committee on Gender Policy in the Parliamentary Committee on Human Rights (Kisselyova and Trokhym 2007, 8). Yet, in 2011, after the change of government as a result of presidential elections of 2010, gender issues were moved again, now to the responsibility of the Ministry of Social Policy. Importantly, such 'political instability leads to high personnel flow and the necessity to teach new people over and over' (NGO employee).

More than one-third of participants mentioned a lack of awareness at all levels of government around gender issues. This was evident in the following observations:

> The government needs to take on gender issues but does not know how. (State official)

> After the presidential decree we have a system of gender advisers, but what can they advise when they don't have information or experience?[9] . . . Our politicians and bureaucrats don't understand why they should pay attention to gender. (Researcher)

> Some politicians are carriers of patriarchal values. This is dangerous for both women and men. They came to the Rada just because they were successful businessmen but now they're making decisions not about business but about the whole society. (NGO employee)

One important reason for the lack of awareness, according to an NGO employee, is that

> whenever the issue of gender is raised, men say that there is Article 24 of the Constitution that guarantees equal rights to everyone, therefore the gender problem is artificial.

Many stories were recollected by the respondents on how resistant those in power are to change. For example, as one NGO employee reported to us:

> A male communist politician said, 'If you [women] become so equal then who will give birth in the country?'

Finally, there is the issue of motivation. One university instructor explained, 'There are no material benefits from gender promotion; therefore, there is no interest among officials.'

One-third of the participants believe, as does an NGO employee, that one of the key remaining obstacles to gender equality 'is women's lack of participation in politics.' After Ukraine's independence, women's participation in politics decreased dramatically. In 1991, it fell from the previous 36 per cent to 3 per cent (Hrycak 2005, 74). In the Rada, formed as a result of the September 2007 early elections, the proportion of women was 7.5 per cent. A former state official similarly observed, 'We don't have women in leadership positions. All the high positions are men.' Indeed, besides the exceptional Yulia Tymoshenko – Ukraine's former prime minister – women do not serve in the Cabinet of Ministers, and only three of twenty-seven parliamentary committees are headed by women. The low number of women in the highest levels of power led some respondents such as one state official, to conclude that 'women in Ukraine are simply not allowed into politics.' A former state official also asserted that 'politicians do not want to share their power; without women the competition is lower.' This extends to women politicians, who as a university professor explained, 'are against feminism because taking such a position prevents further competition with other women.' The implications of this are serious. According to the International Centre for Policy Studies (ICPS), 'Unbalanced representation of women and men in the Rada and local councils contradicts the principles of democracy; it impedes the recognition of international commitments undertaken by Ukraine, and it limits the capacity of elected bodies to comprehensively analyse and reasonably consider social policies' (ICPS 2007, 2).

However, even women who get power are not necessarily supportive of gender equality (Hrycak 2007, 153, 175). As one example, most women deputies were not supportive of the Gender Equality Law. One of them mentioned in reference to the first gender bill proposed in 1999 that Ukraine could not afford this law before it solves the problem of the needy children (Hrycak 2005, 75). Women deputies ridiculed the notion of equal rights legislation, claiming that women are already equal if not over-emancipated and need to devote themselves to motherhood more (Hrycak 2001, 141). One activist interviewee also recalled:

Deputy Lilia Hryhorovych, who considers herself a prominent gender expert, said there was no inequality in our society.

Moving Forward: Suggested Directions for Change

The role of education figured prominently in the recommendations made by the participants. All respondents identified the need for education – at all levels of society and within all sectors – as the most important prerequisite for making any meaningful inroads in terms of gender equality. For example,

You have to work at all levels to make change. (Centre director)

We need to educate all levels of society. (State official)

There is a need for a massive gender literacy campaign at all levels. (University instructor)

What is missing is a balanced, broad, and deep understanding of gender issues. (NGO representative)

Many of those interviewed, as evidenced in the following quote from a state official, also underscored the need to distinguish between gender and feminism in order for Ukrainian society to become more open to gender equality initiatives: 'What is necessary is a general information breakthrough . . . to make people understand that gender is not feminism.' For two-thirds of the respondents, education should begin with the general public, as the following excerpts show:

We need to start with a serious campaign accessible to the people in order to show how GM actually helps each woman and man. (Researcher)

First there needs to be an understanding of gender issues by the people. (NGO representative)

The general public needs to understand what is written in the Gender Equality Law. Society should evolve and the knowledge base should change. (NGO activist)

Developing information that is historically and culturally relevant and accessible to the general public was also underscored in the following statements made by our interviewees:

Information campaigns are often targeting people who are already specializing in the problem, but the regular citizen is not reached. (State official)

Even the little information that exists is not available to the wide masses of people. (University professor)

Two-thirds of the interviewees also identified the need to educate politicians and bureaucrats, saying, for example:

We need to influence the consciousness of public figures. (NGO representative)

Education of the representatives in power by the state itself is essential. (Researcher)

While difficult . . . training for civil servants is very important. (University instructor)

More than one-third emphasized the need to better engage the educational sector. According to a number of experts,

We need to use universities, colleges, and schools to improve gender consciousness. (State official)

We have to launch the educational system, so analysts will be prepared by the state because the state needs them. (Researcher)

Gender themes have to be incorporated into different educational fields: political science, economics, legal studies, and so on. (University professor)

There is a real need to train the trainers; for example, the schoolteachers. (Researcher)

A university professor also called for 'gender expertise of school textbooks and study programs' to stop the reproduction of stereotypes through the educational system.

Even more specifically, respondents highlighted the need to further develop gender studies in Ukraine. For example, a gender research centre employee observed: 'We need an institute for gender studies.' Indeed, there is still no coordinating body for gender studies in Ukraine. The UNDP (2003) made a similar recommendation calling for a national centre that could synthesize gender research in Ukraine, translate research knowledge within and beyond universities to the media and government, facilitate that awareness of gender, and analyse the status and development opportunities of the gender perspective in all areas of society. Importantly, respondents noted that these types of initiatives, even if they are funded by international donors, should be sensitive and responsive to the Ukrainian context. As one NGO representative elaborated, there is a good research centre, but:

it has specific non-Ukrainian orientation, it is oriented towards Russian research potential, and does not pay attention to the Ukrainian context. It is the responsibility of donors to think who they fund.

Focusing efforts on the media was also considered a priority by nearly one-quarter of the respondents. For example, one state official argued:

> We need to get the media interested, develop professional training for journalists who would present gender issues. Informing society begins with informing journalists.

In a similar vein, a university instructor noted that 'there's an urgent need to work with journalists who keep proliferating stereotypes.' Yet, one university professor called for 'gender censorship of ads and TV.' To achieve more accurate coverage of both women and men in the media, similar recommendations have been put forward by the UNDP (2003). They have suggested professional monitoring groups for news media, an ethical code for journalists, planned and regular trainings, and gender courses in journalistic education. As a state official succinctly explained, 'Informing the media, you inform society.'

In recognition that 'wide disparities remain between what has been written on paper and what is practised in reality' (Kisselyova and Trokhym 2007, 3), nearly all respondents spoke of the need for improvement in how laws and gender plans and programs are actually implemented and monitored. This is evidenced in the following excerpts from interviews:

> There is a need to develop a national mechanism of implementing gender policy. (State official)

> The most important step in the future is to strengthen the mechanisms of control and monitoring. (NGO representative)

For example, in terms of the current law on ensuring equal rights and opportunities, there is no mechanism for reviewing cases of discrimination and no procedure for bringing guilty parties to account. Realizing, however, as does an NGO activist that 'the law is not enough,' more than one-third of all respondents identified the need to move beyond judicial mechanisms of protection to develop a stronger overall state infrastructure to promote gender equality. The numerous suggestions on how the overall infrastructure could be improved included the following:

A separate state structure regarding gender. (Researcher)

A state program and good central body to deal with the issue, because the ministry is only preoccupied with the social protection of women which is not enough. (Research centre director)

It would be good to introduce into the Rada a person responsible for gender equality. (State official)

We need a gender lobby in government. (University instructor)

Another theme within these recommendations was that gender issues could not be relegated to one ministry within government. An activist addressed the shortcoming of such an approach by arguing that 'all ministries have to be responsible for gender law and policies.'

In addition to the formal state structures dealing with gender issues, a little more than one-third of the study's participants identified the need to equalize the participation of women and men in the political process and decision making at the highest levels of power. For example, in the words of a former state official, 'We need to reach the 30 per cent of women in the Rada and then it will automatically change everything, we will feel different power, we will feel a change.' Within the group of respondents who advocated the increase of women in formal politics, there was, however, disagreement on how this would be best achieved. Some were strongly in favour of quotas, and as the following statement from a university professor indicates, some argued that there is support among Ukrainian citizens for such an initiative:

Sociological research says that the population of Ukraine is not against the introduction of quotas into the political parties' electoral lists. This includes 60 per cent of women between the ages of thirty and forty. People don't need explanations of what gender quotas are.

Yet not everyone is supportive of this idea, and our respondents were divided on this issue. A parliamentary committee member stated that

quotas will not necessarily make a difference because the elected female deputies

> will be not women but *zhinochky* in the Rada.[10] This is often the situation
> today, therefore it doesn't even make sense to divide the Rada on men and
> women or to count how many women deputies are there.

Indeed, despite the existence of quotas in the Soviet Union and the
presence of the 36 per cent of women in the Ukrainian parliament in
the mid-1980s, no profound improvements to gender equality occurred
(Hrycak 2005).

Another major theme to emerge is the need for better monitoring and
research. One-quarter of respondents emphasized the need to systematically track progress and produce knowledge that will lead to change.
For example, one research centre director said, 'Research and analysis
of progress are needed because the only evaluation done consists of reports to international foundations.' Similarly, according to an institute
director:

> The officials always report that Ukraine fulfils everything; only when
> confronted by facts that they admit that there are problems. That's why
> we need gender research – to build the concrete arguments for politi-
> cians.

Indeed, as recognized in more general GM literature, one of the biggest challenges to gender mainstreaming lies in the danger of its co-
optation by mainstream policy makers (Carney 2003), and one of the
reasons for GM's ineffectiveness is the over-focus of bureaucracies on
indicators as opposed to the tangible results of real equality (Phillips
2005). This fear of GM's co-optation and formalization is especially
relevant in the post-communist development context, where officials
try to maintain a positive image for Western partners while engaging
in a lasting tradition of false reporting – a legacy of the socialist system.
According to the respondents, improved monitoring would include,
for instance:

> Gender analysis of work done by all ministries. (University professor)

> More developed and credible statistics. (Researcher)

And for such statistics to be produced, said one university instructor, 'we must think what markers can be used to evaluate the situation.'

Indeed, significant data gaps that remain impede understanding gender dynamics and taking action on gender inequities. One researcher asserted:

> Only when you give them – politicians and bureaucrats – concrete examples about male mortality, the number of women of childbearing age abroad – only then they recognize its importance.

National statistics 'provide decision makers with relevant facts . . . and because living conditions differ for men and women, there is a need for these fact, statistics, to be disaggregated by gender' (UNDP 2003, 84). In the case of Ukraine, respondents emphasized:

> Gender is not only about subsidies and protection of mothers. (NGO director)

> There are men's problems in gender as well. (NGO employee)

Perhaps, as one state official stated rather pointedly:

> Men are ashamed to report their problems; maybe, the men's matters are even more complicated than women's in practice.

The need to explicitly address men's concerns in Ukraine through the mechanism of gender mainstreaming was described as critical and pressing. Respondents noted that within 'foreign' frameworks of GM there is too much focus on women and even resistance to extending GM to men even though, as one researcher submitted;

> it is now men who are more discriminated against, there is more unemployment among men, more sickness, reduced quality of life, and life expectancy.

In terms of health, this is certainly the case. The average life expectancy for men is ten years less than for women, and this has been identified 'as one of the most alarming health issues in the country' (UNDP 2003, 70). In line with this, one NGO employee pointed out,

'Male . . . mortality rates are now similar to wartime.' Similarly, a university professor noted that 'the death rate among men is three times higher than among women in the 28 to 40 age group.' The gendered difference in mortality rates is a specific problem in Ukraine that any effective GM effort has to acknowledge and address.

Finally, one key to improving GM work in Ukraine is to better connect the work of the state and NGOs. This was emphasized by one state official, who said:

> There is a need for cooperation between the state that now has to work on gender and the NGOs that know how.

Some scholars have argued, for example, that the transformative potential of GM can only be realized when advocacy coalitions have the opportunity to set policy agendas that incorporate the representation of their interests and, indeed, the specificities of their nation states (Jahan 1995). In Ukraine, this is a challenge because of the current weaknesses and fragmentation within women's and equality-seeking organizations and because, as Galligan et al. (2007) submit, 'Women in post-socialist Europe are very rarely involved from the outset in shaping the GM agenda in their countries. Instead, GM initiatives that have been put on the agenda have come from a government decision, usually promoted by the need to comply with EU and international requirements' (p. 120). The need for active participation from the civil sector is essential because GM strategies that fail to account for the differences in societal and political contexts of developed and transitional countries run the risk of falling short of any type of transformative change. At the same time, as put by an NGO representative:

> We can't expect the results from GM overnight. What was established for thousands of years cannot be changed in the blink of an eye.

Conclusions

The findings of this chapter contribute to filling the gap in evaluating the implementation of gender equality instruments in Ukraine. In particular, the research provides insights for assessing the application and applicability of gender mainstreaming in transitional countries, which differ from developed countries because of their distinct histories, cultures, languages, and identities – and also experiences of communism (Galligan et al. 2007, 13). Although before 1995 the discussion of gender was unheard-of in Ukraine, today the government can boast numerous issued documents that target improving the status of women as well as developing gender equality for both men and women. Although a number of positive developments across sectors were mentioned by the project participants, the overall situation is far from ideal.

In response, the study's participants proposed a number of suggestions for moving forward. Primarily, a massive educational campaign targeting various social groups – such as state officials, educators, and the media, as well as the general public – was emphasized. Second, the implementation of the formal documents was identified as crucial. Third, equalizing men's and women's participation in politics was pointed out, although there was no consensus on how this could be achieved. Significantly, the need to create a GM strategy more appropriate to the Ukrainian context was revealed.

Most importantly, through communication with gender-related practitioners on the ground, this study reveals a consistent grievance about the transposition of external GM approaches and concepts by international donors onto the situation in Ukraine. Western approaches, Western terminology, and Western modes of work with both officials and the affected populations are not considered to be effective for Ukraine. This is far from saying that GM in principle is inapplicable for Ukraine. It is clear, however, that the strategic goal of GM can be better achieved in a different – more context-driven – tactical way. In particular, this means that the external pressure to simply translate and apply GM mechanisms and policies developed elsewhere needs to be replaced by an approach that engages a range of local actors and country sectors and is sensitive to Ukraine's sociohistorical context, including specific norms and assumptions regarding language, gender roles, and stereotypes.

NOTES

1 'Mainstreaming a gender perspective,' according to the U.N. Economic and Social Council (1997, 3), 'is the process of assessing the implications for women and men of any planned action, including legislation, policies or programs, in any area and at all levels. It is a strategy for making the

concerns and experiences of women as well as of men an integral part of the design, implementation, monitoring and evaluation of policies and programs in all political, economic and societal spheres, so that women and men benefit equally, and inequality is not perpetuated. The ultimate goal of mainstreaming is to achieve gender equality.'

2 See Chapter 1, in this volume, for an in-depth discussion of this theme.

3 Zakon Ukrayiny, Pro Zabezpechennia Rivnyh Prav ta Mozhlyvostei Zhinok ta Cholovikiv [Law of Ukraine on Ensuring Equal Rights and Opportunities for Women and Men, in *Vidomosti Verkhovnoyi Rady Ukrayiny*, 2005, no. 52, p. 561. Available in Ukrainian at http://zakon.rada.gov.ua/cgi-bin/laws/main.cgi?nreg=2866–15. Translation into English done by the authors.

4 The concept of *Berehynia* entails a traditional Ukrainian woman taking care of her house and family: seeing to food, clothing, and emotional needs. She is a domesticated source of beauty, order, and well-being. Originally Berehynia was a pagan Slavic goddess of earth and fertility, but later she also transformed into a domestic Madonna and a guardian of family and nation (Hubbs 1988, 14–15). Thus, Berehynia represents a 'pagan goddess conjoined with the Virgin Mary' (Rubchak 1996, 320). Today, Berehynia is the 'main symbol of Ukrainian rural culture' and 'the centre of the idyllic world of the lost and adored' (Pavlychko 1992, 91).

5 This quote was originally taken from the news report on the presidential website. Unfortunately, the link to the exact quote is not available anymore, yet a similar and more recent statement can be accessed at http://en.for-ua.com/news/2007/03/05/132530.html.

6 *Osnovy Teoriyi Genderu* [Gender Theory Basics] (Kyiv: KIC, 2004).

7 See Chapter 10 in this volume for an in-depth gender content-analysis of Ukrainian school textbooks.

8 This number used to be even more than 1,200, according to Sydorenko (2001).

9 The function of gender advisers was assigned not to gender specialists but to the deputy ministers and deputy oblast governors on top of their prior work responsibilities and regardless of their educational background.

10 This is the equivalent to 'wifey' – a diminutive of wife, or a 'little woman.'

REFERENCES

Beveridge, F., and S. Nott. 2002. Mainstreaming: A Case for Optimism and Cynicism. *Feminist Legal Studies* 10(3): 299–331.

Booth, C., and C. Bennett. 2002. Gender Mainstreaming in the European Union: Towards a New Conception and Practice of Equal Opportunities? *European Journal of Women's Studies* 9(4): 430–46.

Carney, G. 2003. Communicating or Just Talking? Gender Mainstreaming and the Communication of Global Feminism. *Women and Language* 26(1): 52–60.

Cockerham, W.C., B.P. Hinote, G.B. Cockerham, and P. Abbott. 2006. Health Lifestyles and Political Ideology in Belarus, Russia, and Ukraine. *Social Science Medicine* 62(1): 799–809.

Daly, M. 2005. Gender Mainstreaming in Theory and Practice. *Social Politics: International Studies in Gender, State and Society* 12(3): 433–50.

Einarsdóttir, T. 2003. Challenging the Slow Motion of Gender Equality: The Case of Iceland. Paper presented at the 5th European Feminist Research Conference, Lund University, Sweden, 22–24 August.

Galligan, Y., S. Clavero, and M. Calloni. 2007. *Gender Politics and Democracy in Post-socialist Europe*. Leverkusen: Barbara Burdich Press.

Hafner-Burton, E.M., and M.A. Pollack. 2002. Mainstreaming Gender in Global Governance. *European Journal of International Relations* 8(2): 339–73.

Hankivsky, O. 2005. Gender vs. Diversity Mainstreaming: A Preliminary Examination of the Role and Transformative Potential of Feminist Theory. *Canadian Journal of Political Science* 38(4): 977–1001.

– 2008. Globalization, Trafficking, and Health: A Case Study of Ukraine. In C. Patton and H. Loshny, eds., *Global Science/Women's Health*, 175–99. Amherst: Cambria Press.

Hrycak, A. 2001. The Dilemmas of Civil Revival: Ukrainian Women since Independence. *Journal of Ukrainian Studies* 26(1–2): 135–58..

– 2005. Coping with Chaos: Gender and Politics in a Fragmented State. *Problems of Post-Communism* 52(5): 69–81.

– 2006. Foundation Feminism and the Articulation of Hybrid Feminisms. *Post-Socialist Ukraine East European Politics and Societies* 20: 69–100.

–2007. Gender and the Orange Revolution. *Journal of Communist Studies and Transition Politics* 23(1): 152–79.

Hubbs, J. 1988. *Mother Russia: The Feminine Myth in Russian Culture*. Bloomington: Indiana University Press.

International Centre for Policy Studies (ICPS). 2007. How to Ensure Gender Equality in Politics. *International Center for Policy Studies Newsletter* 17(364), 21 May. Available at: http://www.pasos.org/layout/set/print/www-pasos members-org/news/how-to-ensure-gender-equality-in-politics.

Jahan, R. 1995. *The Elusive Agenda: Mainstreaming Women in Development*. New York: Zed Books.

Johnson, J.E. 2007. *Domestic Violence Politics in Post-Soviet States.* Oxford: Oxford University Press.

Kisselyova, O., and I. Trokhym. 2007. *A Gender Analysis of EU Development Instruments and Policies in Ukraine.* Kyiv: Network of East-West Women, Gender Watch.

Mazey, S. 2002. Gender Mainstreaming Strategies in the EU: Delivering on an Agenda? *Feminist Legal Studies* 10: 227–40.

Pavlychko, S. 1992. Between Feminism and Nationalism: New Women's Groups in Ukraine. In M. Buckley, ed., *Perestroika and Soviet Women,* 82–96. Cambridge: Cambridge University Press.

Phillips, L. 2005. Gender Mainstreaming: The Global Governance of Women? *Canadian Journal of Development Studies* 26: 651–63.

Plotyan, S. 2006. Legislative Securing of Women's Participation in the Process of Decision Making: European Experience for Ukraine. In *Women and Politics in Ukraine,* J. Sverdljuk and S. Oksamytna eds., pp. 106–109. Conference Proceedings Women and Politics in Ukraine: Benefiting from International Experience. Kyiv, 7 October 2005. Full text available at: http://www.dfc.ukma.kiev.ua/books/women_politics_ukr_text.pdf (accessed January 23, 2011).

Pollack, M.A., and E. Hafner-Burton. 2000. Mainstreaming Gender in the European Union. *European Journal of Public Policy* 7(3): 432–56.

Powell, M. 2005. A Rights-Based Approach to Gender Equality and Women's Rights. *Canadian Journal of Development Studies* 26: 605–17.

Predborska, I. 2005. The Social Position of Yong Women in Present-Day Ukraine. *Journal of Youth Studies* 8(3): 349–65.

Pyshchulina, O. 2004. An Evaluation of Ukrainian Legislation to Counter and Criminalize Human Trafficking. In S. Stoecker and L. Shelley, eds., *Human Trafficking and Transnational Crime: Eurasian and American Perspectives,* 115–24. London: Rowman and Littlefield.

Rees, T. 2002. The Politics of 'Mainstreaming' Gender Equality. In E. Breitenbach, A. Brown, F. Mackay, and J. Webb, eds., *The Changing Politics of Gender Equality in Britain,* 45–69. Cambridge: Palgrave.

Rubchak, M. 1996. Christian Virgin or Pagan Goddess? In R. Marsh, ed., *Women in Russia and Ukraine,* 315–30. Cambridge: Cambridge University Press.

Shaw, J. 2005. Mainstreaming Equality and Diversity in European Union Law and Policy. *Current Legal Problems* 58: 255–32.

Shymchyshyn, M. 2005. Ideology and Women's Studies Programs in Ukraine. *NWSA Journal* 17(3): 173–85.

Squires, J. 2005. Is Mainstreaming Transformative? Theorising Mainstreaming in the Context of Diversity and Deliberation. *Social Politics* 12(3): 366–88.

Sydorenko, O. 2001. *Zhinochi Organizatsiyi Ukrayiny: Dovidnyk*. Kyiv: Tsentr Innovatsiyi ta Rozvytku.

United Nations Development Proram (UNDP). 2003. *Gender Issues in Ukraine: Challenges and Opportunities*. Kyiv: UNDP.

United Nations Economic and Social Council. 1997. Coordination of the Policies and Activities of the Specialized Agencies and Other Bodies of the United Nations System. Available at http://www.un.org/womenwatch/osagi/pdf/ECOSOCAC1997.2.PDF.

United Nations in Ukraine (UNU). 2010. Gender Stereotypes Hinder Gender Equality in Ukraine, UNDP-backed Poll says. UNU Website at http://www.un.org.ua/en/information-centre/news/543–2007–08–22 (accessed 23 Feb. 2011).

Veitch, J. 2005. Looking at Gender Mainstreaming in the UK Government. *International Feminist Journal of Politics* 7(4): 600–6.

Walby, S. 2005. Gender Mainstreaming: Productive Tensions in Theory and Practice. *Social Politics* 12(3): 321–43.

Woodrow Wilson International Center for Scholars (WWICS). 2007. Women's NGOs in Ukraine and End of Western Aid. *Kennan Institute U.S. Alumni Series* 14. June. Available at http://www.wilsoncenter.org/index.cfm?fuseaction=events.event_summaryandevent_id=237920 (accessed 21 Aug. 2009).

Woodward, A. 2003. European Gender Mainstreaming: Promises and Pitfalls of Transformative Policy. *Review of Policy Research* 20(1): 65–88.

– 2008. Too Late for Gender Mainstreaming? Taking Stock in Brussels. *Journal of European Policy* 18(3): 289–302.

Yakushko, O. 2005. Ambivalent Sexism and Relationship Patterns among Women and Men in Ukraine. *Sex Roles* 52(9/10): 589–96.

Afterword

OLENA HANKIVSKY AND ANASTASIYA SALNYKOVA

Making this volume happen has not been without its challenges. These included determining the appropriate mix of themes and topics, ensuring that the collection would be primarily shaped by Ukrainian scholars living in Ukraine, dealing with issues of translation and language use, and ultimately responding to various opinions regarding the scholarly merits of contributions, especially those that represented less traditional styles of academic writing. In presenting this wide range of accounts, our intention was to support and accept essays on their own terms, paying close attention to ensuring that the editing process would not impose any uniform system of thought or silence or distort the voices of those who may not conform, as Funk (2006) has cautioned against elsewhere, to the expectations of those who do not live or write in the context of Western feminism. While, in some instances, compromises had to be made – and we are grateful for the cooperation from all our contributors – the purpose was to give, as much as possible, authentic voice to the scholarship of all the contributors and to produce a volume that, despite its inclusion of a wide range of approaches, offers numerous insights.

The chapters in this volume have provided critical, in-depth evaluation of gender issues in a select number of political and social realms in Ukraine. They contribute to the advancement of a gendered analysis of transitional countries by promoting an approach that addresses the effects of change on both differently situated men and women and in the relationships between them. All authors were afforded a general set of guidelines to ensure cohesion across the chapters, while also providing maximum flexibility in the treatment of all themes and topics. Specifically, each of the contributors were asked to detail how her chapter contributes to the understanding of the effects of the post-Soviet transition process on the gender order in Ukraine and to specify the theoretical and methodological approaches of her work. Another requirement was that each chapter engage, as much as possible, with relevant literature on gender and transition in other post-authoritarian states. The final product is a unique mix of contributions that reflect a range of different views from various disciplinary, methodological, and stylistic perspectives on the contemporary situation in Ukraine.

A distinctive feature of this volume is that it pays particular attention to the state, its institutions, and policies across conventional disciplinary boundaries and assesses progress to date on gender equality with an eye to uncovering current gaps in activities and research as well as identifying future challenges in the field. It addresses the issues of political elites and power institutions, education, and newly emerging research and policy areas such as the health dimensions of gender, homelessness, masculinities, fatherhood, and LGBT communities.

In charting the history and aftermath of transition, the chapters in this collection are especially effective in mapping the positive advances in relation to gender equality in Ukraine. It is not widely recognized, for example, that Ukraine was on the forefront of many international and post-Soviet countries in establishing formal constitutional guarantees of gender equality in its 1996 Constitution, and it was the first among the post-communist states to criminalize trafficking and combat domestic violence in 1998. Ukraine was also the first former Soviet republic to repeal criminal responsibility for non-violent male homosexual intercourse between adults. In the past decade, significant developments in gender studies have occurred in Ukraine as evidenced by the growing number of local research centres, publications, and study programs in many regions of the country.

At the same time, the authors in this collection underscore that while state legislation, policies, and programs are progressive, even by any measure of international standards, change in all sectors is hampered by a range of factors including firmly entrenched beliefs, traditions, stereotypes, and assumptions about the lives of women and men and the proper performance of gender within a particular conception of a Ukrainian gender order. Many also highlight the ambivalent effects of democratic advancement for gender equality in Ukraine, illustrating that while in some spheres, improvements have been realized, for the most part, economic hardships related to democratic transition have been crippling. Indeed, this volume demonstrates the extent to which the promises of the Orange Revolution in relation to gender equality have not materialized. Although certain positive developments like the passing of a gender equality law did occur, government retrenchment in terms of funding for gender-related programs occurred almost simultaneously and pro-natalist rhetoric continued. To illustrate the multidimensional and multilayered gendered lived experiences of Ukrainian men and women, several authors draw on first person narratives. As such, they effectively situate individual experiences of gender in the context of social processes and structures. They illuminate how consequential gender is for the real lives of real people, in terms of education, labour market allocation, citizen engagement, economic security, mechanisms for coping with stress, health problems, and overall well-being and life expectancy.

Despite the breadth and depth of the topics addressed, this collection is far from exhaustive. In many ways, the essays and research featured in this volume represent the tip of the iceberg in an ongoing story and struggle of transition. Much more work needs to be done to reflect on and evaluate developments to date and to identify how to move the field of gender equality forward. However, in identifying lessons learned, the contributions in this collection also foreshadow and signal important areas for future investigation as well as areas that will continue to challenge the Ukrainian state and society. Before closing, we felt that it was worth speaking directly to some of these possibilities.

Some fruitful topics for future investigation would include, first, the role of the media in promoting or undermining gender equality. Another topic would be international influences on politics and policy developments with regard to gender in transitional countries, including Ukraine. This would include the effects of Europeanization in terms of discursive power and pragmatic diplomatic pressure, and Western aid with its successes and shortcomings. Other equally important topics that require attention include the following: the gendered effects of migration and trafficking (on men and women); regional differences in relation to gender legislation and equality outcomes (depending on the history, economics, and political power of these regions); mapping the diversity of gender non-governmental organizations in Ukraine and modelling the most effective strategies of their potential cooperation; the expected benefits and shortcomings of the introduction of gender quotas in the Ukrainian political context; labour market discrimination towards women in Ukraine; the effects on the issues of gender of diverse religions which have become more widespread and active after the collapse of the Soviet Union; and better understanding of the gendered health care needs and experiences of women and men, and especially the specific health issues of men whose life expectancy, as we have heard more than once in this volume, is unacceptably low in Ukraine. Moreover, such examinations would benefit from improvements in data collection across all sectors in Ukraine and in-depth comparative analyses with other post-Soviet countries.

The next phase of research should also challenge the confines of a gender-specific approach to include, in an explicit fashion, other intersecting factors and social locations. For example, Snitow (2006) has observed that 'sometimes in Central and East Europe, the category "gender" gains currency as a foreign import that holds out promise as an explanatory model. Often, though, it displaces other models or obscures them – most commonly "class," which in post-communism is still a much-discredited structure of explanation' (pp. 289–90). Arguably, the primary focus on gender can do more than just obscure issues of class; it can also deter one from examining how gender intersects with age, race/ethnicity, geography, sexuality, ability, and religion to create social inequalities and discrimination. Increasingly, gender theory points to the importance of intersectionality for demonstrating that gender cannot be understood as a stand-alone category.

People's lives, experiences, needs, and subject locations are created by intersecting social locations that include but are not limited to considerations of gender. In Ukraine, this is evident in the analyses put forward in a number of the chapters in this collection which considered differences not only between groups of men and women but also among women and men. Further examinations could also be focused on the specific needs of particularly vulnerable populations such as new immigrants to Ukraine, disabled men and women, Tatar women in Ukraine's Crimean peninsula, miners in Donbas, single parents, and men and women living in rural areas experiencing greater poverty and food insecurity. Although this volume starts to touch on these complicating intersections of gender, this is an important line of research that requires further development in the Ukrainian context.

All the chapters in this volume point to the need to move beyond formal legislation, plans, and programs to create an enabling environment for transforming gender relations. They also make an important contribution by furthering the understanding of gender, power, and privilege in the realms of state structures, politics, policy, and society and by providing new directions for responding to inequality and oppression and for working towards gender equality reform in the cultural context of Ukraine. They highlight new opportunities and new challenges as the country continues to navigate its past, present, and future and negotiate its own identity vis-à-vis gender equality amid both Western and Eastern pressures, tendencies, and influences. Such information provides an important backdrop to analysing how the country moves forward on issues of gender. Certainly, important developments continue. For example, in 2010, the newly formed government called a meeting on gender issues and appointed one of the foremost Ukrainian scholars and activists on gender Larysa Kobelianska to the post of the President's Gender Adviser. At the same time, no new national gender equality strategy or plan has been ratified. Any future developments and their overall effects will therefore need to be carefully monitored and evaluated.

In sum, this collection not only fills an important gap in the literature on gender in transitional post-Soviet countries, we hope that this volume will stimulate further debate and discussion that has begun in the region and encourage more comparative scholarship. Most importantly, however, it is our hope that this volume instigates new attention and interest in Ukraine, a country that has not been front and centre in the literature. For those already working on issues of gender in Ukraine, we trust that this collection will inspire them to continue to develop their programs of research in this field.

REFERENCES

Funk, N. 2006. Women's NGOs in Central and Eastern Europe and the Former Soviet Union: The Imperialist Criticism in Women and Citizenship in Central and Eastern Europe. In J. Lukić, J. Regulska, and D. Zaviršek, eds., *Women and Citizenship in Central and Eastern Europe,* 265–86. Aldershot: Ashgate.

Hankivsky, O., and R. Cormier. 2011. Intersectionality and Public Policy: Some Lessons from Existing Models. *Political Research Quarterly* 64(1): 217–29.

Snitow, Ann. 2006. Cautionary Tales. In J. Lukić, J. Regulska, and D. Zavrišek eds., *Women and Citizenship in Central and Eastern Europe,* 287–97. Aldershot: Ashgate.